Community/Public Health Nursing

Promoting the Health of Populations

evolve

To access your Student Resources, visit:

http://evolve.elsevier.com/Nies

Evolve® Student Learning Resources for *Nies/McEwen: Community/Public Health Nursing: Promoting the Health of Populations,* **Fourth Edition** offer the following features:

Student Resources

- **Quiz**
  Multiple-choice review questions with instant scoring and feedback at the click of a button.

- **Case Studies**
  Real-life clinical situations to help you develop your assessment and critical thinking skills, with questions and answers.

- **Glossary**
  Key Terms and their definitions, with search engine. Also available as flashcards.

- **WebLinks**
  Link to hundreds of websites carefully chosen to supplement the content of the textbook. The WebLinks are regularly updated, with new ones added as they develop.

- **Resource Tools**
  Materials such as assessment tools and detailed tables that supplement the chapter content.

- **Content Updates**
  Updates of new trends and developments that occur after publication of the book, to help you stay current in this field of study.

Community/Public Health Nursing

Promoting the Health of Populations

Fourth Edition

MARY A. NIES, PhD, RN, FAAN, FAAHB

Assistant Vice President of Health Sciences for Research in Community Health
Formerly Dean of Stony Brook University's School of Nursing
Professor of Nursing and of Preventive Medicine
Health Sciences Center
State University of New York, Stony Brook
Stony Brook, New York

MELANIE MCEWEN, PhD, RN

Associate Professor
University of Texas Health Science Center at Houston
School of Nursing
Houston, Texas

SAUNDERS

ELSEVIER

11830 Westline Industrial Drive
St. Louis, Missouri 63146

Community/Public Health Nursing: Promoting the Health of Populations

ISBN-13: 978-1-4160-2887-1
ISBN-10: 1-4160-2887-0

Notice

Neither the Publisher nor the Authors assume any responsibility for any loss or injury and/or damage to persons or property arising out of or related to any use of the material contained in this book. It is the responsibility of the treating practitioner, relying on independent expertise and knowledge of the patient, to determine the best treatment and method of application for the patient.

The Publisher

Previous editions copyrighted 2001, 1997, 1993

ISBN-13: 978-1-4160-2887-1
ISBN-10: 1-4160-2887-0

Managing Editor: Linda Thomas
Developmental Editor: Barb Watts
Publishing Services Manager: John Rogers
Senior Project Manager: Beth Hayes
Designer: Julia Dummitt

Printed in Canada

Last digit is the print number: 9   8   7   6   5   4   3   2   1

*I dedicate this book to Phil Yankovich, my husband, companion, and best friend,
whose love, caring, and true support are always there for me.
He provides me with the energy I need to pursue my dreams.*

*To Kara Nies Yankovich, my daughter, for whom I wish a happy and healthy life.
Her energy, joy, and enthusiasm for life give so much to me.*

*To Earl and Lois Nies, my parents,
for their never-ending encouragement and lifelong support.
They helped me develop a foundation for creative thinking,
new ideas, and spirited debate.*

MARY A. NIES

*I dedicate this book to my husband, Scott McEwen, whose love, support,
and encouragement have been my foundation for the past thirty years.
I can't wait to see what happens during the next thirty!*

MELANIE MCEWEN

Authors

Mary A. Nies

Mary A. Nies, PhD, RN, FAAN, FAAHB, is Assistant Vice President of Health Sciences for Research in Community Health and Professor of Nursing and of Preventive Medicine at the State University of New York, Stony Brook. She was formerly the Dean of Stony Brook University's School of Nursing. Dr. Nies received her diploma from Bellin School of Nursing in Green Bay, Wisconsin; her BSN from University of Wisconsin, Madison; her MSN from Loyola University, Chicago; and her PhD in Public Health Nursing, Health Services, and Health Promotion Research at the University of Illinois, Chicago. She completed a postdoctoral research fellowship in health promotion and community health at the University of Michigan, Ann Arbor. She is a Fellow of the American Academy of Nursing and a Fellow of the American Academy of Health Behavior. Dr. Nies co-edited *Community Health Nursing: Promoting the Health of Aggregates*, which received the 1993 Book of the Year award from the *American Journal of Nursing*. Her program of research focuses on the outcomes of health promotion interventions for minority and nonminority women and low-income women in the community. Her research is involved with physical activity and obesity prevention for populations, especially women. Her work also includes consulting in the areas of public and community health and health promotion education, practice, and research.

Melanie McEwen

Melanie McEwen, PhD, RN, is an Associate Professor at the University of Texas Health Science Center at Houston School of Nursing. Dr. McEwen received her BSN from the University of Texas School of Nursing in Austin; her Master's in Community and Public Health Nursing from Louisiana State University Medical Center in New Orleans; and her PhD in Nursing at Texas Woman's University. Dr. McEwen has been a nursing educator for more than 18 years and is also the author of *Community-Based Nursing: An Introduction* (Saunders, 2002) and co-author/editor of *Theoretical Basis for Nursing* (Lippincott, 2006).

Contributors

Margaret M. Andrews, PhD, RN, CTN, FAAN
Director and Professor
Department of Nursing
School of Health Professions and Studies
University of Michigan–Flint
Flint, Michigan
Chapter 12, Cultural Diversity and Community Health Nursing

Barbara Artinian, RN, PhD
Professor Emeritus
School of Nursing
Azusa Pacific University
Azusa, California
Chapter 19, Populations Affected by Disabilities

Joan Teague Bickes, MSN, APRN, BC
Assistant Professor
College of Nursing
Wayne State University
Detroit, Michigan
Chapter 33, Community Health Nursing: Making a Difference

Deborah Godfrey Brown, PhD, MS, RN
Associate Professor
College of Nursing
University of Rhode Island
Kingston, Rhode Island
Chapter 6, Community Health Planning, Implementation, and Evaluation

Tonya J. Broyles, RN
PhD Candidate
College of Nursing
University of Tennessee–Knoxville
Knoxville, Tennessee
Chapter 13, Environmental Health

Patricia M. Burbank, DNSc, RN
Professor
College of Nursing
University of Rhode Island
Kingston, Rhode Island
Chapter 6, Community Health Planning, Implementation, and Evaluation

Glenna Burg, MS, RN, BC
Adjunct Assistant Professor
College of Nursing
Montana State University
Bozeman Montana
Chapter 21, Rural and Migrant Health

Patricia Butterfield, PhD, RN, FAAN
Associate Professor and Director
Occupational and Environmental Health Nursing Program
School of Nursing
University of Washington
Chapter 3, Thinking Upstream: Nursing Theories and Population-Focused Nursing Practice

Mary Brecht Carpenter, MPH, RN
Consultant, Community/Public Health Nursing
Purcellville, Virginia
Chapter 14, Child and Adolescent Health

Holly Cassells, PhD, RN, MPH
Professor
School of Nursing and Health Professions
University of the Incarnate Word
San Antonio, Texas
Chapter 4, Epidemiology
Chapter 5, Community Assessment

Kathleen Chafey, PhD, RN
Professor
College of Nursing
Montana State University–Bozeman
Bozeman, Montana
Chapter 21, Rural and Migrant Health

Tom H. Cook, PhD, RN, FNP
Assistant Professor
School of Nursing
Vanderbilt University
Nashville, Tennessee
Chapter 2, Historical Factors: Community Health Nursing

Nellie S. Droes, DNSc, RN, CS
Associate Professor
School of Nursing
East Carolina University
Greenville, North Carolina
Chapter 20, Homeless Populations

Anita W. Finkelman, MSN, RN
Senior Vice President, Nursing Operations
Orbis Education, Inc.
Faculty, College of Nursing
University of Oklahoma
Oklahoma City, Oklahoma
Chapter 9, The Health Care System

Susan Rumsey Givens, BSN, RN, C, MPH, LCCE
Childbirth Educator
LCCE Certified Lamaze Instructor
Mount Carmel St. Ann's Hospital
Westville, Ohio
Chapter 14, Child and Adolescent Health

Deanna E. Grimes, DrPH, RN, FAAN
Associate Professor
Director, MSN-MPH Program
School of Nursing
University of Texas Health Science Center at Houston
Houston, Texas
Chapter 23, Communicable Disease

Joanne M. Hall, PhD, RN, FAAN
Associate Professor
School of Nursing
University of Tennessee–Knoxville
Knoxville, Tennessee
Chapter 13, Environmental Health
Chapter 24, Substance Abuse

Diane C. Hatton, DNSc, RN, CS
Associate Professor
Hahn School of Nursing and Health Science
University of San Diego
San Diego, California
Chapter 20, Homeless Populations

Wade G. Hill, PhD, RN
Assistant Professor
College of Nursing
Montana State University–Bozeman
Bozeman, Montana
Chapter 21, Rural and Migrant Health

Lisa Jensen, CNM, FNP, MS
Assistant Clinical Professor
School of Nursing
State University of New York, Stony Brook
Stony Brook, New York
Chapter 15, Women's Health

MaryAnne Laffin, RN, MS, FNP, CNM, FACNM
President, New York State Association of Licensed
  Midwives
Bellerose, New York
Chapter 11, Policy, Politics, Legislation, and Community Health Nursing

Jean Cozad Lyon, PhD, APRN, BC
Chief Nursing Officer
Sierra Surgery and Imaging
Carson City, Nevada
Chapter 8, Case Management

Jane Mahoney, DSN, RN
Assistant Professor
School of Nursing
University of Texas Health Science Center at Houston
Houston, Texas
Chapter 22, Populations Affected by Mental Illness

Melanie McEwen, PhD, RN
Associate Professor
School of Nursing
University of Texas Health Science Center at Houston
Houston, Texas
Chapter 1, Health: A Community View
Chapter 22, Populations Affected by Mental Illness
Chapter 33, Community Health Nursing: Making a Difference

Cathy D. Meade, PhD, RN, FAAN
Professor, Department of Interdisciplinary Oncology
College of Medicine
Division of Cancer Prevention and Control
Health Outcomes and Behavior
Adjunct Appointment, College of Nursing
Director, Education Program
H. Lee Moffitt Cancer Center & Research Institute
Tampa, Florida
Chapter 7, Community Health Education

Carrie Morgan, MSN, ARNP
Instructor
School of Nursing
University of Louisville
Louisville, Kentucky
Chapter 10, Economics of Health Care
Chapter 16, Men's Health

Carrie L. Motyka, MS, APRN, BC
Adjunct Instructor, School of Nursing
Oakland University
Rochester, Michigan
Doctoral Candidate, College of Nursing
Wayne State University
Detroit, Michigan
Chapter 31, Home Health and Hospice

Mary A. Nies, PhD, RN, FAAN, FAAHB
Assistant Vice President of Health Sciences for Research
  in Community Health
Formerly Dean of Stony Brook University's School of
  Nursing
Professor of Nursing and of Preventive Medicine
Health Sciences Center
State University of New York, Stony Brook
Stony Brook, New York
Chapter 1, Health: A Community View
Chapter 31, Home Health and Hospice
Chapter 33, Community Health Nursing: Making a Difference

Julie Novak, DNSc, RN, MA, CPNP, FAANP
Professor and Head, School of Nursing
Associate Dean
College of Pharmacy, Nursing, and Health Sciences
Purdue University
West Lafayette, Indiana
Chapter 32, Health in the Global Community

Alice Pappas, RN, PhD
Director for Clinical Education and Research
Children's Medical Center
Dallas, Texas
Chapter 25, Violence

Cathi A. Pourciau, RN, MSN, FNP-C
Louisiana State University Health Sciences Center
Baton Rouge, Louisiana
Chapter 27, School Health

Carolyn Robinson, PhD, MPH, BSN, BA
Associate Professor
University of Tennessee–Knoxville
College of Nursing
Knoxville, Tennessee
Chapter 13, Environmental Health

Bonnie Rogers, DrPH, COHN-S, LNCC, FAAN
Associate Professor
Director, North Carolina Occupational Safety and Health
    Education and Research Center
Director, Occupational Health Nursing Program
School of Public Health
University of North Carolina at Chapel Hill
Chapel Hill, North Carolina
Chapter 28, Occupational Health

Mary Ellen Trail Ross, DrPH, RN, CS
Assistant Professor
University of Texas Health Science Center–Houston
Houston, Texas
Chapter 17, Senior Health

Beverly Cook Siegrist, EdD, RN, CNE
Professor
Department of Nursing
Western Kentucky University
Bowling Green, Kentucky
Chapter 18, Family Health

Angela Snow, MSN, RN
Instructor of Clinical Nursing
School of Nursing
University of Texas Health Science Center at Houston
Houston, Texas
Chapter 29, Forensic and Correctional Health

Denise Snow, JD, CNM, NP, RN
Clinical Assistant Professor
School of Nursing
State University of New York, Stony Brook
Stony Brook, New York
Chapter 11, Policy, Politics, Legislation, and Community Health Nursing

Linda Stevenson, PhD, RN
Assistant Professor
Louise Herrington School of Nursing
Baylor University
Dallas, Texas
Chapter 25, Violence

Edith Summerlin, PhD, RN
Instructor
School of Nursing
University of Texas Health Science Center at Houston
Houston, Texas
Chapter 17, Senior Health
Chapter 26, Natural and Man-Made Disasters

Patricia Hyland Travers, ScM, MS, RN, COHN-S
Global Health Strategies Manager
Global Environmental Health, Safety, and Assurance
Hewlett Packard Company
Marlboro, Massachusetts
Chapter 28, Occupational Health

Linda L. Treloar, PhD, RN, NP-C
Professor of Nursing
Scottsdale Community College
Scottsdale, Arizona
Chapter 19, Populations Affected by Disabilities

Elaine C. Vallette, DrPH, RN
Dean for Nursing and Allied Health
Baton Rouge Community College
Baton Rouge, Louisiana
Chapter 27, School Health

Jo Wade, RN, PhD
Assistant Clinical Professor
College of Nursing
University of Tennessee–Knoxville
Knoxville, Tennessee
Chapter 24, Substance Abuse

ANCILLARY AUTHORS

Jacqueline L. Burchum, DNSc, APRN, BC
Assistant Professor
College of Nursing
University of Tennessee Health Science Center
Memphis, Tennessee
Annotated Learning Objectives
Annotated Lecture Outlines

Penny Y. Leake, PhD, MS, RN
Associate Professor
Luther College
Decorah, Iowa
PowerPoint Lecture Slides
Teaching Strategies

Tommie L. Norris, DNS, RN
Assistant Professor and Director of BSN Program
College of Nursing
University of Tennessee Health Science Center
Memphis, Tennessee
Test Bank

Beverly Cook Siegrist, EdD, RN, CNE
Professor
Department of Nursing
Western Kentucky University
Bowling Green, Kentucky
Quiz

Quiz

Beverly Siegrist was assisted in the development of the
Quiz by several Department of Nursing colleagues at
Western Kentucky University and students in a graduate
nursing education course.

Western Kentucky University Faculty
M. Susan Jones, PhD, RN
Professor

Sheila Atwell, MSN, RN
Assistant Professor

Freda Embry, MSN, RN
Assistant Professor

Terry Jepson, MSN, ARNP
Assistant Professor

Sherry Lovan, MSN, RN
Assistant Professor

Mary Kovar, MSN, RN
Assistant Professor

NURS 520: Teaching in Schools of Nursing
Western Kentucky University, Spring 2006
Professor
Beverly Siegrist, EdD, RN, CNE

Students
Melissa Burkett, RN, BSN
Wendy Clayton, RN, BSN

Elaine Terry, ME, RN, BSN
Michele Simpson, RN, BSN
Elizabeth Strader, RN, BSN
Demara Goodrich, RN, BSN
Angie Harlan, RN, BSN
Angie Atwood, RN, BSN
Billie Shelton, RN, BSN

REVIEWERS

Jo Azzarello, PhD, RN
Assistant Professor
College of Nursing
University of Oklahoma
Oklahoma City, Oklahoma

Carol Brown, PhD, BA
Associate Professor
School of Nursing
Minnesota State University–Mankato
Mankato, Minnesota

Christine Eisenhauer, MSN, BS
Assistant Professor
Division of Nursing
Mount Marty College
Yankton, South Dakota

Mary Ellen Lashley, PhD, RN, CRNP, CS
Department of Nursing
Towson University
Towson, Maryland

Shelly Luger, BSN, BA
Instructor
Division of Nursing
Mount Marty College
Yankton, South Dakota

Brenda Talley, PhD, RN, CNAA
Assistant Professor
School of Nursing
Georgia Southern University
Statesboro, Georgia

Carole E. Torok, PhD, RN, C
Professor
School of Nursing and Health Systems
State University of New York Institute of Technology
   at Utica/Rome
Utica, New York

Preface

More money is spent per capita for health care in the United States than in any other country ($5440 in 2002). However, many countries have far better indices of health, including traditional indicators such as infant mortality rates and longevity for both men and women, than does the United States. The United States is one of the few industrialized countries in the world that lacks a program of national health services or national health insurance. Although the United States spent 14.9% of its gross domestic product on health care expenditures in 2002, a record high of $1553 billion, 14.0% of the population had no health care coverage.

The greater the proportion of money put into health care expenditures in the United States, the less money there is to improve education, jobs, housing, and nutrition. Over the years, the greatest improvements in the health of the population have been achieved through advances in public health using organized community efforts, such as improvements in sanitation, immunizations, and food quality and quantity. The greatest determinants of health are still equated with factors in the community, such as education, employment, housing, and nutrition. Although access to health care services and individual behavioral changes are important, they are only components of the larger determinants of health, such as social and physical environments.

UPSTREAM FOCUS

The traditional focus of many health care professionals, known as a *downstream focus,* has been to deliver health care services to ill people and to encourage needed behavioral change at the individual level. The focus of community health nursing has traditionally been on health promotion and illness prevention by working with individuals and families within the community. A shift is needed to an *upstream focus,* which includes working with aggregates and communities in activities such as organizing and setting health policy. This focus will help aggregates and communities work to create options for healthier environments with essential components of health, including adequate education, housing, employment, and nutrition and provide choices that allow people to make behavioral changes, live and work in safe environments, and access equitable and comprehensive health care.

Grounded in the tenets of public health nursing and the practice of public health nurses such as Lillian Wald, this fourth edition of *Community/Public Health Nursing: Promoting the Health of Populations* builds on the earlier works by highlighting an aggregate focus in addition to the traditional areas of family and community health and thus promotes upstream thinking. The primary focus is on the promotion of the health of aggregates. This approach includes the family as a population and addresses the needs of other aggregates or population subgroups. It conceptualizes the individual as a member of the family and as a member of other aggregates, including organizations and institutions. Furthermore, individuals and families are viewed as a part of a population within an environment (i.e., within a community).

An aggregate is made up of a collective of individuals, be it family or another group that, with others, make up a community. This text emphasizes the aggregate as a unit of focus and how aggregates that make up communities promote their own health. The aggregate is presented within the social context of the community, and students are given the opportunity to define and analyze environmental, economic, political, and legal constraints to the health of these populations.

Community health nurses have traditionally addressed the needs of aggregates, such as families and school, work site, clinic, and community groups. However, community health nursing texts have traditionally defined the unit of care of the community health nurse generalist with undergraduate preparation as limited primarily to the individual and family. These texts have defined the unit of care of the specialist with graduate preparation as primarily other aggregates, the community, or the population. If community health nursing is a synthesis of nursing and public health practice to promote and preserve the health of populations, then all community health nurses carry out this mandate. Diagnosis and treatment of human responses to actual or potential health problems is the nursing component. The ability to prevent disease, prolong life, and promote health through organized community effort is from the public health component.

Community health nursing practice is responsible to the population as a whole. Nursing efforts to promote health and prevent disease are applied to the public, which includes all units in the community, be they individual or collective (e.g., person, family, other aggregate, community, or population). The generalist is competent to practice such at a minimum safe level, and the specialist is expected to have expert competence and knowledge through enhanced education and experience and is given a higher level of autonomy and freedom. Community health nurses at generalist and specialist levels of practice need to promote the full synthesis of nursing and public health practice and increase their alliance with public health to promote and preserve the health of populations.

PURPOSE OF THE TEXT

In this text, the student is encouraged to become a student of the community, learn from families and other aggregates in the community how they define and promote their own health, and learn how to become an advocate of the community by working with the community to initiate change. The student is exposed to the complexity and rich diversity of the community and is shown evidence of how the community organizes to meet change.

The use of language or terminology by clients and agencies varies in different parts of the United States, and it may vary from that used by government officials. The contributors of this text are a diverse group from various parts of the United States. Their terms vary from chapter to chapter and vary from those in use in local communities. For example, some authors refer to African-Americans, some to blacks, some to Euro-Americans, and some to whites. The student must be familiar with a range of terms and, most important, know what is used in his or her local community.

Outstanding features of this fourth edition include its provocative nature as it raises consciousness regarding the social injustices that exist in the United States and how these injustices, embodied in our market-driven health care system, prevent the realization of health as a right for all. With a focus on social justice, this text emphasizes society's rather than the individual's responsibility for the protection of all human life to ensure that all people have their basic needs met, such as adequate health protection and income. Shifts in reimbursement and the growth of managed care have revitalized the notion of the need for population-focused care, or care that covers all people residing within geographic boundaries, rather than only those populations enrolled in insurance plans. Working toward providing health promotion and population-focused care to all requires a dramatic shift in thinking from individual-focused care for the practitioners of the future. The future paradigm for health care is demanding that the focus of nursing move toward community health promotion if we are to forge toward a health-promoting and wellness-achieving nation.

This text is designed to **stimulate critical thinking and challenge students to question and debate issues.** Complex problems demand complex answers; therefore the student is expected to *synthesize prior biophysical, psychosocial, cultural, and ethical arenas of knowledge.* However, experiential knowledge is also necessary and the student is challenged to *enter new environments within the community* and gain new sensory, cognitive, and affective experiences. The authors of this text have integrated the concept of **upstream thinking,** introduced in the first edition, throughout this fourth edition as an important conceptual basis for nursing practice of aggregates and the community. The student is introduced to the individual and aggregate roles of community health nurses as they are engaged in a collective and interdisciplinary manner, working **upstream,** to facilitate the community's promotion of its own health. Students using this text will be better prepared to work with aggregates and communities in health promotion and with individuals and families in illness. Students using this text will also be better prepared to see the need to take responsibility for participation in organized community action targeting inequalities in arenas such as education, jobs, and housing and to participate in targeting individual health-behavioral change. These are important shifts in thinking for future practitioners who must be prepared to function in a community-focused health care system.

The text is also designed to increase the **cultural awareness and competency** of future community health nurses as they prepare to address the needs of culturally diverse populations. Students must be prepared to work with these growing populations as participation in the nursing workforce by ethnically and racially diverse people continues to lag. Various models are introduced to help students understand the growing link between social problems and health status, experienced disproportionately by diverse populations in the United States, and understand the methods of assessment and intervention used to meet the special needs of these populations.

The goals of the text are to provide the student with the ability to assess the complex factors in the community that affect individual, family, and other aggregate responses to health states and actual or potential health problems; and to help students use this ability to plan, implement, and evaluate community health nursing interventions to increase contributions to the promotion of the health of populations.

MAJOR THEMES RELATED TO PROMOTING THE HEALTH OF POPULATIONS

This text is built on the following major themes:

- A social justice ethic of health care in contrast to a market justice ethic of health care in keeping with the philosophy of public health as "health for all"
- A population-focused model of community health nursing as necessary to achieve equity in health for the entire population
- Integration of the concept of *upstream thinking* throughout the text and other appropriate theoretical frameworks related to chapter topics
- The use of population-focused and other community data to develop an assessment, or profile of health, and potential and actual health needs and capabilities of aggregates
- The application of all steps in the nursing process at the individual, family, and aggregate levels
- A focus on identification of needs of the aggregate from common interactions with individuals, families, and communities in traditional environments
- An orientation toward the application of all three levels of prevention at the individual, family, and aggregate levels
- The experience of the underserved aggregate, particularly the economically disenfranchised, including cultural and ethnic groups disproportionately at risk of developing health problems

Themes are developed and related to promoting the health of populations in the following ways:

- The commitment of community health nursing is to an equity model; therefore community health nurses work toward the provision of the unmet health needs of populations in a system that allows access to care only for those who can pay (Chapters 1, 2, and 3).
- The development of a population-focused model is necessary to close the gap between unmet health care needs and

health resources on a geographical basis to the entire population. The contributions of intervention at the aggregate level work toward the realization of such a model (Chapters 3 and 9).

- Contemporary theories provide frameworks for holistic community health nursing practice that help the students conceptualize the reciprocal influence of various components within the community on the health of aggregates and the population (Chapter 3 and throughout).
- The ability to gather population-focused and other community data in developing an assessment of health is a crucial initial step that precedes the identification of nursing diagnoses and plans to meet aggregate responses to potential and actual health problems (Chapters 5 and 6).
- The nursing process includes, in each step, a focus on the aggregate, assessment of the aggregate, nursing diagnosis of the aggregate, planning for the aggregate, and intervention and evaluation at the aggregate level (Units 2, 3, 4, and 5).
- The text discusses development of the ability to gather clues about the needs of aggregates from complex environments, such as during a home visit, with parents in a waiting room of a well-baby clinic, or with elders receiving hypertension screening, and to promote individual, collective, and political action that addresses the health of aggregates (Units 2, 3, 4, 5, 6, and 7).
- Primary, secondary, and tertiary prevention strategies include a major focus at the population level.
- In addition to offering a chapter on cultural influences in the community, the text includes data on and the experience of underserved aggregates at high risk for developing health problems and who are most often in need of community health nursing services (i.e., low and marginal income, cultural, and ethnic groups) throughout.

ORGANIZATION

The text is divided into eight units. *Unit 1, Introduction to Community Health Nursing,* presents an overview of the concept of health, a perspective of health as evolving and as defined by the community, and the concept of community health nursing as the nursing of aggregates from both historical and contemporary mandates. Health is viewed as an individual and collective right, brought about through individual and collective/political action. The definitions of public health and community health nursing and their foci are presented. Current crises in public health and the health care system and consequences for the health of the public frame implications for community health nursing. The historical evolution of public health, the health care system, and community health nursing is presented. The evolution of humans from wanderers and food gatherers to those who live in larger groups is presented. The text also discusses the influence of the group on health, which contrasts with the evolution of a health care system built around the individual person, increasingly fractured into many parts. Community health nurses bring to their practice awareness of the social context; economic, political, and legal constraints from the larger community; and knowledge of the current health care system and its structural constraints and limitations on the care of populations. The theoretical foundations for the text, with a focus on the concept of *upstream thinking,* and the rationale for a population approach to community health nursing are presented.

Unit 2, The Art and Science of Community Health Nursing, describes application of the nursing process—assessment, planning, intervention, and evaluation—to aggregates in the community using selected theory bases. The unit addresses the need for a population focus that includes the public health sciences of biostatistics and epidemiology as key in community assessment and the application of the nursing process to aggregates to promote the health of populations. Application of the art and science of community health nursing to meeting the needs of aggregates is evident in chapters that focus on community health planning and evaluation, community health education, and case management.

Unit 3, Factors That Influence the Health of the Community, examines factors and issues that can both positively and negatively affect health. Beginning with an overview of the health care delivery system, this unit examines the importance of economics and health care financing on the health of individuals, families, and populations. Health policy and legislation are also discussed, focusing on how policy is developed and the effect of past and future legislative changes on how health care is delivered in the United States. Cultural diversity and associated issues are described in detail, showing the importance of consideration of culture when developing health interventions in the community. The influence of the environment on the health of populations is considered, and the reader is led to recognize the multitude of external factors that influence health.

Unit 4, Aggregates in the Community, presents the application of the nursing process to address potential health problems identified in large groups, including children and adolescents, women, men, families, and seniors. The focus is on the major indicators of health (e.g., longevity, mortality, and morbidity), types of common health problems, use of health services, pertinent legislation, health services and resources, selected applications of the community health nursing process to a case study, application of the levels of prevention, selected roles of the community health nurse, and relevant research.

Unit 5, Vulnerable Populations, focuses on those aggregates in the community considered vulnerable: persons with disabilities, the homeless, those living in rural areas including migrant workers, and persons with mental illness. Chapters address the application of the community health nursing process to the special service needs in each of these areas. Basic community health nursing strategies are applied to promoting the health of these vulnerable high-risk aggregates.

Unit 6, Population Health Problems, focuses on health problems that affect large aggregates and their service needs as applied in community health nursing. These problems include communicable disease, violence and associated issues, substance abuse, and a new chapter describing nursing care during disasters.

Unit 7, Community Health Settings, focuses on selected sites or specialties for community health: school health, occupational health, parish health, and home health and hospice. Recognizing a new trend in community health nursing a new chapter on forensic nursing is also included in this chapter, combined with correctional nursing content.

Unit 8, The Future of Community Health Nursing, presents an overview of what may lie ahead. One chapter is dedicated to global health and describes features of the health care systems in developing and developed countries. The final chapter emphasizes the need for community health nursing to show that it "makes a difference," which calls for an accountability-creativity link from community health nurses in all settings.

SPECIAL FEATURES

The following features are presented to enhance student learning:

- **Learning objectives.** Learning objectives set the framework for the content of each chapter.
- **Key terms.** A list of key terms for each chapter is provided at the beginning of the chapter. The terms are highlighted in bold within the chapter. The definitions of these terms are found in the Glossary located on the book's Evolve website.
- **Chapter outline** *(new to this edition).* The major headings of each chapter are provided at the beginning of each chapter to help locate important content.
- **Theoretical frameworks.** The use of theoretical frameworks common to nursing and public health will aid the student in application of familiar and new theory bases to problems and challenges in the community.
- ***Healthy People 2010.*** Goals and objectives of *Healthy People 2010* are presented in a special box throughout the text.
- **Upstream thinking.** This theoretical construct is integrated into chapters throughout the text.
- **Case studies and application of the nursing process at individual, family, and aggregate levels.** The use of case studies and **clinical examples** throughout the text is designed to ground the theory, concepts, and application of the nursing process in practical and manageable examples for the student.
- **Research highlights** *(new to this edition).* The introduction of students to the growing bodies of community health nursing and public health research literature are enhanced by special boxes devoted to specific research studies.
- **Boxed information.** Summaries of content by section, clinical examples, and other pertinent information are presented as in colored text to aid the students' learning by focusing on major points, illustrating concepts, and breaking up sections of "heavy" content.
- **Learning activities.** Selected learning activities are listed at the end of each chapter to enable students to enhance learning about the community and cognitive experiences.
- **Photo novellas.** Numerous stories in photograph form depicting public health care in a variety of settings and with different population groups.

- **Ethical insights boxes** *(new to this edition).* These boxes present situations of ethical dilemmas or considerations pertinent to particular chapters.

NEW CONTENT IN THIS EDITION

- There is a growing recognition of the unique needs and information related to disasters. This edition contains **a new chapter on disaster preparation** that provides clear and concise information on caring for those affected by disasters.
- Forensic nursing is one of the newest subspecialty areas of community and public health nursing and one that is growing in scope and popularity. In recognition of this trend, **a new chapter on forensic nursing** has been included in this edition, combined with the correctional nursing content.
- Reflecting the need for enhanced education and information related to **hospice nursing** and **palliative care,** the chapter on home health includes expanded content and discussion in these areas.
- New and timely information on **emerging infections** (e.g., SARS, West Nile virus) and changing recommendations (e.g., pediatric immunization schedule) are given in the Communicable Disease chapter.
- Most chapters contain **Research Highlights boxes** highlighting timely, relevant examples of the topics from recent nursing literature and **Ethical Insights boxes** that emphasize specific ethical issues.
- Many new full-color **photo novellas** are included, each depicting community/public health nursing care in a discrete clinical area or with a unique population group.
- Chapter 32 presents information on **health, illness, and disease patterns and health care delivery systems in countries around the world.** This information gives students and nurses a new perspective on the health of Americans and the advantages and disadvantages provided by the U.S. health care delivery system.
- **Resource Tools** refer to supplemental content such as assessment tools, summary tables, and various illustrations. These are numbered and referenced throughout the book and are located on the book's evolve website.

TEACHING AND LEARNING PACKAGE

Instructor's Electronic Resource CD-ROM. This resource contains annotated learning objectives, annotated lecture outlines, and teaching strategies for each chapter. It also provides over 300 full-color PowerPoint lecture slides, an image collection, and an 800-question test bank with alternative item questions.

Evolve website: The website at **http://evolve.elsevier.com/ nies/** is devoted exclusively to this text. It provides materials for both instructors and students.

- **For Instructors:** Annotated learning objectives, annotated lecture outlines, teaching strategies, PowerPoint lecture slides, image collection, and 800 test bank questions with alternative item questions.

- **For Students:** Quiz with multiple-choice questions with answers and correct answer rationales, Case Studies with questions and answers, Glossary, WebLinks, Resource Tools (supplemental material), and Content Updates.

ACKNOWLEDGMENTS

Community/Public Health Nursing: Promoting the Health of Populations could not have been written without sharing the experiences, thoughtful critique, and support of many people: individuals, families, groups, and communities. We give special thanks to everyone who made significant contributions to this book.

We are indebted to our contributing authors whose inspiration, untiring hours of work, and persistence have continued to build a new era of community health nursing practice with a focus on the population level. We thank the community health nursing faculty and students who welcomed the previous editions of the text and responded to our inquiries with comments and suggestions for the fourth edition. These people have challenged us to stretch, adapt, and continue to learn throughout our years of work. We also thank our colleagues in our respective work settings for their understanding and support during the writing and editing of this edition.

Finally, an enormous "thank you" to Elsevier editors Linda Thomas and Barb Watts. Their energy, enthusiasm, encouragement, and patience were vital to this project.

Mary A. Nies
Melanie McEwen

Contents

Unit 3
Factors That Influence the Health of the Community

Unit 4
Aggregates in the Community

Unit 6
Population Health Problems

Unit 7
Community Health Settings

Unit 8
The Future of Community Health Nursing

UNIT 1

Introduction to Community Health Nursing

Health: A Community View

Melanie McEwen and Mary A. Nies

MEDIA RESOURCES

Additional Material for Study, Review, and Further Exploration

evolve Website at http://evolve.elsevier.com/Nies

❖ Quiz ❖ Case Studies ❖ Content Updates ❖ Glossary ❖ WebLinks

OBJECTIVES

Upon completion of this chapter, the reader will be able to do the following:

1. Compare and contrast the public health nursing definitions of health.
2. Define and discuss the focus of public health.
3. List the three levels of prevention and give one example of each.
4. Differentiate between the conceptual models of community health nursing as defined by the American Nurses Association and public health nursing as defined by the Public Health Nursing Section of the American Public Health Association.
5. Describe the purpose of *Healthy People 2010* and give examples of the focus areas that encompass national health objectives.
6. Discuss the community health nursing practice in terms of public health's core functions and essential services.
7. Discuss community health nursing interventions as explained by the Intervention Wheel.

KEY TERMS

aggregate	health	population-focused nursing	public health nursing
community health	health promotion	primary prevention	secondary prevention
community health nursing	population	public health	tertiary prevention
disease prevention			

CHAPTER OUTLINE

DEFINITIONS OF HEALTH AND COMMUNITY
    Health
    Community

DETERMINANTS OF HEALTH AND DISEASE

INDICATORS OF HEALTH AND ILLNESS

DEFINITION AND FOCUS OF PUBLIC HEALTH AND COMMUNITY HEALTH

PREVENTIVE APPROACH TO HEALTH
    Health Promotion and Levels of Prevention
    Prevention Versus Cure
    Healthy People 2010

DEFINITION AND FOCUS OF PUBLIC HEALTH NURSING, COMMUNITY HEALTH NURSING, AND COMMUNITY-BASED NURSING
    Public Health Nursing
    Community Health Nursing
    Community-Based Nursing
    Community and Public Health Nursing Practice

POPULATION-FOCUSED PRACTICE AND COMMUNITY/ PUBLIC HEALTH NURSING INTERVENTIONS
    Community Health Interventions
    The Public Health Intervention Wheel

COMMUNITY HEALTH NURSING AND MANAGED CARE

Community/public health nurses are in a position to assist the U.S. health care system in the transition from a disease-oriented system to a health-oriented system. Costs of caring for the sick account for the majority of escalating health care dollars, which increased from 5.7% of the gross domestic product in 1965 to 14.9% in 2002 (National Center for Health Statistics [NCHS], 2004). National annual health care expenditures reached $1,553 billion in 2002, or an astonishing $5,440 per person.

U.S. health expenditures reflect a focus on the care of the sick. In 2002, $.31 of each health care dollar supported hospital care and $.22 supported physician services. Although the majority of these funds provided care for the sick, only $.03 of every health care dollar backed preventive public health activities (NCHS, 2004). Despite high hospital and physician expenditures, U.S. health indicators rate considerably below the health indicators of many other countries. This reflects the severe disproportion of funding for preventive services and social and economic opportunities. Furthermore, the health status of the population within the United States varies markedly across areas of the country and among groups (e.g., the economically disadvantaged and many cultural and ethnic groups).

Nurses constitute the largest group of health care workers; therefore they are instrumental in creating a health care delivery system that will meet the health-oriented needs of the people. According to a recent survey of registered nurses (RNs) conducted by the Health Resources and Services Administration, about 56% of approximately 2.4 million employed RNs in the United States worked in hospitals during 2004 (down from 66.5% in 1992). This survey also found that about 15%, approximately 400,000, of all RNs worked in community, school, or occupational health settings; 11.5% worked in ambulatory care settings; and 6.3% worked in nursing homes or other extended care facilities (U.S. Department of Health and Human Services/Health Resources and Services Administration/Bureau of Health Professions [USDHHS/HRSA/BHP], 2006).

Between 1980 and 2000, the number of nurses employed in community and public health settings increased by 155%, and those employed in ambulatory cares setting increased by 127% (USDHHS/HRSA/BHP, 2002). The decline in the percentage of nurses employed in hospitals and subsequent increase in nurses employed in community settings indicates a shift in focus from illness and institutional-based care to a focus on health promotion and preventive care. This shift will likely continue into the future as alternative delivery systems, such as ambulatory and home care, will employ more nurses (Inglis, 2004).

Community/public health nursing is the synthesis of nursing practice and public health practice. The major goal of community health nursing is to preserve the health of the community and surrounding populations by focusing on health promotion and health maintenance of individuals, families, and groups within the community. Thus, community/public health nursing is associated with health and the identification of populations at risk rather than with an episodical response to patient demand.

The mission of public health is social justice, which entitles all people to basic necessities such as adequate income and health protection and accepts collective burdens to make this possible. Public health, with its egalitarian tradition and vision, conflicts with the predominant U.S. model of market justice that only entitles people to what they have gained through individual efforts. Although market justice respects individual rights, collective action and obligations are minimal. An overinvestment in technology and curative medical services within the market justice system has stifled the evolution of a health system designed to protect and preserve the health of the population. There is a need for an

ethic of social justice, for it is society's responsibility, rather than the individual's, to meet the basic needs of all people. Thus there is a need for public funding of prevention efforts to enhance the health of our population.

Current U.S. health policy advocates changes in personal behaviors that might predispose individuals to chronic disease or accident. This policy promotes exercise, healthy eating, tobacco cessation, and moderate consumption of alcohol. However, simply encouraging the individual to overcome the effects of unhealthy activities lessens focus on collective behaviors necessary to change the determinants of health stemming from such factors as air and water pollution, workplace hazards, and unequal access to health care. Because living arrangements, work/school environment, and other sociocultural constraints affect health and well-being, public policy must address societal and environmental changes, in addition to lifestyle changes, that will positively influence the health of the entire population.

With ongoing changes in the health care system and increased employment in community settings, there will be greater demands on community health nurses to broaden their public health perspective. The American Nurses Association's (ANA) Code of Ethics (2001) promotes social reform by focusing on health policy and legislation to positively affect accessibility, quality, and cost of health care. Community and public health nurses, therefore, must align themselves with public health programs that promote and preserve the health of populations by influencing sociocultural issues such as violation of human rights, homelessness, violence, and stigma of illness. This allows nurses to be positioned to promote the health, welfare, and safety of all individuals.

This chapter examines health from a population-focused, community-based perspective. Therefore it requires understanding of how people identify, define, and describe related concepts. The following section explores six major ideas:
1. Definitions of "health" and "community"
2. Determinants of health and disease
3. Indicators of health and disease
4. Definition and focus of public and community health
5. Description of a preventive approach to health
6. Definition and focus of "public health nursing," "community health nursing" and "community-based nursing"

DEFINITIONS OF HEALTH AND COMMUNITY

Health

The definition of **health** is evolving. The World Health Organization's (WHO) early, classic definition of health set a trend toward describing health in social terms, rather than in medical terms. Indeed, the WHO (1958, p. 1) defined health as "a state of complete physical, mental, and social well-being and not merely the absence of disease or infirmity."

Social means "of or relating to living together in organized groups or similar close aggregates" (*American Heritage,* 1997, p. 1291) and refers to units of people in communities who interact with each other. "Social health" connotes community vitality and is a result of positive interaction among groups within the community with an emphasis on health promotion and illness prevention. For example, community groups may sponsor food banks in churches and civic organizations to help alleviate problems with hunger and nutrition. Other community groups may form to address problems of violence and lack of opportunity, which can negatively affect social health.

In the mid 1980s, the WHO expanded the definition of health to include the following socialized conceptualization of health:

> *The extent to which an individual or group is able, on the one hand, to realize aspirations and satisfy needs; and, on the other hand, to change or cope with the environment. Health is, therefore, seen as a resource for everyday life, not the objective of living; it is a positive concept emphasizing social and personal resources, and physical capacities.*
>
> *(WHO, 1986, p. 73)*

Saylor (2004) pointed out that the WHO definition considers several dimensions of health. These include physical (structure/function), social, role, mental (emotional and intellectual), and general perceptions of health status. It also conceptualizes health from a macro perspective, as a resource to be used rather than a goal in and of itself.

The nursing literature contains many, varied definitions of health. For example, health has been defined as "a state of well-being in which the person is able to use purposeful, adaptive responses and processes physically, mentally, emotionally, spiritually, and socially" (Murray and Zentner, 2001, p. 53); "actualization of inherent and acquired human potential through goal-directed behavior, competent self-care, and satisfying relationships with others" (Pender, 2002, p. 22); and a state of a person that is characterized by soundness or wholeness of developed human structures and of bodily and mental functioning (Orem, 2001).

The variety of characterizations of the word illustrates the difficulty in standardizing the conceptualization of health. Commonalities involve description of "goal-directed" or "purposeful" actions, processes, responses, or behaviors and possessing "soundness," "wholeness," and/or "well-being." Problems can arise when the definition involves a unit of analysis. For example, some authors use the individual or "person" as the unit of analysis and exclude the community. Others many include additional concepts, such as adaptation and environment, in health definitions and then present the environment as static and requiring human adaptation, rather than as changing and enabling human modification.

For many years, community and public health nurses have favored Dunn's (1961) classic concept of wellness, in which family, community, society, and environment are interrelated and have an impact on health. From his viewpoint, illness, health, and peak wellness are on a continuum; health is fluid and changing. Consequently, within a social environment, the state of health depends on the goals, potentials, and performance of individuals, families, communities, and societies.

Community

The definitions of **community** are also numerous and variable. Baldwin and colleagues (1998) outlined the evolution of the definition of community by examining definitions that appeared in community health nursing texts. They determined that before 1996, definitions of community focused on geographical boundaries, combined with social attributes of people. Through citing several sources from the later part of the decade, the authors observed that geographical location became a secondary characteristic in the discussion of what defines a community.

In recent nursing literature, community has been defined as "a collection of people who interact with one another and whose common interests or characteristics form the basis for a sense of unity or belonging" (Allender and Spradley, 2005, p. 6); "a group of people sharing common interests, needs, resources and environment" (Thomas, 2003, p. 6); "a group of people who share some type of bond, who interact with each other, and who function collectively regarding common concerns" (Clark, 2003, pp. 4-5); and "a locality-based entity, composed of systems of formal organizations reflecting society's institutions, informal groups and aggregates" (Shuster and Goeppinger, 2004, p. 344). Maurer and Smith (2005) further addressed the concept of community and identified four defining attributes: people, place, interaction, and common characteristics, interests, or goals. In this text, community is seen as a group or collection of locality-based individuals, interacting in social units and sharing common interests, characteristics, values, and/or goals.

Maurer and Smith (2005) noted that there are two main types of communities: geopolitical communities and phenomenological communities. Geopolitical communities are those most traditionally recognized or imagined when considering the term *community*. Geopolitical communities are defined or formed by both natural and manmade boundaries and include cities, counties, states, and nations. Other commonly recognized geopolitical communities are school districts, census tracts, zip codes, and neighborhoods. Phenomenological communities, on the other hand, refer to relational, interactive groups. In phenomenological communities, the place or setting is more abstract, and people share a group perspective or identity based on culture, values, history, interests, and goals. Examples of phenomenological communities would be schools, colleges, and universities; churches, synagogues, and mosques; and various groups or organizations.

A community of solution is a type of phenomenological community. A community of solution is a collection of people who form a group specifically to address a common need or concern. The Sierra Club, whose members lobby for the preservation of natural resource lands, and a group of disabled people who challenge the owners of an office building to obtain equal access to public buildings, education, jobs, and transportation are examples. These groups or social units work together to realize a level of potential "health" and to address identified actual and potential health threats and health needs.

Population and **aggregate** are related terms that are often used in public health and community health nursing. Population is typically used to denote a group of people having common personal or environmental characteristics. It can also

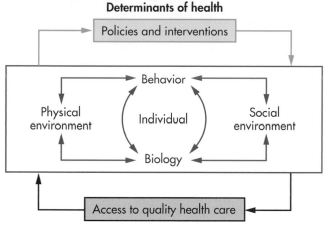

Determinants of health

FIGURE 1-1 *Healthy People 2010*—Determinants of health.

refer to all of the people in a defined community (Maurer and Smith, 2005). Aggregates are subgroups or subpopulations that have some common characteristics or concerns (Clark, 2003). Depending on the situation, needs, and practice parameters, community health nursing interventions may be directed toward a community (e.g., residents of a small town), a population (e.g., all elders in a rural region), or an aggregate (e.g., pregnant teens within a school district).

DETERMINANTS OF HEALTH AND DISEASE

The health status of a community is associated with a number of factors such as health care access, economic conditions, social and environmental issues, and cultural practices, and it is essential for the community health nurse to understand the determinants of health and recognize the interaction of the factors that lead to disease, death, and disability. It has been estimated that individual behaviors and environmental factors are responsible for about 70% of all premature deaths in the United States (USDHHS, 2000). Indeed, individual biology and behaviors influence health through their interaction with each other and with the individual's social and physical environments. In addition, policies and interventions can improve health by targeting detrimental or harmful factors related to individuals and their environment. Figure 1-1 depicts the interaction of these determinants and show how health is influenced.

In a seminal work, McGinnis and Foege (1993) described what they termed "actual causes of death" in the United States. Leading the list was smoking, which was implicated in almost 20% of the annual deaths in the United States—approximately 400,000 individuals. Diet and activity patterns were deemed to account for about 14% of deaths (about 300,000 per year), and alcohol was implicated in about 5% of all deaths because of its association with accidents, suicides, homicides, and cirrhosis and chronic liver disease. While all of these causes of mortality are related to individual lifestyle choices, they can also be strongly influenced by population-focused policy efforts and education. For example, the prevalence of adult smoking has fallen dramatically during the past decade, largely due to

legal efforts (e.g., laws prohibiting sale of tobacco to minors and much higher taxes), organizational policy (e.g., smoke-free workplaces) and education. Likewise, recent concerns about the widespread increase in incidence of overweight and obesity has led to calls for population-based measures to address the issue.

In another important writing, McKeown (2001) observed that health has improved over the past 100 years largely because people become ill less often. He noted that at the population level, health can be largely attributed to higher standards of living, better nutrition, a healthier environment, and having fewer children. Furthermore, public health efforts, such as immunization, and medical care, including management of acute episodic illnesses (e.g., pneumonia, tuberculosis) and chronic disease (e.g., cancer, heart disease), have also contributed significantly to the increase in life expectancy (Rothstein, 2001).

Community and public health nurses should understand these concepts and appreciate that health and illness are influenced by a web of factors, some which can be changed (e.g., individual behaviors, such as tobacco use, diet, activity) and some which cannot (e.g., biology, age, gender). Other factors (e.g., physical and social environment) will require changes that may need to be accomplished from a policy perspective. Community health nurses must work with policy makers and community leaders to identify patterns of disease and death and to advocate for activities and policies that promote health at the individual, family, and community levels.

INDICATORS OF HEALTH AND ILLNESS

A variety of health indicators are used by health providers, policy makers, and community health nurses to measure the health of the community. Local or state health departments, the Centers for Disease Control and Prevention, and the National Center for Health Statistics provide morbidity, mortality, and other health status–related data. State and local health departments are responsible for collecting morbidity and mortality data and forwarding the information to the appropriate federal-level agency, which is often the Centers for Disease Control and Prevention. Some of the more commonly reported indicators are life expectancy, infant mortality, age-adjusted death rates, and cancer incidence rates.

Indicators of mortality illustrate the health status of a community and/or population because changes in mortality reflect a number of social, economic, health service, and related trends (Torrens, 2002). These data may be useful in analyzing health patterns over time, comparing communities from different geographical regions or comparing different aggregates within a community.

When developing the national health objectives for *Healthy People 2010*, a total of 10 leading health indicators were identified that reflected the major public health concerns in the United States. They include individual behaviors (e.g., physical activity, overweight and obesity), physical and social environmental factors (e.g., environmental quality, injury

HEALTHY PEOPLE **2010**	Leading Health Indicators
• Physical Activity	• Mental Health
• Overweight and Obesity	• Injury and Violence
• Tobacco Use	• Environmental Quality
• Substance Abuse	• Immunization
• Responsible Sexual Behavior	• Access to Health Care

From US Department of Health and Human Services: *Healthy People 2010 objectives*, Washington, DC, 2000, The Author.

and violence) and health systems issues (e.g., access to health care). Each of these indicators can affect the health of individuals and communities, and they can be correlated with leading causes of morbidity and mortality. For example, tobacco use is linked to heart disease, stroke, and cancer; substance abuse is linked to accidents, injuries, and violence; irresponsible sexual behaviors can lead to unwanted pregnancy as well as sexually transmitted diseases, including HIV/AIDS; and lack of access to health care can contribute to poor pregnancy outcomes, untreated illness, and disability.

Community health nurses should be aware of health patterns and health indicators within their practice. Nurses should ask many questions, including the following: What are the leading causes of death and disease among various groups served? How do infant mortality rates and teenage pregnancy rates in this community compare with regional, state, and national rates? What are the most serious communicable disease threats? What are the most common environmental risks?

The community health nurse may identify areas for further investigation and intervention through an understanding of health, disease, and mortality patterns. For example, if a school nurse learns that the teenage pregnancy rate in her community is higher than regional and state averages, he or she should address the problem with school officials, parents, and students. Likewise, if an occupational health nurse discovers an apparent high rate of chronic lung disease in an industrial facility, he or she should work with company management, employees, and state and federal officials to identify potential harmful sources. Finally, if a public health nurse works in a state-sponsored AIDS clinic and recognizes an increase in the number of women testing positive for HIV, he or she should report all findings to the designated agencies. The nurse should then participate in investigative efforts to determine what is precipitating the increase and work to remedy the identified threats or risks.

DEFINITION AND FOCUS OF PUBLIC HEALTH AND COMMUNITY HEALTH

C. E. Winslow is known for the following classic definition of public health:

Public health is the Science and Art of (1) preventing disease, (2) prolonging life, and (3) promoting health and efficiency through organized community effort for:

(a) sanitation of the environment,

(b) control of communicable infections,

(c) education of the individual in personal hygiene,

(d) organization of medical and nursing services for the early diagnosis and preventive treatment of disease, and

(e) development of the social machinery to ensure everyone a standard of living adequate for the maintenance of health, so organizing these benefits as to enable every citizen to realize his birthright of health and longevity.

(Hanlon, 1960, p. 23)

A key phrase in this definition of public health is "through organized community effort." The term **public health** connotes organized, legislated, and tax-supported efforts that serve all people through health departments or related governmental agencies.

The public health nursing tradition, begun in the late 1800s by Lillian Wald and her associates, clearly illustrates this phenomenon (Wald, 1971, see Chapter 2). After moving into the immigrant community to provide care for individuals and families, these early public health nurses saw that neither administering bedside clinical nursing nor teaching family members to deliver care in the home adequately addressed the true determinants of health and disease. They resolved that collective political activity should focus on advancing the health of aggregates and improving social and environmental conditions by addressing the social and environmental determinants of health, such as child labor, pollution, and poverty. Wald and her colleagues impacted the health of the community by organizing the community, establishing school nursing, and taking impoverished mothers to testify in Washington, DC (Wald, 1971).

More recently, the Institute of Medicine (1988) identified the following three primary functions of public health: assessment, assurance, and policy development. Box 1-1 depicts each of the three primary functions and describes them briefly. All nurses working in community settings should develop knowledge and skills related to each of these primary functions.

The term **community health** extends the realm of public health to include organized health efforts at the community level through both government *and* private efforts. Participants include privately funded agencies such as the American Heart Association or the American Red Cross. A variety of private and public structures serve community health efforts.

Public health efforts focus on prevention and promotion of population health at the federal, state, and local levels. These efforts at the federal and state levels concentrate on

BOX 1-1 Core Public Health Functions

Assessment: Regular collection, analysis, and information sharing about health conditions, risks, and resources in a community.

Policy development: Use of information gathered during assessment to develop local and state health policies and to direct resources toward those policies.

Assurance: Focuses on the availability of necessary health services throughout the community. It includes maintaining the ability of both public health agencies and private providers to manage day-to-day operations and the capacity to respond to critical situations and emergencies.

From Institute of Medicine: *The future of public health* Washington, DC, 1988, National Academy Press.

BOX 1-2 Essential Public Health Services

➤ Monitor health status to identify community health problems.

➤ Diagnose and investigate health problems and health hazards in the community.

➤ Inform, educate, and empower people about health issues.

➤ Mobilize community partnerships to identify and solve health problems.

➤ Develop policies and plans that support individual and community health efforts.

➤ Enforce laws and regulations that protect health and ensure safety.

➤ Link people to needed personal health services and assure the provision of health care when otherwise unavailable.

➤ Assure a competent public health and personal health care workforce.

➤ Evaluate effectiveness, accessibility, and quality of personal and population-based health services.

➤ Research for new insights and innovative solutions to health problems.

From US Department of Health and Human Services/Public Health Service: *The public health workforce: an agenda for the 21st century,* Washington, DC, 1997, The Author.

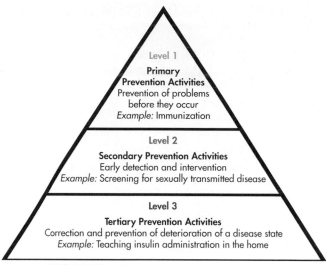

FIGURE 1-2 The three levels of prevention.

providing support and advisory services to public health structures at the local level. The local level structures provide direct services to communities through two avenues:

• Community health services protect the public from hazards such as polluted water and air, tainted food, and unsafe housing.

• Personal health care services such as immunization and family planning services, well-infant care, and STD (sexually transmitted disease) treatment.

Personal health services may be part of the public health effort and often target the populations most at risk and in need of services. Public health efforts are multidisciplinary because they require people with many different skills. Community health nurses work with a diverse team of public health professionals, including epidemiologists, local health officers, and health educators. Public health science methods that assess biostatistics, epidemiology, and population needs provide a method of measuring characteristics and health indicators and disease patterns within a community. In 1994, the American

Public Health Association drafted a list of 10 essential public health services, which the U.S. Department of Health and Human Services (USDHHS, 1997) later adopted. This list appears in Box 1-2.

PREVENTIVE APPROACH TO HEALTH

Health Promotion and Levels of Prevention

Contrasting with "medical care," which focuses on disease management and "cure," public health efforts focus on health promotion and disease prevention. **Health promotion** activities enhance resources directed at improving well-being, whereas **disease prevention** activities protect people from disease and the effects of disease. Leavell and Clark (1958) identified three levels of prevention commonly described in nursing practice: primary prevention, secondary prevention and tertiary prevention (Figure 1-2 and Table 1-1).

Primary prevention relates to activities directed at preventing a problem before it occurs by altering susceptibility or reducing exposure for susceptible individuals. Primary prevention consists of two elements: general health promotion and specific protection. Health promotion efforts enhance resiliency and protective factors and target essentially well populations. Examples include promotion of good nutrition, provision of adequate shelter, and encouraging regular exercise. Specific protection efforts reduce or eliminate risk factors and include such measures as immunization and water purification (Keller et al., 2004; McEwen, 2002;).

Secondary prevention refers to early detection and prompt intervention during the period of early disease pathogenesis. Secondary prevention is implemented after a problem has begun but before signs and symptoms appear and targets those populations who have risk factors (Keller et al., 2004). Mammography, blood pressure screening, scoliosis screening, and Papanicolaou smears are examples of secondary prevention.

TABLE 1-1   Examples of Levels of Prevention and Clients Served in the Community

DEFINITION OF CLIENT SERVED*	LEVEL OF PREVENTION		
	PRIMARY (HEALTH PROMOTION AND SPECIFIC PREVENTION)	SECONDARY (EARLY DIAGNOSIS AND TREATMENT)	TERTIARY (LIMITATION OF DISABILITY AND REHABILITATION)
Individual	Dietary teaching during pregnancy Immunizations	HIV testing Screening for cervical cancer	Teaching new clients with diabetes how to administer insulin Exercise therapy after stroke Skin care for incontinent patients
Family (two or more individuals bound by kinship, law, or living arrangement and with common emotional ties and obligations [see Chapter 18])	Education or counseling regarding smoking, dental care, or nutrition Adequate housing	Dental examinations Tuberculin testing for family at risk	Mental health counseling or referral for family in crisis (e.g., grieving or experiencing a divorce) Dietary instructions and monitoring for family with overweight members
Group or aggregate (interacting people with a common purpose or purposes)	Birthing classes for pregnant teenage mothers AIDS and other STD education for high school students	Vision screening of first-grade class Mammography van for screening of women in a low-income neighborhood Hearing tests at a senior center	Group counseling for grade-school children with asthma Swim therapy for physically disabled elders at a senior center Alcoholics Anonymous and other self-help groups Mental health services for military veterans
Community and populations (aggregate of people sharing space over time within a social system [see Chapter 5]; population groups or aggregates with power relations and common needs or purposes)	Fluoride water supplementation Environmental sanitation Removal of environmental hazards	Organized screening programs for communities (e.g., health fairs) VDRL screening for marriage license applicants in a city Lead screening for children by school district	Shelter and relocation centers for fire or earthquake victims Emergency medical services Community mental health services for chronically mentally ill Home care services for chronically ill

AIDS, Acquired immunodeficiency syndrome; *HIV,* human immunodeficiency virus; *STD,* sexually transmitted disease; *VDRL,* Venereal Disease Research Laboratory.
*Note that terms are used differently in literature of various disciplines. There are not any clear-cut definitions; for example, families may be referred to as an aggregate, and a population and subpopulations may exist within a community.

Tertiary prevention targets populations who have experienced disease or injury and focuses on limitation of disability and rehabilitation. Aims of tertiary prevention are: to keep health problems from getting worse; to reduce the effects of disease and injury; and to restore individuals to their optimal level of functioning (Keller et al., 2004; McEwen, 2002). Examples include teaching how to perform insulin injections and disease management to a diabetic, referral of a spinal cord injury victim for occupational and physical therapy, and leading a support group for grieving parents.

Much of community health nursing practice is directed toward preventing the progression of disease at the earliest period or phase feasible using the appropriate level(s) of prevention. For example, when applying "levels of prevention" to a client with HIV/AIDS, a nurse might perform the following interventions:

- Educate students on the practice of sexual abstinence or "safer sex" by using barrier methods (primary prevention)
- Encourage testing and counseling for clients with known exposure or who are in high-risk groups; provide referrals for follow-up for clients who test positive for HIV (secondary prevention)
- Provide education on management of HIV infection,

advocacy, case management, and other interventions for those who are HIV+ (tertiary prevention) (McEwen, 2002).

The concepts of prevention and population-focused care figure prominently in a conceptual orientation to nursing practice referred to as "thinking upstream." This orientation is derived from an analogy of patients falling into a river upstream and being rescued downstream by health providers overwhelmed with the struggle of responding to disease and illness. The river as an analogy for the natural history of illness was first coined by McKinlay (1979), with a charge to health providers to refocus their efforts toward preventive and "upstream" activities. In a description of the daily challenges of providers to address health from a preventive versus curative focus, McKinlay differentiates the consequences of illness (*downstream* endeavors) from its precursors (*upstream* endeavors). The author then charges health providers to critically examine the relative weight of their activities toward illness response versus the prevention of illness.

Butterfield (1990) adapted McKinlay's upstream analogy to nursing practice by examining preventive health efforts in nursing from a historical and theoretical perspective. In this context, a population-based perspective on health and health determinants is critical to understanding and formulating nursing actions to

ETHICAL Insights

Inequities: Distribution of Resources

In the United States, inequities in the distribution of resources pose a threat to the common good and a challenge for community and public health nurses. Factors that contribute to wide variations in health disparities include education, income, and occupation. Lack of health insurance is a key factor in this issue, as about 20% of non elderly adults and 25% of children in the United States are uninsured. Lack of insurance is damaging to population health, as low-income, uninsured individuals are much less likely than nonpoor insured individuals to received timely physical examinations and preventive dental care.

Public health nurses are regularly confronted with the consequences of the fragmented health care delivery system. They diligently work to improve the circumstances for populations who have not had adequate access to resources largely because of who they are and where they live.

Ethical questions commonly encountered in community and public health nursing practice include the following: Should resources (e.g., free or low-cost immunizations) be offered to all, even those who have insurance that will pay for the care? Should public health nurses serve anyone who meets financial need guidelines, regardless of medical need? Should the health department provide flu shots to persons of all ages or just those most likely to be severely affected by the disease? Should illegal aliens or persons working on "green cards" receive the same level of health care services that are available to citizens?

Social justice in health care is a goal for all. To this end, community and public health nurses must face the challenges and dilemmas related to these and other questions as they assist individuals, families, and communities deal with the uneven distribution of health resources.

From Ervin NE and Bell SE: Social justice issues related to uneven distribution of resources, *Journal of the New York State Nurses Association* 35(1):8-13, 2004.

prevent disease. By examining the origins of disease, nurses identify social, political, environmental, and economic factors that often lead to poor health options for both individuals and populations. The call to refocus the efforts of nurses "upstream, where the real problems lie" (McKinlay, 1979) has been welcomed by community health nurses in a variety of practice settings. For these nurses, this theme provides affirmation of their daily efforts to prevent disease in populations at risk in schools, work sites, and clinics throughout their local communities and in the larger world. ■

Prevention Versus Cure

Spending additional dollars for cure in the form of health care services does not improve the health of a population, whereas spending money on prevention does improve health. Feldstein (2003) and others (Lamarche, 1995; Torrens, 2002) note that there is an absence of convincing evidence that indicates that the amount of money expended for health care improves the health of a population. The real determinants of health, as mentioned, are prevention efforts that provide education, housing, food, a decent minimal income, and safe social and physical environments. The United States spends nearly one seventh of the nation's wealth on health care or "cure" for individuals and could possibly divert money away from the needed resources and services that make a greater impact on health (McKeown, 2001; NCHS, 2004).

U.S. policy makers have not committed to achieving these important health outcomes for the poor, vulnerable, and uninsured populations. With a limited health workforce and monetary resources, the United States cannot continue to spend vast amounts on health care services when the investment fails to improve health outcomes. In industrialized countries, life expectancy at birth is not related to the level of health care expenditures; in developing countries, longevity is closely related to the level of economic development and the education of the population (Feldstein, 2003; Lamarche, 1995).

A continued overexpansion of the current health care system could actually be detrimental to the health of a population. This may deter a large investment of the country's wealth in education and other developmental efforts that positively impact health. Managed care organizations (MCOs) focus on prevention; therefore they have determined that the rate of health care cost increases have slowed among employees of large firms (Torrens and Williams, 2002). Prevention programs may help reduce costs for those enrolled in MCOs, but it is unclear who will provide these services for the uninsured, poor, and other vulnerable populations. In addition, who will provide adequate schooling, housing, meals, wages, and a safe environment for the disadvantaged? Reductions in health care spending would decrease the effects of economic disparities by allowing investments in sufficient housing, jobs, nutrition, and safe environments.

Healthy People 2010

In 1979, the U.S. Department of Health and Human Services published a national prevention initiative titled *Healthy People: The Surgeon General's Report on Health Promotion and Disease Prevention*. The 1979 version established goals that would reduce mortality among infants, children, adolescents and young adults, and adults and increase independence among older adults. In 1990, the mortality of infants, children, and adults declined sufficiently to meet the goal. Adolescent mortality did not reach the 1990 target, and data systems were unable to adequately track the target for older adults (USDHHS, 2000).

Published in 1989, *Healthy People 2000* built upon the first Surgeon General's report. *Healthy People 2000* contained the following broad goals (USDHHS, 1989):

1. Increase the span of healthy life for Americans.
2. Reduce health disparities among Americans.
3. Achieve access to preventive services for all Americans.

The purpose of *Healthy People 2000* was to provide direction for individuals wanting to change personal behaviors and to improve health in communities through health promotion policies. The report assimilated the broad approaches of health promotion, health protection, and preventive services and contained more than 300 objectives organized into 22 priority areas. Although many of the objectives fell short, the initiative was extremely successful in raising providers' awareness of health behaviors and health promotional activities. States, local health departments, and private sector health workers used the objectives to determine the relative health of their community and set goals for the future.

HEALTHY PEOPLE 2010	Focus Areas	
1. Access to quality health services	15. Injury and violence prevention	
2. Arthritis, osteoporosis and chronic back conditions	16. Maternal, infant, and child health	
3. Cancer	17. Medical product safety	
4. Chronic kidney disease	18. Mental health and mental disorders	
5. Diabetes	19. Nutrition and overweight	
6. Disability and secondary conditions	20. Occupational safety and health	
7. Educational and community-based programs	21. Oral health	
8. Environmental health	22. Physical activity and fitness	
9. Family planning	23. Public health infrastructure	
10. Food safety	24. Respiratory disease	
11. Health communication	25. STDs	
12. Heart disease and stroke	26. Substance abuse	
13. HIV	27. Tobacco use	
14. Immunization and infectious diseases	28. Vision and hearing	

From US Department of Health and Human Services: *Healthy People 2010 objectives,* Washington, DC, 2000, The Author.

Healthy People 2010 emerged in January 2000. It expanded upon the objectives from *Healthy People 2000* through a broadened prevention science base, an improved surveillance and data system, and a heightened awareness and demand for preventive health services. This reflects changes in demographics, science, technology, and disease. *Healthy People 2010* lists the following broad goals:

Goal 1: Increase quality and years of healthy life.

Goal 2: Eliminate health disparities.

The first goal moves beyond the idea of increasing life expectancy to incorporate the concept of health-related quality of life (HRQOL). This concept of health includes aspects of physical and mental health and their determinants and measures functional status, participation, and well-being. HRQOL expands the definition of health—beyond simply opposing the negative concepts of disease and death—by integrating mental and physical health concepts (USDHHS, 2000).

In *Healthy People 2010*, some 467 objectives are divided into 28 focus areas. The focus areas are listed in the Healthy People box above. The objectives can help guide health promotion activities and can be used to aid in community-wide initiatives (USDHHS, 2000). All health care practitioners, particularly those working in the community, should review the *Healthy People 2010* objectives and focus on the relevant areas in their practice. Practitioners should incorporate these objectives into programs, events, and publications whenever possible and should use them as a framework to promote healthy cities and communities. Selected relevant objectives are presented throughout this book to acquaint future community health nurses with the scope of the *Healthy People 2010* initiative and to enhance awareness of current health indicators and national goals (see www.healthypeople.gov for more information).

DEFINITION AND FOCUS OF PUBLIC HEALTH NURSING, COMMUNITY HEALTH NURSING, AND COMMUNITY-BASED NURSING

The terms *community health nursing* and *public health nursing* are often synonymous or interchangeable. Like the practice of community/public health nursing, the terms are evolving. In the past debates and discussions, definitions of "community health nursing" and "public health nursing" indicate similar yet distinctive ideologies, visions, or philosophies of nursing. These concepts and a third, related term—*community-based nursing*—are discussed in this section.

Public Health Nursing

Public health nursing has frequently been described as the synthesis of public health and nursing practice. Freeman (1963) provided a classic definition of public health nursing:

Public health nursing may be defined as a field of professional practice in nursing and in public health in which technical nursing, interpersonal, analytical, and organizational skills are applied to problems of health as they affect the community. These skills are applied in concert with those of other persons engaged in health care, through comprehensive nursing care of families and other groups and through measures for evaluation or control of threats to health, for health education of the public, and for mobilization of the public for health action. (p. 34)

More recently, the American Public Health Association (APHA) Committee on Public Health Nursing (1996) stated the following:

Public health nursing is the practice of promoting and protecting the health of populations using knowledge from nursing, social, and public health sciences. Public health nursing practice is a systematic process by which

1. the health and health care needs of a population are assessed in order to identify subpopulations, families, and individuals who would benefit from health promotion or who are at risk of illness, injury, disability or premature death;

2. a plan for intervention is developed with the community to meet identified needs that takes into account available resources, the range of activities that contribute to health and the prevention of illness, injury, disability, and premature death;

3. the plan is implemented effectively, efficiently and equitably;

4. evaluations are conducted to determine the extent to which the interventions have an impact on the health status of individuals and the population;

5. the results of the process are used to influence and direct the current delivery of care, deployment of health resources, and the development of local, regional, state, and national health policy and research to promote health and prevent disease. (pp. 1-2)

Community Health Nursing

In 1980, the ANA defined **community health nursing,** stating that it:

. . . is a synthesis of nursing practice and public health practice applied to promoting and preserving the health of populations. The practice is general and comprehensive. It is not limited to a particular age group or diagnosis and is continuing, not episodic. The dominant responsibility is to the population as a whole; nursing directed to individuals, families, or groups contributes to the health of the total population. Health promotion, health maintenance, health education and management, coordination, and continuity of care are utilized in a holistic approach to the management of the health care of individuals, families, and groups in a community. (ANA, 1980, p. 2)

A common theme of these definitions is the provision of nursing service to the community or population as a whole. Muecke (1984) noted that whereas the ANA definition focused on care to individuals, families, and groups within a community, the APHA definition focused on care to the community as a whole. The APHA considers the individual or single family *only* as part of a risk group. Both definitions are important for addressing the health of aggregates. In the community, individual health and family health are necessary building blocks to the health of populations, but they represent only one facet of health care provision at the aggregate level.

Some nursing authors use *community health nursing* as a global or umbrella term and *public health nursing* as a component or subset. Others, as stated, use the terms interchangeably. This book will use the terms interchangeably; however, it is important to note that, although minor, there are distinctive differences in practice parameters and ideology.

Community-Based Nursing

The term *community-based nursing* has been identified and defined in recent years to differentiate it from what has traditionally been seen as community and public health nursing practice. Community-based nursing practice refers to "application of the nursing process in caring for individuals, families and groups where they live, work or go to school or

RESEARCH **HIGHLIGHTS**

Public Health Nurse Job Satisfaction

A study of 192 public health nurses was recently conducted to describe the characteristics and relationships of organizational structure and job satisfaction among public health nurses. The researchers found that the nurses in the study reported "moderate" levels of job satisfaction. Factors identified that increased job satisfaction were more years of experience at the health department and improved vertical and horizontal decision-making opportunities. Other factors that nurses indicated would improve their job satisfaction were better pay, more input, and better role clarity. The researchers concluded that job satisfaction improves when supervisors and subordinates consult together concerning job tasks and decisions, and when individuals are involved with peers in decision making.

From Campbell, SL, Fowles, ER, and Weber, BJ: Organizational structure and job satisfaction in public health nursing, *Public Health Nursing* 21(6):564-571.

2002, p. 6). Community-based nursing is setting-specific, and the emphasis is on acute and chronic care and includes such practice areas as home health nursing and nursing in out patient or ambulatory settings.

Zotti, Brown, and Stotts (1996) compared community-based nursing and community health nursing and explained that the goals of the two are different. Community health nursing emphasizes preservation and protection of health, and community-based nursing emphasizes managing acute or chronic conditions. In community health nursing, the primary client is the community; in community-based nursing, the primary clients are the individual and the family. Finally, services in community-based nursing are largely direct, and in community health nursing, services are both direct and indirect.

Community and Public Health Nursing Practice

Community and public health nurses practice disease prevention and health promotion. It is important to note that community health nursing practice is collaborative and is based in research and theory. It applies the nursing process to the care of individuals, families, aggregates, and the community. Table 1-2 presents the Standards for Public Health Nursing Practice developed by the Quad Council of Public Health Nursing Organizations. The Quad Council is comprised of representatives from the Association of State and Territorial Directors of Nursing, the Association of Community Health Nursing Educators, the Public Health Nursing Section of the American Public Health Association, and the Community Health Nursing Council of the ANA.

As discussed, the core functions of public health are assessment, policy development, and assurance. In 2003, the Quad Council closely examined the core functions and developed a set of public health nursing competencies; these are summarized in Table 1-3 (Quad Council, 2003). Current and future community health nurses should study these competencies to understand the practice parameters and skills required for public health practice.

TABLE 1-2   Standards of Public Health Nursing Practice

Standards of Care

Standard I. Assessment	The public health nurse assesses the health status of populations using data, community resources identification, input from the population, and professional judgment.
Standard II. Diagnosis	The public health nurse analyzes collected assessment data and partners with the people to attach meaning to those data and determine opportunities and needs.
Standard III. Outcomes Identification	The public health nurse participates with other community partners to identify expected outcomes in the populations and their health status.
Standard IV. Planning	The public health nurse promotes and supports the development of programs, policies, and services that provide interventions that improve the health status of populations.
Standard V. Assurance: Action Component of the Nursing Process for Public Health Nursing	The public health nurse assures access and availability of programs, policies, resources, and services to the population.
Standard VI. Evaluation	The public health nurse evaluates the health status of the population.

Standards of Professional Performance

Standard I. Quality of Care	The public health nurse systematically evaluates the availability, accessibility, acceptability, quality, and effectiveness of nursing practice for the population.
Standard II. Performance Appraisal	The public health nurse evaluates his or her own nursing practice in relation to professional practice standards and relevant statutes and regulations.
Standard III. Education	The public health nurse acquires and maintains current knowledge and competency in public health nursing practice.
Standard IV. Collegiality	The public health nurse establishes collegial partnerships while interacting with healthy care practitioners and others and contributes to the professional development of peers, colleagues, and others.
Standard V. Ethics	The public health nurse applies ethical standards in advocating for health and social policy and delivery of public health programs to promote and preserve the health of the population.
Standard VI. Collaboration	The public health nurse collaborates with the representatives of the population and other health and human service professionals and organizations in providing for and promoting the health of the population.
Standard VII. Research	The public health nurse uses research findings in practice.
Standard VIII. Resource Utilization	The public health nurse considers safety, effectiveness, and cost in the planning and delivery of public health services when using available resources to ensure the maximum possible health benefits to the population.

From Quad Council of Public Health Nursing Organizations: *Scope and standards of public health nursing practice,* Washington, DC, 1999, American Nurses Publishing.

POPULATION-FOCUSED PRACTICE AND COMMUNITY/ PUBLIC HEALTH NURSING INTERVENTIONS

Community/public health nurses must use a population-focused approach to move beyond providing direct care to individuals and families. **Population-focused nursing** concentrates on specific groups of people and focuses on health promotion and disease prevention, regardless of geographical location (Baldwin et al., 1998). Population-focused practice (Minnesota Department of Health, 2003):

* Focuses on the entire population
* Is based on assessment of the populations' health status
* Considers the broad determinants of health
* Emphasizes all levels of prevention
* Intervenes with communities, systems, individuals, and families

While community and public health nurses may be responsible for a specific subpopulation in the community (e.g., a school may be responsible for its pregnant teenagers), population-focused practice is concerned with many distinct and overlapping community subpopulations. The goal of population-focused nursing is to promote healthy communities.

Population-focused community health nurses would not have exclusive interest in one or two subpopulations but would focus on the many subpopulations that make up the entire community. A population focus involves concern for those who do, and for those who do not, receive health services. A population focus also involves a scientific approach to community health nursing: an assessment of the community or population is necessary and basic to planning, intervention, and evaluation for the individual, family, aggregate, and population levels.

Community health nursing practice requires the following types of data for scientific approach and population focus: (1) the epidemiology, or body of knowledge, of a particular problem and its solution and (2) information about the community. Each type of knowledge and its source appears in Table 1-4. To determine the overall patterns of health in a population, data collection for assessment and management decisions within a community should be ongoing, not episodical.

Community Health Interventions

Community health nurses focus on the care of individuals, groups, aggregates, and populations in many settings, including homes, clinics, and schools. In addition to interviewing clients and assessing individual and family health, community health nurses must be able to assess an aggregate's health needs and resources and identify its values. Community health nurses must also work with the community to identify and implement programs that meet health needs and

TABLE 1-3   Summary of Public Health Nursing Competencies

DOMAIN	COMMUNITY AND PUBLIC HEALTH NURSING COMPETENCIES
1. Analytic Assessment Skills	Defines a problem
	Determines appropriate use and limitation of data
	Selects and defines variables relevant to defined public health problems
	Identifies relevant and appropriate data and information sources
	Evaluates the integrity and comparability of data and identifies gaps in data sources
	Applies ethical principles to the collection, maintenance, use, and dissemination of data and information
	Partners with communities to attach meaning to data
	Obtains and interprets information regarding risks and benefits to the community
	Applies data collection processes, information technology, and computer systems storage/retrieval strategies
	Recognizes how the data illuminate ethical, political, scientific, economic, and overall public health issues
2. Policy Development/Program Planning Skills	Collects, summarizes, and interprets information relevant to an issue
	States policy options and writes clear and concise policy statements
	Identifies, interprets, and implements public health laws, regulations, and policies related to specific programs
	Articulates the health, fiscal, administrative, legal, social, and political implications of policy options
	States the feasibility and expected outcomes of each policy option
	Utilizes current techniques in decision analysis and health planning
	Decides on the appropriate course of action
	Develops a plan to implement policy, including goals, outcome and process objectives, and implementation steps
	Translates policy into organizational plans, structures, and programs
	Prepares and implements emergency response plans
	Develops mechanisms to monitor and evaluate programs for effectiveness and quality
3. Communication Skills	Communicates effectively
	Solicits input from individuals and organizations
	Advocates for public health programs and resources
	Leads and participates in groups to address specific issues
	Uses the media, advanced technologies, and community networks to communicate information
	Presents accurate demographic, statistical, programmatic, and scientific information for professional and lay audiences
	Listens to others in an unbiased manner; respects others' points of view; promotes the expression of diverse opinions and perspectives
4. Cultural Competency Skills	Utilizes appropriate methods for interacting sensitively, effectively, and professionally with persons from diverse cultural, socioeconomic, educational, racial, ethnic, and professional backgrounds and with persons of all ages and lifestyle preferences
	Identifies the role of cultural, social, and behavioral factors in determining the delivery of public health services
	Develops and adapts approaches to problems that consider cultural differences
	Understands the dynamic forces contributing to cultural diversity
	Understands the importance of a diverse public health workforce
5. Community Dimensions of Practice Skills	Establishes and maintains linkages with key stakeholders
	Utilizes leadership, team building, negotiation, and conflict resolution skills to build community partnerships
	Collaborates with community partners to promote the health of the population
	Identifies how public and private organizations operate within a community
	Accomplishes effective community engagements
	Identifies community assets and resources
	Develops, implements, and evaluates a community public health assessment
	Describes the role of government in the delivery of community health services
6. Basic Public Health Sciences Skills	Identifies the individual's and organizations' responsibilities within the context of the Essential Public Health Services and core functions
	Defines, assesses, and understands the health status of populations, determinants of health and illness, factors contributing to health promotion and disease prevention, and factors influencing the use of health services
	Understands the historical development, structure, and interaction of public health and health
	Identifies and applies basic research methods used in public health
	Applies the basic public health sciences, including behavioral and social sciences, biostatistics, epidemiology, environmental public health, and prevention of chronic and infectious diseases and injuries
	Identifies and retrieves current relevant scientific evidence
	Identifies the limitations of research and the importance of observations and interrelationships
	Develops a lifelong commitment to rigorous critical thinking
7. Financial Planning and Management Skills	Develops and presents a budget
	Manages programs within budget constraints
	Applies budget processes
	Develops strategies for budget priorities
	Monitors program performance
	Prepares proposals for funding from external sources
	Applies basic human relationship skills to the management of organizations, motivation of personnel, and resolution of conflicts
	Manages information systems for collection, retrieval, and use of data for decision making
	Negotiates and develops contracts and other documents for the provision of population-based services
	Conducts cost-effectiveness, cost-benefit, and cost utility analyses

Continued

TABLE 1-3   Summary of Public Health Nursing Competencies (*cont'd*)

DOMAIN	COMMUNITY AND PUBLIC HEALTH NURSING COMPETENCIES
8. Leadership and Systems Thinking Skills	Creates a culture of ethical standards within organizations and communities
	Helps create key values and shared vision and uses these principles to guide action
	Identifies internal and external issues that may impact delivery of essential public health services
	Facilitates collaboration with internal and external groups to ensure participation of key stakeholders
	Promotes team and organizational learning
	Contributes to development, implementation, and monitoring of organizational performance standards
	Uses the legal and political system to effect change
	Applies theory of organizational structures to professional practice

From Quad Council of Public Health Nursing Organizations: *Public health nursing competencies,* Washington, DC, 2003, Quad Council.

TABLE 1-4   Data Required for Population Focus

BODY OF KNOWLEDGE ABOUT PROBLEM		INFORMATION ABOUT THE COMMUNITY	
DEFINITION	SOURCES	DEFINITION	SOURCES
Cause or etiology	Epidemiological research	Demographic data	Demographics such as age, sex, and socioeconomic and racial distributions
Groups at high risk	Community health nursing research	Health status of the subpopulations	Vital statistics such as mortality and morbidity
Treatment methods	Clinical research in nursing and medicine	Services given to various subpopulations	Annual reports of health care organizations
			Services provided by health planning agencies
Effectiveness of treatment methods	Research in other fields	Measure of effectiveness of services	Computerized information systems for monitoring high-risk populations

From Williams CA: Population-focused practice. In Stanhope M and Lancaster J, editors: *Community health nursing: process and practice for promoting health,* St. Louis, 1984, Mosby.

evaluate the effectiveness of programs following implementation. For example, school nurses were once only responsible for running first aid stations. Now they are actively involved in assessing the needs of their population and defining programs to meet those needs through activities such as health screening and group health education and promotion. The activities of school nurses may be as varied as designing health curricula with a school and community advisory group, leading support groups for elementary school children with chronic illness, and monitoring the health status of teenage mothers.

Similarly, occupational health nurses are no longer required to simply maintain an office or dispensary. They are involved in many different types of activities. These activities might include maintaining records of workers exposed to physical or chemical risks, monitoring compliance with OSHA standards, teaching classes on health issues, and leading support group discussions for workers with health-related problems.

Private associations, such as the American Diabetes Association, employ community health nurses for organizational ability and health-related skill. Other community health nurses work with multidisciplinary groups of professionals, serve on boards of voluntary health associations like the American Heart Association, are members of health planning agencies and councils, and work with nursing organizations directed at major public health problems like the Nurses' Environmental Health Watch.

The Public Health Intervention Wheel

The Public Health Intervention Model was initially proposed in the late 1990s by nurses from the Minnesota Department of Health to describe the breadth and scope of public health nursing practice (Keller et al., 1998). This model was later revised and termed the Intervention Wheel (Figure 1-3) (Keller et al., 2004a; Keller et al., 2004b) and has become increasingly recognized as a framework for community and public health nursing practice.

The Intervention Wheel contains three important elements: (1) it is population-based; (2) it contains three levels of practice (community, systems, and individual/family); and (3) it identifies and defines 17 public health interventions. The levels of practice and interventions are directed at improving population health (Keller et al., 2004a). Within the Intervention Wheel, the 17 health interventions are grouped into 5 "wedges." These interventions are actions taken on behalf of communities, systems, individuals, and families to improve or protect health status. Table 1-5 provides definitions.

The Intervention Wheel is further dissected into levels of practice in which the interventions may be directed at an entire population within a community, a system that would affect the health of a population, and/or the individuals and families within the population. Thus each intervention can and should be applied at each level. For example, within the intervention "disease investigation," a systems-level intervention might be

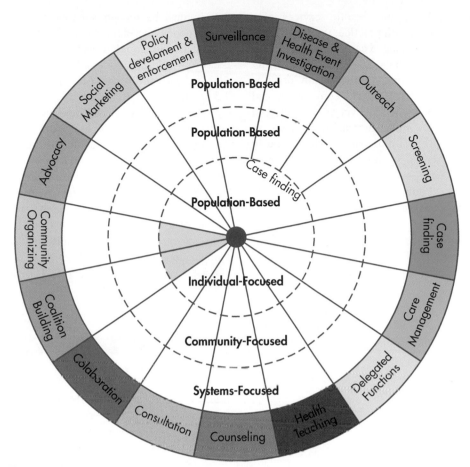

FIGURE 1-3   Public Health Intervention Wheel. (Minnesota Department of Health Center for Public Health Nursing.)

the community health nurse working with the state health department and federal vaccine program to coordinate a response to cases of measles in a migrant population. A population- or community-level intervention for "screening" would be when public health nurses work with area high schools to give each student a profile of their health to promote nutritional and physical activity lifestyle changes to improve their health.

Finally, an individual-level implementation of the intervention "referral and follow-up" would be a nurse who receives a referral to care for an individual with a diagnosed mental illness who would require regular monitoring of his medication compliance to prevent rehospitalization (Keller et al., 2004b).

COMMUNITY HEALTH NURSING AND MANAGED CARE

Shifts in reimbursement and the growth of managed care have revitalized the notion of population-based care. MCOs use financial incentives and organizational structures to increase efficiency and decrease health care costs. The foundation for managed care is management of health care for an enrolled group of individuals. This group of enrollees becomes the population of interest (Torrens and Williams, 2002).

An understanding of enrolled populations and health care patterns is essential for managing health care services and resources effectively. Most MCOs have become sophisticated in identifying key subgroups within the population of enrollees at risk for health problems. Typically, managed care systems target subgroups according to characteristics associated with risk or use of expensive services, such as selected clinical conditions, functional status, and past service use patterns.

Although comprehensive national health reform has not occurred, the dialogue about health care reform continues. Many experts believe that health care reform is occurring at the state level. Market forces and cost-containment efforts help lead the trend toward managed care (Shi and Singh, 2004). In many states, Medicaid populations are becoming part of managed care plans. Nationally, about 50 million people are part of health maintenance organizations (HMOs). A growing number of people are enrolled in HMOs and other types of managed care arrangements. A reformed health care system will include principles of managed care and a population-based approach to public health practice.

The purpose of public health is to improve the health of the public by promoting healthy lifestyles, preventing disease and injury, and protecting the health of communities (Berkowitz, 1995). In the past, shrinking public health resources have supported personal health services over community health. In public health practice, the community is the population of interest. Managed care may consider the served population to be individuals belonging to the HMO and specific HMO client groups. Public health practice continues to focus on public health and community, and managed care focuses on service delivery. The personal health care system will be under increasing pressure to provide the services that health departments previously provided. Traditionally served by public health, the most vulnerable populations will pose tremendous challenges to managed care providers. Public health will be responsible for partnering with managed care to provide service to these populations.

Providing population-based care requires a dramatic shift in thinking from individual-based care. Some of the practical demands of population-based care are the following:

1. It must be recognized that populations are not homogeneous; therefore it is necessary to address the needs of special subpopulations within populations.
2. High-risk and vulnerable subpopulations must be identified early in the care delivery cycle.
3. Nonusers of services often become high-cost users; therefore, it is essential to develop outreach strategies.
4. Quality and cost of all health care services are linked together across the health care continuum.

Nurses in community and public health have an opportunity to share their expertise regarding population-based approaches to health care for groups of individuals across health care settings. Today, health care practitioners require additional skills in assessment, policy development, and assurance to provide community public health practice and population-based service. According to a Pew Health Professions Commission report (1994), essential competencies

TABLE 1-5 Public Health Interventions and Definitions

PUBLIC HEALTH INTERVENTION	DEFINITION
Surveillance	Describes and monitors health events through ongoing and systematic collection, analysis, and interpretation of health data for the purpose of planning, implementing, and evaluating public health interventions
Disease and other health event investigation	Systematically gathers and analyzes data regarding threats to the health of populations, ascertains the source of the threat, identifies cases and others at risk, and determines control measures
Outreach	Locates populations of interest or populations at risk and provides information about the nature of the concern, what can be done about it, and how services can be obtained
Screening	Identifies individuals with unrecognized health risk factors or asymptomatic disease conditions
Case finding	Locates individuals and families with identified risk factors and connects them with resources
Referral and follow-up	Assists individuals, families, groups, organizations, and/or communities to identify and access necessary resources to prevent or resolve problems or concerns
Case management	Optimizes self-care capabilities of individuals and families and the capacity of systems and communities to coordinate and provide services
Delegated functions	Directs care tasks that a registered professional nurse carries out under the authority of a health care practitioner as allowed by law
Health teaching	Communicates facts ideas, and skills that change knowledge, attitudes, values, beliefs, behaviors, and practices of individuals, families, systems, and/or communities
Counseling	Establishes an interpersonal relationship with a community, a system, and a family or individual, with the intention of increasing or enhancing their capacity for self-care and coping
Consultation	Seeks information and generates optional solutions to perceived problems or issues through interactive problem solving with a community system and family or individual.
Collaboration	Commits two or more persons or organization to achieve a common goal through enhancing the capacity of one or more of the members to promote and protect health
Coalition building	Promotes and develops alliances among organizations or constituencies for a common purpose
Community organizing	Helps community groups to identify common problems or goals, mobilize resources, and develop and implement strategies for realizing the goals they collectively have set
Advocacy	Pleads someone's cause or acts on someone's behalf, with a focus on developing the community, system, and individual or family's capacity to plead their own cause or act on their own behalf
Social marketing	Utilizes commercial marketing principles and technologies for programs designed to influence the knowledge, attitudes, values, beliefs, behaviors, and practices of the population of interest
Policy development and enforcement	Places health issues on decision makers' agendas, acquires a plan of resolution, and determines needed resources, resulting in laws, rules, regulations, ordinances, and policies. Policy enforcement compels others to comply with laws, rules, regulations, ordinances, and policies.

From Keller, LO, Strohschein, S, Lia-Hoagberg, B, and Schaffer, MA: Population-based public health interventions: Practice-based and evidence-supported. Part I. Minnesota Department of Health, Center for Public Health Nursing.

necessary for practitioners in managed care include promoting healthy lifestyles, providing preventive and primary care, expanding and ensuring access to cost-effective and technologically appropriate care, participating in coordinated and interdisciplinary care, and involving patients and families in the decision-making process. Public health nurses must work in partnership with colleagues in managed care settings to improve community health. Partnerships may address information management, cultural values, health care system improvement, and the physical environment roles in health and may require complex negotiations to share data across boundaries. The partners may need to develop new community assessment strategies to augment epidemiological methods that often mask the context or meaning of the human experience of vulnerable populations.

SUMMARY

Knowledge and skills enable community health nurses to work in diverse community settings ranging from the isolated rural area to the crowded urban ghetto. To meet the health needs of the population, the community health nurse must work with many individuals and groups within the community. The community health nurse must develop sensitivity to these groups and respect the community and its established method of problem management. This will enable the nurse to become more proficient in helping the community improve overall health.

LEARNING ACTIVITIES

1. Interview several community health nurses and several clients regarding their definitions of health. Share the results with your classmates. Do you agree with their definitions? Why or why not?
2. Interview several community health nurses regarding their opinions on the focus of community health nursing. Do you agree?
3. Ask several neighbors or consumers of health care about their views of the role of public health and community health nursing. Share your results with your classmates.

REFERENCES

Allender JA, Spradley BW: *Community health nursing: Promoting and protecting the public's health,* ed 6, Philadelphia, 2005, Lippincott Williams & Wilkins.

American heritage college dictionary, ed 3, New York, 1997, Houghton Mifflin.

American Nurses Association: *A conceptual model of community health nursing,* Pub No CH-10, Kansas City, Mo, 1980, The Association.

American Nurses Association: *Code of Ethics,* Kansas City, Mo, 2001, The Association.

American Public Health Association: *Ad hoc committee on public health nursing: the definition and role of public health nursing practice in the delivery of health care,* Washington, DC, 1996, The Association.

Baldwin JH et al: Population-focused and community-based nursing: moving toward clarification of concepts, *Public Health Nursing* 15(1):12-18, 1998.

Beauchamp DE: Public health as social justice. In Mappes T, Zembaty J, editors: *Biomedical ethics,* ed 2, New York, 1986, McGraw-Hill.

Berkowitz B: Health system reform: a blueprint for the future of public health, *J Public Health Pract* 1:1-6, 1995.

Butterfield PG: Thinking upstream: nurturing a conceptual understanding of the societal context of health behavior, *Adv Nurs Sci* 12:1-8, 1990.

Campbell, SL, Fowles, ER, Weber, BJ: Organizational structure and job satisfaction in public health nursing, *Public Health Nursing* 21(6):564-571, 2004.

Clark MJ: *Nursing in the community: dimensions of community health nursing,* ed 4, Upper Saddle River, NJ, 2003, Prentice Hall.

Dunn HL: *High level wellness,* Arlington, Va, 1961, RW Beatty, Ltd.

Ervin, NE, Bell SE: Social justice issues related to uneven distribution of resources. *Journal of the New York State Nurses Association* 35(1):8-13, 2004.

Feldstein PJ: *Health policy issues: an economic perspective,* ed 3, Chicago, 2003, Health Administration Press.

Freeman RB: *Public health nursing practice,* ed 3, Philadelphia, 1963, WB Saunders.

Green LW, Anderson CL: *Community health nursing,* St. Louis, 1986, Times Mirror/Mosby College Publishing.

Hanlon JJ: *Principles of public health administration,* ed 3, St. Louis, 1960, Mosby.

Inglis T: Nursing the trends: Nurses have more employment options than ever. *AJN Career Guide, 2004* 104(1):25-32, 2004.

Institute of Medicine: *The future of public health,* Washington, DC, 1988, National Academy Press.

Keller, LO, Strohschein, S, Lia-Hoagberg, B, Schaffer, MA: Population-based public health interventions: a model for practice. *Public Health Nursing* 15(3):207-215, 1998.

Keller, LO, Strohschein, S, Lia-Hoagberg, B, Schaffer, MA: Population-based public health interventions: practice-based and evidence-supported. Part I. *Public Health Nursing* 21(5):453-468, 2004a.

Keller, LO, Strohschein, S, Schaffer, MA, Lia-Hoagberg, B: Population-based public health interventions: innovations in practice, teaching and management. Part II. *Public Health Nursing* 21(5):469-487, 2004b.

Lamarche PA: Our health paradigm in peril, *Public Health Report* 110:556-560, 1995.

Leavell HR, Clark EG: *Preventive medicine for the doctor in his community,* New York, 1958, McGraw-Hill.

Maurer FA, Smith CM: *Community/public health nursing practice: Health for families and populations,* ed 3, St. Louis, 2005, Elsevier.

McGinnis MJ, Foege W: Actual causes of death in the United States. *JAMA* 270(18):2207-2212, 1993.

McKinlay JB. A case for refocusing upstream: the political economy of illness. In Jaco EG, editor: *Patients, physicians, and illness,* ed 3, New York, 1979, The Free Press.

McKeown T: Determinants of health. In Lee PR, Estes CL, editors: *The nation's health,* ed 6, Boston, 2001, Jones & Bartlett.

Minnesota Department of Health: Definitions of population based practice. March, 2003, The Author, http://www.health.state.mn.us/divs/chs/phn/interventionsfull2004.pdf#search ='minnesota%20department%20of%20 health%20division%20of%20community% 20health%20services'.

Muecke MA: Community health diagnosis in nursing, *Public Health Nurs* 1:23-35, 1984.

Murray RB, Zentner JP: *Health promotion strategies through the life span,* ed 7, Upper Saddle River, NJ, 2001, Prentice Hall.

National Center for Health Statistics: *Health: United States, 2004,* Hyattsville, Md, 2004, The Author.

Orem DE: *Nursing: concepts of practice,* ed 6, St. Louis, 2001, Mosby.

Pender NJ: *Health promotion in nursing practice,* ed 4, Upper Saddle River, NJ, 2002, Prentice Hall.

Pew Health Professions Commission: *Current issues in health professions: education and workforce reform,* University of California, San Francisco, 1994, The Author.

Quad Council of Public Health Nursing Organizations: *Scope and standards of public health nursing practice,* Washington, DC, 1999, American Nurses Publishing.

Quad Council of Public Health Nursing Organizations: *Public health nursing competencies,* Washington, DC, 2003, Quad Council.

Rothstein WG: Trends in mortality in the twentieth century. In Lee PR, Estes CL, editors: *The nation's health,* ed 6, Boston, 2001, Jones & Bartlett.

Saylor C: The circle of health: a health definition model, *Journal of Holistic Nursing* 22(2): 98-115, 2004.

Shi L, Singh DA: *Delivering health care in America: a systems approach,* ed 3, Sudbury, MA, 2004, Jones & Bartlett.

Shine KI: Informed joint decision-making, *Public Health Report* 110:555, 1995.

Shuster GR, Goeppinger J: Community as client: using the nursing process to promote health. In Stanhope M, Lancaster J, editors: *Community health nursing: process and practice for promoting health,* ed 6, St. Louis, 2004, Elsevier.

Thomas SA: Caring in community health nursing. In Hitchcock JE, Schubert, PE, Thomas SA, editors: *Community health nursing: caring in action,* ed 2, Clifton Park, NY, 2003, Delmar Learning.

Torrens PR: Historical evolution and overview of health services in the United States. In Williams SJ, Torrens PR, editors: *Introduction to health services,* ed 6, Albany, NY, 2002, Delmar Publishers.

Torrens PR, Williams SJ: Managed care: restructuring the system. In Williams SJ, Torrens PR, editors: *Introduction to health services,* ed 5, Albany, NY, 2002, Delmar Publishers.

US Department of Health and Human Services: *Healthy People 2000 objectives,* Washington, DC, 1989, The Author.

US Department of Health and Human Services: *Healthy People 2010 objectives,* Washington, DC, 2000, The Author.

US Department of Health and Human Services, Health Resources and Services Administration, Bureau of Health Professions, Division of Nursing: *Preliminary finding: 2004 National Sample Survey of Registered Nurses,* The Author, http://bhpr.hrsa.gov/healthworkforce/reports/rnpopulation/preliminaryfindings.htm

US Department of Health and Human Services/ Public Health Service: *The public health workforce: an agenda for the 21st century,* Washington, DC, 1997, The Author.

Wald LD: *The house on Henry Street,* New York, 1971, Dover Publications.

Williams CA: Community-oriented, population-focused practice: the foundation of specialization in public health nursing. In Stanhope M, Lancaster J, editors: *Community health nursing: process and practice for promoting health,* ed 5, St. Louis, 2000, Mosby.

World Health Organization: *Chron WHO* 1:1-2, 1958.

World Health Organization: A discussion document on the concept and principles of health promotion, *Health Promotion* 1:73-78, 1986.

Zotti ME, Brown P, Stotts RC: Community-based nursing versus community health nursing: What does it all mean? *Nursing Outlook* 44(5):211-217, 1996.

2

Historical Factors: Community Health Nursing in Context

Tom H. Cook

MEDIA RESOURCES

Additional Material for Study, Review, and Further Exploration

evolve Website at http://evolve.elsevier.com/Nies

❖ Quiz ❖ Case Studies ❖ Content Updates ❖ Glossary ❖ WebLinks

---

OBJECTIVES

Upon completion of this chapter, the reader will be able to do the following:

1. Describe the impact of aggregate living on population health.
2. Identify approaches to aggregate health from prehistoric to present times.
3. Understand historical events that have influenced a holistic approach to population health.
4. Compare the application of public health principles to the nation's major health problems at the turn of the twentieth

century (i.e., acute disease) with that at the beginning of the twenty-first century (i.e., chronic disease).
5. Describe two leaders in nursing who had a profound impact on addressing aggregate health.
6. Discuss major contemporary issues facing community health nursing and trace the historical roots to the present.

KEY TERMS

Edwin Chadwick	health visiting	Florence Nightingale	Lemuel Shattuck
District Nursing	Edward Jenner	pandemic	John Snow
Elizabethan Poor Law	Robert Koch	Louis Pasteur	stages in disease history
Flexner Report	Joseph Lister	sanitary revolution	Lillian Wald
House on Henry Street			

CHAPTER OUTLINE

EVOLUTION OF HEALTH IN WESTERN POPULATIONS
    Aggregate Impact on Health
    Evolution of Early Public Health Efforts

ADVENT OF MODERN HEALTH CARE
    Evolution of Modern Nursing
    Establishment of Modern Medical Care and Public
      Health Practice
    Establishment of Public Health Nursing

CONSEQUENCES FOR THE HEALTH OF AGGREGATES
    Twenty-First Century

SOCIAL CHANGES AND COMMUNITY HEALTH NURSING

CHALLENGES FOR COMMUNITY HEALTH NURSING

This chapter presents an overview of selected historical factors that have influenced the evolution of community health and explains current health challenges for community health nursing. This text examines the evolving health of Western populations from prehistoric to recent times and the evolution of modern health care and the role of public health nursing. Consequences for the health of aggregates and the challenges for community health nursing are also considered.

EVOLUTION OF HEALTH IN WESTERN POPULATIONS

The study of humankind's evolution has seldom taken into consideration the interrelationship between an individual's health, an individual's environment, and the nature and size of the individual's community. Medical anthropologists use paleontological records and disease descriptions of primitive societies to speculate on the interrelationship between early

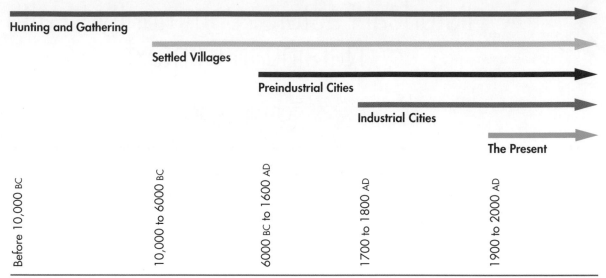

FIGURE 2-1   Stages in the disease history of humankind. Stages overlap and time periods are widely debated in the field of anthropology. Some form of each stage remains evident in the world today.

humans and environment patterns of health and illness (Armelagos and Dewey, 1978). Historians have also documented the existence of public health activity (i.e., an organized community effort to prevent disease, prolong life, and promote health) since prehistoric times. The following section describes how aggregates and early public health efforts impact the health of Western populations.

Aggregate Impact on Health

Polgar (1964) defined the following **stages in the disease history** of humankind: hunting and gathering stage, settled villages stage, preindustrial cities stage, industrial cities stage, and present stage (Figure 2-1). In these stages, increased population, increased population density, and imbalanced human ecology resulted in changes in cultural adaptation. Humans caused this ecological imbalance by altering their environment to accommodate group living. This imbalance had a marked consequence on health.

Although these stages are associated with the evolution of civilization, it is important to note that the information is limited. For example, the stages depict the evolution of Western civilization from the perspective of the Western world. They consist of overlapping historical time periods, which anthropologists widely debate. However, the stages do provide a frame of reference to aid in determining the relationship among humans, disease, and environment from prehistoric times to the present day. The stages chronicle the initiation of each stage in the Western world, but it is important to realize that each stage still exists in civilization today. For example, Australian aborigines continue to hunt and gather food and settled villages are common in Third World countries.

The community nurse must be aware that populations from each stage represent a great variety of people with distinct cultural traditions and a broad range of health care practices and beliefs. For example, a nurse in an American community may have to plan care for immigrants or refugees from a settled village or a preindustrial city. Community nurses must recognize that the environment, the aggregate's health risks, and the host culture's strengths and contributions affect the health status of each particular aggregate. For example, the Hispanic Health and Nutrition Examination Survey (HHANES) collected data between 1982 and 1984 and found that perinatal outcomes among women born in Mexico worsen in correspondence to the length of time they live in the United States (Guendelman et al., 1990). Whereas Mexico's cultural orientation protects mothers from the risk-associated behaviors of drinking and smoking, Mexican descendants born in the United States are more likely to engage in unhealthy behaviors and practices common to other Americans.

Hunting and Gathering Stage

During the Paleolithic period, or Old Stone Age, nomadic and seminomadic people engaged in hunting and gathering. Generations of small aggregate groups wandered in search of food for two million years. Armelagos and Dewey (1978) reviewed how their size, density, and relationship to the environment probably affected their health. These groups may have avoided many contagious diseases because the scattered aggregates were small, nomadic, and separated from other aggregates. Under these conditions, disease would not spread between the groups. Evidently, the disposal of human feces and waste was not a great problem; the nomadic people most likely abandoned the caves they used for shelter once waste accumulated.

Settled Village Stage

Small settlements were characteristic of the Mesolithic period, or Middle Stone Age, and the Neolithic period, or New Stone Age. Wandering people became sedentary and formed small encampments and villages. The concentration of people in these small areas caused new problems. For

TABLE 2-1   Disease Definitions

DISEASE	DEFINITIONS
Endemic	Diseases that are always present in a population (e.g., colds and pneumonia)
Epidemic	Diseases that are not always present in a population but flare up on occasion (e.g., diphtheria and measles)
Pandemic	The existence of disease in a large proportion of the population: a global epidemic (e.g., HIV, AIDS, and annual outbreaks of influenza type A)

example, people began to domesticate animals and live close to their herds, which probably transmitted diseases such as salmonella, anthrax, Q fever, and tuberculosis (TB) (Polgar, 1964). These stationary people also domesticated plants, which may have reduced the range of consumable nutrients and may have led to deficiency disease. They had to secure water and remove wastes, which often resulted in the cross-contamination of the water supply and the spread of waterborne diseases such as dysentery, cholera, typhoid, and hepatitis A.

Preindustrial Cities Stage

In preindustrial times, large urban centers formed to support the expanding population. Populations inhabited smaller areas; therefore, preexisting problems increased. For example, the urban population had to resource increased amounts of food and water and remove increased amounts of waste products. Some cultures developed elaborate water systems. For instance, the Aztec king Ahuitzutl had a stone pipeline built to transport spring water to the inhabitants of Mexico City (Duran, 1964). However, waste removal via the water supply led to diseases such as cholera. With the development of towns, rodent infestation increased and facilitated the spread of plague. People had more frequent close contact with each other; therefore, the transmission of diseases spread by direct contact increased, and diseases such as mumps, measles, influenza, and smallpox became endemic (Polgar, 1964). A population must reach a certain size to maintain a disease in endemic proportions (Table 2-1); for example, approximately 1 million people are needed to sustain measles at an endemic level (Cockburn, 1967).

Industrial Cities Stage

Industrialization caused urban areas to become denser and more heavily populated. Increased industrial wastes, air and water pollution, and harsh working conditions took a toll on health. During the eighteenth and nineteenth centuries, there was an increase in respiratory diseases such as TB, pneumonia, and bronchitis and in epidemics of infectious diseases such as diphtheria, smallpox, typhoid fever, typhus, measles, malaria, and yellow fever (Armelagos and Dewey, 1978). Furthermore, imperialism spread epidemics to susceptible populations throughout the world because settlers, traders, and soldiers moved from one location to another introducing communicable diseases into native population groups.

Present Stage

Although infectious diseases no longer account for a majority of deaths in the Western world, they continue to cause many deaths in the non-Western world. They also remain prevalent among low-income populations and some racial and ethnic groups in the West. People from nonindustrial communities rarely develop Western diseases such as cancer, venous disorders, heart disease, obesity, and diabetes. These diseases usually appear when cultures adopt Western customs (Burkitt, 1978). Western diseases also seem to emerge when cultures transition into urban environments. Epidemiological studies suggest that common disease factors are changes in diet (i.e., increases in refined sugar and fats and lack of fiber) and environmental and occupational hazards. An increase in population and population density also increases mental and behavioral disorders (Garn, 1963).

The disease patterns and environmental demands changed when wandering, hunting, and gathering aggregates grew into large populations and became sedentary. Humans had to adapt to an overpopulated, largely urban existence with marked consequences for health; the leading causes of death changed from infectious diseases to chronic illnesses.

Evolution of Early Public Health Efforts

Traditionally, historians believed that organized public health efforts were eighteenth- and nineteenth-century activities associated with the Sanitary Revolution. However, modern historians have shown that organized community health efforts to prevent disease, prolong life, and promote health have existed since prehistoric times.

Public health efforts developed slowly over time. The following sections briefly trace the evolution of organized public health and highlight the periods of prehistoric times (i.e., before 5000 BC), classical times (i.e., 3000-200 BC), the Middle Ages (i.e., AD 500-1500), the Renaissance (i.e., fifteenth, sixteenth, and seventeenth centuries), the eighteenth century, and the nineteenth century. However, it is important to note that, like the disease history of humankind, public health efforts exist in various stages of development throughout the world. This brief history encapsulates a Western view of organized public health efforts.

Prehistoric Times

Early nomadic humans became domesticated and tended to live in increasingly larger groups. Aggregates ranging from family to community inevitably shared episodes of life, health, sickness, and death. Whether based on superstition or sanitation, health practices evolved to ensure the survival of many aggregates. For example, for hundreds of years, primitive societies used elements of medicine (e.g., voodoo), isolation (e.g., banishment), and fumigation (e.g., smoke) to manage disease and thus protect the community (Hanlon and Pickett, 1990).

BOX 2-1 Romans Provided Public Health Services

The Romans provided public health services that included the following (Rosen, 1958):

➤ A water board to maintain the aqueducts
➤ A supervisor of the public baths
➤ Street cleaners
➤ Supervision of the sale of food

Classical Times

In the early years of 3000 to 1400 BC, the Minoans devised ways to flush water and construct drainage systems. Circa 1000 BC, the Egyptians constructed elaborate drainage systems, developed pharmaceutical preparations, and embalmed the dead. Pollution is an ancient problem. Exodus reported that "all the waters that were in the river stank" and in Leviticus, the Hebrews formulated the first written hygiene code. This hygiene code protected water and food by creating laws that governed personal and community hygiene such as contagion, disinfection, and sanitation.

Greece

Greek literature contains accounts of communicable diseases such as diphtheria, mumps, and malaria (Rosen, 1958). The Hippocratic book *Airs, Waters and Places,* a treatise on the balance between humans and their environment, may have been the only volume on this topic until the development of bacteriology in the late nineteenth century (Rosen, 1958). Diseases that were always present in a population, such as colds and pneumonia, were called endemic. Diseases that were occasionally present, such as diphtheria and measles, were called epidemic (see Table 2-1). The Greeks emphasized the preservation of health, or good living, which the goddess Hygeia personified, and on curative medicine, which the goddess Panacea personified. Life had to be in balance with environmental demands; therefore, the Greeks weighed the importance of exercise, rest, and nutrition according to age, sex, constitution, and climate (Rosen, 1958).

Rome

Although the Romans readily adopted Greek culture, they far surpassed Greek engineering by constructing massive aqueducts, bathhouses, and sewer systems. For example, at the height of the Roman empire, Rome provided its 1 million inhabitants with 40 gallons of water per person per day, which is comparable with modern consumption rates (Rosen, 1958) (Box 2-1). However, inhabitants of the overcrowded Roman slums did not share in public health amenities such as sewer systems and latrines.

The Romans also observed and addressed occupational health threats. In particular, they noted the pallor of the miners, the danger of suffocation, and the smell of caustic fumes (Rosen, 1958). For protection, miners devised safeguards by using bags, sacks, and masks made of membranes and bladder skins.

In the early years of the Roman Republic, priests were believed to mediate diseases and often dispensed medicine.

Public physicians worked in designated towns and earned money to care for the poor. In addition, they were able to charge wealthier patients a service fee. Much like a modern HMO or group practice, several families paid a set fee for yearly services. Hospitals, surgeries, infirmaries, and nursing homes appeared throughout Rome. In the fourth century, a Christian woman named Fabiola established a hospital for the sick poor. Others repeated this model throughout medieval times.

Middle Ages

The decline of Rome, which occurred circa 500 AD, led to the Middle Ages. Monasteries promoted collective activity to protect public health, and the population adopted protective measures such as building wells and fountains, cleaning streets, and disposing of refuse. The commonly occurring communicable diseases were measles, smallpox, diphtheria, leprosy, and bubonic plague. Physicians had little to offer in the management of diseases such as leprosy. The church took over by enforcing the hygienic codes from Leviticus and establishing isolation and leper houses, or leprosaria (Rosen, 1958).

A **pandemic** is the existence of disease in a large proportion of the population (see Table 2-1). One such pandemic, the bubonic plague, ravaged much of the world in the fourteenth century. This plague, or Black Death, claimed close to half the world's population at that time (Hanlon and Pickett, 1990). For centuries, medicine and science did not recognize that fleas, which were attracted to the large number of rodents that inhabited urban areas, were transmitters of plague. Modern public health practices such as isolation, disinfection, and ship quarantines emerged in response to the bubonic plague (Box 2-2).

During the Middle Ages, clergymen acted as physicians and treated kings and noblemen. Monks and nuns provided nursing care in small houses designated as hospitals. Medieval writings contained information on hygiene and addressed such topics as housing, diet, personal cleanliness, and sleep (Rosen, 1958).

Life in an English Household in the Sixteenth Century

In the following account, Erasmus described how life in the sixteenth century must have affected health (Hanlon and Pickett, 1990):

As to floors, they are usually made with clay, covered with rushes that grow in the fens and which are so seldom removed that the lower parts remain sometimes for twenty years and has in it a collection of spittle, vomit, urine of dogs and humans, beer, scraps of fish and other filthiness not to be named. (p. 25)

Such accounts appeared in literature throughout the nineteenth century. ■

The Renaissance

Although the cause of infectious disease remained undiscovered, two events important to public health occurred during the Renaissance. In 1546, Girolamo Fracastoro presented a theory that infection was a cause and epidemic

BOX 2-2 Human Plague Cases Documented in the United States

Plague is an acute, often fatal bacterium that is endemic and occasionally epidemic in Africa, Asia, and South America. The bite of infectious fleas spreads plague, and the WHO estimates an average of 1087 cases each year worldwide. Sanitary precautions ensure a low frequency of human plague in the United States. America averages 13 cases of plague each year; approximately 80% of these cases occur in New Mexico, Arizona, and Colorado. General control measures include public education and plague surveillance in rodents and rodent predators. When this surveillance detects plague, local health care providers and the public should receive an alert about possible risks.

In 2002, two cases of human plague were reported in New York City. The couple was traveling from Santa Fe, New Mexico, when they became ill with fever and unilateral inguinal adenopathy. Blood cultures revealed *Yersinia pestis,* the causative agent for bubonic plague. Measures were taken by public health officials to contain exposure at the New York City hotel, the hospital's emergency department as well as in and around the couple's home in New Mexico.

From Centers for Disease Control and Prevention: Plague home page: http://www.cdc.gov/ncidod/dvbid/plague/index.htm and Centers for Disease Control and Prevention: Imported plague: New York City, 2002, *Morb Mortal Wkly Rep* 52;31, 2003.

was a consequence of the "seeds of disease." Also, in 1676, Anton van Leeuwenhoek described microscopic organisms, but he did not associate them with disease (Rosen, 1958).

The **Elizabethan Poor Law,** enacted in England in 1601, held the parishes responsible for providing relief for the poor. This law governed health care for the poor for more than two centuries and became a prototype for later U.S. laws.

Eighteenth Century
Great Britain
The eighteenth century was marked by imperialism and industrialization. Sanitary conditions remained a great problem. During the Industrial Revolution, a gradual change in industrial productivity occurred. The industrial boom sacrificed many lives for profit. In particular, it forced poor children into labor. Under the Elizabethan Poor Law, parishes established workhouses to employ the poor. Orphaned and poor children were wards of the parish; therefore the parish forced these young children to labor in parish workhouses for long hours (George, 1925). At 12 to 14 years of age, a child became a master's apprentice. Those apprenticed to chimney sweeps reportedly suffered the worst fate because their masters forced them into chimneys at the risk of being burned and suffocated.

Vaccination was a major discovery of the times. In 1796, **Edward Jenner** observed that people who worked around cattle were less likely to have smallpox. He discovered that immunity to smallpox resulted from an inoculation with the cowpox virus. Jenner's contribution was significant because approximately 95% of the population suffered from smallpox and approximately 10% of the population died

from smallpox during the eighteenth century. Frequently, the faces of those who survived the disease were scarred with pockmarks.

Although Europeans like Hume, Voltaire, and Rousseau and Americans like Adams, Jefferson, and Franklin were expounding liberal views on human nature, the **Sanitary Revolution's** public health reforms were beginning to take place throughout Europe and England. In the eighteenth century, scholars used survey methods to study community health problems (Rosen, 1958). The survey mapped "medical topographies," which were geographical factors related to regional health and disease. A health education movement provided books and pamphlets on health to the middle and upper classes, but it neglected "economic factors" and was not concerned with the working classes (Rosen, 1958).

Nineteenth Century
Communicable diseases ravaged the population that lived among unsanitary conditions, and many lives were lost. For example, in the mid 1800s, typhus and typhoid fever claimed twice as many lives each year as the battle of Waterloo (Hanlon and Pickett, 1990).

Edwin Chadwick called attention to the consequences of unsanitary conditions that shortened the life span of the laboring class in particular. Chadwick contended that death rates were high in large industrial cities like Liverpool, where more than half of all children born of working-class parents died by age 5. Laborers lived an average of 16 years. In contrast, tradesmen lived 22 years and the upper classes lived 36 years (Richardson, 1887). In 1842, Chadwick published his famous *Report on an Inquiry Into the Sanitary Conditions of the Laboring Population of Great Britain*. The report furthered the establishment of the General Board of Health for England in 1848. Legislation for social reform followed, which concerned child welfare; factory management; education; and care for the elderly, sick, and mentally ill. Clean water, sewers, fireplugs, and sidewalks emerged as a result.

In 1849, a pathologist named Rudolf Virchow argued for social action—bettering the lives of the people through improving economic, social, and environmental conditions—to attack the root social causes of disease. He proposed "a theory of epidemic disease as a manifestation of social and cultural maladjustment" (Rosen, 1958, p. 86). He further argued that the public was responsible for the health of the people; social and economic conditions heavily affected health and disease; efforts to promote health and fight disease must be social, economic, and medical; and the study of social and economic determinants of health and disease would yield knowledge to guide appropriate action.

In a significant development, in 1854, an English physician, anesthetist, and epidemiologist named **John Snow** demonstrated that cholera was transmissible through contaminated water. In a large population afflicted with cholera, he shut down the community's water resource by removing the pump handle from a well and carefully documented changes as the number of cholera cases fell dramatically (Rosen, 1958).

United States

In the United States during the nineteenth century, waves of epidemics continued to spread. Diseases such as yellow fever, smallpox, cholera, typhoid fever, and typhus particularly impacted the poor. These illnesses spread because cities grew and the poor crowded into inadequate housing with unsanitary conditions.

Lemuel Shattuck, a Boston bookseller and publisher with an interest in public health, organized the American Statistical Society in 1839 and issued a *Census of Boston* in 1845. The census showed high overall mortality and very high infant and maternal mortality rates. Living conditions for the poor were inadequate, and communicable diseases were widely prevalent (Rosen, 1958). Shattuck's 1850 *Report of the Massachusetts Sanitary Commission* outlined the findings and recommended modern public health reforms that included keeping vital statistics and providing environmental, food, drug, and communicable disease control information. Shattuck called for well-infant, well-child, and school-age child health care; mental health care; vaccination; and health education. Unfortunately, the report fell on deaf ears and little was done to improve population health for many years. For example, a state board of health was not formed until 19 years later. Around the same time, the National Institute, a Washington, DC, scientific organization, asked the newly formed American Medical Association (AMA) to establish a committee to uniformly collect vital statistics.

ADVENT OF MODERN HEALTH CARE

Early public health efforts evolved further in the mid nineteenth century. Administrative efforts, initial legislation, and debate regarding the determinants of health and approaches to health management began to appear on a social, economic, and medical level. The advent of "modern" health care occurred around this time, and nursing made a large contribution to the progress of health care. The following sections discuss the evolution of modern nursing, the evolution of modern medical care and public health practice, the evolution of the community caregiver, and the establishment of public health nursing.

Evolution of Modern Nursing

Florence Nightingale, the woman credited with establishing "modern nursing," began her work during the mid-nineteenth century. Historians remember Florence Nightingale for contributing to the health of British soldiers during the Crimean War and establishing nursing education. However, most historians failed to recognize her remarkable use of public health principles and distinguished scientific contributions to health care reform (Cohen, 1984; Dossey, 2000; Grier and Grier, 1978). The following review of Nightingale's work emphasizes her concern for environmental determinants of health; her focus on the aggregate of British soldiers through emphasis on sanitation, community assessment, and analysis; the development of the use of gra-

phically depicted statistics; and political advocacy to benefit populations.

Nightingale was from a wealthy English family, was well educated, and traveled extensively. Her father tutored her in mathematics and many other subjects. Nightingale later studied with Adolphe Quetelet, a Belgian statistician. Quetelet influenced her profoundly and taught her the discipline of social inquiry (Goodnow, 1933). Nightingale also had a passion for hygiene and health. In 1851, at the age of 31 years, she trained in nursing at Kaiserswerth Hospital in Germany. She later studied the organization and discipline of the Sisters of Charity in Paris. Nightingale wrote extensively and published her analyses of the many nursing systems she studied in France, Austria, Italy, and Germany (Dock and Stewart, 1925).

In 1854, Nightingale responded to distressing accounts of a lack of care for wounded soldiers during the Crimean War. She and 40 other nurses (lay nurses, Roman Catholic sisters, and Anglican sisters) traveled to Scutari, which, at the time, was part of the Ottoman Empire. Upon their arrival, they learned that the British army's management method for treating the sick and wounded had created conditions that resulted in extraordinarily high death rates among soldiers. One of Nightingale's greatest achievements was improving the management of ill and wounded soldiers.

Nightingale faced an assignment in The Barrack Hospital, which had been built for 1700 patients. In 4 miles of beds, she found 3000 to 4000 patients separated by only 18 inches of space (Goodnow, 1933, pp. 55-56).

The beds were mostly of straw, and many were laid directly on the floor. The few sheets to be had were of canvas and so rough that the men begged not to have them used. Practically no laundry was being done; there was no hospital clothing; and the patients were still in their uniforms, stiff with blood and covered with filth. There was no soap, no towels, no basins, and very few utensils of any sort. Every place swarmed with vermin. Men ate half-cooked food with their fingers because utensils did not exist.

During the Crimean War, cholera and "contagious fever" were rampant. An equal number of men died from disease and battlefield injury (Cohen, 1984). Nightingale found that allocated supplies were bound in bureaucratic red tape; for example, supplies were "sent to the wrong ports or were buried under munitions and could not be got" (Goodnow, 1933, p. 86).

Nightingale encountered problems reforming the army's methods for care of the sick because she had to work through eight military affairs departments related to her assignment. She sent reports of the appalling conditions of the hospitals to London, and with resultant government money and donated funds sent her way, she immediately set up diet kitchens and a laundry and provided food, clothing, dressings, and laboratory equipment (Dock and Stewart, 1925).

Major reforms occurred during the first 2 months of her assignment. Aware that an interest in keeping social statistics was emerging, Nightingale realized that her most forceful argument would be statistical in nature. She reorganized the methods of keeping statistics and was the first to use shaded and colored Coxcomb graphs of wedges, circles, and squares to illustrate the preventable deaths of soldiers. Nightingale compared the deaths of soldiers in hospitals during the Crimean War to the average annual mortality in Manchester and to the deaths of soldiers in military hospitals in and near London at the time (Figure 2-2). Through her reforms, she also showed that, by the end of the war, the death rate among ill soldiers during the Crimean War was no higher than that among well soldiers in Britain (Cohen, 1984). Indeed, Nightingale's careful statistics revealed that the death rate for treated soldiers decreased from 42% to 2%. Furthermore, she established community services and activities to improve the quality of life for recovering soldiers. These included rest and recreation facilities, study opportunities, a savings fund, and a post office. She also organized care for the families of the soldiers (Dock and Stewart, 1925).

After returning to London at the close of the war in 1856, Nightingale devoted her efforts to sanitary reform. At home, she surmised that if the sanitary neglect of the soldiers existed in the battle area, it probably existed also at home in London. She prepared statistical tables to support her suspicions (Table 2-2).

In one study comparing the mortality of men aged 25 to 35 years in the army barracks of England with that of men the same age in civilian life, Nightingale found the mortality of the soldiers was nearly twice that of the civilians. In one of her reports, she stated, "Our soldiers enlist to death in the barracks" (Kopf, 1978, p. 95). Further, she believed that allowing a young soldier to die needlessly from unsanitary conditions was equivalent to taking him out, lining him up, and shooting him (Kopf, 1978). She was very political and distributed her reports to members of Parliament and to the medical and commanding officers of the army (Kopf, 1978). Prominent male leaders of the time challenged her reports. Undaunted, she rewrote them in greater depth and redistributed them.

In her efforts to compare the hospital systems in European countries, Nightingale discovered that each hospital kept incomparable data and that many hospitals used various names and classifications for diseases. She noted that these differences prevented the collection of similar statistics from larger geographical areas. These statistics would create a regional health-illness profile and allow for comparison with other regions. She printed common statistical forms that some hospitals in London adopted on an experimental basis. A study of the tabulated results revealed the promise of this strategy (Kopf, 1978) (Box 2-3).

In 1861, Nightingale lobbied officials to add two areas of data collection to the census. She asked officials to include the number of sick and infirm in the population and data depicting the housing of the population (Kopf, 1978), stating the following:

The connection between the health and the dwellings of the population is one of the most important that exists. The "diseases" can be approximated also. In all the more important—such as smallpox, fevers, measles, heart disease, etc., all those which affect the national health, there will be very little error. Where there is error, in these things, the error is uniform . . . and corrects itself. (p. 98)

Although census officials did not adopt her recommendations linking illness and housing to health, Nightingale's

suggestions were visionary. It is interesting to note, however, that the paradigm for nursing practice and nursing education that evolved through Nightingale's work did not incorporate her emphasis on statistics and a sound research base. It is also curious why nursing education did not consult her writings and stress the importance of determining health's social and environmental determinants until much later.

Establishment of Modern Medical Care and Public Health Practice

To place Nightingale's work in perspective, it is necessary to consider the development of medical care in light of common education and practice during the late nineteenth and early twentieth centuries. Goodnow (1933) called this time a "dark age." Medical sciences were underdeveloped and bacteriology was unknown. Few medical schools existed at the time, so apprenticeship was the path to medical education. The majority of physicians believed in the "spontaneous generation" theory of disease causation, which stated that disease organisms grew from nothing (Najman, 1990). Typical medical treatment included bloodletting, starving, using leeches, and prescribing large doses of metals such as mercury and antimony (Goodnow, 1933).

Nightingale's uniform classification of hospital statistics noted the need to tabulate the classification of diseases in hospital patients and the need to note the diseases patients contracted in the hospital. These diseases, such as gangrene and septicemia, were later called *iatrogenic* diseases (Kopf, 1978). Considering the lack of surgical sanitation in hospitals at the time, it is not surprising that iatrogenic infection was rampant. For example, Goodnow (1933) illustrates the following unsanitary operating procedures:

Before an operation the surgeon turned up the sleeves of his coat to save the coat, and would often not trouble to wash his hands, knowing how soiled they soon would be! The area of the operation would sometimes be washed with soap and water, but not always, for the inevitability of corruption made it seem useless. The silk or thread used for stitches or ligatures was hung over a button of the surgeon's coat, and during the operation a convenient place for the knife to rest was between his lips. Instruments . . . used for . . . lancing abscesses were kept in the vest pocket and often only wiped with a piece of rag as the surgeon went from one patient to another. (pp. 471-472)

During the nineteenth century, the following important scientists were born: **Louis Pasteur** in 1822, **Joseph Lister** in 1827, and **Robert Koch** in 1843. Their research also had a profound impact on health care, medicine, and nursing. Pasteur was a chemist, not a physician. While experimenting with wine production in 1854, he proposed the theory of the existence of germs. Although his colleagues ridiculed him at first, Pasteur applied his theories and developed his methods for handling and studying bacteria. Subsequently, Pasteur's colleagues gave him acknowledgment for his work.

Lister, whose father perfected the microscope, observed the healing processes of fractures. When the bone was broken but the skin was not, he noted that recovery was uneventful. However, when both the bone and the skin were broken, fever, infection, and even death were frequent. He

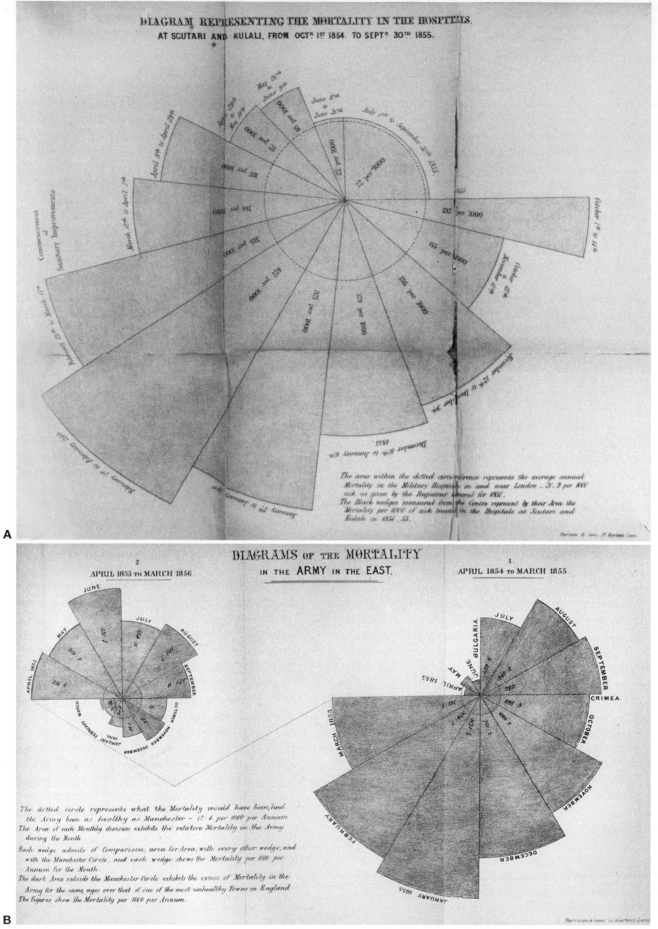

FIGURE 2-2 Coxcomb charts by Florence Nightingale. (From Nightingale F: *Notes on matters affecting the health, efficiency and hospitalization of the British army,* London, 1858, Harrison and Sons.)

Photographs of large, fold-out charts from an original preserved at the University of Chicago. Library (Public domain; courtesy University of Chicago Library.)

TABLE 2-2   Nightingale's Crimean War Mortality Statistics: Nursing Research that Made a Difference

YEAR	DEATHS THAT WOULD HAVE OCCURRED IN HEALTHY DISTRICTS AMONG MALES OF THE SOLDIERS' AGES*	ACTUAL DEATHS OF NONCOMMISSIONED OFFICERS AND MEN	EXCESS OF DEATHS AMONG NONCOMMISSIONED OFFICERS AND MEN
1832	763	2914	2151
1840	829	3300	2471
1841	857	4167	3310
1842	888	5052	4164
1843	914	5270	4356
1844	920	3867	2947
1845	911	4587	3676
1846	930	5125	4195
1847	981	4232	3251
1848	987	3213	2226
1849	954	4052	3098
1850	919	3119	2200
1851	901	2729	1828
1852	915	3120	2205
1853	920	3392	2472
Total	13,589	58,139	44,550

From Grier B, Grier M: Contributions of the passionate statistician, *Res Nurs Health* 1:103-109, 1978. Copyright © 1978 by John Wiley & Sons, Inc. Reprinted by permission of John Wiley & Sons, Inc.
Number of deaths of noncommissioned officers and men also shows the number of deaths that would have occurred if the mortality were 7.7 per 1000—such as it was among Englishmen of the soldiers' age in healthy districts, in the years 1849 to 1853—which fairly represent the average mortality.
*The exact mortality in the healthy districts is 0.0077122, using the logarithm of 3.8871801.

BOX 2-3   Nightingale's Use of Statistical Methods in Community Assessment

London's Southeastern Railway planned to remove St. Thomas Hospital to increase the railway's right-of-way between London Bridge and Charing Cross. Nightingale applied her statistical method to the health needs of the community by conducting a *community assessment*. She plotted the cases served by the hospital, analyzed the proportion by distance, and calculated the probable impact on the community if the hospital were relocated to the proposed site. In her view, hospitals were a part of the wider community that served the needs of humanity. Kopf (1978) noted that this method of health planning and matching resources to the needs of the population was visionary and was not reapplied until the twentieth century.

found the proposed answer to his observation through Pasteur's work. Something outside the body entered the wound through the broken skin, causing the infection (Goodnow, 1933). Lister's surgical successes eventually improved when he soaked the dressings and instruments in mixtures of carbolic acid (i.e., phenol) and oil.

In 1882, Koch discovered the causative agent for cholera and the tubercle bacillus. Pasteur discovered immunization in 1881 and the rabies vaccine in 1885. These discoveries were significant to the development of public health and medicine. However, physicians accepted these discoveries slowly (Rosen, 1958). For example, TB was a major cause of death in late nineteenth-century America and often plagued

its victims with chronic illness and disability. It was a highly stigmatized disease, and most physicians thought it was a hereditary, constitutional disease associated with poor environmental conditions. Hospitalization for TB was rare because the stigma caused families to hide their infected relatives. Without treatment, the communicability of the disease increased. Common treatment was a change of climate (Rosen, 1958) Although Koch had announced the discovery of the tubercle bacillus in 1882, it was 10 years before the emergence of the first organized community campaign to stop the spread of the disease.

The case of puerperal (i.e., childbirth) fever illustrates another example of slow innovation stemming from scientific discoveries. Although Pasteur showed that *Streptococcus* caused puerperal fever, it was years before physicians accepted his discovery. However, medical practice eventually changed, and physicians no longer delivered infants after performing autopsies on puerperal fever cases without washing their hands (Goodnow, 1933).

Debate over the causes of disease occurred throughout the nineteenth century. Scientists discovered organisms during the latter part of the century, which supported the theory that specific contagious entities caused disease. This discovery challenged the earlier, miasmic theory that environment and atmospheric conditions caused disease (Greifinger and Sidel, 1981). The new scientific discoveries had a major impact on the development of public health and medical practice. The emergence of germ theory of disease focused diagnosis and treatment on the individual organism and the individual disease.

State and local governments felt increasingly responsible for controlling the spread of disease. A community outcry for social reform forced state and local governments to take notice of the deplorable living conditions in the cities. In the New York City riots of 1863, the populace expressed their disgust for overcrowding; filthy streets; lack of provisions for the poor; and lack of adequate food, water, and housing for the people. Local boards of health formed and took responsibility for safeguarding food and water stores and managed the sewage and quarantine operation for victims of contagious diseases (Greifinger and Sidel, 1981).

The New York Metropolitan Board of Health formed in 1866, and state health departments formed shortly thereafter. States built large public hospitals that treated TB and mental disease with rest, diet, and quarantine. In 1889, the New York City Health Department recommended the surveillance of TB and TB health education, but physicians did not welcome either recommendation (Rosen, 1958). Despite their objections, the New York City Health Department required institutions to report cases of TB in 1894 and required physicians to do the same in 1897.

In the later part of the nineteenth century, the National Tuberculosis Association attempted to control TB by "enlisting community support and action through a systematic and organized campaign of public health education" (Rosen, 1958, p. 390). Many voluntary health organizations followed with organized efforts to "further community health through education, demonstrating ways of improving health services, advancing related research or legislation, and guarding and representing the public interest in this field" (Rosen, 1958, p. 384).

In 1883, The Johns Hopkins University Medical School in Baltimore, Maryland, formed under the German model that promoted medical education on the principles of scientific discovery. In the United States, the Carnegie Commission appointed Abraham Flexner to evaluate medical schools throughout the country based on the German model. In 1910, the **Flexner Report** outlined the shortcomings of U.S. medical schools that did not use this model. Within a few years, the report caused philanthropic organizations such as the Rockefeller and Carnegie Foundations to withdraw funding of these schools, which ensured the closure of scientifically "inadequate" medical schools (Greifinger and Sidel, 1981). A new breed of physicians emerged, who had been taught that germ theory was the "single agent theory" of disease causation (Greifinger and Sidel 1981, p. 132) (Box 2-4).

Philanthropic foundations continued to influence health care efforts. For example, the Rockefeller Sanitary Commission for the Eradication of Hookworm formed in 1909. Hookworm was an occupational hazard among southern workers. The discovery of preventive efforts to eradicate hookworm kept the workers healthy and thus proved to be a great industrial benefit. The model was so successful that the Rockefeller Foundation established the first school of public health, The Johns Hopkins School of Hygiene and Public Health, in 1916. The focus of this institution was the preservation and improvement of individual and community health and the prevention of disease through multidisciplinary

---

BOX 2-4 Scientific Theory/Single Agent Theory

The emphasis on the use of scientific theory, or single agent theory, in medical care developed into a focus on disease and symptoms rather than a focus on the prevention of disability and care for the "whole person." The old-fashioned family doctor viewed patients in relation to their families and communities and apparently helped people cope with problems in personal life, family, and society. American medicine adopted science with such vigor that these qualities faded away. Science allowed the physician to deal with tissues and organs, which were much easier to comprehend than the dynamics of human relationships or the complexities of disease prevention. Many physicians made efforts to integrate the various roles, but society was pushing toward academic science.

---

efforts. The faculty came from a broad range of sciences including biological, physical, social, and behavioral. Foundations made additional efforts, which led to the formation of the International Health Commission, schools of tropical medicine, and medical research institutes in foreign ports.

Historical Methodology for Nursing Research

Historiography is the methodology of historical research. It involves specialized techniques, principles, and theories that pertain to historical matters. Historical research involves interpreting history and contributing to understanding through data synthesis. It relies on existing sources or data and requires the researcher to gain access to sources such as libraries, librarians, and databases.

Historical research should be descriptive. It should answer the questions of who, what, when, where, how, and the interpretive why. Historians reconstruct an era using primary sources and interpret the story from that perspective. Historical research in nursing will enhance the understanding of current nursing practice and will help prepare for the future.

From Lusk B: Historical methodology for nursing research, Image J Nurs Sch 29(4):355-359, 1997. ■

Establishment of Public Health Nursing

Public health nursing as a holistic approach to care developed in the late nineteenth and early twentieth centuries. Public health nursing and community health nursing evolved from home nursing practice, community organizations, and political interventions on behalf of aggregates.

England

Public health nursing developed from providing nursing care to the sick poor and providing information and channels of community organization that enable the poor to improve their own health status.

District Nursing

District nursing, which stemmed from the first tradition, developed in England. Between 1854 and 1856, the Epidemiological Society of London developed a plan that trained selected poor women to provide nursing care to the community's sick poor. The society theorized that nurses belonging to their patient's social class would be more effective caregivers and that more nurses would be available in the community (Rosen, 1958).

A similar plan implemented in Liverpool in 1859 was more successful. After experiencing the excellent care a nurse gave his sick wife in his home, William Rathbone, a Quaker, strongly believed that nurses could offer the same care throughout the community. He developed a plan that divided the community into 18 districts and assigned a nurse and a social worker to each district. This team met the needs of their communities in nursing, social work, and health education. The community widely accepted the plan. To further strengthen it, Rathbone consulted Nightingale about educating the nurses. She assisted him by providing training for the district nurses, referring to them as "health nurses." The model was successful, and, eventually, voluntary agencies on the national level adopted the plan (Rosen, 1958).

Health Visiting

Health visiting to provide information for improved health is a parallel service based on the district nursing tradition. The Ladies Section of the Manchester and Salford Sanitary Association originated health visiting in Manchester in 1862. Health pamphlets alone had little effect; therefore, this service enlisted home visitors to distribute health information to the poor.

In 1893, Nightingale pointed out that the district nurse should be a health teacher and a nurse for the sick in the home. She felt that teachers should educate "health missioners" for this purpose. However, the model charged the district nurse with providing care for the sick in the home and the health visitor with providing health information in the home. Eventually, government agencies sponsored health visitors, medical health officers supervised them, and the municipality paid them. Thus, a collaborative model developed between government and voluntary agencies and exists in the United States today.

United States

In the United States, public health nursing also developed from the traditions of district nursing and home nursing. In 1877, the Women's Board of the New York City Mission sent a graduate nurse named Francis Root into homes to provide care for the sick. The innovation spread and nursing associations, later called visiting nurse associations, were implemented in Buffalo in 1885 and in Boston and Philadelphia in 1886.

In 1893, nurses **Lillian Wald** and Mary Brewster established a district nursing service on the Lower East Side of New York City called the **House on Henry Street.** This was a crowded area teeming with unemployed and homeless immigrants who needed health care. This organization, later called the Visiting Nurse Association of New York City, played an important role in establishing public health nursing in the United States. Box 2-5 contains Wald's compelling account of her early exposure to the community where she identified public health nursing needs.

Wald described a range of services that evolved from the house at Henry Street. Nurses provided home visits and patients paid carfare or a cursory fee. Physicians were con-

sultants to Henry Street, and families could arrange a visit by calling the nurse directly or a physician could call the nurse on the family's behalf. The nursing service adopted the philosophy of meeting the health needs of aggregates, which included the many evident social, economic, and environmental determinants of health. By necessity, this involved an aggregate approach that empowered people of the community.

Helen Hall, who later directed the House at Henry Street, wrote that the settlement's role was "one of helping people to help themselves" (Wald, 1971, p. 4) through the development of centers of social action aimed at meeting the needs of the community and the individual. Community organization led to the formation of a great variety of programs including youth clubs, a juvenile program, sex education for local school-teachers, and support programs for immigrants. A community studies department carried out systematical community assessments "so that we could tell our neighbors' story where it would do the most good" (Wald, 1971, p. vi). Mothers from the settlement went to Washington, DC, and testified about raising children in "decaying tenements." Neighbors of the settlement entered a democratic process that took them from the steps of city hall to the nation's capital to speak out on behalf of the needs of the aggregate. They spoke out for necessities like traffic lights, schools, garbage collection services, unemployment insurance, and health care. The Children's Bureau and the Social Security Act Legislation formed as a result of these efforts. The testimony had an impact on the formation of Medicare in 1963.

Aggregate programs like school nursing were based on individual observations and interventions. Wald reported the following incident that preceded her successful trial of school nursing (1971):

I had been downtown only a short time when I met Louis. An open door in a rear tenement revealed a woman standing over a washtub, a fretting baby on her left arm, while with her right she rubbed at the butcher's aprons which she washed for a living.

"Louis," she explained, "was bad." He did not "cure his head of lice and what would become of him, for they would not take him into the school because of it?" Louis said he had been to the dispensary many times. He knew it was awful for a twelve-year-old boy not to know how to read the names of the streets on the lamp-posts, but "every time I go to school Teacher tells me to go home."

It needed only intelligent application of the dispensary ointments to cure the affected area, and in September, I had the joy of securing the boy's admittance to school for the first time in his life. The next day, at the noon recess, he fairly rushed up our five flights of stairs in the Jefferson Street tenement to spell the elementary words he had acquired that morning. (pp. 46-47)

Overcrowded schools, an uninformed and uninterested public, and an unaware department of health all contributed to this neglect. Wald and the nursing staff at the settlement kept anecdotal notes on the sick children teachers excluded from school. One nurse found a boy in school whose skin was desquamating from scarlet fever and took him to the president of the Department of Health in an attempt to place physicians in schools. A later program had physicians screen children in school for one hour each day; however, this program suffered because it was not comprehensive.

BOX 2-5 Lillian Wald: *The House on Henry Street*

The following highlights from *The House on Henry Street*, published in 1915, bring Lillian Wald's experience to life:

A sick woman in a squalid rear tenement, so wretched and so pitiful that, in all the years since, I have not seen anything more appalling, determined me, within half an hour, to live on the East Side.

I had spent two years in a New York training-school for nurses. . . . After graduation, I supplemented the theoretical instruction, which was casual and inconsequential in the hospital classes twenty-five years ago, by a period of study at a medical college. It was while at the college that a great opportunity came to me.

While there, the long hours "on duty" and the exhausting demands of the ward work scarcely admitted freedom for keeping informed as to what was happening in the world outside. The nurses had no time for general reading; visits to and from friends were brief; we were out of the current and saw little of life saved as it flowed into the hospital wards. It is not strange, therefore that I should have been ignorant of the various movements which reflected the awakening of the social conscience at the time.

Remembering the families who came to visit patients in the wards, I outlined a course of instruction in home nursing adapted to their needs, and gave it in an old building in Henry Street, then used as a technical school and now part of the settlement. Henry Street then as now was the center of a dense industrial population.

From the schoolroom where I had been giving a lesson in bedmaking, a little girl led me one drizzling March morning. She had told me of her sick mother, and gathering from her incoherent account that a child had been born, I caught up the paraphernalia of the bedmaking lesson and carried it with me.

The child led me over broken roadways—there was no asphalt, although its use was well established in other parts of the city—over dirty mattresses and heaps of refuse—it was before Colonel Waring had shown the possibility of clean streets even in that quarter—between tall, reeking houses whose laden fire-escapes, useless for their appointed purpose, bulged with household goods of every description. The rain added to the dismal appearance of the streets and to the discomfort of the crowds which thronged them, intensifying the odors which assailed me from every side. Through Hester and Division street we went to the end of Ludlow; past odorous fishstands, for the streets were a market-place, unregulated, unsupervised, unclean; past evil-smelling, uncovered garbage-cans; and—perhaps worst of all, where so many little children played—past the trucks brought down from more fastidious quarters and stalled on these already overcrowded streets, lending themselves inevitably to many forms of indecency.

The child led me on through a tenement hallway, across a court where open and unscreened closets were promiscuously used by men and women, up into a rear tenement, by slimy steps whose accumulated dirt was augmented that day by the mud of the streets, and finally into the sickroom.

All the maladjustments of our social and economic relations seemed epitomized in this brief journey and what was found at the end of it. The family to which the child led me was neither criminal nor vicious. Although the husband was a cripple, one of those who stand on street corners exhibiting deformities to enlist compassion, and masking the begging of alms by a pretense at selling; although the family of seven shared their two rooms with boarders—who were literally boarders, since a piece of timber was placed over the floor for them to sleep on—and although the sick woman lay on a wretched, unclean bed, soiled with a hemorrhage two days old, they were not degraded human beings, judged by any measure of moral values.

In fact, it was very plain that they were sensitive to their condition, and when, at the end of my ministrations, they kissed my hands (those who have undergone similar experiences will, I am sure, understand), it would have been some solace if by any conviction of the moral unworthiness of the family I could have defended myself as a part of a society which permitted such conditions to exist. Indeed, my subsequent acquaintance with them revealed the fact that, miserable as their state was, they were not without ideals for the family life, and for society, of which they were so unloved and unlovely a part.

That morning's experience was a baptism of fire. Deserted were the laboratory and the academic work of the college. I never returned to them. On my way from the sickroom to my comfortable student quarters my mind was intent on my own responsibility. To my inexperience it seemed certain that conditions such as these were allowed because people did not know, and for me there was a challenge to know and to tell. When early morning found me still awake, my naive conviction remained that, if people knew things—and "things" meant everything implied in the condition of this family—such horrors would cease to exist, and I rejoiced that I had had a training in the care of the sick that in itself would give me an organic relationship to the neighborhood in which this awakening had come.

To the first sympathetic friend to whom I poured forth my story, I found myself presenting a plan which had been developing almost without conscious mental direction on my part.

Within a day or two a comrade from the training-school, Mary Brewster, agreed to share in the venture. We were to live in the neighborhood as nurses, identify ourselves with it socially, and, in brief, contribute to it our citizenship.

I should like to make it clear that from the beginning we were most profoundly moved by the wretched industrial conditions which were constantly forced upon us. . . . I hope to tell of the constructive programmes that the people them-selves have evolved out of their own hard lives, of the ameliorative measures, ripened out of sympathetic comprehension, and finally, of the social the new compunction of the community. (pp. 1-9)

From Wald L: *The house on Henry Street*, New York, 1971, Dover Publications. (Original work published 1915, Henry Holt.)

Twentieth Century

In 1902, Wald convinced the Commissioner of Health in New York City, to try a school nursing experiment. Henry Street loaned a public health nurse named Linda Rogers to the New York City Health Department to work in a school (Dock and Stewart, 1925). The experiment was successful, and schools adopted nursing on a widespread basis. These early school nurses performed physical assessments, treated minor infections, and taught health to pupils and parents.

Example of Historical Nursing Research

Fairman's (1996) review of 150 fictional novels from 1850 to 1995 revealed how the image of nursing has changed over the past 140 years. The results showed that the image of nursing improved dramatically from the negative perception of the 1850s. Trained nurses became more common in the early 1900s, and the novels began to depict strong, independent, female nurses. The positive image continued until the 1960s and 1970s when novels presented the negative image of "bed hopping honeys." Popular literature showed the most negative image of nurse, and classics and children's literature showed a more positive image.

From Fairman PL: Analysis of the image of nursing and nurses as portrayed in fictional literature from 1850 to 1995, dissertation, 1996, University of San Francisco. ∎

In 1909, Wald mentioned the efficacy of home nursing to one of the officials of the Metropolitan Life Insurance Company. The company decided to provide home nursing to its industrial policyholders, and soon the United States and Canada used the successful program (Wald, 1971).

The increasing demand for public health nursing was hard to satisfy. In 1910, the Department of Nursing and Health formed at the Teachers College of Columbia University in New York City. A course in visiting nursing placed nurses at the Henry Street settlement for fieldwork. In 1912, the newly formed National Organization of Public Health Nursing elected Lillian Wald its first president. This organization was open to public health nurses and to those interested in public health nursing. In 1913, the Los Angeles Department of Health formed the first Bureau of Public Health Nursing (Rosen, 1958). That same year, the National Organization of Public Health Nursing appointed its first public health nurse.

At first, many public health nursing programs used nurses in specialized areas such as school nursing, TB nursing, maternal-child health nursing, and communicable disease nursing. In subsequent years, a more generalized program became commonplace. In this model, a nurse hired by an official agency covered the population of one district and provided prevention, health promotion, and health maintenance care. Visiting nurses worked with voluntary home health agencies, such as the Visiting Nurse Association, to provide care to the homebound ill through physician referral.

In the twenty-first century, the focus is on cost containment and the provision of health care services under managed care. Change is taking place in the traditional models of public health nursing and visiting nursing and other home health agencies. The focus of care is increasing within the community, and new models that use nursing in the community to contain costs are appearing with variation among states and areas within a state. For example, some models focus on providing care to rural populations (VanderMeer, Savage, and Davis, 2001) and disease management (Gorski and Johnson, 2003), whereas others focus on specialized areas like medically fragile children (Mentro, 2003) and clients with disabilities (Kodner and Kyriacou, 2003). Box 2-6 shows one contemporary model.

CONSEQUENCES FOR THE HEALTH OF AGGREGATES

An understanding of the consequences of the health care delivery system's impact on aggregate health is necessary to form conclusions about community health nursing from a historical perspective. Implications for the health of aggre-

BOX 2-6 A Model of District Nursing

In an ethnohistorical study of the development of public health nursing in rural New England, Dreher (1984) unexpectedly found a model of population-based nursing that may meet the nation's current and future health concerns. Dreher collected data from public records; the census; direct observations; and interviews with town residents, public officials, medical care providers, and active and retired public health nurses. The health model of the 1920s used a district nurse, or "town hall" nurse, which exists today. The findings show that the district nurse provided health education and services to people in four neighboring towns. The district nurse's activities were under local administration, and property tax revenues paid for the services; patients and third-party reimbursement did not contribute funds. The district nurse provided a full range of community nursing services to people in need, whether or not the patients were able to pay or were covered by insurance. The nurse performed school nursing, health promotion and prevention, and home health care. The district nurse held weekly office hours in the town halls of the four communities, performed blood pressure screening, and gave routine parenteral medications and health counseling. Mobility was not an issue because the district nurse performed home visits for patients confined to their homes. The district nurse conducted routine screening in schools and planned and carried out programs that addressed identified needs. The annual cost per visit from the district nurse was far less than the nurse services from a nearby home health agency. This model exemplifies a way of addressing the nation's health problems through prevention, promotion, and maintenance care.

gates relate to new causes of mortality and additional theories of disease causation.

Twenty-First Century

New Causes of Mortality

Over the last 100 years, the causes of mortality in Western societies have changed from mostly infectious diseases to chronic diseases. Increased food production and better nutrition during the nineteenth and early twentieth centuries contributed to the decline in infectious disease–related deaths. Other factors include better sanitation through water purification, sewage disposal, improved food handling, and milk pasteurization. According to McKeown (1981) and Evans, Barer, and Marmor (1994), "modern" medicine such as antibiotics and immunization had little effect on health until well into the twentieth century. Indeed, improved vaccination programs began in the 1920s, and powerful antibiotics came into use after 1935.

The advent of chronic disease in Western populations puts selected aggregates at risk, and those aggregates need health education, screening, and programs to ensure occupational and environmental safety. Too often, modern medicine focuses on the single cause of disease (i.e., germ theory) and treating the acutely ill. Health providers have treated the chronically ill with an acute care approach although preventive care, health promotion, and restorative care are necessary to combat escalating rates of chronic disease. This expanded approach may develop under new systems of cost containment.

SOCIAL CHANGES AND COMMUNITY HEALTH NURSING

Several social and political changes have occurred in the United States that have affected the development of community health nursing practice. During the twentieth century, the health of the aggregate client, nursing, health, and environment were influenced by the development of health insurance, problems caused by discrimination and racism, the advancement of feminism, and, in the twenty-first century, terrorism. The following material reviews these developments and highlights their importance to community health nursing practice.

Changes in health insurance changed the course of health care delivery. The greatest health concerns at the beginning of the twentieth century were lost wages associated with illness. The cost of health care was so low that there was little need for health insurance. In the early twentieth century, there was little technology, and treatments available at the time, including surgery, were often performed in private homes.

During the 1920s and 1930s, the costs of health care increased. As the population moved from rural to urban living, the number of large private homes, the delivery point for health care, decreased. Increased technology, the acceptance of medicine as a science, and the closure of several medical schools during the 1920s increased the demand and therefore raised the cost of health care (Faulkner, 1960; Rosenberg, 1987).

As hospitals began to organize, they formed the American Hospital Association, whose leaders encouraged the development of health insurance plans. During the 1930s, health insurance plans that were unique to individual hospitals merged under the name of Blue Cross (Anderson, 1944; Eilers, 1963; Thomasson, 2002). Increases in medical technology and the fact that employers began to offer health insurance in place of employee compensation during and after World War II contributed to the growth of private health insurance (Health Insurance Institute, 1961). Federal and state movements during the 1960s supported the development of health insurance for the poor and the elderly populations (Oliver, Lee, and Lipton, 2004).

Discrimination and racism have affected the development of community health in America (Gamble, 1997). The American Nurses Association Position Statement on Discrimination and Racism in Health Care (ANA, 1998) states "differential access to resources limits basic and preventive health care to members of some groups. An equal distribution of health care resources results in morbidity and mortality rates that vary substantially among racial and ethnic categories and economic classes." Current community health initiatives need to continue to address historical traditions and practices to ensure the absence of both discrimination and racism in current community health nursing practice.

The historical concept of feminism can be traced to the eighteenth century. Whereas feminism means many things to different people, the philosophy of feminism embraces gender issues, economics, politics, and the humanities. Its basic premise is that people are inherently equal and deserve equal opportunities. In health care, feminism focuses on reproductive freedom for women. Feminists, regardless of focus, support the equality of all and are united against innate stereotypes.

Feminism has affected health care delivery in two important ways. First, the feminist perspective has encouraged the involvement of people, especially women, in all dimensions of economic life. Employment and career opportunities based on qualifications, not gender, provide women with multiple career opportunities. Second, the feminist perspective of equality is in direct opposition to discrimination in health care delivery.

Terrorism against the United States is a recent historical event that will affect public health and nursing practice well into the twenty-first century. In response to terrorism against the United States on September 11, 2001, the health system is considered a resource in the country's arsenal against terrorist activities. Bioterrorism preparedness is a new concept in health care. It is the responsibility of community health leaders to successfully prepare the nation's health system to respond to any future bioterrorist attack.

There are vulnerable areas of defense that remain within the U.S. public health response efforts which need continual attention (Century Foundation, 2005). In the event of future terrorism against the United States, increased numbers of community health practitioners would be needed to distribute vaccines and antibodies in an emergency. Additionally, public health laboratories would require additional capabilities to respond to a chemical terrorism threat, increased electronic tracking of disease outbreak information, and adequate crisis response plans by state. Currently, community health priorities are being met with limited and often inadequate resources (Trust for America's Health, 2005).

Viewing Immigrants as Assets: A Glimpse Into Australia's Public Health History

Like the United States and Canada, Australia is a land of immigration with its own unique public health history. In 1788—18 years after Captain Cook claimed the continent for Britain—the British began using Australia as a settlement for England's convicts and continued doing so until 1825. From 1826 to 1850, Australia held England's excess population. After 1850, the living conditions in England improved significantly and caused the level of British emigration to drop dramatically. Populating the Australian colony turned into a public health disaster for England because the journey was a difficult 6 to 8 months at sea.

The first few convict fleets barely survived the journey. By the time the immigrants arrived in Australia, they were plagued with disease and unable to build a settlement. British historical records show that the second English fleet contained 1260 convicts. By the time the fleet reached Australia, 267 convicts perished. Shortly after arriving, 124 of the survivors died in the Sydney hospital. For the next 25 years, the surviving convicts were limited in their ability to help England build a settlement because they were starved and diseased. Overcrowding and reduced food and water rations made the journey difficult to survive. These poor travel conditions were related to the overall negligence and corruption of the private contractors who put priority on valuable cargo.

The British authorities realized that they needed to ensure the convicts' safe arrival. William Redfern, the assistant surgeon and former convict of New South Wales, advised Governor Macquarie to regulate the shipping contractors and supervise the convicts' health. Redfern recommended placing a convict surgeon aboard each ship to improve traveling conditions. Specifically, he recommended that the surgeons air out passenger cabins and bedding daily, make more drinking water available, provide full rations and articles of comfort, install bathing and cleaning facilities, and regularly fumigate the ship with nitric or muriatic acid. After Macquarie installed these regulations, the death rate among convicts on ships to Australia plummeted between 1788 and 1868; it was much lower in comparison to the passenger deaths on similar private fleets making the shorter trip from Europe to North America.

The Australian government believed that it was even more important that settlers, rather than convicts, arrive healthy and ready to work; therefore these public health standards were extended to ships that carried assisted immigrants. The Australian government prepaid the fares for assisted immigrants. Regulations from London mandated that surgeons and matrons be responsible for the hygiene, medical care, welfare, and discipline of the passengers. This measure, called the Passenger Act, created a marked improvement in the health of young children and all immigrants by placing a doctor and nurse aboard each ship. The British Board of Trade controlled the health conditions on all passenger ships and made the passage to Australia "so safe that it was looked upon as a holiday by many immigrants, who arrived healthier than when they had left England (Jupp, 1990).

This glimpse into Australia's immigration policy exemplifies one development in the history of public health. Whether they coerced the convicts or assisted passage for settlers, the Australian government populated its country through the belief that immigrants are assets and proved that the health of immigrants is a public responsibility.

Data from Jupp J: Two hundred years of immigration. In Reid J and Trompf R, editors: The health of immigrant Australia, Orlando, 1990, Harcourt Brace. ∎

CHALLENGES FOR COMMUNITY AND PUBLIC HEALTH NURSING

Community health nurses face the challenge of promoting the health of populations. They must accomplish this with an "inclusive" understanding of the multiple causes of morbidity and mortality. The specialization of medicine and nursing has affected the delivery of nursing and medical care. Well-prepared nurses must be aware of the increased technological advances specialization has instigated. These advances resulted in an increase in the number and percentage of advanced practice nurses in the past two decades. In 2000, 10% of registered nurses (RNs) in the United States were prepared at the master's or doctoral level (USDHHS, 2002), and most of these advance practice nurses were specialists. However, the

past decade has also seen an increase in the number and percentage of RNs working in community settings. In 2000, approximately 41% of all RNs worked in community settings such as occupational health, public health departments, physician's offices, and schools (USDHHS, 2002).

The need for education in community health nursing calls for a primary care curriculum that prepares students to meet the needs of aggregates through population-based strategies, such as those that promote literacy, nutrition programs, decent housing and income, education, and safe social and physical environments. Health care services alone cannot solve today's health problems. All health care workers must learn to work with, and on behalf of, aggregates and help them build a constituency for the consumer issues they face.

A population focus for nursing addresses the health of all in the population through the careful gathering of information and statistics. A population focus will better enable community health nurses to contribute to the ethic of social justice by emphasizing society's responsibility for health (Beauchamp, 1986). Helping aggregates to help themselves will empower the people and create avenues for addressing their concerns.

Example of Historical Nursing Research

In 1909, a "preventorium" for poor children considered to be at risk for developing TB was opened in the suburbs of New York City. This institution was the result of years of international study and consensus that determined that programs to manage TB should focus more on preventing active disease than on treating it. The idea was to send infected children to the country to prevent them from developing clinically active disease.

Although the causative agent of TB was identified in 1882, there was no effective treatment until decades later. In the early twentieth century, public health officials were seeking ways to arrest the spread of TB and saw the preventorium as a way of addressing "pretuberculosis." The consensus was that "delicate, weak, wan, malnourished, or pale . . . urban children between the ages of four and 14, with at least one parent with active tuberculosis, could have their health restored in the preventorium" (p. 143). The highly regimented program included good nutrition, rest, exercise, sunlight, and prolonged exposure to the open air. Children typically stayed 3 to 6 months and most were followed for years after discharge. Similar preventoria opened throughout the United States into the 1920s, until falling incidence and better treatment options led health officials to conclude that they were no longer needed.

From Connolly C: Pale, poor and "pretubercular" children: A history of pediatric antituberculosis efforts in France, Germany and the United States, 1899-1929, Nurs Inquiry, 11:138-147, 2004. ∎

SUMMARY

Western civilization evolved from the Paleolithic period to the present, and people began to live in increasingly closer proximity to each other; therefore, they experienced a change in the nature of their health problems.

In the mid nineteenth and early twentieth centuries, public health efforts and the precursors of modern and public health nursing began to improve societal health. Nursing pioneers, such as Nightingale in England and Wald in the United States, focused on the collection and analysis of statistical data, health care reforms, home nursing, community empowerment, and nursing education. They established the groundwork for today's community health nursing.

Modern community health nurses must grapple with an array of philosophical controversies that affect their practice. These controversies include different opinions about what "intervention" means, a focus on both the individual and the aggregate, discrimination, feminism, the very real potential for additional terrorism in America, and the best way to solve the critical problem of runaway health care costs.

LEARNING ACTIVITIES

1. Research the history of the health department or Visiting Nurse Association in a particular city or county.
2. Find two recent articles about Florence Nightingale. After reading the articles, list Nightingale's contributions to public health, public health nursing, and community health nursing.
3. Discuss with peers how Lillian Wald's approach to individual and community health care provides an understanding of how to facilitate the empowerment of aggregates in the community.
4. Obtain copies of early articles from nursing journals (e.g., *American Journal of Nursing* dates from 1900). Discuss the health problems, medical care, and nursing practice these articles illustrated.
5. Collect copies of early nursing textbooks. Discuss the evolution of thoughts on pathology, illness management, and health promotion.

REFERENCES

Amaro H, Whitaker R, Coffman G, Heeren T: Acculturation and marijuana and cocaine use: findings from NHANES 1982-84, *Am J Public Health* 80(suppl):54 60, 1990.

American Nurses Association: Discrimination and racism in health care, The Author, https://www.nursingworld.org/readroom/position/ethics/etdisrac.htm, 1998.

Anderson OW: *State enabling legislation for non-profit hospital and medical plans,* Ann Arbor, 1944, University of Michigan Press.

Armelagos GK, Dewcy JR: Evolutionary response to human infectious diseases. In Logan MH, Hunt EE, editors: *Health and the human condition,* North Scituate, Mass, 1978, Duxbury Press.

Beauchamp DE: Public health as social justice. In Mappes T, Zembaty J, editors: *Biomedical ethics,* ed 2, New York, 1986, McGraw-Hill.

Hunt EE, editors: *Health and the human condition,* North Scituate, Mass, 1978, Duxbury Press.

Burkitt DP: Some diseases characteristic of modern western civilization. In Logan MH, Hunt EE, editors: *Health and the human condition,* North Scituate, Mass, 1978, Duxbury Press.

Centers for Disease Control and Prevention: Prevention of plague: recommendations of the Advisory Committee on Immunization Practices, *Morb Mortal Wkly Rep* 45(RR-14):1-15, 1996.

Centers for Disease Control and Prevention: Plague home page: http://www.cdc.gov/ncidod/dvbid/plague/index.htm and Centers for Disease Control and Prevention: Imported plague: New York City, 2002, *Morb Mortal Wkly Rep* 52:31, 2003.

Century Foundation: Breathing easier? The report of the Centruy Foundation Working group on Bioterrorism Preparedness, The

Author, http://www.tcf.org/Events/1-13-05/breathingtranscript.pdf.

Cockburn TA: The evolution of human infectious diseases. In Cockburn T, editor: *Infectious diseases: their evolution and eradication,* Springfield, Ill, 1967, Charles C Thomas.

Cohen IB: Florence Nightingale, *Sci Am* 250:128-137, 1984.

Connolly C: Pale, poor and "protubercular" children: A history of pediatric antituberculosis efforts in France, Germany and the United States, 1899-1929, *Nurs Inquiry* 11:138-147, 2004.

Dock LL, Stewart IM: *A short history of nursing: from the earliest times to the present day,* New York, 1925, Putnam.

Dossey BM: *Florence Nightingale: mystic, visionary, reformer,* Springhouse, Pa, Springhouse Publishing, 2000.

Dreher M: District nursing: the cost benefits of a population-based practice, *Am J Public Health* 74:1107-1111, 1984.

Duffus RL: *Lillian Wald: neighbor and crusader,* New York, 1938, Macmillan.

Duran FD: *The Aztecs: the history of the Indies of New Spain,* New York, 1964, Orion Press (Translated, with notes, by Heyden D and Horcasitas F).

Ehrenreich B, English D: *Witches, midwives, and nurses: a history of women healers,* Old Westbury, NY, 1973, The Feminist Press.

Eilers RD: *Regulation of Blue Cross and Blue Shield plans,* Homewood, Ill, 1963, Richard D. Irwin, Inc.

Evans RG, Barer ML, Marmor TR: *Why are some people healthy and others not? The determinants of health of* populations, Hawthorne, NY, 1994, Aldine de Gruyter.

Fairman PL: Analysis of the image of nursing and nurses as portrayed in fictional literature

from 1850 to 1995, dissertation, 1996, University of San Francisco.

Faulkner EJ: *Health insurance,* New York, 1960, McGraw-Hill.

From Centers for Disease Control and Prevention: Plague home page: http://www.cdc.gov/ncidod/dvbid/plague/index.htm and Centers for Disease Control and Prevention: Imported plague: New York City, 2002, *Morb Mortal Wkly Rep* 52:31, 2003.

Gamble VN: Under the shadow of Tuskegee: African Americans and health care, *Am J Public Health* 11:1773-1778, 1997.

Garn SM: Culture and the direction of human evolution, *Hum Biol* 35:221-236, 1963.

George MD: *London life in the XVIIIth century,* New York, 1925, Knopf.

Goodnow M: *Outlines of nursing history,* Philadelphia, 1933, WB Saunders.

Gorski LA, Johnson K: A disease management program for heart failure, *Home Healthcare Nurse* 21:734-744, 2003.

Greifinger RB, Sidel VW: American medicine: charity begins at home. In Lee P, Brown N, Red I, editors: *The nation's health,* San Francisco, 1981, Boyd and Fraser.

Grier B, Grier M: Contributions of the passionate statistician, *Res Nurs Health* 1.103-109, 1978.

Guendelman S et al: Generational differences in perinatal health among the Mexican American population: findings from HHANES 1982-84, *Am J Public Health* 80(suppl):61-65, 1990.

Hanlon JJ, Pickett GE: *Public health administration and practice,* ed 9, St. Louis, 1990, Mosby.

Health Insurance Institute: *Source book of health insurance data, 1960,* New York, 1961, The Author.

Hughes CC: Medical care: ethnomedicine. In Logan MH, Hunt EE, editors: *Health and the human condition,* North Scituate, Mass, 1978, Duxbury Press.

Hume EE: *Max von Pettenkofer,* New York, 1927, Hoeber.

Jupp J: Two hundred years of immigration. In Reid J, Trompf R, editors: *The health of immigrant Australia,* Orlando, Fla, 1990, Harcourt Brace & Co.

Kodner DL, Kyriacou CK: Bringing managed care home to people with chronic, disabling conditions, *J Aging Health* 15:189-222, 2003.

Kopf EW: Florence Nightingale as statistician, *Res Nurs Health* 1:93-102, 1978.

Lamarche PA: Our health paradigm in peril, *Public Health Rep* 110:556-560, 1995.

Lee PR, Brown N, Red I, editors: *The nation's health,* San Francisco, 1981, Boyd and Fraser.

Leininger M: *Transcultural health care issues and conditions,* Philadelphia, 1976, FA Davis.

Logan MH, Hunt EE, editors: *Health and the human condition,* North Scituate, Mass, 1978, Duxbury Press.

Lusk B: Historical methodology for nursing research, *Image J Nurs Sch* 29(4):355-359, 1997.

McDermott W, Deuschle KW, Barnett CR: Health care experiment at Many Farms. *Science* 175:23-31, 1972.

McKeown T: Determinants of health. In Lee P, Brown N, Red I, editors: *The nation's health,* San Francisco, 1981, Boyd and Fraser.

Mentro AM: Health care policy for medically fragile children *J Pediatr Nurs* 18:225-232, 2003.

Mullan DF, Machiaveli, Hood R: Public health practice: past and present, *Am J Public Health* 90:702-706, 2000.

Najman JM: Theories of disease causation and the concept of a general susceptibility: a review, *Soc Sci Med* 14A:231-237, 1990.

Newbern VB: Women as caregivers in the South: 1900-1945, *Public Health Nurs* 11:247-254, 1994.

Nightingale F: *Notes on matters affecting the health, efficiency and hospitalization of the British army,* London, 1858, Harrison and Sons.

Oliver TR, Lee PR, Lipton HL: A political history of Medicare and prescription drug coverage, *Milbank Q* 82(2):283-354, 2004.

Polgar S: Evolution and the ills of mankind. In Tax S, editor: *Horizons of anthropology,* Chicago, 1964, Aldine de Gruyter.

Richardson BW: *The health of nations: a review of the works of Edwin Chadwick,* vol 2, London, 1887, Longmans, Green.

Rosen G: *A history of public health,* New York, 1958, MD Publications.

Rosenberg CE: *The care of strangers,* New York, 1987, Basic Books.

Smith FB: *The people's health 1830-1910,* London, 1979, Croom Helm.

Thomasson, MA: The importance of group coverage: how tax policy shaped U.S. health insurance, *Expl Econ Hist* 39:233-253, July 2002.

Trust for America's Health: Ready or not? Protecting the public's health form disease and bioterrorism, The Author, http://healthy-americans.org/reports/bioterror05.

U.S. Department of Health and Human Services, Health Resources and Services Administration, Bureau of Health Professions, Division of Nursing: *The registered nurse population: findings from the National Sample Survey of Registered Nurses, March 2000,* Rockville, Md, 2002, The Author.

US Department of Health and Human Services, Health Resources and Services Administration, Bureau of Health Professions, National Center for Health Workforce: *United States health workforce personnel factbook,* Rockville, Md, 2003, The Author.

VanderMeer JL, Savage GT, Davis JA: Restructuring rural health care: expanding the PACE for rural elders, *Online J Rural Nurs Health Care* 2(1), 2001.

Versluysen MC: Old wives' tales? Women healers in English history. In Davies C, editor: *Rewriting nursing history,* Totowa, NJ, 1980, Barnes and Noble.

Wald L: *The house on Henry Street,* New York, 1971, Dover Publications. (Original work published 1915, Henry Holt)

3

Thinking Upstream: Nursing Theories and Population-Focused Nursing Practice

Patricia G. Butterfield

MEDIA RESOURCES

Additional Material for Study, Review, and Further Exploration

evolve Website at http://evolve.elsevier.com/Nies

❖ Quiz ❖ Case Studies ❖ Content Updates ❖ Glossary ❖ WebLinks

---

OBJECTIVES

Upon completion of this chapter, the reader will be able to do the following:

1. Describe different theories and their application to community/public health nursing.
2. Differentiate between upstream interventions, which are designed to alter the precursors of poor health, and downstream interventions, which are characterized by efforts to modify individuals' perceptions of health.
3. Critique a theory in regard to its relevance to population health issues.
4. Explain how theory-based practice achieves the goals of community/public health nursing by protecting and promoting the public's health.

KEY TERMS

conservative scope of practice
critical social theory

health belief model (HBM)
macroscopic
microscopic

Milio's framework for prevention
self-care deficit theory

theory
upstream thinking

CHAPTER OUTLINE

THINKING UPSTREAM: EXAMINING THE ROOT CAUSES OF POOR HEALTH

HISTORICAL PERSPECTIVES ON NURSING THEORY

HOW THEORY PROVIDES DIRECTION TO NURSING

MICROSCOPIC VERSUS MACROSCOPIC APPROACHES TO THE CONCEPTUALIZATION OF COMMUNITY HEALTH PROBLEMS

ASSESSING A THEORY'S SCOPE IN RELATION TO COMMUNITY HEALTH NURSING

REVIEW OF THEORETICAL APPROACHES
    The Individual Is the Locus of Change
    The Upstream View: Society Is the Locus of Change

HEALTHY PEOPLE 2010

It seems as though many community health problems are so complex, so multifaceted, and so deep that it is impossible for a nurse to make substantial improvements in health. Although we see persons who have just been diagnosed with cancer, cardiovascular disease, or pulmonary disease, we know that their diseases began years or even decades ago. In many cases, genetic risks for diseases are interwoven with social, economic, and environmental risks in ways that are difficult to understand and more difficult to change. In the face of all these challenges, how can we as nurses hope to affect the health of the public in a significant way? How can the actions we take today reduce the current burden of illness and prevent illness in the next generation of citizens?

When nurses work on a complex community health problem, they need to think strategically. They need to know where to focus their time, energy, and programmatic resources. Most likely they will be up against health problems that have existed for years, with other layers of foundational problems that may have existed for generations. If nurses use organizational resources in an unfocused manner, they will not solve the problem at hand and may create new problems along the way. If they do not build strong relationships with community partners (e.g., parent groups, ministers, local activists), they will fail. If nurses are unable to advocate for their constituencies in a scientifically responsible, logical, and persuasive manner, they will fail. In the face of these challenges and many more, how can nurses succeed in their goal to improve public health?

Fortunately, there are road maps for success. Some of those road maps can be found by reading a nursing history book or archival work that tell the story of a nurse who succeeded in improving health by leveraging diplomacy skills or neighborhood power; Lillian Wald is one example of such a nurse. Other road maps may be found in "success stories" that provide an overview of how a nurse approached a problem, mobilized their resources, and moved strategically to promote change. This chapter addresses another road map for success: the ability to think conceptually, almost like a chess player, to formulate a plan to solve complex problems. Thinking conceptually is a subtle skill that requires you to understand the world at an abstract level, seeing the manifestations of power, oppression, justice, and access as they exist within our communities. Most of all, thinking conceptually means that you develop a "critical eye" for the community and understand how change happens at micro and macro levels.

This chapter begins with a brief overview of nursing theory followed by a discussion of the scope of community health nursing in addressing population health concerns. Several theoretical approaches are compared to demonstrate how different conceptualizations can lead to different conclusions about the range of interventions available to the nurse. The text uses the analogy of upstream versus downstream thinking to differentiate between population-directed strategies and individual-directed strategies.

THINKING UPSTREAM: EXAMINING THE ROOT CAUSES OF POOR HEALTH

In his description of the frustrations in medical practice, McKinlay (1979) used the image of a swiftly flowing river to represent illness. In this analogy, physicians are so busy rescuing victims from the river that they fail to look upstream to see who is pushing patients into the perilous waters. McKinlay used this story to illustrate the ultimate futility of "downstream endeavors," which are characterized by short-term, individual-based interventions, and challenged health care providers to focus more of their energies "upstream, where the real problems lie" (McKinlay, 1979, p. 9). **Upstream thinking** actions focus on modifying economic, political, and environmental factors that are the precursors of poor health throughout the world. Although the story cites medical practice, it is equally fitting to the dilemmas of nursing practice. Although nursing has a rich history of providing preventive and population-based care, the current health system emphasizes episodic and individual-based care. This system has done little to stem the tide of chronic illness to which 70% of American deaths can be attributed (Centers for Disease Control and Prevention, 2004).

HISTORICAL PERSPECTIVES ON NURSING THEORY

Many scholars agree that Florence Nightingale was the first nurse to formulate a conceptual foundation for nursing practice. However, in the years after her leadership, nursing practice became largely atheoretical and was based primarily on reacting to the immediacy of patient situations and medical staff. Thus, hospital and medical personnel defined the boundaries of nursing practice. Once nursing leaders saw that others were defining their profession, they began to take proactive action to advance the theoretical and scientific foundation of nursing practice. Some of the early nursing theories were extremely myopic and depicted health care situations that involved only one nurse and one patient. Family members and other health professionals were noticeably absent from the context of care. Historically, this characterization may have been an appropriate response to the constraints of nursing practice and the need to emphasize the medically independent activities of the nursing profession.

Although somewhat valuable, theories that address health from a microscopic rather than a macroscopic perspective have limited applicability to community/public health nursing. Such perspectives are inadequate because they do not address social, political, and environmental factors that are central to an understanding of communities. More recent advances in nursing theory development address the dynamic nature of health sustaining and/or damaging environments and address the nature of a collective (e.g., school, worksite) versus an individual client.

HOW THEORY PROVIDES DIRECTION TO NURSING

The goal of theory is to improve nursing practice. Chinn and Kramer (1999) stated that using theories or parts of theoretical frameworks to guide practice best achieves this goal. Students often find theory intellectually burdensome and cannot see the care benefits of something so seemingly obtuse. Theory-based practice guides data collection and interpretation in a clear and organized manner; therefore it is easier for the nurse to diagnose and address health problems. Through the process of integrating theory and practice, the student can focus on factors that are critical to understanding the situation. The student also has an opportunity to analyze the realities of nursing practice in relation to a specific theoretical perspective, in a process of ruling in and ruling out the fit of particular concepts (Schwartz-Barcott et al., 2002). Barnum (1990) stated, "A theory is like a map of a territory as opposed to an aerial photograph. The map does not give the full terrain (i.e., the full picture); instead it picks out those parts that are important for its given purpose" (p. 1). Using a theoretical perspective to plan nursing care guides the student in assessing a nursing situation and allows the student "to plan and not get lost in the details or sidetracked in the alleys" (J. M. Swanson, personal communication, May 1992).

Like other abstract concepts, different nursing authors have defined and interpreted theory in different ways. Several authors' definitions of **theory** are listed in Box 3-1. The lack of uniformity among these definitions reflects the evolution of thought and the individual differences in the understanding of relationships among theory, practice, and research. The definitions also reflect the difficult job of describing complex and diverse theories within the constraints of a single definition. Reading several definitions can foster an appreciation for the richness of theory and help the reader identify one or two particularly meaningful definitions. Within the profession, definitions of theory typically refer to a set of concepts and relational statements and the purpose of the theory. This chapter presents theoretical perspectives that are congruent with a broad interpretation of theory and correspond with the definitions proposed by Dickoff and James (1968), Torres (1986), and Chinn and Kramer (1999).

MICROSCOPIC VERSUS MACROSCOPIC APPROACHES TO THE CONCEPTUALIZATION OF COMMUNITY HEALTH PROBLEMS

In many ways, each nurse must find their own way of interpreting the complex forces that shape societies to understand population health. The nurse can best achieve this

Box 3-1   Definitions of Theory Proposed by Nursing Theorists

➤ "A systematic vision of reality; a set of interrelated concepts that is useful for prediction and control" (Woods and Catanzaro, 1988, p. 568).
➤ "A conceptual system or framework invented for some purpose; and as the purpose varies so too must the structure and complexity of the system" (Dickoff and James, 1968, p. 19).
➤ "A creative and rigorous structuring of ideas that projects a tentative, purposeful, and systematic view of phenomena" (Chinn and Kramer, 1999, p. 51).
➤ "A set of ideas, hunches, or hypotheses that provides some degree of prediction and/or explanation of the world" (Pryjmachuk, 1996, p. 679).
➤ "Theory organizes the relationships between the complex events that occur in a nursing situation so that we can assist human beings. Simply stated, theory provides a way of thinking about and looking at the world around us" (Torres, 1986, p. 19).

transformation by integrating population-based practice and theoretical perspectives to conceptualize health from a macroscopic versus microscopic perspective. Table 3-1 differentiates between these two approaches to conceptualizing health problems.

It is helpful to use the example of a target to understand the concept of **microscopic** versus **macroscopic**. The individual is the bull's eye; this center contains the health problem of interest (e.g., pediatric exposure to lead compounds). In this context, a microscopic approach to assessment would focus exclusively on individual children with lead poisoning. Nursing interventions would focus on the identification and removal of lead sources in the home. However, the nurse can broaden his or her view of this problem by addressing individual health threats and by examining interpersonal and intercommunity factors that perpetuate lead poisoning on a national scale. This approach would include the bull's eye and the concentric circles that extend from the center of the target. A macroscopic approach to lead exposure may incorporate the following activities: examining trends in the prevalence of lead poisoning over time, estimating the percentage of older homes in a neighborhood that may contain lead pipes or lead-based paint surfaces, and locating industrial sources of lead emissions. These efforts usually involve the collaborative efforts of nurses from school, occupational, and other community settings. Doty (1996) notes that macro-level perspectives provide nurses with the conceptual tools that empower clients to make health decisions based on their own interests and the interests of the community at large.

One common dilemma in community health practice is the tension between working on behalf of individuals and working on behalf of a population. For many nurses, this tension is exemplified by the need to reconcile and prioritize multiple daily tasks. Population-directed actions are often more global than the immediate demands of ill people; therefore they may sink to the bottom of the priority list. A community health nurse or nursing administrator may plan to spend the day on a community project directed at preventive efforts, such as screening programs, updating the surveillance program, or meeting with key community members about a specific preventive program. However, the nurse may actually end up spending the day responding to the emergency of the day. This type of reactive rather than proactive nursing practice prevents progress toward "big picture" initiatives and population-based programs. When faced with multiple

TABLE 3-1   Microscopic Versus Macroscopic Approaches to the Delineation of Community Health Nursing Problems

MICROSCOPIC APPROACH	MACROSCOPIC APPROACH
Examines individual, and sometimes family, responses to health and illness.	Examines interfamily and intercommunity themes in health and illness.
	Delineates factors in the population that perpetuate the development of illness or foster the development of health.
Often emphasizes behavioral responses to individual's illness or lifestyle patterns.	Emphasizes social, economic, and environmental precursors of illness.
Nursing interventions are often aimed at modifying individual's behavior through changing his or her perceptions or belief system.	Nursing interventions may include modifying social or environmental variables (i.e., working to remove care barriers and improving sanitation or living conditions).
	May involve social or political action.

demands, nurses must be vigilant in devoting a sustained effort toward population-focused projects. Daily pressures can easily distract the nurse from a population-based nursing practice. The Quad Council of Public Health Nursing Organizations emphasizes "systems thinking" in daily practice and the importance of improving health through the design and implementation of population-based interventions (American Public Health Association, 2003).

A theoretical focus on the individual can preclude understanding of a larger perspective. Dreher (1982) used the term **conservative scope of practice** in describing frameworks that focus energy exclusively on intrapatient and nurse-patient factors. She stated that such frameworks often adopt psychological explanations of patient behavior. This mode of thinking attributes low compliance, missed appointments, and reluctant participation to problems in patient motivation or attitude. Nurses are responsible for altering patient attitudes toward health rather than altering the system itself "even though such negative attitudes may well be a realistic appraisal of health care" (Dreher, 1982, p. 505). This perspective does not entertain the possibility of altering the system or empowering patients to make changes.

ASSESSING A THEORY'S SCOPE IN RELATION TO COMMUNITY HEALTH NURSING

Theoretical scope is especially important to community health nursing because there are many levels of practice within this specialty area. For example, a home health nurse who is caring for ill people after hospitalization has a very different scope of practice than a nurse epidemiologist or health planner. Although it is important that all nurses practice with an understanding of population health, this understanding is critical for nurses whose practice is founded on inter-population rather than intrapopulation dynamics. Unless a given theory is broad enough in scope to address health and the determinants of health from a population perspective, the theory will not be very useful to community health nurses. Although the past 25 years yielded much advancement in the development of nursing theory, there continues to be a lack of clarity about community health nursing's theoretical foundation (Batra, 1991). Applying the terms *microscopic* and *macroscopic* to health situations may help nurses fill this void and stimulate theory development in community health nursing.

Although the concept of macroscopic is similar to the upstream analogy, the term *macroscopic* refers to a broad scope that incorporates many variables to aid in understanding a health problem. Upstream thinking would fall within this domain. Viewing a problem from this perspective emphasizes the variables that precede or play a role in the development of health problems. Macroscopic is the broad concept and upstream is a more specific concept. These related concepts and their meanings can help nurses develop a critical eye in evaluating a theory's relevance to population health.

REVIEW OF THEORETICAL APPROACHES

The differences among theoretical approaches demonstrate how a nurse may draw very diverse conclusions about the reasons for client behavior and the range of available interventions. The following section uses two theories to exemplify individual microscopic approaches to community health nursing problems; one originates within nursing and one is based in social psychology. Two other theories demonstrate the examination of nursing problems from a macroscopic perspective; one originates from nursing and another has roots in phenomenology. The format for this review is as follows:

1. The individual is the locus of change (i.e., microscopic)
   a. Orem's self-care deficit theory of nursing
   b. The health belief model (HBM)
2. Thinking upstream: Society is the locus of change (i.e., macroscopic)
   a. Milio's framework for prevention
   b. Critical social theory

The Individual Is the Locus of Change

Orem's Self-Care Deficit Theory of Nursing

Dorothea Orem was a staff and private duty nurse and later worked in the faculty at Catholic University of America. Her combined experience provided the basis for her self-care deficit theory of nursing. In 1958, Orem began to formalize her insights about the purpose of nursing activities and why individuals required nursing care (Eben et al., 1986; Fawcett, 2001). The theory is based on the assumption that self-care needs and activities are the primary focus of nursing practice. Orem outlined her general theory of nursing and stated that this general theory is actually a composite of the following related constructs: the theory of self-care deficits, which provides criteria for identifying those who need nursing; the theory of self-care, which explains self-care and why it is necessary; and the theory of nursing systems, which specifies nursing's role in the delivery of care and how nursing helps people. Major concepts from Orem's **self-care deficit theory** are listed in Box 3-2.

The basic concepts of this theory evolved from observing the chronology of illness in hospitalized patients. The theory is based on the premise that nursing is a response to a sick person's inability to administer self-care. Nursing assumes the role of providing some or all self-care activities on the patient's behalf (Orem, 2001). This focus makes the content and scope of the theory most useful to nurses practicing within an institutionalized setting. Orem briefly specified the role of population-based nursing in the sixth edition of her book, *Nursing: Concepts of Practice* (2001). However, the concepts of wholly compensatory, partially compensatory, and supportive-developmental are so embedded in an individual orientation to disease that applying these concepts to a population can be awkward at best. Patient deficits (and nurses' efforts to address them) are central to this theory; thus, its

Box 3-2 Concepts From Orem's Self-Care Deficit Theory

➤ *Self-care:* "The production of actions directed to self or to the environment in order to regulate one's functioning in the interest of one's life, integrated functioning, and well-being."

➤ *Therapeutic self-care demand:* "The measures of care required at moments in time in order to meet existent requisites for regulatory action to maintain life and to maintain or promote health, development, and general well-being."

➤ *Self-care agency:* "The complex capability for action that is activated in the performance of the actions or operations of self-care."

➤ *Self-care deficit:* "A relationship between self-care agency and therapeutic self-care demand in which self-care agency is not adequate to meet the known therapeutic self-care demand."

➤ *Nursing agency:* "The complex capability for action that is activated by nurses in their determination of needs for, design of, and production of nursing for people with a range of types of self-care deficits."

➤ *Nursing system:* "A continuing series of actions produced when nurses link one way or a number of ways of helping to meet their own actions or the actions of people under care that are directed to meet these persons' therapeutic self-care demands or to regulate their self-care agency."

From Orem DE: *Nursing: concepts of practice*, ed 6, New York, 2001, Mosby, p. 31.

ability to inform community-level problems and health promotion strategies is limited.

Application of Self-care Deficit Theory

During a discussion about theory-based initiatives, a British nurse lamented over her nursing supervisors' intention to adopt Orem's self-care deficit theory. It would become the primary theory for her specialty area of occupational health nursing. She was frustrated and argued that much of the model's assumptions seemed incongruous with the realities of her daily practice. Kennedy (1989) maintained that the self-care deficit theory assumes that people are able to exert purposeful control over their environments in the pursuit of health; however, people may have little control over the physical or social aspects of their work environment. On the basis of this thesis, she concluded that the self-care model is incompatible with the practice domain of occupational health nursing.

Kennedy exemplified the dissonance that nurses feel when a particular theory is inappropriately imposed in a work setting. Although it is easy to recognize the importance of Orem's concepts to many arenas of nursing practice, it is also apparent that her perspective would not lend itself well to understanding the diverse health needs of people in a worksite. Kennedy (1989) clearly articulated this position when she stated that "the many facets of the occupational health nurse's role may 'fit in comfortably with Orem's self-care model.' But will Orem's model fit into the many facets of the occupational health nurse's role? That is the key question we should be asking" (p. 354).

The Health Belief Model

The second theory that focuses on the individual as the locus of change is the **health belief model (HBM).** The model evolved from the premise that the world of the perceiver determines action. The model had its inceptions during the late 1950s when America was breathing a collective sigh of relief after the development of the polio vaccine. Although a lifesaving vaccine finally came into existence, health professionals were stymied when some people chose not to bring themselves or their children into clinics for immunization. Social psychologists and other public health workers recognized the need to develop a more complete understanding of factors that influence preventive health behaviors. Their efforts resulted in the HBM.

Kurt Lewin's work lent itself to the model's core dimensions. He proposed that behavior is based on current dynamics confronting an individual rather than prior experiences (Maiman and Becker, 1974). Within this framework, diseases are regions of negative valence, which act to repel the individual. Figure 3-1 outlines the variables and relationships in the HBM. The model assumes that the major determinant of preventive health behavior is disease avoidance. Major concepts include perceived susceptibility to disease "X," perceived seriousness of disease "X," modifying factors, cues to action, perceived benefits minus perceived barriers to preventive health action, perceived threat of disease "X," and the likelihood of taking a recommended health action; the arrows specify the direction between concepts. Disease "X" represents a particular disorder that a health action may prevent. Importantly, actions that relate to breast cancer will be different from those relating to measles. For example, in breast cancer, a cue to action may involve a public service advertisement encouraging women to make an appointment for a mammogram. However, for measles, a cue to action may be news of a measles outbreak in a neighboring town.

Application of the Health Belief Model

Over the years, a number of authors have proposed broadening the scope of the HBM to address health promotion and illness behaviors (Kirscht, 1974; Pender, 1987) and to merge its concepts with other theories that describe health behavior (Cummings, Becker, and Malie, 1980). This conceptualization of health and health behaviors represented my first encounter with the power of theory-based practice. The following section contains a brief personal account of my perceptions addressing the strengths and limitations of the model.

My first class in nursing theory followed a format similar to many other courses throughout the country. Each week, students considered a new theoretical perspective. Faculty and classmates explored the theorist's background and the theory's assumptions, concepts, and relational statements and discussed the theory's application to nursing practice. Like many other students, I was experiencing mixed feelings about the class. Most of the content was intellectually interesting, but I found it difficult applying the concepts to patients in neighborhood clinics and those at home. Several weeks into the class, we reviewed the HBM. My interest was immediately piqued; the model captured a perspective on health that was different from any other framework or nursing theory. After the seminar, I went to the library and checked out *The Health Belief Model and Personal Health*

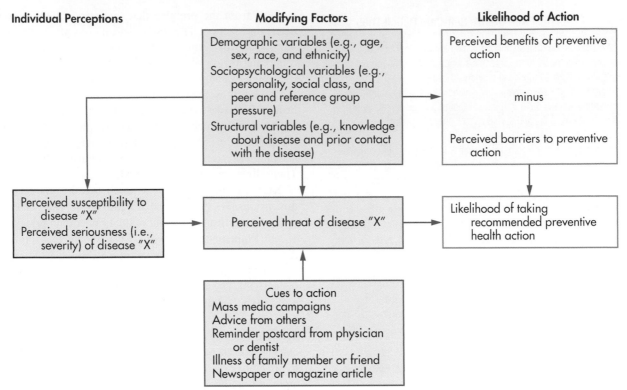

Individual Perceptions   **Modifying Factors**   **Likelihood of Action**

Demographic variables (e.g., age, sex, race, and ethnicity)
Sociopsychological variables (e.g., personality, social class, and peer and reference group pressure)
Structural variables (e.g., knowledge about disease and prior contact with the disease)

Perceived benefits of preventive action

minus

Perceived barriers to preventive action

Perceived susceptibility to disease "X"
Perceived seriousness (i.e., severity) of disease "X"

Perceived threat of disease "X"

Likelihood of taking recommended preventive health action

Cues to action
Mass media campaigns
Advice from others
Reminder postcard from physician or dentist
Illness of family member or friend
Newspaper or magazine article

FIGURE 3-1   Variables and relationships in the HBM. (Redrawn from Rosenstock IM: Historical origins of the health belief model. In Becker MH, editor: *The health belief model and personal health behavior,* Thorofare, NJ, 1974, Charles B. Slack).

Behavior by Marshall Becker (1974) and became absorbed in the book.

The model's focus on compliance was something that many nurses could relate to in their own clinical practice. For the first time, the HBM offered me some insight into patient behavior and helped me organize ideas about why people choose to disregard the instructions of well-intended nurses and doctors. I was intrigued by the way the model interpreted behaviors from the patient's perspective rather than the nurse's perspective. Concepts such as "perceived seriousness," "perceived susceptibility," and "cue to action" afforded new insights into the dynamics of health decision making. The HBM provided answers to problems that many nurses encountered in their everyday clinical practice.

I began to apply the model's concepts to guide my clinical work with some families in the community. One such family had never immunized their 18-month-old son. The father owned a health food store and shunned the use of anything deemed "unnatural." The family believed that childhood immunization for polio, tetanus, measles, and such belonged in the "unnatural" group. In my assessment, I concluded that the family failed to immunize the child because the parents did not perceive the susceptibility and seriousness of childhood illnesses; they belonged to a reference group that disdained most traditional medical practices and favored inaction over action. During the next few weeks, I mapped out a strategy that would focus on raising the parents' awareness of children's susceptibility to childhood illnesses by providing them with information about communicable diseases. During the next three visits, I inundated the family

with literature and pictures that graphically demonstrated the sequelae of diphtheria, polio, and pertussis. Eventually the parents took their son to an immunization clinic for his first shot.

Twenty years later, I still have mixed feelings about the means I used to drive this family's compliance to the accepted standard of pediatric health care. For the most part, the family's actions were not based on any true insight into the risks and benefits of childhood immunization; they wanted to please me and avoid further criticism. My training in community health nursing provided me with a very real understanding of the risks incurred when children are not protected against communicable diseases. It is also important to understand that infectious disease prevention is only effective at the population level if the decision to immunize originates within a collective understanding of families within the community. Nurses can be most effective when they work within schools, industries, and civic organizations to provide education and a supportive environment that promotes healthy choices. ■

In the years since this experience, I have become more skilled in assessing and labeling patient problems and have gained a better appreciation for the strengths and limitations that any theoretical framework imposes on a situation.

Limitations of the Health Belief Model

The HBM places the burden of action exclusively on the client. It assumes that only those clients who have distorted or negative perceptions of the specified disease or recommended health action will fail to act. In practice, this model focuses the nurse's energies on interventions designed to modify the client's distorted perceptions.

True to its historical roots, the model offers an explanation of health behaviors that is similar to a mechanical system. Consulting the HBM, a nurse may induce compliance by using model variables as catalysts to stimulate action. For example, an intervention study based on HBM precepts sought to increase follow-up in hypertensive clients by increasing their perceived susceptibility and seriousness to the dangers of hypertension (Jones, Jones, and Katz, 1987). In addition, the study provided patients with education over the telephone or in the emergency department, which was designed to increase their perception of the benefits of follow-up. According to the authors, the interventions resulted in a dramatic increase in compliance. However, they noted that several patient groups failed to respond to the intervention. In particular, a small group of patients without available child care failed to comply. Studies such as these, which have been conducted by behavioral researchers for more than 25 years, demonstrate the predictive abilities and the limitations of HBM concepts (Lajunen and Rasanen, 2004; Mirotznik et al., 1998).

The HBM may effectively promote behavior change by altering patients' perspectives, but it does not acknowledge the health professional's responsibility to reduce or ameliorate health care barriers. The model reflects the type of theoretical perspective that dominated nursing education and behavioral health for many years. The narrow scope of the model is its strength and its limitation: The nurse is not challenged to examine to the root causes of health opportunities and behaviors in the communities we serve.

The Upstream View: Society Is the Locus of Change

Milio's Framework for Prevention

Milio's framework for prevention (1976) provides a thought-provoking complement to the HBM and provides a mechanism for directing attention upstream and examining opportunities for nursing intervention at the population level. Milio outlined six propositions that relate an individual's ability to improve healthful behavior to a society's ability to provide accessible and socially affirming options for healthy choices. Milio used these propositions to move the focus of attention upstream. She conceded that the range of available health choices is critical in shaping a society's overall health status. In addition, she stated that policy decisions in governmental and private organizations shape the range of choices available to individuals. She believed that national-level policy making was the best way to favorably impact the health of most Americans rather than concentrating efforts on imparting information to change individual patterns of behavior.

Milio (1976) proposed that health deficits often result from an imbalance between a population's health needs and its health-sustaining resources. She stated that the diseases associated with excess (i.e., obesity and alcoholism) afflict affluent societies, and the diseases that result from inadequate or unsafe food, shelter, and water afflict the poor. Within this context, the poor in affluent societies may experience the least

Box 3-3 Set of Propositions Proposed by Milio

➤ "The health status of populations is the result of deprivation and/or excess of critical health-sustaining resources."

➤ "Behavior patterns of populations are a result of habitual selection from limited choices and these habits of choice are related to: (a) actual and perceived options available; (b) beliefs and expectations developed and refined over time by socialization, formal learning, and immediate experience."

➤ "Organizational behavior (decisions or policy-choices made by governmental/nongovernmental, national/non-national; not-profit/for-profit, formal/non-formal organizations) sets the range of options available to individuals for their personal choice-making."

➤ "The choice-making of individuals at a given point in time concerning potentially health-promoting or health-damaging selections is affected by their effort to maximize valued resources."

➤ "Social change may be thought of as changes in patterns of behavior resulting from shifts in the choice-making of significant numbers of people within a population."

➤ "Health education, as the process of teaching and learning health-supporting information, can have little significantly extensive impact on behavior patterns, that is, on personal choice-making of groups of people, without the easy availability of new, or newly-perceived alternative health-promoting options for investing personal resources."

From Milio N: A framework for prevention: changing health-damaging to health-generating life patterns, *Am J Public Health* 66:435-439, 1976.

desirable combination of factors. Milio (1976) cited the socioeconomic realities that deprive many Americans of a health-sustaining environment despite the fact that "cigarettes, sucrose, pollutants, and tensions are readily available to the poor" (p. 436). Propositions proposed by Milio are listed in Box 3-3.

Personal and societal resources affect the range of health-promoting or health-damaging choices available to individuals. Personal resources include the individual's awareness, knowledge, beliefs, and the beliefs of the individual's family and friends. Money, time, and the urgency of other priorities are also personal resources. Community and national locale strongly influence societal resources. These resources include the availability and cost of health services, environmental protection, safe shelter, and the penalties or rewards for failure to select the given options.

Milio (1976) challenged health education's assumption that knowledge of health-generating behaviors implies an act in accordance with that knowledge. She cited the lifestyles of health professionals to support her argument. She proposed that "most human beings, professional or nonprofessional, provider or consumer, make the easiest choices available to them most of the time" (p. 435). Health-promoting choices must be more readily available and less costly than health-damaging options for individuals to gain health and for society to improve health status. Milio's framework can enable a nurse to reframe this view by understanding the historic play of social forces that have limited the choices available to the parties involved.

Comparison of the Health Belief Model and Milio's Conceptualizations of Health

Milio's health resources bear some resemblance to the concepts in the HBM. The purpose of the HBM is to provide the nurse with an understanding of the dynamics of personal health behaviors. The HBM specifies broader contextual variables, such as the constraints of the health care system, and their influence on the individual's decision-making processes. In contrast, Milio based her framework on an assessment of community resources and their availability to individuals. This differs from the HBM, which may assume that each person has unlimited access to health resources and free will. By assessing such factors up front, the nurse is able to gain a more thorough understanding of the resources people actually have. Milio offered a different set of insights into the health behavior arena by proposing that many low-income individuals are acting within the constraints of their limited resources. Furthermore, she investigated beyond downstream focus and population health by examining the choices of significant numbers of people within a population.

Compared to the HBM, Milio's framework provides for the inclusion of economic, political, and environmental health determinants; therefore, the nurse is given broader range in the diagnosis and interpretation of health problems. Whereas the HBM allows only two possible outcomes (i.e., "acts" or "fails to act" according to the recommended health action), Milio's framework encourages the nurse to understand health behaviors in the context of their societal milieu.

Implications of Milio's Framework for Current Health Delivery Systems

Through its broader scope, Milio's model provides direction for nursing interventions at many levels. Nurses may use this model to assess the personal and societal resources of individual patients and analyze social and economic factors that may inhibit healthy choices in populations. Population-based interventions may include such diverse activities as working to improve the nutritional content of school lunches and encouraging political activity on behalf of health care reform (Hobbs et al., 2004; Milio, 2001).

Overall, current health care delivery systems perform best when responding to people with diagnostic-intensive and acute illnesses. Those people who experience chronic debilitation or have less intriguing diagnoses generally fare worse in the health care system despite efforts by community- and home-based care to "fill the gaps." Nurses in both hospital and community-based systems often feel constrained by profound financial and service restrictions imposed by third-party payers. These third parties often terminate nursing care after the resolution of the latest immediate health crisis and fail to cover care aimed toward long-term health improvements. Many health systems use nursing standards and reimbursement mechanisms that originate from a narrow, compartmentalized view of health; therefore it is imperative to practice nursing from a broader understanding of health, illness, and suffering.

Nursing and health service literature often focus on health care access issues. This topic is interesting because tremendous access disparities exist between insured and uninsured people in the United States. Access to care is associated with economic, social, and political factors, and, depending on individual and population needs, it can be a primary determinant of health status and survival. Structural variables, such as race-ethnicity, educational status, gender, and income, may be highly predictive of health status. These types of factors, which are also strongly grounded in the sociopolitical and economic milieu, identify risk factors for poor health and opportunities for community-based interventions.

> Personal behavior patterns are not simply "free" choices about "lifestyle" that are isolated from their personal and economic context. Lifestyles are patterns of choices made from available alternatives according to people's socioeconomic circumstances and how easily they are able to choose some over others (Milio, 1981). ■

Critical Social Theory

Milio used societal awareness to aid in the understanding of health behaviors. Similarly, **critical social theory** uses societal awareness to expose social inequalities that keep people from reaching their full potential. This theoretical approach is devised from the belief that social meanings structure life through social domination. Proponents of this theoretical approach maintain that social exchanges that are not distorted from power imbalances will stimulate the evolution of a more just society (Allen, Diekelmann, and Benner, 1986). Critical theory assumes that truth standards are socially determined and that no form of scientific inquiry is value free. Allen and colleagues (1986) stated, "One cannot separate theory and value, as the empiricist claims. Every theory is penetrated by value interests" (p. 34).

Application of Critical Social Theory

Application of critical social theory uses the processes of inductive reasoning. Rather than superimposing concepts onto a situation, the nurse discovers relevant concepts through an ongoing process of data collection and analysis. Sources of data may include interviews with critical informants, news articles, and transcripts of governmental proceedings. For example, if the domain of interest involves child care options for employees of a large microcomputer manufacturer, data sources may initially include the age and gender distribution of the workers, a review of worksite policies on parental leave, and interviews with both workers and administrative officials. Further into the analysis, the nurse may choose to incorporate additional sources of data, such as interviews with shift workers that address the difficulties in accessing evening and nighttime child care or statistics on job turnover among child care workers.

The methodological approaches adopted in critical social theory may also differ from those suggested by other nursing theories. The theory does not mandate a specific method of analysis. It chooses methods that are congruent with the focus of study. The dialectic can be a methodological tool; the

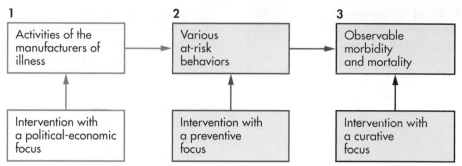

FIGURE 3-2   Continuum of health behaviors and corresponding intervention foci. (From McKinlay JB: A case for refocusing upstream: the political economy of illness. In *Proceedings of an American Heart Association Conference: applying behavioral science to cardiovascular risk,* Seattle, June 17-19, 1979. Reproduced with permission. Copyright © American Heart Association).

investigator seeks understanding by examining contradictions within the phenomenon of interest. In this context, the nurse may examine how the concepts of power and empowerment influence access to quality child care (Kuokkanen and Leino-Kilpi, 2000). The nurse may contrast an organization's policies with interviews from workers who believe the organization is an impediment to achieving quality child care. Data analysis may also include an examination of the interests of workers and administration in promoting social change versus maintaining the status quo.

Wild (1993) used critical social theory to analyze the social, political, and economic conditions associated with the cost of prescription analgesics and the corresponding financial burden of clients who require these medications. Wild compared the trends in pharmaceutical pricing with the inflation rates of other commodities. The study stated that pharmaceutical sales techniques, which market directly to physicians, distance the needs of ill clients from the pharmaceutical industry. A critique of this issue from a client perspective revealed limited access to information addressing the extreme variations in cost among different analgesics (e.g., greater than a tenfold difference in cost among similar drug formulations). Wild's analysis specified nursing actions that a downstream analysis would not consider, such as challenging pricing policies on behalf of client groups.

Challenging Assumptions About Preventive Health Through Critical Social Theory

The HBM and Milio's prevention model focus on personal health behaviors from a disease avoidance or preventive health perspective; nurses may also analyze this phenomenon using critical social theory. Again, McKinlay's upstream analogy refers to health workers who were so busy fishing sick people out of the river that they did not look upstream to see who was pushing the sick into the water. Later in the same article, McKinlay (1979) used his upstream analogy to ask the rhetorical question, "How preventive is prevention?" (p. 22). He used this tactic to critically examine different intervention strategies aimed at enhancing preventive behavior. Figure 3-2 illustrates McKinlay's model, which contrasts the different modes of prevention. He linked health professionals' curative and lifestyle modification interventions to a downstream conceptualization of health; the majority of alleged preventive

actions fail to alter the process of illness at its origin. Political-economic interventions remain the most effective way to address population determinants of health and ameliorate illness at its source.

McKinlay (1979) further delineated the activities of the "manufacturers of illness—those individuals, interest groups, and organizations which, in addition to producing material goods and services, also produce, as an inevitable byproduct, widespread morbidity and mortality" (pp. 9-10). The manufacturers of illness embed desired behaviors in the dominant cultural norm and thus foster the habituation of high-risk behavior in the population. Unhealthy consumption patterns are integrated into everyday lives; for example, the American holiday dinner table offers concrete examples of "the binding of at-riskness to culture" (p. 12). The existing health care system devotes its efforts in a misguided attempt to change the products of the illness manufacturers and neglects the processes that create the products.

Waitzkin (1983) continued this theme by asserting that the health care system's emphasis on lifestyle diverts attention from important sources of illness in the capitalist industrial environment and "it also puts the burden of health squarely on the individual rather than seeking collective solutions to health problems" (p. 664). Salmon (1987) supported this position by noting that the basic tenets of Western medicine promote an understanding of individual health and illness factors and obscure the exploration of their social and economic roots. He stated that critical social theory "can aid in uncovering larger dimensions impacting health that are usually unseen or misrepresented by ideological biases. Thus the social reality of health conditions can be both understood and changed" (p. 75).

Nurses in all practice settings face the challenge of understanding and responding to collective health within the context of a health system that allocates resources at the individual level. The Tavistock Group (1999) released a set of ethical principles that summarizes this juxtaposition by noting that "the care of individuals is at the center of health care delivery, but must be viewed and practiced within the overall context of continuing work to generate the greatest possible health gains for groups and populations" (pp. 2-3). This perspective is an accurate reflection of Western-oriented thought, which generally gives individual health precedence

Social Injustice in Community-Based Practice

Chafey (1996) refers to "putting justice to work in community-based practice" and notes that nursing has a rich historic legacy in social justice activities Although social justice activities are alive and well in nursing practice, many leaders think that the continuing struggle for resources is taking its toll on the scope of social action within community health systems. In addition, the policies of the current federal administration often emphasize market justice values over social justice values. Market justice refers to the principle that people are entitled to valued ends (e.g., status, income) when they acquire them through fair rules of entitlement. In contrast, social justice refers to the principle that all citizens bear equitably in the benefits and burdens of society (Drevdahl et al., 2001). These are complex concepts and cannot be easily distilled into a clear set of rules or nursing policies. However, in the context of community health nursing, health (and consequently health care) is considered a right rather than a privilege. To the extent that certain citizens, by virtue of their income, race, health needs, or any other attribute, are unable to access health care, our society as a whole suffers. Nurses are well positioned to "stand on the shoulders" of yesterday's nursing leaders and act on behalf of justice in health care access for all citizens.

over collective health. Although nurses can appreciate the concept of individual care at the center of health delivery, they should also consider transposing this principle. This allows the nurse to consider a health care system that places the community in the center of health care and holds the goal of generating health gains for individuals. Fortunately, these worldviews of health delivery systems are not mutually exclusive and nurses can understand the duality of health care needs in individuals and populations.

HEALTHY PEOPLE 2010

The *Healthy People 2010* documents provide health professionals with a broad mandate to save lives by thinking and acting strategically. Within the nursing profession, theories, models, and frameworks empower nurses to think and act strategically. The *Healthy People 2010* documents are classified into 28 focal areas that address specific diseases (e.g., diabetes, cancer, chronic kidney disease), care systems (e.g., health care access), and cross-cutting issues in public health (e.g., persons with disabilities, family planning). As opposed to many other chapters in this book, this chapter addresses all the focal areas rather than one or two of them. Each of the focal areas specified by the Centers for Disease Control and Prevention and in the *Healthy People 2010* documents encompasses a complex and multifaceted problem, one that can only be addressed by "looking upstream." By thinking about the root causes of health problems, we begin to understand the importance of directing nursing efforts toward the antecedents of poor health and lost opportunities. There is simply no other way to bring positive changes to the more than 290 million U.S. and 6 billion global citizens that inhabit our planet.

The following photos present environmental health issues and efforts being taken by nurses to address them.

SUMMARY

Community health nurses have been instrumental in making many of the lifesaving advances in sanitation, communicable disease, and environmental conditions that today's society takes for granted. Community health practice helps develop a broad context of nursing practice because community environments are inherently less restrictive than hospital settings. Clarke and Cody (1994) compared the environmental characteristics in community-based settings to those in hospital-based settings. They proposed that the dynamic nature of community settings lends itself best to the education of professional nurses (Clarke and Cody, 1994).

In a discussion addressing the future of community health nursing, Bellack (1998) differentiates between "nursing in the community" and "nursing with the community." This subtle reframing of the nursing role reinforces the notion that the health agenda originates from natural leaders, church members, local officials, parents, children, teens, and other community members. Forming and advancing a shared vision of health can be a formidable challenge for the nurse; like any other complex issue, multiple viewpoints are the norm. Even "naming" health problems can be difficult, because different constituents are likely to see issues differently and pursue different lines of reasoning. However, allowing the genesis of change to occur from within the community is the essential challenge of nursing "with" the community. "Nursing with the community" efforts allow the nurse to create agendas that arise from community members rather than those imposed upon community members. Listening, being patient, providing accurate and scientifically sound information, and respecting the experiences of community members are essential to the success of these efforts.

The nursing profession has advanced and with it so has the need to develop nursing theories that formalize the scientific base of community health nursing. The richness of community health nursing comes from the challenge of conceptualizing and implementing strategies that will enhance the health of many people. Likewise, nurses in this practice area must have access to theoretical perspectives that address the social, political, and environmental determinants of population health. The integration of population-based theory and practice gives nurses the means to favorably impact the health of the global community.

LEARNING ACTIVITIES

1. Select a theory or conceptual model. Evaluate its potential for understanding health in individuals, families, a population of 400 children in an elementary school, a community of 50,000 residents, and 2000 workers within a corporate setting.
2. Identify one health problem (e.g., substance abuse, domestic violence, or cardiovascular disease) that is prevalent in the community or city. Analyze the problem using two different theories or conceptual models. One should emphasize individual determinants of health and another should emphasize population determinants of health.

Open mine waste in the rural West can pose continuing threat to local citizens. Nurses have been involved in advocacy efforts to ensure that citizens receive periodic screening for exposure to lead. Nurses can be active in policy efforts to prevent environmental disasters in the future.

A public health nurse inspects the site of an asphalt spill off of a rural railway car. Hazardous materials spills often occur in remote areas away from health care services. Broad conceptual frameworks allow nurses to think upstream and incorporate environmental risks into the consideration of community health issues.

Citizens can be unaware of biologic and chemical contaminants in their drinking water. Nurses are playing more active roles in water testing and in communicating the results of such test to community members. When health is conceptualized broadly, nurses understand and view risk in new ways.

A public health nurse teaches a class on environmental health for local nurses. Environmental health is an important part of community health nursing's expanding practice.

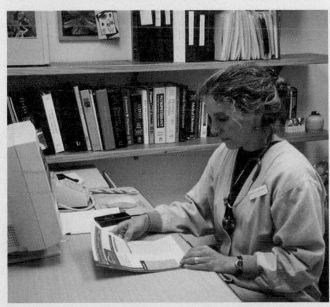

A nurse practitioner reviews educational materials addressing occupational and environmental health risks. By providing guidance for her clients, she is working to reduce risks and empowering her clients to act to reduce their personal and community-based risks.

What are some differences in the way these different perspectives inform nursing practice?

3. Review the American Nurses Association's definition of community health nursing practice and the American Public Health Association's definition of public health nursing practice. What do these definitions indicate about the theoretical basis of community health nursing? How does the theoretical basis of community health nursing practice differ from that of other nursing specialty areas?

REFERENCES

Allen DG, Diekelmann N, Benner P: Three paradigms for nursing research: methodologic implications. In Chinn P, editor: *Nursing research methodology: issues and implementation,* Rockville, Md, 1986, Aspen Publishers.

American Public Health Association, Public Health Nursing Section: *Quad council PHN competencies,* The Author, http://www.csu-chico.edu/~horst/about/competencies.html.

Barnum BJS: *Nursing theory: analysis, application, evaluation,* Glenview, Ill, 1990, Scott, Foresman/Little, Brown Higher Education.

Batra C: Professional issues: the future of community health nursing. In Cookfair JM, editor: *Nursing process and practice in the community,* St. Louis, 1991, Mosby.

Becker MH, editor: *The health belief model and personal health behavior,* Thorofare, NJ, 1974, Charles B. Slack.

Bellack JP: Community-based nursing practice: necessary but not sufficient, *J Nurs Educ* 37(3):99-100, 1998 (guest editorial).

Centers for Disease Control and Prevention, National Center for Chronic Disease Prevention and Health Promotion: Chronic disease prevention, 2004, The Author, http://www.cdc.gov/nccdphp/power_prevention/pop_epidemic.htm.

Chafey K: Caring is not enough: ethical paradigms for community-based care, *N HC Perspect Community* 17(1):10-15, 1996.

Chinn PL, Kramer MK: *Theory and nursing: integrated knowledge development,* ed 5, St. Louis, 1999, Mosby.

Clarke PN, Cody WK: Nursing theory-based practice in the home and community: the crux of professional nursing education, *Adv Nurs Sci* 17(2):41-53, 1994.

Cummings KM, Becker MH, Malie MC: Bringing the models together: an empirical approach to combining variables to explain health actions, *J Behav Med* 3:123-145, 1980.

Dickoff J, James P: A theory of theories: a position paper, *Nurs Res* 17:197-203, 1968.

Doty RE: Alternative theoretical perspectives: essential knowledge for the advanced practice nurse in the promotion of rural family health, *Clin Nurs Specialist* 10(5):217-219, 1996.

Dreher MC: The conflict of conservatism in public health nursing education, *Nurs Outlook* 30(9):504-509, 1982.

Drevdahl D, Kneipp SM, Canales MK, Dorcy KS: Reinvesting in social justice: a capital idea for public health nursing? *ANS Adv Nurs Sci* 24(2):19-31, 2001.

Eben JD et al: Self-care deficit theory of nursing. In Marriner A, editor: *Nursing theorists and their work,* St. Louis, 1986, Mosby.

Fawcett J: The nurse theorists: 21st-century updates—Dorothea E. Orem, *Nurs Sci Q* 14(1):34-38, 2001.

Hobbs SH, Ricketts TC, Dodds JM, Milio N: Analysis of interest group influence on federal school meals regulations 1992 to 1996, *J Nutr Educ Behav* 36(2):90-98, 2004.

Jones PK, Jones SL, Katz J: Improving follow-up among hypertensive patients using a health belief model intervention, *Arch Intern Med* 147:1557-1560, 1987.

Kennedy A: How relevant are nursing models? *Occup Health* 41(12):352-354, 1989.

Kirscht JP: The health belief model and illness behavior. In Becker MH, editor: *The health belief model and personal health behavior,* Thorofare, NJ, 1974, Charles B. Slack.

Kuokkanen L, Leino-Kilpi H: Power and empowerment in nursing: three theoretical approaches. *J Adv Nurs* 31(1):235-241, 2000.

Lajunen T, Rasanen M; Can social psychological models be used to promote bicycle helmet use among teenagers? A comparison of the health belief model, theory of planned behavior and the locus of control, *J Safety Res* 35(1):115-123, 2004.

Maiman LA, Becker MH: The health belief model: origins and correlates in psychological theory. In Becker MH, editor: *The health belief model and personal health behavior,* Thorofare, NJ, 1974, Charles B. Slack.

McKinlay JB: A case for refocusing upstream: the political economy of illness. In *Proceedings of an American Heart Association Conference: applying behavioral science to cardiovascular risk,* Seattle, June 17-19, 1979.

Milio N: A framework for prevention: changing health-damaging to health-generating life patterns, *Am J Public Health* 66:435-439, 1976.

Milio N: *Promoting health through public policy,* Philadelphia, 1981, FA Davis.

Mirotznik J, Ginzler E, Zagon G, Baptiste A: Using the health belief model to explain clinic appointment-keeping for the management of a chronic disease condition, *J Community Health* 23(3):195-210, 1998.

Orem DE: *Nursing: Concepts of practice,* ed 6, New York, 2001, Mosby.

Pender NJ: *Health promotion in nursing practice,* ed 2, Norwalk, Conn, 1987, Appleton-Century-Crofts.

Pryjmachuk S: A nursing perspective on the interrelationship between theory, research, and practice, *J Adv Nurs* 23:679-684, 1996.

Rosenstock IM: Historical origins of the health belief model. In Becker MH, editor: *The health belief model and personal health behavior,* Thorofare, NJ, 1974, Charles B. Slack.

Salmon JW: Dilemmas in studying social change versus individual change: considerations from political economy. In Duffy M, Pender NJ, editors: *Conceptual issues in health promotion: a report of proceedings of a Wingspread Conference,* Indianapolis, Ind, 1987, Sigma Theta Tau.

Schwartz-Barcott D, Patterson BJ, Lusardi P, Farmer BC: From practice to theory: tightening the link via three fieldwork strategies, *J Adv Nurs* 39(3):281-289, 2002.

Tavistock Group: A shared statement of ethical principles for those who shape and give health care: a working draft from the Tavistock Group, *Image J Nurs Sch* 31:2-3, 1999.

Torres G: *Theoretical foundations of nursing,* Norwalk, Conn, 1986, Appleton-Century-Crofts.

Waitzkin H: A Marxist view of health and health care. In Mechanic D, editor: *Handbook of health, health care, and the health professions,* New York, 1983, Free Press.

Wild LR: Caveat emptor: a critical analysis of the costs of drugs used for pain management, *Adv Nurs Sci* 16:52-61, 1993.

Woods NF, Catanzaro M: *Nursing research: theory and practice,* St. Louis, 1988, Mosby.

UNIT 2

The Art and Science of Community Health Nursing

4

Epidemiology

Holly Cassells

MEDIA RESOURCES

Additional Material for Study, Review, and Further Exploration

evolve Website at http://evolve.elsevier.com/Nies

❖ Quiz ❖ Case Studies ❖ Content Updates ❖ Glossary ❖ WebLinks

OBJECTIVES

Upon completion of this chapter, the reader will be able to do the following:

1. Identify epidemiological models used to explain disease and health patterns in populations.
2. Use epidemiological methods to describe the state of health in a community or aggregate.
3. Calculate epidemiological rates in order to characterize population health.
4. Understand the use of epidemiological methods in primary, secondary, and tertiary prevention.
5. Evaluate epidemiological study designs for researching health problems.

KEY TERMS

age-adjustment of rates
age-specific rates
analytic epidemiology
attack rate
cause and effect relationship
crude rates

descriptive epidemiology
ecosocial epidemiology
epidemiological triangle
epidemiology
incidence rates
morbidity rates

mortality rates
natural history of disease
person-place-time model
prevalence rate
proportionate mortality ratio
rates

risk
risk factor
screening programs
standardization of rates
surveillance
web of causation

CHAPTER OUTLINE

USE OF EPIDEMIOLOGY IN DISEASE CONTROL AND PREVENTION

CALCULATION OF RATES
    Morbidity: Incidence and Prevalence Rates
    Other Rates

CONCEPT OF RISK

USE OF EPIDEMIOLOGY IN DISEASE PREVENTION
    Primary Prevention
    Secondary and Tertiary Prevention

    Establishing Causality
    Screening
    Surveillance

USE OF EPIDEMIOLOGY IN HEALTH SERVICES

EPIDEMIOLOGICAL METHODS
    Descriptive Epidemiology
    Analytic Epidemiology

Epidemiology is the study of the distribution and determinants of health and disease in human populations (Harkness, 1995) and is the principal science of community health practice. It entails a body of knowledge derived from epidemiological research and specialized epidemiological methods and approaches to scientific research. Community health nurses use epidemiological concepts to improve the health of population groups by identifying risk factors and optimal approaches that reduce disease risk. Epidemiological methods are important for accurate community assessment

BOX 4-1   Person-Place-Time Model

Person: "Who" factors, such as demographic characteristics, health, and disease status.
Place: "Where" factors, such as geographical location, climate and environmental conditions, and political and social environment.
Time: "When" factors, such as time of day, week, or month and secular trends over months and years.

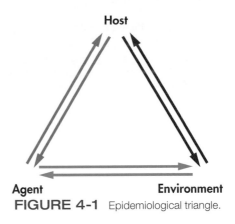

FIGURE 4-1   Epidemiological triangle.

and diagnosis, and in planning and evaluating effective community interventions. This chapter discusses the uses of epidemiology and its specialized methodologies.

USE OF EPIDEMIOLOGY IN DISEASE CONTROL AND PREVENTION

Although epidemiology originated in ancient times, formal epidemiological techniques developed in the nineteenth century. Early applications focused on identifying factors associated with infectious diseases and the epidemic spread of disease in the community. Public health practitioners hoped to improve preventive strategies by identifying critical factors in disease development.

Specifically, investigators attempted to identify characteristics of people who suffered from a disease such as cholera or plague and compare them with characteristics of those who remained healthy. These differences might include a broad range of personal factors such as age, socioeconomic status, and health status. Investigators also questioned whether there were differences in the location or living environment of ill people, compared with healthy individuals, and whether these factors influenced disease development. Finally, researchers examined whether common time factors existed (i.e., when people acquired disease). Use of this **person-place-time model** organized epidemiologists' investigations of the disease pattern in the community (Box 4-1). This study of the amount and distribution of disease constitutes **descriptive epidemiology.** Identified patterns frequently indicate possible causes of disease that epidemiologists can examine with more advanced epidemiological methods.

In addition to investigating the person, place, and time factors related to disease, epidemiologists examine complex relationships among the many determinants of disease. This investigation of the causes of disease, or etiology, is called analytic epidemiology.

Even before the identification of bacterial agents, public health practitioners recognized that single factors were insufficient to cause disease. For example, while exploring the cholera epidemics in London in 1855, Dr. John Snow collected data about social and physical environmental conditions that might favor disease development. He specifically examined the contamination of local water systems. Snow also gathered information about people who became ill; this included their living patterns, their water sources, their socioeconomic characteristics, and their health status. A comprehensive database helped him develop a theory about

the possible cause of the epidemic. Snow suspected that a single biological agent was responsible for the cholera infection, although the organism, *Vibrio cholerae,* was undiscovered. He compared the death rates among individuals using one source of water with those among people using a different water source. This suggested an association between cholera and water quality.

The epidemiologist examines the interrelationships between host and environmental characteristics and uses an organized method of inquiry to derive an explanation of disease. This model of investigation is called the **epidemiological triangle** because the epidemiologist must analyze the following three elements: agent, host, and environment (Figure 4-1). The development of disease is dependent upon the extent of the host's exposure to an agent, the strength or virulence of the agent, and the host's genetic or immunological susceptibility. Disease is also dependent upon the environmental conditions existing at the time of exposure, which include the biological, social, political, and physical environment (Table 4-1). The model implies that the rate of disease will change when the balance among these three factors is altered. By examining each of the three elements, a community health nurse can methodically assess a health problem, determine protective factors, and evaluate the factors that make the host vulnerable to disease.

Conditions linked to clearly identifiable agents such as bacteria, chemicals, toxins, and other exposure factors are readily explained by the epidemiological triangle. However, other models that stress the multiplicity of host and environmental interactions have developed, and understanding of disease has progressed. The "wheel model" is an example of such a model (Figure 4-2). The wheel consists of a hub that represents the host and its human characteristics such as genetic makeup, personality, and immunity. The surrounding wheel represents the environment and comprises biological, social, and physical dimensions. The relative size of each component in the wheel depends on the health problem. A relatively large genetic core represents health conditions associated with heredity. Origins of other health conditions may be more dependent upon environmental factors (Mausner and Kramer, 1985). This model subscribes to multiple-causation rather than single-causation disease theory; therefore it is more useful for analyzing complex

TABLE 4-1   A Classification of Agent, Host, and Environmental Factors That Determine the Occurrence of Diseases in Human Populations

AGENTS OF DISEASE—ETIOLOGICAL FACTORS	EXAMPLES
A. Nutritive elements	
Excesses	Cholesterol
Deficiencies	Vitamins, proteins
B. Chemical agents	
Poisons	Carbon monoxide, carbon tetrachloride, drugs
Allergens	Ragweed, poison ivy, medications
C. Physical agents	Ionizing radiation, mechanical
D. Infectious agents	
Metazoa	Hookworm, schistosomiasis, onchocerciasis
Protozoa	Amoebae, malaria
Bacteria	Rheumatic fever, lobar pneumonia, typhoid, TB, syphilis
Fungi	Histoplasmosis, athlete's foot
Rickettsia	Rocky Mountain spotted fever, typhus, Lyme disease
Viruses	Measles, mumps, chickenpox, smallpox, poliomyelitis, rabies, yellow fever, human immunodeficiency virus

HOST FACTORS (i.e., INTRINSIC FACTORS)—INFLUENCE EXPOSURE, SUSCEPTIBILITY, OR RESPONSE TO AGENT	EXAMPLE
A. Genetic	Cystic fibrosis, Huntington's disease
B. Age	Alzheimer's disease
C. Sex	Rheumatoid arthritis
D. Ethnic group	Tay-Sachs disease, sickle cell disease
E. Physiological state	Fatigue, pregnancy, puberty, stress, nutritional state
F. Prior immunological experience	Hypersensitivity, protection
Active	Prior infection, immunization
Passive	Maternal antibodies, gamma globulin prophylaxis
G. Intercurrent or preexisting disease	
H. Human behavior	Personal hygiene, food handling, diet, interpersonal contact, occupation, recreation, use of health resources, tobacco use

ENVIRONMENTAL FACTORS (i.e., EXTRINSIC FACTORS)—INFLUENCE EXISTENCE OF THE AGENT, EXPOSURE, OR SUSCEPTIBILITY TO AGENT	EXAMPLES
A. Physical environment	Geology, climate
B. Biological environment	
Human populations	Density
Flora	Sources of food, influence on vertebrates and arthropods, as a source of agents
Fauna	Food sources, vertebrate hosts, arthropod vectors
C. Socioeconomic environment	
Occupation	Exposure to chemical agents
Urbanization and economic development	Urban crowding, tension and pressures, cooperative efforts in health and education
Disruption	Wars, floods

Modified from Lilienfeld DE, Stoley PD: *Foundations of epidemiology*, New York, 1994, Oxford University Press.

chronic conditions and identifying factors that are amenable to intervention.

Example of the Epidemiological Approach

An early example of the epidemiological approach is John Snow's investigation of a cholera epidemic in the 1850s. He analyzed the distribution of person, place, and time factors by comparing the death rates among people living in different geographical sectors of London.

Snow noted that people using a particular water pump had significantly higher mortality rates resulting from cholera than people using other water sources in the city. Although the cholera organism was yet unidentified, the clustering of disease cases around one neighborhood pump suggested new prevention strategies to public health officials (i.e., that cholera might be reduced in a community by controlling contaminated drinking water sources) (Snow, 1936). ■

Following the discovery of the causative agents of many infectious diseases, public health interventions eventually resulted in a decline in widespread epidemic mortality, particularly in developed countries. This caused the focus of

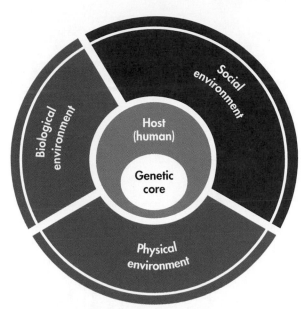

FIGURE 4-2 Wheel model of human-environment interaction. (Redrawn from Mausner JS, Kramer S: *Mausner and Bahn epidemiology: an introductory text,* ed 2, Philadelphia, 1985, WB Saunders.)

BOX 4-2 Coronary Heart Disease Risk Factors Supported by Epidemiological Data From the Framingham Study

➤ Age
➤ Gender (male)
➤ Current cigarette smoking
➤ Hypertension
➤ High LDL cholesterol
➤ Low HDL cholesterol
➤ (Diabetes)*

From Executive summary of the third report of the National Cholesterol Education Program (NCEP) expert panel on detection, evaluation, and treatment of high blood cholesterol in adults (adult treatment panel III), *JAMA* 285:2486-2497, 2001.
*Diabetes is not included in the Framingham Global Risk Score but is now considered to be a coronary heart disease risk equivalent, meaning that persons with diabetes will be treated as intensively as those with coronary heart disease.
LDL, Low-density lipoprotein; *HDL,* high-density lipoprotein.

---

public health to shift to chronic diseases such as cancer, coronary heart disease, and diabetes during the past few decades. These chronic diseases tend to have multiple interrelated factors associated with their development rather than a single causative agent.

In studying chronic diseases, epidemiologists use methods that are similar to those used in infectious disease investigation, thereby developing theories about chronic disease control. Risk factor identification is of particular importance to chronic disease reduction. Risk factors are variables that increase the rate of disease in people who have them (e.g., a genetic predisposition) or in people exposed to them (e.g., an infectious agent or a diet high in saturated fat). Therefore their identification is critical to identifying specific prevention and intervention approaches that effectively and efficiently reduce chronic disease morbidity and mortality. For example, the identification of cardiovascular disease risk factors has suggested a number of lifestyle modifications that could reduce the morbidity risk before disease onset. Primary prevention strategies, such as dietary saturated fat reduction, smoking cessation, and hypertension control, were developed in response to previous epidemiological studies that identified these risk factors (Box 4-2). The **web of causation** model illustrates the complexity of relationships among causal variables for heart disease (Figure 4-3).

Recently a new paradigm, **ecosocial epidemiology,** challenges both the more individually focused risk factor approach to understanding disease origins and the growing interest in molecular epidemiology, exemplified by the sequencing of genes to determine individual susceptibility to various diseases (MacDonald, 2004). This ecological approach emphasizes the role of evolving macro-level socioenvironmental factors, including complex political and economic forces and microbiological processes, in under-

standing health and illness. Investigating the context of health will necessitate alternative research approaches, such as qualitative and ecological studies and studies of social institutions and processes. In turn, the examination of social and contextual origins will enlighten the interventions of public health practitioners. For example, Lorion (2001) analyzed pervasive community violence as a "contextual pathogen" that can migrate from community streets to the school setting. This context of violence is responsible for altering student and staff emotional and physical health, and for a continuing escalation of risk from small acts of hassling and threats leading to assault and homicide in the school setting. In addition to understanding the effects of exposure to violence on individuals, public health practitioners must examine violence as a larger contextual factor that, as Lorion describes, is "contagious, contaminating, and corrosive" to the community's health.

CALCULATION OF RATES

The community health nurse must analyze data about the health of the community to determine the pattern of disease in a community. The nurse may collect data by conducting surveys or compiling data from existing records (e.g., data from clinic facilities or vital statistics records). Assessment data often are in the form of counts or simple frequencies of events (e.g., the number of people with a specific health condition). Community health practitioners interpret these raw counts by transforming them into rates.

Rates are arithmetic expressions that help practitioners consider a count of an event relative to the size of the population from which it is extracted (e.g., the population at risk). Rates are population proportions or fractions in which the numerator is the number of events occurring in a specified period of time. The denominator consists of those in the population at the specified time period (e.g., per day, per week, or per year). This proportion is multiplied by a constant (k) that is a multiple of 10, such as 1000, 10,000, or 100,000. The constant usually converts the resultant number to a whole

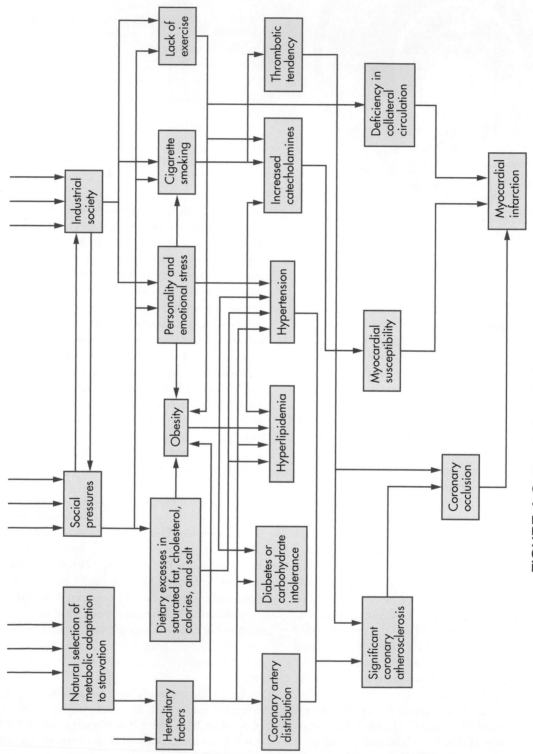

FIGURE 4-3 The web of causation for myocardial infarction: a current view. (From Friedman GD: *Primer of epidemiology*, ed 4, New York, 1994, McGraw-Hill.)

number, which is larger and easier to interpret. Thus, a rate can be the number of cases of a disease occurring for every 1000, 10,000 or 100,000 people in the population.

$$Rate = \frac{Numerator}{Denominator} =$$

$$\frac{Number\ of\ health\ events\ in\ a\ specified\ period}{Population\ in\ same\ area\ in\ same\ specified\ period} \times k$$

When raw counts are converted to rates, the community health nurse can make meaningful comparisons with rates from other districts or states, from the nation, and from previous time periods. These analyses assist the nurse in determining the magnitude of a public health problem in a given area and allow more reliable tracking of trends in the community over time (Box 4-3).

Sometimes a ratio is used to express a relationship between two variables. A ratio is obtained by dividing one quantity by another, and the numerator is not necessarily part of the denominator. For example, a ratio could contrast the number of male births to that of female births. Proportions can describe characteristics of a population. A proportion is often a percentage, and it represents the numerator as part of the denominator.

Morbidity: Incidence and Prevalence Rates

The two principal types of **morbidity rates,** or rates of illness, in public health are incidence rates and prevalence rates. **Incidence rates** describe the occurrence of new cases of a disease or condition (e.g., teen pregnancy) in a community over a period of time relative to the size of the population at risk for that disease or condition during that same time period. The denominator consists of only those at risk for the disease or condition; therefore, known cases or those not susceptible (e.g., those immunized against a disease) are subtracted from the total population (Table 4-2.)

$$Incidence\ rate = \frac{\begin{array}{c}Number\ of\ new\ cases\ or\ events \\ occurring\ in\ the\ population\ in\ a \\ specified\ period\end{array}}{\begin{array}{c}Population\ at\ risk\ during\ same \\ specified\ period\end{array}} \times k$$

The incidence rate may be the most sensitive indicator of the changing health of a community because it captures the fluctuations of disease in a population. Although incidence rates are valuable for monitoring trends in chronic disease, they are particularly useful for detecting short-term acute disease changes—such as those that occur with infectious hepatitis or measles—when the duration of the disease is typically short.

If a population is exposed to an infectious disease at a given time and place, the nurse may calculate the attack rate, a specialized form of the incidence rate. Attack rates document the number of new cases of a disease in those exposed to the disease. A common example of the application of the **attack rate** is food poisoning; the denominator is the number of people exposed to a suspect food, and the numerator is the number of people who were exposed and became ill. The nurse can calculate and compare the attack rates of illness among those exposed to specific foods to identify the critical food sources or exposure variables.

BOX 4-3 Using Rates in Everyday Community Health Nursing Practice

The following school situation exemplifies the value of rates:

A community health nurse screened 500 students for TB in Southside School and identified 15 students with newly positive tuberculin tests. The proportion of Southside School students affected was 15/500, or 0.03 (3%), or a rate of 30/1000 students at risk for TB. Concurrently, the nurse conducted screening in Northside School and again identified 15 positive tuberculin tests. However, this school was much larger than the Southside School and had 900 potentially at-risk students. To place the number of affected students in perspective relative to the size of the Northside School, the nurse calculated a proportion of 15/900, or 0.017 (1.7%), or a rate of 17/1000 students at risk.

On the basis of this comparison, the nurse concluded that although both schools had equal numbers of tuberculin conversions, Southside School had the greater rate of tuberculin test conversions. Based on this information, the nurse could then explore reasons for the difference in these rates.

TABLE 4-2 Examples of Rate Calculations

MORBIDITY RATES	CRUDE DEATH RATE
Incidence Rate	**Crude Rates**
$\dfrac{Number\ of\ new\ cases\ in\ given\ time\ period}{Population\ at\ risk\ in\ same\ time\ period} \times 1000 =$	$\dfrac{Number\ of\ deaths\ in\ year}{Total\ population\ size} \times 100,000$
$\dfrac{75}{4,000-250\ old\ cases} = .02$	$\dfrac{1720}{200,000} = .0086$
$.02 \times 1000 = 20$ per 1000 per time period	$.0086 \times 100,000 = 860$ per 100,000 per year
Prevalence Rate	**Crude Birth Rate**
$\dfrac{Number\ of\ existing\ cases}{Total\ Population} \times 1000 =$	$\dfrac{Number\ of\ births\ in\ year}{Total\ population\ size} \times 100,000$
$\dfrac{250}{4000} = .0625$	$\dfrac{2900}{200,000} = .0450$
$.0625 \times 1000 = 62.5$ per 1000	$.0145 \times 100,000 = 1450$ per 100,000 per year

A **prevalence rate** is the number of all cases of a specific disease or condition (e.g., deafness) in a population at a given point in time relative to the population at the same point in time.

$$Prevalence\ rate = \frac{Number\ of\ existing\ cases\ in\ population\ at\ a\ specified\ point\ in\ time}{Population\ at\ same\ specified\ point\ in\ time} \times k$$

When prevalence rates describe the number of people with the disease at a specific point in time, they are sometimes called point prevalences. For this reason, cross-sectional studies frequently use them. Period prevalences represent the number of existing cases during a specified period or interval of time and include old cases and new cases that develop within the same period of time.

The following factors influence prevalence rates: the number of people who experience a particular condition (i.e., incidence) and the duration of the condition. A nurse can derive the prevalence rate by multiplying incidence by duration ($P = I \times D$). An increase in the incidence rate or the duration of a disease increases the prevalence rate of a disease. With the advent of life-prolonging therapies (e.g., insulin for treatment of type 1 diabetes mellitus), the prevalence of a disease may increase without a change in the incidence rate. Those who survive a chronic disease without cure remain in the "prevalence pot" (Figure 4-4). For conditions such as cataracts, surgical removal permits many people to recover and thereby move out of the prevalence pot. Although the incidence has not necessarily changed, the reduced duration of the disease lowers the prevalence rate of cataracts in the population.

Morbidity rates are not available for many conditions because surveillance of many chronic diseases is not widely

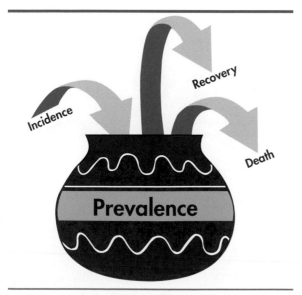

FIGURE 4-4 Prevalence pot: the relationship between incidence and prevalence. (Redrawn from Morton RF, Hebel JR, McCarter RJ: *A study guide to epidemiology and biostatistics,* ed 3, Gaithersburg, Md, 1990, Aspen Publishers.)

conducted. Furthermore, morbidity rates may be subject to underreporting when they are available. Routinely collected birth and death rates, or **mortality rates,** are more widely available. Table 4-2 provides examples of calculating selected rates.

Other Rates

Numerous other rates are useful in characterizing the health of a population. For example, **crude rates** summarize the occurrence of births (i.e., crude birth rate), mortality (i.e., crude death rates), or diseases (i.e., crude disease rates) in the general population. The numerator is the number of events, and the denominator is the average population size or the population size at midyear (i.e., usually July 1) multiplied by a constant.

The denominators of crude rates represent the total population and not the population at risk for a given event; therefore, these rates are subject to certain biases in interpretation. Crude death rates are sensitive to the number of people at the highest risk for dying. A relatively older population will probably produce a higher crude death rate than a population with a more evenly distributed age range. Conversely, a young population will have a somewhat lower crude death rate. Similar biases can occur for crude birth rates (e.g., higher birth rates in young populations). This distortion occurs because the denominator reflects the entire population and not exclusively the population at risk for giving birth. Age is one of the most common confounding factors that can mask the true distribution of variables. However, many variables, such as race and socioeconomic status, also can bias the interpretation of biostatistical data. Therefore, the nurse may use several approaches for removing the confounding effect of these variables on rates.

Age-specific rates characterize a particular age-group in the population and usually consider deaths and births. Determining the rate for specific subgroups of a population and using a denominator that reflects only that subgroup removes age bias.

$$Age\text{-}specific\ rate = \frac{Number\ of\ cases\ in\ a\ specific\ age\ category\ in\ population\ at\ a\ specified\ time}{Population\ in\ the\ same\ age\ category\ at\ the\ same\ specified\ time} \times k$$

To characterize a total population using age-specific rates, rates for each category must be computed because a single summary rate, such as a mean, is not used to characterize a total population using age-specific rates. Specific rates for other variables can be determined in a similar fashion (e.g., race-specific or gender-specific rates) (Table 4-3).

Age-adjustment or **standardization of rates** is another method of reducing bias when there is a difference between the age distributions of two populations. The nurse uses either the direct method or the indirect standardization method. The direct method selects a standard population, which is often the population distribution of the United States. This method essentially converts age-specific rates for age categories of the two populations to those of the standard population, and it calculates a summary age-adjusted rate for each of the two populations of interest. This enables the nurse to compare the two rates as if both had the standard population's age structure (i.e., without the prior problem of age distortion). Tables 4-4, 4-5, and 4-6 give examples of the computations.

The second method, indirect standardization, allows the nurse to compare two populations as though they possessed similar age distributions (i.e., it removes the effect of age). This is helpful especially when age-specific rates are unknown or, in direct adjustment, when the nurse must compare many strata. Indirect adjustment involves the calculation of a standardized mortality ratio (SMR), which is a single age-adjusted death ratio that compares the observed deaths with those that would be expected if the population of interest had the mortality experience of the standard population.

$$SMR = \frac{Total\ observed\ deaths}{Total\ expected\ deaths}$$

A ratio of 1 indicates that observed deaths and expected deaths were equal. A ratio greater than 1 indicates that more deaths occurred in the population of interest than expected, based on the standard population's rates. A ratio of less than 1 indicates that fewer deaths occurred in the population of interest than expected based on the standard population's rates. Standardized rations and rates adjusted using the direct method can be produced for other rates (e.g., birth or morbidity rates) and for other variables (e.g., income or birth weight).

The procedure for calculating a SMR is essentially the reverse of direct standardization (Tables 4-7 and 4-8). First, the nurse applies age-specific rates from a standard population to each age category of the two populations of interest to produce expected deaths for each stratum. The standard population may be the U.S. population, like direct adjustment, or it may be the larger or more stable of the two populations. Second, the nurse divides the actual number of observed deaths by the sum of expected deaths for each population to produce a SMR for each population. Note that age-adjusted rates are actually not "real" death rates; rather, they are representations of the experience of populations if their age distributions were similar to the standard population.

The **proportionate mortality ratio** (PMR) method also describes mortality. It represents the percentage of deaths resulting from a specific cause relative to deaths from all causes. It is often helpful in identifying areas in which public health programs might make significant contributions in reducing deaths. In some situations, a high PMR may reflect a low overall mortality or reduced number of deaths resulting from other causes. Therefore the PMR requires consideration in the context of the mortality experience of the population.

TABLE 4-3 Comparison of U.S. Mortality Rates—2003 (Preliminary)

DEATH RATE	RATE PER 100,000
Crude death rate	840.4
Age-adjusted death rate	831.2
Age-specific death rates	
Under 1 Year	710.1
1 to 4	31.1
5-14	16.8
15-24	80.2
25-34	102.2
35-44	199.3
45-54	430.3
55-64	937.3
65-74	2,253.5
75-84	5,460.1
85 and over	14,595.6

From Center for Disease Control and Prevention National Center for Health Statistics: Hyattsville-Deaths: Preliminary data for 2003, Nat Vital Stat Rep 53(15), 2003, http://www.ede.gov/nc.hs/data /nvsr/nvsr53/nrsr53_15.pdf

TABLE 4-4 Direct Standardizations of Mortality Rates by Age for "South Community" and "North Community"

AGE (YR)	SIZE OF POPULATION (A)	PERCENT OF POPULATION	NUMBER OF DEATHS (B)	AGE-SPECIFIC DEATH RATE PER 1000 (B/A)
South Community*				
<15	5400	30.4	10	1.85/1000
15 to 44	7300	41.1	16	2.19/1000
45 to 64	3400	19.2	38	11.18/1000
>65	1650	9.3	84	50.91/1000
Total	17,750	100	148	
North Community†				
<15	1030	34.2	2	1.94/1000
15 to 44	1500	49.8	4	2.67/1000
45 to 64	407	13.5	4	9.83/1000
>65	75	2.5	4	53.33/1000
Total	3012	100	14	

Step 1: Determine age-specific death rates. Divide the number of deaths by the population size for each age category.

*Crude death rate = $\frac{148}{17,750}$ = $\frac{8.34}{1000}$

†Crude death rate = $\frac{14}{3012}$ = $\frac{4.64}{1000}$

TABLE 4-5   Direct Standardizations of Mortality Rates

| | UNITED STATES 1990 | | SOUTH COMMUNITY† | | NORTH COMMUNITY‡ | |
AGE (YR)	SIZE OF POPULATION	PERCENT OF POPULATION (A)*	AGE-SPECIFIC DEATH RATE PER 1000 (B₁)	EXPECTED NO. OF DEATHS PER 1000 (A × B₁)	AGE-SPECIFIC DEATH RATE PER 1000 (B₂)	EXPECTED NO. OF DEATHS PER 1000 (A × B₂)
<15	55,961,000	21.9	1.85	0.405	1.94	0.425
15 to 44	118,490,000	46.5	2.19	1.018	2.67	1.242
45 to 64	48,345,000	19.0	11.18	2.124	9.83	1.868
>65	32,283,000	12.7	50.91	6.466	53.33	6.773
Totals	255,079,000	100		10.013		10.308

Step 2: Compute expected number of deaths by multiplying proportion of U.S by age-specific death rates. Sum expected deaths to produce age-adjusted death rate.
*Convert to decimal before computing product **A** × **B**.

†Age-adjusted mortality rate = $\dfrac{10.013}{1000}$ (sum of A = B₁)

‡Age-adjusted mortality rate = $\dfrac{10.308}{1000}$ (sum of A = B₂).

TABLE 4-6   Summary of Tables 4-4 and 4-5

AREA	CRUDE MORTALITY RATE	AGE-ADJUSTED MORTALITY RATE
South Community	8.34 per 1000	10.013 per 1000
North Community	4.64 per 1000	10.308 per 1000

* When the confounding effect of different age distributions is removed through age adjustment, mortality rates for the two communities are similar.

TABLE 4-7   Indirect Standardization of Mortality Rates

| | | POPULATION SIZE (B) | | EXPECTED DEATHS (A × B)/100,000 | |
AGE (YR)	AGE-SPECIFIC U.S. DEATH RATES (A)*	SOUTH COMMUNITY	NORTH COMMUNITY	SOUTH COMMUNITY	NORTH COMMUNITY
<15	95.18	5400	1030	5.14	0.98
15 to 44	155.40	7300	1500	11.34	2.33
45 to 64	788.76	3400	407	26.82	3.21
>65	4922.32	1650	75	81.22	3.69

*1991 data from US Census Bureau: *Statistical abstract of the United States: 1994,* ed 114, Washington, DC, 1994, The Author. U.S. age-specific mortality rates are multiplied by population of each community to produce expected deaths. These are then summed and standard mortality ratios are calculated as shown in Table 4.8. Death rates are per 100,000 population.

TABLE 4-8   SMR Based on Data From Tables 4-7 and 4-4

VARIABLE	SOUTH COMMUNITY	NORTH COMMUNITY
Total expected deaths	124.52	10.21
Total observed deaths (from Table 4-4)	148	14
SMR of death (observed to expected)	1.19	1.37

SMRs of greater than 1 indicate that more deaths were observed in both communities than would be expected based on the morality experience of the overall U.S. population. When mortality data for the two communities are standardized to a third or standard population, the SMRs indicate a similar mortality experience.

$$PMR = \frac{\text{Number of deaths resulting from a specific cause in a specific time period}}{\text{Total number of deaths in time period}}$$

Table 4-9 summarizes the advantages and disadvantages of crude, specific, and adjusted rates. Numerous other rates assess particular segments of the population. Table 4-10 provides a summary of the major public health rates. A standard epidemiology textbook contains more information.

CONCEPT OF RISK

The concepts of risk and risk factor are familiar to community health nurses whose practices focus on disease prevention. **Risk** refers to the probability of an adverse event (i.e., the likelihood that healthy people exposed to a specific factor will acquire a specific disease). **Risk factor** refers to the specific exposure factor, such as cigarette smoke, excessive stress, high

TABLE 4-9   Advantages and Disadvantages of Crude, Specific, and Adjusted Rates

RATE	ADVANTAGES	DISADVANTAGES
Crude	Actual summary rates Readily calculable for international comparisons (widely used despite limitations)	Populations vary in composition (e.g., age): therefore differences in crude rates are difficult to interpret
Specific	Homogeneous subgroup Detailed rates useful for epidemiological and public health purposes	Cumbersome to compare many subgroups of two or more populations
Adjusted	Summary statements Differences in composition of group "removed," permitting unbiased comparison	Fictional rates Absolute magnitude dependent on chosen standard population Opposing trends in subgroups masked

Modified from Mausner JS, Kramer S: *Mausner and Bahn epidemiology: an introductory text,* ed 2, Philadelphia, 1985, WB Saunders.

TABLE 4-10   Major Public Health Rates

RATE DENOMINATOR	RATES	USUAL	FACTOR RATE FOR UNITED STATES, 2002
Total population	Crude birth rate = number of live births during the year/average (midyear) population	Per 1000 population	13.9
	Crude death rate = number of deaths during the year/average (midyear) population	Per 1000 population	8.5
	Age-specific death rate = number of deaths among people of a given age-group in 1 year/average (midyear) population in specified age-group	Per 1000 population	0.17 (5 to 14 yr) 4.30 (45 to 54 yr) 23.15 (65 to 74 yr)
	Cause-specific death rate = number of deaths from a stated cause in 1 year/average (midyear) population	Per 100,000 population	240.8 (heart diseases) 193.2 (malignant neoplasms)
Women aged 15 to 44	Fertility rate = number of live births during 1 year/number of women aged 15 to 44 in same year	Per 1000 women aged 15 to 44	64.8
Live births	Infant mortality rate = number of deaths in 1 year of children younger than 1 year/number of live births in same year	Per 1000 live births	7.0
	Neonatal mortality rate = number of deaths in 1 year of children younger than 28 days/number of live births in same year	Per 1000 live birth	4.7
	Maternal mortality rate (puerperal) = number of deaths from puerperal causes in 1 year/number of live births in same year	Per 100,000 live births	7.6
Live births and fetal deaths	Fetal death rate = number of fetal deaths in 1 year/number of live births in same year	Per 1000 live births and fetal deaths	6.4
	Perinatal mortality rate = number of fetal deaths (>28 weeks plus infant deaths <7 days)/number of live births and fetal deaths (>28 weeks during the same year)	Per 1000 live births and fetal deaths	6.9

Modified from Mausner JS, Kramer S: *Mausner and Bahn epidemiology: an introductory text,* ed 2, Philadelphia, 1985, WB Saunders. Rates from National Center for Health Statistics: Health, United States, 2004, http://www.cdc.gov/nchs/data/hus/hus04trend.pdf#022

noise levels, or environmental chemicals. Frequently, the exposure factor is external to the individual. Risk factors may include fixed characteristics of people, such as age, sex, or genetic makeup. Although these intrinsic factors are not alterable, certain lifestyle changes may reduce the effect of these risk factors. For example, positive dietary practices and exercise regimens may modify the effects of the risk factor of aging for certain health conditions. Specifically, calcium and hormonal supplements may reduce the risk of osteoporosis for susceptible women.

Epidemiologists describe disease patterns in aggregates and quantify the effects of exposure to particular factors on the disease rates. To identify specific risk factors, epidemiologists compare rates of disease for those exposed with those nonexposed. One method for comparing two rates is subtracting the rate of nonexposed individuals from the exposed. This measure of risk is called the *attributable risk;* it is the estimate of the disease burden in a population. For example, if the rate of non–insulin-dependent diabetes were 5000 per 100,000 people in the obese population (i.e., those weighing more than 120% of ideal body weight) and 1000 per 100,000 people in the non-obese population, the attributable risk of non–insulin-dependent diabetes resulting from obesity would be 4000 per 100,000 people (i.e., $\frac{5000}{100,000} - \frac{1000}{100,000}$).

This means that 4000 cases per 100,000 people may be attributed to obesity. Thus a prevention program designed to reduce obesity could theoretically eliminate 4000 cases per

100,000 people in the population. Attributable risks are particularly important in describing the potential impact of a public health intervention in a community.

A second measure of the excess risk caused by a factor is the *relative risk ratio.* The relative risk is calculated by dividing the incidence rate of disease in the exposed population by the incidence rate of disease in the nonexposed population. In the previous example, a relative risk of 5 was obtained by dividing 5000/100,000 by 1000/100,000. This risk ratio suggests that an obese individual has a fivefold greater risk of diabetes than a non-obese individual. In general, a relative risk of 1 indicates no excessive risk from exposure to a factor; a relative risk of 1.5 indicates a 50% increase in risk; a relative risk of 2 indicates twice the risk; and a relative risk of less than 1 suggests a factor may have a protective effect associated with a reduced disease rate.

The relative risk ratio forms the statistical basis for the risk factor concept. Relative risks are valuable indicators of the excess risk incurred by exposure to certain factors. They have been used extensively in identifying the major causal factors of many common diseases and direct public health practitioners' efforts to reduce health risks.

Community health nurses may apply the concept of relative risk to suspected exposure variables to isolate risk factors associated with community health problems. For example, a community health nurse might investigate an outbreak of probable food-borne illness. The nurse may compare the incidence rate among those exposed to potato salad in a school cafeteria with the incidence rate among those unexposed. The relative risk calculated from the ratio of these two incidence rates indicates the amount of excess risk for disease incurred by eating the potato salad. A community health nurse might also determine the relative risks for other suspected foods and compare them with the relative risk for potato salad. Attack rates are the calculated incidence rates for foods involved in food-borne illnesses. A food with a markedly higher relative risk than other foods might be the causal agent in a food-borne epidemic. The identification of the causal agent, or specific food, is critical to the implementation of an effective prevention program such as teaching proper food-handling techniques.

USE OF EPIDEMIOLOGY IN DISEASE PREVENTION

Primary Prevention

The central goals of epidemiology are describing the disease patterns, identifying the etiological factors in disease development, and taking the most effective preventive measures. These preventive measures are specific to the stage of disease progression or the **natural history of disease,** from prepathogenesis through resolution of the disease process. When interventions occur before disease development, they are called *primary prevention.* Primary prevention relies on epidemiological information to indicate those behaviors that are protective, or those that will not contribute to an increase in disease, and those that are associated with increased risk.

Two types of activities constitute primary prevention. Those actions that are general in nature and designed to foster healthful lifestyles and a safe environment are called *health promotion.* Actions aimed at reducing the risk of specific diseases are called *specific protection.* Public health practitioners use epidemiological research to understand practices that are likely to reduce or increase disease rates. For example, numerous research studies have confirmed that regular exercise is an important health promotion activity that has positive effects on general, physical, and mental health. Immunizations exemplify specific protection measures that reduce the incidence of particular diseases.

Secondary and Tertiary Prevention

Secondary prevention occurs after pathogenesis. Those measures designed to detect disease at its earliest stage, namely screening and physical examinations that are aimed at early diagnosis, are secondary prevention. Interventions that provide for early treatment and cure of disease are also in this category. Again, epidemiological data and clinical trials determining effective treatments are crucial in disease identification. Mammography, guaiac testing of feces, and the treatment of infections and dental caries are all examples of secondary prevention. *Tertiary prevention* includes the limitation of disability and the rehabilitation of those with irreversible disease such as diabetes and spinal cord injury. Epidemiological studies examine risk factors affecting function and suggest optimal strategies in the care of patients with chronic advanced disease.

Establishing Causality

As discussed earlier, a principal goal of classic epidemiology is to identify etiological factors of diseases to encourage the most effective primary prevention activities and develop treatment modalities. During the last few decades, researchers recognized that many diseases have not one but multiple causes. Epidemiologists who examine disease rates and conduct population-focused research often find multiple factors associated with health problems. For example, cardiovascular disease rates may vary by location, ethnicity, and smoking status. Even infectious diseases often require not only an organism but also certain behaviors or conditions to cause exposure. Determining the extent that these correlates represent associative or causal relationships is important for public health practitioners who seek to prevent, diagnose, and treat disease.

The following six criteria establish the existence of a **cause and effect relationship:**

1. *Strength of association:* Rates of morbidity or mortality must be higher in the exposed group than in the nonexposed group. Relative risk ratios, or odds ratios, and correlation coefficients indicate whether the relationship between the exposure variable and the outcome is causal. For example, epidemiological studies demonstrated an elevated relative risk for heart disease among smokers compared with nonsmokers (Doll and Hill, 1956).

2. *Dose-response relationship:* An increased exposure to the risk factor causes a concomitant increase in disease rate. The risk of heart disease mortality is higher for heavy smokers compared with light smokers (Mattson, Pollack, and Cullen, 1987).

3. *Temporally correct relationship:* Exposure to the causal factor must occur before the effect, or disease. For heart disease, smoking history must precede disease development.

4. *Biological plausibility:* The data must make biological sense and represent a coherent explanation for the relationship. Nicotine and other tobacco-derived chemicals are toxic to the vascular endothelium. In addition to raising low-density lipoprotein (LDL) and decreasing high-density lipoprotein (HDL) cholesterol levels, cigarette smoking causes arterial vasoconstriction and platelet reactivity, which contributes to platelet thrombus formation.

5. *Consistency with other studies:* Varying types of studies in other populations must observe similar associations. Numerous studies of different designs have repeatedly supported the relationship between smoking and heart disease.

6. *Specificity:* The exposure variable must be necessary and sufficient to cause disease; there is only one causal factor. Although specificity may be strong causal evidence, this criterion is less important today. Diseases do not have single causes; they have multifactorial origins.

The exposure variable of smoking is one of several risk factors for heart disease. Few factors are linked to a single condition. Smoking is not specific to heart disease alone. It is a causal factor for other diseases like lung and oral cancers. Further, smoking is not "necessary and sufficient" to the development of heart disease because there are nonsmokers who also experience coronary heart disease. Therefore the causal criterion of specificity more frequently pertains to infectious diseases.

Although these criteria are useful in evaluating epidemiological evidence, it is important to note that causality can never be proven and is always a matter of judgment. In reality, absolute causality is only rarely established. Rather, epidemiologists more commonly refer to suggested causal and associated factors. The effect of confounding variables makes it difficult to ascertain true relationships between the exposure and outcome variables. Confounding variables are independently related to both the dependent variable and the independent variable. Therefore, confounding variables may mask the true relationship between the dependent and independent variables. For example, Buring and Lee (1995) discussed the need to control dietary fat when examining the relationship between physical activity and coronary heart disease. This is necessary because studies have shown that dietary fat is independently related to both physical exercise (Simoes et al., 1995) and heart disease (Willett, 1990) in some populations. The apparent association between physical activity and heart disease may be attributable to the difference in fat intake between those with and without heart disease. Those with heart disease may tend to have a higher fat intake and a decreased activity level than those without heart disease. The outcome is not solely attributable to exercise. On the other hand, Buring and Lee (1995) provided an example in which dietary fat is not a confounding variable despite its relation to physical activity. Dietary fat is not a confounder of the relationship of physical exercise and osteoporosis because dietary fat is not a risk factor for the dependent variable of osteoporosis.

By measuring the confounding variable, the researcher can statistically account for its effect in the analysis (e.g., by using multiple logistical regression analysis or stratification). A biostatistics text contains a discussion of these methods. Alternatively, matching subjects in treatment and control groups with respect to the confounding variable minimizes the effects of the confounder. Again, standardization for variables such as age is another method for managing spurious associations, which makes true relationships more apparent. An understanding of such relationships facilitates the practitioners' interpretation and application of findings.

Screening

Again, a central aim of epidemiology is to describe the course of disease according to person, place, and time. Observations of the disease process may suggest factors that aggravate or ameliorate its progress. This information also assists in determining effective treatment and rehabilitation options (i.e., secondary or tertiary prevention approaches).

The purpose of **screening programs** is to identify risk factors and diseases in their earliest stages. Screening is usually a secondary prevention activity because disease appears *after* a pathological change has occurred, or ideally, early in the disease process. In all forms of secondary and tertiary prevention, the identification of illness prompts the nurse to consider which forms of upstream prevention could have affected disease development.

Community health nurses commonly conduct screening programs. A community health nurse may devote a large portion of his or her work activities to performing physical examinations, promoting client self-examination, or conducting screening programs in schools, clinics, or community settings. Although these secondary prevention activities are important services that provide vital information on community health status, they focus on detecting existing disease. Nurses should contrast secondary prevention activities with primary prevention and anticipatory guidance, which are hallmarks of community health nursing practice.

There are several guidelines community health nurses should consider for screening programs. First, nurses must plan and execute adequate and appropriate follow-up treatment for patients with disease. Health fairs have been criticized for the lack of consistent follow-up of screening activities. Second, in the planning phase, the nurse should determine if early disease diagnosis constitutes a real benefit to clients in terms of increased life expectancy or quality of life. Third, a critical prerequisite to screening is the existence of acceptable and medically sound treatment and follow-up.

BOX 4-4 Guidelines for Screening Programs

➤ Screen for conditions in which early detection and treatment can improve disease outcome and quality of life.
➤ Screen populations that have risk factors or are more susceptible to the disease.
➤ Select a screening method that is simple, safe, inexpensive to administer, acceptable to clients, and has acceptable sensitivity and specificity.
➤ Plan for the timely referral and follow-up of positive cases.
➤ Identify referral sources that are appropriate, cost-effective, and convenient for clients.

TABLE 4-11 Sensitivity and Specificity of a Screening Test

SCREENING TEST	THOSE WITH DISEASE	THOSE WITHOUT DISEASE
Positive	True positives (a)	False positives (b)
Negative	False negatives (c)	True negatives (d)

$$\text{Sensitivity (in percent)} = \frac{\text{True positives}}{\text{All with disease}} - \frac{(a)}{(a + c)} \times 100$$

$$\text{Specificity (in percent)} = \frac{\text{True negatives}}{\text{All with disease}} - \frac{(d)}{(b + d)} \times 100$$

In the past, public health providers have debated the ethical and practical arguments for implementing human immunodeficiency virus (HIV) screening. Concern exists regarding the potential for stigma and discrimination against those who screen positively for a test; therefore, those implementing screening programs should establish procedures for ensuring confidentiality. These procedures, in conjunction with the development of azidothymidine (AZT) and other antiviral treatments, have encouraged earlier identification of HIV-positive individuals.

A screening program's procedures must also be cost effective and acceptable to clients. Although sigmoidoscopy is a common and effective screening procedure for colon cancer, it is not a simple and inexpensive test. Consequently, it is primarily those who demonstrate a high risk for colon cancer that undergo the examination. Finally, a nurse should consider whether or not to screen a population based on the significant costs for screening programs and procedures, follow-up for clients who test positive, and subsequent medical care (Box 4-4).

When developing a screening program, the community health nurse also must evaluate issues specific to the validity of the screening test. Detecting clients with disease is the purpose of screening, and *sensitivity* is the test's ability to do this correctly. Conversely, *specificity* is the extent to which a test can correctly identify those who do not have disease. To obtain estimates of these two dimensions, the nurse must compare screening results with those of some definitive diagnostic procedure (Mausner and Kramer, 1985). For a given test, the sensitivity and specificity tend to be inversely related to each other. When a test is highly sensitive, individuals without disease may be labeled positive. These false-positive tests may cause stress and worry for clients and require further diagnostic testing to confirm a diagnosis. With a highly sensitive test, specificity may be lower and the test may not detect disease in some clients. These false-negative test results mean that some individuals may receive false reassurance and will not receive follow-up care.

Optimally, a screening test should be maximally sensitive and specific. To a large extent, this depends on the stringency of the cut-off point established for determining a positive disease case. For example, with an established high blood pressure criterion of 140/90, more people will have high blood pressure than with a cut-off of 150/90. The lower cut-off is more sensitive and will lead to more false positives. The higher criterion may be more specific, and although fewer people will be hypertensive, there will be fewer false-positive cases than with the lower cut-off level. Table 4-11 includes the formula for calculating sensitivity and specificity.

Sensitivity and specificity reflect the *yield* of a screening test, which is the amount of detected disease. One measure of yield is the *positive predictive value* of a test, which is the proportion of true positive results relative to all positive test results. On the basis of Table 4-11, the formula is $\frac{a}{a + b}$. The positive predictive value is dependent on the prevalence of undetected disease in a population. Screening for a rare disease such as phenylketonuria will yield a lower predictive value and more false-positive results. In phenylketonuria, a low predictive value is acceptable because the false-negative result has such serious consequences. The predictive value is also affected by the nature of the screened population. Screening only the individuals at high risk for a disease will produce a higher predictive value and can be a more efficient way to identify those with health problems. For example, diabetes screening in a Mexican-American or African-American adult population should produce a higher predictive value than screening the general adult population.

Surveillance

In addition to screening, **surveillance** is a mechanism for the ongoing collection of community health information. Monitoring for changes in disease frequency is essential to effective and responsive public health programs. Identifying trends in disease incidence or identifying risk factor status by location and population subgroup over time allows the community health nurse to evaluate the effectiveness of existing programs and implement interventions targeted to high-risk groups. Again, identifying new cases for calculating incidence rates is particularly useful in evaluating morbidity trends. However, this form of surveillance data is more difficult to collect, and public health practitioners can only access the data for selected diseases. Prevalence rates, mortality data, risk factor data, and hospital and health service data can help indicate a program's successes or deficiencies.

HEALTHY PEOPLE 2010 | Objectives for Surveillance

Objective	Baseline Data	Target Data
23-1: Increase the proportion of public health agencies that provide Internet and e-mail access to at least 75% of their employees. Teach employees to use Internet and other electronic information systems to apply data and other information to public health practice.		
23-2: Increase the proportion of health agencies that have made information available to the public in the past year on the Leading Health Indicators, Health Status Indicators, and Priority Data Needs.		
23-3: Increase the proportion of all major health data systems that use geo-coding to promote nationwide use of geographic information systems (GIS) at all levels.	45% have geo-coded records	90%
23-4: Increase the proportion of population-based *Healthy People 2010* objectives for which national data are available for all population groups identified for the objective.	11%	100%
23-5: Increase the proportion of Leading Health Indicators, Health Status Indicators, and Primary Data Needs for which data—especially for select populations—are available at the tribal, state, and local levels.		
23-6: Increase the proportion of *Healthy People 2010* objectives that are tracked regularly at the national level.	82%	100%
23-14: Increase the proportion of public health agencies that provide comprehensive epidemiology services to support essential public health service.		
23-17: Increase the proportion of public health agencies that conduct or collaborate on population-based prevention research.		

US Department of Health and Human Services: *Healthy people 2010*, Conference edition, Washington DC, 2000, US Government Printing Office.

RESEARCH HIGHLIGHTS

Reducing Infant Mortality Rates Using the Perinatal Periods of Risk Model

Infant mortality rates are an accepted indicator for measuring a nation's health. The rate is representative of the health status and social well-being of any nation. Despite decreases in the past 50 years, infant mortality rates in the United States remain higher than in other industrialized countries. Using overall infant mortality rates to determine the effectiveness of interventions does not help communities focus on particular underlying factors contributing to the rates. Targeting interventions to the factors most responsible for the infant mortality rate should help reduce the rate more rapidly and effectively. This study was designed to determine and rank contributing factors to fetal-infant mortality in a specific community using the Perinatal Periods of Risk (PPOR) model.

The PPOR model provides direction, focus, and suggestions for effective interventions. The model helps users identify and rank four factors as they contribute to the overall infant mortality rate: (a) mother's health before and between pregnancies, (b) maternal health care systems, (c) neonatal health care systems, and (d) infant health during the first year of life. The PPOR model is based on two major theoretical constructs: age of fetus-infant at death and birthweight. The PPOR model maps each death in a geographic region based on birthweight and age at death, including fetal, neonatal, and postneonatal periods. The lowest birthweight infant deaths are combined into one cell named the maternal health cell. The three remaining groups are put into cells suggesting the primary preventive focus for that group: maternal health, newborn health, and infant health. Multiple interventions are important in reducing infant mortality, and the PPOR model guides prioritizing interventions based on the cell contributing the most to infant mortality rates.

The PPOR model was used to map fetal-infant mortality for 1995 to 1998 in the Tulsa County, Oklahoma, as compared to traditional calculation methods. The overall fetal-infant mortality rate using the PPOR model was 12.7 compared to 7.11 calculated using the traditional method. The PPOR calculation helped clearly distinguish which factor was contributing the most to the overall fetal-infant mortality rate. The maternal health cell was contributing 42% to the overall rate in Tulsa County. Because the highest infant mortality was in the maternal health cell, intervention strategies were designed to promote the health of women prior to and between pregnancies. The PPOR model is a useful tool for community partnerships to use in targeting actions for the population groups contributing most to infant mortality rates.

Burns PG: Reducing infant mortality rates using the perinatal periods of risk model, *Public Health Nursing* 22(1): 2-7, 2005.

The U.S. Public Health Service coordinates a system of data collection among federal, state, and local agencies. These groups compile numerous sets of data and base some of these data sets on the entire population (e.g., vital statistics data) and other collections on subsamples of the population (e.g., the National Health Interview Survey). The completeness of data reporting is variable because not all diseases are reportable. For example, practitioners are required to report only four sexually transmitted diseases (i.e., acquired immunodeficiency syndrome [AIDS], syphilis, gonorrhea, and chlamydia) to local and state health departments. Furthermore, not all practitioners report cases on a regular basis and not all people with sexually transmitted diseases actually seek care. Studies have indicated that practitioners also underreport childhood communicable diseases, such as chicken pox and mumps. The Centers for Disease Control and Prevention conducts studies that estimate the magnitude of this underreporting problem.

Practitioners have a continuing need for comprehensive and systematically collected surveillance data that describe the health status of national and local subgroups. They use this information to evaluate the impact of programs on specific groups in a community. For example, the effectiveness of *Healthy People 2000* and *Healthy People 2010* depends on the availability of reliable baseline and continuing data to characterize health problems and evaluate goal achievement as listed in the *Healthy People 2010* table.

Healthy People 2010 (U.S. Department of Health and Human Services, 2000) recognizes the ongoing need to extend the inclusiveness of such surveillance systems. For example, simply documenting children's mortality rates resulting from injury is insufficient for the development of specific methods of injury prevention. Data on the number of injured children and the nature of injury across the nation would increase the usefulness of surveillance information.

Nurses need to describe trends in health and illness by a community's locale, demographics, and risk factor status to intervene effectively on behalf of communities. They must compare the data for their locale with those of a relevant neighboring area (e.g., a census tract, city, county, state, or nation) to gain perspective on the magnitude of a local problem. Ideally, the nurse should have access to surveillance data at several different levels over a period of time. In some instances, community health nurses find it necessary to construct their own surveillance systems that are tailored to specific health conditions or programs in a community. These smaller data collection systems help nurses evaluate programs when the data are readily accessible and compatible with data from large city or statewide surveillance systems.

CLINICAL EXAMPLE

In April 1991, a cluster of six neural tube defects (NTDs) occurred in babies born in Brownsville, Texas, within a span of 6 weeks. Further investigation in Cameron County indicated a rate of 27.1 cases per 10,000 live births compared to 14.7 for babies conceived from 1986 to 1989 and compared to the U.S. rate of approximately 8 per 10,000. This rate was more than three times the national rate and represented an increased risk in Hispanic women. This increased risk was partially attributable to cultural and environmental factors, including lower socioeconomic status and migrant farm work. The investigators implemented a surveillance program that included fetuses of less than 20 weeks' gestation, which obtained more accurate population-based data. Additionally, the program implemented folic acid supplementation in Texas counties along the Mexican border. From 1993 to 1996, NTD rates dropped to 13 per 10,000 following supplementation.

Research suggests that 50% to 70% of NTDs may be preventable with folic acid supplementation. This finding supports the fortification of bread and cereal products; in January 1998, the Food and Drug Administration mandated the addition of 140 mcg of vitamin B per 100 g of most grain products. Dietary intake alone may be insufficient; therefore, the Centers for Disease Control and Prevention recommends that all women of reproductive age consume 400 mcg (0.4 mg) of folic acid daily from a combination of dietary sources such as cereal or grain products, leafy green vegetables, and vitamin supplements.

Data from Centers for Disease Control and Prevention: Neural tube defects in Texas, *Dis Prev News* 58(2):5-6, 1998; Centers for Disease Control and Prevention: Neural tube defect surveillance and folic acid intervention: Texas-Mexico border, 1993-1998, *MMWR Morb Mortality Wkly Rep* 49(01):1-4, 2000, http://www.cdc.gov/mmwr/preview/mmwrhtml/mm4901a1.htm. ∎

Again, epidemiologists describe the course of disease over time. These secular trends are changes that occur over years or decades, such as the decline in uterine cancer and the increase in breast cancer. Frequently, epidemiologists document the associated patterns of treatment and intervention. In many instances, studies conducted by clinical epidemiologists provide this information. Cancer registries are a form of surveillance that document the prevalence and incidence of cancer in a community and document its course, treatment, and associated survival rates. The Surveillance, Epidemiology, and End Results (SEER) program of the National Cancer Institute compiles national cancer data from existing cancer registries covering approximately 26% of the U.S. population (National Cancer Institute, 2005).

Public health practitioners need to conduct community surveys of population segments to plan for the sector's health. For example, a survey of the disabled population that assesses prevalence may also evaluate the adequacy of present services and project future needs.

USE OF EPIDEMIOLOGY IN HEALTH SERVICES

Presented epidemiological approaches can be used to describe the distribution of disease and its determinants in populations. However, epidemiological principles are also useful in studying population health care delivery and in describing and evaluating the use of community health services. For example, determining the ratio of health care providers to population size helps assess the system's ability to provide care. The clients' reasons for seeking care, the clients' payment methods, and the clients' satisfaction are also informative. Regardless of whether community health nurses or health services researchers collected these data, the information is essential for those who strive to improve clients' access to quality health care.

Health Services Epidemiology

Health services epidemiology focuses on the population's health care patterns. In particular, public health practitioners are concerned with the accessibility and affordability of services and the barriers that may contribute to excess morbidity in at-risk groups. Traditionally, children are a vulnerable group, and they are a particular focus of health services research. Studies examining poverty rates and care access have underscored the need to expand insurance coverage to those who do not have private medical insurance and do not qualify for Medicaid programs. ■

Community health nurses can use epidemiological studies to evaluate the quality of care. A comparative study of a special geriatric inpatient evaluation ward, which used an interdisciplinary elderly care program, exemplifies this approach (Rubenstein et al., 1984). The study compared the outcomes of interdisciplinary care with the outcomes of typical elderly care in the hospital ward. Patients in the special unit had lower mortality rates, lower morbidity rates, and higher satisfaction levels. Furthermore, clients incurred lower costs on the special unit compared with other units. This important finding suggests another aspect of health service epidemiology, which is evaluating the cost-effectiveness of health care and specific interventions or modes of delivery.

Ultimately, nurses must apply epidemiological findings in the practice arena. It is essential that they incorporate study results into prevention programs for communities and at-risk populations. Further, the philosophy of public health and epidemiology dictates that nurses extend its application into major health policy decisions, because the aim of health policy planning is to achieve positive health goals and outcomes for improved societal health.

A goal of policy development is to bring about desirable social changes. Epidemiological factors, history, politics, economics, culture, and technology influence policy development. The complex interaction of these factors may explain the slow application of epidemiological knowledge. Lung disease in the United States exemplifies the incomplete progress in implementing effective health policy. In the early 1950s, studies identified and conclusively linked cigarette smoking to lung cancer and heart disease (Doll and Hill, 1952). Since the 1950s, protective public policies have included cigarette taxes, cigarette warning labels, and smoking restrictions in public areas. Nevertheless, until the late 1990s, advertising continued to promote cigarette smoking. Indeed, during the 1980s and 1990s, there was a proliferation of billboard and media advertisements targeted to vulnerable segments of the population (i.e., adolescents and black and Hispanic males). Community forums vigorously protested and debated this practice, and individual states began to hold the tobacco industry legally accountable for cigarette-related disease and death.

In 1976, Milio suggested that public policy also failed to keep pace with epidemiological research findings in other areas. She asserted that consumer health would benefit significantly from a public policy that provides healthier consumer options such as improved workplace safeguards, higher environmental standards, higher quality nutritious food, and improved incentives to reduce alcohol consumption. These goals continue to be primary concerns of public health professionals (Milio, 1976).

In summary, there remain many public policies that public health practitioners and epidemiologists have yet to modify in the interest of improved health. Community health nurses should exercise "societal responsibility" in applying epidemiological findings, but this will require the active involvement of the citizen consumer. Community health nurses collaborating with community members can combine epidemiological knowledge and aggregate-level strategies to affect change on the broadest scale.

EPIDEMIOLOGICAL METHODS

Descriptive Epidemiology

Descriptive epidemiology focuses on the amount and distribution of health and health problems within a population. Its purpose is to describe the characteristics of both people who are protected from disease and those who have a disease. Factors of particular interest include age, sex, ethnicity or race, socioeconomic status, occupation, and family status. Epidemiologists use morbidity and mortality rates to describe the extent of disease and to determine the risk factors that make certain groups prone to acquiring disease.

In addition to "person" characteristics, the place of occurrence describes disease frequency. For example, certain parasitic diseases, such as malaria and schistosomiasis, occur in tropical areas. Other diseases may occur in certain geopolitical entities. For example, gastroenteritis outbreaks often occur in communities with lax water quality standards. Time is the third parameter that helps define disease patterns. Epidemiologists may track incidence rates over a period of days or weeks (e.g., epidemics of infectious disease) or over an extended period of years (e.g., secular trends in the cancer death rate).

These person, place, and time factors can form a framework for disease analysis and may suggest variables associated with high versus low disease rates. Descriptive epidemiology can then generate hypotheses about the cause of disease, and analytic epidemiology approaches can test these hypotheses (Box 4-5).

Analytic Epidemiology

Analytic epidemiology investigates the causes of disease by determining why a disease rate is lower in one population group than in another. This method tests hypotheses generated from descriptive data and either accepts or rejects them on the basis of analytic research. The epidemiologist seeks to establish a cause and effect relationship between a preexisting condition or event, and the disease (see pre-

BOX 4-5 An Example of Descriptive Epidemiology
States

➤ The **P**erson-**P**lace-**T**ime **M**odel is illustrated by an outbreak of tuberculosis (TB) and its rapid spread in an HIV-infected prison population and into the outside community.

➤ *Person:* An index case-patient was connected through DNA fingerprinting of *Mycobacterium* TB isolates to TB disease in 14 other inmates and to the spouse who visited the prisoner. Nine prison employees also had skin test conversions. Secondary transmission occurred from the wife of the index case to a young daughter who had no contact with her father.

➤ *Place:* A 500-person housing unit for HIV-infected inmates at a correctional institution in California.

➤ *Time:* Initial case entered the prison in May 1995 and was diagnosed with TB in August. Follow-up of contacts occurred from September through April 1996.

From Centers for Disease Control and Prevention: Tuberculosis outbreaks in prison housing units for HIV-infected inmates: California, 1995-1996, *MMWR Morb Mortality Wkly Rep* 48(4): 79-82, 1999, http://www.cdc.gov/nchstp/od/mmwr/tuberculosis_outbreaks_in_prison.htm.

vious section on causality). To determine this relationship, the epidemiologist may undertake two major types of research studies, which are *observational* and *experimental* studies.

Observational Studies

Epidemiologists frequently use *observational studies* for descriptive purposes, but they also use them to discover the etiology of disease. The investigator can begin to understand the factors that contribute to disease by observing disease rates in groups of people differentiated by experience or exposure. For example, differences in disease rates may occur in the obese compared with the non-obese, in smokers compared with nonsmokers, and in those with high stress levels compared with those with low stress levels. These characteristics (i.e., obesity, smoking, and stress) are called *exposure* variables.

Unlike experimental studies, observational studies do not allow the investigator to manipulate the specific exposure or experience or to control or limit the effects of other extraneous factors that may influence disease development. For example, life stress is related to depression. People with low socioeconomic status also have high depression rates. People with low socioeconomic status frequently experience greater life stresses; therefore, the confounding factor of socioeconomic status makes it more difficult to demonstrate the effect of stress on depression. The three major study designs used in observational research are cross-sectional, retrospective, and prospective studies.

Cross-Sectional Studies

Cross-sectional studies, sometimes called *prevalence* or *correlational* studies, examine relationships between potential causal factors and disease at a specific time (Figure 4-5). Surveys that simultaneously collect information about risk factors and disease exemplify this design. For example, both

the National Health and Nutrition Examination Survey (NHANES) and the subsequent Hispanic HANES, collected cross-sectional data regarding current dietary practices and physical status on people ranging from 1 to 72 years of age (Delgado et al., 1990). Data from the third NHANES survey showed that the prevalence of the metabolic syndrome as defined by the National Cholesterol Education Program–Adult Treatment Panel III criteria, was 23% of the U.S. population and increased markedly with age (Ford et al., 2002).

Although a cross-sectional study can identify associations among disease and specific factors, it is impossible to make causal inferences because the study cannot establish the temporal sequence of events (i.e., the cause preceded the effect). For example, the NHANES was unable to determine whether high salt intake precedes hypertension—thus making it the causal factor—or whether the reverse is true. Therefore cross-sectional studies have limitations in discovering etiological factors of disease. These studies can help identify preliminary relationships that other analytic designs may explore further; therefore, they are hypothesis-generating studies.

Retrospective Studies

Retrospective studies compare individuals with a particular condition or disease with those who do not have the disease. These studies determine whether cases, or a diseased group, differ in their exposure to a specific factor or characteristic relative to controls, or a nondiseased group. To make unambiguous comparisons, investigators select the cases according to explicitly defined criteria regarding the type of case and the stage of disease. Investigators also select a control group from the general population, which is characteristically similar to the cases (Figure 4-6).

Frequently, people hospitalized for diseases that are not under study become controls if they do not share the exposure or risk factor under study. For example, a researcher may select heart disease patients to be controls in a study of lung cancer patients. However, this may introduce serious bias because these patients often share the risk factor of smoking. The methods of data collection must be the same for both groups to prevent further introduction of bias into the study. Therefore it is desirable for interviewers to remain unaware of which subjects are cases and which are controls.

In retrospective studies, data collection extends back in time to determine previous exposure or risk factors. Investigators analyze study data by comparing the proportion of subjects with disease, or cases, who possess the exposure or risk factors with the corresponding proportion in the control group. A greater proportion of exposed cases than controls suggests a relationship between the disease and the risk factor.

Investigators often use retrospective study designs because these designs address the question of causality better than cross-sectional studies. Retrospective studies also require fewer resources and less data collection time than prospective studies. Many examples of *retrospective,* or *case-control,* studies exist in the literature. One classic example is Doll and Hill's (1952) investigation of risk factors for lung cancer.

Time Dimension

Present

Sample: Subjects sampled
from population-at-large at
one point in time

Advantages	Disadvantages
Quick to plan and conduct	Cannot calculate relative risk with prevalence data
Relatively inexpensive	
	Temporal sequence of factor and outcome unknown
May provide preliminary indication of whether an association between a risk factor and disease exists	
Provides prevalence data needed for planning health services	
Hypothesis generating	

FIGURE 4-5 Cross-sectional, or prevalence, study.

Time Dimension

Past

Sample: Subjects sampled
with regard to disease and
condition

Disease

No Disease

History of exposure
(i.e., risk factors)

Exposed   Not exposed   Exposed   Not exposed
(a)   (c)   (b)   (d)

Advantages	Disadvantages
Can calculate odds ratio (OR), which is an estimate of relative risk: 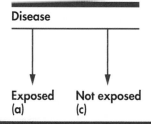 (*If disease is rare.)	Incidence of disease cannot be calculated
	Selection of control group is difficult
Requires fewer subjects than prospective designs	Relies on recall or records for exposure information that is subject to bias
Possible to study multiple risk factors presumed to be related to a disease	Exposure ascertained after disease occurs (i.e., temporal relationship)
Less expensive and difficult to conduct than a prospective study	

$$OR = \frac{a}{a+c} \div \frac{b}{b+d} \stackrel{*}{=} \frac{ad}{bc}$$

FIGURE 4-6 Retrospective, or case-control, study.

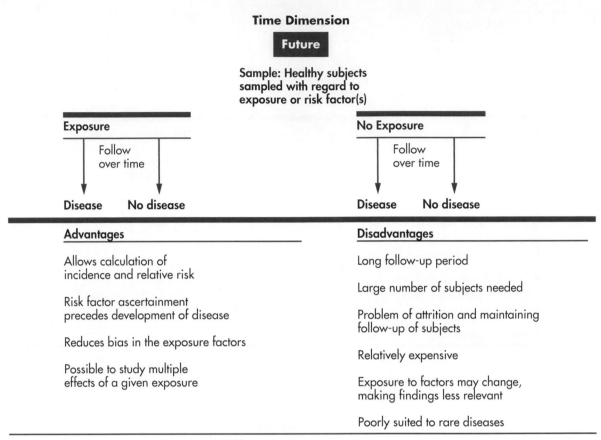

Time Dimension

Future

Sample: Healthy subjects
sampled with regard to
exposure or risk factor(s)

Exposure	No Exposure
Follow over time	Follow over time
Disease No disease	Disease No disease

Advantages	Disadvantages
Allows calculation of incidence and relative risk	Long follow-up period
Risk factor ascertainment precedes development of disease	Large number of subjects needed
Reduces bias in the exposure factors	Problem of attrition and maintaining follow-up of subjects
Possible to study multiple effects of a given exposure	Relatively expensive
	Exposure to factors may change, making findings less relevant
	Poorly suited to rare diseases

FIGURE 4-7   Prospective, or cohort, study.

They compared exposure rates for cases diagnosed with lung cancer with those in the control group diagnosed with cancer outside the chest and oral cavity. Doll and Hill recorded detailed smoking histories on all subjects. Compared with the controls, a significantly higher proportion of lung cancer cases smoked. This study yielded the hypothesis that smoking may be etiologically related to lung cancer.

Prospective Studies

Prospective studies monitor a group of disease-free individuals to determine if and when disease occurs (Figure 4-7). These individuals, or the cohort, share a common experience within a defined time period. For example, a birth cohort consists of all people born within a given time period. The study assesses the cohort with respect to an exposure factor associated with the disease and thus classifies it at the beginning of the study. The study then monitors the cohort for disease development. The investigator compares the disease rates for those with a known exposure with rates for those who remain unexposed. The study observes subjects prospectively; therefore it summarizes data collected over time by the incidence rates of new cases (Box 4-6). Again, comparing two incidence rates produces a measure of relative risk.

$$Relative\ risk = \frac{Incidence\ rate\ among\ exposed}{Incidence\ rate\ among\ unexposed}$$

The relative risk indicates the extent of excess risk incurred by exposure relative to nonexposure. A relative risk of one suggests no excess risk resulting from exposure,

BOX 4-6 Comparison of Time Factors in Retrospective and Prospective Study Design

Cohort Study

Girls with bacteriuria	→	Women with renal disease
Girls with sterile urine	→	Women without renal disease

Case-Control Study

Girls with bacteriuria	←	Women with renal disease
Girls with sterile urine	←	Women without renal disease

PAST -------------- PRESENT (BEGINNING) -------------- FUTURE

Comparison of time factors in prospective design (i.e., cohort) and retrospective design (i.e. case-control) approaches to studying the possible effect of childhood bacteriuria on renal disease in adult women.

whereas a relative risk of two suggests twice the risk of experiencing disease from exposure.

Prospective studies, or *longitudinal, cohort,* or *incidence* studies, are advantageous because they obtain more reliable information about the cause of disease than do other study methodologies. These studies establish a stronger temporal

ETHICAL Insights

The Tuskegee Syphilis Study

In 1932 the U.S. Public Health Service (PHS) began a longitudinal-experimental study of 600 African-American sharecroppers, 399 of whom had syphilis and 201 without the disease. Conducted in one of the poorest counties of Alabama, the subjects were unaware that they had syphilis but were told they were being treated for "bad blood." Enticed by the promise of free medical care and meals, the subjects joined the study without knowledge of their disease, its treatment, or the study procedures. The experimental group was initially treated with ineffective doses of the treatments of the time, bismuth or mercury, and later with aspirin. Even when penicillin became available in the late 1940s, they were actively denied treatment. For 40 years, these men were followed by PHS investigators affiliated with the Tuskegee Institute and hospital who claimed to observe the differences in the progression of the disease in blacks, compared to the control group. During the course of the study, many died of syphilis or other causes, numerous wives became infected, and children were born with congenital syphilis. In 1972, a former venereal disease interviewer, Peter Buxtun, blew the whistle on the study, and reports were published in newspapers. Only after the public became outraged about the unethical nature of the study did the Centers for Disease Control and Prevention and the PHS move to end the study. In 1973, the National Association for the Advancement of Colored People (NAACP) won a $10 million class action suit on behalf the subjects. In 1997, President Bill Clinton formally apologized to the few survivors and their families for the harm inflicted on these men and their families in the name of public health research. The Tuskegee Study raises questions about how a study could proceed without informing and seeking consent of participants, how available treatment could be withheld, and how government researchers could pursue an unethical research plan without periodic review and questioning. Furthermore, the racial and discriminatory issues suggest disturbing questions for researchers and practicing nurses to contemplate, one being that Tuskegee contributes to a legacy of distrust that minorities may harbor toward both the health care delivery system and research programs.

From Centers for Disease Control and Prevention, National Center for HIV, STD, and TB Prevention: The Tuskegee timeline, 2005, http://www.cdc.gov/nchstp/od/uskegee/time.htm; Infoplease: The Tuskegee syphilis experiment, 2005, Pearson Education, http://www.infoplease.com/ipa/A0762136.html.

relationship between the presumed causal factors and the effect than do retrospective and cross-sectional studies. Calculations of incidence rates and relative risks provide a valuable indicator of the level of risk that exposure creates.

However, certain disadvantages are inherent in the prospective design. It is costly in terms of resources and staff to monitor a cohort over time, and lengthy studies result in subject attrition. Problems arising from the nature of chronic diseases may compound these logistical dilemmas. Frequently, chronic diseases have long latency periods between exposure and symptom manifestation. Furthermore, the onset of chronic conditions may be sufficiently insidious, which makes it extremely difficult to document the incidence of disease. In addition, many diseases do not have a unifactorial cause (i.e., single variable) because many interacting factors influence disease. These problems do not negate the benefits of prospectively designed epidemiological studies; rather, they suggest a need to carefully plan and tailor the study specifically to the disease and the study's purpose.

The literature contains numerous prospective studies. In many cases, these studies have been instrumental in substantiating causal links between specific risk factors and disease. A classic example is an early Doll and Hill cohort study of lung cancer deaths (1956). Doll and Hill originally completed questionnaires on a cohort of physicians in Great Britain. Next, they classified the subjects according to several variables, emphasizing the number of cigarettes smoked. In $4\frac{1}{2}$ years, they accessed death certificate data. These data revealed a higher mortality rate resulting from lung cancer and coronary thrombosis among smoking physicians compared with nonsmokers. The death rate for heavy smokers was 166 per 100,000 versus 7 per 100,000 for nonsmokers. Combining these two incidence rates in a measure of excess risk indicated that heavy smokers were 23.7 times more likely to develop lung cancer than nonsmokers (relative risk = $\frac{166}{100,000} \div \frac{7}{100,000}$, or 23.7).

These findings in a prospective study provided strong epidemiological support for smoking as a risk factor for lung cancer.

Another well-known prospective study is the Framingham Heart Study, which has followed an essentially healthy cohort of Framingham, Massachusetts, residents for over 50 years. Findings suggest that serum cholesterol level and other risk factors are associated with the future development of cardiovascular disease (Grundy et al., 1998; Kannel et al., 1971). The Framingham Study was one cohort study that formed the basis for later experimental studies aimed at reducing serum cholesterol through diet modification or drug therapy to ultimately lower the incidence rate of coronary heart disease.

The Nurses' Health Study, another continuing longitudinal study, began to follow female registered nurses in 1976. This study monitored nurses' changing health status and risk factors and examined factors associated with the development of numerous health conditions such as breast cancer and heart disease. An analysis of food-frequency data suggested the protective value of whole grain intake on the development of coronary heart disease (Liu et al., 1999). Another report from the Nurses' Health Study suggested that women who walk briskly three or more hours a week experience a reduction in coronary events similar to women who perform regular vigorous exercise (Manson et al., 1999). Sometimes, however, even well-designed epidemiological studies are not confirmed by clinical trials. For example, the Nurses' Health Study suggested that postmenopausal hormone use was associated with a reduction in coronary heart disease (Stampfer et al., 1991). However, in 2001, a randomized clinical trial conducted by the Women's Health Initiative found that postmenopausal hormone use might actually cause an increase in heart

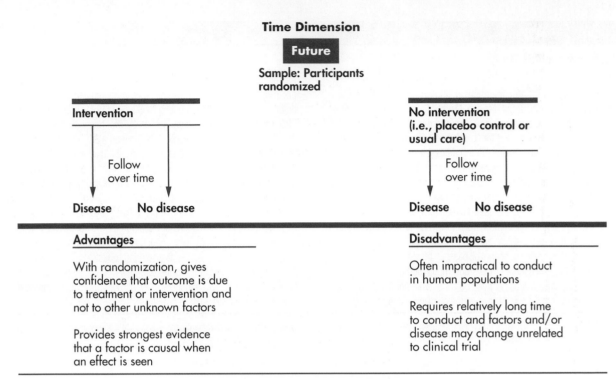

FIGURE 4-8   Experimental, or clinical trial, study.

disease (Writing Group for the Women's Health Initiative, 2002).

Experimental Studies

Another type of analytic study is the experimental design (Figure 4-8). Epidemiological investigations apply experimental methods to test treatment and prevention strategies. The investigator randomly assigns subjects at risk for a particular disease to an experimental or a control group. The investigator observes both groups for the occurrence of disease over time, but only the experimental group receives intervention.

Theoretically, it is possible to introduce an exposure or risk factor as the experimental factor; however, ethical considerations usually prohibit the use of human subjects for these purposes. For example, it is unacceptable to require an experimental group to smoke cigarettes in an experiment; therefore the investigator uses case-control or cohort epidemiological designs. This limitation usually restricts experimental epidemiological studies to prophylactic and therapeutic clinical trials. For example, experimental studies commonly test vaccines and medications for safety and efficacy.

The experimental design is also useful for investigating chronic disease prevention. The Diabetes Prevention Program (DPP) study tested the effect of an intensive behavioral intervention, including both caloric restriction and an increase in physical activity. An average of a 5% weight loss was associated with a 58% reduction in the incidence of type 2 diabetes (DPP Research Group, 2002). The DPP was a primary prevention study, in contrast to the Heart Protection Study, which examined an intervention in subjects with preexisting vascular disease or diabetes. This secondary prevention trial showed that a cholesterol-lowering drug (Simvastatin 40 mg), compared to a placebo, reduced the risk of vascular disease (Heart Protection Study Collaborative Group, 2002). Thus experimental studies help determine which of many preventive programs to implement. Although these studies are medical, experimental designs may help evaluate community health nursing interventions. For example, they may help determine the effectiveness of a sex education program in preventing high rates of teenage pregnancy or the feasibility of an AIDS prevention program among intravenous drug users. For 5 years, nurses participated in a randomized trial of telephone interventions directed toward high-risk prenatal clients. The trial's findings were the impetus for several community-based programs to reduce the incidence or preterm and low-birth-weight babies (Moore, 1999).

SUMMARY

Epidemiology offers the community health nurse methods to quantify the extent of health problems in the community and provides a body of knowledge about risk factors and their association with disease. At each step of the nursing process, epidemiological applications support the practice of the community health nurse. Compiling descriptive data from surveys or studies contributes to understanding the community's health level. In assessing community problems, epidemiological rates describe the magnitude of disease and provide support for community diagnoses. Epidemiological studies suggest interventions and their potential efficacy, information that is useful in planning prevention and intervention approaches. Evaluation studies using epidemiological methods, either reported in literature or conducted by community health nurses, are essential for providing optimal research-based care.

CASE STUDY

Using an Epidemiological and Public Health Approach to Managing a Food-Borne Outbreak

Nurses working in schools, day care centers, camps, and other facilities where food is served must be cognizant of safe food-handling principles. Further, they must be aware of the potential for transmitting disease if proper procedures are not followed. Outbreaks of food-borne illness must be assessed and managed, and often it is the community health nurse who initiates and participates in this process. The following is a scenario in which the nurse utilized the nursing process to analyze and intervene in such an epidemic.

ASSESSMENT

On Wednesday, October 4, the school nurse at Greenly Elementary School saw 8 students who complained of abdominal cramping, diarrhea, and fever. Parents of the sick students were called, and the students were sent home. On Thursday, the nurse was alerted to a large number of absent students. Specifically, 62 students and 10 teachers were absent. Most reported diarrhea symptoms. Because the absentee rate of 10% exceeded the average daily rate of 4% for the 620-student school, and because the nurse determined that the large number of diarrhea cases

suggested an epidemic, the local public health department was notified. Public health officials arrived at the school and began to assess students still at school and those who were recovering at home. Stool cultures were collected and sent to the state laboratory. Results indicated that the organism causing illness was in most cases *Shigella sonnei,* the most commonly found form of the bacteria. Persons with severe symptoms were referred to their physicians for possible antibiotic therapy. Food histories of meals eaten both at school and outside of school were taken.

Friday saw a continuing increase in absenteeism of students and staff reporting gastrointestinal illness. Public health specialists defined the criteria for identifying cases based primarily on positive laboratory results, symptoms of diarrhea or vomiting, fever with nausea or abdominal pain, or all of these. Cafeteria staff were interviewed, and it was determined that one staff member had experienced diarrhea over the previous weekend but had returned to work on Monday. Public health staff continued to take dietary histories on affected and unaffected persons and constructed rates of illness for all foods served in the cafeteria beginning on Friday of the previous week. These data are displayed in the following table.

Number of Exposed by Meal and Food Item (n = 143)

EXPOSURE VARIABLE (FOOD EATEN)	NO. WHO ATE		NO. WHO DID NOT EAT		ODDS RATIO*
	ILL (A)	NOT ILL (B)	ILL (C)	NOT ILL (D)	
Ate on Monday	47	60	18	18	0.78
Ate on Tuesday	63	57	3	20	**7.37**
Fajitas	57	52	8	26	**4.56**
Salad	44	21	24	54	**4.7**
Salsa	26	29	40	48	1.07
Tortillas	48	53	16	26	1.47
Beans	29	32	34	48	1.28
Milk	53	56	11	23	1.98
Ate on Wednesday	21	64	43	15	0.11

*Odds ratios were calculated with the formula: ad ÷ bd.
Modified from Texas Department of Health, *Shigella* outbreak in an elementary school. *Dis Prev News,* 55(6), 1-3, 1995.

From the data, it can be seen that students who ate lunch at school on Tuesday and ate fajitas and salad had higher rates of illness than those who did not. Therefore it was concluded that the outbreak of *Shigella* could be attributed to a food source.

DIAGNOSIS

Determining the likely cause of the outbreak was important in specifying a diagnosis and directing the planning of an intervention. The following diagnosis was formulated:

Increased risk for infectious diarrhea among elementary school children related to inadequate hygiene and food handling practices as evidenced by a 19% increase in reported cases within a 4-day period.

PLANNING

The school nurse, in conjunction with public health specialists, determined that several groups should be targeted in order to eliminate the further spread of disease. They identified a need to assist families in understanding the nature of the disease, how to care for their children who were ill, and how to prevent the spread at home. Within the school, there was a need to review food handling practices and the training that cafeteria workers received. Staff, including teachers, also required information about *Shigella* and how it should be prevented in the everyday lives of students. Needs of special ages and developmental levels of children were also important. A formal plan of what needed to be done, by whom, and when was drawn up. Research into the nature and

Continued

prevention of *Shigella* was gathered from the CDC and the local health department, among other sources. Health department staff developed a plan to release information to the public about the prevention of gastrointestinal illnesses, as many of these diseases are easily spread and so many students were already ill.

Long-Term Goal
• An absence of cases of infectious diarrhea

Short-Term Goals
• Treatment and recovery of all identified cases of diarrhea
• Implementation of an effective program of hygienic practices among students and staff
• Implementation of a food-handler program for all cafeteria workers
• Adequately inform larger community in order to prevent spread of the epidemic

INTERVENTION

The school nurse took a central leadership role directing action within the school aimed at staff, students, and student families. Teaching of appropriate hand washing was stressed. Hand washing supplies and facilities for inspected for soap and running water. Food preparation guidelines were reviewed with staff, and policies regarding remaining at home when ill were reiterated. The health department staff provided technical assistance and made recommendations. They informed community physicians about surveillance and reporting requirements and provided information regarding identifying cases and treatment regimens. Day care centers and preschools were advised to watch for diarrhea outbreaks and to adhere to strict hand washing and diaper handling practices, as these facilities tend to be high risk areas for the transmission of organisms like *Shigella*. The media were contacted to elicit their help in disseminating correct and useful information to the community.

EVALUATION

Immediate evaluation involved monitoring the decline in *Shigella* cases both within the school and in the larger community. The school nurse noted that rates of absenteeism returned to normal on the following Monday. She determined that all classes had had hygiene instruction within the following 2 weeks and that all teachers had received a flyer with specific information about *Shigella*, its care, and prevention. She observed that bathrooms had filled soap dispensers, that a friendly sign reminding students to wash hands was posted near sinks, and that students were given the opportunity to wash hands before lunch and snacks. The public health department, likewise, continued surveillance activities after encouraging physicians to collect and submit stool cultures for suspected cases and to report cases to the health department. Rates of diarrhea declined rapidly in the week after the school outbreak. The infection did not spread to other schools or community groups. This outcome can be attributed to successful epidemic management, yet surveillance remains critical if the public's health is to be protected.

LEVELS OF PREVENTION

Primary
• Teach students and staff about hand washing and hygienic practices.
• Maintain a system that promotes safe food-handling practices.
• Exclude those with symptoms from school or food handling.

Secondary
• Culture all symptomatic individuals.
• Treat those with advanced diarrhea symptoms with antibiotics.
• Exclude those with positive cultures from food handling, and those with symptoms from school.
• Advise families and individuals in the care of those with diarrhea.

Tertiary
• Treat and counsel those determined to be carriers of *Shigella*.

Information on *Shigella* infections available at http://www.cdc.gov/ncidod/dbmd/diseaseinfo/shigellosis_g.htm#What%20is%20shigellosis.

LEARNING ACTIVITIES

1. Compile a database of relevant demographic and epidemiological data for your community by examining census reports, vital statistics reports, city records, and other sources in libraries and agencies.

2. Using numerators from vital statistics and denominators from census data, compute crude death and birth rates for your community.

3. Compare morbidity and mortality rates for your community with those of the state and the nation. Determine whether your community rates are higher

or lower and hypothesize about reasons for any disparities.

4. Consult *Healthy People 2010* to find the national goals for selected causes of morbidity and mortality. Identify groups at an increased risk for these selected diseases. What are the approaches suggested by these documents for reducing the rates of disease? How can this information be useful in planning for your community?

REFERENCES

Buring JE, Lee I-M: Annotation: confounding in epidemiologic research, *Am J Public Health* 85:164-165, 1995.

Burns PG: Reducing infant mortality rates using the perinatal periods of risk model, *Public Health Nurs* 22(1):2-7, 2005.

Centers for Disease Control and Prevention: Neural tube defects in Texas, *Dis Prev News* 58(2):5-6, 1998.

Centers for Disease Control and Prevention: Tuberculosis outbreaks in prison housing units for HIV-infected inmates: California, 1995-1996, *MMWR Morb Mortal Wkly Rep* 48(4):79-82, 1999, The Author, http://www.cdc.gov/nchstp/od/mmwr/tuberculosis_outbreaks_in_prison.htm.

Centers for Disease Control and Prevention: Neural tube defect surveillance and folic acid intervention: Texas-Mexico border, 1993-1998, *MMWR Morb Mortal Wkly Rep* 49(01):1-4, 2000, The Author, http://www.cdc.gov/mmwr/preview/mmwrhtml/mm4901a1.htm.

Centers for Disease Control and Prevention, National Center for Health Statistics: Deaths: preliminary data for 2003, *Nat Vital Stat Rep* 53(15), 2003, The Author, http://www.cdc.gov/nchs/data/nvsr/nvsr53/nvsr53_15.pdf.

Centers for Disease Control and Prevention, National Center for HIV, STD, and TB Prevention: The Tuskegee Timeline, 2005, The Author, http://www.cdc.gov/nchstp/od/tuskegee/time.htm.

Delgado JL et al: Hispanic Health and Nutrition Examination Survey: methodological considerations, *Am J Public Health* 80(suppl):6-10, 1990.

Diabetes Prevention Program Research Group: Reduction in the incidence of type 2 diabetes with lifestyle intervention or metformin, *New Engl J Med* 346(6):393-403, 2002.

Doll R, Hill AB: Study of the aetiology of carcinoma of the lung, *BMJ* 2:1271-1285, 1952.

Doll R, Hill AB: Lung cancer and other causes of death in relation to smoking, *BMJ* 2:1071-1081, 1956.

Executive summary of the third report of the National Cholesterol Education Program (NCEP) Expert panel on detection, evaluation, and treatment of high blood cholesterol in adults (Adult Treatment Panel III), *JAMA* 285:2486-2497, 2001.

Ford ES, Giles WH, Dietz: Prevalence of the metabolic syndrome among US adults: findings from the Third National Health and Nutrition Examination Survey. *JAMA* 287:356-359, 2002.

Friedman GD: *Primer of epidemiology,* ed 4, New York, 1994, McGraw-Hill.

Grundy SM et al: Primary prevention of coronary heart disease: guidance from Framingham: a statement for healthcare professionals from the AHA Task Force on Risk Reduction, *Circulation* 97(18):1876-1887, 1998.

Harkness G: *Epidemiology in nursing practice,* St. Louis, 1995, Mosby.

Heart Protection Study Collaborative Group: MRC/BHF Heart Protection Study of cholesterol lowering with simvastatin in 20,536 high-risk individuals: a randomized placebo-controlled trial, *Lancet* 360:7-22, 2002.

Infoplease. *The Tuskegee Syphilis Experiment,* 2005, Pearson Education, http://www.infoplease.com/ipa/A0762136.html.

Lorion, RP: Exposure to urban violence: shifting from an individual to an ecological perspective. In Schneiderman N et al, editor: *Integrating behavioral and social science with public health,* Washington, DC, 2001, American Psychological Association.

Kannel WB et al: Serum cholesterol, lipoproteins and the risk of coronary heart disease: The Framingham Study, *Ann Intern Med* 74:1-12, 1971.

Lilienfeld DE, Stoley PD: *Foundations of epidemiology,* New York, 1994, Oxford University Press.

Liu S et al: Whole-grain consumption and risk of coronary heart disease: results from the Nurses' Health Study, *Am J Clin Nutr* 70:412-419, 1999.

MacDonald, MA: From miasma to fractals: the epidemiology revolution and public health nursing, *Public Health Nurs* 21:380-391, 2004.

Manson JE et al: A prospective study of walking as compared with vigorous exercise in the prevention of coronary heart disease in women, *N Engl J Med* 341(9):650-658, 1999.

Mattson ME, Pollack ES, Cullen JW: What are the odds that smoking will kill you? *Am J Public Health* 77:425-431, 1987.

Mausner JS, Kramer S: *Mausner and Bahn epidemiology: an introductory text,* ed 2, Philadelphia, 1985, WB Saunders.

Milio N: A framework for prevention: changing health-damaging to health-generating life patterns, *Am J Public Health* 66:435-439, 1976.

Moore ML: From randomized trial to community-focused practice, *Image J Nurs Sch* 31(4):349-354, 1999.

Morton RF, Hebel JR, McCarter RJ: *A study guide to epidemiology and biostatistics,* ed 3, Gaithersburg, Md, 1990, Aspen Publishers.

National Cancer Institute: Surveillance, epidemiology and end results, 2005, The Author, http://seer.cancer.gov/about/.

National Center for Health Statistics: Health, United States, 2004, The Author, http://www.cdc.gov/nchs/data/hus/hus04trend.pdf#022.

Rubenstein L et al: Effectiveness of a geriatric evaluation unit, *N Engl J Med* 311:1664-1670, 1984.

Simoes EJ et al: The association between leisure-time physical activity and dietary fat in American adults, *Am J Public Health* 85:240-244, 1995.

Snow J: *On the mode of communication of cholera,* ed 2, London, 1855, Churchill. Reproduced in *Snow on cholera,* New York, 1936, Commonwealth Fund.

Stampfer MJ et al: Postmenopausal estrogen therapy and cardiovascular disease: ten-year follow-up from the Nurses' Health Study, *N Engl J Med* 325(11):756-762, 1991.

Texas Department of Health, *Shigella* outbreak in an elementary school. *Dis Prev News,* 55(6): 1-3, 1995.

US Department of Health and Human Services: *Healthy people 2010,* Conference edition, Washington DC, 2000, US Government Printing Office.

Willett W: Diet and coronary heart disease. In Willett W, editor: *Nutritional epidemiology,* New York, 1990, Oxford University Press.

Writing Group for the Women's Health Initiative Investigators: Risks and benefits of estrogen plus progestin in healthy postmenopausal women: principal results from the Women's Health Initiative randomized controlled trial, *JAMA* 288:321-333, 2002.

Community Assessment

Holly Cassells

OBJECTIVES

Upon completion of this chapter, the reader will be able to do the following:

1. Discuss the major dimensions of a community.
2. Identify sources of information about a community's health.
3. Describe the process of conducting a community assessment.
4. Formulate community and aggregate diagnoses.
5. Identify uses for epidemiological data at each step of the nursing process.

KEY TERMS

aggregate
census tracts
community diagnosis

community of solution
Healthy Cities and Healthy
    Communities

metropolitan statistical areas
needs assessment
social system

vital statistics
windshield survey

CHAPTER OUTLINE

THE NATURE OF COMMUNITY
    Aggregate of People
    Location in Space and Time
    Social System

HEALTHY COMMUNITIES

ASSESSING THE COMMUNITY: SOURCES OF DATA
    Census Data
    Vital Statistics
    Other Sources of Health Data

NEEDS ASSESSMENT

DIAGNOSING HEALTH PROBLEMS

The primary concern of community health nurses is to improve the health of the community. To address this concern, community health nurses use all the principles and skills of nursing and public health practice. This involves using demographic and epidemiological methods to assess the community's health and diagnose its health needs.

Before beginning this process, the community health nurse must define the community. The nurse may wonder how he or she can provide services to such a large and nontraditional "client," but there are smaller and more circumscribed entities that comprise a community than towns and cities. A major aspect of public health practice is the application of

approaches and solutions to health problems that ensure the majority of people receive the maximum benefit. To this end, the nurse works to use time and resources efficiently.

Despite the desire to provide services to each individual in a community, the community health nurse recognizes the impracticality of this task. An alternative approach considers the community itself to be the unit of service, and works collaboratively with the community using the steps of the nursing process. Therefore, the community is not only the context or place where community health nursing occurs; it is the focus of community health nursing care. The nurse partners with community members to identify community problems and develop solutions to ultimately improve the community's health.

Another central goal of public health practitioners is primary prevention, which protects the public's health and prevents disease development. Chapter 3 discussed how these "upstream efforts" are intended to reduce the pain, suffering, and huge expenditures that occur when significant segments of the population essentially "fall into the river" and require downstream resources to resolve their health problems. In a society greatly concerned about increasingly high health care costs, the need to prevent health problems becomes dire. In addition to reducing the occurrence of disease in individuals, community health nurses must examine the larger aggregate—its structures, environments, and shared health risks—to develop improved upstream prevention programs.

This chapter addresses the first steps in adopting a community- or population-oriented practice. A community health nurse must define a community and describe its characteristics before applying the nursing process. Then, the nurse can launch the assessment and diagnosis phase of the nursing process at the aggregate level and incorporate epidemiological approaches. Comprehensive assessment data are essential to directing effective primary prevention interventions within a community.

Gathering these data is one of the core public health functions identified in the Institute of Medicine's (1988) report on the future of public health. The community health nurse participates in assessing the community's health and its ability to deal with health needs. With sound data, the nurse makes a valuable contribution to health policy development (Keppel, 1995).

THE NATURE OF COMMUNITY

Many dimensions describe the nature of community. These include an aggregate of people, a location in space and time, and a social system (Box 5-1).

Aggregate of People

An **aggregate** is a community composed of people who share common characteristics. For example, members of a community may share residence in the same city, membership in the same religious organization, or similar demographic characteristics such as age or ethnic background. The aggregate of senior citizens, for example, comprises primarily retirees who frequently share common ages, economic pressures, life experiences, interests, and concerns. This group lived through the many societal changes of the past 50 years; therefore, they may possess similar perspectives on current issues and trends. Many elderly people share concern for the maintenance of good health, the pursuit of an active lifestyle, and the security of needed services to support a quality life. These shared interests translate into common goals and activities, which also are defining attributes of a community. Communities also may consist of overlapping aggregates, in which case some community members belong to multiple aggregates.

Many human factors help delineate a community. Health-

BOX 5-1   Major Features of a Community

➤ Aggregate of people
 The "who": personal characteristics and risks
➤ Location in space and time
 The "where" and "when": physical location frequently delineated by boundaries and influenced by the passage of time
➤ Social system
 The "why" and "how": interrelationships of aggregates fulfilling community functions

---

related traits, or *risk factors,* are one aspect of "people factors" to be considered. People who have impaired health or a shared predisposition to disease may join together in a group, or community, to learn from and support each other. Parents of disabled infants, people with AIDS, or those at risk for a second myocardial infarction may consider themselves a community. Even when these individuals are not organized, the nurse may recognize that their unique needs constitute a form of community, or aggregate.

A **community of solution** may form when a common problem unites individuals. Although people may have little else in common with each other, their desire to redress problems brings them together. Such problems may include a shared hazard from environmental contamination, a shared health problem arising from a soaring rate of teenage suicide, or a shared political concern about an upcoming city council election. The community of solution often disbands after problem resolution, but it may subsequently identify other common issues.

Each of these shared features may exist among people who are geographically dispersed or in close proximity to each other. However, in many situations, proximity facilitates the recognition of commonality and the development of cohesion among members. This active sharing of features fosters a sense of community among individuals.

Location in Space and Time
Regardless of shared features, geographical or physical location may define communities of people. Traditionally, community is an entity delineated by geopolitical boundaries; this view best exemplifies the dimension of location. These boundaries demarcate the periphery of cities, counties, states, and nations. Voting precincts, school districts, water districts, and fire and police protection precincts set less visible boundary lines.

Census tracts subdivide larger communities. The U.S. Census Bureau uses them for data collection and population assessment. Census tracts facilitate the organization of resident information in specific community geographical locales. In densely populated urban areas, the size of tracts tends to be small; therefore, data for one or more census tracts frequently describe neighborhood residents. Although residents may not be aware of their census tract's boundaries, census tract data help define and describe neighborhood communities.

The geographical dimension encompasses less formalized types of community that lack official geopolitical boundaries.

Geographical Mapping of Unmarried Teen Births and Selected Sociodemographic Variables

Approximately one million teenagers in the United States become pregnant each year, and 80% of these teens will not be married at the time of their child's birth. Despite the recent declines in unmarried teen birth rates, there has been an increase in the proportion of births to unmarried teens. The rise in nonmarital births becomes a social concern if it contributes to adverse consequences for the teen mothers and their children.

The purpose of this retrospective exploratory study was to analyze and map sociodemographic variables associated with unmarried teen childbirth. It was hypothesized that selected sociodemographic variables would be related to the unmarried teen birth rates. Texas is one of five states in the United States in which teen pregnancies exceed 70 per 1000 females aged 15 to 17 years. Correlational analysis was employed to ascertain the relationship between the sociodemographic variables and the unmarried

teen birth rates for 81 zip codes in Dallas County, Texas. The births occurred between January 1, 1995, and December 31, 1996.

Geographic Information System (GIS) software was used to map the unmarried teen birth rates and the demographic variables. The maps illustrated the spatial distribution of the unmarried teen birth rates in conjunction with sociodemographic variables extracted from the 1990 U.S. Census Bureau. The results indicate that unmarried teen births are positively related to low socioeconomic status, single-parent households, and minority populations. Mapping supports the quantitative relationships between the variables. Maps can be used to identify communities where teens most vulnerable to unmarried pregnancy and childbirth reside and provide policy makers with explicit information about their constituents so that they can develop and implement population-specific interventions.

Blake BJ, Bentov L: Geographical mapping of unmarried teen births and selected sociodemographic variables, *Public Health Nursing* 18(1):33-39, 2001.

A geographical landmark may define neighborhoods (e.g., the East Lake section of town or the North Shore area). A particular building style or a common development era also may identify community neighborhoods. Similarly, a dormitory, a communal home, or a summer camp may be a community because each facility shares a close geographical proximity. Geographical location, including the urban or rural nature of a community, strongly influences the nature of the health problems a community health nurse might find there. Public health is increasingly recognizing that the interaction of humans with the natural environment and with constructed environments, consisting of buildings and spaces for example, is critical to healthy behavior and quality of life.

Location and the dimension of time define communities. The community's character and health problems evolve over time. Although some communities are very stable, most tend to change with the members' health status and demographics and the larger community's development or decline. For example, the presence of an emerging young workforce may attract new industry, which can alter a neighborhood's health and environment. A community's history illustrates its ability to change and how well it addresses health problems over time.

Social System

The third major feature of a community is the relationships that community members form with each other. Community members fulfill the essential functions of community by interacting in groups. These functions provide socialization, role fulfillment, goal achievement, and member support. Therefore, a community is a complex **social system,** and its interacting members comprise various subsystems within the community. These subsystems are interrelated and interdependent (i.e., the subsystems affect each other and affect various internal and external stimuli). These stimuli consist of a broad range of events, values, conditions, and needs.

A health care system is an example of a complex system that consists of smaller, interrelated subsystems. A health

care system can also be a subsystem because it interacts and depends on larger systems like the city government. Changes in the larger system can cause repercussions in many subsystems. For example, when local economic pressures cause a health department to scale back its operations, this affects many subsystems. The health department may eliminate or reduce programs, limit service to other health care providers, reduce access to groups that normally use the system, and deny needed care to families who constitute subsystems in society. Almost every subsystem in the community must react and readjust to such a financial constraint.

Example of Systems Interrelationships

Health problems can have a severe impact on multiple systems. For example, the AIDS (acquired immunodeficiency syndome) epidemic has required significant funds for AIDS clients and public AIDS education and prevention. It has made unrelenting demands on many communities that are already strapped for funds to meet its citizens' basic health needs. In San Francisco, the allocation of funds for AIDS programs has reduced funding for other programs, such as immunizations, family planning, and well-child care. ■

HEALTHY COMMUNITIES

Complex community systems receive many varied stimuli. The community's ability to respond effectively to changing dynamics and meet the needs of its members indicates productive functioning. Examining the community's functions and subsystems provides clues to existing and potential health problems. Examples of a community's functions include the provision of accessible and acceptable health services, educational opportunities, and safe, crime-free environments.

The model in Figure 5-1 suggests assessment dimensions that can help a nurse develop a more complete list of critical community functions. The community health nurse can then prioritize these functions from a particular community's perspective. For example, a study of Americans' views on

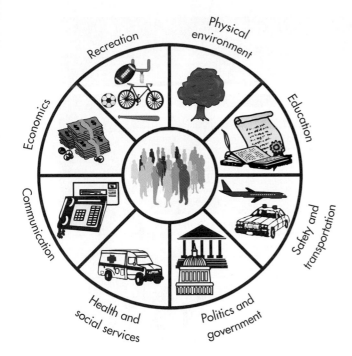

FIGURE 5-1 Diagram of assessment parameters. (From Anderson FT, McFarlane JM: *Community as partner: theory and practice in nursing,* ed 3, Philadelphia, 2000, Lippincott Williams & Wilkins.)

health and healthy communities, conducted for the Healthcare Forum, suggested that the public is more concerned with quality of life issues than the absence of disease. Figure 5-2 indicates that the most important determinants of a healthy community are low crime rates and a child-friendly neighborhood environment (Healthcare Forum, 1994).

The movement called **Healthy Cities and Healthy Communities** helps community members bring about positive health changes. It stresses that interconnectedness among people and among public and private sectors is essential for a community to address the causes of poor health (Flynn, 1992). However, each community and aggregate presumably will have a unique perspective on critical health qualities. Indeed, a community or aggregate may have a divergent definition of health from that of the community health nurse.

ASSESSING THE COMMUNITY: SOURCES OF DATA

The community health nurse becomes familiar with the community and begins to understand its nature by traveling through the area. The nurse begins to establish certain hunches or hypotheses about the community's health, strengths, and potential health problems through this down-to-earth approach, called "shoe leather epidemiology." The community health nurse must substantiate these initial assessments and impressions with more concrete or defined data before he or she can formulate a community diagnosis and plan.

Community health nurses often perform a community **windshield survey** by driving or walking through an area

and making organized observations. The nurse can gain an understanding of the environmental layout, including geographical features, the location of agencies, services, businesses, and industries, and can locate possible areas of environmental concern through "sight, sense, and sound." The windshield survey offers the nurse an opportunity to observe people and their role in the community. Box 5-2 provides examples of a windshield survey assessment. See illustrations depicting an actual "windshield survey" on p. 80.

In addition to direct observational methods, certain public health tools become essential to an aggregate-focused nursing practice. The analysis of demographic information and statistical data provides descriptive information about the population. Epidemiology involves the analysis of these data to discover the patterns of health and illness distribution in a population. Epidemiology also involves conducting research to explain the nature of health problems and identify the aggregates at increased risk. The rest of this section provides data sources and describes how the community health nurse can use demographic and epidemiological data to assess the aggregate.

Census Data

Every 10 years, the U.S. Census Bureau undertakes a massive survey of all American families. In addition to this decennial census, intermediate surveys collect specific types of information. These collections of statistical data describe the population characteristics of the nation within progressively smaller geopolitical entities (e.g., states, counties, and census tracts). The census also describes large metropolitan areas that extend beyond formal city boundaries, called **metropolitan statistical areas.** These areas consist of a central city with more than 50,000 people and include the associated suburban or adjacent counties, which yields a total metropolitan area with more than 100,000 people. Cities and their associated counties with a population of one million or more constitute consolidated statistical areas. A census tract is one of the smallest reporting units. It usually consists of 3000 to 6000 people who share similar characteristics such as ethnicity, socioeconomic status, or housing class.

The census is extremely helpful to community health nurses familiarizing themselves with a new community. The census tabulates many demographic variables including population size, socioeconomic status, housing characteristics, and the distribution of age, sex, race, and ethnicity. Variables that describe the community's health are not part of census data. However, census numbers can be denominators for morbidity and mortality rates (see the Calculation of Rates section in Chapter 4). Public and university libraries generally maintain census data and all data following the 1990 census are available on CD-ROM or on the Internet at www.census.gov. Computerization of the data allows the nurse to view several variables in combination (e.g., age and ethnicity) and easily construct a community profile.

The nurse analyzes and interprets data by comparing current and local census data with previous data and information from various locations. The nurse can identify the attributes that make each community unique by

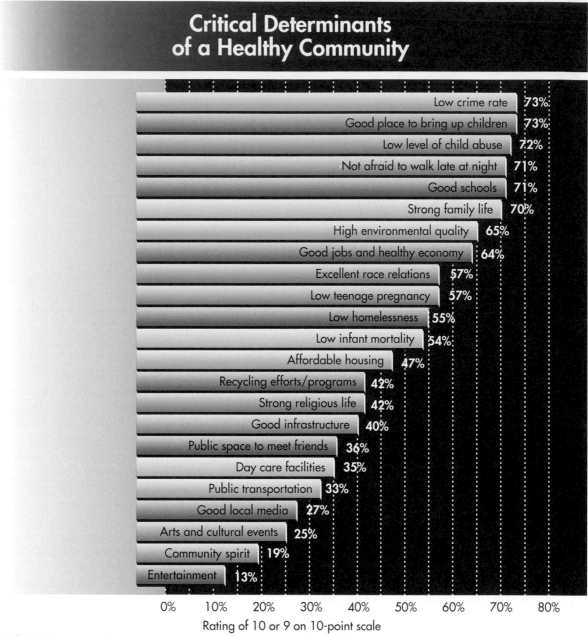

Critical Determinants of a Healthy Community

Determinant	Rating
Low crime rate	73%
Good place to bring up children	73%
Low level of child abuse	72%
Not afraid to walk late at night	71%
Good schools	71%
Strong family life	70%
High environmental quality	65%
Good jobs and healthy economy	64%
Excellent race relations	57%
Low teenage pregnancy	57%
Low homelessness	55%
Low infant mortality	54%
Affordable housing	47%
Recycling efforts/programs	42%
Strong religious life	42%
Good infrastructure	40%
Public space to meet friends	36%
Day care facilities	35%
Public transportation	33%
Good local media	27%
Arts and cultural events	25%
Community spirit	19%
Entertainment	13%

Rating of 10 or 9 on 10-point scale

FIGURE 5-2   What makes a healthy community. (From Healthcare Forum: *What creates health? Individuals and communities respond,* A national study conducted by DYG, Inc., for the Healthcare Forum, San Francisco, 1994, The Author.)

comparing data for one census unit, such as a census tract or a city, with those of another community or the entire nation. These attributes provide clues to the community's potential vulnerabilities or health risks. For example, a community health nurse may review census reports and discover that a district has many elderly people. This directs the nurse toward further assessment of the social resources (i.e., housing, transportation, and community centers), health resources (i.e., hospitals, nursing homes, and geriatric clinics), and health problems common to aging people. By identifying the trends in the population over time, the community health nurse can modify public health programs to meet the changing needs of the community.

Vital Statistics

The official registration records of births, deaths, marriages, divorces, and adoptions form the basis of data in **vital statistics.** Every year, city, county, and state health departments aggregate and report these events for the preceding year. When compared with previous years, vital statistics provide indicators of population growth or reduction. In addition to supplying information about the number of births and deaths, registration certificates record the cause of death, which is useful in determining morbidity and mortality trends. Similarly, birth certificates document birth information (e.g., cesarean delivery and teen mothers) and the occurrence of any congenital malformations. This

BOX 5-2 Questions to Guide Community Observations During a Windshield Survey

1. Community Vitality
   - Are people visible in the community? What are they doing?
   - Who are the people living in the neighborhood? What is their age range? What is the predominant age (e.g., elderly, preschoolers, young mothers, or school age children)?
   - What ethnicity or race is most common?
   - What is the general appearance of those you observed? Do they appear healthy? Do you notice any obvious disabilities, such as those with walkers or wheelchairs, or those with mental or emotional disabilities? Where do they live?
   - Do you notice residents who are well nourished or malnourished, thin or obese, vigorous or frail, unkempt or scantily dressed, or well dressed and clean?
   - Do you notice tourists or visitors to the community?
   - Do you observe any people who appear to be under the influence of drugs or alcohol?
   - Do you see any pregnant women? Do you see women with strollers and young children?

2. Indicators of Social and Economic Conditions
   - What is the general condition of the homes you observe? Are these single-family homes or multifamily structures? Is there any evidence of dilapidated housing or of areas undergoing urban renewal? What forms of transportation do people seem to be using? Is there public transit? Are there adequate bus stops with benches and shade? Is transportation to health care resources available?
   - Is there public housing? What is its condition?
   - Are there any indicators of the kinds of work available to residents? Are there job opportunities nearby, such as factories, small businesses, or military installations? Are there unemployed people visible, such as homeless people?
   - Do you see men congregating in groups on the street? What do they look like and what are they doing?
   - Is this a rural area? Are there farms or agricultural businesses?
   - Do you note any seasonal workers, such as migrant or day laborers?
   - Do you see any women hanging out along the streets? What are they doing?
   - Do you observe any children or adolescents out of school during the daytime?
   - Do you observe any interest in political campaigns or issues, such as campaign signs?
   - Do you see any evidence of health education on billboards, advertisements, signs, radio stations, or television stations? Do these methods seem appropriate for the people you observed?
   - What kinds of schools and day care centers are available?

3. Health Resources
   - Do you notice any hospitals? What kind are they? Where are they located?
   - Are there any clinics? Whom do they serve? Are there any family planning services?
   - Are there doctors and dentists offices? Are they specialists or generalists?
   - Do you notice any nursing homes, rehabilitation centers, mental health clinics, alcohol or drug treatment centers, homeless or abused shelters, wellness clinics, health department facilities, family planning services, or pharmacies?
   - Are these resources appropriate and sufficient to address the kinds of problems that exist in this community?

4. Environmental Conditions Related to Health
   - Do you see evidence of anything that might make you suspicious of ground, water, or air pollutants?
   - What is the sanitary condition of the housing? Is housing overcrowded, dirty, or in need of repair? Are windows screened?
   - What is the condition of the roads? Are potholes present? Are drainage systems in place? Are there low water crossings, and do they have warning signals? Are there adequate traffic lights, signs, sidewalks, and curbs? Are railroad crossings fitted with warnings and barriers? Are streets and parking lots well lit? Is this a heavily trafficked area, or are roads rural? Are there curves or features that make the roads hazardous?
   - Is there handicapped access to buildings, sidewalks, and streets?
   - Do you observe recreational facilities and playgrounds? Are they being used? Is there a YMCA or community center? Are there any day care facilities or preschools?
   - Are children playing in the streets, alleys, yards, or parks?
   - Do you see any restaurants?
   - Is food sold on the streets? Are people eating in public areas? Are there trash receptacles and places for people to sit? Are public restrooms available?
   - What evidence of any nuisances such as ants, flies, mosquitoes, or rodents do you observe?

5. Social Functioning
   - Do you observe any families in the neighborhoods? Can you observe their structure or functioning? Who is caring for the children? What kind of supervision do they have? Is more than one generation present?
   - Are there any identifiable subgroups related to each other either socially or geographically?
   - What evidence of a sense of neighborliness can you observe?
   - What evidence of community cohesiveness can you observe? Are there any group efforts in the neighborhood to improve the living conditions or the neighborhood? Is there a neighborhood watch? Do community groups post signs for neighborhood meetings?
   - How many and what type of churches, synagogues, or places of worship are there?
   - Can you observe anything that would make you suspicious of social problems such as gang activity, juvenile delinquency, drug or alcohol abuse, or adolescent pregnancy?

6. Attitude Toward Health and Health Care
   - Do you observe any evidence of folk medicine practice, such as a botanical or herbal medicine shop? Are there any alternative medicine practitioners?
   - Do you observe that health resources are well utilized or underutilized?
   - Is there evidence of preventive or wellness care?
   - Do you observe any efforts to improve the neighborhood's health? Do you notice any health fairs? Do you see advertisements for health-related events, clinics, or lectures?

Bookshire is a town of about 3,500 in Southeast Texas.

The economy of the town is predominaely agriculture and processing.

Sugar mills and farms are the source of most jobs.

The car's thermometer shows 99 degress, evidence of a pervasive health threat in the summertime.

Accessible and affordable health care is a challenge. This van provides services to unskilled workers and area elders.

Much of the housing is substandard and suggests low-income families.

Many people live in small homes on multiple acre lots.

ETHICAL Insights

Attending to Nondominant Trends: "Hidden Pockets" of Need

Whereas most public health practitioners are attuned to the leading indicators or dominant trends in data, vital statistics or census data can suggest the existence of small "hidden pockets" of people with special needs. One nurse initially assessed her community as in an upper-middle-class bracket. She was surprised to find 20 families living below the poverty level and 3 families living without running water. Although these 20 families made up far less than 1% of the community population, they nevertheless necessitated the attention of the community health nurse. Some may view a focus on such a minority segment as insignificant and in conflict with the "Rule of Utility," which posits "the greatest good for the greatest number." However, community health nursing practice combines principles of beneficence and social justice with utilitarianism, and thus small vulnerable segments of the community are considered legitimate clients of community health nursing. Indeed, social justice not only "gives moral privilege to the needs of the most vulnerable" but also suggests the amelioration of conditions that create social and economic disparities (Boutain, 2005). Furthermore, nurses recognize that this "hidden pocket" is a small piece of the total community and, as such, contributes to its overall health. By attending to these families' health needs, the health of the whole is positively affected.

information also is important in assessing the community health status.

Other Sources of Health Data

The U.S. Census Bureau conducts numerous surveys on subjects of government interest such as crime, housing, and labor. Results of these surveys, the census reports, and vital statistics reports are usually available through public libraries and on the Internet. The National Center for Health Statistics (NCHS) compiles annual National Health Survey data, which describe health trends in a national sample. The NCHS publishes reports on the prevalence of disability, illness, and other health-related variables. Specifically, the Behavioral Risk Factor Surveillance System is the world's largest telephone survey of U.S. citizens' health behaviors and risk factors. It tracks trends by nation, state, and year, with the goal of identifying emerging health problems. Data also are used to evaluate achievement of health objectives and develop prevention strategies. A user-friendly Web site allows one to compile graphs and maps to describe specific risk behaviors by state. See the book's Evolve website at http://evolve.elsevier.com/Nies.

In addition to accessing these important sources of information, community health nurses also can access a broad range of local, regional, and state government reports that contribute to the comprehensive assessment of a population. Local agencies, chambers of commerce, and health and hospital districts collect invaluable information on their community's health. Local health planning agencies also compile and analyze statistical data during the planning process. The community health nurse can use all of these formal and informal resources in learning about a community or aggregate (Table 5-1). Box 5-3 lists additional information about sources of population health data.

Formal data collection does not exist for all community aspects; therefore many community health nurses must perform additional data collection, compilation, and analysis. For example, school nurses regularly use aggregate data from student records to learn about the demographic composition of their population. They conduct ongoing surveys of classroom attendance and causes of illness, which are essential to an effective school health program. Sometimes the nurse must screen the entire school population to discover the extent of a disease. Thus the school nurse is both a consumer of existent data and a researcher who collects new data for the assessment of the school community.

NEEDS ASSESSMENT

The nurse must understand the community's perspective on health status, the services used or required, and concerns. Most official data do not capture this type of information. Data collected directly from an aggregate may be more insightful and accurate; therefore community health nurses sometimes conduct community needs assessments. There are several approaches to gathering subjective data; however, a nurse's careful planning of the process will contribute to its reliability and utility regardless of the method. Box 5-4 presents the required steps in conducting a **needs assessment.**

Selecting a strategy for collecting needs assessment data is dependent upon the size and nature of the aggregate, the purpose for collecting information, and the resources available to the nurse. In some cases, the nurse may survey a small sample of clients to measure their satisfaction with a program. In other situations, a large-scale community needs assessment may help the nurse determine gaps in service. Although the process of needs assessment can indicate a program's strengths and weaknesses, it can also raise expectations for new services on the part of community members (Timmreck, 1995).

A first approach to gathering data is to interview key *community informants.* These may be knowledgeable residents, elected officials, or health care providers. It is essential that the community health nurse recognize that the views of these people may not reflect the views of all residents. A second approach is to hold a *community forum* to discuss selected questions. It is important for the nurse to carefully plan the meeting in advance to gain the most useful information. The community health nurse can also mail surveys to community members to elicit information from a more diverse group of people who may be unwilling or unable to attend a community forum. *Focus groups* are a third approach; these can be very effective in gathering community views, particularly for remote and vulnerable segments of a community and for those with underdeveloped opinions (Hildebrandt, 1999). Nurses who conduct focus groups must carefully select participants, formulate questions, and analyze recorded sessions. These sessions can produce greater interaction and expression of ideas than surveys and may provide more insight into an aggregate's opinions. In addition to encouraging community participation in the identification of

TABLE 5-1   Community Assessment Parameters

PARAMETERS	IMPORTANCE TO CHN	SOURCE OF INFORMATION
Geography Topography Climate (e.g., extreme heat or cold)	Influences nature of health problems and access to health care	Almanac Chamber of Commerce
Population Size Demographic character (e.g., aged or young) Trends Migration Density	Describes population served; suggests their health risks and needs Suggests growth or decline Increases stress; may increase exposure to communicable disease	Census documents Chamber of Commerce Local documents
Environment Water (e.g., source; fluoridated) Sewage and waste disposal Air quality (e.g., ozone; pollutants) Food quality and access Housing (e.g., single-family or multifamily dwellings) Animal control (e.g., exposure to rabies and other zoonotic diseases)	Affects quality of life and nature of environmental health problems Reflects community resources Suggests socioeconomic issues	Local and state health departments Newspapers Local environmental action group Census documents
Industry Employment levels Manufacturing White vs. blue collar Income levels	Affects social class, access to health care, and resources Influences nature of health problems	Chamber of Commerce Almanac Employment commission Census documents
Education Schools (e.g., physical plant; playground safety) Types of education Literacy rates Special education Health services Sex education School lunch programs (e.g., nutritious diets) After-school programs Day care Access to higher education	Influences socioeconomic status, access to health care, and ability to read and understand health information	Census documents School districts and nurse
Recreation Parks and playgrounds Libraries Public and private recreation Special facilities	Reflects quality of life, resources available to community, and concern for the young and disadvantaged	Parks and recreation departments Newspapers
Religion Churches and synagogues Denominations Community programs Health-related programs and parish health programs Community organizations	Influences values in community by organizing common interests and concerns Reflects involvement of members, community skills, and resources for community needs	Chamber of Commerce Newspapers Community center newsletters
Communication Newspapers Neighborhood news Radio and television Telephone Hotlines Medical media Public services announcements	Reflects concerns and needs of the community Networks and resources available for health-related use	Local libraries Newspapers Local health department Medical and nursing society
Transportation Intercity and intracity Handicapped Emergency transport	Affects access to services, food, and other resources Reflects resources available to community	Local bus and train service Local hospital emergency service
Public services Fire protection Police protection Emergency medical services Rape treatment centers Utilities	Affects community security Reflects available resources	Local police department

TABLE 5-1   Community Assessment Parameters (*cont'd*)

PARAMETERS	IMPORTANCE TO CHN	SOURCE OF INFORMATION
Political organization Structure Method for filing positions Responsibilities of positions Sources of revenue Voter registration	Reflects level of citizen activism, involvement, values, and concerns Mechanism for nurse activism and lobbying	Newspapers Local political party organization Local board of elections Local representatives
Community development or planning Activities Major issues	Reflects community needs and concerns Affect level of professionals' involvement in issues	Newspapers Local and state planning board Local community organizations
Disaster programs American Red Cross Disaster plans Potential sources of disaster	Offers a level of preparedness, coordination, and available resources Influences resources and plans	Local American Red Cross office Local emergency coordinating council Local fire department
Health statistics Mortality Morbidity Leading causes of death Births	Reflects health problems, trends, and state of community health Affects resources needed and CHN services provided	Local and state health department Health facilities and programs National vital statistics reports NCHS reports *MMWR*
Social problems Mental health Alcoholism and drug abuse Suicide Crime School dropout Unemployment Gangs	Affects health problems and amounts of required services Influences CHN program priorities	Local and state department of social services Local mental health centers Local hotlines Libraries
Health manpower Number of physicians, dentists, and nurses per population	Influences available health resources and nature of CHN practice	Local and state health planning agency Health professioal organizations Telephone directory Community service directory
Health professional organizations	Provides support for CHN practice	
Community services (e.g., cost and eligibility, accessibility, and acceptability) Institutional care (e.g., hospitals and nursing homes) Mental health care Ambulatory care Preventive health services Nursing services Welfare services	Reflect available resources	Local United Way organization Local voluntary service directory County hospital Local health department Telephone directory

CHN, Community health nursing.

assets and needs, focus groups may lay the groundwork for community involvement in planning the solutions to identified problems (Clark et al., 2003).

DIAGNOSING HEALTH PROBLEMS

The next step of the nursing process is synthesizing assessment data into diagnostic statements about the community's health. These statements specify the nature and cause of the actual or potential community health problem and direct the community health nurses' plans to resolve the problem. Muecke (1984) developed a format that assists in writing a **community diagnosis.** The diagnosis consists of four components: the identification of the health problem or risk,

the affected aggregate or community, the etiological or causal statement, and the evidence or support for the diagnosis (Figure 5-3). Each of these components has an important role to play in the nursing process. The problem represents a synthesis of all assessment data. The "among" phrase specifies the aggregate that will be the beneficiary of the nurse's action plan, and whose health is at risk. The "related to" phrase describes the cause of the health problem and directs the focus of the intervention. All plans and interventions will be aimed at addressing this underlying cause. Lastly, the health indicators are the supporting data, drawn from the completed assessment.

With a clear statement of problem in the form of a diagnosis, the community health nurse is ready to begin the planning phase of the nursing process. Inherent in this phase is

---

BOX 5-3 Retrieval of Data

Current data on U.S. population health are stored in many places. Finding the latest statistics at the local, state, or national level can be a challenging experience for a student, community health nurse, graduate student, or nurse researcher. However, statistics provide a necessary comparison in identifying the health status of an aggregate or population in a community. The following guidelines suggest places to begin a search.

Visit the book's Evolve Web site at http://evolve.elsevier.com/Nies to obtain contact information for the specific agencies listed below.

➤ *Reference librarian:* The best place to start is in a school or community library or in a large university's health sciences library. Cultivate a relationship with the reference librarian and learn how to access the literature of interest (e.g., government documents) or how to perform computer-guided literature searches.

➤ *Government documents:* Local libraries have a listing of government depository libraries, which house government documents for the public. If the government document is not available at a local library, ask the reference librarian to contact a regional or state library for an interlibrary loan. The Library of Congress in Washington, DC, has a Directory of United States Government Depository Libraries.

➤ *Health: United States, 2005:* This is an annual publication of the NCHS (2005), which reports the latest health statistics for the United States. It presents statistics in areas such as maternal-child health indicators (e.g., prenatal care, low birthweight, and infant mortality), life expectancy, mortality, morbidity (e.g., cancer incidence and survival, AIDS, and diabetes), environmental health

indicators (e.g., air pollution and noise exposure), and health system use (e.g., national health expenditures, health insurance coverage, physician contacts, and diagnostic and surgical procedures). Graphs and tables are easy to read and interpret with accompanying texts. Many statistics include a selected number of years to illustrate trends. Some statistics compare themselves with other countries and U.S. minority populations.

➤ *Morbidity and Mortality Weekly Report (MMWR):* The Centers for Disease Control and Prevention (CDC) in Atlanta, Georgia, prepares this publication. State health departments compile weekly reports for the publication, which outline the numbers of cases of notifiable diseases such as AIDS, gonorrhea, hepatitis, measles (rubeola), pertussis, rubella, syphilis, TB, and rabies and reports the deaths in 121 U.S. cities by age. It also reports accounts of interesting cases, environmental hazards, disease outbreaks, or other public health problems. Local and state health departments and many local and health sciences libraries house this weekly publication. A subscription is available at the CDC website, www.cdc.gov/mmwr.

➤ *CDC:* The CDC compiles information on a range of topics including health behavior, educational and community-based programs, unintentional injuries, occupational safety and health, environmental health, oral health, diabetes and chronic disabling conditions, communicable disease, immunizations, clinical preventive services, and surveillance and data systems. Data are reported in several publications and on their website, www.cdc.gov.

BOX 5-4 Steps in the Needs Assessment Process

1. Identify aggregate for assessment.
2. Identify required information.
3. Select method of data gathering.
4. Develop questionnaire or interview questions.
5. Develop procedures for data collection.
6. Train data collectors.
7. Arrange for a sample representative of the aggregate.
8. Conduct needs assessment.
9. Tabulate and analyze data.
10. Identify needs suggested by data.
11. Develop an action plan.

Increased risk of _____
                              (disability, disease, etc.)

among _____ related to
              (community or population)

_____ as demonstrated
              (etiological statement)

in _____ .
              (health indicators)

FIGURE 5-3 Format for community health diagnosis. (Redrawn from Muecke MA: Community health diagnosis in nursing, *Public Health Nurs* 1:23-35, 1984. Used with permission of Blackwell Scientific Publications.)

---

a plan for the intervention and its evaluation. Once again, epidemiological data can be useful as a basis for determining success. By comparing baseline data, national and local data, and other relevant indicators, the nurse can construct benchmarks to gauge achievement of program objectives. This may entail the calculation of incidence rates, if the goal is to reduce the development of disease, or primary prevention. Comparing data to national rates or to prevalence rates found in a local community may be other indicators of success. Reducing the presence of risk factors and documenting patterns of healthy behavior are other objective indices of successful programs.

It is evident that epidemiological data and methods are essential to each phase of the nursing process. The community health nurse compiles a range of assessment data that support the nursing diagnosis. Epidemiological studies support program planning by establishing the effectiveness of certain interventions and their specificity for different aggregates. Finally, epidemiological data are important for the community health nurse's documentation of a program's long-term effectiveness. Box 5-5 provides an evaluation example.

BOX 5-5 Example of Evaluation

Comprehensive Perinatal Program Improves Birth Outcomes in Teenage Medicaid Clients

A collaborative project among a graduate nursing student, a graduate public health student, and a private, nonprofit, community-based medical center using an epidemiological design (i.e., retrospective and cross-sectional) was carried out to evaluate the effect of enrollment in two special perinatal programs—the Comprehensive Perinatal Services Program (CPSP) and the school-based Comprehensive Teenage Pregnancy and Parenting Program (CTAPPP)—on the occurrence of adverse perinatal outcomes in teenage Medicaid clients who delivered at the medical center. The project was in response to staff nurses' observations of a recurring clinical problem: questionable perinatal outcomes among teenage girls giving birth at the medical center, a clinical problem with implications for the health of the community.

The CPSP is a comprehensive program that provides perinatal services including medical, nursing, nutritional, psychosocial, childbirth, and parenting educational interventions that must be provided by a physician or a certified nurse midwife, a certified nutritionist, a social worker with a master's degree, and a certified nurse educator, respectively. The CTAPPP offers academic, health, nutrition, perinatal, and parenting education support and case management services to pregnant and parenting teenagers.

Using historical data, pregnancy outcomes were compiled on 312 Medicaid, largely African-American (75.9%) clients, aged 12 to 18 years, who delivered at the medical center between June 1991 and June 1992. Adverse perinatal outcomes including low birthweight, gestational age less than 37 weeks, and admission to neonatal intensive care unit were found in 10.9% of the study sample; 35% received substandard prenatal care. Enrollment in CPSP was associated with reduced adverse perinatal outcomes; however, enrollment in CTAPPP was not. A more comprehensive prenatal program, such as CPSP, may improve birth outcomes in high-risk teenage populations. The project presents a model for linking data on birth outcomes to data on program participation among Medicaid clients to assess the efficacy of existing programs.

From Perkocha VA et al: The efficacy of two comprehensive perinatal programs on reducing adverse perinatal outcomes, *Am J Prev Med* 11(suppl 1):21-29, 1995.

CASE STUDY   Application of the Nursing Process Assessment and Diagnosis

The following example demonstrates the process of collecting and analyzing data and deriving community diagnoses. It also exemplifies the multiple care levels within which community health nurses function: the individual client, the family, and the aggregate or community levels. In this scenario, the nurse identified an individual client health problem during a home visit, which provided the initial impetus for an aggregate health education program. Data collection expanded from the assessment of the individual to a broad range of literature and data about the nature of the problem in populations. The nurse then formulated a community-level diagnosis to direct the ensuing plan. This was subsequently implemented at the aggregate level and then evaluated.

School nurses frequently address a broad range of student health problems. In the West San Antonio School District, school nurses generally reserve several hours a week for home visits. In a recent case, a teacher expressed concern for a high school junior named "John," whose brother was dying from cancer. In a health class, John shared his personal fears about cancer, which caused his classmates to question their own cancer risks and how they might reduce their risks.

ASSESSMENT

The school nurse visited John's family and learned that their 25-year-old son had testicular cancer. Since his diagnosis 1 year earlier, he had undergone a range of therapies that were palliative but not curative; the cancer was advanced at the time of diagnosis. The nurse spent time with the family discussing care, answering questions, and exploring available support for the entire family.

At a school nurse staff meeting, the nurse inquired about her colleagues' experiences with other young clients with this type of cancer. Only one nurse remembered a young man with testicular cancer. The nurses were not familiar with its prevalence, incidence, risk factors, prevention strategies, or early detection approaches. The nurse recognized the high probability that high school students would have similar questions and could benefit from reliable information.

The school nurse embarked on a community assessment to answer these questions. The nurse first collected information about testicular cancer. Second, the nurse reviewed the nursing and medical literature for key articles discussing client care, diagnosis, and treatment. Epidemiological studies provided additional data regarding testicular cancer's distribution pattern in the population and associated risk factors.

The nurse learned that young men aged 20 to 35 years were at the greatest risk. Other major risk factors were not identified. It was learned that healthy young men do not seek testicular cancer screening and regular health care; they may be apprehensive about conditions affecting sexual function. These factors contribute to delayed detection and treatment. Although only an estimated 8010 new cases of testicular cancer were diagnosed in the United States in 2005, it was one of the most common tumors in young men. Furthermore, this cancer is amenable to treatment with early diagnosis (American Cancer Society, 2005).

Based on these facts, the nurse reasoned that a prevention program would benefit high school students. However, to perform a comprehensive assessment, it was important that the nurse clarify what students did know, how comfortable they were discussing sexual health, and how much the subject interested them. Therefore the nurse approached the junior and senior high school students and administered a questionnaire to elicit this information. The nurse also queried the health teacher about the amount of pertinent cancer and sexual development information the students received in the

Continued

CASE STUDY Application of the Nursing Process Assessment and Diagnosis *(cont'd)*

classroom. The nurse considered the latter an important prerequisite to dealing with the sensitive subject of sexual health. According to the health teacher, the students did receive instruction about physical development and psychosexual issues. Students expressed a strong desire for more classroom instruction on these subjects and more information on cancer prevention. However, they did not have sufficient knowledge of the beneficial health practices related to cancer prevention and early detection.

Key Assessment Data
- Health status of John's brother
- Knowledge, coping, and support resources of family
- Testicular cancer, its natural history, treatment and prevention, incidence, prevalence, mortality and risk factors
- High school students' knowledge about cancer and its prevention
- Students' comfort level discussing sexual health issues

Community
There is an increased risk of undetected testicular cancer among young men related to insufficient knowledge about the disease and the methods for preventing and detecting it at an early stage as demonstrated by high rates of late initiation of treatment.

PLANNING

Clarifying the problem and its cause helped the nurse direct the planning phase of the nursing process and determine both long-term and short-term goals.

Long-Term Goal
- Students will identify testicular lesions at an early stage and seek care promptly.

Short-Term Goals
- Students will understand testicular cancer and self-detection techniques.
- Students will exhibit comfort with sexual health issues by asking questions.
- Male students will report regular testicular self-examination.

Planning encompassed several activities, including the discovery of recommended health care practices regarding testicular cancer. The nurse also sought to determine the most effective and appropriate educational approaches for male and female high school students. Identifying helpful community agencies was also an essential part of the process. The local chapter of the American Cancer Society provided valuable information, materials, and consultative services. A nearby nursing school's media center and faculty were also very supportive of the program.

After formalizing her objectives and plan, the nurse presented the project to the high school's teaching coordinator and principal. Their approval was necessary before the nurse could implement the project. After eliciting their enthusiastic support, the nurse proceeded with more detailed plans. She selected and developed classroom instruction methods and activities that would maximize high school students' involvement. The nurse also ordered a film and physical models for demonstrating and practicing testicular self-examination. She prepared group exercises designed to relax and assist students in being comfortable with the sensitive subject matter. The nurse scheduled two 40-minute sessions dealing with testicular cancer for the junior-level health class. In a final step of the planning phase, she designed evaluation tools that assessed knowledge levels after each class session and measured the extent to which students integrated these health practices into their lifestyles at the end of their junior and senior years.

The nurse was now ready to proceed with the implementation of a testicular cancer prevention and screening program. She initiated the assessment phase by identifying an individual client and family with a health need, and she extended the assessment to the high school aggregate. Her data collection at the aggregate level, for both the general and local high school populations, assisted in her community diagnosis. The diagnosis directed the development of a community-specific health intervention program and its subsequent implementation and evaluation.

INTERVENTION

The nurse conducted the two sessions in a health education class. At the beginning of the class period, students participated in a group exercise and the nurse asked them about their knowledge of testicular cancer. The nurse showed a film and led a discussion about cancer screening. In the second session, she demonstrated the self-examination procedure using testicular models and supervised the students while they practiced the procedure on the models. The nurse advised the male students about the frequency of self-examination. With the females, she discussed the need for young men to be aware of their increased risk, drawing a parallel to breast self-examination.

EVALUATION

After completing the class sessions, the nurse administered the questionnaires she developed for evaluation purposes. Analysis of the questionnaires indicated that knowledge levels were very high immediately after the classes. Students were pleased with the frank discussion, the opportunity to ask questions, and the clear responses to a sensitive subject. Teachers also offered positive feedback. Consequently, the nurse became a knowledgeable health resource in the high school.

Intermediate-term evaluation occurred at the end of the students' junior and senior years. The nurse arranged a 15-minute evaluation during other classes, which assessed the

Continued

CASE STUDY Application of the Nursing Process Assessment and Diagnosis (*cont'd*)

integration of positive health practices and testicular self-examinations into the students' lifestyles. At the end of the school year, the prevalence of regular self-assessment was significantly lower than knowledge levels. However, 30% of male students reported regularly practicing self-examinations at the end of 1 year, and 70% reported they had performed a self-examination at least once during the past year.

The compilation of incidence data is ideal for long-term evaluation and it documents the reduction of a community health problem. Testicular cancer is very rare; therefore, incidence data are not reliable and may not be feasible to collect. However, for more prevalent conditions, objective statistics help reveal increases and decreases in disease rates, and these may be related to the strengths and deficiencies of health programs.

LEVELS OF PREVENTION

The following are examples of the three levels of prevention as applied to this case study.

Primary
- Promotion of healthy lifestyles and attitudes toward sexuality
- Education about sexual health and the care of one's body

Secondary
- Self-examination to detect testicular cancer in its earliest stage
- Referral for medical care as soon as a lump or symptom is discovered
- Medical and surgical care to treat and cure testicular cancer

Tertiary
- Advanced care, including hospice services for those with incurable disease
- Support services and grief counseling to help families cope with loss of a loved one

SUMMARY

Communities form for a variety of reasons and can be homogeneous or heterogeneous in their composition. To help assess the nature of a given community, community health nurses study and interpret data from sources such as local government agencies, census reports, morbidity and mortality reports, and vital statistics. Nurses can gather valuable information about the causes and prevalence of health and disease in a community through epidemiological studies. Based on this information, the community health nurse can apply the nursing process, expanding assessment, diagnosis, planning, intervention, and evaluation from the individual client level to a targeted aggregate in the community.

LEARNING ACTIVITIES

1. Walk through a neighborhood and compile a list of variables that are important to describe with demographic and epidemiological data. Write down hunches or preconceived notions about the nature of the community's population. Compare ideas with the collected statistical data.
2. Walk through a neighborhood and describe the sensory information (i.e., smells, sounds, and sights). How does each relate to the community's health?
3. Compile a range of relevant demographic and epidemiological data for the community by examining census reports, vital statistics reports, city records, and other library and agency sources.
4. Using the collected data, identify three community health problems and formulate three community health diagnoses.

REFERENCES

American Cancer Society: *Cancer reference information: Overview: Testicular cancer*, 2005, The Author, http://www.cancer.org/docroot/CRI/CRI_2_1x.asp?rnav=criov&dt=41.

Anderson ET, McFarlane JM: *Community as partner: theory and practice in nursing*, ed 3, Philadelphia, 2000, Lippincott Williams & Wilkins.

Blake BJ, Bentov L: Geographical mapping of unmarried teen births and selected sociodemographic variables, *Public Health Nursing* 18(1): 33-39, 2001.

Boutain D: Social justice in nursing: A review of the literature. In de Chesnay M, editor: *Caring for the vulnerable*, Boston, 2005, Jones and Bartlett.

Clark MJ et al: Involving communities in community assessment, *Public Health Nurs* 20:456-463, 2003.

Flynn BC: Healthy cities: a model of community change, *Fam Com Health* 15(1):13-23, 1992.

Healthcare Forum: *What creates health? Individuals and communities respond*, A national study conducted by DYG, Inc., for the Healthcare Forum, San Francisco, 1994, The Author.

Hildebrandt E: Focus groups and vulnerable populations: insight into client strengths and needs in complex community health care environments, *Nurs Health Care Perspect* 20(5):256-259, 1999.

Institute of Medicine: *The future of public health*, Washington, DC, 1988, National Academy Press.

Keppel KG: What is assessment? *J Public Health Manage Pract* 1(2):1-7, 1995.

Muecke MA: Community health diagnosis in nursing, *Public Health Nurs* 1:23-35, 1984.

National Center for Health Statistics: *Health: United States, 2005*, The Author, http://www.cdc.gov/nchs/hus.htm.

Perkocha VA et al: The efficacy of two comprehensive perinatal programs on reducing adverse perinatal outcomes, *Am J Prev Med* 11(suppl 1):21-29, 1995.

Timmreck TC: *Planning, program development, and evaluation: a handbook for health promotion, aging, and health services,* Boston, 1995, Jones and Bartlett.

US Department of Health and Human Services: *Healthy People 2010,* Conference edition, Washington DC, 2000, US Government Printing Office.

CHAPTER 6

Community Health Planning, Implementation, and Evaluation

Deborah Godfrey Brown ▪ Patricia M. Burbank

MEDIA RESOURCES

Additional Material for Study, Review, and Further Exploration

evolve Website at http://evolve.elsevier.com/Nies

❖ Quiz ❖ Case Studies ❖ Content Updates ❖ Glossary ❖ WebLinks

OBJECTIVES

Upon completion of this chapter, the reader will be able to do the following:

1. Describe the concept "community as client."
2. Apply the nursing process to the larger aggregate within a system's framework.
3. Describe the steps in the health planning model.
4. Identify the appropriate prevention level and system level for nursing interventions in families, groups, aggregates, and communities.
5. Recognize major health planning legislation.
6. Analyze factors that have contributed to the failure of health planning legislation to control health care costs.
7. Describe the community health nurse's role in health planning, implementation, and evaluation.

KEY TERMS

certificate of need (CON)
community as client
health planning

Health Planning Model
Hill-Burton Act
key informant

National Health Planning and
  Resources Development
  Act

Partnership for Health
  Program (PHP)
Regional Medical Programs
  (RMPs)

CHAPTER OUTLINE

OVERVIEW OF HEALTH PLANNING

HEALTH PLANNING MODEL
  Assessment
  Planning
  Intervention
  Evaluation

HEALTH PLANNING PROJECTS
  Successful Projects
  Unsuccessful Projects
  Discussion

HEALTH PLANNING FEDERAL LEGISLATION
  Early History
  Hill-Burton Act
  Regional Medical Programs
  Comprehensive Health Planning
  Certificate of Need
  National Health Planning and Resources Development
    Act
  Changing Focus of Health Planning

NURSING IMPLICATIONS

Health planning for and with the community is an essential component of community health nursing practice. The term **health planning** seems simple, but the underlying concept is quite complex. Like many of the other components of community health nursing, health planning tends to vary at the different aggregate levels. Health planning with an individual or a family may focus on direct care needs or self-care responsibilities. At the group level, the primary goal may be health education, and at the community level, health planning may involve population disease prevention or environmental hazard control. The following example illustrates the interaction of community health nursing roles with health planning at a variety of aggregate levels.

CLINICAL EXAMPLE

Bianca Tesch is an RN in a suburban high school. During the course of the school year, she noted an increasing incidence of pregnancy-related dropouts. A nurse at the junior high school confirmed a corresponding increase in withdrawal among younger pregnant teenagers. After reviewing information in nursing journals, other professional journals, and the general media, Bianca discovered a national epidemic of unwed pregnant teenagers.

Bianca questioned the reason for the increased pregnancies. Her assessment of the problem included several findings. Sexually active teenagers do not use contraception regularly because they want their actions to seem "spontaneous" and not "planned." Also, a variety of sexual misconceptions led teens to believe they were invulnerable to pregnancy. For example, a typical misconception among female students was "I will not become pregnant if I do not have regular periods or if my boyfriend does not ejaculate inside me." Teenagers also find it difficult or embarrassing to obtain certain contraceptives. The suburb does not have a local family planning clinic, and area physicians are reluctant to counsel teenagers or prescribe contraceptives without parental permission. The nurse also discovered that several years earlier, a group of parents stopped an attempt by the local school board to establish sex education in the school system. The parents believed this responsibility belonged in the home.

Bianca considered all of these factors in developing her plan of action. She met with teachers, officials, and parents. Teachers and school officials were willing to deal with this sensitive issue if parents could recognize its validity. In meetings, many parents revealed they were uncomfortable discussing sexuality with their teenaged children and welcomed assistance. However, they were concerned that teachers might introduce the mechanics of reproduction without giving proper attention to the moral decisions and obligations involved in relationships. The parents expressed their desire to participate in curriculum planning and to meet with the teachers instead of following a previous plan that required parents to sign a consent form for each teenager. In support of the parents, Bianca asked a nearby metropolitan family planning agency to consider opening a part-time clinic in the suburb. The local school board proposed instituting a home-tutoring program for pregnant teenagers, which would encourage their return to school. ■

Implementing such a comprehensive plan is time consuming and requires community involvement and resources. The nurse enlisted the aid of school officials and other community professionals. Time will reveal the plan's long-term effectiveness in reducing teen pregnancy.

This example shows how nurses can and should become involved in health planning. Teen pregnancy is a significant health problem and often results in lower education and lower socioeconomic status, which can lead to further health problems. The nurse's assessment and planned interventions involved individual teenagers, parents and families, the school system, and community resources.

This chapter provides an overview of health planning and evaluation from a nursing perspective. It also describes a model for student involvement in health planning projects and a review of significant health planning legislation.

OVERVIEW OF HEALTH PLANNING

One of the major criticisms of community health nursing practice involves the shift in focus from the community and larger aggregate to family caseload management or agency responsibilities. When focusing on the individual or family, nurses must remember that these clients are members of a larger population group or community, and environmental factors influence them. Nurses can identify these factors and plan health interventions by implementing an assessment of the entire aggregate or community. Figure 6-1 illustrates this process.

The concept of "community as client" is not new. Lillian Wald's work at New York City's Henry Street settlement in the late 1800s exemplifies this concept. At the Henry Street settlement, Miss Wald, Mary Brewster, and other public health nurses worked with extremely poor immigrants.

The "case" element in Wald's early reports received less and less emphasis; she instinctively went beyond the symptoms to appraise the whole individual. She observed that one could not understand the individual without understanding the family and saw that the family was in the grip of larger social and economic forces, which it could not control (Duffus, 1938).

The early beginnings of public health nursing incorporated visits to the homebound ill and applied the nursing process to larger aggregates and communities to improve health for the greatest number of people. Wald's goals, and those of other public health nurses, were health promotion and disease prevention for the entire community (Silverstein, 1985). Health planning at the aggregate or community level is necessary to accomplish these goals.

Through the 1950s, public health nursing adopted Wald's nursing concepts, which focused on mobilizing communities to solve local problems, treat the poor, and improve the environmental conditions that fostered disease. During the 1950s, social changes such as suburbanization, increased family mobility, and enhanced government health expenditures updated nursing roles. Since the mid 1960s, there has been a shift from public health nursing, which emphasizes community care, to community health nursing, which includes all nonhospital nursing activities. New trends constantly emerge through health care reform debates. It has become more important to use nurses as primary care providers in the health care system. Home health care services are a very significant component of the health care system. A continued shift into the community requires that community health nurses become increasingly visible and vocal leaders of health care reform.

The increased focus on community-based nursing practice yields a greater emphasis on the aggregate becoming the client or care unit. However, the community health nurse should not neglect nursing care at the individual and family levels by focusing on health care only at the aggregate level. Rather, the nurse can use this community information to help understand individual and family health problems and improve their health status. Table 6-1 illustrates the differences in

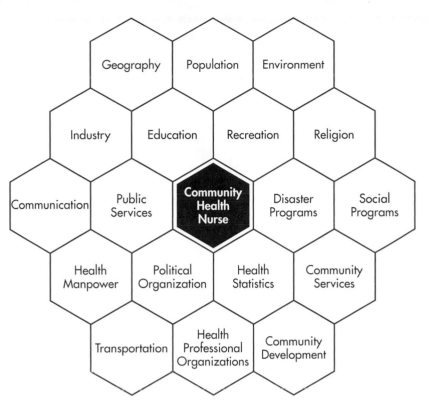

FIGURE 6-1 The community as client. Chapter 5, Table 5-1 (pp. 82-83), provides assessment parameters that help identify the client's assets and needs.

TABLE 6-1   Levels of Community Health Nursing Practice

CLIENT	EXAMPLE	CHARACTERISTICS	HEALTH ASSESSMENT	NURSING INVOLVEMENT
Individual	Lisa McDonald	An individual with various needs	Individual strengths, problems, and needs	Client-nurse interaction
Family	Moniz family	A family system with individual and group needs	Individual and family strengths, problems, and needs	Interactions with individuals and the family group
Group	Boy Scout troop Alzheimer's support group	Common interests, problems, and needs Interdependency	Group dynamics Fulfillment of goals	Group member and leader
Population group	AIDS patients in a given state Pregnant adolescents in a school district	Large, unorganized group with common interests, problems, and needs	Assessment of common problems, needs, and vital statistics	Application of nursing process to identified needs
Organization	A work place A school	Organized group in a common location with shared governance and goals	Relationship of goals, structure, communication, patterns of organization to its strengths, problems, and needs	Consultant and/or employee application of nursing process to identified needs
Community	Italian neighborhood Anytown, USA	An aggregate of people in a common location with organized social systems	Analysis of systems, strengths, characteristics, problems, and needs	Community leader, participant, and health care provider

community health nursing practice at the individual, family, and community levels.

However, before nurses can participate in health care planning, they must be knowledgeable about the process and comfortable with the concept of **community as client** or care focus. It is essential that undergraduate and graduate nursing programs integrate these concepts into the curricula. If basic and advanced nursing education includes health planning, the student becomes aware of the process and the professional involvement opportunities.

Early efforts to provide students with learning experiences in community health investigation included Hegge's (1973) use of learning packets for independent study and Ruybal's opportunities for students to apply epidemiological concepts in community program planning and evaluation (Ruybal, Bauwens, and Fasla, 1975). However, neither of these approaches presented a complete model that incorporated the nursing process into a health planning framework. More recently, Ammerman and Parks (1998) stressed that "asset assessment" is an important component of community

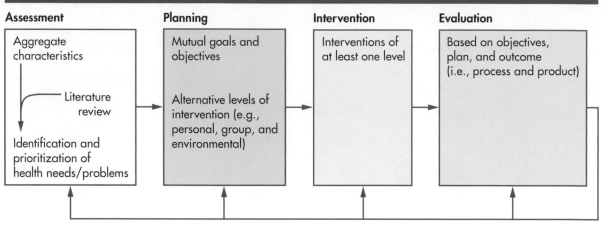

FIGURE 6-2   Health Planning Model.

planning and intervention. Several other authors, including Budgen and Cameron (2003), Shuster and Goeppinger (2004), and Doerr et al. (1998), described the community health planning process. However, none of these models uses practical examples for actual student implementation throughout the entire process.

HEALTH PLANNING MODEL

A model based on Hogue's (1985) group intervention model was developed in response to this need for population focus. The **Health Planning Model** aims to improve aggregate health and applies the nursing process to the larger aggregate within a systems framework. Figure 6-2 depicts this model. Incorporated into a health planning project, the model can help students view larger client aggregates and gain knowledge and experience in the health planning process. Nurses must carefully consider each step in the process, using this model. Box 6-1 outlines these steps. In addition, Box 6-2 provides the systems framework premises that nurses should incorporate.

Several considerations affect how nurses choose a specific aggregate for study. The community may have extensive or limited opportunities appropriate for nursing involvement. Additionally, each community offers different possibilities for health intervention. For example, an urban area might have a variety of industrial and business settings that need assistance, whereas a suburban community may offer a choice of family-oriented organizations like boys and girls clubs and parent-teacher associations that would benefit from intervention.

A nurse should also consider personal interests and strengths in selecting an aggregate for intervention. For example, the nurse should consider whether he or she has an interest in teaching health promotion and preventive health or in planning for organizational change; whether his or her communication skills are better suited to large or small groups; and whether he or she has a preference for working with the elderly or with children. Thoughtful consideration of these and other variables will facilitate assessment and planning.

Assessment

To establish a professional relationship with the chosen aggregate, a community health nurse must first gain entry into the group. Good communication skills are essential to make a positive first impression. The nurse should make an appointment with the group leaders to set up the first meeting.

The nurse must initially clarify his or her position, organizational affiliation, knowledge, and skills. The nurse should also clarify mutual expectations and available times. Once entry is established, the nurse continues negotiation to maintain a mutually beneficial relationship.

Meeting with the aggregate on a regular basis will allow the nurse to make an in-depth assessment. Determining sociodemographic characteristics (e.g., distribution of age, sex, and race) may help the nurse ascertain health needs and develop appropriate intervention methods. For example, adolescents need information regarding nutrition, abuse of drugs and alcohol, and relationships with the opposite sex. They usually do not enjoy lectures in a classroom environment, but the nurse must possess skills to initiate small-group involvement and participation. An adult group's average educational level will affect the group's knowledge base and their comfort with formal versus informal learning settings. The nurse may find it more difficult to coordinate time and energy commitments if an organization is the focus group, because the aggregate members may be more diverse.

The nurse may gather information about sociodemographic characteristics from a variety of sources. These sources include observing the aggregate, consulting with other aggregate workers (e.g., the factory or school nurse, a Head Start teacher, or the resident manager of a high-rise senior citizen apartment building), reviewing available records or charts, and interviewing members of the aggregate (i.e., verbally or via a short questionnaire).

In assessing the aggregate's health status, the nurse must consider both the positive and negative factors. Unemployment or the presence of disease may suggest specific health problems, but low rates of absenteeism at work or school may suggest a need to focus more on preventive interventions. The specific aggregate determines the

BOX 6-1 Health Planning Project Objectives

I. Assessment
   A. Specify the aggregate level for study (e.g., group, population group, or organization). Identify and provide a general orientation to the aggregate (e.g., characteristics of the aggregate system, suprasystem, and subsystems). Include the reasons for selecting this aggregate and the method for gaining entry.
   B. Describe specific characteristics of the aggregate.
      1. *Sociodemographic characteristics:* Including age, sex, race or ethnic group, religion, educational background and level, occupation, income, and marital status.
      2. *Health status:* Work or school attendance, disease categories, mortality, health care use, and population growth and population pressure measurements (e.g., rates of birth and death, divorce, unemployment, and drug and alcohol abuse). Select indicators appropriate for the chosen aggregate.
      3. *Suprasystem influences:* Existing health services to improve aggregate health and the existing or potential positive and negative impact of other community-level social system variables on the aggregate. Identify the data collection methods.
   C. Provide relevant information from the literature review, especially in terms of the characteristics, problems, or needs within this type of aggregate. Compare the health status of the aggregate with similar aggregates, the community, the state, and the nation.
   D. Identify the specific aggregate's health problems and needs based on comparative data collection analysis and interpretation and literature review. Include input from clients regarding their need perceptions. Give priorities to health problems and needs, and indicate how to determine these priorities.
II. Planning
   A. Select one health problem or need, and identify the ultimate goal of intervention. Identify specific, measurable objectives as mutually agreed upon by the student and aggregate.
   B. Describe the alternative interventions that are necessary to accomplish the objectives. Consider interventions at each system level where appropriate (e.g., aggregate system, suprasystem, and subsystems). Select and validate the intervention(s) with the highest probability of success. Interventions may use existing resources, or they may require the development of new resources.
III. Intervention
   A. Implement at least one level of planned intervention when possible.
   B. If intervention was not implemented, provide reasons.
IV. Evaluation
   A. Evaluate the plan, objectives, and outcomes of the intervention(s). Include the aggregate's evaluation of the project. Evaluation should consider the process, product, appropriateness, and effectiveness.
   B. Make recommendations for further action based on the evaluation, and communicate these to the appropriate individuals or system levels. Discuss implications for community health nursing.

BOX 6-2 Systems Framework Premises

I. Each system is a goal-directed collection of interacting or interdependent parts, or subsystems.
II. The whole system is continually interacting with and adapting to the environment, or suprasystem.
III. There is a hierarchical structure (suprasystem → system → subsystems).
IV. Each system is characterized by the following:
   A. *Structure:* Arrangement and organization of parts, or subsystems
      1. Organization and configuration (e.g., traditional vs. non-traditional; greater variability [no right or wrong and no proper vs. improper form])
      2. Boundaries (open vs. closed; regulate input and output)
      3. Territory (spatial and behavioral)
      4. Role allocation
   B. *Functions:* Goals and purpose of system and activities necessary to ensure survival, continuity, and growth of system
      1. General
         a. *Physical:* Food, clothing, shelter, protection from danger, and provision for health and illness care
         b. *Affectional:* Meeting the emotional needs of affection and security
         c. *Social:* Identity, affiliation, socialization, and controls
      2. *Specific:* Each family, group, or aggregate has its own individual agenda regarding values, aspirations, and cultural obligations
   C. *Process and dynamics*
      1. *Adaptation:* Attempt to establish and maintain equilibrium; balance between stability, differentiation, and growth; self-regulation and adaptation (equilibrium and homeostasis)
         a. *Internal:* Families, groups, or aggregates
         b. *External:* Interaction with suprasystem
      2. *Integration:* Unity and ability to communicate
      3. *Decision making:* Power distribution, consensus, accommodation, and authority

The aggregate's suprasystem may facilitate or impede health status. Different organizations and communities provide various resources and services to their members. Some are obviously health related, such as the presence or absence of hospitals, clinics, private practitioners, emergency facilities, health centers, home health agencies, and health departments. Support services and facilities such as group meal sites or Meals on Wheels (MOW) for the elderly and recreational facilities and programs for children, adolescents, and adults are also important. Transportation availability, reimbursement mechanisms or sliding-scale fees, and community-based volunteer groups may determine the use of services. An assessment of these factors requires researching public records (e.g., town halls, telephone directories, and community services directories) and interviewing health professionals, volunteers, and **key informants** (i.e., someone who is familiar with the community) in the community. The nurse should augment existing resources or create a new service rather than duplicating what is already available to the aggregate. (See also Figure 5-1, p. 77.)

A literature review is an important means of comparing the aggregate with the norm. For example, children in a Head Start setting, day care center, or elementary school

appropriate health status measures. Immunization levels are an important index for children, but nurses rarely collect this information for adults. However, the nurse should consider the need for influenza and/or pneumonia vaccines with the elderly. Similarly, the nurse would expect a lower incidence of chronic disease among children, whereas the elderly have higher rates of long-term morbidity and mortality.

may exhibit a high rate of upper respiratory tract infections during the winter. The nurse should review the pediatric literature and determine the normal incidence for this age range in group environments. Further, the nurse should research potential problems in an especially healthy aggregate (e.g., developmental stresses for adolescents or work or family stresses for adults) or determine whether a factory's experience with work-related injury is within an average range. Comparing the foregoing assessment with research reports, statistics, and health information will help determine and prioritize the aggregate's health problems and needs.

The last phase of the initial assessment is identifying and prioritizing the specific aggregate's health problems and needs. This phase should relate directly to the assessment and the literature review and should include a comparative analysis of the two. Most importantly, this step should reflect the aggregate's perceptions of need. Depending on the aggregate, the nurse may consult the aggregate members directly or interview others who work with the aggregate (e.g., a Head Start teacher). Interventions are seldom successful if the nurse omits or ignores the clients' input.

Finally, the nurse must prioritize the identified problems and needs to create an effective plan. The nurse should consider the following factors when determining priorities:
- Aggregate's preferences
- Number of individuals in the aggregate affected by the health problem
- Severity of the health need or problem
- Availability of potential solutions to the problem
- Practical considerations such as individual skills, time limitations, and available resources

In addition, the nurse may further refine the priorities by applying a framework like Maslow's (1968) hierarchy of needs (i.e., lower level needs have priority over higher level needs) or Leavell and Clark's (1965) levels of prevention (i.e., primary prevention may take priority for children, whereas tertiary prevention may take higher priority for the elderly).

Assessment and data collection are ongoing throughout the nurse's relationship with the aggregate. However, the nurse should proceed to the planning stage once the initial assessment is complete. It is particularly important to link the assessment stage with other stages at this step in the process. Planning should stem directly and logically from the assessment, and implementation should be realistic.

Planning

Again, the nurse should determine which problems or needs require intervention in conjunction with the aggregate's perception of its health problems and needs, and based on the outcomes of prioritization. Then the nurse must identify the desired outcome or ultimate goal of the intervention. For example, the nurse should determine whether to increase the aggregate's knowledge level and whether an intervention will cause a change in health behavior. It is important to have specific and measurable goals and desired outcomes. This will facilitate planning the nursing interventions and determining the evaluation process.

Planning interventions is a multistep process. First, the nurse must determine the intervention levels (e.g., subsystem, aggregate system, and/or suprasystem). A system is a set of interacting and interdependent parts (subsystems), organized as a whole with a specific purpose. Just like the human body can be viewed as a set of interacting subsystems (circulatory, neurological, integumentary, etc.), a family, a worksite, or a senior high rise can also be viewed as a system. Each system then interacts with, and is further influenced by, its physical and social environment, or suprasystem (for example, the larger community).

Second, the nurse should plan interventions for each system level, which may center on the primary, secondary, or tertiary levels of prevention. These levels apply to aggregates, communities, and individuals. Primary prevention consists of health promotion and activities that protect the client from illness or dysfunction. Secondary prevention includes early diagnosis and treatment to reduce the duration and severity of disease or dysfunction. Tertiary prevention applies to irreversible disability or damage and aims to rehabilitate and restore an optimal level of functioning (see also Table 1-1, p. 8). Plans should include goals and activities that reflect the identified problem's prevention level.

Third, the nurse should validate the practicality of the planned interventions according to available personal, aggregate, and suprasystem resources. Although teaching is often a major component of community health nursing, the nurse should consider other potential forms of intervention (e.g., personal counseling, game therapy, or community service development). Input from other disciplines or community agencies may also be helpful. Finally, the nurse should coordinate the planned interventions with the aggregate's input to maximize participation.

Intervention

The intervention stage may be the most enjoyable stage for the nurse and the clients. The nurse's careful preliminary assessment and planning should help ensure the aggregate's positive response to the intervention. Although implementation should follow the initial plan, the nurse should prepare for unexpected problems (e.g., bad weather, transportation problems, poor attendance, or competing events). If the nurse is unable to complete the intervention, the reasons for its failure should be analyzed.

Evaluation

Evaluation is an important component for understanding the success or failure of a project. The evaluation should include the participant's verbal or written feedback and the nurse's detailed analysis. Evaluation includes reflecting on each previous stage to determine the plan's strengths and weaknesses (the process). It is also important to evaluate both positive and negative aspects of each experience honestly and comprehensively, and whether the desired outcomes were achieved (the product). During this stage, the nurse may ask the following questions:
- Were plans based on an incomplete assessment?
- Did the plan allow adequate client involvement?

TABLE 6-2 Interventions by Type of Aggregate and System Level

PROJECT	TYPE OF AGGREGATE	SYSTEM LEVEL FOR INTERVENTION
Rehabilitation group	Group, organization	Subsystem and aggregate system
Textile industry	Population group	Aggregate system and suprasystem
Crime watch	Group, organization, and population group	Aggregate system and suprasystem
Bilingual students (case study)	Community	Aggregate system and suprasystem

- Were the interventions realistic or unrealistic in terms of available resources?
- Did the plan consider all levels of prevention?
- Were the stated goals and objectives accomplished?
- Were the participants satisfied with the interventions?
- Did the plan advance the knowledge level of the aggregate and the nurse?

The intervention may have limited impact if the nurse fails to communicate follow-up recommendations to the aggregate upon completion of the project. Although follow-up activity is not necessary for every plan, most require additional interventions within the aggregate using community agencies and resources. A comprehensive health planning project involves a close working relationship with the aggregate and careful consideration of each step. Long-term evaluation may need to be done by those professionals working continuously with the aggregate, to determine behavior changes and/or changes in health status.

HEALTH PLANNING PROJECTS

Successful Projects

Student projects have used this health planning model with group, organization, population group, and community aggregates. Table 6-2 describes interventions with these aggregates at the subsystem, aggregate system, and suprasystem levels.

Textile Industry
CLINICAL EXAMPLE

A nursing student studied a textile plant that had approximately 470 employees but did not have an occupational health nurse. The student nurse collected data and identified three major problems or needs by collaborating with management and union representatives. First, the student nurse observed that the most common, costly, and chronic work-related injury in plant workers was lower back injury. Second, employees had concern about possible undetected hypertension. Third, the first-aid facilities were disorganized and without an accurate inventory system. The student nurse planned and implemented interventions for all three areas.

On the suprasystem level, the student nurse formulated plans with the company's physicians and lobbied management to enact an employee-training program on proper lifting techniques. The student nurse proposed creating specific and concise job descriptions and requirements to facilitate potential employees' medical assessment. In addition, the student nurse organized and clearly labeled the first-aid supplies and developed an inventory system. On the aggregate system

level, the student nurse planned and conducted a hypertension screening program. Approximately 85% of the employees underwent screening, and 10 people had elevated blood pressure readings. These 10 people were subsequently diagnosed as hypertensive.

In evaluating the project, management representatives recognized that a variety of nursing interventions could improve or maintain workers health. Consequently, management hired the student nurse upon graduation to be the occupational health nurse. ■

Crime Watch
CLINICAL EXAMPLE

Another nursing student was concerned with the rising incidence of crime in a community and organized a crime watch program. The student nurse met periodically with the police and local residents, or aggregate system. Interventions included posting crime watch signs in the neighborhood and establishing more frequent police patrols at the suprasystem level. Evaluation of the program revealed that the residents had increased awareness and concern for neighborhood safety. ■

Rehabilitation Group
CLINICAL EXAMPLE

After working at a senior citizens center for a few weeks, a student nurse began a careful assessment of the center's clients. The student nurse interviewed the center's clients and visited its homebound clients served by social workers and the MOW program. Several of the homebound clients identified a need for socialization and rehabilitation. The center had recently purchased a van equipped to transport handicapped people in wheelchairs, which was a necessary factor in fulfilling this need. After the student nurse assessed the clients' health and functional status and determined mutual goals, four of these homebound clients expressed a desire to attend a rehabilitation program at the center. The student nurse and the center's management initiated a weekly program based on the clients' needs, which included van transportation, a coffee hour, a noontime meal, an exercise class, and a craft class. Although some members were initially reluctant to participate and one man withdrew from the group, the group ultimately functioned very well. In evaluating this new program, it was clear that the student nurse made progress in meeting the goals of increased socialization and rehabilitation. ■

Unsuccessful Projects

Project failure is usually caused by problems with one or more steps of the nursing process. Usually the student does not discover problems until the evaluation phase. The following unsuccessful projects illustrate failures at

TABLE 6-3 Unsuccessful Projects

PROJECT	PROBLEMATIC STEP OF NURSING PROCESS
Group home for mentally retarded	Assessment (i.e., mutual identification of health problems and needs)
Safe Rides program	Planning (i.e., mutual identification of goals and objectives)
	Evaluation (i.e., recommendations for follow-up)
Manufacturing plant	Implementation

TABLE 6-4 Level of Prevention for Each Project

PRIMARY PREVENTION	SECONDARY PREVENTION	TERTIARY PREVENTION
Textile industry	Textile industry Group home for mentally retarded	Rehabilitation group
Crime watch Manufacturing plant Safe Rides program		

different steps in the nursing process. Table 6-3 summarizes the identified problem areas for these examples.

Group Home for Mentally Retarded Adults
CLINICAL EXAMPLE
A nursing student worked with an aggregate of six women living in a group home for mentally retarded citizens. The nursing student observed that the clients were all overweight, and she decided to establish a weight reduction program. She proceeded to meet with the women, chart their weight, and discuss their food choices on a weekly basis. After eight weeks, her evaluation revealed that none of the women had lost weight and a few had gained weight. During the assessment phase the student failed to consider the women's perceptions of need and priority. The women did not consider their weight a problem, and their boyfriends provided positive reinforcement regarding their appearance.

Safe Rides Program
CLINICAL EXAMPLE
One student nurse assessed a university student community through a questionnaire and identified a drinking and driving problem. Of those she surveyed, 77% admitted to driving under the influence of alcohol, and 16.5% stated they were involved in an alcohol-related car accident. After identifying the problem and determining student interest, the student nurse worked with the campus alcohol and drug resource center to plan and implement a program called Safe Rides. In this program, student volunteers would work a hot line and dispatch "on call" drivers to pick up students who are unsafe to drive.

The student nurse resolved many potential complications before implementation (e.g., liability coverage for all participating individuals and expense funds for gasoline). The student nurse formulated a 12-hour training program that lasted three weeks to prepare student volunteers for the Safe Rides program. By the end of the semester, Safe Rides was ready to begin. However, the student nurse graduated at the semester's end and her commitment was the program's prime motivating force. Although others were committed and involved, the student nurse did not arrange for a replacement to coordinate and continue the program upon her departure. The Safe Rides program required ongoing coordination efforts, and no one fully implemented the program in the student's absence. ■

Manufacturing Plant
CLINICAL EXAMPLE
Even careful planning cannot always eliminate potential obstacles. For example, one student nurse chose to work in an occupational setting involving heavy industry. The occupational health nurse and the nurse's personnel supervisor both approved the student nurse's entry into the organization. After reviewing the literature, working with the nurse for several weeks, and assessing the organization and its employees, the student nurse concluded that back injury risk was a primary problem. She planned to decrease the risk factors involved in back injuries by distributing information about proper body mechanics in a teaching session.

However, the personnel manager resisted this plan. Although he recognized the need for education, he was initially unwilling to allow employees to attend the session on company time. The student and manager reached a compromise by allowing attendance during extended coffee breaks. However, the personnel manager canceled the program before the student nurse could implement the class; negotiations for a new union contract were forming, and there was high probability of a strike. This caused management to deny any changes in the usual routine.

The student nurse proceeded appropriately and received clearance from the proper officials, but she could not anticipate or circumvent union problems. The student nurse could only share her information and concern with the nurse and the personnel manager and encourage them to implement her plan when contract negotiations were complete. ■

Discussion
Each of these projects attempted to address a particular level of prevention. Most of these examples focused on primary prevention and health promotion because they were student conducted and time limited. Table 6-4 lists these projects and their prevention levels. However, the full-time community health nurse working with an aggregate (e.g., in the occupational health setting) would target interventions for all three levels of prevention at a variety of system levels. It is useful to view nursing interventions with aggregates within a matrix structure to address all intervention opportunities. The matrix in Table 6-5 gives examples of how the occupational health nurse may intervene at all system levels and all prevention levels.

In practice, most interventions occur at the individual level and include all prevention levels. Interventions at the

TABLE 6-5 Occupational Health: Levels of Prevention for System Levels

SYSTEM LEVEL	PRIMARY PREVENTION	SECONDARY PREVENTION	TERTIARY PREVENTION
Subsystem	Yearly physical examination for each employee	Regular blood pressure monitoring and diet counseling for each employee with elevated blood pressure	Referral for job retraining for employee with a back injury
Aggregate and group system	Incentive program to encourage departments to use safety devices	Weight reduction group for overweight employees	Support group for employees who are recovering from problems with alcohol or drug use
Suprasystem	Health fair open to the community and employees	Counseling and referral of community members with elevated blood pressure or cholesterol on the basis of health fair findings	Media advertising to encourage people with substance abuse problems to seek help and use community resources that provide assistance

aggregate level are usually less frequent. For many occupational health nurses, time does not allow intervention at the suprasystem level. However, industries are integral parts of the community system. Factors that affect community health also affect employee health and vice versa. Some industries take their reciprocal relationship with the surrounding community quite seriously. For nurses in these industries, interventions at the suprasystem level may become a reality and improve the health of the community and the workers. This is a good example of refocusing upstream by addressing the real source of problems. Although the chosen example is occupational health nursing, any nurse working with aggregate systems can construct a similar matrix for interventions.

These projects illustrate the variety of available opportunities for aggregate health planning. In addition, they exemplify the application of the nursing process within various aggregate types, at different systems levels, and at each prevention level. These examples demonstrate the vital importance of each step of the nursing process.

1. Aggregate assessments must be thorough. The textile industry project exemplifies this point. Assessments should elicit answers to key questions about the aggregate's health and demographic profile and should compare this information with similar aggregates presented in the literature.
2. The nurse must complete careful planning and set goals that the nurse and the aggregate accept. The rehabilitation group project illustrates the importance of mutual planning.
3. Interventions must include aggregate participation and must meet the mutual goals. The Crime Watch project exemplifies this point.
4. Evaluation must include process and product evaluation and aggregate input.

HEALTH PLANNING FEDERAL LEGISLATION

Health planning at the national, state, and local levels is another example of aggregate planning. Planning at any of these levels can be a broader extension of the suprasystem level and affects the individual, family, group, population, and organization levels. Again, upstream change can occur on these levels; for example, individual consumers and consumer groups have protested some managed care practices at the

suprasystem level, because health policy can directly affect patient care.

Historically, nurses have influenced health planning only minimally at the community level, but health planning has a tremendous effect on nurses and nursing practice. It is necessary to understand planning on a suprasystem level; therefore the following section contains a review of past health planning efforts with projections for the future.

Early History

Although health planning activities existed in the United States before the 1940s, they usually addressed specific health problems (e.g., services for maternal and child health and provision of health care activities). Furthermore, private, nongovernmental agencies such as the American Public Health Association or the American Cancer Society usually initiated these activities. The federal government only had limited involvement. For example, in the 1930s, Blue Cross and the United Fund in New York City were responsible for initiating local health planning, and the Health and Planning Council of New York was formed for its implementation. In addition, most of these efforts were provider oriented.

The federal government's involvement in health planning changed at the end of World War II when it turned its attention to issues in the private sector. At this point, there was a general shortage of hospital beds and a lack of coordination among hospitals. In particular, rural areas needed hospital beds and medical personnel (Kovner, 2002; Lee and Benjamin, 2002).

Hill-Burton Act

In 1946, Congress passed the Hospital Survey and Construction Act (Hill-Burton Act, PL 79-725) to address the need for better hospital access. This Act provided federal aid to states for hospital facilities. A state had to submit a plan documenting available resources and need estimates to qualify for hospital construction and modernization funds under the **Hill-Burton Act** (Shonick, 1995). In addition, each state had to designate a single agency for the development and implementation of the hospital construction plan. The Hill-Burton Act caused the expenditure of vast sums of money and resulted in an increase in the number of beds, especially in general hospitals. Although the Act and its amendments focused only on construction, it improved the quality of care in rural areas and introduced systematic statewide planning (Kovner, 2002).

Regional Medical Programs

The Hill-Burton Act provided construction-related planning, but it did not address coordination and care delivery directly. In response to recommendations from Dr. Michael DeBakey's national commission, Heart Disease, Cancer, and Stroke Amendments of 1965 (PL 89-239) were enacted. This legislation was more comprehensive and established regional medical programs.

The **Regional Medical Programs (RMPs)** intended to make the latest technology for the diagnosis and treatment of heart disease, cancer, stroke, and related diseases available to community health care providers through the establishment of regional cooperative arrangements among medical schools, research institutions, and hospitals. The goals of these cooperative arrangements were "to improve generally the health manpower and facilities available to the nation and to accomplish these ends without interfering with the patterns, or the methods of financing, or patient care or professional practice, or with the administration of hospitals" (Heart Disease, Cancer, and Stroke Amendments of 1965, p. 901).

Although RMPs have been credited with the regionalization of certain services and the introduction of innovative approaches to organization and care delivery, some observers believed the reforms were not comprehensive enough. The RMPs did not partner with the existing federal and state programs; therefore, there were gaps and duplication in service delivery, personnel training, and research (Kovner, 2002).

Comprehensive Health Planning

Congress signed the Comprehensive Health Planning and Public Health Services Amendments of 1966 (PL 89-749) into law to broaden the previous legislation's categorical approach to health planning. Combined with the Partnership for Health Amendments of 1967 (PL 90-174), these amendments created the **Partnership for Health Program (PHP)**. The PHP provided federal grants to states to establish and administer a local agency program to enact local comprehensive health care planning. The PHP's objectives were promoting and ensuring the highest level of health for every person and not interfering with the existing private practice patterns (Shonick, 1995).

To meet these objectives, the PHP formulated a two-level planning system. Under this system, each state had to designate a single health planning agency, or "A" agency. To play a statewide coordinating role, the "A" agency had to partner with an advisory council, which consisted largely of health care consumers. Meanwhile, the local "B" agencies formulated plans to meet designated local community needs, which could be any public or nonprofit private agency or organization. "A" agencies were to encourage the formation of local, comprehensive, health planning "B" agencies, and federal grants were made available for that purpose (Shonick, 1995).

Although the comprehensive health plans were the first of these programs to mandate consumer involvement, they may have failed in their basic intent. The possible failure may have resulted from funding shortage, conflict avoidance in policy formulation and goal establishment, political absence, and provider opposition (e.g., American Medical Association, American Hospital Association, and major medical centers). The mission appeared to be a discussion of the shortfalls of health care delivery rather than the provision of mechanisms for action (DeBella, Martin, and Siddall, 1986; Shonick, 1995).

Certificate of Need

In response to increased capital investments and budgetary pressures, state governments developed the idea of obtaining prior governmental approval for certain projects through the use of a **certificate of need (CON)**. New York State passed the first CON law in 1964, which required government approval of hospitals' and nursing homes' major capital investments. Eventually all states supported this CON requirement, and it ultimately became a component of health legislation (PL 93-641). In practice, state CON programs differ in structure and goals. These differences include program focus, decision-making levels, review standard scope, and appeals process exemption (Thorpe, 2002).

National Health Planning and Resources Development Act

Given the perceived failure of the comprehensive health planning programs, the federal government focused on a new approach to health planning. The federal government was greatly concerned with the cost of health care, which escalated dramatically following the end of World War II; the uneven distribution of services; the general lack of knowledge of personal health practices; and the emphasis on more costly modalities of care. The **National Health Planning and Resources Development Act** of 1974 (PL 93-641) combined the strengths of the Hill-Burton Act, RMPs, and the comprehensive health planning program to forge a new system of single-state and areawide health planning agencies (Shonick, 1995).

The goals and purposes of the new law were an increase in accessibility, acceptability, continuity, and quality of health services; control over the rising costs of health care services; and prevention of unnecessary duplication of health resources. The new law addressed the needs of the underserved and provided quality health care. The provider and consumer were to be involved in planning and improving health services, and it placed the system of private practice under scrutiny.

At the center of the program was a network of local health planning agencies, which developed a health systems plan for its geographical service area. The local agencies then submitted these plans to a state health planning and development agency, which integrated the plans into a preliminary state plan. The state agency presented this preliminary plan to a statewide health coordinating council for approval. The law required that the council consist of at least 16 governor-appointed members and that 50% of these members represent health system agencies and 50% represent consumers. One major function of this council was to prepare a state health plan that reflected the goals and purposes of the Act. Once the council formulated a tentative plan, they presented it at public hearings throughout the state for discussion and possible revisions (Shonick, 1995; Thorpe, 2002).

Despite careful deliberations by health planners with input from consumers, not all states accepted the health system plan at the grassroots level. For example, federal officials commended Rhode Island's state health plan, which was released to the community in late 1979. The officials considered it a substantial achievement and delivered high praise. However, when the council first presented the plan at seven public hearings throughout the state in early 1980, many of the near 10,000 people in attendance protested two of the recommendations. One recommendation would have established a smaller number of larger hospitals, and the second would have reduced the number of hospital beds. In Newport, people argued vehemently that if the local hospital closed and women had to deliver their babies in other communities, native Newporters would cease to exist. The same recommendations precipitated a candlelight march in the suburban community of Westerly, where protesters chanted "Save our hospital" and carried signs that read, "Don't risk losing your health care services" (Coyle, 1980).

It is difficult to understand why a plan aimed at "promoting quality of care while constraining costs" met such resistance. In retrospect, planners agreed that although they spent an abundance of time and care developing the plan, the public was not prepared for the ambitious recommendations. Furthermore, many believed that the council had more power than it actually held, and members of the hospital community attempted to discredit the plan. The council presented a second state health plan in 1983, which substantially modified the two previous recommendations, and the public offered little or no opposition. By this time, the public better understood the council's function and the recommendations were more conservative.

The problems that the recommendations encountered in Rhode Island were symptoms of the legislation's overall failure to effect major change in the health care system. A significant problem was that legislation grandfathered the entire health care system (i.e., health care delivery methods did not change). Although legislation mandated consumer involvement in the health system agency, it was often difficult to implement this aspect. In addition, hospitals and other facilities had greater resources to influence the political process. Despite the mandated efforts by CON and required reviews, costs continued to rise, and the health care system remained essentially unchanged (Kronenfeld, 1997; Thorpe, 2002).

Changing Focus of Health Planning

Health planning legislation is heavily influenced by the politics of the administration in power at any given time. The Reagan administration encouraged competition within the health care system. During the 1980s, the administration emphasized cost shifting and cost reduction with greater state power, less centralization of functions, and less national control. This approach represented the government's philosophical shift and combined it with a funding cutback from the Omnibus Budget Reconciliation Act in 1981. This combination dealt a deathblow to federal health planning (Mueller, 1993). The cutbacks caused health system agencies to redefine their role, and the federal government recommended eliminating these agencies.

A reduction in federal funding and the influence of medical lobbies caused the closure of some health system agencies. Those that remained open experienced a decrease in staff, a resulting decrease in overall board functioning, and a reordering of priorities. In an effort to compensate for the decrease in federal funding, some health system agencies sought nonfederal funding or built coalitions to provide the necessary power base for change. Although the administration did not renew federal health planning legislation in the 1980s, it used other regulatory approaches to control costs. These included basing payments to Medicare on diagnosis-related groups and, in the 1990s, many individual states requiring their Medicaid recipients to enroll in HMOs (health maintenance organizations).

The Clinton administration's plan for health care reform would have revitalized planning at the national level. The failure of Congress to pass the plan in 1994 gave planning efforts back to state and local agencies. In autumn 1998, 29 states and the District of Columbia were involved in some form of health planning. Of these states, seven had statewide health plans, local health plans, and some other type of local health planning; two states had statewide and local health plans; six states had statewide health plans and some other local health planning entity; three states had local health plans and some other local health planning entity; eight states and the District of Columbia had statewide health plans exclusively; and three states had some type of local health planning entity (American Health Planning Association [AHPA], 2004).

New York State's Long Term Care Financing and Integration Act of 1997 is an example of state health planning legislation. This piece of legislation allowed New York State's Partnership for Long Term Care to develop continuing care retirement communities and manage long-term care plans. Other examples of state health planning legislation include the following:

- Louisiana set a moratorium on nursing home beds in 1996 and extended it to 2001.
- Arkansas added Act 396 (hospice facility and agency services) and Act 1360 (child health management services clinics).
- Missouri passed legislation in 1996 that no longer requires CON review for hospitals, ambulatory surgical centers, and dialysis centers after 2001 (AHPA, 2004).

At the beginning of the twenty-first century, 36 states and the District of Columbia still require CON reviews for selected expenditures that include nursing homes, psychiatric facilities, and expensive equipment (AHPA, 2004).

Student nurses can support the health planning process to improve aggregate health care with awareness of, and involvement in, the political process. This can involve following health care legislation at the state and national levels, being an informed voter, contacting legislators on issues of concern, and participating in special events.

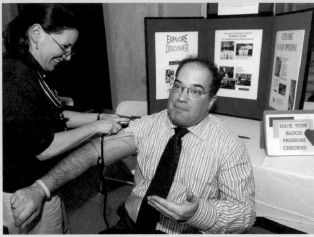

Student nurses attend "higher Ed Day" at the state house to highlight their accomplishments and their participation in the improvement of the health of the state's residents. This student nurse is taking an individual's blood pressure while providing educational information about hypertension identification, referral, and treatment.
(Courtesy Michael Salerno.)

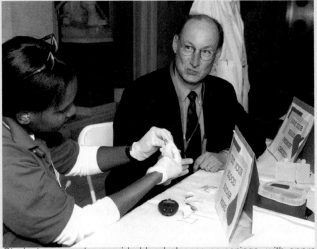

Student nurses also provide blood glucose screenings, with appropriate educational information regarding normal ranges, diet-controlled diabetes, and appropriate referral and treatment when necessary.
(Courtesy Michael Salerno.)

Rhode Island Board of Governors
for Higher Education
301 Promenade Street
Providence, Rhode Island 02908–5748

Telephone 401 222-6560
Facsimile 401 222-6111
TDD 401 222-1350

RIBGHE

April 14, 2005

Professor Debby Godfrey Brown
Nursing
University of Rhode Island
White Hall, Room 233
Kingston, RI 02881

Dear Professor Brown:

During the 2004 session of the General Assembly, legislative leaders appropriated $800,000 to increase enrollment in our three nursing programs. This decision proved to be a prudent investment. Your participation in Higher Education Day at the State House received rave reviews. The blood pressure and glucose screenings were services that virtually every legislator and policymaker could identify with. Thank you for your participation and please extend my thanks to the future nurses as well.

Sincerely,

Jack R. Warner

They knew we were here! Positive feedback helps the student nurses to recognize the importance of their participation and nursing actions. In addition, their role modeling can have an influence on other legislation such as funding for their nursing program.

CASE STUDY   Application of the Nursing Process

A bilingual community health nursing student named José Mendez worked with the school system in a community that had a large Portuguese subsystem. His aggregate was the students enrolled in the town's bilingual program. His contacts included the school nurse and the program teachers.

ASSESSMENT

José included the specific group of students, the members of the school system's organizational level, and the population group of the town's Portuguese-speaking residents in his assessment of the aggregate's health needs. José identified the subsystem's lack of primary disease prevention, specifically related to hygiene, dental care, nutrition, and lifestyle choices, by observing the children, interviewing teachers and community residents, and reviewing the literature. José's continued assessment and prioritization revealed that the problem was related to a lack of knowledge and not a lack of concern.

DIAGNOSIS

Individual
- Inadequate preparation at home regarding basic hygiene, dental care, nutrition, and healthy lifestyles

Family
- Inadequate knowledge base regarding basic hygiene, dental care, nutrition, and healthy lifestyles

Community
Inadequate resources for communicating basics of hygiene, dental care, nutrition, and healthy lifestyles to the Portuguese community

PLANNING

The teachers and staff of the bilingual program helped contract and set goals, which reinforced the need for mutuality at this step in the process. A variety of alternative interventions were necessary to accomplish the following goals:

Individual
Long-Term Goal
- Students will regularly practice good hygiene, preventive dental care, good nutrition, exercise, and adequate sleep habits.

Short-Term Goal
- Students will learn the basics of good hygiene, preventive dental care, good nutrition, exercise, and adequate sleep habits.

Family
Long-Term Goal
- Families will regularly practice and teach their children good hygiene, preventive dental care, good nutrition, exercise, and adequate sleep habits.

Short-Term Goal
- Families will learn the basics of good hygiene, preventive dental care, good nutrition, exercise, and adequate sleep habits.

Community
Long-Term Goal
- Systematic programs will provide families and their children with education and information regarding the basics of good hygiene, preventive dental care, good nutrition, exercise, and adequate sleep habits.

Short-Term Goal
- Bilingual personnel will translate information into Portuguese, and program teachers will distribute it to families. This information will cover the basics of good hygiene, preventive dental care, good nutrition, exercise, and adequate sleep habits.

INTERVENTION

Sometimes nursing students' projects are more limited than the planning stage's ideal; in this case, interventions only assessed one grade level.

Individual
- The student nurse taught children many healthy lifestyle basics, including nutrition, hygiene, and dental care. Classes presented information in Portuguese and English.

Family
- All parents received a summary of the class content in both languages and in pictures.

Community
- The local teachers communicated the student nurse's activities to their state-level coordinators, and the coordinators incorporated the student nurse's materials into the bilingual program throughout the state.

EVALUATION

Individual, Family, Community
This community health planning project had an impact on the individuals in the specific aggregate and had broader implications for the family systems and the community suprasystem. The outcomes, or product, were hugely successful. Mutually identified goals and objectives influenced the development of the process and incorporated input from a variety of sources. The student nurse believed the resources and support for the bilingual program were adequate. Although the student nurse only addressed primary prevention, the continuing nature of the project will allow the teachers, the school nurse, and the families to assess problems related to the program's content. Future implementation may address secondary and tertiary prevention.

Continued

However, within these programs, requirements for approval are more liberal, expedited reviews are conducted, and certain projects are exempted from review, which weakens the CON cost containment mandate. For example, the CON review threshold for capital expenditures in hospitals and nursing homes varies from none in Florida to $4,000,000 in Hawaii. In Nevada, CON review applies only to new construction costing more than $2,000,000 in rural counties (AHPA, 2004).

CON reviews for new equipment are required in 27 states. In these states, the threshold varies from $400,000 in New Hampshire to $3,000,000 in Delaware and New York; however, the mental hygiene threshold is $1,000,000 in New York. Only 12 of the 36 states and District of Columbia require a CON review for all or any new services. The remaining 24 states limit the services CON may review (AHPA, 2004).

Newer high-technology services (i.e., lithotripsy, gamma knives, and position emission tomography) still need CON review in most states. Furthermore, it is anticipated that state CON programs will assume a stronger role because states must increasingly monitor and report the quality, cost, and access to health care that managed care promised (Piper, 1999).

During the 2004 presidential election campaign, candidates George W. Bush and John F. Kerry both offered proposals for the expansion of health insurance coverage for people currently lacking health insurance. While their goals were similar, the plans for achieving these goals differed in scope. The Bush plan incorporated tax incentives to support the expansion of private sector insurance, while Kerry's plan focused on expanding enrollments in existing federal programs to extend health insurance coverage to more individuals (Sheils, 2004).

Experts in the health planning area believe there will be a paradigm shift from an emphasis on medical care to an emphasis on health care and local, community-based approaches to health issues. The *Healthy People 2010* objectives are a good example of this (see Table 11-1, p. 187). To help achieve improved health status for all, health planning needs a coordinated approach that combines public and private cooperation with an emphasis on supplies and services. Advances in planning models and the sophistication level of planners will impact future health planning efforts (Thomas, 1999).

Nurses must work collaboratively with health planners to improve aggregate health. Nurses can influence health planning at the local and state, or community, level by fusing current technology with their knowledge of health care needs and skills gained through working with individuals, families, groups, and population groups. This is an example of "upstream interventions": The nurse presents group needs or concerns to health planning boards. The nurse may become directly involved in the planning process by participating in CON reviews or gaining membership on health planning councils. Even as students, nurses can begin to participate by engaging in aggregate-level projects, such as those outlined in this chapter, and by tracking health care legislation and contacting their legislators about important issues.

NURSING IMPLICATIONS

Increased nursing involvement is one method of strengthening local and national health planning. Nurses can use this health planning model to facilitate a systematic approach to improve aggregate health care. Nurses can assess aggregates from small groups through population groups; identify the group's health needs; and perform planning, intervention, and evaluations by applying this model. The health of individuals, families, and groups would improve if nurses reemphasized the larger aggregate.

SUMMARY

Community health nurses are responsible for incorporating health planning into their practice. Nurses' unique talents and skills, augmented by the comprehensive application of the nursing process, can facilitate population health improvement at various aggregate levels. Health planning policy and process constitute part of the knowledge base of the baccalaureate-prepared nurse. Systems theory provides one framework for nursing process application in the community. Interventions are possible at subsystem, system, and suprasystem levels using all three levels of prevention.

LEARNING ACTIVITIES

1. Assess a neighborhood or local community using the following exploratory techniques: Perform a windshield survey by driving through the area and identifying types of houses, schools, churches, health-related agencies, and businesses, and looking for potential environmental and safety hazards; interview a town hall clerk, a senior citizen at a meal site or day care center, a newspaper reporter, a visiting nurse, a police officer, a social worker, or a school nurse regarding the community; call the local, county, or state health department for morbidity and mortality statistics; or attend a town council or school committee meeting. Compare and contrast these findings with classmates' findings.

2. Construct a matrix similar to Table 6-5 using interventions from the school nurse setting.

3. In class, identify 10 to 15 questions that will elicit important health information from young adults. Each student must write answers to these questions. Tally the student responses, and draw conclusions from this assessment. Identify problems or potential problem areas, and construct a plan to solve or prevent these problems.

4. Attend a state or local health planning meeting. Observe the number of health care providers and consumers in attendance. Compare the meeting's issues with the goals of improving care quality and reducing health care costs.

5. Interview a health planner at the state or local level to determine the status of health planning and CON review in the community or state.

REFERENCES

American Health Planning Association: *National directory of health planning, policy, and regulatory agencies,* ed 15, Washington, DC, 2004, The Association.

Ammerman A, Parks C: Preparing students for more effective community interventions: assets assessment, *Fam Commmunity Health* 21(1):32-46, 1998.

Budgen C, Cameron G: Program planning implementation and evaluation. In Hitchcock JE, Schubert PE, and Thomas SA, editors: *Community health nursing: caring in action,* ed 4, Clifton Park, NY, 2003, Delmar.

Comprehensive Health Planning and Public Health Services Amendments of 1966, PL 89-749, 1966.

Coyle P: Music, sirens, voices raised in protest against RI health plan, *The Westerly Sun* January 3, 1980.

DeBella S, Martin L, Siddall S: *Nurses' role in health care planning,* Norwalk, Conn, 1986, Appleton-Century-Crofts.

Doerr B et al: Beyond community assessment into the real world of learning aggregate practice, *Nurs Health Care Perspect* 19(5): 214-220, 1998.

Duffus RL: *Lillian Wald: neighbor and crusader,* New York, 1938, Macmillan.

Heart Disease, Cancer, and Stroke Amendments of 1965, PL 89-239, 1965.

Hegge ML: Independent study in community health nursing, *Nurs Outlook* 21:652-654, 1973.

Hogue C: An epidemiologic approach to distributive nursing practice. In Hall JE, Weaver BR, editors: *Distributive nursing practice: a systems approach to community health,* ed 2, Philadelphia, 1985, Lippincott Williams & Wilkins.

Hospital Survey and Construction Act of 1946 (Hill-Burton Act), PL 79-725, 1946.

Kovner AR: Hospitals. In Kovner AR, Jonas S, editors: *Health care delivery system in the United States,* ed 7, New York, 2002, Springer.

Kronenfeld J: *The changing federal role in health care policy,* Westport, Conn, 1997, Praeger.

Leavell HR, Clark EG: *Preventive medicine for the doctor in his community,* New York, 1965, McGraw-Hill.

Lee P, Benjamin AE: Health policy and the politics of health care. In Williams SJ, Torrens PR, editors: *Introduction to health services,* ed 6, Albany, NY, 2002, Delmar.

Maslow AH: *Toward a psychology of being,* New York, 1968, Van Nostrand Reinhold.

Mueller K: *Health care policy in the United States,* Lincoln, Neb, 1993, University of Nebraska Press.

National Health Planning and Resources Development Act of 1974, PL 93-641, 1974.

Partnership for Health Amendments of 1967, PL 90-174, 1967.

Piper T: *CON trends in America: a panorama of change,* The Author, www.aphanet.org/articles.html, 1999.

Ruybal SE, Bauwens E, Fasla MJ: Community assessment: an epidemiological approach, *Nurs Outlook* 23:365-368, 1975.

Sheils J: Bush and Kerry health care proposals: cost and coverage compared, September 2004, The Lewin Group, 2005, from http://www.lewin.com/Spotlights/Features/Lewin_Candidates_Health_Plan_Analysis.htm.

Shonick W: *Government and health services,* New York, 1995, Oxford University Press.

Shuster GF, Goeppinger J: Community as client: assessment and analysis. In Stanhope M, Lancaster J, editors: *Community and public health nursing,* ed 6, St. Louis, 2004, Mosby.

Silverstein NG: Lillian Wald at Henry Street: 1893-1895, *ANS Adv Nurs Sci* 7:1-12, 1985.

Thomas R: *New health planning for the new millennium,* The Author, www.ahpanet.org/articles.html, 1999.

Thorpe K: Cost containment. In Kovner A, Jonas S, editors: *Health care delivery in the Untied States,* ed 7, New York, 2002, Springer.

CHAPTER

7

Community Health Education

Cathy D. Meade

MEDIA RESOURCES

Additional Material for Study, Review, and Further Exploration

evolve Website at http://evolve.elsevier.com/Nies

❖ Quiz ❖ Case Studies ❖ Content Updates ❖ Glossary ❖ WebLinks ❖ Resource Tools

7A Learning Theories and Their Relationship to Health Education, **7B** Framework for Developing Health Communications, **7C** Patient Communication: Testicular Self-Examination (TSE), **7D** SMOG Formula for Estimating Readability Grade Level of Printed Text

---

OBJECTIVES

Upon completion of this chapter, the reader will be able to do the following:

1. Describe the goals of health education within the community setting.
2. Examine the nurse's role in community education within a sociopolitical and cultural context.
3. Select a learning theory and describe its application to the individual, family, or aggregate.
4. Examine effective teaching and learning strategies that exemplify community-centered health education for the individual, family, or aggregate.
5. Compare and contrast Freire's approach to health education with an individualistic health education model.

6. Examine the importance of community partnerships and collaborations having an impact on health disparities.
7. Outline a systematic process for developing relevant health education materials, messages, media, and programs.
8. Relate and apply factors that enhance the suitability of health education materials, messages, media, and programs for an intended audience.
9. Prepare an appropriate teaching plan and evaluation criteria for the individual, family, and group.

KEY TERMS

behavioral theory
cognitive theory
community-based
  participatory methods

community empowerment
culturally effective care
health disparities
health education

health literacy
humanistic theory
learner verification
learning

materials and media
participatory action research
problem-solving education
social learning theory

CHAPTER OUTLINE

CONNECTING WITH EVERYDAY REALITIES

HEALTH EDUCATION IN THE COMMUNITY

LEARNING THEORIES, PRINCIPLES, AND HEALTH EDUCATION MODELS
  Learning Theories
  Knowles' Assumptions About Adult Learners
  Health Education Models
  Models of Individual Behavior
  Model of Health Education Empowerment
  Community Empowerment

THE NURSE'S ROLE IN HEALTH EDUCATION

ENHANCING COMMUNICATION

FRAMEWORK FOR DEVELOPING HEALTH COMMUNICATIONS
  Stage I: Planning and Strategy Development
  Stage II: Developing and Pretesting Concepts, Messages, and Materials
  Stage III: Implementing the Program
  Stage IV: Assessing Effectiveness and Making Refinements

HEALTH EDUCATION RESOURCES
  Literacy and Health
  Assess Materials: Become a Wise Consumer and User
  Assessing the Relevancy of Health Materials

CONNECTING WITH EVERYDAY REALITIES

The nurse may be tempted to often ask the following questions:

- Why does this woman keep smoking when she is pregnant?
- Why does this young man not take his diabetic medications (insulin) each day?
- Why don't the parents immunize their kids on time?
- Why don't more men and women attend the clinic's prostate and mammography screenings—they're free!
- Why does the community have such an alarming rate of obesity?

Although these questions represent the nurse's intense desire to understand the link between health behavior and health education, they do not yield answers or empower individuals or families. In fact, such questions do not address the root health issues and create a "blaming the victim" approach (Israel et al., 1994). The nurse might reframe the previous questions to better get at the root reasons and, in turn, empower individuals, families, and groups. Instead, ask the following questions:

- What life stressors are getting in the way of the expectant mom from quitting smoking for good?
- How does the young man with diabetes prefer to learn? What makes it difficult for him to know when to take his meds? What could the nurse do to better connect the lifesaving instructions about insulin to his everyday activities?
- What types of barriers might prevent the family from getting their kids immunized on time? Do they understand the schedule? Could the nurse do a better job of explaining the importance of immunizations? Could a personalized chart record help?
- What kinds of outreach methods might better attract community members to the free cancer screenings? In what way could sustained relationships with community stakeholders and community members make a difference?
- What role might the nurse play in developing links with grocery stores, senior centers, and churches to reach community members with nutrition messages that are easy to understand and that fit their cultural background? What social, physical, cultural, linguistic, or structural factors should be considered when developing such messages?

HEALTH EDUCATION IN THE COMMUNITY

Historically, teaching has been a significant nursing responsibility since Florence Nightingale's (1859) early work. Gardner (1936) emphasized that health teaching is one of the most fundamental nursing principles and that "a nurse, in even the most obscure position must be a teacher of no mean order." There is much support for the nurse's involvement in health education, including the Nurse Practice Acts, professional statements of the American Nurses Association (ANA) (1975), the American Hospital Association's (AHA) (1972) patient's bill of rights, the Joint Commission on Accreditation of Healthcare Organizations (JCAHO) (1995), the Office of Minority Health's (OMH) national standards on Culturally and Linguistically Appropriate Services (OMH, 1999), and the U.S. Department of Health and Human Services (USDHHS) *Healthy People 2010* objectives (USDHHS, 2000). Health education is an integral part of the nurse's role in the community for promoting health, preventing disease, and maintaining optimal wellness (Box 7-1). Moreover, the community is a vital link for the delivery of effective and equitable health care and offers the nurse multiple opportunities for providing appropriate health education within the context of a setting that is familiar to community members (Meade, 2002a).

The role of the nurse as health educator is especially important in light of the increasing diversity and demographically changing population in the United States, the increasingly technological advancements in health care, and the need to reduce the disconnect between scientific discovery to the delivery of interventions in the community (Freeman, 2004). More than ever before, health education activities and services are taking place outside the walls of

---

BOX 7-1   Health Education Roles and Activities of the Nurse in the Community

- Advocate
- Caregiver
- Case manager
- Collaborator
- Community care agent
- Consultant
- Counselor
- Culture broker
- Educator
- Facilitator of health-promoting behaviors
- Information agent and broker
- Innovator
- Liaison
- Mediator
- Negotiator
- Policy analyst, policy maker, or change agent
- Promoter of collaborative partnerships
- Promoter of self-care and self-efficacy
- Referral resource
- Recognizes dimensions of health choices
- Researcher
- Sensitizer
- Social activist

Based on data from Clark, 2003; Jezewski, 1993; Rankin and Stallings, 2000; Redman, 2001.

hospital in such settings as missions, beauty and barber shops, grocery stores, homeless shelters, community-based clinics, health maintenance organizations, schools, work sites, senior centers, mobile health units. Women, Infants, and Children (WIC) sites, and homes At the core of health education is the development of trusting relationships based on nurturing interactions, the use of **community-based participatory methods** that highlight community strengths, and the creation of sustainable collaborations and partnerships (Leung, Yen, and Minkler, 2004; Meade and Calvo, 2001; Minkler, 2005; Olshansky et al., 2005; Smedley et al., 2003).

Health education's goal is to understand health behavior and to translate knowledge into relevant interventions and strategies for health enhancement, disease prevention, and chronic illness management. Health education aims to enhance wellness and decrease disability and attempts to actualize the health potential of individuals, families, communities, and society and includes a broad and varied set of strategies aimed at influencing individuals within their social environment for improved health and well-being (Green and Kreuter, 2005). The nurse is in an ideal position to bring together the necessary skills, knowledge, and community resources to impact the health of the community.

> **Health education** *is any combination of learning experiences designed to predispose, enable, and reinforce voluntary behavior conducive to health in individuals, groups or communities. (Green and Kreuter, 2005)*

Over the past decade, health education has increasingly become viewed as an instrument of change (Glanz et al., 2002). Steuart and Kark (1962) state that "health education must achieve its ends through means that leave inviolate the rights of self-determination of the individuals and their community." A major challenge for community health nurse educators is to address the complex sociopolitical conditions that affect community health by placing value on the contributions of community members and building on their strengths. The lasting effect of cognitive and behavioral changes relies heavily on learner participation to influence change in health behaviors and practices (Green and Kreuter, 2005; Leung et al., 2004; MacLeod and Zimmer, 2005; Wallerstein, 2002). In this manner, nurses alone cannot set individual, family, or community priorities. Rather, learners (community members) must be involved in determining their health education needs and priorities.

In Chapter 3, Butterfield cogently indicates that most literature focuses on individual relationships that shape a patient's health behaviors. She purports that downstream thinking seriously restricts a nurse's ability to consider the multitude of external factors that influence behavior (e.g., environment, culture, social roles, and socioeconomics). Upstream endeavors, or macroscopic perspectives, help nurses gain insight into a more global perspective on behavior and helps address the complexity of the larger, more powerful systems that influence behavior. Upstream thinking emphasizes variables that precede or play a role in the development of health problems. When nurses view human responses to health

and illness within the sociopolitical-economic framework, they can identify and understand power imbalances within the community that prohibit groups from achieving full potential. Butterfield suggests that social critical theory helps nurses explore societal, political, and environmental forces that impact global community health.

Community health education is based on practical, relevant, and scientifically sound methods and widely accessible technology. In the late 1970s, Kleinman (1978) described a social and cultural community health care system that related external factors (e.g., economical, political, and epidemiological) to internal factors (e.g., behavioral and communicative). This view of a sociocultural health care system grounds health education activities within sociopolitical structures, especially within local environmental settings, and views the community as client (Brackley et al., 2003; Giachello et al., 2003; Horowitz et al., 2004; Klinedinst, 2005; Meade et al., 2003; Petersen et al., 2004; Villarruel et al., 2004). Moreover, the creation and delivery of relevant health education interventions and communications within the community setting is a national imperative as outlined by *Healthy People 2010,* OMH's Standards for the Provision of Culturally Competent Health Care (1999), and several Institute of Medicine reports (e.g., Nielsen-Bohlman et al., 2004; Smedley et al., 2003). Nurses are uniquely qualified to influence the health and well-being of community members' health behaviors through innovative activities that incorporate culturally, linguistically, and educationally relevant health education and outreach communications (Meade, 2003; Watters, 2003).

LEARNING THEORIES, PRINCIPLES, AND HEALTH EDUCATION MODELS

Learning Theories

Learning theories are helpful in understanding how individuals, families, and groups learn. The field of psychology provides the basis for these theories and illustrates how environmental stimuli elicit specific responses. Theories can aid nurses to recognize the mechanisms that potentially modify knowledge, attitude, and behavior. Bigge and Shermis (2004) asserts that **learning** is an enduring change that may involve the modification of insights, behaviors, perceptions, or motivations. Although psychology textbooks describe learning theories in great detail, the following broad categories relate to the nursing application in a community setting: stimulus-response (S-R) conditioning (i.e., behavioristic), cognitive, humanistic, and social learning. **Resource Tool 7A** Learning Theories and Their Relationship to Health Education on the book's evolve website at http://evolve.elsevier.com/Nies outlines these learning theories.

The nurse needs to remember that theories are not completely right or wrong. Different theories work well in different situations. Knowles (1989) relates that behaviorists program individuals through S-R mechanisms to behave in a certain fashion. **Humanistic theories** help an individual

RESEARCH HIGHLIGHTS

Linking Theory to Practice: An Example of an HIV/STD Risk Reduction Intervention for African American and Latino Adolescent Girls

An educational, skill-based HIV/STD (human immunodeficiency virus/sexually transmitted disease) risk-reduction intervention was designed and evaluated using a randomized controlled trial among African American and Latina adolescent girls. The primary outcome of interest was change in self-reported unprotected sexual intercourse; secondary outcomes included the frequency of sexual intercourse while intoxicated, the number of sexual partners, number of biologically confirmed STDs, and theoretical mediators such as intent/belief about condoms. The sample (N = 682) was drawn from an adolescent clinic. Participants took part in one 25-minute intervention (group discussion, videotapes, games, exercises) based on cognitive-behavioral theory. The study had three groups: (1) the information-based HIV/STD intervention that offered safe-sex information; (2) a skills-based HIV/STD group offering information plus skills for practicing safer sex, for example, roleplaying, handling condoms, and so on; and (3) control (health promotion issues unrelated to sexual behavior). Results show no significant difference between the information intervention and the health control intervention. However, the skills-intervention participants reported less unprotected sexual intercourse at the 12-month follow-up than did the information-only group. At the 12-month follow-up, participants in the skills intervention reported fewer sexual partners compared with the health control group and were less likely to test positive for STDs than the control group. No differences in number of partners or frequency of partners among the groups were observed at the 3- and 6-month follow-up points. The information-based group gave higher rating for liking the intervention than either the health-promotion control intervention or other skills-based intervention. Analyses showed no differences in efficacy of the intervention among African Americans and Latinas on STD rates, sexual risk behavior, or evaluation of the interventions. Overall, the skill-based intervention was significantly more effective among the Latinas than among the African Americans in increasing the use of condoms ($p = .02$) and with condom negotiation skills ($p = .05$).

Results suggest that a behavioral intervention, which combines information and skills training, has the potential to reduce unprotected intercourse and STD rate among adolescent girls. The effects of the intervention were significant primarily at the 12-month follow-up, and not at short-term follow-up periods, which may indicate that adolescents were able to implement those practices with new partners over time. A limitation of the study is the use of self-report measures. One important direction for HIV/STD prevention education is to determine the extent to which the same intervention can be applied among different groups that differ in race/ethnicity. Although continued research is necessary to further validate and refine efficacy-enhancing strategies, the study reinforces the importance of the nurse in using theoretical variables in planning, designing, and testing health education interventions (Jemmott et al., 2005).

Jemmott JB et al: HIV/STD risk reduction interventions for African American and Latino adolescent girls at an adolescent medicine clinic, *Arch Pediatr Adolesc Med* 159:440-449, 2005

develop his or her potential in a self-directing and holistic manner. Cognitive theorists recognize the brain's ability to think, feel, learn, and solve problems and they train the brain to maximize these functions. Although social learning theory is largely a **cognitive theory**, it also includes elements of behaviorism (Bandura, 1977b). **Social learning theory's premise is based on behavior explaining and enhancing learning through the concepts of efficacy, outcome expectation, and incentives.**

CLINICAL EXAMPLE

Application of Characteristics of Adult Learners to the Development of a Community Support Group

In the 1980s, the author and a colleague began a community support group for individuals with amyotrophic lateral sclerosis (ALS). The support group was also open to family members and friends. ALS is an incurable degenerative neuromuscular disease that affects nerve and muscle function and the brain's ability to control muscle movement. It is more commonly referred to as Lou Gehrig disease. Community members provided feedback and identified the need for education and support for ALS. At that time, southeast Wisconsin did not have a support group. This initial dialogue provided the organizing framework for the inception of the support group and based on observations and interactions at the monthly meetings, an illustration of Knowles' assumptions follows:

Need to know: At the support group, the facilitator-nurse introduces topics by describing the reason for the discussion and rationale for the selected subject (e.g., common concerns of patients and family members and informal assessments based on conversations). To prepare for discussion, group members introduce themselves, and the nurse asks what they hope to learn from the presentation. In some cases, members are unsure why they desire more information on a given topic but indicate that they want to listen. Progression of the disease is variable; therefore the need to know is facilitated by the nurse and other patients who have already noted the importance of specific learning tasks (e.g., need for assistive walking device, need for financial planning, or need for information on assistive breathing devices).

Self-Concept: A comfortable, informal environment allows patients to express emotions and frustrations about this disease. Participants are encouraged to express themselves. Participants cultivate mutual respect and trust and hugs are common. Members understand that others share similar situations and concerns. Group members have an opportunity to speak out about ways to manage their disease (e.g., decisions about life support and feeding tubes). Even if the choices are not congruent with others, participants recognize and acknowledge these decisions without imposing their own value judgments. Facilitators and group members are equal partners in the learning process.

Experiences: Some patients and family members have gone through other difficult life experiences (e.g., other illnesses or deaths in the family) and can help others cope with the management of ALS. Patients share the strengths gained from such experiences with other members. Additionally, individuals and family members who are going through varying stages of the disease process can share their experiences (e.g., obtaining home care, selecting a computer, and managing breathing difficulties). They share tips and timesaving strategies with each other and newly diagnosed families and learn from those previously diagnosed.

Readiness to Learn: Family members often assume many roles when someone is ill, especially with a chronic illness such as ALS. The redefinition of roles creates learning opportunities; however, this may hinder learning if it is too overwhelming. For example, the well spouse may assume the roles of caregiver, parent, and financial supporter. It is helpful to identify resources to help the family cope with new roles (e.g., respite care).

Orientation to Learning: Learning a variety of psychomotor skills is necessary to care for the ALS patient (e.g., suctioning, positioning, using a feeding tube, and toileting). The time frame for learning such skills varies depending on the course of illness. Presenting information about such skills too early in the course of the disease may cause fear and anxiety. Families are often resistant to learning such tasks until the need is apparent. In some cases, this may be evident at a crisis point (e.g., a fall, a choking incident, or severe respiratory distress). However, facilitators introduce these topics slowly by providing information via the support group, newsletter, printed brochures, and personal one-on-one discussions.

Motivation: Individuals and families experience a shift in life goals when facing ALS. Such shifts may create learning opportunities aimed at enhancing quality of life, survivorship, and maintaining self-esteem. For example, a college professor with ALS kept his link to the university. He was highly motivated to continue his research work and supervise his graduate students. To continue his academic work, he learned to manage his breathing by using a ventilator, arranging transportation to the university, obtaining nursing care, and creating communication methods by using a computer.

Today, there are more than eight ALS support/caregiver groups in Wisconsin that grew from just a few who recognized an unmet need in the community. The ALS Association Wisconsin Chapter evolved from a local support group and became an official ALSA chapter in 1987. The Chapter has four primary goals: (1) provide education, guidance, services, and support to ALS patients, their families, and their caregivers; (2 promote public awareness of ALS; (3) raise funds for ALS research; and (4) establish an ALS-certified, multidisciplinary clinic to provide the highest level of care to the patients served by the Chapter. For more information on services, go to http://alsawi.org/hopeline.php ∎

Knowles' Assumptions About Adult Learners

Knowles (1980, 1989) outlined several assumptions about adult learners. He contends that adults, like children, learn better in a facilitative, nonrestrictive, and nonstructured environment. Nurses who are familiar with these assumptions can develop teaching strategies that motivate and interest individuals, families, and groups and encourage active participation in the learning process. Nurses can help to create a self-directing, self-empowering learning environment. The following characteristics impact learning: the client's need to know, concept of self, readiness to learn, orientation to learning, experience, and motivation. Table 7-1 and Research Highlights, Application of Characteristics of Adult Learners to the Development of a Community Support Group, expand upon these characteristics.

Health Education Models

In addition to learning theories, applying education theories and principles to situations involving individuals, families, and groups illustrates how ideas fit together, offers explanations for health behaviors or actions, and helps direct community nursing interventions. Such theoretical elements form the basis of understanding health behavior. Glanz and colleagues (2002) state that theories give educators the power to assess an intervention's strength and impact, and they serve to enrich, inform, and complement practice. Theoretical frameworks offer nurses an intervention blueprint that promotes learning and provides them with an organized approach to explaining concept relationships (Padilla and Bulcavage, 1991).

> *What the nurse needs is often not a single theory that would explain all that he or she hears, but rather a framework with meaningful hooks and rubrics on which to hang the new variables and insights offered by different theories. With this customized metatheory or framework, the nurse can triage new ideas into categories that have personal utility in his or her practice and everyday realities. (Green, 1998, p. 2)*

Models of Individual Behavior

Two models that explain preventive behavior determinants are the Health Belief Model (HBM), which is presented in Table 7-2 (Becker et al., 1977; Hochbaum, 1958; Kegeles et al., 1965; Rosenstock, 1966), and the Health Promotion Model (HPM) (Pender, Murdaugh, and Parsons, 2005). Both models are multifactorial, based on value expectancy, and address individual perceptions, modifying factors, and likelihood of action. Glanz and colleagues (1997) conducted an extensive search of the health behavior literature from mid 1992 to mid 1994 and found that 526 of 1174 relevant articles, or 44.8%, used at least one theory or model. The HBM was the most commonly cited theory.

The HBM is based on social psychology and has undergone much empirical testing to predict compliance on singular preventive measures. The initial purpose of the HBM was to explain why people did not participate in health education programs to prevent or detect disease, in particular, tuberculosis (TB) screening programs (Hochbaum, 1958). Subsequent studies addressed other preventive actions and factors related to adherence to medical regimens (Becker, 1974). Primarily, the HBM is a value expectancy theory that addresses factors that promote health-enhancing behavior. It is disease specific and focuses on avoidance orientation. The HBM considers perceived susceptibility, perceived severity, perceived benefits, perceived barriers, and other sociopsychological and structural variables. In an early review of 46 studies using the HBM, perceived benefits was found to be the most powerful predictive element within the model, whereas perceived severity had the lowest associative value (Janz and Becker, 1984). Self-efficacy, or the notion that an individual can act successfully on a given behavior to produce the desired outcome (Bandura, 1977a, 1977b), was later added to the HBM (Rosenstock, Strecher, and Becker, 1988; Strecher et al., 1986).

TABLE 7-1 Characteristics of Adult Learners

CHARACTERISTICS	APPLICATION TO HEALTH EDUCATION
Need to know Adults must know why they need to learn. Self-Concept Adults have a self-concept that developed from dependence to independence. It moves from other's direction to self-direction. Adults want to be capable of self-direction.	The nurse explores why individuals, families, and groups want to learn. The nurse helps individuals recognize their need to learn. The nurse acknowledges that individuals, families, and groups are able to make choices and decisions. The nurse creates an environment in which patients can express themselves. The nurse recognizes that individuals, families, and groups can learn from their selected actions and can take self-direction and responsibility for such behaviors.
Experience Adults may draw upon many life experiences. Such experiences are enriching and are powerful learning resources.	The nurse assesses individuals, families, and groups for life experiences related to health issues. The nurse helps facilitate connections between previous and present experiences. The nurse allows individuals, families, and groups to share experiences with others in a supportive manner. Experiential methods, problem solving, case methods, and discussion can help uncover the learner's experiences. The nurse clarifies previous and present experiences; this is especially helpful with negative or biased experiences.
Readiness to learn Developmental tasks and social roles affect readiness to learn. The timing learning experiences with developmental tasks is important.	The nurse assesses and identies individual, family, and group roles (e.g., caregivers or single parents) and key developmental tasks. The nurse seeks to understand the impact of roles and tasks on learning. The nurse creates role-modeling experiences.
Orientation to learning Learning is present oriented and "now" based. Learning is directed to the immediate need and is problem centered.	The nurse assesses the learning needs of individuals, families, and groups on the basis of their priority. The nurse recognizes everyday stresses and hassles and addresses them within their learning context. The nurse provides health information, gives responses to their immediate needs, and offers provides health information, gives responses to their immediate needs, and offers problem-solving skills.
Motivation Internal drivers and factors are powerful motivators (e.g., self-esteem, life goals, quality of life, and responsibility).	The nurse determines individual, family, and group motivators. The nurse assesses for barriers that block motivation (e.g., poor self-esteem or lack of resources) and provides appropriate education, counseling, and referrals.

Modified from Knowles MS: *The making of an adult educator: an autobiographical journey,* San Francisco, 1989, Jossey-Bass; and Knowles MS: *The modern practice of adult education: from pedagogy to andragogy,* Chicago, 1980, Association Press/Follett.

TABLE 7-2 Health Belief Model

COMPONENTS	EXAMPLE AND EXPLANATION
Perceived susceptibility	Belief that disease state is present or likely to occur
Perceived severity	Perception that disease state or condition is harmful and has serious consequences
Perceived benefits	Belief that health action is of value and has efficacy
Perceived barriers	Belief that health action would be associated with hindrances (e.g., cost)
Self-efficacy	Belief that actions can be performed to achieve the desired outcome (one's confidence)
Demographics	Age, sex, and ethnicity
Cues to action	Influencing factors to get ready for action (e.g., billboards, reminder cues, newspapers)

For a more detailed description of the HBM, see Becker (1974).

Janz, Champion, and Strecher (2002) later point out several deficits of the HBM, which include the inconsistent measurement of HBM concepts and the lack of establishing validity and reliability of the measures prior to testing. For example, applying similar construct measures across different behaviors, such as barriers for mammography and colonoscopy, may be quite different. Although the past decade has produced some good examples of HBM scale development (Champion, 1999; Rawl et al., 2000), caution should be taken when applying the HBM in multicultural settings. It would be important to determine if the overall assumptions of the HBM—assumptions related to the value of health and illness—are similar to those of the particular racial/ethnic group under study. Further, checking wording for cultural distinctions is critical to the model's usefulness (Janz et al., 2002). Although the HBM identifies an array of variables important in explaining individual health, nurses should view these variables within a larger societal perspective.

Pender's Health Promotion Model (HPM) is a competence or approach-oriented model and, unlike the HBM, does not rely on personal threat as a motivating factor. The HPM brings together a number of constructs from expectancy-value theory and social cognitive theory within a holistic nursing framework (Pender et al., 2005). Gillis (1993) reviewed 23 studies conducted between 1983 and 1992 and reported that Pender's HPM was the most common theoretical framework in health promotion studies. Gillis identified that self-efficacy was the strongest determinant of participation in a health-promoting lifestyle, followed by social support, perceived benefits, perceived barriers, and an individual's definition of health education. Locus of control was the least important determinant, although it is the most studied.

The HPM is meant to provide an organizing framework to explain why individuals engage in health actions. It is applicable across the lifespan and has been used to examine the multidimensional nature of persons interacting with their physical and interpersonal environments, such as the use of bicycle helmet use (Lohse, 2003) or health-promoting behaviors among Hispanics (Hulme et al., 2003). Table 7-3 lists the main HPM components with behavioral action as the desired output.

The HBM and HPM can assist community health nurses in examining an individual's health choices and decisions for influencing health-related behaviors. The models offer nurses a cluster of variables that provide interesting insights into explaining health behavior. These variables are helpful cues; the nurse should consider them in planning and interacting with health education interventions but not try to fit an individual into all the categories. Simply put, models are aids that guide nurses in assessing patients and in developing, selecting, and implementing relevant educational interventions. In applying the models, a nurse or nursing student might consider the following questions in relation to his or her own health behavior:

- Do you strive for improved health?
- Are you or your family susceptible to heart disease or obesity?
- Does a family history of cardiovascular disease motivate you or your family to exercise?
- Does looking fit and toned and having energy motivate you to exercise?
- Do work, school, or family get in the way of your exercise plans?
- Has a family member, friend, or health professional recently reminded you of the benefits of exercise and encouraged you to start exercising?
- Do you believe you can initiate and incorporate an exercise program into your lifestyle, or do you need external reinforcement and cues?
- Do money, safety, and time pose barriers to planning an exercise program?
- Do you see any benefits to exercise, for example, looking and feeling better and more energized?

In modifying your health behaviors, how important is exercise compared with other behaviors (e.g., cutting down on snacks, getting relief from work and school stresses, spending quality time with your family)?

Think about these questions and consider your answers. Talk about these issues with a colleague and try to develop an action plan tailored to your own priorities, needs, and capabilities.

Model of Health Education Empowerment

The HBM and HPM focus on individual strategies for achieving optimal health and well-being. The models are

TABLE 7-3 Health Promotion Model Components and Outputs

COGNITIVE-PERCEPTUAL FACTORS	EXAMPLE AND EXPLANATION
Importance of health	Perceived value of health to functioning and life
Perceived control of health	Perceived ability to control health (external, internal, or chance)
Perceived self-efficacy	Perceived ability to perform the necessary behaviors to achieve an outcome
Definition of health	Views of what health means for the individual May vary from absence of illness to self-actualization
Perceived health status	Perception of how the individual view health May range from wellness to illness
Perceived benefits of health-promoting behaviors	Perception of positive outcomes that can occur from health-promoting behavior (e.g., feel fit and toned)
Perceived barriers to health-promoting behaviors	Perception of things that obstruct health-promoting behaviors (e.g., money and transportation)

MODIFYING FACTORS	EXAMPLE AND EXPLANATION
Demographics	Age, sex, and race
Biological	Weight and body fat
Interpersonal influences	Interactions with family and nurses
Situational factors	Environmental determinants that make health promoting options available
Behavioral	Previous knowledge or skills
Cues to action	Influencing factors such as internal cues (e.g., good self-image) and external cues (e.g., mass media)

For a more comprehensive description and explanation of the HPM, see Pender et al. (2005).

similar in that they are multifactorial, are based on the idea of value expectancy, and address individual perceptions, modifying factors, and likelihood of action. Although such approaches may be appropriate in changing individual behaviors, they do not address the complex relationships among social, structural, and physical factors in the environment, such as racism, lack of social support systems, and inaccessible health services (Israel et al., 1998; Smedley et al., 2003). Van Wyk (1999) suggests that nurses cannot assign power and control to the individual within the community but rather that the "power" must be taken on by the individual with the nurse *guiding* the dynamic process. This process includes examining race, ethnicity, education/literacy, gender, and class and recognizing the structural and foundational changes that are needed to elicit change for socially and politically disenfranchised groups. Although information dissemination for behavior change has been the mainstay of traditional health education, Travers (1997) describes this alternative conceptualization as simply "health education for social change." This means people become involved in collective action to create healthy lifestyles and environments.

Features of a more appropriate health education model is one that embraces a broader definition of health that address social, political, and economic aspects of health. This view of the health care system as a sociocultural system can better ground health education interventions within the sociopolitical structure, especially within local environmental settings (Goodman et al., 1998; Labonte, 1994). Such a theoretical perspective is congruent with community health education because it supports learner participation and involvement and emphasizes empowerment.

Empowerment is the total sum of efforts that are defined as "gaining controls over decision-making at the individual, family, community, and societal levels." Empowerment and literacy are two concepts that share a common history: The concept of empowerment can be traced back to Paulo Freire, a Brazilian educator in the 1950s who sought to promote literacy among the poorest of the poor, most oppressed members of the population. He based his work on a problem-solving approach to education, which contrasts with the banking education approach that places the learner in a passive role. **Problem-solving education** allows active participation and ongoing dialogue and encourages learners to be critical and reflective about health issues. Freire suggested that when individuals assume the role of *objects,* they become powerless and allow the environment to control them. However, when individuals become *subjects*, they influence environmental factors that affect their lives and community. Thus community members, or subjects, are the best resources to elicit change (Freire, 1970, 1973).

His methodology, often referred to as critical consciousness, involves not only education but also activism on the part of the educator. The basic tenets of Freire's work centers on empowerment, the contextualization of peoples' daily experiences and collaborative, collegial dialogue in adult education. Freire's work speaks to a variety of action research applications, including those that relate to improving community health of marginalized populations.

Freire's approach to health education increases health knowledge through a participatory group process. This process explores the problem's nature and addresses the problem's deeper issues. The nurse, or facilitator-educator, is a resource person and is an equal partner with the other group members. Listening is the first phase and is essential to understanding the issues. The exchange of ideas and concerns creates a problem-posing dialogue and identifies root problems or generative themes. The group discusses and explores the problem's root causes. Finally, group members create relevant action plans that are congruent with their own reality (Freire, 1973).

The goal of participatory action research (PAR) is social change. It is consistent with the role and responsibilities of the community nurse (Olshansky et al., 2005) and embraces the use of community-based participatory methods. What this means is that participation and action from stakeholders and important knowledge about conditions and issues gained facilitates strategies reached collectively (e.g., access to care, access to information, etc.). In this manner, the value of communities' experiential knowledge is affirmed (Leung et al., 2004). Examples of the use of PAR include Horowitz et al. (2004), who describe the use of combining local and academic expertise to study health disparities and create

peer-led classes to improve chronic disease management in East and Central Harlem; Edgren and colleagues (2005), who offered suggestions for involving the community in fighting against asthma; English et al. (2004), who developed the REACH 2010 program to build a public health community capacity program with a tribal community in the Southwest; and Giachello et al. (2003), who addressed the disproportionately high rate of diabetes in southeast Chicago through community-led activities.

At the core of empowerment are *information, communication,* and *health education* (WHO, 1994). When nurses involve individuals, families, and groups in their learning, it validates their role and helps ensure the intervention's relevance (Leung et al., 2004; Meade, 2003; Minkler and Wallerstein, 2002; Olshansky et al., 2005). Nurses can use empowerment strategies to help people develop skills in problem solving, networking, negotiating, lobbying, and information seeking to enhance health. Freire's approach may seem similar to health education's emphasis on helping people take responsibility for their health by providing them with information, skills, reinforcement, and support. However, Freire purports that knowledge imparted by the collective group is significantly more powerful than information provided by health educators. Freire's approach attempts to uncover the social and political aspects of problems and encourages group members to define and develop action strategies. Health changes are complex and usually do not have immediate solutions; therefore the term problem *posing,* rather than problem *solving,* may better describe this empowerment process (Minkler and Wallerstein, 2002).

Examples of Empowerment Education and Participatory Methods

1a. Wang and Burris (1994) first described the use of photovoice as an empowerment strategy that uses photographs or pictures to tell a story or teach literacy. This participatory process integrates empowerment education, feminist theory, and documentary photography to fuel critical consciousness and document a community's strengths and problems directly. Photovoice allows people to identify, represent, and enhance their community through specific photographic techniques. Community members explore issues related to the social, economic, cultural, and biomedical factors that affect them by documenting their everyday lives. The images become educational tools that increase their health status knowledge individually and collectively, empower them to mobilize for social change, and communicate their situation to policy makers. Facilitated group discussions validate concerns about family, self, and community; aid in problem identification; and challenge members to create action strategies.

Participatory involvement may be a diagnostic tool for readdressing inadequate assumptions. For example, photovoice revealed that the major issues for rural women in China were the lack of transportation, water, and child care—not a lack of knowledge. Thus empowerment resulted in access to resources and networks and knowledge based on "real needs."

1b. López and colleagues (2005) further relate how photovoice was used as a participatory action research method with African American breast cancer survivors in rural east North Carolina, referred to as the "inspirational images project." The aim of the study was to use this research method to allow women to convey the social and cultural meaning of silence about breast cancer and to voice their survivorship concerns so that relevant interventions could be developed to meet their needs. The task of the women was to take at least six pictures of people, places, or things that they enjoyed in life; significant things they encountered as a survivor; and what was used to cope. Discussion of photographs (e.g., picture of church) led to discussions including a six-step inductive questioning technique suggested by Wallerstein and Bernstein (1988), which helps participants in framing educational strategies:

- What do you SEE in this photograph?
- What is HAPPENING in the photograph?
- How does this relate to OUR lives?
- WHY do these issues exist?
- How can we become EMPOWERED by our new social understanding?
- What can we DO to address these issues?

The use of photovoice offers an important and creative way to facilitate shared knowledge to achieve social change.

2. Chang, Li, and Liu (2004) report the use of an empowering process using Freire's dialogical interviewing among 15 newly diagnosed cancer patients over three months in Taiwan. Data collection among 15 cancer patients included the use of open-ended questions and participatory observation. Emergent themes derived from ongoing and constant analysis revealed the following empowered outcomes: redefinition of health, feelings of confidence, active involvement, revitalization of self and desire to live, negotiating care goals, and having strength to help others. A key nursing implication for health education showed that an essential element of empowerment was helping clients to think critically to make their lives meaningful in times of difficulty.

Community Empowerment

Robertson and Minkler (1994) indicate that although empowerment education, community participation, and a broader socialized health definition fit the new definition of health promotion, this definition may potentially undervalue individual empowerment. Although this approach provides a socialized conceptualization of health and separates individuals from their health status, it also minimizes the associations between people and their daily difficulties in managing health and illness. This strong push to embrace collective empowerment may negate the value of professionally based direct health services. Rather, Wallerstein and Minkler (2002) suggest that an empowerment continuum be

used that acknowledges the value and interdependence of individual and political action strategies aimed at the collective while maintaining the community organization as central.

Community organization reinforces one of the fields underlying premises as outlined by Nyswander (1956): "Start where the people are." Moreover, Labonte (1994) states that the community is the engine of health promotion and a vehicle of empowerment. He describes five spheres of an empowerment model, which focus on the following levels of social organization: interpersonal (personal empowerment), intragroup (small group development), intergroup (community), interorganizational (coalition building), and political action. Meade et al. (2001a) points out that attention must be given to collective rather than individual efforts to ensure that the outcomes reflect the voices of the community and truly make a difference in people's lives.

Labonte's (1994) multilevel empowerment model allows us to consider both macro-level and micro-level forces that combine to create both health and disease. Therefore, it seems that both micro and macro viewpoints on health education provide nurses with multiple opportunities for intervention across a broad continuum. In summary, health education activities that respond to McKinlay's (1979) call to study "upstream," that examine the underlying causes of health inequalities, through multilevel education and research allows nurses to be informed by critical perspectives from education, anthropology, and public health. For more extensive readings on this topic, see *Methods in Community-based Participatory Research for Health* (Israel et al., 2005).

To effect change at the community level, nurses must be knowledgeable about key concepts central to community organization (Table 7-4). This approach is an effective methodological tool that enables nurses to partner with the community, identify common goals, develop strategies, and mobilize resources to increase community empowerment, capacity, and community competence. Key concepts inherent in community health education programming are empowerment, community competence, issue selection, principle of relevance, principle of participation, and creation of critical consciousness (Minkler and Wallerstein, 2002).

Keck (1994) indicated that successful community health relies on empowering citizens to make decisions about individual and community health. Empowering citizens causes power to shift from health providers to community members in addressing health priorities. The basic tenets of community empowerment are not new; however, the belief that this framework is valuable and important is new. Collaboration and cooperation among community members, academicians, clinicians, health agencies, and businesses help ensure that scientific advances, community needs, sociopolitical needs, and environmental needs converge in a humanistic manner. The development of LUNA (Latinas Unidas por un Nuevo Amanecer, Inc.) in Tampa, Florida, illustrates how the basic tenets of community need and organization fueled the development of a locally initiated group. LUNA represents a grassroots initiative to meet the needs of Hispanic breast cancer survivors and serves as a

TABLE 7-4   Community Organization Practice

KEY CONCEPTS	APPLICATION TO HEALTH EDUCATION (NURSING ACTIONS)
Empowerment Help individuals, families, and groups gain insight and mastery over life situations through problem solving and dialogue	The nurse works with community members in identifying and defining issues and creates mechanisms for discussion and problem solving and identification of other factors that have an impact on everyday lives.
Community competence Help the community achieve desired goals through collaboration	The nurse names key leaders and members to work collaboratively to identify and set goals and priorities. The nurse contact social and political leaders and networks. The nurse allows community members to define their own issues and helps them focus on their objectives.
Principle of relevancy Know what issues are important to community members (these may differ from the issues important to nurses)	The nurse holds town hall meetings and group discussions to allow members to share concerns and important issues. The nurse encourages the community to define issues. The nurse facilitates community members to make decisions about health programs and messages.
Principle of participation Learn by doing	The nurse encourages group support. The nurse recognizes that active vs. passive participation results in greater likelihood of attitude and behavior changes.
Issue selection Identify community problems that the community believes are specific, meaningful, and attainable	The nurse uses problem-solving techniques to help group members identify relevant issues vs. troubling problems (e.g., door-to-door surveys and group process activities).
Creation of critical consciousness Encourage relationships of equality and mutual respect among group members and educators to identify root problems and generate appropriate action plans.	The nurse uses problem-posing dialogue (Freire, 1973) to understand root issues and devises creative and innovative methods to transform situations.

Modified from Minkler M, Wallerstein N: Improving health through community organization and community building. In Glanz K, Rimer BK, Lewis, FM, editors: *Health behavior and education: theory, research, and practice,* ed 3, San Francisco, 2002, Jossey-Bass, pp. 279-311.

model for nurses, researchers, and community advocates working with underserved groups of cancer survivors.

EXAMPLE OF COMMUNITY EMPOWERMENT-COLLABORATION-PARTICIPATION: LUNA

In 2002, a Latina nurse (Melba Martinez, R.N., B.S.N), who was diagnosed with breast cancer in 1995, started the first grassroots support group for Latinas with breast cancer in West Central Florida. The group began with five members and within the first year had 38 active members who attended monthly meetings. The group was initiated in response to an unmet need in the Tampa Bay area, that is, lack of education services for Latinas diagnosed with breast cancer who primarily spoke Spanish. Over the years, LUNA has created a network of over 80 Latina survivors and has grown and become *Latinas Unidas por un Nuevo Amanecer,* Inc., a non-profit organization whose mission is to provide support and offer culturally and linguistically relevant education to Hispanic breast cancer survivors and their families, friends, and caregivers. The organization primarily serves underserved, immigrant, low-income Latinas with limited English proficiency, assists with navigating the health care system and serves as a community resource. LUNA draws on the tenets of community organization and empowerment fueled by problem-posing education. The three components of the LUNA model are: (1) education (e.g., classes and presentations, Spanish cancer information, health care navigation, community outreach); (2) support (e.g., peer to peer, home, hospital and phone visits, communications); and (3) social reintegration (e.g., celebration of life events such as birthdays, cancer camps, walks, and other social events).

Outcomes from LUNA

1. Campamento Alegria: The first ever oncology camp for Latina breast cancer survivors. An annual program designed to provide Latinas diagnosed with cancer a positive and unforgettable experience through a variety of activities that help sustain them through their cancer journey.

2. Community education and outreach: Attendance at various community events and health fairs to increase breast cancer screening awareness and provide cancer information and resources in Spanish.

3. Ongoing monthly educational meetings: Presentations and classes provided by Spanish-speaking health professionals on various survivorship issues and cancer-related topics.

4. Development of two new LUNA support groups in the last year (in Clearwater and Brandon, Florida).

The process for creating LUNA began with one nurse who through dedication and dialogue with others in the same situation began taking charge of the situation. From both her nursing and personal experiences she knew how hard it was for Hispanic women diagnosed with cancer to navigate the health care system, how difficult it was to take time for self-care, and how challenging it was for Hispanic women to talk about their fears. She recognized that Latinas with breast cancer should reach out to each other with understanding and compassion in their own language to move toward self-education and self-actualization. Since its inception, LUNA has partnered with various community-based organizations, hospitals, academic centers, churches, and other social support services to create a strong web of support. LUNA represents a ground up effort, which got its start by addressing an unmet need of Hispanic breast cancer survivors. It serves as an excellent model and reminder for nurses, researchers, and community advocates that the best ideas come from the soul. For more information: http://hispanicbreastcancer.org/ (in Spanish).

Acknowledgments: Melba Martinez, RN, BSN, and Dinorah (Dina) Martinez, MA, MPH.

"Never doubt that a small, group of thoughtful, committed citizens can change the world. Indeed, it is the only thing that ever has." Margaret Mead ■

THE NURSE'S ROLE IN HEALTH EDUCATION

Although learning theories and health education models provide a useful framework for planning health interventions, the nurse's ability to facilitate the education process and become a partner with individuals and communities is key to the method's application. At the core of health education is the therapeutic relationship between the nurse and individuals, families, and the community. Nurses hold the process together and are catalysts for change in delivering humanistic care. Nurses can activate ideas, offer appropriate interventions, identify resources, and facilitate group empowerment. Rankin and Stallings (2000) describe the following key characteristics of nurses in facilitating the teacher–learner process: confidence, competence, caring, and communication. It is beyond the scope of this chapter to describe communication techniques in detail, but it reminds the reader about the value of establishing inclusion and trust before content.

CLINICAL EXAMPLE

Mr. Chen often visits the neighborhood senior center weekly to play cards and have lunch with several of his longtime friends. Once a month he takes part in the blood pressure clinic offered by the health department. The health department's outreach services offers clinics in community-based centers, and an increased number of community members use this free service on an ongoing basis. Mr. Chen has limited resources, so the clinic provides him with valuable access to health information. On his first visit to the clinic, his blood pressure is 178/88. On his second visit, his reading is 188/94. He states that the city hospital has treated him for high blood pressure for over 5 years and that doctors prescribed several medications 6 months earlier.

The nurse's assessment reveals that Mr. Chen takes his medication only when he does not "feel so good." He said his doctor advises him to take his medicines regularly, and he states that he takes them faithfully when he doesn't feel well. He tells the nurse that he remembers getting some booklets about his medications and "blood," but he found them too long and tiring to read. The nurse's educational assessment reveals that Mr. Chen has completed 8 years of schooling, does not read much, enjoys television over print, and prefers to learn from pictures or from other people in groups. His low reading skills impact his ability to get health instructions in a meaningful way. He has taken the health instruction literally (e.g., he interprets "take regularly" to mean take consistently when "I don't feel right" vs. take the pills on a regular schedule).

To facilitate learning, the nurse establishes a teaching plan with Mr. Chen's input. This plan involves communicating health instructions in more relevant ways (e.g., using pictures, drawings, mnemonics, videotapes) and puts him in touch with county resources to buy his medicines. The nurse also establishes a follow-up plan and verifies

with Mr. Chen his understanding of how to take his meds by asking him to repeat back in his own words when/how he takes his meds. She also plans to develop a series of health education group classes for the seniors about health and wellness, with high blood pressure being one of the topics of discussion. ■

ENHANCING COMMUNICATION

The critical step of inclusion establishes the base for possible health action; it sets the relationship. The nurse enhances inclusion by greeting individuals, families, and groups in a warm fashion, offering comfort, and attending to immediate concerns or stresses. Education does not begin with the first instructional word. Rather, education begins with establishing an atmosphere conducive to learning. Simply put, a therapeutic relationship involves trust and building a relationship. If the nurse attends to inclusion first, individuals, families, and groups begin to trust the nurse, thereby trusting the health education message. This trust is evident through active participation and commitment in the education process. If the content or health message is positive, proactive, and personalized, it is more likely that participants will receive the message within the context of their everyday realities. Nurses are essential in creating and delivering appropriate health messages and programs and must address sociopolitical and environmental forces within appropriate cultural, literacy, and linguistic expressions (Meade et al., 2002a).

While Chapter 12 contains a detailed perspective on cultural diversity and community health nursing, it is important to note that the ongoing enhancement and refinement of nursing knowledge and skills for providing **culturally effective care** is critical to community health education. Meleis (1999) cogently describes culturally competent care as care that exhibits sensitivity to the differences in individuals based on their vast experiences and responses due to their backgrounds, sexual orientation, socioeconomic status, ethnicity, literacy, and cultural background. She depicts several properties that make up the "essence of health nurses" who deliver culturally competent care. First, they possess an explanatory system that values diversity. This is a system that is not drained by the constant attempt to interpret symbols but rather is energized by the variations. Second, they show expert assessment skills to discern different and similar patterns of responses that help to plan appropriate educational interventions. Third, culturally competent nurses are aware of the diversity of communication patterns and how language and communication influence "trust within the relationship." Culturally effective professionals also recognize how marginalization may increase health risks for individuals and that using the expertise of insiders in the culture is a highly valued skill. Last, nurses who deliver culturally effective care readily acknowledge differences and do not tolerate inequities.

For detailed information on the provision of culturally appropriate health care, consult the Office of Minority

ETHICAL Insights

Ethical Issues Related to Health Education

➤ **Individual versus collective/societal rights and responsibility for health:** What factors should the nurse consider when balancing the health education needs of the individual versus collective (e.g., family and community)?

➤ **Allocation of resources:** In what way do policies promote and/or hinder promotion of health? Do national/local government and corporate/institutional policies impact the availability of resources? How can the nurse get involved in shaping and redirecting health policy and moving policy into practice?

➤ **Social justice and equity:** Do all community members enjoy equity in their access to health education and information? What strategies, programs, and interventions can be implemented to reduce the discovery to delivery disconnect?

➤ **Health literacy:** Do community members understand the plethora of printed and electronic health messages communicated to them in terms of language, ease of reading, and linguistics? Nurses should assess their roles as information brokers, advocates, translators, facilitators, collaborative problem solvers, and navigators.

➤ **Cultural effectiveness:** What skills, knowledge, and experiences are necessary when planning health education within the context of people's history and everyday realities? The nurse should assess his/her abilities to approach health education tasks with confidence, compassion, competence and cultural humility.

Health's national standards for Culturally and Linguistically Appropriate Services (CLAS) (OMH, 1999). The standards, published in 1999, reinforce the ability of health care providers and organizations to understand and respond effectively to the cultural and linguistic needs brought by patients and community members to the health care setting. Several standards have particular relevance to community nursing. Standard 2 relates that consumers should receive, from all staff members, effective, understandable, and respectful care that is provided in a manner compatible with their cultural health beliefs and practices and preferred language (Standard 1). Standard 12 states that health care organizations should develop participatory, collaborative partnerships with communities and utilize a variety of formal and informal mechanisms to facilitate community and patient/consumer involvement in designing and implementing CLAS-related activities.

As each nurse addresses diversity and strives for culturally effective care, it is key that issues are identified and alternatives explored that are empowering and affirming to all involved. This requires self-awareness and recognizing that diversity development, attention to the cultural and linguistic appropriate care, and cultural effectiveness are a process, not a program. Consider for a moment how you exhibit nursing leadership skills related to this issue (Swanson, 2004). Consider also some of the ethical issues that you might confront in the community.

As an example, consider the following nursing research study by Strickland and colleagues (1999), who addressed religion in the design and delivery of a culturally and linguistically appropriate cervical health promotion program for eastern Washington's Yakama Indian women. The investigators conducted personal interviews with spiritual leaders and male and female members of the Wa'Shat Longhouse religion and obtained religious influences by asking questions about life views, communication channels, and leadership. Results showed that program goals must be holistic, teaching methods must include circular symbols, and intentions must be linked with natural communication patterns and must involve elders. Results revealed that storytelling, talking circles, role models, and multiple sensory modalities were important teaching approaches. For example, the circle symbol of unity connected the people and the earth. The group facilitator needs to be an equal learner who respects the wisdom, experiences, and contributions of each member. Also, time is loosely structured among the Yakama; therefore, an educational session may require an entire morning. The investigators also found that, unlike other cultures, the Yakama culture values information directly from the elders over the dissemination of prevention information.

FRAMEWORK FOR DEVELOPING HEALTH COMMUNICATIONS

Within the community, the nurse's intended audience may be an individual, family, group, or many segments of the community. Using a systematic approach to the development, design, and delivery of health education programs, messages and media provide the nurse with an organized, user-friendly approach to health message delivery. Although nurses may use a variety of educational models, theoretical frameworks, and teaching and learning principles, the National Cancer Institute suggests the "Framework for Developing Health Communications" to create a variety of health education messages and programs (USDHHS, 2002). **See Resource Tool 7B,** Framework for Developing Health Communications, on the book's evolve website at http://evolve.elsevier. com/Nies.

This organizing framework has four stages (simplified from six) and is depicted by a circular loop that offers the opportunity for continuous assessment, feedback, and improvement. The framework has been used widely by the author when developing cancer education materials and media on such topics as smoking, prostate cancer, breast and cervical cancer, and stress management (Brandon et al., 2004; Jacobsen et al., 2002; Meade, 1994; Meade, Meade et al., 2002; Schapira, Meade, and Nattinger, 1997). This framework can be easily adapted to the design and development of all types of health education topics such as diabetes, hypertension, nutrition, and so forth.

This framework is based on the principles of social marketing, health education, and mass communication theories and relies on intended audience assessment to guide the process. It is highly congruent with Freire's model of empowerment education, which encourages ongoing dialogue with potential consumers and users of health education services. Although this model focuses on communication strategies aimed at the programmatic level, the basic elements are applicable to individual, family, and group systems. The nurse should not expect to apply the model in a linear manner but rather to move back and forth between the stages. These stages mirror the nursing process (assessment, planning, implementation, and evaluation) and provide a sequential path for continuous assessment, feedback, and improvement for achieving a successful communication program.

The ideas contained in this "Framework for Developing Health Communications" model are a practical schema for planning and implementing health education communications programs. Nurses should use the model as a guide to planning health education messages and programs. It is also suggested that the nurse use an organized and systematic approach rather than attempt to fit his or her health education plan into every step (see "Launching a Breast Education and Outreach Screening Program").

Stage I: Planning and Strategy Development

The planning stage provides the foundation for the communication program's planning process and is crucial in setting the stage for communications. Understanding the intended audience's learning needs and targeting the program or message to the audience is key to activating effective health education. This step reinforces Freire's philosophical tenets of ascertaining the intended audience's needs and creating an open dialogue. This stage also reduces expensive alterations once the program is under way.

Questions to Ask
- Who is the intended audience?
- What is known about the audience and from what sources?
- What are the communication and education objectives and goals?
- What evaluation strategies will the nurse use?
- What is the health issue of interest?

Collaborative Actions to Take
- Review available data from health statistics, census data, local sources, libraries, newspapers, and local or community stakeholders.
- Think about and get partners involved.
- Obtain new data (i.e., interviews and focus groups using problem-posing dialogue format).
- Determine the intended group's needs and perceptions of health problems (i.e., identify audiences).
  - Physical (e.g., gender, age, health history)
  - Behavioral (e.g., lifestyle characteristics and health-related activities)
  - Demographic (e.g., income, years of schooling, language and cultural characteristics)
  - Psychographics (e.g., beliefs, values, and attitudes)
- Identify issues behind the issues and identify health knowledge gaps.
- Establish goals and objectives that are specific, attainable, prioritized, and time specific.
- Assess resources (e.g., money, staff, and materials).

Launching a Breast Education and Outreach Screening Program

In 1993, the H. Lee Moffitt Cancer Center and Research Institute, or Moffitt, formed a partnership with Suncoast Community Health Centers, Inc., or Suncoast, in rural Hillsborough County, Florida. The partnership brought breast cancer education and screening services to Hispanic migrant and seasonal farmworkers and low-income rural women via Moffitt's Lifetime Cancer Screening Mobile Unit. In 1993, a cancer center physician visited Suncoast, which is a federally funded, community-based center located about 30 miles south of Tampa. He was moved by the center's services and impressed with the clinic's dedication to reaching medically underserved populations. Suncoast consists of three comprehensive health care clinics in Plant City, Ruskin, and Dover, Florida, and offers services to Hillsborough County's low-income rural populations, which includes farmworkers. Suncoast provides a range of medical services, but they do not have mammography facilities. Moffitt was expanding its community outreach initiatives through mobile outreach services. Moffitt is a freestanding, private, nonprofit institution affiliated with, and located at, the University of South Florida campus in Tampa. Moffitt is a National Cancer Institute–designated comprehensive cancer center in Florida and is widely known for state-of-the-art treatment, outpatient and ambulatory services, and advanced screening modalities. After a series of meetings between Suncoast and Moffitt's Lifetime Cancer Screening Center, the groups formed a partnership based on a shared goal, that is, improving the breast health of high-risk and medically underserved women. Both parties determined that the goal was to develop and offer the community culturally appropriate education, accessible mammography service, and follow-up care. This program continues to be a sustainable initiative through the community education and outreach program. ■

Description of Health Issue and Intended Audience

Despite progress in the fight against cancer, many communities continue to bear a disproportionate share of the cancer burden. Such communities often include racially and ethnically and culturally diverse populations with low levels of income and education, families with inadequate medical insurance, and individuals who experience barriers in differing cultural beliefs and practices or limited literacy or language abilities (American Cancer Society, 2005; Freeman, 2004). Cancer is the leading cause of premature death in women, and breast cancer accounts for approximately one third of all malignancies, especially in women with low incomes. Low rates of early detection cause treatment delays and poor prognoses in rural women, especially those with breast cancer (Bradley, Given, and Roberts, 2002; Shinagawa, 2000). Nurses must reach at-risk populations with effective, appro-

TABLE 7-5 Teaching-Learning Formats

TEACHING FORMAT	APPLICATION TO HEALTH EDUCATION
Brainstorming session	Allows participants the freedom to generate ideas and discuss them in a group setting. Cultivates creativity. Fosters empowerment to allow members to identify the issue and find solutions.
Community-wide programs	Can reach large numbers of community members through a systematic plan. May include individual or group approaches with a defined intended audience.
Demonstration	Effective in learning perceptual motor skills. Aids in visual identification.
Group discussion	Members can learn from each other and receive support. Nurses can tailor teaching content to group needs. Ideal for groups combining patients and families. Nurses, health professionals, or lay members can lead the groups. Facilitator must be comfortable with group method and familiar with group characteristics.
Lecture	Varying group sizes can use formal oral presentations. Group member share expertise and experiences. Presenter must be comfortable and possess speaking ability. Requires organizational skills and ability to highlight key points in interesting and creative ways. A combination of lecture media may enhance learning. Audience participation is linked to the presenter's speaking style and ability. Audience feedback is limited.
Personal discussion (i.e., individual and one-on-one)	Allows individual assessment and identification of cultural barriers, physical impairments, learning needs, literacy, and anxiety. Promotes the tailoring of health education plans. Ideal to capture "teachable moments." Does not allow sharing and support from others. High cost of staff time.
Role playing	Effective in influencing attitudes and opinions. Encourages problem-solving and critical thinking skills. Enhances learner participation. Some members may be hesitant to become involved.
Task force committee	Join individuals with diverse backgrounds and expertise to achieve a goal. May represent many interests and perspectives.
Town hall meetings	Can offer shared experience in a familiar setting.

Data from Rankin and Stallings, 2001; Redman, 2001; USDHHS, 2002.

priate, and measurable methods to reduce cancer morbidity and mortality.

The lack of mammography screening and education for rural Hillsborough County's medically underserved women represented a health service gap (Meade et al., 2002a). In particular, Hispanic farmworkers represent a particular subgroup of women who face a number of potential barriers to acceptable mammography services. These barriers are lack of insurance, limited access to health care, low levels of education and literacy, cultural and linguistic differences, and immigrant status. Educational interventions and tools that address (a) unique value systems, (b) cultural and linguistic factors, and (c) access issues, as well as capitalize on the strengths of the women, are needed (Meade and Calvo, 2001). The women want and need health information about breast health, but they also experience everyday survival issues and struggles. What was needed in Hillsborough County was the delivery of a culturally relevant health service in a geographically convenient area. Women aged 40 and older were eligible for this service. The intended audience was primarily Hispanic migrant and seasonal farmworkers but also included women from diverse ethnic backgrounds who were medically underserved.

Goal: To prevent premature death and disability from breast cancer through early detection, screening, and culturally and linguistically relevant education.

Objectives: To increase education, mammograms, clinical breast examinations, and follow-up programs among medically underserved women in rural Hillsborough County. ■

Stage II: Developing and Pretesting Concepts, Messages, and Materials

The nurse's decisions in Stage I can help guide him or her in selecting appropriate communication channels and producing effective and relevant materials. The nurse must consider how to reach the intended audience and use supporting materials and media. "Channel" refers to how the nurse will reach communication sites (i.e., churches, clinics, nurses, or community-based organizations). "Format" refers to how the nurse will communicate the health message (e.g., through individual or group discussion) (Table 7-5). **Materials and media** are the program's tools, not the program itself (Table 7-6). Education is a human activity and should not focus on audiovisuals exclusively. To ensure that the messages are relevant and meaningful, the nurse can engage in qualitative research methods (pretesting) to obtain feedback about the understandability and acceptability of the materials. Learning now what works and doesn't work saves time later.

Questions to Ask

- What channels are best?
- What formats should be used?
- Are there existing resources?
- How can the nurse present the message?
- How will the intended audience react to the message?

TABLE 7-6 **Materials and Media**

MEDIA	CONSIDERATIONS IN HEALTH EDUCATION SETTINGS
Audiotapes	Do not requires reading
	Portable and small
	Individuals can use them at home in a comfortable setting and can replay and use them at their own pace
	Economical
	Helpful for individuals with visual difficulties or low literacy skills
Bulletin boards	Inexpensive and easy to develop
	Direct attention to a specific message; uses few words
Exhibits and displays	Graphics offer appeal
	Placement in high-traffic areas (e.g., waiting rooms and examination rooms reach wide audiences)
Flip charts and chalkboards	Excellent format to enlarge teaching concepts or cue reader to salient points; may add graphics and diagrams
	Chalkboards are reusable; flip charts have replacement pads
	Inexpensive
Games and simulations	Involve patients in a fun manner; involve the entire family
	Highly effective with children
Graphics	Can convey important points in salient and visual fashion
Drawings and visuals	Can aid understanding for low-literacy audiences
	Visuals messages should be pretested to ensure acceptability and understanding
Interactive videotapes (i.e., multimedia)	A variety of computer programs, interactive videodisks, and computer-assisted instructions are available and are undergoing testing
	Algorithms and branching decisions aid patients in decision making, problem solving, and fact acquisition (Holmes-Rovner et al., 2005; Hahn et al., 2004)
	Interactive patient education is becoming more common via kiosks in waiting rooms
	Nurses should assess computer comfort level
	Software development may be time intensive and costly
Models and real objects	Bring the teaching concept to the patient in a familiar way
Demonstrations	Helpful when conveying psychomotor skills; encourage patient involvement and tactile learning (e.g., penis model for condom placement or breast model to show breast self-exam)
	No reading needed
Storytelling	Reading is minimal
	Encourages questions and elicits insights (Werle, 2004)
	Helpful in individual and group instruction
	Nurses can incorporate models and real objects into displays or fairs
Overheads	Useful in small and large group settings
	Highlights key points and helps patient focus ideas
	Use of color and advance organizers, large type, and key points are recommended; avoid busy and cluttered overheads
	Can be prepared in advance
	Inexpensive
Photographs, picture books, and slide series (i.e., PowerPoint slides); photoessay and photovoice/photonovella	Help promote understanding by showing realistic images and real situations
	Help patients make connections to their life
	Photographs may appear alone or in combination with other photographs or slides or placed in an album (Paskett et al., 1996; Wang and Burris, 1997; Lopéz et al., 2005)
	PowerPoint slides are easily updated
	Helpful for patients with limited literacy skills; offers visual presentation of concepts
	Effective with an individual and with small groups (i.e., self-study or reflection)
	Easily updated.
Printed materials (brochures, leaflets, or booklets)	Portable, widely available, and economical
	Useful in reinforcing health concepts and interactions
	Patients can set and adjust the pace and refer back to information later
	Can be effective with individuals, families, groups, or community-wide dissemination
	Materials written at simple levels can be effective and acceptable for both low-level and high-level readers (Doak et al., 1998; Meade et al., 1989)
	Personalized materials are highly effective (Skinner et al., 1999) and are a promising strategy for health education (Kreuter et al., 1999)
	Nurses should assess issues of readability, design, layout, cultural relevance, and appropriateness of content (Guidry and Walker, 1999; Kreuter and McClure, 2004; Michielutte et al., 1999)
Programmed materials, self-help guides, slides and tape programs	May involve printed materials combined with visuals to allow self-pacing
	Helpful to learn facts
	Nurse should assess individual or group to determine whether independent learning style is preferred
	Storytelling (Werle, 2004)
Teaching cards	Portable, use few words, and offer visual interpretations
Flashcards	The nurse can create them economically and update them easily
	Effective with individual, small group, or family instruction
Radio and newspapers	Reach large audiences within the community
	Effective in conveying general health information in a user-friendly manner
	Nurses can play an active role in disseminating health information (Meade, 1992)

Continued

TABLE 7-6 Materials and Media (cont'd)

MEDIA	CONSIDERATIONS IN HEALTH EDUCATION SETTINGS
Television and cable television	Reach large audiences within the community Can help enhance community members' general health and well-being Effective in influencing attitudes and behaviors Offer a familiar medium for viewer to learn about health topics Nurses can play key roles in reaching the community (Meade, 1992)
Videotapes, DVDs	Combine audio and visual medium to convey realistic images (Meade, 1996). Videotapes DVDs should incorporate role modeling concept (Gagliano, 1998) Expensive to produce and update; requires access to audiovisual equipment and viewing sites Videotapes DVDs may be costly to produce and purchase, but with computerized digital editing are easily updated
Online resources (i.e., Internet, simple dial-up services, and World Wide Web)	Electronic information sources can link individuals, families, and groups to health information, databases, and bulletin board and chat services (Bush, 1999) Common Internet providers are America Online and Earthlink Can reach large audiences rapidly Must access World Wide Web sites for accuracy, credibility, and relevancy New technologies can help consumers find health information, advice, and support

Data from USDHHS, 2002.

- Will the audience understand, accept, and use the message?
- What changes may improve the message?

Collaborative Actions to Take

- Identify messages and materials.
- Decide whether to use existing materials or produce new ones.
- Select channels and formats.
- Develop relevant materials with the target audience.
- Pretest the message and materials and obtain audience feedback (e.g., through interviews, questionnaires, focus groups, and readability testing). Pretesting helps ensure comprehension, acceptability, and personal relevance.

Selecting Channels and Methods

Nurses selected a combination of channels to communicate health information about breast cancer, screenings, and early detection methods (e.g., community-based clinics, missions, social service agencies, health events, and fairs). Nurses conducted individual interactions at the mobile site.

Nurses collected a variety of health materials and media about breast cancer from national, state, and local sources and determined that many of the printed materials were not culturally or educationally suited for the individuals the nurse were serving; for example, the materials were geared toward high reading levels, and few Spanish-language materials were available. ■

Developing Materials

In 1994, through a grant from Avon, or the National Alliance of Breast Cancer Organizations (NABCO), Suncoast and Moffitt designed bilingual English and Spanish materials to educate and encourage women to practice self-breast examinations and receive screening. A series of focus groups and pretesting measures ensured the materials were culturally and educationally relevant. Additionally, a grant from the Cancer Research Foundation of America, Inc., funded the development of a 14-minute Spanish videotape on breast and cervical cancer. Women now view this tape in the mobile unit while waiting for their appointments.

Community agencies, missions, and clinics received printed service schedules. Although translators were sporadically present in the van, it became apparent that a permanent bilingual staff was necessary. Ongoing dialogue with community members and clinics helped refine the screening process, the education component, and the follow-up services to ensure effectiveness, efficiency, appropriateness, and timely follow-up. All mobile runs now have bilingual and bicultural staff. ■

Stage III: Implementing the Program

At this stage, the nurse introduces the health education message and program to the intended audience and reviews and revises necessary components. The nurse also analyzes the program and health message for effectiveness and tracks the mechanisms using process evaluation. This type of managing the implementation process examines the procedures and tasks involved in the program or message, such as monitoring media, identifying the intended audience's interim reactions, and addressing internal functioning (e.g., work schedules and expenditures).

Questions to Ask

- How should the health education program/message get launched?

- How do we maintain interest and sustainability?
- How can we use process evaluation?
- What are the strengths of the health program?
- How can we be sure that we keep on track within the timeline and budget?
- How can we find out if we have reached the intended audience?
- How well did each step work (i.e., process evaluation)?
- Are we maintaining good relationships with our partners?

Collaborative Actions to Take

- Work with community organizations, businesses, media, and other health agencies to enhance effectiveness.
- Monitor and track progress.
- Establish process evaluation measures (e.g., follow-up with users of the service, number of community members who used the service, and expenditures).

Implementation

The mass media introduced the service at a press conference and continues to publish human-interest stories, especially during October—Breast Awareness Month. The outreach worker posts flyers at a variety of sites (e.g., beauty shops, laundromats, grocery stores, unemployment offices, and community centers). Twice per month, the mobile unit travels to rural areas. There, the staff greet women and answer questions about the procedure and follow-up. Staff consists of the outreach worker, nurse practitioner, mammography technician, and outreach worker. ■

Stage IV: Assessing Effectiveness and Making Refinements

Outcome evaluation examines whether changes in knowledge, attitudes, and behavior did or did not occur as a result of the program. Together with the process evaluation, examination of data on how well the program is functioning results and directs modifications. The nurse prepares for a new development cycle using information gained from audience feedback, communication channels, and the program's intended effect. This phase helps to continually refine the health message and respond to the intended audience's needs. New information helps to validate the programs' strengths and allow for necessary modifications. Feedback is necessary to continually refine the message.

Questions to Ask

- What was learned?
- How can outcome evaluation be used to assess effectiveness?
- What worked well, and what did not work well?
- Has anything changed within the intended audience?
- How might we refine the methods, channels, or formats?
- Overall, what lessons were learned, and what modifications could strengthen the health education activity?

Collaborative Actions to Take

- Conduct outcome evaluations (e.g., randomized experiment, evaluation studies, define data needed for data collection).
- Reassess and revise goals and objectives.
- Modify unsuccessful strategies or activities.
- Generate continual support from businesses, health care agencies, and other community groups for ongoing collaboration and partnerships.
- Provide justification for continuing or ending the program.
- Summarize the health education program or message in an evaluation report.
- The reader should consider how to plan health education messages or programs using this model. The exercise in Figure 7-1 will help the reader organize ideas systematically.

Assessing Efficiency

Process Evaluation: A number of newspaper, television, and radio advertisements publicized the free or low-cost mammography service and highlighted the importance of breast health. Also, several human-interest stories emerged, which communicated the screening services to a wider audience. Since 1993, an increase in the number of staff involved in the program and the number of funded projects that support the program enhanced the breadth and depth of the services. The on-site service logistics have made continual improvements, most notably in adding a dedicated outreach worker to the program.

In the first few years of operation, a total of 200 women underwent screening, which is a modest number. Assessment revealed that many women failed to appear for breast screenings because they had a "fear of cancer" and were uncertain how to navigate the health care system. Typically, many women from the community did not seek preventive health care; they sought care only for acute illness. Assessment showed that peer outreach was necessary to ensure participation. Therefore, a subsequent request to Avon-NABCO in 1997 aimed to link 350 women to screening by proposing an outreach component, which consisted of a bilingual lay worker who would provide customized recruitment, culturally and linguistically appropriate instruction, and follow-up care.

In 1998, the program implemented stronger outreach and education elements to reach 400 women. Peer outreach continued to be the program's key component. During 1998, the program exceeded its goal by linking 471 women to screening and follow-up. In 1999, the program produced over 600 screenings. In 2005 (the last full year of data), over 1,000 women were outreached.

Women expressed gratitude for the sensitivity and personal attention given by the peer outreach worker and mobile unit staff. Formal and informal feedback reveals that women respond well to the services and are especially satisfied with the Spanish-language educational materials.

Outcome Evaluation: During the program's first 6 years, fewer than 200 women received screening per year. The number of women screened now approaches over 1000 per year. The number of community partners has increased considerably, a

Instructions: Think about a target group that you are currently working with and
planning to deliver/create a health education program or message.
Complete the exercise by asking yourself the following questions:

Questions to Ask	Action Plan
• What is the overall intended message/goal? What are my reasons for planning this message? How do I know that it is needed or wanted by the audience?	
• Who is the intended audience? (Write a brief statement describing the characteristics of the group.)	
• What are the benefits of this message to the group?	
• What channels will I use to deliver the message? Provide a rationale.	
• Will I need to create materials? Are there available materials that are appropriate for the group?	
• How will I know if my message gets across to the audience? Did the audience respond? How many people were reached? Who responded?	
• Was there change? What are the reasons the message was or was not effective? What can be modified to strengthen the message?	

FIGURE 7-1 Planning your health education message.

reflection of enhanced community capacity. Regular health fairs and health events are scheduled, and continual refinement of services and follow-up are ongoing. ■

Feedback

Reports describing process and outcome evaluation and analysis provide a point of reference for continual improvements. Such reports apply knowledge and outline methods to enhance and improve the service's efficiency and effectiveness. Lifetime's mobile mammography van continues to provide service to women in rural Hillsborough County. Each year, the number of women receiving service increases. The program exists under the auspices of the cancer center's Community Education and Outreach Program in collaboration with Lifetime Cancer Screening and Prevention Center. Ongoing funding opportunities sustain the program as well as institutional support.

The program has incorporated a network of outreach and educational components to reach rural migrant and seasonal farmworkers and low-income elderly women in south and east

Hillsborough County. The program's leaders aim to extend its reach into surrounding counties, such as rural Pasco. Although the program provides desired links to screening services and formed successful community partnerships, it is important to develop and refine **community empowerment** strategies through outreach and education to sustain and widely disseminate the program. Building on this successful model of education and outreach (see Meade et al., 2002b), we have applied lessons learned for outreaching to other high-risk populations such as Haitian and African-American women. ■

HEALTH EDUCATION RESOURCES

A variety of health education materials and resources are available from local, state, and national organizations and agencies. Such associations provide helpful information about services, educational materials, and links to support groups or self-help groups. Often, printed and electronic materials are available for free or for a nominal cost. Nurses can help individuals, families, and groups access materials, services, or equipment loan programs and become knowledgeable about available community resources. Additionally, identifying gaps in services or resources may help nurses create the necessary services or materials. Some examples of resources follow:

- Local and regional hospitals, clinics, libraries, health education centers, and businesses
- Local and state governmental sources (e.g., health departments and social service agencies); check the Yellow Pages or Internet for listings
- Community-based organizations (i.e., advertised, non-advertised, and those recommended by community leaders and stakeholders, National Association of Community Health Centers)
- Universities and colleges, community colleges, and academic nursing centers
- Professional organizations (e.g., American Public Health Association, National Association of Hispanic Nurses, National Black Nurses Association, National Student Nurses Association)
- Commercial organizations (e.g., pharmaceutical companies, medical supply companies, and patient and health education companies); printed and electronic sources are often available
- Federal government sources (e.g., National Institutes of Health [NIH]; National Cancer Institute; National Heart, Lung, Blood Institute; Office of Minority Health [OMH]; Centers for Disease Control [CDC]; National AIDS Clearinghouse; and Office on Smoking and Health)
- Voluntary agencies and their local affiliates (e.g., American Heart Association, Amyotrophic Lateral Sclerosis Association, Susan G. Komen Breast Cancer Foundation, Lance Armstrong Foundation, American Diabetes Association, American Council for Drug Disorders, American Dairy Council, and American Lung Association)
- Internet searches
- Medline Plus Health Information (i.e., a service of the National Library of Medicine for patient and consumer information)

Can you think of another organization that you or your family recently obtained information from relating to a health need? The book's evolve website (http://evolve.elsevier.com/nies/) contains a summary of major organizations and resources. Also, university or college libraries often provide information on beginning and advanced search strategies and are one of the most credible and accessible forms of information. The National Library of Medicine, at http://www.nlm.nih.gov/hinfo.html, maintains extensive health-related bibliographies and offers links to databases such as Medline Plus Health Information, Household Products Database, Office of the Surgeon General, NIH Senior Health, and more.

The nurse can locate many health resources through a variety of search engines on the Internet. As the Web continues to evolve as a major source of information exchange, an assessment of the quantity, quality, and broad nature of information must be undertaken as well. Key to the plethora of resources is gauging the appropriateness of the materials and media in consideration of literacy (see next section).

Literacy and Health

In her 1944 text, *The Public Health Nurse in the Community,* Rue stated that the community's illiteracy level is an important factor in health program planning. This factor remains a significant issue in planning health education programs and materials. Low literacy is a problem of great magnitude in the United States and has serious implications across the continuum of the health care. Literacy is operationally defined as the ability to read and write at the fifth-grade reading level in any language and can be measured according to a continuum (National Literacy Act, 1991). Health literacy is about empowerment, that is, having access to information, knowledge, and innovations. It is increasingly important for social, economic, and health development and is a key public health issue in the delivery of effective safe health care. If not addressed by nurses, the community will suffer (Kickbush, 2001; Nielsen-Bohlman et al., 2004).

Health literacy involves a constellation of skills, including the ability to perform the basic reading tasks required to function in the health care environment, and involves knowing when and where to go for cancer screenings, reading labels on prescription bottles, understanding public health messages about mammography or colon cancer screening, completing health insurance forms, recognizing how to read food labels, or being aware of the expectations of prevention trials (Williams et al., 1995). Consider the following clinical example.

CLINICAL EXAMPLE

A 2-year-old is diagnosed with an inner ear infection and prescribed an antibiotic. Her mother understands that her daughter should take the prescribed medication twice a day. After carefully studying the label on the bottle and deciding that it does not tell how take the medicine, she fills the teaspoon and pours the antibiotic into her daughter's ear (Parker et al., 2003). ■

Thus, the nurse in a community setting who sees a sick child at the pediatric clinic should ask the following questions:

- Will the parents know what to do if their infant gets a fever?
- Do the parents know how to read a thermometer? Did I show them? Were they able to "show me back"?
- Will the parents know what action to take in case of a very high fever at 1:00 AM in the morning?
- Does the family know whom to call and under what conditions, should their baby's condition worsen? Does the family have an understanding of what constitutes *worsen?*
- Do the parents have an understanding of the names of the medicines for their baby, how they work, and how and when to give them?

Early research shows serious disparities between the reading levels of materials and patient's reading skills (Alexander, 2000; Gazmararian et al., 1999a, 1999b; Glazer, Kirk, and Bosler, 1996; Guidry and Walker, 1999; Kirsch et al., 1993; Macario et al., 1998; Meade, 1999; Meade and Byrd, 1989; Meade et al., 1994; Mohrmann et al., 2000; Weiss and Coyne, 1997; Wells et al., 1994; Williams et al., 1995, 1998a). Additionally, materials often fail to incorporate the intended audience's cultural beliefs, values, languages, and attitudes (C. C. Doak et al., 1998; Guidry and Walker, 1999; Meade et al., 2003; Powe et al., 2005; Wilson et al., 2003). Studies show that low literacy increases the use of health care services (Baker et al., 1998); decreases self-esteem and increases shame (Parikh et al., 1996); is a better predictor than race/ethnicity or age of disease for advanced stage of prostate cancer presentation (Bennett et al., 1998); and is a better predictor of cervical cancer screening knowledge than ethnicity or education (Lindau et al., 2002). Other studies show that low literacy is independently associated with worse glycemic control (Schillinger et al., 2002); creates barriers to understanding HIV safer sex practices (Wolf et al., 2004); and leads to health care and linguistic isolation that places individuals at risk for developing health complications (Davis et al., 2002; Estrada et al., 2004; Holmes-Rovner et al., 2005; Sharp et al., 2002).

While the past decade has seen unprecedented advances in translating research findings into public health practices to reduce health risks, such successes has not been realized by all members of society representing various age, race and ethnic, and socioeconomic groups. It continues to be seen that community members who are unable to read well enough to cope with the persistent reading demands of an increasingly complicated health care system often fall behind more literate groups in adopting and using health education and promotion procedures and interventions (Davis et al., 2002; Davis and Wolf, 2004; Dolan et al., 2004; Wilson et al., 2003; Wolf et al., 2004). Although the exact relational mechanisms between literacy and health are unclear, it is known that individuals with very low literacy skills are at an increased risk for poor health. A number of recent systematic reviews of health literacy studies (Dewalt et al., 2004; Nielsen-Bohlman et al., 2004; Paasche-Orlow et al., 2005) show evidence of the high prevalence of limited health literacy, increasingly complex medical systems, and need for high-level navigation skills for self-management of acute and chronic disease and promotion of health. Simply put, health instructions not read and interventions poorly understood influence self-care abilities and health and wellness.

In 1999, the American Medical Association's Report of the Council on Scientific Affairs revealed that patients with the most health care needs were often the least able to read and understand information to function successfully within the health care system. It was recommended that a broad policy agenda on health literacy be crafted to involve decision makers from the public and private sector. The recognition of this topic as a serious health issue subsequently resulted in the naming of a specific objective within the *Healthy People 2010* document, which states that a public health goal "is to improve the health literacy of persons with inadequate or marginal literacy skills" (Objective 11.2) (USDHHS, 2000). The document goes on to state that low health literacy prevents many individuals from gaining the full benefits of health care and suggests that health literacy is linked to health promotion and preventive behaviors.

In 2004, the Institute of Medicine (IOM) published a landmark report titled *Health Literacy: A Prescription to End Confusion* that relates that millions of U.S. adults are unable to read and act on the plethora of health instructions and messages (Nielsen-Bohlman et al., 2004). The definition of health literacy adopted by the IOM report is consistent with the *Healthy People 2010* document and is as follows: "the capacity to obtain, interpret and understand basic health information and services and the competence to use such information and services to enhance health." The IOM report lists a series of recommendations that offer the nurse a blueprint of action. Several recommendations emphasize the need for clear communication, stress the importance of involving consumers in the development of the health communications process, and relate the need to create culturally and linguistically appropriate health information. For information on the report and other health literacy related resources, go to the IOM's website, http://www.iom.edu/, and search for the term *health literacy*.

The Doaks (Leonard and Cecelia), who brought the literacy issue to the forefront in public health, describe the health community as a written culture. Unfortunately, many written instructions are over the heads of patients. There is a serious mismatch between the readability levels of health instructions and the reading skills of patients, but nurses can adapt the literacy levels of their instructions and reduce this mismatch. Techniques to reduce this mismatch are cogently outlined in the book *Teaching Patients With Low Literacy Skills* (C. C. Doak, Doak, and Root, 1996), which offers practical suggestions for preparing and evaluating materials.

Within Stage I of the "Framework for Developing Health Communications" model, the nurse can use assessment skills to determine the reading level of the intended audience. For example, the nurse could employ a number of informal and formal assessment measures to assess an individual's literacy skills. Informal measures include asking a series of simple questions to provide a better indication of their reading skills, for example, Do you enjoy reading? What do you read? How often do you read? Where do you get your health information? Although years of schooling completed can serve as a gauge of literacy, previous studies suggest that a three to four grade level difference often exists between individual's literacy level and years of education completed. The nurse could ask patients to read a paragraph from a health material aloud.

Skilled readers enjoy reading, are fluent readers, understand content, interpret the meaning of words, and look up unfamiliar words. Limited readers read slowly, miss the intended meaning, take words literally, tire quickly from reading, and skip over uncommon words. Also, the nurse should ask the patients a few questions about the information they read. Readers should be able to answer questions about the material's content. Although these strategies are especially helpful with individuals with low literacy, people at all literacy levels prefer and better understand simply written, concise materials and are more motivated by materials that are relevant to their learning needs (C. C. Doak et al., 1998; L. G. Doak et al., 1996).

Such informal assessment techniques can be coupled with formal but easy-to-administer assessment methods to create a reading profile. Formal instruments that have been used in health care settings to estimate reading level include the Wide-Range Achievement Test, Level III (Jastak and Wilkinson, 1999) and the Rapid Estimate of Adult Literacy in Medicine (REALM—Figure 7-2) (Davis et al., 1993). Although these instruments take only minutes to administer, they are unavailable in Spanish. To date, the Test of Functional Health Literacy in Adults (TOFHLA) (Parker et al., 1995) is the only tool that has been used in a variety of health settings with English-speaking/reading subjects (Gazmararian et al., 1999; Kalichman et al., 2000; Williams et al., 1998b) and, to a limited degree, with Spanish-speaking subjects (Kalichman and Rompa, 2000; Schillinger et al., 2002). While the use of formal tools to measure reading level may be helpful to assess literacy, the time to administer it in community-based settings greatly limits its use. Rather, Meade and Calvo (2001) suggest asking people a series of simple questions, including years of schooling, to obtain an indication of health literacy. Ongoing research is needed to develop a relevant health literacy index (Kickbush, 2001; Nielsen-Bohlman et al., 2004) that shows a composite of health literacy capabilities for positive health, social, and economic outcomes.

Helpful Tips for Effective Teaching

- Assess reading skills using informal and formal methods.
- Determine what your patient wants to know
- Stick with the essentials. Limit the number of concepts or key points. Focus on key critical and survival skills.
- Set realistic goals and objectives. Take cues from your patients about what they want to learn and how to help them learn.
- Use clear and concise language. Avoid technical terms if possible. For example, substitute the word *problem* for *complication*. Use the term *high blood pressure* instead of the word *hypertension*, or use the word *chance* instead of *possibility*. Do not needlessly simplify if the intended meaning is lost. Although the words *insulin* and *infection* are polysyllabic words, people with diabetes are often quite familiar with them (Box 7-2).
- Consider developing a glossary or vocabulary list for common words on the health topic. For example, in

teaching a family about dental health, create a list of common words about the topic and words that might substitute well (e.g., flossing, toothbrush, cavity, decay, check-ups, x-rays).
- Space your teaching out over time if possible. Incorporate health education activities into other activities. For example, ask women about their smoking habits at each prenatal visit. Relate teaching to their everyday concerns. Introduce human papillomavirus (HPV) education into women and men's health visits.
- Personalize health messages. Use the active voice. For example, instead of saying, "It is important that patients read labels if they want to cut down on fat and sodium intake," say "Read the labels on foods to know what is in them. This helps to cut down on the your fat and salt intake" **See Resource Tool 7C,** Patient Communication: Testicular Self-exam (TSE), on the book's evolve website at http://evolve.elsevier.com/Nies.
- Incorporate methods of illustration, demonstration, and real-life examples. Connect the health message to everyday events and real-life situations.
- Give and get. Review information often. Ask the patient questions before, during, and after teaching.
- Summarize often. Provide the patient with feedback. Obtain feedback from the patient.
- Be creative. Use your imagination to convey difficult concepts (e.g., use picture cards, drawings, objects, videos, flipcharts, multimedia decision aids, photographs, storytelling).
- Use appropriate resources and materials to enhance teaching and convey ideas (e.g., videotapes, computer-based interactive programs, and bulletin boards).

BOX 7-2 PATIENT COMMUNICATION: Prostate Cancer and Treatment Options

Version A (harder to grasp)

The doctor has recently communicated to the patient that he has localized prostate cancer, commonly labeled Stage I. In addition to managing the anxieties associated with a life-threatening illness, patients with this disease must carefully consider the available treatment modalities and account for the potential effect each one may have on quality of life. Patients must seriously evaluate the benefits and adverse side effects of each treatment modality and determine the most efficacious intervention for their lifestyle.

Version B (easier to grasp)

You have just been told that you have early-stage prostate cancer. Choosing a treatment is hard, but it is important. Besides dealing with fears that go along with having cancer, you need to know about your treatment options.
- Get to know the benefits and side effects of each treatment.
- Think about how each treatment may affect your life.
- Ask questions. Write them down. Talk with your family.
- Choose the best treatment for you.

Rapid Estimate of Adult Literacy in Medicine (REALM)©
Terry Davis, PhD • Michael Crouch, MD • Sandy Long, PhD

Patient's name/
Subject #_____
Date_____Clinic_____

Reading   Grade
Level _____Completed_____
Date of Birth_____
Examiner_____

List 1		List 2		List 3	
fat	_____	fatigue	_____	allergic	_____
flu	_____	pelvic	_____	menstrual	_____
pill	_____	jaundice	_____	testicle	_____
dose	_____	infection	_____	colitis	_____
eye	_____	exercise	_____	emergency	_____
stress	_____	behavior	_____	medication	_____
smear	_____	prescription	_____	occupation	_____
nerves	_____	notify	_____	sexually	_____
germs	_____	gallbladder	_____	alcoholism	_____
meals	_____	calories	_____	irritation	_____
disease	_____	depression	_____	constipation	_____
cancer	_____	miscarriage	_____	gonorrhea	_____
caffeine	_____	pregnancy	_____	inflammatory	_____
attack	_____	arthritis	_____	diabetes	_____
kidney	_____	nutrition	_____	hepatitis	_____
hormones	_____	menopause	_____	antibiotics	_____
herpes	_____	appendix	_____	diagnosis	_____
seizure	_____	abnormal	_____	potassium	_____
bowel	_____	syphilis	_____	anemia	_____
asthma	_____	hemorrhoids	_____	obesity	_____
rectal	_____	nausea	_____	osteoporosis	_____
incest	_____	directed	_____	impetigo	_____

Score
List 1 _____
List 2 _____
List 3 _____
Raw Score _____

Directions:
1. Give the patient a laminated copy of the Realm and score answers on an unlaminated copy that is attached to a clipboard. Hold the clipboard at an angle so that the patient is not distracted by your scoring procedure. Say:
"I want to hear you read as many words as you can from this list. Begin with the first word on List 1 and read aloud. When you come to a word you cannot read, do the best you can or say 'blank' and go on to the next word."
2. If the patient takes more than five seconds on a word, say "blank" and point to the next word, if necessary, to move the patient along. If the patient begins to miss every word, have him/her pronounce only known words.
3. Count as an error any word not attempted or mispronounced. Score by marking a plus (+) after each correct word, a check (v) after each mispronounced word, and a minus (−) after words not attempted. Count as correct any self-corrected words.
4. Count the number of correct words for each list and record the numbers in the "Score" box. Total the numbers and match the total score with its grade equivalent in the table below.

Grade Equivalent	
Raw Score	**Grade Range**
0 to 18	**3rd Grade and Below** Will not be able to read most low literacy materials; will need repeated oral instructions, materials composed primarily of illustrations, or audiotapes or videotapes.
19 to 44	**4th to 6th Grade** Will need low literacy materials; may not be able to read prescription labels.
45 to 60	**7th to 8th Grade** Will struggle with most patient education materials; will not be offended by low literacy materials.
61 to 66	**High School** Will be able to read most patient education materials.

FIGURE 7-2 The Rapid Estimate of Adult Literacy in Medicine (REALM) is a screening instrument to assess and adult patient's ability to read common medical words and lay terms for body parts and illnesses. It is designed to assist medical professionals in estimating a patient's literacy level to use the appropriate level of patient education materials or oral instructions. The test takes 2 to 3 minutes to administer and score (Reprinted with permission of Dr. Terry Davis, Louisiana State University. From Davis TC et al: Rapid estimate of adult literacy in medicine: a shortened screening instrument, *Fam Med* 25:56-57, 1993).

TABLE 7-7 Components of Learner Verification

(Checks the suitability of the message with community members)

COMPONENTS	DESCRIPTION
Attraction	Readers should be attracted to the message. For example, the cover should stimulate interest, and, when possible, pictures should foster an identification that "tells me that this is important for my situation." *Example: Is this material attractive/pleasing to you?* *Overall, would you be likely to pick up and read this brochure?*
Comprehension	Readers should be able to summarize the main points in their own words, not the vocabulary of the instruction. *Example: What do you feel is the main point?* *Are there any words that you might not understand?*
Acceptance	Readers need to perceive that the information is culturally acceptable for their lifestyle, situation, and background. *Example: Is there anything that bothers you about this booklet?* *In your opinion, who is this booklet for?*
Persuasion	Readers need to feel that the instruction is significant for them. *Example: Do you think that the message in this book is important for you?*
Self-efficacy	Is the message doable, and does the reader feel confident in carrying it out? *Example: Do you think you could do what is suggested in this booklet?*

Modified from C. C. Doak et al., 1996.

- Put patients at ease. Focus on inclusion and trust before delivering content.
- Praise patients, but do not patronize them. Let them know what they are doing right. Focus on their strengths and assets and what they bring to the teaching encounter.
- Be encouraging throughout the educational steps. We all like to be told what we are doing right.
- Allow time for patients and family members to think and ask questions.
- Remember that comprehension and understanding requires time and practice. Ongoing feedback helps refocus the teaching encounter and can keep you on track.
- Conduct learner verification (i.e., process that checks suitability of information) to ensure understanding (Table 7-7)
- Evaluate the teaching plan and keep adding new information to the interaction.

Assess Materials: Become a Wise Consumer and User

Materials are collected, stored, and disseminated within community sites. In many instances, nurses distribute pamphlets, but patients either do not read them or they review them only superficially.

People of this country have had so much pamphlet materials passed out to them free that some have lost respect for free literature. Health educators may have contributed to this delinquency by passing out health literature carelessly and indiscriminately. The nurse who expects the pamphlet to take the place of the health teacher is employing weak measures in the health education program. (Rue, 1944, p. 215)

This statement continues to be true today. It is important that nurses evaluate health materials before they disseminate them to individuals, families, or the general public. Such steps need to be applied to the review and assessment of Web sites as well (Ademiluyi et al., 2003; Bock et al., 2004). Health materials should strengthen previous teaching and be used as an adjunct to health instruction.

Assessing the Relevancy of Health Materials

It is critical that nurses find and use materials and media that are appropriate for the intended target audience in community health education initiatives. Some questions that the nurse should ask include the following:

- Do the materials match the intended audience?
- Are the materials appealing and culturally and linguistically relevant?
- Do they convey accurate and up-to-date information?
- Are the messages clear and understandable?
- Do the messages promote self-efficacy and motivation?

Figure 7-3 provides an assessment guide for reviewing health materials that this author has used for gauging the appropriateness of materials. The nurse can use this guide in critiquing printed materials. Similarly, the nurse can make slight modifications in assessing other types of health resources (e.g., videotapes, websites, and multimedia interactive modules). The tool allows the nurse to review health materials systematically for appropriateness within the intended target audience. The material assessment should focus on the following criteria: format-layout, type, verbal content, visual content, and aesthetic quality.

Format/layout

- Is the information organized clearly? Does it make sense?
- Do headers or advance organizers cue the reader? Headers help the reader visualize what is next.
- Is there a 50% to 50% allocation of white and black space? This gives the reader breathing space.
- Is the information easy to read and uncluttered?

Type

- Is the type or font a readable size? Consider the age of your intended group and whether visual difficulties are likely.

Verbal content

- Is the information current, accurate, and relevant to the intended group?
- Is the information culturally acceptable?
- Are difficult terms defined?

Assessment of Health Education Materials

Name of material/media _____

Author _____

Intended target audience _____

Cost/availability/producer _____

> **Directions:** Assess your printed material using the following tool. Use the rating scale of 1-4 for each item in a major category.   *1 = poor   2 = fair   3 = good   4 = very good   N/A = not applicable.*
>
> For each category, give it an overall category rating of: *(+) effective or (−) not effective, (X) unsure*

Category/criteria Comments	Rating
	1 = Poor; 2 = Fair; 3 = Good; 4 = Very Good
Format/Layout	
Organizational style	_____
White/black space	_____
Margins	_____
Grouping of elements	_____
Use of headers/advance organizers	_____
Overall category rating of:	
(+) effective _____ (−) not effective _____ (X) unsure _____	
Type	
Size	_____
Style	_____
Spacing	_____
Overall category rating of:	
(+) effective _____ (−) not effective _____ (X) unsure _____	
Verbal Content	
Clarity	_____
Quantity	_____
Relevancy to intended group	_____
e.g., age, gender, race/ethnicity	_____
Use of active voice	_____
Difficulty/readability level	_____
Grade level	_____
Accuracy	_____
Currency	_____
Overall category rating of:	
(+) effective _____ (−) not effective _____ (X) unsure _____	

Category/criteria	Rating Comments
	1 = Poor; 2 = Fair; 3 = Good; 4 = Very Good
Visual Content	
Tone/mood	_____
Clarity	_____
Cueing	_____
Relevancy to intended group	_____
e.g., age, gender, race/ethnicity	
Currency	_____
Accuracy	_____
Detail	_____
Overall category rating of:	
(+) effective _____ (−) not effective _____ (X) unsure _____	
Aesthetic Quality/Appeal	
Attractiveness	_____
Color	_____
Quality of production	_____
Personalized instructions	_____
Overall category rating of:	
(+) effective _____ (−) not effective _____ (X) unsure _____	
Comments:	

Overall, based on your scoring of 1 to 4 and an evaluation of its effectiveness with the intended target audience, how suitable would you rate this educational tool? Circle one.

1 = poor: probably won't work with my intended audience. I would probably not ever use it.

2 = fair: has a low likelihood of success with my intended audience. I would use it rarely and only in combination with other sources

3 = good: has a good likelihood of being suitable and relevant for about half of my intended audience. I would use it sometimes.

4 = very good: has a high likelihood of being suitable and relevant for most of my intended audience. I would most definitely use it!

FIGURE 7-3   Form for assessing health education materials. (Modified from EPET, 1981; Meade 2001). Assessment guide to review health materials. (Modified from University of Kentucky: *Assessment guide to review health materials,* Patient Education Materials Workshop, 1980.)

CASE STUDY   Application of the Nursing Process

The following case study and teaching plan provide an example of selected teaching approaches and learning needs for the individual, family, and community.

Emma Jackson, aged 29, receives ongoing health care at her neighborhood's community-based clinic, a federally funded community clinic. She visits the nurse practitioner, and the nurse confirms that Mrs. Jackson is 2 months pregnant. She is married and has a 6-year-old son. Emma tells the nurse she smokes and wants to quit, but she has been unable to quit since her last pregnancy. She tells the nurse, "I smoke when I get stressed. I have so many things on my mind." Her husband is also a smoker and has tried to quit at times as well. The nurse refers Mrs. Jackson to a community nursing student named Irene Green for counseling, education, and follow-up.

ASSESSMENT

Irene recognizes that smoking during pregnancy is detrimental for the unborn infant, unhealthy for Mrs. Jackson, and harmful for the 4-year-old child who breathes the secondhand smoke (Castles et al., 1999; DiFranza and Lew, 1995; Fang et al., 2004; Tuthill et al., 1999; USDHHS, 2004). Irene also knows that smokers often experience stages of readiness in their attempts to quit, and relapse is often part of the process (Prochaska and DiClemente, 1983). She notes that family and community support systems are important.

Irene assesses Mrs. Jackson on an individual level, which follows:
- Smoking history, smoking patterns, and previous attempts to quit
- Support systems (e.g., family, friends, and peers)
- Perceived barriers to quitting
- Perceived benefits to quitting
- Perceived priority in addressing this health issue versus other everyday stresses
- Perceived effect of smoking behavior on family communication patterns
- Confidence and perceived efficacy in ability to quit

Assessment of other groups includes families, neighborhoods, churches, community organizations, and environmental messages that promote smoking cessation.

DIAGNOSIS

Individual
- Altered health maintenance (tobacco use) in response to personal stressors, unawareness of available resources, and insufficient support systems
- Ineffective individual coping related to inadequate resources and support networks, evidenced by unsuccessful management of stressors
- Decisional conflict related to previous unsuccessful attempts (lack of confidence in ability to quit smoking and stay quit)

- Health-seeking behavior (desire to quit smoking) for individual and family

Family
- Potential for altered family processes related to lack of agreement about household smoking patterns

Community
- Inadequate organized smoking cessation programs and initiatives for populations at risk related to lack of economic resources and community-building coalitions

PLANNING

Individual
Long-Term Goal
- Mrs. Jackson will quit smoking.

Short-Term Goals
- Mrs. Jackson will recognize that continued smoking is unhealthy for herself, her unborn infant, her young child, and her family.
- Mrs. Jackson will become aware of ways to enhance her confidence during smoking cessation.
- Mrs. Jackson will identify situations and stressors that influence her smoking patterns.
- Mrs. Jackson will learn two strategies to cope with stressful situations and apply those strategies.

Family
Long-Term Goal
- Mr. and Mrs. Jackson will quit smoking and become a smoke-free family.

Short-Term Goals
- Mr. and Mrs. Jackson acknowledge the benefits of a smoke-free environment.
- Mr. Jackson recognizes the need to quit smoking.
- The couple recognizes the need to support each other in smoking cessation.
- Mr. and Mrs. Jackson identify and discuss specific supportive actions during the smoking cessation phases. The couple enlists the support of another person or network.

Community
Long-Term Goals
- The community will support and endorse a smoke-free environment and publicize these efforts through billboards and other media.
- Community agencies and organizations will integrate smoking cessation and relapse programs and messages into their existing health-related activities.
- Cigarette advertising will cease.

CASE STUDY   Application of the Nursing Process (cont'd)

Short-Term Goals

- A coalition of community members will develop and implement policies to support smoking cessation and relapse strategies.
- A consortium of health care agencies and community-based organizations recognize the need to develop partnerships in creating smoking cessation strategies for the community and for high-risk groups.

INTERVENTION

Individual

Planning and interventions encourage expression, promote the use of adaptive coping mechanisms, offer positive reinforcement, disseminate appropriate smoking cessation strategies and provide culturally and educationally relevant materials and media. The nurse applies the five As approach to smoking cessation counseling (Ask, Advise, Assess, Assist, and Arrange). Irene offers empowerment strategies to help Mrs. Jackson cope with her smoking cessation attempts and identifies daily hassles and stressors. Irene gives tailored smoking cessation messages and culturally and educationally appropriate materials and initiates a follow-up plan that is acceptable and doable based on ongoing assessment and feedback (Chalmers et al., 2004; DiClemente et al., 2000; Melvin et al., 2000; Quinn et al., 2005).

Family

Planning and interventions recognize the need for strong support systems within families. Irene provided education and counseling to promote family self-care and recognized that she must address and incorporate Mr. Jackson's support, or lack thereof, into the care plan. Irene makes links to community resources (e.g., health classes, support groups, and networking with other expectant moms who quit or are attempting to quit) to build Mrs. Jackson's support system.

Community

Planning and interventions implemented on an aggregate level identify key community leaders, agencies, legislators, and lay members who are committed to supporting smoking cessation/relapse initiatives at a sociopolitical level (e.g., creating smoking cessation/relapse initiatives at various community channels). Program initiatives assist community members in defining issues and solutions to the effects of smoking on individuals, families, and community groups. Developing coalitions and partnerships among community-based organizations, health care groups, governmental agencies, and intended audience members through dialogue and increased awareness is essential.

EVALUATION

Evaluation is systematic and continuous and focuses on the individual, family, and community.

Individual

An evaluation of Mrs. Jackson's smoking habits occurs within the health system and the community (clinics and WIC). These groups address both process (decrease in number of cigarettes smoked) and outcome (quit or not quit) endpoints. Mrs. Jackson experiences an increase in her coping skills and support system, which is evident in her personalized care plan.

- Irene tailors smoking cessation messages to Mrs. Jackson to fit her everyday life.
- Irene provides Mrs. Jackson with follow-up (e.g., telephone, letter, and follow-up visits).

Family

Care plans include support pattern development with family or significant other in smoking cessation initiatives

- Irene assesses family health patterns and screened for other at-risk behaviors.
- Irene identifies and addresses family support and communication patterns in the care plan.

Community

Irene introduces smoking cessation and relapse programs and smoking prevention initiatives to at least two channels of dissemination (e.g., churches, schools, work sites, and community-based clinics).

- Smoking cessation/relapse messages are infused throughout the community through radio, television, and billboards.
- Community task forces and coalitions demonstrate a collaborative partnership among lay members, community leaders, organizers, and legislators to address smoking-related health issues.

- Does the text reflect the racial and ethnic diversity of the intended audience?
- What is the reading level?

Visual content

- Are the graphics accurate, current, and relevant to the intended group?

- Does cueing help the reader connect the printed words and pictures?
- Will the reader understand the intended meanings of the pictures?
- Is the information culturally acceptable?
- Are the pictures on the cover reflective of the material inside?

- Do the pictures reflect the target audience's racial and ethnic diversity?

Aesthetic quality and appeal
- Is the material appealing?
- Are there helpful special features (e.g., glossary, space for notes, and useful telephone numbers)?

Assessment of Reading Level

Part of the written material's assessment is reading level. Many formulas are available to estimate the printed text's readability and grade level, including the SMOG readability formula. **See Resource Tool 7D,** SMOG Formula for Estimating Readability Grade Level of Printed Text, on the book's evolve website at http://evolve.elsevier.com/Nies.

Readability formulas are objective, quantitative tools that measure sentence and word variables. However, they do not consider factors such as motivation, experience, or need for information (Meade and Smith, 1991). These formulas do estimate reading ease and provide guidelines for assessing and rewriting health information. The Flesch-Kincaid Formula (Flesch, 1948) is another broad estimate of reading and is programmed into most computer software programs' grammar editing tools.

Learner Verification

The best way to identify material suitability is to deliver the materials to the intended audience and obtain feedback about acceptability, understanding, and usefulness. **Learner verification** engages intended members in dialogue and helps uncover unsuitable aspects of the material (i.e., content, visuals, or format) (Doak et al., 1996). If the nurse discovers a need for new educational materials or media, he or she may incorporate Freirean principles to produce empowering products. The Freire approach supports learner participation in the development process, ensures the learner is the active subject of the educational experience, and allows learners to define content and outcomes. Freire's approach focuses on people's experiences and ideas and creates themes to address them.

The process of learner verification helps to identify the likelihood if the message is well suited to the audience. It involves verifying or checking if certain elements work well together to result in a good match of information for the learner. See Table 7-7 for a description of the specific elements and sample questions associated with each one. For example, the chapter author used a learner verification processes to develop education toolboxes on breast and cervical and prostate cancer for Hispanic migrant and seasonal farmworker and African-American women and men, respectively. Following the conduct of a series of focus groups with members of the intended audience to elicit themes about health, illness, cancer, and prevention, we then conducted a series of learner verification measures. Through a series of systematic questions and interviewing processes, we were able to collect information in the intended audience's own words to help shape and refocus the cancer issues (breast, cervical, and prostate from their own perspective (African-American men and women and Hispanic men and women farmworkers). Such verifying checks help to assess the understanding of words and pictures, the acceptability of music and narrator and pictures, the efficacy and persuasion of the message and overall attractiveness of the tools (e.g., videotape, flipchart, and booklet). Similarly, this approach was used to adapt smoking-relapse prevention materials for pregnant and postpartum women (Quinn et al., 2005). The use of learner verification fits well within the framework of community-based participatory research methods as outlined earlier in this chapter.

SUMMARY

Teaching is a significant component of community health nursing, and it impacts virtually every nursing activity. The goal of health education is to facilitate a process that allows individuals, families, and groups to make well-informed decisions about health practices. An understanding of learning and the theoretical frameworks that explain behaviors and health actions is inherent in community health education. No single theory explains human behavior; the nurse must apply multiple theories and approaches.

Nurses must be knowledgeable about sociopolitical, cultural, environmental, and ecological forces affecting community health to ensure the success of health education strategies. Health education, which is relevant for an intended group, is based on individual variables and social, structural, political, cultural, and economic factors within the larger community context. Nurses develop relevant teaching interventions by assessing their audience and their characteristics thoroughly and by using an organized and systematic approach to delivering health messages and programs. Implementing social action strategies such as advocating health-promoting lifestyles, creating an environment for problem-posing dialogue, and providing links to appropriate health resources supports the philosophy of critical consciousness. Nurses can facilitate the principle of social justice by mastering health information delivery and committing themselves to creating empowerment strategies that equip individuals, families, and communities with knowledge and navigation skills for healthy lifestyles and environments.

Nurses can use a variety of methods, materials, and media to support health education activities, including electronic and Web-based information. The nurse should review and evaluate these resources for their cultural, linguistic, and literacy suitability for the intended group. Embracing the notion that health education is an ongoing interactive process influenced by many internal and external factors is key to meeting the needs of individuals, families, and communities. Nurses can make important contributions to the prevention of disease and the promotion of personal and community health with knowledge, spirit, and commitment to empowerment strategies.

LEARNING ACTIVITIES

1. In groups of two to four students, describe how theoretical frameworks help explain health behavior. Identify the strengths and limitations of models that focus on individual health determinants versus models that encompass sociopolitical factors.
2. Discuss the role of the nurse in health education. Outline specific activities and roles that the community nurse can perform with regard to health education issues. Share with each other a particular experience relating to cultural effectiveness that would enhance/impede this role.
3. Identify a specific intended group in the community (e.g., homeless, seniors). Describe the group's characteristics and identify the methods for obtaining this information.
4. Select an aggregate (e.g., students, elderly, pregnant women, homeless, deaf children, new immigrants).
   a. Describe the group's characteristics, learning needs, and strengths.
   b. Identify the methods for obtaining this information.
   c. Next, describe the application of Freire's empowerment education model to address health issues.
5. Identify an issue of concern among community members (e.g., obesity, access to care). Discuss sociopolitical issues that impact this health issue. Outline specific community-based participatory activities and roles that the community nurse can perform that might help address this health issue.
6. Select a health education brochure or health website. Apply the assessment criteria presented to assess its appropriateness for the intended audience. Evaluate the relative strengths of the printed material or website and potential areas for improvement using learner verification questions.

REFERENCES

Ademiluyi G et al: Evaluating the reliability and validity of three tools to assess the quality of health information on the internet, *Patient Educ Couns* 50:151-155, 2003.

Alexander DE: Readability of published dental educational materials, *J Am Dent Assoc* 131:937-942, 2000.

American Cancer Society: *Cancer facts and figures: 2005,* Atlanta, 2005, The Author.

American Hospital Association: *A patient's bill of rights in hospitals,* Chicago, 1972, The Author.

American Medical Association, Ad Hoc Committee on Health Literacy for the Council on Scientific Affairs: Health literacy: report of the council on scientific affairs, *JAMA* 281:552-557, 1999.

American Nurses Association: *The professional nurse and health education,* Kansas City, Mo, 1975, The Author.

Babcock DE, Miller MA: *Client education: theory and practice,* St. Louis, 1994, Mosby.

Baker DW et al: Health literacy and the risk of hospital admission, *J Gen Intern Med* 13(12):791-798, 1998.

Bandura A: Self-efficacy: toward a unifying theory of behavioral change, *Psychol Rev* 84:191-215, 1977a.

Bandura A: *Social learning theory,* Englewood Cliffs, NJ, 1977b, Prentice Hall.

Becker MH, editor: *The health belief model and personal health behavior,* Thorofare, NJ, 1974, Charles B. Slack.

Becker MH et al: The health belief model and prediction of dietary compliance: a field experiment, *J Health Soc Behav* 18:348-366, 1977.

Bennett CL et al: Relationship between literacy, race, and stage of presentation among low-income patients with prostate cancer, *J Clin Oncol* 16:3101-3104, 1998.

Bigge ML, Shermis SS: *Learning theories for teachers,* ed 6, Boston, 2004, Pearson/Allyn and Bacon.

Bock B et al: Smoking cessation treatment on the Internet: content, quality, and usability, *Nicotine Tob Res* 6:207-219, 2004.

Brackley M et al: Community readiness to prevent intimate partner violence in Bexar County, Texas, *J Transcul Nurs* 14:227-236, 2003.

Bradley CJ, Given CW, Roberts C: Race, socio-economic status, and breast cancer treatment and survival, *J Natl Cancer Inst* 3:490-496, 2002.

Brandon TM et al: Efficacy and cost-effectiveness of minimal intervention to prevent smoking relapse: dismantling the effects of content versus contact, *J Consult Clin Psych* 20:797-808, 2004.

Breckon DJ, Harvey JR, Lancaster RB: *Community health education: settings, roles, and skills for the 21st century,* ed 4, Gaithersburg, Md, 1998, Aspen.

Burns PG: Reducing infant mortality using the perinatal periods of risk model, *Public Health Nurs* 22(1):2-7, 2005.

Champion VL: Revised susceptibility, benefits, and barriers scale for mammography screening, *Res Nurs Health* 22:341-348, 1999.

Chang L-C, Li I-C, Liu C-H: A study of the empowerment process for cancer patients using Freire's dialogical interviewing, *J Nurs Res* 12:41-49, 2004.

Clark MJD: *Community health nursing: caring for populations,* ed 4, Stamford, Conn, 2003, Appleton & Lange.

Davis TC, Wolf MS: Health literacy: implications for family medicine, *Fam Med* 36:595-598, 2004.

Davis TC et al: Rapid estimate of adult literacy in medicine: a shortened screening instrument, *Fam Med* 25:56-57, 1993.

Davis TC et al: Health literacy and cancer communication, *CA Cancer J Clin* 52:134-149, 2002.

Dewalt DA et al: Literacy and health outcomes: a systematic review of the literature, *J Gen Intern Med* 19:1228-1239, 2004.

Doak CC, Doak LG, Root JH: *Teaching patients with low literacy skills,* ed 2, Philadelphia, 1996, Lippincott Williams & Wilkins.

Doak CC et al: Improving comprehension for cancer patients with low literacy skills: strategies for clinicians, *CA Cancer J Clin* 48:151-162, 1998.

Doak LG et al: Strategies to develop effective cancer education materials, *Oncol Nurs Forum* 23:1305-1312, 1996.

Dolan NC et al: Colorectal cancer screening knowledge, attitudes and beliefs among veterans: does literacy make a difference? *J Clin Oncol* 22:2617-2622, 2004.

Edgren KK et al: Community involvement in the conduct of a health education and research project: community against asthma, *Health Prom Pract* 6:263-269, 2005.

English KC et al: Intermediate outcomes of a tribal community public health infrastructure assessment, *Ethn Dis* 14: S1-61-S1-69, 2004.

Estrada CA et al: Literacy and numeracy skills and anticoagulation control, *Am J Med Sci* 328:88-93, 2004.

Freeman HP: Poverty, culture, and social injustice: Determinants of cancer disparities, *CA Cancer J Clin* 54:72-77, 2004.

Freire P: *Pedagogy of the oppressed,* New York, 1970, Herder and Herder (Translated from original manuscript, 1968). (New York, 2000, Continuum)

Freire P: *Education for critical consciousness,* New York, 1973, Seabury Press.

Gardner MS: *Public health nursing,* ed 3, New York, MacMillan, 1936.

Gazmararian JA et al: Health literacy among Medicare enrollees in a managed care organization, *JAMA* 281:545-551, 1999a.

Gazmararian JA et al: Reading skills and family planning knowledge and practices in a low-income managed care population, *Obstet Gynecol* 93:239-244, 1999b.

Giachello AL et al: Reducing diabetes health disparities through community-based participatory action research: the Chicago southeast diabetes community action coalition, *Pub Health Rep* 118:309-323, 2003.

Gillis AJ: Determinants of a health-promoting lifestyle: an integrative review, *J Adv Nurs* 18:345-353, 1993.

Glanz K et al, editors: *Health behavior and health education: theory, research and practice,* ed 2, San Francisco, 1997, Jossey-Bass, 1997.

Glanz K et al, editors: *Health behavior and health education: theory, research and practice,* ed 3, San Francisco, 2002, Jossey-Bass.

Glazer HR, Kirk LM, Bosler FE: Patient education pamphlets about prevention, detection, and treatment of breast cancer for low literacy women, *Patient Educ Couns* 27:185-189, 1996.

Goodman RM et al: Identifying and defining the dimensions of community capacity to provide a basis for measurement, *Health Educ Behav* 25:358-378, 1998.

Green L: Introduction to behavior change and maintenance: theory and measurement. In Schumaker S, Schron EB, Ockene JK, editors: *The handbook of health behavior change,* New York, 1998, Springer.

Green LW, Kreuter MW: *Health program planning: an educational and ecological approach,* ed 4, New York, 2005, McGraw-Hill.

Guidry JJ, Walker VD: Assessing cultural sensitivity in printed cancer materials, *Cancer Prac* 7:291-296, 1999.

Hochbaum GM: *Public participation in medical screening programs: a sociopsychological study,* US Public Health Service Pub No 572, Washington, DC, 1958, US Government Printing Office.

Holmes-Rovner M et al: Evidence based patient choice: a prostate cancer decision aid in plain Language, *BMC Med Informat Dec Making* 5:1-11, 2005.

Horowitz CR et al: Using community-based participatory research to reduce health disparities in East and Central Harlem, *Mt. Sinai J Med* 71:368-374, 2004.

Hulme PA et al: Health-promoting lifestyle behaviors of Spanish-speaking Hispanic adults, *J Transcult Nurs* 14:244-254, 2003.

Israel BA et al: Health education and community empowerment: conceptualizing and measuring perceptions of individual, organization, and community control, *Health Educ Q* 32:149-170, 1994.

Israel BA et al: Review of community-based research: assessing partnership approaches to improve public health, *Annu Rev Public Health* 19:173-202, 1998.

Israel BA et al, editors: *Methods in community-based participatory research for health,* San Francisco, 2005, Jossey-Bass.

Jacobsen PB et al: Efficacy and costs of two forms of stress management training for cancer patients undergoing chemotherapy, *J Clin Oncol* 20:2851-2862, 2002.

Janz NK, Becker MH: The health belief model: a decade later, *Health Educ Q* 11:1-47, 1984.

Janz NK, Champion VL, Strecher VJ: The health belief model. In Glanz K, Rimer BK, Lewis FM, editors: *Health behavior and education: theory, research and practice,* ed 3, Jossey-Bass, 2002, San Francisco, pp. 45-66.

Jastak S, Wilkinson GS: *The wide-range achievement test III: revised administration manual,* Wilmington, Del, 1999, Jastak Associates.

Jemmott JB et al: HIV/STD risk reduction interventions for African American and Latino adolescent girls at an adolescent medicine clinic, *Arch Pediatr Adolesc Med* 159:440-449, 2005.

Jezewski MA: Culture brokering as a model for advocacy, *Nurs Health Care* 14:78-85, 1993.

Joint Commission on Accreditation of Healthcare Organizations: *1996 accreditation manual for hospitals,* vol 1, Oak Brook, Ill, 1995, The Author.

Kalichman SC, Rompa D: Functional health literacy is associated with health status and health-related knowledge in people living with HIV-AIDS, *J Acquir Immune Defic Syndr* 25:337-344, 2000.

Kalichman SC et al: Health literacy and health-related knowledge among persons living with HIV/AIDS, *Am J Prev Med* 18:325-331, 2000.

Keck CW: Community health: our common challenge, *Fam Community Health* 172:1-9, 1994.

Kegeles SS et al: Survey of beliefs about cancer detection and Papanicolaou tests, *Public Health Rep* 80:815-823, 1965.

Kickbush IS: Health literacy: addressing the health and education divide, *Health Prom Intern* 16:289-297, 2001.

Kirsch et al: *Adult literacy in America: a first look at the findings of the national adult literacy survey,* Washington DC, National Center for Education Statistics, 1993, US Department of Education.

Kleinman A: Concepts and a model for the comparison of medical systems as cultural systems, *Soc Sci Med* 12:85-93, 1978.

Klinedinst NJ: Effects of a nutrition education program for urban, low-income, older adults: a collaborative program among nurses and nursing students, *J Community Health Nurs* 22:93-104, 2005.

Knowles MS: *The modern practice of adult education: from pedagogy to andragogy,* Chicago, 1980, Association Press/Follett.

Knowles MS: *The making of an adult educator: an autobiographical journey,* San Francisco, 1989, Jossey-Bass.

Kreuter MW, McClure SM: The role of culture in health communication, *Annu Rev Public Health,* 25:439-455, 2004.

Kreuter MW, Strecher VJ, Glassman B: One size does not fit all: the case for tailoring print materials, *Ann Behav Med* 21:276-283, 1999.

Kreuter MW et al: Effectiveness of individually tailored calendars in promoting childhood immunization in urban public health centers, *Am J Public Health* 94:122-127, 2004.

Labonte R: Health promotion and empowerment: reflections on professional practice, *Health Educ Q* 21:253-268, 1994.

Leung MW, Yen IH, Minkler M: Community-based participatory research: a promising approach for increasing epidemiology's relevance in the 21st century, *Intern J Epidemiol* 33:499-506, 2004.

Lindau ST et al: The association of health literacy with cervical cancer prevention knowledge and health behaviors in a multiethnic cohort of women, *Am J Obstet Gynecol* 186:938-943, 2002.

Lohse JL: A bicycle safety education program for parents of young children, *J Sch Nurs* 19:100-110, 2003.

López EDS et al: Photovoice as a community-based participatory action method: a case study with African American breast cancer survivors in rural eastern North Carolina. In Israel BA, Eng E, Schulz AJ, Parker EA, editors: *Methods in community-based participatory research for health,* San Francisco, 2005, Jossey-Bass, pp. 326-358.

Macario E et al: Factors influencing nutrition education for patients with low literacy skills, *J Am Diet Assoc* 98:559-564, 1998.

MacLeod ML, Zimmer LV: Rethinking emancipation and empowerment in action research: lessons from small rural hospitals, *Can J Nurs Res* 37:78-84, 2005.

Maslow AH: *Motivation and personality,* ed 3, Harper and Row, 1987, New York.

McKinlay JB: Epidemiological and political determinants of social policies regarding the publichealth *Soc Sci Med* 13A:541-558, 1979.

McLaughlin HG: SMOG-grading: a new readability formula, *J Reading* 12:204-206, 1969.

Meade CD: Approaching the media with confidence, *Public Health Nurs* 9:209-214, 1992.

Meade CD: Producing videotapes for cancer education: methods and examples, *Oncol Nurs Forum* 23: 837-846, 1996.

Meade CD: Improving understanding of the informed consent process and document, *Semin Oncol Nurs* 15:124-137, 1999.

Meade CD: Cancer care for diverse populations: relevant communications and research, *Cancer Control* 10:1-2, 2003.

Meade CD, Byrd JC: Patient literacy and the readability of smoking education literature, *Am J Public Health* 79:204-206, 1989.

Meade CD, Byrd JC, Lee M: Improving patient comprehension of literature on smoking, *Am J Public Health* 79:1411-1412, 1989.

Meade CD, Calvo A: Developing community-academic partnerships to enhance breast health among rural and Hispanic migrant and seasonal farmworkers, *Oncol Nurs Forum* 28:1577-1584, 2001.

Meade CD, McKinney WP, Barnas G: Educating patients with limited literacy skills: The effectiveness of printed and videotaped materials about colon cancer, *Am J Public Health* 84:119-121, 1994.

Meade CD, Smith CF: Readability formulas: cautions and criteria, *Patient Educ Couns* 17:153-158, 1991.

Meade CD et al: Readability of American Cancer Society patient education literature, *Oncol Nurs Forum* 19:51-55, 1992.

Meade CD et al: Impact of culturally, linguistically and literacy relevant videotaped cancer information among Hispanic farmworker women, *J Canc Educ* 17:50-54, 2002a.

Meade CD et al: Screening and community outreach programs for priority populations: considerations for oncology managers, *J Oncol Management* Sept/Oct 11(5):14-22, 2002b.

Meade CD et al: Focus groups in the design of prostate cancer screening information for Hispanic farmworkers and African American men, *Onc Nurs Forum* 30:967-975, 2003.

Meleis AI: Culturally competent care, *J Transcult Nurs* 10:12, 1999.

Minkler M: Community-based research partnerships: challenges and opportunities, *J Urban Health* 82(2 Suppl 2):ii3-ii12, 2005.

Minkler M, Wallerstein N: Improving health through community organization and community building. In Glanz K, Rimer BK, Lewis, FM, editors, *Health behavior and education: theory, research, and practice,* ed 3, San Francisco, 2002, Jossey-Bass, pp. 279-311.

Mohrmann CC et al: An analysis of printed breast cancer information for African American women, *J Cancer Educ* 15:23-27, 2000.

The National Literacy Act of 1991, PL 102-73, 1991.

Nielsen-Bohlman L et al, editors: *Health literacy: a prescription to end confusion* [Institute of Medicine report], Washington, DC, 2004, The National Academies Press.

Nightingale F: *Notes on nursing,* New York, 1859, Appleton-Century Crofts.

Nyswander DB: Education for health: Some principles and their application, *Health Educ Mono* 14:65-70, 1956.

Office of Minority Health: *Assuring cultural competence in health care: recommendations for national standards and an outcomes-focused research agenda* 1999, The Author, http://www.omhrc.gov/clas/cultural1a.htm.

Olshansky E et al: Participatory action research to understand and reduce health disparities, *Nurs Outlook* 53:121-126, 2005.

Paasche-Orlow MK et al: The prevalence of limited literacy, *J Gen Intern Med* 20: 175-184, 2005.

Padilla GV, Bulcavage LM: Theories used in patient/health education, *Semin Oncol Nurs* 7:87-96, 1991.

Parikh NS et al: Shame and health literacy: the unspoken connection, *Patient Educ Couns* 27:33-39, 1996.

Parker EA et al: Community action against asthma: examining the partnership process of a community-based participatory research project, *J Gen Intern Med* 18:558-567, 2003.

Parker RM et al: The test of functional health literacy in adults: a new instrument for measuring patients' literacy skills, *J Gen Intern Med* 10:537-541, 1995.

Paskett ED, et al: Use of a photo essay to teach low-income African-American women about mammography, *J Cancer Educ* 11:216–220, 1996.

Pavlov IP: *Experimental psychology, and other essays,* New York, 1957, Philosophical Library.

Pender NJ, Murdaugh CL, Parsons MA: *Health promotion in nursing practice,* ed 5, Upper Saddle River, NJ, 2005, Pearson Education.

Petersen R et al: Moving beyond disclosure: women's perspectives on barriers and motivators to seeking assistance for intimate partner violence, *Women Health* 40:63-76, 2004.

Piaget J: *Adaptation and intelligence: organic selection and phenocopy,* 1980, Chicago, University of Chicago.

Powe BD et al: Perceptions about breast cancer among African American women: do selected educational materials challenge them? *Patient Educ Couns* 56:197-204, 2005.

Prochaska JO, DiClemente CC: Stages and processes of self-change of smoking: toward an integrative model of change, *J Consult Clin Psychol* 51:390-395, 1983.

Quinn G, Brandon T, Ellison BB, Meade CD, Roach N, Lopez E, Albrecht T, Brandon TH. Adapting smoking relapse-prevention materials for pregnant and postpartum women: formative research. *Matern Child Health J* 10:1-11, 2005.

Rankin SH, Stallings KD: *Patient education: principles and practices,* ed 4, New York, 2000, Lippincott Williams & Wilkins.

Rawl SM et al: The impact of age and race on mammography practices, *Health Care Women Int* 21:583-597, 2000.

Redman BK: *The practice of patient education,* ed 9, St. Louis, 2001, Mosby.

Robertson A, Minkler M: New health promotion movement: a critical examination, *Health Educ Q* 21:295-312, 1994.

Rogers CR: *A Carl Rogers reader,* Boston, 1989, Houghton Mifflin.

Rosenstock I: Why people use health services, *Milbank Memorial Fund Q* 44:94-127, 1966.

Rosenstock IM, Strecher VJ, Becker MH: Social learning theory and the health belief model, *Health Educ Q* 15(2):175-183, 1988.

Rue CB: *The public health nurse in the community,* Philadelphia, 1944, WB Saunders.

Salazar MK: Hispanic women's beliefs about breast cancer and mammography, *Cancer Nurs* 19:437-446, 1996.

Schapira MM, Meade C, Nattinger AB: Enhanced decision-making: the use of a videotape decision-aid for patients with prostate cancer, *Patient Educ Couns* 30(2):119-127, 1997.

Schillinger D et al: Association of health literacy with diabetes outcomes, *JAMA* 288:475-482, 2002.

Sharp LK et al: Health literacy, cervical cancer risk factors, and distress in low-income African-American women seeking colposcopy, *Ethn Dis* 12:541-546, 2002.

Shinagawa SM: The excess burden of breast carcinoma in minority and medically underserved communities: application, research, and redressing institutional racism, *Cancer* 88(5 Suppl), 1217-1223, 2000.

Skinner BF: *About behaviorism,* New York, 1976, Vintage Books, Random House.

Smedley BD et al, editors: *Unequal treatment: confronting racial and ethnic disparities in health care,* Washington, DC: 2003, National Academies Press.

Steuart GW, Kark SO: *A practice of social medicine: a South African team's experiences in different African communities,* Edinburgh, 1962, Livingstone.

Strickland J et al: Health promotion in cervical cancer prevention among the Yakama Indian women of the Wa'Shat Longhouse, *J Transcult Nurs* 10:190-196, 1999.

Swanson J: Diversity: Creating an environment of inclusiveness, *Nursing Adm Q* 28:207-211, 2004.

Travers KD: Reducing inequities through participatory research and community empowerment, *Health Educ Behav* 24:344-356, 1997.

US Department of Health and Human Services, Public Health Services: *Healthy People 2010,* ed 2, Vol 1: *Understanding and improving health;* Vol 2: *Objectives for improving health,* Washington DC, 2000, US Government Printing Office.

US Department of Health and Human Services, Centers for Disease Control and Prevention, National Center for Chronic Disease Prevention and Health Promotion: *The health consequences of smoking: a report of the surgeon general,* Atlanta, 2004, Office on Smoking and Health.

US Department of Health Human Services: *Making health communication programs work,* NIH Pub No 02-5145, Bethesda, Md, 2002, Office of Cancer Communications, National Cancer Institute.

US Public Health Service: *Treating tobacco use and dependence: clinical practice guideline.* Bethesda, Md, US Department of Health and Human Services.

Van Wyk NC: Health education as education of the oppressed, *Curationis* 22:29-34, 1999.

Villarruel AM et al: Predictors of sexual intercourse and a use intentions among Spanish-dominant Latino youth; a test of the planned behavior theory, *Nurs Res* 53:172-181, 2004.

Wallerstein N: Empowerment to reduce health disparities, *Scand J Public Health Suppl* 59:72-77, 2002.

Wallerstein N, Bernstein E: Empowerment education: Freire's ideas adapted to health education, *Health Educ Q* 15:379-394, 1988.

Wang C, Burris MA: Empowerment through photo novella: portraits of participation, *Health Educ Q* 21:171-186, 1994.

Wang C, Burris MA: Photovoice: concept, methodology, and use for participatory needs assessment, *Health Educ Behav* 24:369-387, 1997.

Watters EK: Literacy for health: an interdisciplinary model, *J Transcult Nurs* 14:48-54, 2003.

Weiss BC, Coyne C: Communicating with patients who cannot read, *N Engl J Med* 337:272-274, 1997.

Wells JA et al: Literacy of women attending family planning clinics in Virginia and reading levels of brochures on HIV prevention, *Fam Plann Perspect* 26:113-131, 1994.

Williams MV et al: Inadequate functional health literacy among patients at 2 public hospitals, *JAMA* 274:1677-1682, 1995.

Williams MV et al: Inadequate literacy is a barrier to asthma knowledge and self-care, *Chest* 114:1008-1015, 1998a.

Williams MV et al: Relationship of functional health literacy to patients' knowledge of their chronic disease: a study of patients with hypertension or diabetes, *Arch Intern Med* 158:166-172, 1998b.

Wilson FL et al: Literacy, readability and cultural barriers: critical factors to consider when educating older African Americans about anticoagulation therapy, *J Clin Nurs* 12:275-292, 2003.

Wolf MS et al: Health literacy and patient knowledge in a Southern US HIV clinic, *Int J STD AIDS* 15:747-752, 2004.

World Health Organization: Health promotion and community action in developing countries, Geneva, 1994, The Author.

Case Management

Jean Cozad Lyon

MEDIA RESOURCES

Additional Material for Study, Review, and Further Exploration

evolve Website at http://evolve.elsevier.com/Nies

❖ Quiz ❖ Case Studies ❖ Content Updates ❖ Glossary ❖ WebLinks

---

OBJECTIVES

Upon completion of this chapter, the reader will be able to do the following:

1. Define case management.
2. Discuss the purpose of providing case management services.
3. Identify the origin and purpose of case management.
4. Discuss trends that influence the development of case management programs.
5. Incorporate case management concepts into clinical practice settings.
6. Identify educational preparation and skills recommended for case managers.

KEY TERMS

case management
client-centered case management
continuum of care

discharge planning
system-centered case management
utilization review

CHAPTER OUTLINE

OVERVIEW OF NURSING CASE MANAGEMENT

Case management is a term that describes a wide variety of patient care coordination programs in acute hospital and community settings. The term *case management* applies to community health settings, which include public and mental health settings and population groups of all ages.

Since the late 1980s and the 1990s, a variety of case management programs have emerged (Huber, 2002). From 1990 to 2005, case management evolved rapidly in response to changes in the health care environment and increased managed care programs. Client service use reflects a greater emphasis on health care costs; therefore third-party payers evaluate the appropriate use of health care resources such as diagnostic tests, laboratory tests, length of hospital visits, and duration of home health care services. Managed care organizations (MCOs) may deny reimbursement to health care providers who exceed the expected costs. Health care providers must closely monitor their use of resources; therefore they introduced various forms of case management programs.

The development of case management models in acute hospital and community settings created confusion over what programs and services compose case management and how case management differs from other services like social services and **discharge planning.** A single definition of case management does not exist. The Case Management Society of America (CMSA) (1995) offers the following definition of case management:

> *Case management is a collaborative process, which assesses, plans, implements, coordinates, monitors, and evaluates options and services to meet an individual's health needs through communication and available resources to promote quality cost-effective outcomes. (p. 2)*

The philosophy statement from the CMSA (2005) says:

> *Case management is not a profession in itself, but an area of practice within one's profession. Its underlying premise is that when an individual reaches the optimum level of wellness and functional capability, everyone benefits: the individuals being served, their support systems, the health care delivery systems and the various reimbursement sources.*

According to the American Nurses Association, nursing case management is "a health care delivery process whose goals are to provide quality health care, decrease fragmentation, enhance the client's quality of life, and contain costs" (1992).

Many labels describe case management within a profession. In addition to case management, other titles include case coordination, continuing care coordination, service integration, care management, service integration, continuity coordination, and service coordination. Multiple case management labels cause further confusion among health care professionals and heath care consumers. Case management takes on many forms depending on the level, discipline, organization, situation, and basic client care needs that are addressed (Huber, 2002).

Some hospitals, health maintenance organizations (HMOs), and other insurance companies inaccurately use the term

BOX 8-1 Possible Case Management Functions

> ➤ Identifying the target population
> ➤ Determining screening and eligibility
> ➤ Arranging services
> ➤ Monitoring and follow-up
> ➤ Assessing
> ➤ Planning care
> ➤ Reassessing
> ➤ Assisting clients through a complex, fragmented health care system
> ➤ Care coordination and continuity

case management to describe "utilization management," "managed care," or the method of monitoring and controlling service use within a system or care episode to control cost. Many of these providers have case management programs that transcend use control and monitor the patient following hospital discharge. Some of the programs provide continued services to high-risk clients for an indefinite time, regardless of the client's location (Box 8-1).

Case management programs aim to provide a service delivery approach to ensure the following: cost-effective care, alternatives to institutionalization, access to care, coordinated services, and patient's improved functional capacity (Lyon, 1993). These goals apply to community health and acute care settings.

ORIGINS OF CASE MANAGEMENT

Case management has a long history with the mentally ill, elderly patients, and the community setting (Steinberg and Carter, 1983). Public health, mental health, and long-term care settings have implemented and studied case management services and have reported them in the literature for many years (Mahn and Spross, 1996; Weil and Karls, 1985).

Public Health

Community service coordination, which was a forerunner of case management, appeared in public health programs in the early 1900s. During this time, health care providers reported these community service and case management programs in the nursing literature. Programs focused on community education in sanitation, nutrition, and disease prevention became prevalent. Lillian Wald conducted many of these programs at the Henry Street Settlement House in New York City. The Metropolitan Life Insurance Company later expanded nursing services for individuals, families, and the community (Conger, 1999) to include disease prevention and health promotion.

The concept of **continuum of care** originated following World War II to describe the long-term services required for discharged psychiatric patients (Grau, 1984). Service coordination evolved into case management; this term first appeared in social welfare literature during the early 1970s.

Case Management in Mental Health

During the late 1960s and early 1970s, mental health care emphasized moving patients from mental health institutions back into the community (Crosby, 1987; Pittman, 1989). The Community Mental Health Center Act of 1963 placed federal approbation on deinstitutionalization, which emphasized the importance of community mental health services. Mental health providers began to move patients from large state institutions to the community.

Several problems resulted from the deinstitutionalization of mentally ill patients. In 1977, Congress acknowledged that many disabled people were deinstitutionalized without basic needs, proper follow-up, or health care monitoring. Congress further recognized that a systematic approach to service delivery could have prevented many state hospital readmissions. Case management in community mental health helped avoid client service fragmentation (Pittman, 1989).

Case Management and the Elderly

Specific elderly services recognized that age-generic programs do not adequately assist older people. Many older people have special, population-specific health care needs. Thus, case management services frequently target the elderly population, specifically homebound individuals, or those with complex problems. However, not all older people who subscribe to multiple services require a case manager. Older adults may not need a case manager if they possess adequate functional status and can coordinate and access services for themselves, if they have family support, or if they have formal or informal caregivers who provide these functions for them These individuals require information about options, available services, and follow-up assistance (Lyon et al., 1995).

Disease-Specific Case Management

Case management services are often provided for individuals who are identified as having medical conditions that are high-cost or high-volume acute and chronic illnesses. Examples of these illnesses include chronic obstructive pulmonary disease and chronic cardiac conditions such as congestive heart failure. The goal of disease-specific case management is to keep these individuals as healthy as possible and stable in their home environment. One particular goal is to decrease the frequency and length of hospital stays and consequently decrease health care costs.

PURPOSE OF CASE MANAGEMENT

Case management is client centered and system centered. **Client-centered case management** assists the client or patient through a complex, fragmented, and often confusing health care delivery system and achieves specific client-centered goals. **System-centered case management** recognizes that health care resources are finite. The upward spiral in health care costs causes third-party payers such as Medicare, MCOs, and insurance companies to demand cost-effective

---

> ### ETHICAL Insights
>
> **Ethical Issues in Case Management**
>
> There are several ethical considerations that a case manager should take into consideration when working with populations. Some of these include:
> 1. Confidentiality of clients served must be maintained. Communicating patient information to others who are involved with the client's care must be done only with the client's knowledge and permission.
> 2. Health care resources are expensive and limited in number. The case manager needs to remain aware of this and identify resources that are appropriate to individual clients or to groups of clients with the same identified needs.
> 3. Respect for the client's right to be informed about their care and services, and that the client has a right to choose to receive services or not.

health care. Client consumers insist on cost-effective, quality care. This demand forces health care providers to reevaluate the way they administer care, to emphasize quality improvement, and to focus on decreasing cost. Health care resources then become allocated to those populations with the greatest needs.

Case management assists patients and families who need care coordination to access necessary resources in a time-efficient manner (Bower, 1992). For hospitalized patients, health care service coordination begins either upon the patient's admission or shortly thereafter and continues following the patient's discharge for an unspecified time. The patient's physical and psychosocial status and the plan's success will determine the length of the case manager's evaluation and intervention (Lyon, 1993; Lyon et al., 1995).

UTILIZATION REVIEW AND MANAGED CARE

Equity and cost-effectiveness require management and allocation of available resources in a hospital, community, city, state, or particular health care client population. System-centered case management rations and sets priorities for those in a larger group or population who could benefit from specific services.

Case management programs are often motivated by the need to evaluate, use, and allocate health care resources. Many case management programs evolved from utilization review departments. These departments showed that monitoring service use alone is insufficient for managing patient populations with diverse resource needs. Over time, the **utilization review** nurses assumed the additional case manager responsibilities.

TRENDS THAT INFLUENCE CASE MANAGEMENT

Numerous trends influenced case management programs. During the 1970s, hospitals billed Medicare, Medicaid, and other third-party payers for client services and received reimbursement. Health care costs skyrocketed and rapidly became the basis for discussion and concern throughout the health care industry and the country. In 1983, PL 98-21 of the Social Security Amendments introduced the prospective payment system (PPS) in the acute care setting. Under the PPS, health care providers receive a fixed amount of money based on the relative cost of resources they use to treat Medicare patients within each diagnosis-related group. Other third-party payers followed this example and negotiated reimbursement schedules through preferred provider programs or managed care contracts (U.S. Department of Commerce, 1990).

Health care costs continue to escalate, the population is aging, and the elderly population is increasing. Many elderly suffer from chronic illness and require health care resources. These issues influenced, and still influence, the introduction of case management services to control costs and distribute health care resources in a variety of settings.

CASE MANAGER EDUCATION PREPARATION

It is essential to determine what classification of health care provider is best qualified to provide case management services. Traditionally, case managers were social workers (SWs) who assumed the role of discharge planner. Client health care needs have become more complex, the need for ongoing patient assessment has emerged, and available resources have become more numerous and diverse; therefore nurses have become case managers. Several health care organizations exclusively employ SWs in case manager roles, others exclusively employ nurses in case management, and others use a combination of SWs and nurses, depending on the client population's needs. Combining the strength and knowledge of the nurse's clinical background with the SW's community service background is a combination that can efficiently move a client through the complex health care system (Lyon et al., 1995).

Nurse Case Managers

Although both nurses and SWs have proven themselves to be excellent case managers, this chapter focuses on the nurse case manager in discussing educational requirements. A nurse case manager's optimum education level is debatable. Basic nursing education for case managers required by employers can vary. Some may require a baccalaureate degree and others may not. In some settings, a master's degree may be required. Some programs are more interested in prior experience, continuing education, and case management certification than the entry-level nursing degree. Education and experience requirements may vary depending on the program's geographical location, specific client needs, and available staff.

Nurses with master's degrees and a focus in case management are readily available in urban settings. This gives facilities the opportunity to hire case managers who are academically prepared in theory and clinical experience. Rural areas that do not have master's-level academic programs are at a great disadvantage in recruiting and hiring qualified nurses. To fill the case manager role, rural facilities promote nurses to case management positions, provide them with continuing education programs, and offer them necessary job-related experience. Although this is not the ideal solution, it is often the only option for smaller facilities and those in more remote parts of the United States.

Regardless of the educational requirements in the individual case management program, case managers need a minimum skill level to ensure success in the role. These skills include sound knowledge of reimbursement structures; knowledge of available resources within the institution, organization, or community; working knowledge of the identification and evaluation of quality outcomes; the ability to perform cost-benefit ratios; and an understanding of financial strategies. In addition to the required knowledge, the nurse case manager needs the following characteristics: flexibility, creativity, excellent communication skills, and the ability to work autonomously.

Certification as a case manager is now available through the Case Management Society of America. Certification can be specific to case management (Certified Case Manager) or utilization review case management (CPUM). According to the CMSA (2005), applicants for certification as a Certified Case Manager must:

- Possess a good moral character.
- Meet acceptable standards of practice.
- Accomplish specific educational requirements, including a postsecondary degree program in a field that promotes the psychosocial or vocational well-being of consumers.
- Provide a job description for each case management position held.
- Meet the continuum of care requirement.
- Hold a license that is based upon the applicant having taken an examination in the area of educational specialization.
- Ensure that the license grants the ability to practice without the supervision of another licensed professional.
- Perform the six essential activities of case management:
  1. Assessment
  2. Coordination
  3. Planning
  4. Monitoring
  5. Implementation
  6. Evaluation in multiple environments over a minimum of five of the six core components, which include process and relationships, health care management, community resources and support, service delivery, psychosocial intervention, and rehabilitation case management

Several other organizations also offer certification in specialty case management. A few of these include certification in disability management, healthcare quality, utilization management, managed care and case management administrator certification. Case management professionals who are interested in obtaining certification should carefully research the options available for certification and select the credentialing program that fits their work performed, education, and future career goals (CMSA, 2005).

CASE MANAGER SERVICES

Although case management programs differ in structure and design, case managers provide some services regardless of the program's location. There appears to be a consensus in the literature that there are six core functions or activities that delineate case management: assessment, coordination, planning, monitoring, implementation, and evaluation in multiple environments. The focus of each of these functions varies depending on the case management model (CMSA, 2005).

Case managers help clients and families who need care coordination across the health care continuum access necessary resources in a time-efficient manner (Bower, 1992). Examples of care coordination include assisting the client or family member with medical appointments, equipment acquisition, home meal delivery, home follow-up services (e.g., home health or public health nursing), appointment transportation, and medical insurance or Medicare form completion. The types of services differ depending on the location of the case management program, the population of clients, and the scope of case management services. Some case managers in managed care environments monitor whether the patient keeps medical appointments and follows the prescribed course of treatment.

The coordination of health care services for hospitalized patients begins at admission or shortly thereafter and continues after discharge for an unspecified time (Ethridge and Lamb, 1989; Lyon, 1991). Depending on the setting, community case management services continue for varying lengths of time. Some programs continue service coordination indefinitely for populations like the high-risk elderly or the chronically ill. Other programs move patients' case management status from active to inactive when the patient no longer requires services. However, these clients become active again if their condition changes. Case management services continue in the home health care setting until the client is discharged from the program. It is widely recognized that early intervention on the part of a case manager and appropriate referrals prevent costly complications and can result in better health outcomes (Thurkettle and Noji, 2003).

CASE MANAGER ROLES AND CHARACTERISTICS

The individual case manager's role will vary depending on the specific program's services. The literature includes little information about the role or characteristics of nurse case managers, and most studies and articles discuss patient outcomes and organizational program designs.

Conti's (1996) study of 59 nurse case managers reported that their most frequently used skills were business knowledge, efficiency and effectiveness skills integration, influential communication, and clinical knowledge. In a study of 413 case managers and staff nurses, Crabtree-Tonges (1998) found that nurse case managers thought that the need for higher levels of role autonomy and collaboration are essential. Novak (1998) evaluated the opinions of nurse case managers regarding their professional roles. She found that nurse case managers believed critical thinking and prioritizing are the highest rated personal attributes in their roles; the critical function of coordinating a multidisciplinary care plan was the second highest rated response.

Meisler and Midyette (1994) identified the following distinct roles of the nurse case manager: manager, clinician, consultant, educator, and researcher. The manager is responsible for evaluating and monitoring costs and resources. The clinician develops and manages the care plan for a patient or a population. The consultant works closely and collaboratively with a multidisciplinary team, patient, and family. The educator teaches the health care team and notifies the staff of any practice or program changes. The researcher performs continuing evaluation research and observation, and monitors and evaluates identified quality outcomes and costs.

Nurse case managers must be flexible. The health care environment experiences rapid change, and new regulations and reimbursement schedules frequently emerge. The health care provider must respond to these changes rapidly to remain competitive. It is an ideal job for the self-directed nurse who enjoys being involved in a larger health care team within the organization and in the larger community.

CASE IDENTIFICATION

Identification of case management clients occurs in many ways, and each program should determine the criteria for eligibility for case management services. These criteria depend on the services provided, the service's location, the population served, and whether the service is in an acute care or community setting. Some programs are diagnosis based and use many community health care resources; for example, clients with chronic obstructive pulmonary disease often require numerous hospitalizations. Programs may focus on a particular population (e.g., the elderly) and establish criteria to identify which clients to target for services (e.g., the high-risk elderly who are chronically ill or frail and would benefit from case management services).

All clients referred for case management must undergo screening to determine their appropriateness for inclusion in the program. Not all referred clients need the services of a nurse case manager. Often, a nurse can arrange community services or instruct the client and family in the most appropriate follow-up based on client need and program design. The screening instrument must be comprehensive enough to determine which clients meet the program's criteria and user friendly enough to allow the screener to evaluate the clients rapidly to determine their appropriateness for the program. The screener should refer clients to more suitable services within the community if they are not appropriate candidates for a particular case management program. For example, a nurse may refer an HIV-positive client to a case management program for high-risk clients in the community, but the program may not accept HIV and AIDS clients because the community already has a program for HIV-positive clients.

Instead, the nurse should refer the client to a case management program that focuses exclusively on comprehensive service coordination for HIV and AIDS clients.

THE REFERRAL PROCESS

The nurse may perform program referrals in a variety of ways. In the acute care hospital setting, referrals are usually based on patient diagnosis or other criteria that trigger a nurse case manager referral (e.g., patient rehospitalization). Internal mechanisms alert the case manager of the patient's admission (e.g., a computerized list).

In community settings, referrals originate from a variety of sources such as a client's family, a primary care provider, or a hospital case manager. These referrals may be written or verbal. Staff in community agencies can also make service referrals; for example, the American Heart Association or American Cancer Society may receive calls from clients and families requesting information and assistance.

CASE MANAGEMENT MODELS

The literature has reported a variety of case management models. These models may be hospital based or community based, and some provide client services across the health care continuum. Further, case management models are designed for a variety of populations.

Hospital-Based Case Management

The acute care setting uses the following essential models of case management: the New England model, the discharge planner and arbitrator model, and the geriatric specialist model. In these models, the case manager provides patient services during hospitalization and performs short-term or limited intervention after discharge.

New England Model

The New England model of case management is a primary nursing care delivery system operated within the hospital (Bower, 1992; Zander, 1988, 1990). In this client-centered model, a registered nurse (RN) provides primary nursing care to one patient group and case management to another patient group. The nurse may or may not provide primary nursing care to the case management group. In the case management role, the nurse is responsible for clinical nursing care and the financial outcome of each managed care patient. The nurse measures the financial outcome through critical paths and aims to discharge each patient within the allotted number of hospital days under the PPS (Bower, 1992; Zander, 1988, 1990).

The New England model resembles a modified primary nursing model with additional managed care responsibilities more closely than case management because the primary nurse provides direct patient care and financial managed care responsibilities. An essential part of the nurse's responsibilities includes use of critical paths to determine the patient's progress and monitor consumed resources (a utilization review or managed care function). The nurse performs a limited telephone follow-up after discharge and may make a single home visit. Using staff nurses for patient follow-up after discharge can create problems. Administration must find replacements for staff nurses in the acute-care setting when staff performs phone calls or home visits. They must also consider the education and experience level of the staff nurse acting in the community health nursing role.

Discharge Planner and Arbitrator Case Management Model

In this model, the RN patient care provider is the discharge planner and the manager of utilization review strategies and quality assurance activities. A multidisciplinary utilization review team also maximizes resource use and discharge planning services. The program's quality assurance component incorporates an evaluation process of patient outcomes that results from the community service discharge referrals from all discharge planning sources (Bair, Griswold, and Head, 1989).

Geriatric Clinical Nurse Specialist Model

The case managers in this model are master's-prepared geriatric clinical nurse specialists who augment the staff nurses' basic care. The case managers use a comprehensive discharge planning protocol for hospitalized elderly patients, whom the staff nurses follow (Naylor, 1990; Neidlinger, Scroggins, and Kennedy, 1987). This protocol includes a comprehensive patient assessment and a comprehensive discharge plan for post hospital care. The protocol may include assessment of the patient's health status, orientation level, skill level, motivation level, sociodemographic data, health status knowledge, and perception levels. The discharge plan is based on patient assessment. Case managers often monitor patients on a short-term basis through telephone or home visits for at least 2 weeks following discharge.

Private Pay Case Management

Private pay case management is another type of service offered in many communities. In this program, a nurse case manager or SW offers case management services on a contract basis or in conjunction with an existing program. If the client does not meet the criteria for an existing case management program or if an existing program's services expire before the client is satisfied, the client or family must pay for the case manager's services. Families who need service coordination assistance often request this service. The length of time the case manager provides these services depends on the client's needs.

Pharmacy Model of Case Management

Pharmacy case management has a focus on medication management for clients with chronic illness who take multiple medications (Huber, 2002). The goal of pharmacy case management is to manage the client's polypharmacy to ensure the correct medications are taken by clients in the correct doses and frequency.

Case Management Models Across the Health Care Continuum

Some models provide patient discharge services from the acute hospital setting and continue with long-term case management services in the community setting after discharge. The Arizona model is one example of this case management model.

Arizona Model

In this case management model, nurse administrators, educators, researchers, and clinicians are case managers. They are responsible for patients during hospitalization and refer patients to appropriate community services following discharge (Ethridge, 1991; Ethridge and Johnson, 1996; Ethridge and Lamb, 1989). For several months or years, nurse case managers may work with chronically ill individuals who have frequent exacerbations or are entering terminal phases of their disease (Bower, 1992).

Community Case Management Models

Some case managers provide services exclusively in the community setting after discharge. Proponents argue that discharge planning and case management should be two separate and distinct functions with separate staff, procedures, and accountability. Supporters of this model believe case management's purpose is much broader than discharge planning and includes alternative planning to institutionalization, which ensures cost-effective care, access to comprehensive care, coordinating services, and improved client functional capacity (Simmons and White, 1988). The Denver model and the Indianapolis model are two exclusively community-based case management models.

CLINICAL EXAMPLE: DENVER CASE MANAGEMENT MODEL

In 1989, the Denver Regional Council of Governments evaluated counselor-facilitated hospital discharges in five metro-area Colorado hospitals. The sample included 1040 people aged 75 or older and continued for eight weeks after discharge. The counselor intervention system resulted in fewer deaths, a 21% decrease in the number of discharged individuals in nursing homes, and an increase in those released into their homes rather than institutions. The research supported the trend toward case management services and services in the home for high risk, high-cost cases in particular (Denver Regional Council of Governments, 1989). ■

CLINICAL EXAMPLE: INDIANAPOLIS CASE MANAGEMENT MODEL

In 1985, a randomized control study stratified 1001 newly discharged patients by varying admission risk (low, medium, or high) and assigned them to intervention or control groups (Weinberger et al., 1988). Nurses in the outpatient setting closely monitored patients in the intervention, distributed appointment reminders, and rescheduled missed appointments. High-risk patients in the intervention group had higher outpatient costs ($131 per month compared with $107) and lower inpatient costs ($535 per month compared with $800). Shorter, less intensive hospital stays contributed to the high-risk intervention group's reduced inpatient

costs. The Arizona model of case management produced similar results (Ethridge and Lamb, 1989). ■

APPLICATION OF CASE MANAGEMENT IN COMMUNITY HEALTH

Case management can be used in all community health settings, with interventions at the primary, secondary and tertiary levels of prevention, based on the community program and population served. Nurses working as case managers in the community setting will have diverse roles and responsibilities.

Public Health Clinic Settings

Depending on the services provided in the public health setting, the nurse has an opportunity to provide education, screening and referrals as needed to the clients served. Examples of primary prevention can include an ante partum clinic, where the nurse interacts with women and can teach about pregnancy, diet, and exercise during pregnancy.

Working with parents in pediatric settings, the nurse case manager can teach nutrition, growth and development and provide anticipatory guidance (primary level of prevention). The nurse can also screen children for growth and development and make referrals as needed to the Women, Infants, and Children (WIC) program, and other specialty programs available in the area for the clients' needs (secondary prevention).

Nurses can also serve as case manager working with elderly, providing nutrition education (primary prevention), screening for hypertension (secondary prevention), and even assistance with medication management and care of chronic diseases (tertiary prevention). The opportunities for community health nurses to provide case management services are vast, depending upon the location, populations served, and resources available in the community.

Occupational Health Settings

More employers are providing health screening and education to their employees to keep their work force healthy. Community health nurses who work occupational health settings are in a position to provide primary prevention in health education classes designed for the needs of the employees. These classes can be designed based on the health status of workers, to prevent the types of injuries that they are prone. The nurse in this setting can also provide primary prevention by offering flu shots and other immunizations to keep the employees healthy.

Secondary prevention can be provided to employees through screening clinics for hypertension, and other potential chronic illnesses or health problems that the employees may be more susceptible due to the nature of work performed. Referrals can be made as needed for follow-up with these employees. The occupational health nurse would continue to follow these employees and case manage any health issues that could impact the employees ability to perform the duties of the job.

Case management for tertiary prevention can include keeping in touch with injured employees, monitoring their recovery, therapy, or other services that are provided to the employee in the process of returning to health and their jobs. The occupational health nurse who provides case management services to these employees offers them education, referrals as needed, and assistance in their recovery process.

High-Risk Clinic Settings

There are many examples of health care settings that provide services to high-risk clients in which the nurse serves as case manager. A few examples include HIV clinics, settings that provide health care services to high risk perinatal clients, clients who have received transplants, dialysis settings, oncology clinics and infusion centers. The case management services offered by the nurse are determined by the specific needs of the clients seen in these settings. The models of case management are also developed for the needs of the clients.

Clients With Chronic Diseases

The community health nurse who interacts with clients with chronic diseases can be instrumental in monitoring the client in the community, monitoring medication management, assessing clients to identify problems early and intervene with the physician to modify therapy (Box 8-2). With patients with chronic obstructive pulmonary disease (COPD), hypertension, or congestive heart failure, early intervention on the part of the nurse can decrease the need for hospitalization and if hospitalized, ensure early hospitalization with a shorter length of stay.

Home Health and Hospice Settings

The community health nurse working in home health or hospice services are often assigned a case load of clients for whom they provide case management services. In both of these settings, the nurse case manager provides primary, secondary and tertiary prevention to clients. These services are designed base on the individual needs of clients and their families. Coordination of care, referrals, assessment, medication management, patient and family education, and the development of plans of care are just a few of the nursing functions that are provided through a case management model.

RESEARCH IN CASE MANAGEMENT

Results of case management research are scarce in the literature; the documented studies describe the implemented programs and evaluate the program outcomes. An example is given in the Research Highlights box.

Case management programs in all settings require further study. Terms used in case management programs should be defined for comparison across clinical sites. Programs with similar organizational structures and services can then be compared across settings. Critical to the success of case management programs is the inclusion of costs and cost

RESEARCH HIGHLIGHTS

Case Management: A Randomized Clinical Control Trial

Lyon et al. (1995) conducted a randomized clinical control trial in a multidisciplinary case management program of HMO clients. The study consisted of 156 adults who were aged 65 and older, lived at home with limited social support, and had multidimensional problems. The program provided comprehensive geriatric assessment and care coordination services to eligible adults enrolled in the HMO. Hospital discharge planners, outpatient clinic staff, home health nurses, and family members provided referrals for the program. After the case manager received the referral, he or she randomly assigned the client to either the control group for regular HMO services, or to one of two treatment groups. Group 1 received a detailed assessment and health care plan and Group 2 received a detailed assessment and continuing case management services. Clients enrolled in Group 2, the case management group, had fewer HMO and non-HMO hospital admissions and shorter stays compared with Group 1, the control group. The differences in the number of admissions to long-term care facilities or mortality among the two treatment groups were insignificant. A detailed cost analysis showed that Group 2, the case management group, had a 1-year savings to the HMO of $187,504.

Lyon JC et al: *Case management for high risk elderly.* Paper presented at the 123rd annual meeting of the American Public Health Association, San Diego, 1995.

BOX 8-2 Case Management Goals: Chronic Diseases and Conditions

Case management services to improve the health of clients with:
➤ Chronic mental illness
➤ Chronic physical illness
  1. Heart disease
  2. Stroke
  3. HIV
➤ Diabetes
➤ Disabilities

savings. The researcher or case manager must report the program's description, and the case manager's role and professional background. Well-defined patient and program outcomes are essential to the evaluation of case management programs. With the implementation of well designed research with measurable outcomes, management in health care settings across the continuum of care can identify the most cost-effective programs for specific populations served.

SUMMARY

Case management programs will continue to emerge in all health care settings. These programs will change as the needs of the population change. A common need among all programs is to collect data on the efficacy of programs, measuring client and program outcomes to ensure that the services that are offered are meeting targeted goals.

Staff who work as case managers should consider obtaining certification to develop common knowledge and skills among case management providers and better validate the services provided.

CASE STUDY   Application of the Nursing Process

The following case study is an example of a comprehensive case management program. Case management programs and the served populations are diverse; this is only one example of case management implementation.

Judy, the case manager at an HIV early intervention program, received a call from Don, a white male aged 29. Don had just moved from a neighboring state, where he recently discovered he was HIV-positive. A clinic administered his HIV test, and he did not receive any health services. He found the HIV clinic's phone number in the phone book and did not have a local health care provider. He was a construction worker before he moved, but the company laid him off. He moved to Reno to find work because new building and growth abounded in the area. He moved into a local motel and paid rent for the following 2 weeks. He did not have health insurance, but he was eligible for continued health insurance coverage through the Consolidated Omnibus Budget Reconciliation Act (COBRA). Unfortunately, he could not afford to pay the COBRA premium because he was unemployed. He felt desperate, alone, isolated, and depressed, and he needed help.

Judy performed an intake screening and assisted Don in receiving needed services. She scheduled appointments with the clinic's health care providers and met with him to identify the services he needed. Judy completed her assessment after Don attended the clinical appointment and met with her for case management.

ASSESSMENT

Don was HIV-positive, but he did not have any symptoms of AIDS. He took medication, ate well, maintained good physical condition and dentition, and owned a car. Although he had limited finances, he paid his rent for 2 weeks. He did not have health insurance and could not afford medications or laboratory tests. Judy developed the following plan:

Individual

Judy used Ryan White grant funds to finance Don's services through the clinic. She applied for housing assistance and scheduled an appointment with the clinic's SW to discuss his financial situation and job prospects. The pharmacist provided his medications, which were funded by the clinic, explained the drugs in detail, and offered to answer questions.

Family

Don was estranged from his family. His mother, who lived 2000 miles away, was aged 65, widowed, and retired. Don had not visited his two siblings in 10 years and chose not to have family contact. Although Don had friends at his last job, he had not made friends in Reno. Before moving, he was in a relationship with a woman for 2 years. After the relationship ended, he did not know where she lived.

Community

Judy knew Don could access a solid network of community services. Don was new in the community and he did not have social support; therefore Judy identified that he needed to contact job placement services and attend an HIV support group.

DIAGNOSIS

Judy developed the following nursing diagnoses for Don:

Individual

- Knowledge deficit related to HIV, including knowledge of the disease, medications, and available resources
- Inadequate income from unemployment

Family

- Lack of family and social support
- Poor family communication patterns

Community

- Adequate services through the HIV clinic
- Coordination of services through case management

PLANNING

Judy made the following plan, which is open for modification, and established goals with Don.

Individual

Short-Term Goals
- Don will find employment within 2 months. If his employer does not provide health care benefits, the clinic program will continue to provide them.
- If Don does not find work and cannot pay rent, local HIV funding will be used to provide housing assistance.

Long-Term Goal
- The clinic will provide health care services, medications, laboratory tests, and other outpatient services.

Family

Short-Term Goal
- Don was not interested in communicating with his family. Judy respected his wishes and did not pursue the issue in the short term.

Long-Term Goal
- Judy will ask Don again if he is interested in having contact with his family. Judy will offer Don the opportunity of family counseling to explore his feelings regarding his family and allow Don to determine if he wants to communicate with any of his family members.

Continued

CASE STUDY · Application of the Nursing Process (cont'd)

Community

Short-Term Goal
• Judy will collect information on available community resources to share with Don.

Long-Term Goal
• Judy will evaluate Don's involvement in using community resources. As needed, Judy will offer Don more options of resources that are available that are appropriate.

INTERVENTION

Individual

Acting as his case manager, Judy connected Don with job opportunities, housing, and community support groups. Judy explained the available programs and allowed Don to choose his services.

Don had to attend his scheduled clinic appointments, take his medication, and contact his case manager regularly.

Family

Judy knows that Don is estranged from his family. As appropriate, Judy will continue to approach Don about exploring his feelings about his family with a professional counselor. If Don is interested in making contact with any of his family members, Judy will assist in the coordination of this process.

Community

The plan supplemented the services that Don could not afford. The plan focused on Don's individual needs in health care, employment, housing, and support groups. Judy will provide Don with available services in the Community. As new programs become available, Judy will contact Don to explain the services, and make referrals to services that both she and Don feel are appropriate.

EVALUATION

Individual

Judy evaluated the results of Don's comprehensive case management plan on a continuing basis. If Don obtained employment in construction, he could support himself adequately and would require financial assistance primarily with his medications. If he did not find a job, or if his health status changed and he was unable to work in construction, then Judy would need to modify the plan.

Family

Judy evaluates Don's interest in getting in touch with his family. She will assist him in getting referred for family therapy. When and if Don wishes to contact any of his family, Judy will assist him in making arrangements.

Community

Judy will need to connect Don with community support groups to establish friendships and gain social support.

LEARNING ACTIVITIES

1. Contact case management programs in the community and acute care setting.
2. Interview case management program directors. Ask them about their program's structure and process, the program's acceptance criteria, and their referral sources.
3. Ask the directors what data they collect on their clients and what is reported to their administration.
4. Ask the directors about their program's required education and experience levels for case managers.
5. Spend a day with a case manager and ask about their various roles and services.
6. Participate in a client/family interview.

REFERENCES

American Nurses Association: *Case management by nurses,* Washington, DC, 1992, The Association.

Bair NL, Griswold JT, Head JL: Clinical RN involvement in bedside-centered case management, *Nurs Econ* 7(3):150-154, 1989.

Bower KA: *Case management by nurses,* Washington, DC, 1992, American Nurses Publishing.

Calhoun, J, Casey P: Redesigning case management in managed care: an eclectic approach—from city to ranch, *Lippincotts Case Manage* 7(5):180-188, 2002.

Case Management Society of America: *Standards of practice for case management,* Little Rock, Ark, 1995, The Author.

Case Management Society of America: *Philosophy of case management,* 2005, The Author, http://www.cmsa.org/ABOUTUS/Definitionof CaseManagement/tabid/104/Default.aspx.

Conger MM: Nursing case management: a managed care organizational strategy. In Conger MM, editor: *Managed care: practice strategies for nursing,* Thousand Oaks, Calif, 1999, Sage Publications.

Conti RM: Nurse case manager roles: implications for practice and education, *Nurs Adm Q* 21(1):67-80, 1996.

Crabtree-Tonges M: Job design for nurse case managers intended and unintended effects on satisfaction and wellbeing, *Nurs Case Manage* 3:11-23, 1998.

Crosby RL: Community care of the chronically mentally ill, *J Psychosoc Nurs* 25(1):33-37, 1987.

Denver Regional Council of Governments: *DRCOG study may trigger new national policy,* Denver, 1989, The Author.

Ethridge PA: Nursing HMO: Carondelet St. Mary's experience, *Nurs Manage* 22(7):22-27, 1991.

Ethridge PA, Johnson S: The influence of reimbursement on nurse case management practice: Carondelet's experience. In Cohen EL, editor: *Nurse case management in the 21st century,* St. Louis, 1996, Mosby.

Ethridge PA, Lamb GS: Professional nursing case management improves quality, access, and costs, *Nurs Manage* 20(3):30-35, 1989.

Grau L: Case management and the nurse, *Geriatr Nurs* 5(8):372-375, 1984.

Huber, DL: The diversity of case management models, *Lippincotts Case Manage* 7(6):212-220, 2002.

Lyon JC: *Descriptive study of models of discharge planning and case management in California,* doctoral dissertation, Ann Arbor, Mich, 1991, University of California, San Francisco, University Microfilms International.

Lyon JC: Models of nursing care delivery and case management: clarification of terms, *Nurs Econ* 11(3):163-169, 1993.

Lyon JC et al: *Case management for high risk elderly,* Paper presented at the 123rd annual meeting of the American Public Health Association, San Diego, 1995.

Mahn VA, Spross JA: Nursing case management as an advanced practice role. In Hamric AB, Spross JA, Hanson CM, editors: *Advanced nursing practice: an integrative approach,* Philadelphia, 1996, Saunders.

Meisler N, Midyette P: CNS to case manager: broadening the scope, *Nurs Manage* 25(11):44-46, 1994.

Naylor MD: Comprehensive discharge planning for hospitalized elderly: a pilot study, *Nurs Res* 39(3):156-161, 1990.

Neidlinger SH, Scroggins K, Kennedy LM: Cost evaluation of discharge planning for hospitalized elderly, *Nurs Econ* 5(5):225-230, 1987.

Novak DA: Nurse case managers' opinions of their role, *Nurs Case Manag* 3(6):231-237, 1998.

Pittman DC: Nursing case management: holistic care for the deinstitutionalized mentally ill, *J Psychosoc Nurs* 27(11):23-27, 1989.

Simmons WJ, White M: Case management and discharge planning: two different worlds. In Volland P, editor: *Discharge planning: an interdisciplinary approach to continuity of care,* Owings Mills, Md, 1988, National Health Publication.

Steinberg RM, Carter GW: *Case management and the elderly,* Lexington, Mass, 1983, Lexington Books, DC Health.

Thurkettle, MA, Noji, A: Shifting the healthcare paradigm: The case manager's opportunity and responsibility, *Lippincotts Case Manag,* 8(4):160-165, 2003.

US Department of Commerce/International Trade Administration: *Health and medical services: US industrial outlook,* US Document, Washington, DC, 1990, The Author.

Weil M, Karls J: *Case management in human service practice,* San Francisco, 1985, Jossey-Bass.

Weinberger M et al: The cost-effectiveness of intensive post discharge care: a randomized trial, *Med Care* 26(11):1092-1101, 1988.

Zander KS: Managed care and nursing case management. In Mayer GG, Madden MJ, Lawrenz E, editors: *Patient care delivery models,* Gaithersburg, Md, 1990, Aspen.

Zander KS: Nursing case management: strategic management of cost and quality outcomes, *J Nurs Admin* 18(5):23-30, 1988.

UNIT 3

Factors That Influence the Health of the Community

The Health Care System

Anita W. Finkelman

MEDIA RESOURCES

Additional Material for Study, Review, and Further Exploration

evolve Web Site at http://evolve.elsevier.com/Nies

❖ Quiz ❖ Case Studies ❖ Content Updates ❖ Glossary ❖ WebLinks ❖ Resource Tools

9A The President's Advisory Commission on Consumer Protection and Quality in the Health Care Industry: Recommendations

OBJECTIVES

Upon completion of this chapter, the reader will be able to do the following:

1. Analyze landmark health care legislation and its influence on the delivery system.
2. Describe the organization of the public health care subsystem at the federal, state, and local levels.
3. Compare and contrast the scope of the private health care subsystem and the public health care subsystem.
4. Describe the roles of the members of the health care team.
5. Discuss the relationship of critical health care issues to the health care organization and health care providers.
6. Discuss future concerns for the health care delivery system.

KEY TERMS

accreditation
alternative therapies
client rights
downsizing
health care reform

managed care
managed care organizations
 (MCOs)
Medicaid
Medicare

outcomes measures
provider organizations
public health
quality care
redesigning

reengineering
reregulating
rightsizing
telehealth

CHAPTER OUTLINE

MAJOR LEGISLATIVE ACTIONS AND THE HEALTH CARE SYSTEM
  Federal Legislation
  State Legislative Role
  Legislation Influencing Managed Care

COMPONENTS OF THE HEALTH CARE SYSTEM
  Private Health Care Subsystem
  Public Health Subsystem
  Federal Level Subsystem
  State Level Subsystem
  Local Health Department Subsystems
  Health Care Providers

CRITICAL ISSUES IN HEALTH CARE DELIVERY
  Managed Care
  Quality Care
  Fraud and Abuse
  Information Technology
  Consumerism, Advocacy, and Client Rights
  Coordination and Access to Health Care
  Disparity in Health Care Delivery
  Health Care Reform: The Clinton Health Reform Initiative

FUTURE OF PUBLIC HEALTH AND HEALTH CARE SYSTEM

The health care system of the United States is dynamic, multifaceted, and not comparable with any other health care system in the world. It is regularly praised for its technological breakthroughs, frequently criticized for its high costs, and often difficult to access by those most in need. This chapter describes landmark health care legislation, the components of the health care system, critical health care organization and provider issues, the role of government in public health, and health care reform and presents a futuristic perspective.

MAJOR LEGISLATIVE ACTIONS AND THE HEALTH CARE SYSTEM

An examination of the major legislative actions that federal and state governments have taken and recognition of their influence on health and health care delivery are critical to understand the evolution of the health care system in the United States. Throughout the twentieth century, the United States Congress enacted bills that had a major influence on the private and public health care subsystems. Legislation pertaining to health increased in scope in each decade of the twentieth century, with the goal of improving the health of populations and coping with changing health care needs. During the last two decades, concerns about an increase in health care costs and the growth of managed care stimulated even more legislation.

Federal Legislation

The following discussion describes some of the landmark federal laws that have influenced health services and health care professionals. These are summarized in Table 9-1.

- *Pure Food and Drugs Act of 1906:* This Act established a program to supervise and control the manufacture, labeling, and sale of food. Subsequent legislation included meat and dairy products, pharmaceuticals, cosmetics, toys, and household products. Since 1927, the Food and Drug Administration (FDA) has administered elements of this Act.
- *Children's Bureau Act of 1912:* The Children's Bureau was founded to protect children from the unhealthy child labor practices of the time and to enact programs that had a positive effect on children's health. In 1921, the Sheppard-Towner Act extended children's health care programs by providing funds for the health and welfare of infants.
- *Social Security Act of 1935 and its amendments (1965, 1972):* The Social Security Act and its subsequent amendments have had a far-reaching effect on health care for many groups. The Social Security Administration (SSA) provides welfare for high-risk mothers and children. Benefits were later expanded to include health care provisions for older adults and the handicapped. This major governmental action was the enactment of legislation for Medicare and Medicaid.
- *Medicare, Title XVIII Social Security Amendment (1965):* This federal program, administered by the Centers for Medicare and Medical Services (formerly Health Care

TABLE 9-1   Critical Federal Legislation Related to Health Care

DATE	LEGISLATION
1906	Pure Food and Drugs Act
1912	Children's Bureau Act
1921	Shepard-Towner Act
1935	Social Security Act
1944	Public Health Act
1945	McCarren-Ferguson Act
1946	Hill-Burton Act
1953	Department of Health, Education, and Welfare as a cabinet-status agency; in 1979 divided into US Department of Education and USDHHS
1956	Health Amendments Act
1964	Nurse Training Act
1965	Social Security Act amendments: Title XVIII Medicare; Title XIX Medicaid
1970	Occupational Safety and Health Act
1972	Social Security Act amendments: Professional Standards Review Organization; further benefits under Medicare and Medicaid, including dialysis
1973	Health Maintenance Act
1974	National Health Planning Resources Act
1981, 1987, 1989, 1990	Omnibus Budget Reconciliation Acts
1982	Tax Equity and Fiscal Responsibility Act
1985	Consolidated Omnibus Budget Reconciliation Act
1988	Family Support Act
1990	Health Objectives Planning Act
1996	Health Insurance Portability and Accountability Act
1996	Welfare Act
2003	Medicare Reinvestment Act
2004	Nurse Reinvestment Act

Financing Administration [HCFA]), pays specified health care services for all people 65 years of age and older who are eligible to receive Social Security benefits. People with permanent disabilities and those with end-stage renal disease are also covered. The objective of Medicare is to protect older adults and the disabled against large medical outlays. The program is funded through a payroll tax of most working citizens. Private funds in the form of payroll taxes go to the federal government. Individuals or providers may submit payment requests for health care services and are paid according to Medicare regulations. See Chapter 10 for more information on Medicare.

- *Medicaid, Title XIX Social Security Amendment (1965):* This combined federal and state program provides access to care for the poor and medically needy of all ages. Each state is allocated federal dollars on a matching basis (i.e., 50% of costs are paid with federal dollars). Each state has the responsibility and right to determine services to be provided and the dollar amount allocated to the program. Basic services (i.e., ambulatory and inpatient hospital care, physical therapy, laboratory, radiography, skilled nursing, and home health care) are required to be eligible for matching federal dollars. States may choose from a wide range of optional services including drugs, eyeglasses, intermediate care, inpatient psychiatric care, and dental care. Limits are placed on the amount and duration of

TABLE 9-2 2006 Health and Human Services Poverty Guidelines

SIZE OF FAMILY UNIT	48 CONTIGUOUS STATES AND DC	ALASKA	HAWAII
1	$9,800	$12,250	$11,270
2	13,200	16,500	15,180
3	16,600	20,750	19,090
4	20,000	25,000	23,000
5	23,400	29,250	26,910
6	26,800	33,500	30,820
7	30,200	37,750	34,730
8	33,600	42,000	38,640
For each additional person, add	$2,820	$3,520	$3,240

From Annual update of the HHS poverty guidelines. *Federal Register* 7(15): 3848-3849, January 24, 2006.

service. Unlike Medicare, Medicaid provides long-term care services (e.g., nursing home and home health) and personal care services (e.g., chores and homemaking). In addition, Medicaid has eligibility criteria based on level of income. Table 9-2 provides the U.S. Department of Health and Human Services (USDHHS) poverty guidelines for 2006. Medicaid is also turning to managed care, but it is still unclear how successful this will be. The Medicaid population has complex needs, and managed care organizations may not be able to provide optimum services to these beneficiaries. See Chapter 10 for more information on Medicaid.

- *Public Health Act of 1944:* The Public Health Act consolidated all existing public health legislation into one law. Since then, many new pieces of legislation have become amendments. Examples of some of its provisions, either in the original law or in amendments, provided for or established the following:
  - Health services for migratory workers
  - Family planning services
  - Health research facilities
  - National Institutes of Health (NIH)
  - Nurse training acts
  - Traineeships for graduate students in public health
  - Home health services for people with Alzheimer's disease
  - Prevention and primary care services
  - Rural health clinics
  - Communicable disease control
- *McCarren-Ferguson Act of 1945:* The McCarren-Ferguson Act has had a major influence on the insurance industry by giving states the exclusive right to regulate health insurance plans (Knight, 1998). No federal government agency is solely responsible for monitoring insurance. Some federal agencies are involved in insurance reimbursement; however, the structure of the benefit program for federal employees and military personnel, Medicare, and Medicaid allows Congress to pass laws that can override state laws if the laws meet certain criteria.

- *Hill-Burton Act of 1946:* The Hill-Burton Act authorized federal assistance in the construction of hospitals and health centers with stipulations about services for the uninsured. As a result, hospitals with obligations to care for the uninsured were built in towns and cities across the United States. Through these measures, hospital care became more accessible, but by the late 1990s, the high cost of health care, combined with decreasing lengths of stay and increasing use of primary care, forced the closure of many of the hospitals built with Hill-Burton funds.
- *Health Amendments Act of 1956:* The Health Amendments Act, Title II, authorizes funds to aid registered nurses (RNs) in full-time study of administration, supervision, or teaching. In 1963, the Surgeon General's Consultant Group on Nursing noted that there were still too few nursing schools, nursing personnel were not put to good use, and there was limited nursing research. As a result, in 1964, the Nurse Training Act provided funds for loans and scholarships for full-time study for nurses and funds for construction of nursing schools.
- *Occupational Safety and Health Act of 1970:* The Occupational Safety and Health Act focuses on the health needs and risks in the workplace and environment. It continues to provide critical programs important to the workplace and the community. See Chapter 28 for more information on both the Occupational Safety and Health Act and the Occupational Safety and Health Administration.
- *Health Maintenance Organization Act of 1973:* The HMO Act provides grants for HMO development. The Act requires that employers offer federally qualified HMOs as a health care coverage option to employees and established that states were responsible for the oversight of HMOs. Although initially it was not successful in stimulating HMO growth, this legislation has had a long-term effect on the growth of managed care.
- *National Health Planning and Resources Act of 1974:* The National Health Planning and Resources Act assigned health planning responsibility to the states and local health systems agencies. In addition, it requires health care facilities to obtain prior approval from the state for expansion in the form of a certificate of need (CON).
- *Omnibus Budget Reconciliation Acts (1981, 1987, 1989, and 1990):* The Omnibus Budget Reconciliation Acts were each enacted in response to the huge federal deficit. They have influenced funding for nursing homes, home health agencies, and hospitals and set up guidelines and regulations about several issues, including a move from process to outcome evaluation, use of restraints, and prescription drugs for Medicaid recipients.
- *Tax Equity and Fiscal Responsibility Act of 1982:* The Tax Equity and Fiscal Responsibility Act was a major amendment to the Social Security Act of 1935, establishing the prospective payment system (PPS) for Medicare, the diagnosis-related group (DRG) system. This law changed health care radically by introducing a new reimbursement method. See Chapter 10 for more information on DRGs.

- *Consolidated Omnibus Budget Reconciliation Act of 1985:* COBRA is a federal law that affects health care delivery and reimbursement. It requires all hospitals with emergency services that participate in Medicare to treat any client in their emergency services, whether or not that client is covered by Medicare or has the ability to pay. This legislation includes requirements for Medicaid services for prenatal and postnatal care to low-income women in two-parent families in which the primary spouse is unemployed. Another important requirement of COBRA focuses on the problem of the loss of insurance when a person loses his or her job. Employers who terminate an employee must now continue benefits for the employee and dependents for a specified period of time if the employee had health benefits before the termination. COBRA is an example of how a federal law can affect state health care practices. The federal government must determine who receives federal Medicare funds; therefore COBRA provides the opportunity for the federal government to legislate health care delivery at the state level.

- *Family Support Act of 1988:* The Family Support Act expanded coverage for poor women and children and required states to extend Medicaid coverage for 12 months to families who have increased earnings but are no longer receiving cash assistance. This Act also required states to expand Aid to Families with Dependent Children (AFDC) coverage to two-parent families when the principal wage earner is unemployed.

- *Health Objectives Planning Act of 1990:* The Health Objectives Planning Act was initiated in response to the 1979 report *Healthy People. The Surgeon General's Report on Health Promotion and Disease Prevention.* After that report, the federal government began to take a directive approach in identifying and monitoring national health care goals. *Healthy People 2000* and *Healthy People 2010* are also results of the Health Objectives Planning Act.

- *Health Insurance Portability and Accountability Act of 1996:* The Health Insurance Portability and Accountability Act (HIPAA) addressed several insurance issues. Critical issues were the portability of coverage and preexisting conditions. This law established that insurers cannot set limits on coverage of longer than 12 months. This is a complex law, but it is important for consumers with preexisting conditions.

- *Welfare Reform Act of 1996:* The Welfare Reform Act placed restrictions on eligibility for AFDC, Medicaid, and other federally funded welfare programs. This law decreased the number of people on welfare and forced many individuals to take low-paying jobs, many of which do not offer health insurance. Between 1994 and March 1999, welfare roles dropped 47% (DeParle, 1999). Many individuals, particularly underserved women and children, subsequently lost Medicaid coverage.

- *Medicare Modernization Act of 2003:* The Medicare Modernization Act is the most significant law in 40 years for senior health care, though there is disagreement as to whether or not it will positively address serious concerns about prescription coverage for seniors. The law provides seniors and people living with disabilities with some prescription drug benefit coverage and more choice and better benefits. Medicare prescription drug coverage was added to benefits effective January 1, 2006.

- *Nurse Reinvestment Act of 2003:* The Nurse Reinvestment Act is significant because it is a response to the critical nursing shortage that is present across the country. Funding is provided to increase enrollments and number of practicing nurses.

The thrust of federal legislation has been on either prevention of illness through influencing the environment (e.g., Occupational Safety and Health Act of 1970) or provision of funding to support programs that influence health care (e.g., Social Security Act of 1935). Beginning with the Shepard-Towner Act of 1921 and continuing to the present, federal grants have increased the involvement of state and local governments in health care. The involvement of the federal government through fiscal allocations to state and local governments provided money for programs not previously available to state and local areas. Similar services became available in all states. Funds supporting these services were accompanied by regulations that applied to all recipients. Many state and local government programs were developed based on availability of federal funds. The involvement of the federal government through funding has served to standardize the public health policy in the United States (Pickett and Hanlon, 1990). With the rising number of uninsured and underinsured, universal coverage continues to be a critical concern that has not been solved, despite multiple bills proposed in the Congress between 2001 and 2003.

State Legislative Role

State governments are also directly involved in health care policy, legislation, and regulation. State governments focus particularly on financing and delivery of services and oversight of insurance. The latter has become important as managed care has grown. The states have major input in the following basic health care areas (Robert Wood Johnson Foundation, 1997):

- *Public health and safety:* States are responsible for protecting public welfare through such areas as prevention and treatment of communicable diseases, monitoring of environmental health conditions, prevention of harm from violence, and prevention of workplace accidents.

- *Provision of indigent care:* Most state constitutions require that the state, either alone or with local governments, provide health care to those who cannot pay for it. This is usually provided by facilities run by state or local governments.

- *Purchase care:* Many states have been changing from the role of provider of health care to purchaser of care. States must purchase care, or contract for care, for state employees and for Medicaid beneficiaries.

- *Regulation:* States are responsible for licensing and credentialing facilities and professionals to ensure safety and quality. They are also responsible for regulation of

FIGURE 9-1 U.S. health care system.

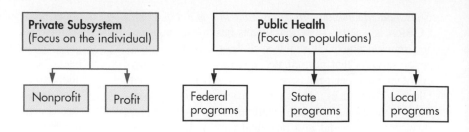

insurers. States use CONs to control health care costs, particularly those related to long-term care facilities and specialized technology. CONs require that the health care organization meet certain criteria to receive approval to build or expand physical facilities and to purchase expensive equipment (e.g., computed tomography and magnetic resonance imaging equipment).

- *Resource allocation:* Traditionally states have not been responsible for financial support of medical and nursing education, which has been primarily through federal funding. However, states are more involved in identifying need (e.g., number of health care professionals that the state needs to graduate to meet state health care needs). Some states still assist in funding some public health care facilities.

Legislation Influencing Managed Care

Much of the recent legislation (i.e., usually state level) influencing **managed care organizations** (MCOs) is in response to consumers' concerns about MCOs' efforts to control costs. Considerable variability exists across states in MCO legislation, and usually these acts are in response to consumer calls for reform (Levy, 2002). The following examples describe a growing number of legislative acts that provide more control over managed care:

- *Provider protection initiatives (PPIs):* The need for the removal of "gag rules" has been one area of concern for providers and clients. MCOs use gag rules to control what their providers discuss with clients about all treatment options. Additionally, many MCOs provide financial incentives to providers to control costs. These incentives are paid to providers based on their performance data (e.g., number of hospital admissions, length of stay, types of treatment, and types and number of prescriptions ordered).
- *Any willing provider initiatives:* Provider panels are the lists of providers that are approved by an MCO for reimbursement. These initiatives require that MCOs accept any provider on their provider panels who meets plan requirements and is willing to agree to the contract.
- *Direct access legislation:* Client freedom-of-choice legislation is rapidly growing as clients become more concerned about their lack of provider choice and want direct access to providers without obtaining prior approval.
- *Mandated benefits requirement:* This legislation mandates specific minimum health care benefits. Examples of these are the designation of specific basic services, emergency care without prior approval, coverage for experimental

treatments, mental health parity, diabetes management, prostate screening, chiropractic treatment, and hospice services.

- *Consumer rights:* Consumers are demanding more rights than just provider choice. Examples include coverage for specific benefits, such as emergency services without prior approval; longer lengths of stay (e.g., obstetric and mastectomy); detailed disclosure of benefits and plan procedures; provider choice; and impartial mechanism for grievances (Mariner, 1996). Efforts have been made to pass a national patients' rights bill, but this has not occurred even though many states passed this type of legislation by early 2006.

COMPONENTS OF THE HEALTH CARE SYSTEM

The current health care system consists of private and public health care subsystems (Figure 9-1). The private health care subsystem includes personal care services from various sources, both nonprofit and profit, and numerous voluntary agencies. The major focus of the public health subsystem is prevention of disease and illness. These subsystems are not always mutually exclusive, and their functions sometimes overlap.

With the rapid growth of technology and increased demands on the private and public health care subsystems, health care costs have become prohibitive. Cost-effectiveness and cost containment have become a critical driving force as health care delivery system changes are made, and cost-effectiveness often conflicts with the provision of quality care.

Community health nursing requires an understanding of the mission, organization, and role of the private and the public health care subsystems and the contexts within which they function to effectively collaborate with health care organizations to reach community health goals. An organizational framework in which private and voluntary organizations and the government work collaboratively to prevent disease and promote health is essential. Public health and community health nurses are in a unique position to provide leadership and facilitate change in the health care system.

Private Health Care Subsystem

Most personal health care services are provided in the private sector. Services in the private subsystem include health promotion, prevention and early detection of disease, diagnosis and treatment of disease with a focus on cure, rehabilitative-restorative care, and custodial care. These services are provided in clinics, physicians' offices, hospitals, hospital ambulatory centers, skilled care facilities, and homes. Increasingly, these private sector services are available through MCOs.

Private health care services in the United States began with a simple model. Physicians provided care in their offices and made home visits. Clients were admitted to hospitals for general care if they experienced serious complications during the course of their illness. Currently, a variety of highly skilled health care professionals provide comprehensive, preventive, restorative, rehabilitative, and palliative care. A broad array of services is available, which range from general to highly specialized with multidelivery configurations.

Personal care provided by physicians is delivered under the following five basic models:

1. The solo practice of a physician in an office continues to be present in some communities.
2. The single specialty group model consists of physicians in the same specialty, who pool expenses, income, and offices.
3. Multispecialty group practice provides for interaction across specialty areas.
4. The integrated health maintenance model has prepaid multispecialty physicians.
5. The community health center, developed through federal funds in the 1960s, addresses broader inputs into health such as education and housing.

Managed care has become the dominant paradigm in health care, affecting all aspects of health care delivery. Managed care involves capitated payments for care rather than fee-for-service. Health care providers, including physicians, hospitals, community clinics, and home care providers, are integrated in a system such as an HMO. See Chapter 10 for a more detailed discussion of managed care and reimbursement.

Voluntary Agencies

Voluntary or nonofficial agencies are a part of the private health care system of the United States and developed at the same time that the government was assuming responsibility for public health. In the United States during the 1700s and early 1800s, voluntary efforts to improve health were virtually nonexistent because early settlers from Western Europe were not accustomed to participating in organized charity. Immigration expanded to include slaves from Africa and people from Eastern Europe, and their well-being received little attention.

Toward the end of the nineteenth century, new immigrants brought a heritage of social protest and reform. Wealthy business people, such as the Rockefellers, Carnegies, and Mellons, responded to the needs and set up foundations that provided health and welfare money for charitable endeavors. District nurses, such as Lillian Wald, established nursing practices in the large cities for the poor and destitute. Services did not just focus on illness but also on work conditions, health, communicable diseases, living conditions, and language skills.

Voluntary agencies can be classified into the following categories (Hanlon and Pickett, 1990):

1. Specific diseases, such as the American Diabetes Association, American Cancer Society, and Multiple Sclerosis Society
2. Organ or body structures, such as the National Kidney Foundation or the American Heart Association
3. Health and welfare of special groups, such as the National Council on Aging
4. Particular phases of health, such as the Planned Parenthood Federation of America

Philanthropic groups also support research and programs. Many professional organizations, such as the American Medical Association and the American Nurses Association, have a significant role in advocacy and in providing professional expertise.

Voluntary organizations provide major sources of help in prevention of disease, promotion of health, treatment of illness, advocacy, consumer education, and research. For example, private and voluntary organizations currently support clients with acquired immunodeficiency syndrome (AIDS). In many cities, the Chicken Soup Brigade provides meals for clients with AIDS who are unable to cook for themselves, and AIDS support groups exist in most larger communities.

Overlap of services often occurs among the numerous private, voluntary, and public agencies. The private and public agencies provide a wide array of services, but sometimes duplication causes them not to be cost-effective. Without voluntary and official agencies, the array of services would be less than what is currently available.

The future is somewhat uncertain for voluntary agencies because major changes are occurring in health care. In the mid-1990s, the Pew Health Professions Commission projected that the emerging health care system would be an amalgam of different public and private forces that would work together to provide integrated, resource-conscious, population-based services (O'Neil and Pew Health Professions Commission, 1998). It was projected that the system would also be more innovative and diverse in how it responded to health needs and more concerned with disease prevention and promotion of health. The Pew Health Professions Commission's projection has not yet been fully realized.

Public Health Subsystem

The U.S. Constitution mandates that the federal government "promote the general welfare of its citizens." The public health subsystem is required by law to address the health of populations. Activities are covered by legal provisions at the local, state, and federal levels of government. At the federal level, Congress enacts laws and writes rules and regulations. The various departments of the executive branch implement and administer them. Interpretations of, and amendments to, the Constitution and Supreme Court decisions over time have changed and increased the role of the federal government in health activities.

Federal policies and practices have had an increasing influence on local and state governments in meeting health and social problems, and many laws have been enacted to respond to changing health needs. Coordination of federal services under several agencies culminated in the establishment of the Department of Health Education and Welfare under President Eisenhower in 1953. In 1979, this department was separated into the Department of Education and the USDHHS. The USDHHS is currently the second largest department of the federal government; only the Department of Defense is larger.

Public health refers to the efforts organized by society to protect, promote, and restore the people's health. Public health programs, services, and institutions emphasize the prevention of disease and address the health needs of the population as a whole. Public health activities typically respond to changing technology and social values, but the goals remain the same (i.e., to reduce the amount of disease, premature death, and disease-produced discomfort and disability).

The public health subsystem is concerned with the health of the population and a healthy environment. The scope of public health is broad and encompasses activities that promote good health. The public health subsystem is organized into multiple levels (i.e., federal, state, and local) to more effectively provide services to those who are unable to obtain health care without assistance and to establish laws, rules, and regulations to protect the public.

Federal Level Subsystem

Most health-related activities at the federal level are implemented and administered by the USDHHS. This department is directed by the Secretary of the USDHHS, numerous undersecretaries, and assistant secretaries. The Surgeon General is the principal deputy to the assistant secretary of the USDHHS. The USDHHS has 11 major agencies (Box 9-1).

Other federal agencies perform activities related to health. For example, the Department of Education is involved with health education and school health. The Department of Agriculture administers the inspection of meat and milk and provides funds for the Women, Infants, and Children program (supplemental nutrition), the food stamp program, and the school-based nutrition program.

Scope of Health Services of the Federal Level Subsystem

The federal government targets the following major health areas: the general population, special populations, and international health. For the general population, federal activities include protection against hazards, maintenance of vital and health statistics, advancement of scientific knowledge through research, and provision of disaster relief. In recent years, public health efforts have been directed toward changing behaviors by fostering healthy eating habits, exercise, and preventing tobacco, drug, and alcohol use. Other programs have provided nutritional food and food stamps to individuals and families to ensure adequate food intake.

Services for special populations include protection of workers against hazardous occupations and work conditions and health care for veterans, American Indians, Alaskan natives, federal prisoners, and members of the armed services. In addition, the federal government provides special services

---

BOX 9-1 Structure of the U.S. Department of Health and Human Services

The USDHHS is composed of several agencies that provide different services related to U.S. health care. Among them are:

➤ The **Administration on Aging** is the agency responsible for coordinating home and community based services for older persons and their caregivers.

➤ The **Centers for Medicare and Medicaid Services** administers those programs.

➤ The **Administration for Children and Families** provides family assistance (welfare), child support, Head Start and other programs to strengthen the family unit.

➤ The **Centers for Disease Control and Prevention (CDC)** conducts and supports programs directed to prevent and control infectious diseases; they assist states during epidemics. In addition, they provide services related to health promotion and education and professional development and training.

➤ The **Food and Drug Administration** provides surveillance over the safety and efficacy of foods, pharmaceuticals, and other consumer goods.

➤ The **Health Resources and Services Administration** is concerned with the development of health services programs and facilities. The Division of Nursing is in this unit. A major focus of this agency is funding grants for nursing education and training. The **Indian Health Service** is also in this unit, providing health services for Native Americans and Alaskan Natives.

➤ The **National Institutes of Health** perform and support research programs. The focus of their efforts is to develop and extend the scientific knowledge base related to their respective areas. The National Institute for Nursing Research is part of NIH, and it focuses on nursing research.

➤ The **Substance Abuse and Mental Health Services Administration** awards grants and funds research related to problems with substance abuse and mental health.

➤ The **Agency for Healthcare Quality and Research** works to improve quality, safety, efficiency and effectiveness of health care services for all Americans.

➤ The **Agency for Toxic Substances and Disease Registry** serves the public by using the best science, taking responsive public health actions, and providing trusted health information to prevent harmful exposures and diseases related to toxic substances.

---

for children, older adults, the mentally ill, and the vocationally handicapped.

In the international arena, the federal government works with other countries and international health organizations (e.g., the World Health Organization and the Red Cross) to promote various health programs throughout the world.

State Level Subsystem

States are responsible for the health of their citizens and are the central authorities in the public health care system. The organization and activities of public health services vary widely among the states. Most state agencies are directed by a health commissioner or secretary of health who is typically appointed by the governor. Each state also has a health officer, who is usually a physician with a degree and experience in public health. In some states, the health officer directs the health department. Many states have boards of health, which determine policies and priorities for allocation of funds. Staffing of the state agency varies among states; however, compared with other state programs, state health programs usually have a large staff.

The state level, however, does not stand alone. It is highly dependent on the federal level for resources and guidance. For example, funds that the federal government contributes to Medicaid, which is jointly funded by the federal government and states, have been reduced. This has had a major impact on services that states can provide to their most vulnerable citizens. Cooperation between the state and federal levels has also been brought to the forefront with efforts to plan for bioterrorism, an event that would necessitate cooperation and sharing. The United States requires an integrated system so that both federal and state levels work to the benefit of all citizens.

Scope of Health Services of the State Level Subsystem

Each state is responsible for its own public health laws; therefore state policy is widely varied. Factors that affect the level of state services include per capita income, political factors related to division of power between state and local health departments (LHDs), and competition among officials, providers, and the business community.

As discussed in Chapter 1, the three core functions of public health are assessment, policy development, and assurance (Institute of Medicine [IOM], 1988). Assessment activities include the collection of data pertaining to vital statistics, health facilities, and human resources; epidemiological activities, such as communicable disease control, health screening, and laboratory analyses; and participation in research projects. In the area of policy development, states formulate goals, develop health plans, and set standards for local health agencies. Assurance activities involve inspection in a variety of areas, licensing, health education, environmental safety, personal health services, and resource development.

Nurses represent the largest group of professionals providing health services. State legislatures determine licensure requirements and enact nurse practice acts. State boards of nursing are the administrative arm for implementation of these laws and regulations.

Local Health Department Subsystems

LHDs are generally responsible for the direct delivery of public health services and protection of the health of citizens though not all communities/counties have LHDs. State and local governments (i.e., city and county) delegate the authority to conduct these activities. The organization of LHDs varies widely depending on community size, economics, partnerships with the private health care system, health care facilities, business support, health care needs, transportation, and the number of citizens requiring public health care. Some LHDs function as district offices of the state health department, others are responsible to local government and the state, and still others are autonomous, particularly those

in large cities. LHDs may be a separate agency or a division within an agency, such as the USDHHS.

A health officer or administrator appointed by local government directs the LHDs. At least half of the states require that the health officer of an LHD have a medical degree. An interdisciplinary team carries out the activities of the department. Public health nurses and health inspectors represent the two largest groups of professional staff members. Other professional staff members include dentists, social workers, epidemiologists, nutritionists, and health educators.

Scope of Services of the Local Health Department Subsystem

LHDs are responsible for determining the health status and needs of their constituents. This involves identifying unmet needs and taking actions to meet these needs. Most services to groups and individuals are provided at the local level. These services fall into the following four major categories:

1. *Community health services* include control of communicable disease (i.e., surveillance and immunizations), maternal-child health programs, nutrition services, and education. Health promotion education is directed toward changing behavior; individuals are encouraged to eat healthy foods, increase their amount of exercise, and decrease their use of tobacco, drugs, and alcohol. Other programs provide nutritional food and food stamps to individuals and families. Preventive screening for potential problems throughout the lifespan is a major activity of LHDs.
2. *Environmental health services* include food hygiene (e.g., inspection of food-producing and food-processing plants and restaurants); protection from hazardous substances; control of waste, air, noise, and water pollution; and occupational health. The objective of these activities is to provide a safe environment.
3. *Personal health services* provide care to individuals and families in clinics, schools, and prisons. In many areas, home health care services are provided through the LHD.
4. *Mental health services* are provided through the LHDs in many communities. These services are supported by funds offered by local and regional mental health and mental retardation facilities and programs. See Chapter 22 for more information on community-based mental health care.

In the preceding description of the three government levels that provide public health services (i.e., local, state, and federal), distinctive and overlapping roles have been discussed. The federal government has been assuming a larger role in the protection of the population through regulation and funding. It finances specific programs (e.g., Medicare and categorical programs for mothers and infants) and provides direct care to special populations (e.g., veterans). States establish health codes, regulate the insurance industry, and license health care facilities and personnel. States also provide funds for services offered through Medicaid. Direct care activities funded by state health departments may include care in mental hospitals, state medical schools, and associated hospitals. LHDs are the primary agencies that provide direct services to communities, families, and individuals.

LHDs establish local health codes, fund public hospitals (i.e., city-county), and provide services to populations and individuals at risk. Programs and services for state health departments and LHDs vary across jurisdictions. The services provided reflect the values of the residents and officials, available resources, and perceived needs of their respective populations within their state and local area. Although the goals of the public health subsystem do not change, the programs and services change to meet the changing needs of the public.

Health Care Providers

Providers of health care are individuals, groups, and organizations that deliver or support health care services. This section describes health care providers, including provider organizations, health care professionals, and nontraditional providers.

Provider Organizations

The following are examples of health care **provider organizations:**

- Hospital
- Clinic
- Physician practice
- Ambulatory care center
- Home health agency
- Long-term care facility
- Skilled nursing facility
- Rehabilitation center
- Hospice service
- Public health department
- School health clinic
- Birthing center
- Ambulatory surgical center
- Occupational health clinic
- Crisis clinic
- Any other type of organization that provides health care to the community

Health care provider organizations are undergoing tremendous changes. This is particularly true of hospitals, which are merging, consolidating, and closing. As discussed previously, the Hill-Burton Act provided funds to increase hospital beds and accomplished this goal. However, currently there are too many beds. With the increasing shift to ambulatory and primary care, hospital stays have shortened, and the clients who are admitted to the hospital are more acutely ill and require more intensive care. Consequently, decreased hospital stays cause more home care admissions or more discharges from long-term care facilities for short-term recovery and rehabilitation. Figure 9-2 provides data about length of hospital stays.

The terms that are used to describe these changes are *reengineering; redesigning, rightsizing,* and *downsizing* the workforce; and *reregulating* professional practice.

Reengineering

Reengineering is a management technique that was borrowed from industry and recently applied to the health care delivery system. Reengineering involves more than a few simple

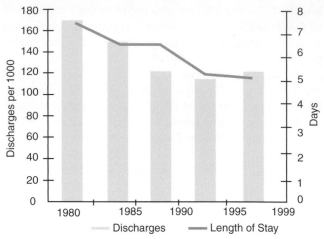

FIGURE 9-2   Discharge and length of stay for all payers. (From U.S. National Center for Health Statistics: *Vital and health Statistics,* series 13, Washington, D.C., The Author.

changes in an organization. It requires a reinvention or re-creation of processes, work, and systems.

Reengineering has become common in health care because the consumer has demanded it. The consumer in the current managed care environment is not just the client but also businesses that contract for employee health care, all levels of government, third-party payers, and MCOs. Another important factor is competition among all the providers as they seek managed care contracts to increase client volume.

To be successful, reengineering needs to include a cross-functional approach, emphasizing that people do not work in isolation. This has resulted in many organizations that are cross-training staff to work in several roles or settings. It emphasizes efficiency, effectiveness, role redesign, and the knowledge of staff to provide the best care or product available (Beyers, 1999; Flarey and Smith, 1999; Hammer and Champy, 1993; Turner, 1999).

Redesigning, Rightsizing, and Downsizing

Redesigning, rightsizing, and **downsizing** the workforce are terms that typically cause nurses to become alert and concerned. Staffing levels in health care organizations dropped during the 1990s, and the effect that this has had on care is of great concern to consumers and health care professionals, particularly nurses and physicians. Managed care demanded cost-effectiveness, which placed health care organizations in the position of increasing their productivity. The most common method used to increase productivity is to cut staff members; however, the result is not always improved productivity. Staff members may then be overworked, quality suffers, and morale drops, all of which affect overall productivity. However, staff roles need to be carefully assessed and redesigned. More research needs to be done about the effects of staffing, delivery models, and use of unlicensed assistive personnel (UAP). Strategies that help make redesigning, rightsizing, and downsizing more successful are education,

ETHICAL Insights

Mandatory Staffing Levels

Nurses are speaking out about their concerns through their professional organizations and their state legislative process. California nurses initiated a major effort to affect staffing levels in their hospitals. In October 1999, California passed a law requiring California hospitals to meet fixed nurse-to-client ratios. This landmark legislation was the first in the United States. This law is important because California is the state that has experienced the influence of managed care for the longest period of time, and it is recognizing critical concerns about the effects of some managed care approaches (Purdon, 1999). As of 2006, California is struggling with the implementation of the legislation at a time when there is a nursing shortage. This has clearly had an impact on the success of the law.

empowerment and involvement in the process, communication, teamwork, support and reward, and evaluation (Doran et al., 2002; Laschinger, Almost, and Tuer-Hodes, 2003; Laschinger and Finegan, 2005; Perla, 2002).

Now, the country faces a severe shortage of nursing staff. The earlier cutbacks affected some communities in that nurses refused to return to hospitals that earlier had terminated them. In addition, enrollment in nursing programs decreased; although the Nurse Reinvestment Act of 2003 and other methods used to increase interest in nursing as a profession have begun to affect enrollment, it is still not enough. Other critical factors affecting the problem are nursing faculty shortage, which makes it difficult for schools of nursing to increase enrollment, and the need for more clinical sites. The aging nursing workforce who are nearing retirement is another concern, one that will need to be faced very soon. Redesigning, rightsizing, and downsizing were responses to problems about costs and the need to do things differently, but now the delivery system faces the consequences of these approaches and some new problems, too.

Reregulating

The Pew report (O'Neil and Pew Health Professions Commission, 1998) identifies **reregulating** professional practice as a critical issue. Currently, health care delivery is less and less limited by boundaries, particularly state boundaries. Large medical centers have satellite delivery centers that may cross state boundaries and, in some cases, international boundaries; staff members may be expected to move from one medical center to another. Home health agencies may have clients in adjacent states. Telehealth has eliminated all boundaries as long as the equipment is available. Mobility and globalization will have effects on the health care organization and health care professionals. In 1998, the Pew Health Professions Commission identified critical health care professional competencies for the twenty-first century, which have been used to improve nursing education as the competencies help to identify critical content areas and experiences (Box 9-2).

Health Care Professionals

The health care team has been growing and changing over the last few years with new types of health care professionals

BOX 9-2 Health Care Professional Competencies for the Twenty-First Century

- ➤ Embrace a personal ethic of social responsibility and service.
- ➤ Exhibit ethical behavior in all professional activities.
- ➤ Provide evidence-based, clinically competent care.
- ➤ Incorporate the multiple determinants of health in clinical care.
- ➤ Apply knowledge of the new sciences.
- ➤ Demonstrate critical thinking, reflection, and problem-solving skills.
- ➤ Understand the role of primary care.
- ➤ Rigorously practice preventive health care.
- ➤ Integrate population-based care and services into practice.
- ➤ Improve access to health care for those with unmet health needs.
- ➤ Practice relationship-centered care with individuals and families.
- ➤ Provide culturally sensitive care to a diverse society.
- ➤ Partner with communities in health care decisions.
- ➤ Use communication and information technology effectively and appropriately.
- ➤ Work in interdisciplinary teams.
- ➤ Ensure care that balances individual, professional, system, and societal needs.
- ➤ Practice leadership.
- ➤ Take responsibility for quality of care and health outcomes at all levels.
- ➤ Contribute to continuous improvement of the health care system.
- ➤ Advocate for public policy that promotes and protects the health of the public.
- ➤ Continue to learn and help others learn.

From O'Neil E, Pew Health Professions Commission: *Recreating health professional practice for a new century,* San Francisco, 1998, Pew Health Professions Commission.

added and other members of the team taking on new responsibilities. The following is a brief review of the major types of professional and nonprofessional members of the health care team:

- *Registered nurse (RN):* This appears to be a simple designation that should be familiar to the reader. However, different educational routes exist to obtain a license to practice nursing, including diploma, associate degree, and baccalaureate degree. In addition, many nurses now obtain master's degrees and doctorates. These advanced degrees provide them with the opportunity to do more independent practice, teach, and conduct research. RNs practice in all types of health settings.
- *Nurse practitioner (NP):* This is a nurse who has obtained education beyond a baccalaureate degree and has studied content related to primary care. An NP specializes in such areas as adult health, pediatrics, neonatology, gerontology, and psychiatric nursing. NPs may work in clinics, the community, a private practice, the home, the hospital, and long-term care facilities (i.e., any setting in which health care is provided).
- *Nurse midwife (NM):* This is a nurse who has completed an additional educational program focused on midwifery. NMs work in all types of settings in which women's health and obstetrical services are provided.
- *Licensed practical nurse or licensed vocational nurse (LPN or LVN):* LPNs and LVNs perform some specific nursing

functions and play a critical role in providing direct client care. They have high school degrees and additional training. They work in all types of settings, typically under the direct supervision of an RN or a physician.

- *Physician (MD or DO):* A physician has a medical degree and typically specializes in a specific area of practice (e.g., internal medicine, surgery, pediatrics, and gynecology). Currently, many physicians are specializing in primary practice or family practice because managed care has increased the need for physicians who will act as the primary care provider for clients. In this role, the physician acts as the "gatekeeper" for the client. Many insurance plans require that the client first see his or her primary care provider before seeing a specialist to receive reimbursement for the care. Some insurers are now allowing NPs and NMs to act as primary care providers.
- *Physician assistant (PA):* The PA is a "physician extender" who provides medical services under the supervision of a licensed physician. The role was developed in the 1960s in response to a shortage of primary care physicians in certain areas. PAs generally work in primary care.
- *Registered dietitian (RD):* This health care professional assesses the client's nutritional status and needs. RDs work in hospitals, long-term care facilities, clinics, community health, and homes. An RD has knowledge about nutrition and food and, in a community setting, would recommend healthy diets and provide nutrition counseling and education.
- *Social worker (SW):* SWs assist clients and their families with problems related to reimbursement, access to care, housing, care in the home, transportation, and social problems. They have been used as discharge planners, particularly in acute care facilities or hospitals, often as case managers; however, they work in all types of settings.
- *Occupational therapist (OT):* OTs assist clients with impaired functions to reach the clients' maximum level of physical and psychosocial independence. They work in all types of settings.
- *Speech-language pathologist:* Speech-language pathologists assist clients who need rehabilitative services related to speech and hearing. They work in all types of settings.
- *Physical therapist (PT):* PTs focus on assisting clients who are experiencing musculoskeletal problems. PTs typically work in rehabilitation and focus on maximizing physical functioning. They work in all types of settings.
- *Pharmacist:* Pharmacists prepare and dispense medications. Pharmacists have become much more involved in client education about medications and in monitoring and evaluating the effects of medications. They work in all types of settings, including the local drug store, where they play a critical role in ensuring safe prescriptions and providing consumer education.
- *Respiratory therapist (RT):* RTs provide care to clients with respiratory illnesses. They use oxygen therapy, intermittent positive pressure respirators, artificial mechanical ventilators, and inhalation therapy. Most RTs work in hospitals and long-term care, but they are becoming more common in home health care.

- *Chiropractor:* Chiropractors are concerned with improving the function of the clients' nervous system with various treatment modalities (e.g., spinal manipulation, diet, exercise, and massage). Interest in using chiropractors has been increasing as the consumer has become more interested in nontraditional medical interventions. Chiropractors are mostly community based.
- *Paramedical technologists:* Paramedical technologists work in various medical technology areas (e.g., radiology, nuclear medicine, and other laboratories).
- *Unlicensed assistive personnel (UAP):* This member of the health care team has caused some controversy in last few years; however, the UAP is a critical member of the team. Aides and assistants have been in existence for a long time. Their responsibilities have changed over the years, and they are currently providing more direct client care. They are supervised by RNs, who must ensure that they are able to provide safe care to the client. The amount of education and training of UAPs is highly variable, and this has caused much concern about practice parameters and the effect on the quality of care.

Nontraditional Health Care Providers

Nontraditional health care providers deliver alternative or complementary therapies. Consumers have become more interested in this type of care and have demanded that it be available (Burcham, 1999; Korczyk and Witte, 1998).

Although many large medical centers are now developing programs and centers that offer complementary therapies, reimbursement for these services is still lagging. The NIH agreed to conduct research focused on a wide array of alternative therapies and their effects on health and disease. In 1998, the NIH established the National Center for Complementary and Alternative Therapies to meet the need. This represents a major change in the scientific and medical communities.

Alternative therapies, provided by a variety of health care providers, include massage therapy, herbal therapy, healing touch, energetic healing, acupuncture, and acupressure. Ethnic healers, such as *curanderos,* and folk healers are also found in some communities. Training and licensure requirements vary but will probably become more standard as their care becomes more accepted in established medical practice. Many nurses have incorporated alternative therapies in their practice and are seeking continuing education on this topic.

CRITICAL ISSUES IN HEALTH CARE DELIVERY

Managed Care

Managed care refers to any method of health care delivery designed to reduce unnecessary use of services, increase cost containment or cost-effectiveness, and ensure high quality care. Managed care is currently the most dominant force in health care delivery. It affects health care organizations, health care providers, and reimbursement. It has a direct influence on what care is provided and by whom, where, when, and whether it is to be provided.

Managed care is complex and many MCO models exist. These include HMOs, preferred provider organizations (PPOs), integrated delivery systems (IDSs), and physician hospital organizations (PHOs). Each of these models has different characteristics, and often clients can choose their health policy from several different models. For example, an employer may offer employees the option of choosing an HMO plan or a PPO plan. See Chapter 10 for additional information on managed care and reimbursement.

Quality Care

Accreditation is one means to assess the quality of services and care of the organization. Specific minimum standards must be met by an organization to obtain accreditation. Many groups provide accreditation for health care providers and MCOs. The JCAHO accredits hospitals, home care agencies, long-term care facilities, ambulatory care centers, and MCOs. The National Committee on Quality Assurance accredits MCOs and uses the Health Plan Employer Data Information Set (HEDIS) to collect data about plans and consumer satisfaction. Medicare also uses HEDIS. The American Healthcare Commission also accredits MCOs (Diamond, 1998; O'Malley, 1997; Snowden, 1998).

Purchasers of care are also concerned about the accreditation status of MCOs when they negotiate MCO contracts. Insurers and MCOs are concerned about the accreditation status of health care provider organizations, as are nursing schools that use clinical sites for educational purposes. Health care providers should also be concerned about the accreditation status of their employers. The Consumer Assessment of Health Plans (CAHPS) is a new survey and reporting tool sponsored by the Agency for Health Care Policy and Research (AHCPR), Harvard Medical School, the Research Triangle Institute, and RAND. CAHPS collects data and reports on consumer experience with specific aspects of their health plans. This type of survey provides data that help purchasers of plans compare and contrast plans (AHCPR et al., 1998).

Currently, quality care monitoring focuses on improvement. With the improvement approach, **outcomes measures** have moved to the forefront. Accrediting organizations require outcomes data and use them to assess overall performance. Practitioners use outcomes to identify the treatment goals with the client. Report cards are used to compare and contrast health care organizations and health care plans. These report cards are available to the consumer, providers, and insurers. Quality data are no longer hidden and will continue to be available as new methods are developed to assess improvement based on outcomes (Beyers, 2003; McCarthy, 2002).

Despite all these efforts to evaluate and accredit to ensure quality care, the United States has not really been all that successful. There is still discussion about what constitutes quality care, and how to best assess quality.

Quality care has been a concern of consumers and providers for many years. Quality care is a difficult concept to define and more difficult to measure. In 1996, President Clinton established the Advisory Commission on Consumer Protection and Quality in the Health Care Industry, and its final report was published in 1999 (The President's Advisory Commission on Consumer Protection and Quality in the Health Care Industry, 1999). As identified in this report, "the purpose of the health care system must be to continuously reduce the impact and burden of illness, injury, and disability and to improve the health and functioning of the people of the United States." The report strongly supports public-private partnerships, strong leadership with clearly defined goals for improvement, an increase in consumer strength and rights, a focus on vulnerable populations, promotion of accountability, reduction in errors and an increase in health care safety, fostering of evidence-based practice, adaptation of organizations for change, an increase in health care workforce involvement, and investment in information systems. For additional information found in the report, visit the book's website at http://elsevier.com/Nies and see **Resource Tool 9A.**

The report from the President's Advisory Commission on Consumer Protection and Quality in the Health Care Industry (1999) had a major impact in that it stimulated a series of more in-depth explorations of the health care delivery system, which resulted in a series of reports developed by the Institute of Medicine (IOM). The IOM defines quality as "the degree to which health services for individuals and populations increase the likelihood of desired health outcomes and are consistent with current professional knowledge" (Chassin and Galvin, 1998, p. 1000). The following is a brief description of the content of these important reports that are changing health care delivery.

To Err Is Human: Building a Safer Health System

The first report, *To Err Is Human: Building a Safer Health System* (Kohn, Carrigan, and Donaldson, 1999), focused on safety within the health care delivery system. Data indicated that there have been, and continue to be, serious safety problems. Examples include the following:

- When data from one study was extrapolated, the findings indicated that at least 44,000 Americans die each year as a result of a medication error, and another study indicated the number could be as high as 98,000 (American Hospital Association Statistics, 1999; as cited in Kohn et al., 1999).
- In a given year more people die as a result of medical errors than from motor vehicle accidents (43,458), breast cancer (42,297), or AIDS (16,516) (CDC, 1998; as cited in Kohn et al., 1999).
- Health care costs represent over 50% of total national costs, which includes lost income, lost household production, disability, and health care costs (Thomas et al., 1999; as cited in Kohn et al., 1999).

There are clear problems, and, to date, the focus has only been on hospital errors. This, however, does not negate the presence of medical errors in community, home care, long-term care, ambulatory care or primary care areas, and other health care settings. These are settings that require further exploration.

The report on safety clearly states that there is no one answer to solving this problem. This report defines safety as "freedom from accidental injury" and defines error as "the failure of a planned action to be completed as intended or the use of a wrong plan to achieve an aim" (Kohn et al., 1999, p. 3). Errors are directly related to outcomes, which is a significant concern in quality improvement efforts. Patient safety is a critical component of quality (Kohn et al., 1999).

This initiative represents a collaborative effort from a health care professional organization, an accrediting organization, and consumers. Getting the patient involved is a very important strategy; however, the critical next step is listening to the patient. JCAHO also developed a safety focus, which was implemented in 2003 accreditation cycle. It focuses on accurate patient identification, effective communication, safe use of high-alert medications, elimination of wrong site surgery, safe use of infusion pumps, and safe use of clinical alarms, all of which are discussed in this IOM report (Kirkpatrick, 2003). Worker safety is also a concern, and occupational health is an important component of community health. Patient safety and worker safety are connected. Though worker safety was not a focus of this report, "the committee believes that creating a safe environment for patients will go a long way in addressing issues of worker safety as well" (Kohn et al., 1999, p. 20). The four key messages from this report are

> first, the magnitude of harm that results from medical errors is great; second, errors result largely from systems' failures, not individual failures; third, voluntary and mandatory reporting programs are needed now to improve patient safety; and fourth, the IOM committee and others call on health care systems to focus on error reduction as an important part of their operations and to embrace organizational change needed to reorient error-ridden systems and process. (Maddox, Wakefield, and Bull, 2001, p. 9)

Crossing the Quality Chasm

The second major report, *Crossing the Quality Chasm* (IOM, 2001), focuses on developing a new health care system for the twenty-first century, one that improves care. The first conclusion from the report is that the system is in need of fundamental improvement. The report emphasizes the impact of the rapid change in the health care system: new medical science, new technology, rapid availability of information, and so on. Health care providers cannot keep up, and "performance of the health care system varies considerably" (IOM, 2001, p. 3). As was noted in *To Err Is Human,* the system is fragmented, poorly organized, and does not make the best use of its resources. Another conclusion from the report is the impact that the increase of chronic conditions has had on the system. With people living longer, mostly due to the advances in medical science and technology, more are living with chronic conditions. Many of these patients also have comorbid conditions—complicated problems that require collaborative treatment efforts. The health care system is ineffective in dealing with these problems. To address these multiple concerns, the report supports

changes that were identified by Wagner, Austin, and Von Korff (1996):

1. Need for evidence-based, planned care
2. Reorganization of practices to meet the needs of patients who require more time, a broad array of resources, and closer follow-up
3. Systematic attention to patients' need for information and behavioral change
4. Ready access to necessary clinical expertise
5. Supportive information systems

The report recommendations for an agenda for crossing the quality chasm, which are directly related to nursing, include the following:

- All health care constituents, including policy makers, purchasers, regulators, health professionals, health care trustees and management, and consumers, commit to a national statement of purpose for the health care systems as a whole and to a shared agenda.
- Clinicians and patients and the health care organizations that support care delivery adopt a new set of principles to guide the redesign of care processes.
- The USDHHS identifies a set of priority conditions to focus initial efforts, provide resources to stimulate innovation, and initiate the change process. (See comments about the report, *Priority Areas for National Action,* later in this section. This report followed the *Crossing the Quality Chasm* report, and it does identify specific conditions.)
- Health care organizations design and implement more effective organizational support processes to make change in the delivery of care possible.
- Purchasers, regulators, health professions, educational institutions, and the USDHHS create an environment that fosters and rewards improvement by (1) creating an infrastructure to support evidence-based practice, (2) facilitating the use of information technology, (3) aligning payment incentives, and (4) preparing the workforce to better serve patients in a world of expanding knowledge and rapid change. (IOM, 2001, p. 5)

Envisioning the National Health Care Quality Report

Much has been said about the lack of health care quality. To pursue improvement means that the United States needs methods to determine if care has been improved. The goal of *Envisioning the National Health Care Quality Report* (Hurtado, Swift, and Corrigan, 2001) is to develop these methods, which should complement other reports on quality as well as *Healthy People 2010,* which identifies public health objectives (USDHHS, 2000). To be effective, there needs to be effective communication and collaboration among the quality efforts. The report recommends that there be a classification matrix of measures, which includes two dimensions: (1) the consumer perspective and (2) components of health care quality. "The matrix is a tool to visualize possible combinations of the two dimensions (consumer perspectives and components of health care quality) of the framework and better understand how various aspects of framework relate to one another" (Hurtado et al., 2001, p. 8). In order to develop a national health quality report and analyze data, there needs to be a new health infrastructure with uniform data standards and computerized clinical data systems. How would a national health care quality report affect efforts to improve quality?

* Supply a common understanding of quality and how to measure it that reflects the best current approaches and practices.
* Identify aspects of the health care system that improve or impede quality.
* Generate data associated with major quality initiatives.
* Educate the public, the media, and other audiences about the importance of health care quality and the current level of quality.
* Identify, for policy makers, the problem areas in health care quality that most need their attention and action, with the understanding that these priorities may change over time and differ by geographic location.
* Provide policy makers, purchasers, health care providers, and others with realistic benchmarks for quality of care in the form of national, regional, and population comparisons.
* Make it easier to compare the quality of the U.S. health care system with that of other nations.
* Stimulate the refinement of existing measures and the development of new ones.
* Stimulate data collection efforts at the state and local levels (mirroring the national effort) to facilitate targeted quality improvements.
* Incorporate improved measures as they become available and practicable.
* Clarify the many aspects of health care quality and how they affect one another and quality as a whole.
* Encourage data collection efforts needed to refine and develop quality measures and, ultimately, stimulate the development of a health information infrastructure to support quality measurement and reporting. (Hurtado et al., 2001, p. 31)

Leadership by Example

This report, requested by Congress, examines the federal government's quality enhancement processes (Corrigan, Eden, and Smith, 2003). It focuses on six government programs: Medicare, Medicaid, The State Children's Health Insurance Program, the Department of Defense TRICARE and TRICARE for life programs, the Veterans Administration program, and the Indian Health Services program, all of which have a direct impact on community health. Approximately 100 million people are covered by these programs. The report's conclusion is improvement in this process is particularly needed.

1. There is a lack of consistent performance measurement across and within programs.
2. The usefulness of quality information has been questioned.
3. There is a lack of a conceptual framework to guide the evaluation.
4. There is a lack of computerized clinical data.
5. There is a lack of commitment to guide decisions.
6. There is a lack of a systematic approach for assessing the quality enhancement activities.

Each one of these problems will require substantial changes in the health care delivery system. The report notes that

federal leadership is needed because the federal government is in a unique position to assume a lead role in developing a national health care quality improvement initiative. The federal government is a "regulator; purchaser; health care provider; and sponsor of research, education, and training" (Hurtado et al., 2001, p. 6). It is the largest purchaser of care, and, thus, it could have a major impact on many people. It provides direct care to many: military personnel and their families, Native Americans, and veterans. Through these programs, the federal government could establish models to improve care. This has already been demonstrated through Medicare and Medicaid. As a regulator, it also can affect many health care providers who are not in the federal system; for example, health care organizations that accept Medicare or Medicaid funds must comply with federal regulations. It should be noted that regulation is not the best way to make improvement changes because the "the regulatory approach is a blunt tool that generally fails to differentiate among grades of quality" (Hurtado et al., 2001, p. 7). Regulation should not be relied on as the only approach to the problem. Through sponsorship of research, education, and training, however, the federal government can have a major impact. The report's conclusions recommend that the federal government lead by example and coordinate government roles in improving health care quality. In doing this, the government will have an impact on all parts of the health care delivery system.

Who Will Keep the Public Healthy?

This report brings public health into the forefront, which is badly needed. It addresses the needs for public health in a world that is affected by globalization, rapid travel, scientific and technological advances, and demographic changes. To address public health problems, there is a great need for public health professionals who are prepared to deal with the problems. "A public health professional is a person educated in public health or a related discipline who is employed to improve health through a population focus" (Gebbie, Rosenstock, and Hernandez, 2003, p. 4). The eight content areas that are important for today's and future public health professions are informatics, genomics, communication, cultural competence, community-based participatory research, global health, policy and law, and public health ethics. These areas are in addition to the long-held core components of public health: epidemiology, biostatistics, environmental health, health services administration, and social and behavioral science. This report provides an in-depth exploration of the educational needs for improved public health.

Health Professions Education

In the report *Health Professions Education* (Greiner and Knebel, 2003) the education of health professionals is viewed as a bridge to quality care. This discussion does not focus just on education but also on the need to have qualified, competent staff in order to improve health care. The report indicates that health professions education is in need of change to meet the growing demands of the health care system today. "All health professionals should be educated to deliver patient-centered care as members of an interdisciplinary team, emphasizing evidence-based practice, quality improvement approaches, and informatics" (Greiner and Knebel, 2003, p. 3). All of these critical areas have been discussed in this text because they are very relevant to nurses and nursing care.

Priority Areas for National Action: Transforming Health Care Quality

The IOM report *Crossing the Quality Chasm* (2001) identifies that the first step the United States needs to take to address quality of care is to conduct a systematic identification of the priority areas for quality improvement in order to make the changes that are necessary (Adams and Corrigan, 2003). The *Priority Areas for National Action* (Adams and Corrigan, 2003) developed this list by identifying 19 priority areas. The first two areas are to promote care coordination and self-management/health literacy, both of which affect a broad range of groups. The other areas are concerned with the continuum of care across the lifespan, preventive care, inpatient/surgical care, chronic conditions, end-of-life care, and behavioral care. The 19 areas that Adams and Corrigan identified are:

- Care coordination
- Self-management/health literacy
- Asthma—appropriate treatment for persons with mild/moderate persistent asthma
- Cancer screening that is evidence based—focus on co-lorectal and cervical cancer
- Children with special health care needs (are at increased risk for chronic physical, developmental, behavioral condition)
- Diabetes—focus on appropriate management of early disease
- End-of-life with advanced organ system failure—focus on congestive heart failure and chronic obstructive pulmonary disease
- Frailty associated with old age—preventing falls and pressure ulcers, maximizing function, and developing advanced care plans
- Hypertension—focus on appropriate treatment of early disease
- Immunization—children and adult
- Ischemic heart disease—prevention, reduction of recurring events, and optimization of functional capacity
- Major depression—screening and treatment
- Medical management—preventing medication errors and overuse of antibiotics
- Nosocomial infections—prevention and surveillance
- Pain control in advanced cancer
- Pregnancy and childbirth—appropriate prenatal and intra-partum care
- Severe and persistent mental illness—focus on treatment in the public sector
- Stroke—early treatment in the public sector
- Tobacco dependence treatment in adults
- Obesity (emerging area)

(Adams and Corrigan, 2003, p. 3)

These areas should be used as a guide by health care providers as they develop their QI programs and should be of concern as community health is addressed. Communities can use this list to develop their community health focus and thus improve the quality of life and care of populations in the community.

Keeping Patients Safe: Transforming the Work Environment of Nurses

The IOM report *Keeping Patients Safe: Transforming the Work Environment of Nurses* (Page, 2004) clearly is an important report for nurses in all types of settings. This extensive report addresses critical quality and safety issues with a particular focus on nursing care and nurses and examines these issues from the perspective of the work environment. As the report states, "When we are hospitalized, in a nursing home, or managing a chronic condition in our own homes—at some of our most vulnerable moments—nurses are the health care providers we are most likely to encounter, spend the greatest amount of time with, and be dependent upon for our recovery" (Page, 2004, p. ix). From the review of the critical work environment, the report then discusses methods for designing the work environment so that nurses may provide safer patient care. The content identifies concerns related to the nursing shortage, health care errors, patient safety risk factors, the central role of the nurse in patient safety, and work environment threats to patient safety. Recommendations for resolving these concerns include patient safety defenses; evidence-based model for safety defenses; reengineering issues; transformational leadership and evidence-based management; maximizing workforce capability through safe staffing levels, need for knowledge and skills and clinical decision making, and interdisciplinary collaboration; workspace design; and building and creating a culture of safety. This report will undoubtedly have a major impact on the practice of nursing, health care delivery, and how nursing is taught.

Patient Safety: Achieving a New Standard of Care

This IOM report expands the work done on safety in earlier reports (Aspden et al., 2004). It emphasizes the need to establish a national health information infrastructure and need for data standards. Why is this important? It is impossible to monitor and then address safety issues without data, and the goal is to have national data as patients receive care from multiple providers. The ultimate goal should be prevention of errors and not resolution of errors after they have occurred. Routine use of electronic health records would give health care providers and patients immediate access to complete patient information as well as tools to guide decision making and help prevent errors (Aspden et al., 2004).

Fraud and Abuse

Health care fraud is widespread. The billions of dollars spent on health care and struggles for control between providers, consumers, and MCOs have provided an arena that lends itself to fraud and abuse. Officials estimate that up to 10% of the total health care expenditures in 2003, or about $170 billion, was lost to fraud and abuse (National Health Care Anti-Fraud Association [NHCAA], 2005). Indeed, in 1994, a U.S. congressional committee concluded that an effective antifraud program was crucial to stopping fraud throughout the health care system (U.S. House of Representatives, 1994). In response, a number of actions have been taken to combat the problem. Among them are the False Claims Act Amendments (1986), which allow private citizens to collect a percentage of recovered funds if they report fraudulent Medicare claims and monies are recovered as a result (Stanton, 2001). The Health Insurance Portability and Accountability Act of 1996 (HIPAA) contains a set of provisions that address fraud, including a Fraud and Abuse Control Program, the Medicare Integrity Program, and the Health Care Fraud and Abuse Data Collection Program. Each of these programs is designed to address concerns over health care fraud. In addition, HIPAA dramatically increased funding for fraud enforcement activities (Michael, 2003).

Major health care fraud and abuse incidents have influenced the most vulnerable of the population (i.e., the mentally ill and older adults). In the 1980s and 1990s, a major psychiatric scandal occurred, involving large sums of money and abuse of clients (Meier, 1997; Mohr, 1996, 1997). This scandal involved many patient abuses, including inappropriate admissions, administration of medications and treatment that were not required, unsafe physical restraint for long periods of time, verbal abuse, and denial of patient rights. Hospitals falsified documentation to receive higher levels of reimbursement and discharged patients as soon as their insurance ran out, with limited or no discharge planning. Another major incident concerning fraud included a case involving Columbia/HCA, in which federal investigations found widespread fraud, overcharges, and substandard care (Eichenwald, 1997).

In recent years, overbilling and unnecessary visits in home health care were reported across the United States, which resulted in widespread reforms to Medicare reimbursement for home health services (Infante and McAnaney, 2004; Michael, 2003). As an example, one hospital in South Carolina was recently forced to repay $9.5 million to Medicare due to overbilling for its home health, hospice, and durable medical equipment programs throughout the 1990s (Healthcare Risk Management, 2004).

Also recently, a very large number of cases have been prosecuted involving overbilling of insurance companies by both physicians and chiropractors; in many cases, tens of millions of dollars were involved. These cases involved services that were not performed, services that were performed but unnecessary, and more expensive services or procedures than were actually provided or performed (NHCAA, 2005; Taylor, 2003).

Many nurses have been directly influenced by fraud and abuse by participating in it, by trying to fight it, and by their apathy. Nurses need to assert their role as advocates and know how to cope with unethical behavior in health care organizations (Camunas, 1998; Michael, 2003).

Information Technology

The development of information technology over the last decade has been phenomenal. Clinical staff members use computers in all health care settings. **Telehealth** is growing, which means that clients can receive care via technology, such as computer, video, or interactive television. The Internet has opened doors for consumers and providers, and health information has exploded. Although information availability has been enhanced to millions of people, which resulted in an explosion of knowledge regarding health and health issues, the quality of this information is sometimes questionable. Providers must address the source and content of Internet information (Brody, 1999).

Consumerism, Advocacy, and Client Rights

The growth of managed care has increased the strength of consumerism. Over the past decade, the baby boom generation has been subsidizing the health care system and paying more in premiums than it has taken out in claims. However, growing concern exists that as this generation ages, it will demand more care than previous generations. Consumers are now critical of the health care system and demanding changes as they encounter problems. MCOs and providers are recognizing the importance of the consumer voice and the need for explanations. *Client-* or *customer-centered health care* is a term that has become commonly used in health care, and more effort has been made to provide the consumer with information.

Client rights are now an important health care issue that individual states and the federal government have been addressing through legislation. In fall 1999, the House and Senate passed bills that focused on client rights in the managed care environment (Pear, 1999a). There is no doubt that this will be a critical issue in the future. Client rights issues that are vitally important are information disclosure, physician and provider choice, direct access to specialists, reimbursement for emergency care, and reimbursement denial. As has been discussed, there is still no national patients' bill of rights.

Coordination and Access to Health Care

The social justice foundation of public health is yet to be realized because many inequalities in access to health care still exist. The United States has more than 43 million uninsured individuals (Pear, 1999b). Characteristics of uninsured people reflect a wide range of incomes, races, and occupations, although children, minorities, the poor, and those with less education are overrepresented.

Health care providers often function in isolation from one another and provide fragmented services. Although multiple services are available for the wellness–serious illness continuum, coordination is lacking. Services range from office-clinic, home care, adult day care, acute care institutions, and specialized institutions to skilled nursing facilities. The services provided by one agency or one provider do not help the individual transit, or move, across boundary lines and receive services offered by others. In addition, the services tend to be geographically separated, and each agency has different criteria for access. The focus of services has not kept pace with the changing needs of individuals and populations. Millions of Americans lack access to health care services, and inadequate financial resources are a deterrent to available health services.

The current health care system is pluralistic and competitive, and it provides fragmented and uncoordinated care. Private care agencies and institutions are in competition with one another for clients, health professionals, and resources. Even with recent reforms, two hospitals in the same geographical area may be competing for the same clients while other communities may not have a hospital at all, have only minimal services, or lack essential services such as obstetrics. Hospital home care programs are in direct competition with private home care agencies. Hospitals diversify services to become economically viable; therefore, they comzpete with HMOs for the ambulatory market. Public health services can be viewed as indirectly competing for resources. This fragmentation and duplication must be overcome to provide coordinated, collaborative, and accessible service to all citizens.

Disparity in Health Care Delivery

Disparity in health care delivery is certainly related to the number of uninsured and underinsured, but it is also more than this. The IOM (2002) report *Unequal Treatment: Confronting Racial and Ethnic Disparities in Health Care* addressed factors that might provide causes of disparities in health care. The report indicates that bias, prejudice, and stereotyping on the part of health care providers might be major factors in explaining differences in care. Disparities were particularly found in cancer, cardiovascular disease, HIV/AIDS, diabetes, and mental illness. To address this problem, there needs to be more cross-cultural education for health care professionals to improve awareness of cultural and social factors and their impact on health care. Nursing education has included more content and learning experiences related to cross-cultural issues. There also needs to be greater standardization of data collection to gain more understanding of the problem. Nurses need to be leaders in providing direction for this data collection, as these are data that affect their practice. A third strategy that needs consideration is the development of policies that look at the entire health care system to decrease fragmentation in the delivery system and education of health care professionals. Fragmented delivery affects nursing care; for example, patients may be more acutely ill when admitted to a hospital or come to a clinic because previous care was not coordinated effectively.

Health Care Reform: The Clinton Health Reform Initiative

The United States appeared to be ready for **health care reform** when the Clinton administration took office (Skocpol,

---

1994). By 1990, support for reform had reached a 40-year high in the polls, and the election of Bill Clinton in 1992 brought the health care debate onto the national agenda. Believing reform of the health care system to be part of his election mandate, the new president assembled an ambitious plan to produce legislation for national reform of the health care system. The process was initially supported by diverse sectors of the system. As the shape of the Clinton proposals began to emerge, some participants began to distance themselves and ultimately opposed the reform approach. This was true in the case of many major power constituents (i.e., businesses, physicians, and insurance companies). The insurance sector was probably the most vocal in making its objections known.

The approach used by the administration was inclusive, with strong support for public health. The bill eventually proposed in Congress included a version of the core functions outlined in the 1988 IOM study *The Future of Public Health*. Public health's inclusion in the reform agenda fostered a renewed interest in prevention and health promotion. The focus was to improve health status and contain costs. After defeat of the reform bills in 1994, the consensus emerged that despite the American public's recognition of the need for reform, little recognition existed that such reform would have specific consequences for individual Americans in terms of cost and choice.

FUTURE OF PUBLIC HEALTH AND THE HEALTH CARE SYSTEM

The debate continues as the new century begins.
- What health care services should be provided?
- Who should have access to health care services?
- Who should pay for health care services?
- How should health care be delivered?
- What is the role of the government?

Changes in the health care system are necessary to meet the changing needs of populations. The private care subsystem needs to set limits on the care provided, setting criteria for use of technology and determining which conditions will be treated, which interventions are effective, and who should receive the care (Banta, 1990). Managed care has pressured the private care subsystem into focusing more on health promotion and prevention; however, the success of this pressure is unclear.

It is difficult to speculate on the role of community health as the health care delivery system changes, but it is clear it will be part of the change. However, the community health focus on health promotion, disease prevention, and a population-based approach to health care is finding a new audience. *Healthy People 2010* is having some impact. The IOM reports indicate a need for improvement in all sectors of the health care delivery system. There is recognition of the need for an electronic medical record, which, to be effective, would have to incorporate care provided in the community. The growing concern over bioterrorism and roles of health care organizations, practitioners, and the government must address the community health components of the system. Local, state, and national political leaders must begin to grapple with the health of the population and the need to reduce the levels of health care expenditures in a voluntary environment.

Futurists rarely identify the public health subsystem as a component of the health care system, but this is changing. Perhaps the history of the public health subsystem's involvement with the poor and disenfranchised is a major influence in inattention to their problems. The assumptions underlying the ecological model demand that attention be paid to the poor and underserved, but the political aspects of health care frequently demand a focus in another direction. Furthermore, focus on environmental influences on the population is critical for the future health of any nation.

Predicting future trends in human values is more difficult than predicting scientific discoveries or the patterns of disease. However, Koop (1989) stated that the ultimate test of the public health subsystem is whether it effectively serves the people by their measurements, not those of the public health profession. Since the beginning of the 1990s, a significant shift has occurred in thinking about the future of the health care system. Consumer rights and further efforts to control or limit managed care will be critical issues to be resolved in the future. How these decisions will affect public health is unclear.

SUMMARY

The health care system is complex and changes quickly. Federal, state, and local legislation and policies affect the system, and understanding the legislation and its effect on the health care delivery system is critical for any nurse. In addition, the development of managed care has demonstrated how important it is for health care providers to understand the reimbursement system and to learn how to advocate for their clients.

The many different types of health care organizations and health care providers also affect the health care system. Interdisciplinary care will be necessary for success in the system and to ensure that the client receives cost-effective, quality care. There are many concerns about health care, including cost, access, the number of uninsured, quality, and health care fraud and abuse. Resolving these problems will not be an easy task, but it must be done. Understanding the system helps as health care providers learn to function in the rapidly changing system.

LEARNING ACTIVITIES

1. Describe the organization of the state and local health departments.
2. Visit the LHD and learn what services are provided. How do these services relate to *Healthy People 2010* objectives?
3. Identify regional and state health services.
4. Visit a voluntary agency. Determine the services they offer and how the agency collaborates with the local public health agency. Does the agency have a Web site? If so, visit it and find out what information is available to consumers and professionals.
5. Discuss how critical health care issues (e.g., managed care, quality care, fraud and abuse, diversity and disparity) affect health care organizations in the community.
6. Site examples of health care consumerism in the local community. What are their histories?
7. Give a personal reaction to health care fraud and abuse. How should the principles found in the Code for Nurses apply in practice?
8. Visit the website for the Agency for Healthcare Research and Quality (http://www.ahrq.gov) and search for practice guidelines related to community health. Select one and review it. How might the guideline apply to a community health nurse?

REFERENCES

Adams K, Corrigan J, editors: *Priority areas for national action: transforming health care quality.* Washington, DC, 2003, National Academies Press.

Agency for Health Care Policy and Research, Harvard Medical School, Research Triangle Institute, RAND: *Consumer assessment of health plans,* Washington, DC, 1998, AHCPR.

Annual update of the HHS poverty guidelines, *Fed Reg* 64(52):13428-13430, March 18, 1999.

American Hospital Association: *Hospital statistics.* Chicago, 1999, The Author.

Aspden P et al, editors: *Patient safety: achieving a new standard for care.* Washington, DC, 2004, National Academies Press.

Banta H: What is health care? In Kovner A, editor: *Health care delivery in the United States,* ed 4, New York, 1990, Springer.

Beyers M: Re-engineering patient care in a multi-institutional system. In Smith S, Flarey D, editors: *Process-centered health care organization,* Gaithersburg, Md, 1999, Aspen.

Beyers M: Viewpoint: Report cards are here to stay. *Patient care management* 19(1):10-11, 2003.

Brody J: The health hazards of point-and-click medicine, *New York Times,* August 3, 1999.

Burcham M: Credentialing alternative medicine: a challenge for managed care organizations, *Managed Care Q* 7(2):39, 1999.

Cammas C: Ethical dilemmas of nurse executives, *J Nurs Admin* 24(7-8):45, 1998.

DeParle J: States struggle to use windfall born of shifts in welfare law, *New York Times,* August 29, 1999.

Centers for Disease Control and Prevention, National Center for Health Statistics: Births and deaths: preliminary data for 1998. *Nat Vital Stat Rep* 47(25):6, 1998.

Chassin M, Galvin R: The urgent need to improve health care quality. *JAMA* 280(2): 1000–1005, 1998.

Corrigan J, Eden J, Smith B, editors: *Leadership by example.* Washington, DC, 2003, National Academies Press.

Diamond F: NCQA adds performance to accreditation reviews, *Manage Care* 8(5), 1998, The Author, www.managedcaremag.com.

Doran DI et al: An empirical test of the nursing role effectiveness model. *J Adv Nurs* 38(1): 29-39, 2002.

Eichenwald K: Hospital chain cheated U.S. on expenses, documents show, *New York Times,* August 22, 1997.

Flarey D, Smith S: Re-engineering: the journey to a process-centered organization. In Smith S, Flarey D, editors: *Process-centered health care organization,* Gaithersburg, Md, 1999, Aspen.

Gebbie K, Rosenstock L, Hernandez L, editors: *Who will keep the public healthy?* Washington, DC, 2003, National Academies Press.

Greiner A, Knebel E, editors: *Health professions education.* Washington, DC, 2003, National Academies Press.

Hammer M, Champy J: *Re-engineering the corporation: a manifesto for business revolution,* New York, 1993, Harper Business.

Hanlon G, Pickett J: *Public health administration and practice*, ed 9, St. Louis, 1990, Mosby.

Healthcare Risk Management: Hospital to pay $9.5 million for Medicare billing issues, *Healthcare Risk Manage,* 2004.

Horn SD: Improving quality of care. In Kovner AR, Jonas S, editors: *Health care delivery in the United States,* ed 7, New York, 2002, Springer.

Hurtado M, Swift E, Corrigan J, editors: *Envisioning the national health care quality report,* Washington, DC, 2001, National Academies Press.

Infante M, McAnaney K: Home health agencies can avoid fraud charges with compliance plans, *Hosp Home Health* 21(5):49-51, 2004.

Institute of Medicine: *The future of public health,* Washington, DC, 1988, National Academies Press.

Institute of Medicine: *Crossing the quality chasm.* Washington, DC, 2001, National Academies Press.

Institute of Medicine: *Unequal treatment: confronting racial and ethnic disparities in health.* Washington, DC, 2002, National Academies Press.

Kirkpatrick C: Safety first. The JCAHO introduces new patient safety goals. *Nurse Week* 2(4):18-20, 2003.

Knight W: Managed care: what it is and how it works, Gaithersburg, Md, 1998, Aspen.

Kohn L, Corrigan J, Donaldson M, editors: *To err is human: building a safer health system.* Washington, DC, 1999, National Academies Press.

Koop CE: An agenda for public health, *J Public Health Policy* 10:7, 1989.

Korczyk S, Witte H: *The complete idiot's guide to managed health care,* New York, 1998, Alpha Books.

Laschinger HK, Almost J, Tuer-Hodes D: Workplace empowerment and magnet hospital characteristics. *J Nurs Admin* 33(7):410-420, 2003.

Laschinger HK, Finegan J: Using empowerment to build trust and respect n the workplace: a strategy for addressing the nursing shortage. *Nurs Econ* 23(1):6-17, 2005.

Levy D, editor: *2002 state by state guide to managed care law,* Gaithersburg, Md, 2002, Aspen.

Maddox P, Wakefield M, Bull, J: Patient safety and the need for professional and educational change. *Nurs Outlook* 49(1):8-13, 2001.

Mariner W: State regulation of managed care and the Employer Retirement Income Security Act, *N Engl J Med* 335(26):1986, 1996.

McCarthy M: U.S. government releases nursing home report cards. *Lancet* 360(9346):1670, 2002.

Meier B: For-profit care's human cost: Tenet Health Care to settle some old accounts, *New York Times,* August 8, 1997.

Michael JE: What home healthcare nurses should know about fraud and abuse. *Home Healthcare Nurse* 21(8):523-530, 2003.

Mohr W: Dirty hands: the underside of marketplace health care, *Adv Nurs Sci* 19(1):28, 1996.

Mohr W: Outcomes of corporate greed, *Image* 29(1):39, 1997.

National Health Care Anti-Fraud Association (NHCAA): *Health care fraud: a serious and costly reality for all Americans.* The Author, http://www.nhcaa.org/pdf/all_about_hcf. pdf.

O'Malley C: Quality measurement for health systems: accreditation and report cards, *Am J Health Syst Pharm* 54(7):1528, 1997.

O'Neil E, Pew Health Professions Commission: *Recreating health professional practice for a new century,* San Francisco, 1998, Pew Health Professions Commission.

Page A, editor: *Keeping patients safe: transforming the work environment of nurses.* Washington, DC, 2004, Institute of Medicine of the National Academies Press.

Pear R: House passes bill to expand rights on medical care, *New York Times,* October 8, 1999a.

Pear R: Insurers ask government to extend health plans, *New York Times,* May 23, 1999b.

Perla L: The future roles of nurses. *J Nurse Staff Dev* 18(4):194-197, 2002.

Pickett G, Hanlon JJ: *Public health administration and practice,* ed 9, St. Louis, 1990, Mosby.

Purdon T: California to set level of staffing for nursing care, *New York Times,* October 12, 1999.

Robert Wood Johnson Foundation: *State health care reform: looking back toward the future,* Princeton, NJ, 1997, The Author.

Shindul-Rothschild J, Berry D, Long-Middleton E: Where have all the nurses gone? Final results of our patient care survey, *Am J Nurs* 96(11):25, 1996.

Skocpol T: From social security to health security? *J Health Polit Policy Law* 19:239, 1994.

Snowden F: National benchmarking is on the way, *Inside Case Manage* 5(9):2, 1998.

Stanton TH: Fraud and abuse enforcement in Medicare: finding middle ground. *Health Affairs* 20(4):28-38, 2001.

Taylor M: Storm warning. *Modern Healthcare* 33(46):26-30, 2003.

The President's Advisory Commission on Consumer Protection and Quality in the Health Care Industry: *Quality first: better health care for all Americans*, Washington, DC, 1999, US Government Printing Office.

Thomas E et al: Costs of medical injuries in Utah and Colorado. *Inquiry* 36:255-264, 1999.

Turner S: *The nurse's guide to managed care,* Gaithersburg, Md, 1999, Aspen.

US Census Bureau: *Statistical abstract of the United States,* Washington, DC, 1996, US Government Printing Office.

US Department of Health and Human Services: *Healthy People 2010,* Washington, DC, 2000, US Government Printing Office.

US House of Representatives: *Deceit that sickens America: health care fraud and its innocent victims.* Hearings before the Subcommittee on Crime and Criminal Justice of the Committee on the Judiciary House of Representatives, One Hundred and Third Congress, Second Session, Washington, DC, 1994, US Government Printing Office.

Wagner E, Austin B, Von Korff M: Organizing care for patients with chronic illness. *Milbank Q* 74(4):511-542, 1996.

Economics of Health Care

Carrie Morgan

MEDIA RESOURCES

Additional Material for Study, Review, and Further Exploration

evolve Website at http://evolve.elsevier.com/Nies

❖ Quiz ❖ Case Studies ❖ Content Updates ❖ Glossary ❖ WebLinks

OBJECTIVES

Upon completion of this chapter, the reader will be able to do the following:

1. Discuss factors that influence the cost of health care.
2. Identify terms used in the financing of health care.
3. Discuss public financing of health care.
4. Discuss private financing of health care.
5. Discuss health insurance plans.
6. Describe trends in health care financing.
7. Describe the effects of economics on health care access.
8. Identify the future of health care economics.

KEY TERMS

access
actuarial classification
adverse selection
ambulatory care
capitated reimbursement
carrier
carve-out service
co-insurance
co-payment
cost containment

cost shifting
current procedural
  terminology (CPT
  codes)
deductible
diagnosis-related group (DRG)
effectiveness
flexible spending account
gatekeeper
health care provider

health insurance plan
indemnity plan
health maintenance
  organization (HMO)
managed care plan
managed care groups
mandate
Medicaid
Medicare
Medigap insurance

out-of-pocket expenses
outcome
preferred provider
  organization (PPO)
premium
primary care provider
prospective payment
  system

CHAPTER OUTLINE

FACTORS INFLUENCING HEALTH CARE COSTS
  Historical Perspective
  Use of Health Care
  Lack of Preventive Care
  Lifestyle/Health Behaviors
  Societal Beliefs
  Technological Advances
  Aging of Society
  Pharmaceuticals
  Shift to For-Profit

PUBLIC FINANCING OF HEALTH CARE
  Medicare
  Medicaid
  Effect of Medicare and Medicaid on Health Economics
  Governmental Grants

PHILANTHROPIC FINANCING OF HEALTH CARE

HEALTH INSURANCE PLANS
  Historical Perspective
  Types of Health Care Plans
  Reimbursement Mechanisms of Insurance Plans
  Covered Services
  National Health Insurance

ACCESS TO HEALTH CARE
  Universal Coverage

COST CONTAINMENT
  Historical Perspective of Cost Containment
  Current Trends in Cost Containment

CARING FOR THE UNINSURED
  Historical Perspective
  Societal Perceptions
  Ethical Dilemmas

TRENDS IN HEALTH FINANCING
Cost Sharing
Health Care Alliances
Self-Insurance
Flexible Spending Accounts
Health Promotion/Disease Prevention

ROLES OF THE COMMUNITY HEALTH NURSE
IN THE ECONOMICS OF HEALTH CARE
Researcher
Educator
Provider of Care
Advocate

Economics represents the science of allocation of resources. Resources are commonly known as goods or services, for example, health care services. Economics affects all aspects of health care. Nurses have traditionally avoided the arena of health care economics, preferring to focus on the actual, direct care of the client. So strong is the feeling of social justice that some nurses express a reluctance to be informed of the individual client's health care financing source for fear that this knowledge will influence their care. Community health nurses who deal with the medically underserved have had more experience in this area. However, even these nurses may have only rudimentary knowledge.

Health care costs continue to rise and consume a greater percentage of our nation's resources. Nursing can no longer ignore the intricacies of health care financing. The health of individuals, families, and aggregates are influenced by economics. Economically disadvantaged individuals who have difficulty obtaining the basics, such as food and shelter, are less likely to have access to health care. Financing for health promotion/disease prevention is limited.

This chapter focuses on the economics of health care. It specifically discusses factors that influence health care costs, terminology of health care financing, and future trends of health care economics. This chapter also addresses the future of health care financing. Table 10-1 presents terms and definitions that are important to the discussion of these topics.

FACTORS INFLUENCING HEALTH CARE COSTS

Historical Perspective
Until the 1930s, the predominant method of health care financing in the United States was private payment. **Health care providers** charged a fee for the services they rendered, and the patient paid these **out-of-pocket expenses.** The price of the service was under the control of the provider and generally represented the cost of providing that service. A certain amount of "charity" services was expected. The assumption was that those who could pay would pay and those who couldn't pay should receive care and pay what they could.

The following types of hospitals existed:
1. Public hospitals, which received public funds and served the health care needs of the entire population regardless of ability to pay
2. Private hospitals, which cared mainly for those whose ability to pay was greater than the general population

3. For-profit hospitals, which were limited in number, received funds from investors, and cared for those who could definitely pay

This system worked well as long as the number of those who could pay outnumbered those who could not. During the Great Depression, with more than 25% of the population out of work, the number of those capable of financing the health care system was greatly reduced. Public financing of health care was limited. Hospitals and physicians went bankrupt because they were no longer able to collect fees.

In 1929, Texas school teachers negotiated a prepaid health provision contract with Baylor Hospital. The teachers paid a sum of money each month, which guaranteed them access to health care through Baylor Hospital. The concept of insurance for health care proved extremely successful for Baylor Hospital. Other hospitals began to develop and enter into these types of insurance plans.

Health insurance, or the idea of paying a small fee for guaranteed health care, appealed to the public. During World War II, faced with a limited workforce and government restrictions on wages, employers began to see health insurance as a means of supplementing their workers' benefits without granting a wage increase. Workers viewed health insurance as freedom from fear that illness would impoverish them. Societal concerns were mainly focused on sick care and acquisitions of curative therapies whenever needed. Health care providers envisioned guaranteed payment for their services (Higgins, 1997). These types of insurance plans were indemnity plans.

To extend this same "insurance" to the general population, the Social Security Act of 1935 was amended in 1965 to create Medicare and Medicaid. Medicare provided indemnity insurance to those over the age of 65, and Medicaid, a state-administered health insurance plan, provided a health care payer source for the poor and the disabled.

As a result of these health care resources, the majority of the population was protected by indemnity health care insurances from various sources. Indemnity plans lacked an incentive for limitation of use and little or no provisions for health promotion. The emphasis was placed on illness care, providers received a fee only when a service was rendered, and all costs of services were reimbursed. Insulated from rising health care costs, health care consumers demanded complex and technologically advanced services whenever illness struck. These demands for costly services represented the major driving force in rising health care costs.

TABLE 10-1   Terminology Used In Health Care Financing

The financing of health care has given rise to new terminology. Nurses, as providers of care and consumers of services, need to be knowledgeable about these terms to increase their understanding of health care financing. These terms are in bold within the chapter.

Terms Pertaining to Consumers

Access: Ability to obtain health care services in a timely manner, at a reasonable cost, by a qualified practitioner, and at an accessible location.

Carve-out service: A service (i.e., mental health care) provided within a standard benefit package, but delivered exclusively by a designated provider or group.

Charges: The posted prices of provider services.

Coinsurance: Cost sharing required by a health plan whereby the individual is responsible for a set percentage of the charge for each service.

Copayment: Cost sharing required by the health plan whereby the individual must pay a fixed dollar amount for each service.

Deductible: Cost sharing whereby the individual pays a specified amount before the health plan pays for covered services.

Fee schedule: List of predetermined payment rates for medical services.

Flexible spending account (FSA): A mechanism by which an employee may pay for uncovered health care expenses through payroll deductions.

Gatekeeper: Person in a MCO who decides whether a patient will be referred for specialty care. Doctors, nurses, NPs, and PAs function as gatekeepers.

Health care provider: An individual or institution that provides medical services (e.g., physicians, hospitals, or laboratories).

Health plan: A health insurance plan that pays a predetermined amount for covered services.

Indemnity plan: A health plan that pays covered services on a fee-for-service basis.

Health maintenance organization (HMO): A managed care plan that acts as an insurer and sometimes a provider for a fixed prepaid premium. HMOs usually employ physicians.

Managed care plan: A health plan that uses financial incentives to encourage enrollees to use selected providers who have contracted with the plan.

Medicaid: Joint federal- and state-funded programs that provide health care services for low-income people.

Medicare: A health insurance program for people over 65 years of age, those who are disabled, and sufferers of end-stage renal disease.

Medicare+Choice: Medicare recipients may choose to enroll in a coordinated care plan, private fee-for-service, or medical savings account plan created by the Balanced Budget Act of 1997.

Medigap insurance: Privately purchased individual or group health insurance plan designed to supplement Medicare coverage.

Out-of-pocket expenses: Payment made by the individual for medical services.

Point of service (POS): A managed care plan that combines prepaid and fee-for-service plans. Enrollees may choose to use the services of an uncontracted provider by paying an increased copayment.

Portability: An individual changing jobs is guaranteed coverage with the new employer without a waiting period or having to meet additional deductible requirements.

Preferred provider organization (PPO): A health plan that contracts with providers to furnish services to the enrollees of the plan. Usually no insurance copayment is required.

Premium: Amount paid periodically to purchase health insurance benefits.

Primary care provider: A generalist physician, typically family physicians, internists, gynecologists, and pediatricians, who provides comprehensive medical services.

Terms Pertaining to Providers

Ambulatory care: Medical services provided on an outpatient basis in a hospital or clinic setting.

Capitation: Payment mechanism that pays health care providers a fixed amount per enrollee to cover a defined set of services over a specified time period regardless of actual services provided.

Care management: Process used to improve quality of care by analyzing variations in and outcomes for current practice in the care of specific health conditions.

Cost containment: Reduction of inefficiencies in the consumption, allocation, or production of health care services.

Customary charge: Physician payment based on a median charge for a given service within a 12-month period.

Diagnosis-related group (DRG): A system of payment classification for inpatient hospital services based on the principal diagnosis, procedure, age and gender of the patient, and complications.

Effectiveness: Net health benefit provided by a medical service or technology for a typical patient in community practice.

Fully capitated: A stipulated dollar amount established to cover the cost of all health care services delivered for a person.

Maximum allowable costs: Specified cost level established by the health plan.

Outcome: The consequences of a medical intervention on a patient.

Physician's current procedural terminology (CPT) codes: A list of codes for medical services and procedures performed by physicians and other health care providers that has become the health care industry's standard for reporting physician procedures and services.

Practice guidelines: An explicit statement of what is known and believed about the benefits, risks and costs of particular courses of medical action intended to assit decisions made by practitioners, patients, and others about appropriate health care for specific and clinical conditions.

Utilization review: A formal prospective, concurrent, or retrospective assessment of the medical necessity, efficiency, and appropriateness of health care services.

Terms Pertaining to Third-Party Payers

Actuarial classification: Classification of enrollees that is determined by use of the mathematics of insurance, including probabilities to ensure adequacy of the premium to provide future payment.

Administrative costs: Costs that the insurer incurs for utilization review, marketing, medical underwriting, agents' commissions, premium collection, claims processing, insurer profit, quality assurance activities, medical libraries, and risk management.

Adverse selection: Larger proportion of people with poorer health status enroll in specific plans or options. Plans that enroll a subpopulation with lower-than-average costs are favorably selected.

Capital cost: Depreciation, interest, leases and rentals, taxes, and insurance on tangible assets.

Carrier: An organization that contracts with the HCFA to administer claims processing and make Medicare payments to health care providers.

Cost contract: Arrangement between a managed health care plan and the HCFA for reimbursement of the costs of services provided.

Cost shifting: The cost of uncompensated care is passed on to the insured, resulting in higher costs for those with insurance coverage.

Mandate: A state or federal statute or regulation that requires coverage for certain health services.

Risk assessment: Statistical method used to estimate claims costs of enrollees.

The spiraling health care costs were fueled by the presence of technologic advances, society's sense of entitlement to these therapies, a guaranteed payer, and the prevailing medical orientation toward curative measures. National health care expenditures in 1996 were 38.4 times that of expenditures in 1960. The biggest raise of 26 times occurred between 1960 and 1990 (Centers for Medicare and Medicaid Services [CMMS] 2003).

By the 1980s, the first efforts to curtail these costs were made by the federal government. Medicare hospital reimbursement was based on a **prospective payment system.** Hospital reimbursement would be based on a classification system that identified costs according to diagnosis and client characteristics. The age of managed care, the prevailing method of health care financing for the twentieth century, had begun. The effort to manage rising health care costs has taken many different forms.

Use of Health Care

According to economic principles, use is influenced by the existence of a desirable product, the demand for the product, and the availability of financial funding for a product. Health care is the product, and the demand for this product increases when funding is available. This is the phenomenon that has occurred in the United States. In 2002, health care expenditures represented 14.9% of the gross domestic product. This is twice as much as in other industrialized nations.

In an attempt to reduce unnecessary utilization, insurance plans began to limit coverage for certain services and people. Restrictions on use of health care, such as the establishment of a "gatekeeper" that requires preauthorization, limited coverage for preexisting illnesses, and exclusion of those participants whose use was deemed exorbitant, have been instituted. These moves have sparked resentment and resistance by the general public. Protests and legal torts involving denied services began to emerge.

These restrictions have had limited success in curbing health care costs. In 2002, health care expenditures were $1.5 trillion, or a 9.3% increase from 2000. Expenses for health care vary according to types of care and sources of funding (Table 10-2). In 1960, out-of-pocket expenditure for physicians' fees was 61.6% compared to 7.2% governmental expenditure for these fees. In 2002, the out-of-pocket expenditure for physicians' fees was 10.1%, and governmental expenditure had risen to 33.8%.

Lack of Preventive Care

Until recently, little to no incentive has existed to prevent illness or promote health. Curative measures have traditionally been the focus of health care. Soaring health care costs and an improved knowledge of health have heightened the public's awareness of their obligation to assume responsibility for their health by amending many unhealthy behaviors. As a result, more people are demanding preventive health care from the provider and their health care contractors. Public financing of health care has increased funding for such preventive care as screening tests, periodic examinations, and immunizations. Use of these preventive health services has increased, but disparities exist relating to ethnic background and economic status (National Center for Health Statistics [NCHS], 2004). There continues to be a wide gap between the amount of funding available for preventive treatment modalities and funding for curative treatments. Traditionally funding for preventive measures such as immunization, communicable disease investigation, and health education was provided to the communities through grants awarded based on requests. Awards for these funds is politically influenced.

Lifestyle and Health Behaviors

A healthy lifestyle does not ensure everlasting good health. However, the leading causes of death and illness can be positively affected by changes in lifestyle. Recent studies have found that a low-fat diet, exercise, and stress reduction will curtail the development of cardiovascular disease, the leading cause of death. Smoking cessation reduces the incidence of lung cancer. Seat belt use reduces the severity of injuries incurred during moving vehicle accidents. Effective treatment of illness must be coupled with a change in lifestyle. In the near future, access to expensive and unique medical treatment will probably be influenced less by the patient's ability to pay and more by the person's commitment to compulsory lifestyle changes. Legislation has levied "sin taxes" on products whose use has been associated with chronic illnesses. The Commonwealth of Kentucky has the highest rate of adult smoking in the country. To offset the cost of Medicaid care, the legislature has levied a $0.30 per package cigarette tax. This income will be utilized to fund care for, prevention of, and research on chronic illness (Commonwealth of Kentucky Department of Revenue, 2005).

Old movies dramatize the change in lifestyle that has taken place in the past 30 years. The current "smoke-free" environment appears shockingly contrasted to the nonchalant attitude toward smoking that was pervasive 30 years ago. The advent of the Health Belief Model and Pender's Health Prevention Model has given rise to numerous studies into methods of achieving lifestyle changes. The total effects of these changes are just now being seen. Meanwhile, the health care system must continue to contend with the results of years of unhealthy lifestyles.

Health care funding has changed to provide funding for preventive services. Some insurance plans provide monetary incentives, such as reduction in insurance premiums, for those who participate in behavioral changes toward a healthier lifestyle. Medicare will pay for some screening procedures performed for specific persons at specified times (CMMS, 2003). Funding for behavioral changes is limited, inadequate, or unavailable. Weight loss programs, support groups for smoking cessation, or participation in relaxation programs are not considered reimbursable treatment regimens. Pharmaceutical interventions are reimbursable.

TABLE 10-2   Personal Health Care Expenditures, According to Type of Expenditure and Source of Funds: United States, Selected Years 1960-2002

[Data are compiled from various sources by the Centers for Medicare and Medicaid Services]

Type of personal health care expenditures and source of funds

	1960	1970	1980	1990	1995	1999	2000	2001	2002
Amount per capita	$126	$301	$931	$2,398	$3,233	$3,835	$4,049	$4,352	$4,695
Amount in billions									
All personal health care expenditures	$23.4	$63.2	$214.6	$609.4	$865.7	$1,065.0	$1,135.3	$1,231.4	$1,340.2
Percent distribution									
All sources of funds	100.0	100.0	100.0	100.0	100.0	100.0	100.0	100.0	100.0
Out-of-pocket payments	55.2	39.7	27.1	22.5	16.9	17.3	17.0	16.3	15.9
Private health insurance	21.4	22.3	28.3	33.4	33.4	34.4	35.1	35.5	35.8
Other private funds	2.0	2.8	4.3	5.0	5.1	5.3	4.8	4.4	4.2
Government	21.4	35.2	40.3	39.0	44.6	43.0	43.1	43.8	44.2
Federal	8.7	22.9	29.3	28.6	34.1	32.6	32.8	33.5	33.6
State and local	12.6	12.3	11.1	10.5	10.5	10.3	10.4	10.4	10.6
Amount in billions									
Hospital care expenditures	$9.2	$27.6	$101.5	$253.9	$343.6	$393.5	$413.2	$444.3	$486.5
Percent distribution									
All sources of funds	100.0	100.0	100.0	100.0	100.0	100.0	100.0	100.0	100.0
Out-of-pocket payments	0.8	9.1	5.2	4.4	3.1	3.2	3.1	2.9	3.0
Private health insurance	35.8	32.6	35.6	38.3	32.5	32.5	33.3	33.6	33.9
Other private funds	1.2	3.3	4.9	4.1	4.3	5.2	4.9	4.3	4.2
Government	42.2	55.1	54.3	53.2	60.1	59.1	58.8	59.1	58.9
Medicaid	9.6	10.4	10.9	15.9	16.8	16.9	16.9	17.1	
Medicare	19.4	26.0	26.7	31.2	31.2	30.7	30.9	30.7	
Amount in billions									
Physician services expenditures	$5.4	$14.0	$47.1	$157.5	$220.5	$270.9	$290.3	$315.1	$339.5
Percent distribution									
All sources of funds	100.0	100.0	100.0	100.0	100.0	100.0	100.0	100.0	100.0
Out-of-pocket payments	61.6	46.1	30.2	19.3	11.9	11.7	11.1	10.5	10.1
Private health insurance	29.8	30.1	35.3	43.0	48.5	47.6	48.5	48.7	49.1
Other private funds	1.4	1.6	3.9	7.2	8.0	8.3	7.3	7.1	6.9
Government	7.2	22.2	30.5	30.6	31.6	32.4	33.1	33.8	33.8
Medicaid		4.6	5.2	4.5	6.7	6.5	6.6	6.9	7.2
Medicare	11.8	17.4	19.1	19.0	20.1	20.4	20.6	20.3	
Amount in billions									
Nursing home expenditures	$0.8	$4.2	$17.7	$52.7	$74.6	$89.6	$93.8	$99.1	$103.2
Percent distribution									
All sources of funds	100.0	100.0	100.0	100.0	100.0	100.0	100.0	100.0	100.0
Out-of-pocket payments	77.9	53.6	40.0	37.5	26.9	28.1	27.9	26.9	25.1
Private health insurance	0.0	0.2	1.2	5.8	7.5	8.4	7.8	7.7	7.5
Other private funds	6.3	4.9	4.5	7.5	6.4	5.0	4.4	3.8	3.4
Government	15.7	41.2	54.2	49.2	59.1	58.5	59.8	61.7	64.0
Medicaid	22.3	50.2	43.9	47.5	46.7	47.5	47.3	49.3	
Medicare	3.4	1.7	3.2	9.3	9.7	10.1	12.1	12.5	
Amount in billions									
Prescription drug expenditures	$2.7	$5.5	$12.0	$40.3	$60.8	$104.4	$121.5	$140.8	$162.4
Percent distribution									
All sources of funds	100.0	100.0	100.0	100.0	100.0	100.0	100.0	100.0	100.0
Out-of-pocket payments	96.0	82.4	69.4	59.1	42.7	32.9	31.5	30.2	29.9
Private health insurance	1.3	8.8	16.7	24.4	37.1	45.8	46.5	47.5	47.8
Government	2.7	8.8	13.9	16.6	20.1	21.3	21.9	22.4	22.3
Medicaid		7.6	11.7	12.6	16.0	16.5	17.1	17.5	17.5
Medicare				0.5	1.3	2.0	1.9	1.7	1.6
Amount in billions									
All other personal health care expenditures	$5.3	$11.9	$36.3	$104.9	$166.2	$206.6	$216.5	$232.0	$248.6
Percent distribution									
All sources of funds	100.0	100.0	100.0	100.0	100.0	100.0	100.0	100.0	100.0
Out-of-pocket payments	84.2	78.6	64.3	49.6	38.3	39.1	38.4	36.7	35.8
Private health insurance	1.6	3.3	15.5	24.7	25.2	26.3	26.1	25.8	25.0
Other private funds	4.2	3.6	4.3	4.7	4.3	4.2	4.0	3.7	3.5

Continued

TABLE 10-2   Personal Health Care Expenditures, According to Type of Expenditure and Source of Funds: United States, Selected Years 1960-2002 (cont'd)

	1960	1970	1980	1990	1995	1999	2000	2001	2002
Government	10.1	14.5	16.0	20.9	32.2	30.4	31.5	33.8	35.6
Medicaid	3.3	3.9	6.5	12.5	14.9	15.7	16.9	18.3	
Medicare	1.1	3.8	7.1	13.1	8.9	9.0	9.7	10.2	

From Centers for Medicare and Medicaid Services, Office of the Actuary: National health accounts, National health expenditures, 2002, The Author, http://www.cms.hhs.gov/statistics/nhe.

Societal Beliefs

With the advent of such wonders as penicillin, society began to believe that the eradication of disease was just a few years away. More and more resources were dedicated to this illusive search. Armed with the belief that disease would soon be eliminated, societal interest in preventive care was limited. The general belief was that more money available for health care meant better health care and the greater likelihood that illness would be cured.

Health care professionals also were slow to embrace preventive care. Most efforts were directed toward curing illness. With what seemed to be an unending source of financing for curative care, illness prevention seemed counterproductive.

As health care costs accelerated at an alarming rate and technological advances did not keep up with the increase in illnesses, the health of society had to become a collaborative effort between society itself and the health care industry. Although United States spends more money on health care than any other industrialized country, it ranks seventh in health status when compared with other countries (NCHS, 2004). In other countries, workers are often paid to take "holiday" time for stress reduction. Health care insurance was meant to provide protection from financial disaster resulting from a serious illness. As health care insurance increased coverage of the services provided, society considered it to represent a source of financial protection for an individual's entire health. Society views insurance as an economic shield protecting against all disease and illness. The belief in cure rather than prevention, combined with this financial safety net, encouraged society to become a passive participant in health care. The feeling "I don't have to worry, I have insurance" became the pervasive societal thought (Sloan, 2004).

This belief that the client remains a passive participant in health care has become outmoded. People still expect the health care industry to cure them when they are ill, but there is an increase in preventive care interest. Interest in health education, health promotion, and behavioral changes has increased. Resistance to behavior change remains high among minorities and those of lower socioeconomic status and lower education levels (NCHS, 2003). Funding for these preventive measures remains limited.

Technological Advances

Modern society has come to expect miraculous technological advances. In response to this demand, and supplied with funding from various sources, technological advances have become too numerous to mention. The United States leads the world in laboratory and clinical research. People come from all over the world for education and to train in leading American centers for excellence (Weintraub and Shine, 2004). Available technological advances can save the lives of people who would otherwise die. These advances, although remarkable, are expensive and result in 20% of the population consuming 80% of the health care resources. In 2002, hospital stays with at least one operation on vessels of the heart performed on individuals older than 75 years increased by 170% (NCHS, 2004). As the health care dollar shrinks, these advances raise ethical questions involving health care access and rationing. The availability of these technological advances also contributes to health care use. In countries such as Canada and Germany, the latest technology, such as MRI (magnetic resonance imaging), is available only in large hospitals. In contrast, most community hospitals in the United States provide a wide variety of tertiary services, including the most current technological advances.

Availability restriction on technology has resulted in significantly reduced cost of health care; however, the delays, inconvenience, and lack of care that plague these countries would not be tolerated by the American public (Vermont Medical Roundtable, 1999).

Aging of Society

Health care expenditures increase with age. According to the 2000 U.S. Census, individuals older than 65 years constituted 12.4% of the total population. This population is expected to increase by 20% by the year 2050 (U.S. Census Bureau, 2004). The percentage of those older than 85 years will increase from the present level of 1.9% of the total population to 5% of the total population. The average Medicare spending enrollees aged 65 to 75 was $4400 in the year 2003, compared to $8500 for those 85 years and older (NCHS, 2004). The number of persons aged 20 to 64 will decrease from 58.1% to 53.4% (Figure 10-1). This means that the number of those consuming the greatest amount of health care resources will increase more rapidly than those who provide the monetary support for these resources. Per capita lifetime expenditure is $316,600. Nearly one third of life expenditures are incurred during middle age; half will be incurred during the senior years; and for those older than 85 years, one third will be incurred during the last year of life (Alemayehu and Warner, 2004).

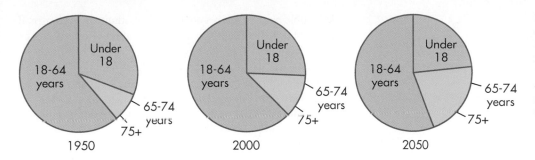

FIGURE 10-1 Percentage of population in four age-groups: United States, 1950, 2000, and 2050. (From National Center for Health Statistics: *Health, United States: 2004*, Hyattsville, Md, 2004, The Author, http://www.cdc.gov/nchs/data/hus/hus04.pdf.)

Pharmaceuticals

A relatively new phenomenon that has influenced health care economics is the utilization of drugs, both over-the-counter and prescription drugs. New drugs are improving health outcomes and quality of life. These new drugs and new uses for older drugs are curing some illnesses, preventing or delaying other chronic diseases, and hastening recovery from other illnesses. In 2003, Medicare added a pharmaceutical benefit for enrollees. The Medicare Prescription Drug and Modernization Act provides $600 toward prescription drugs for persons with $12,124 (couples $16,363) income per year. In 2006, all Medicare recipients are eligible for this prescription drug benefit (Weintraub and Shine, 2004). As with other health care services, once a funding source has been established, utilization and costs increase.

Between the years 1995 to 1996 and 2001 to 2002, physician visits or hospital outpatient visits in which five or more prescriptions were ordered increased from 4% to 7%. The largest increase was for those individuals older than 75 years, from 13% in 1995 to 1996 to 20% in 2001 to 2002 (NCHS, 2004) (Figure 10-2).

Prescriptions drug expenses increased from $2.7 million in 1960 to $162.4 million in 2002. In 1960, 96% of these expenses were paid by the individual, out of pocket. By 2002, this figure is down to 30%, with insurance and government providing reimbursement for 47.8% and 22.3%, respectively. Drugs have been a required service of Medicaid since its beginning, which may explain why it covers 17.5% of the government's cost (see Table 10-2).

Shift to For-Profit

The final contributor to the increase in health care costs is a national shift from non-profit health care to for-profit health care. This has given rise to the new phrase "health care industry." More and more large-profit organizations are taking over smaller community organizations. As the emphasis is on profit, mechanisms of achieving higher reimbursement have been developed.

The prospective reimbursement rates are based on diagnoses and patient characteristics. These are represented by codes, following the International Classification and Diagnosis, 9th edition, or ICD-9. Physician services are coded according to **current procedural terminology (CPT)** codes. Coding of the patient's illness can result in an increase in reimbursement. Specialists in coding are employed by both third-party payers and service providers. Third-party payers' code specialists

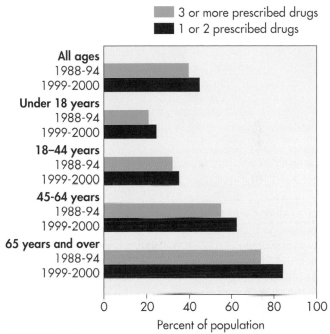

3 or more prescribed drugs
1 or 2 prescribed drugs

FIGURE 10-2 Percentage of persons reporting prescription drug use in the past month by age: United States, 1988-1994 and 1999-2000. (From National Center for Health Statistics: *Health, United States, 2004*, Hyattsville, Md, 2004, The Author, Ahttp://www.cdc.gov/nchs/data/hus/hus04.pdf.)

scrutinize the claims for the appropriated data to support the code. Service provider code specialists are paid to ensure that the code is as accurate as possible to obtain the higher reimbursement. The appropriateness of services is based on the diagnosis code. For example, spirometry is appropriate (reimbursable) when the patient's diagnosis code indicates a variety of pulmonary and nonpulmonary conditions. Specialists in coding can quickly identify these codes, thus increasing payment for services. This has changed health care practices to the utilization of services that are low in costs and higher in reimbursement. High-cost services are limited or not offered.

Insurance plans have begun to target only the healthiest persons as enrollees. Known as "cherry picking," this practice by insurance plans excludes coverage of conditions such as chronic illnesses or limits coverage for services related to these conditions. **Carve-out services** might be designated for those who need these services the least (Schur, Berg, and Yegian, 2004).

BOX 1O-1 Medicare Fraud

What is fraud?
- ➤ Billing Medicare for services not received
- ➤ Billing Medicare for services other than those received
- ➤ Use of another's Medicare card to obtain services

Be suspicious if provider tells you:
- ➤ Medicare wants you to have this service
- ➤ They know how to get Medicare to pay for service
- ➤ The more services provided, the cheaper they are

Be suspicious if provider:
- ➤ Changes co-payment of Medicare-approved services
- ➤ Advertises "free" consultations to those with Medicare
- ➤ Claim they represent Medicare
- ➤ Use pressure to persuade you of need for high-priced services
- ➤ Use telemarketing as a marketing tool

Whenever you receive a Medicare payment notice, review it for errors. Make sure Medicare was not billed for services not received.

Modified from Centers for Medicare and Medicaid Services: *Medicare fraud: Detection and prevention tips,* Baltimore, no date, The Author, http://www.medicare.gov/FraudAbuse/Tips.asp.

Fraudulent claims are another source of health care cost increase. Medicare and Medicaid fraud is estimated to cost these programs millions of dollars each year. Consumers are asked to help identify fraud by closely scrutinizing their health care bills for charges for services not delivered (Box 10-1).

PUBLIC FINANCING OF HEALTH CARE

As the popularity and benefits of employer-provided insurance plans were recognized, it became evident that the health care of some segments of society was being neglected. The 1960s, with a pervasive thrust for social justice in the public and political arenas, presented the ideal opportunity for governmental participation in health care financing. In 1965, the federal government enacted the first movement toward universal health care coverage. Titles XVIII and XIX of the Social Security Act created Medicare and Medicaid, respectively.

Medicare

Medicare was intended to provide health care to the growing population of those 65 years of age or older. Medicare Part A coverage is an entitlement program, which rendered services free of charge to people 65 years of age and older and people who are disabled or suffer from end-stage renal disease. Services covered by Medicare Part A include inpatient care in hospitals and skilled nursing facilities (not unskilled or long-term care). It also covers hospice care and some home health care. In 2002, 41 million persons were enrolled in Medicare Part A. Of the $266 billion expenditures of Medicare, 57% was for hospitalization and 3% was for home health services. Although this is an entitlement program, the enrollee must pay a **deductible** for health services. The

deductible paid by the beneficiary when admitted as a hospital inpatient was $912 in 2005, an increase of $36 from the year's $876 deductible. The Part A deductible is the beneficiary's only cost for up to 60 days of Medicare-covered inpatient hospital care in a benefit period. Beneficiaries must pay an additional $228 per day for Days 61 through 90 in 2005, and $456 per day for hospital stays beyond the 90th day in a benefit period (CMMS, 2003).

Medicare does not pay for all health care costs of enrollees. There are costs that must be paid by the individual. These costs are called "gaps" in Medicare coverage. Individuals often decide to consider buying a medigap policy to cover these gaps in Medicare coverage. For those eligible for Medicare Part A, another plan, Medicare Part B, may be purchased for a monthly fee. Medicare Part B is a type of **medigap insurance**. About 93% of Medicare's 41.8 million beneficiaries are enrolled in Part B, which helps pay for physician services, hospital outpatient care, durable medical equipment and other services, including some home health care. Participation in Medicare Part B is not compulsory. The monthly premium paid by beneficiaries enrolled in Medicare Part B, which covers physician services, outpatient hospital services, certain home health services, durable medical equipment, and other items, will be $78.20, an increase of $11.60 over the $66.60 premium in 2004 (CMMS, 2003) (Table 10-3).

Among persons 65 years old and older, 63% had Medicare and private medigap insurance, whereas 24% had Medicare alone. Within this age-group, 27% of those who are financially disadvantaged are covered by both Medicare and Medicaid (NCHS, 2004).

Medicaid

Medicaid provides universal health care coverage for the indigent and children. A joint state and federal venture, eligibility to this program is dependent on the size and income of the family. The created purpose of this program is support for the health care needs of the medically indigent. Priority participation is given to children, pregnant women, and the disabled.

The federal government sets baseline eligibility requirements. State governments who wish to provide care to more of its citizens through this program can lower the eligibility requirements. For example, the federal government may set 100% of poverty as an eligibility requirement, but Kentucky may set the requirement as 110% of poverty. This means that a family living in Kentucky can have an income slightly above the federal standard and still qualify for Medicaid. The federal government **mandates** covered services, but state governments may provide more services.

In 2001, the average expenditure per eligible recipient of Medicaid was $4560. Amount varies from state to state with the lowest expenditure of $2405 in California to $8904 in New York (CMMS, 2003).

Children under the age of 12 years are more likely to be covered by Medicaid than persons belonging to other age-groups. Four out of 10 financially disadvantaged persons under the age of 65 years are covered by Medicaid (see Table 10-2).

TABLE 10-3   Medicare Benefits: 2004

	ORIGINAL MEDICARE	STERLING LIFE INSURANCE COMPANY (FORMERLY MEDICARE ADVANCE)
Premium	Medicare Part B: $66.60/mo	Medicare Part B: $66.60/mo plus $78 per month
Inpatient care	Days 1-60: Initial deductible $876	Days 1-5: $150/day
	Days 61-90: $219/day	Days 6-365: $0/day
	Days 91-150: $438	
Skilled nursing facility	Following 3 days in hospital	Following 3 days in hospital
	Day 1-20: $0/day	Days 1-10: $0/day
	Day 21-100: 109.5/day	Days 11-100: $25/day
	100-day limit	100-day limit
Home health	No co-payment for covered visits	25% of costs for covered visits
Doctor's office visits	20% of approved amounts	$15 for primary care physician
		$35 for specialist visit
Ambulance services	20% of approved amounts	$100 for approved charges
Preventive services		
Bone mass measurements	20% of approved amounts	No co-payment if approved
Colorectal screening	20% of approved amounts	No co-payment if approved
Immunizations	No co-payment for flu/pneumonia	No co-payment if approved
	20% of approved amounts	
Mammograms	20% of approved amounts	No co-payment if approved
Pap smear/pelvic examination	No co-payment pap smear	No co-payment if approved
		20% of approved amount for pelvic examination
Prostate cancer screening	No co-payment for lab service	No co-payment if approved
	20% of approved amount for related service	
Routine physical examinations	$0	No co-payment for 1 year
Health/wellness education	$0	Covered for nursing hotline/disease management

Modified from Centers for Medicare and Medicaid Services: *Health care directory for people with Medicare*, Baltimore, 2003, The Author, http://www.medicare.gov/Library/PDFNavigation/ PDFInterim.asp?Language=English&Type=Pub&PubID=02231.

Effect of Medicare and Medicaid on Health Care Economics

The enactment of Medicare and Medicaid created an unprecedented demand for services. By the end of the first 5 years, Medicare costs had more than doubled the original estimates (Vermont Medical Roundtable, 1999). The cost-based reimbursement used by these programs established a new source of funding that dramatically influenced hospital use. By 1975, the average length of stay for Medicare patients was twice that of their younger insured counterparts (Turner, 1999). Medicare reimbursement rates generally became the standard for all insurance **carriers.**

Government funding of health care has admirably provided more people with access to high quality care who otherwise could not afford it, but the cost of this care amounts to $350 billion dollars per year. Approximately 47% of the total cost of health care in the United States is paid by the government, but Medicare and Medicaid recipients represent less than 40% of the population. Persons under the age of 65 years and covered by Medicaid are twice as likely to be hospitalized as those with private insurance (NCHS, 2004).

Governmental Grants

The bulk of health promotion and disease preventive measures have long been limited to the arena of public health care. Funding for these foundation public health services is provided from the government on different levels related to priorities such as the 2010 Health Objectives. These health grants are administered through the public health department at each govenmental level or community. The federal government provided funding to the states through "block grants." These are amounts of money given to the states to provide care to the populace based on a variety of sources. There are specific restrictions as to how these monies can be spent including limitations in the populace that receive the services and what types of programs are to be funded. The states use these monies to provide for the care of the public within these restrictions. Depending on the health needs of the state, these monies may be spent to provide prenatal care for the underinsured or uninsured, smoking cessation education, or child safety. The state may set aside a specific amount of money to fund certain types of health care. Even the local government may make funds available for a specific need of the members of the community.

To ensure that the needs of the community are being addressed, health care providers and programs may be required to compete for these funds. Submission of proposals, grant applications, or requests must be submitted, reviewed, and prioritized. Allocation of funds are provided based on need and program merit. This type of funding is directed toward the populace in general and not to specific individuals. When the funding is no longer provided, the programs cease, which can results in lack of continuity of care.

Currently, the funding priorities are closely related to the achievement of the *Healthy People 2010* objectives. Limitations on the amounts provided are related to governmental resources.

PHILANTHROPIC FINANCING OF HEALTH CARE

A limited amount of the nation's estimated $1.5 trillion health care bill is paid by philanthropic funding whose services are usually capricious and research or disease oriented. Eligibility for services through these associations is generally limited to the specific disease or population of interest, as with the American Heart Association. Few direct services are rendered, and these are awarded on individual case consideration. Ancillary health care needs such as transportation, parental housing, or wigs may be addressed. Informational and research activities constitute the majority of services provided by these types of organizations. The organizations fund many educational programs that increase awareness of specific diseases, screening procedures, and preventive measures (Chattopadhyay and Carande-Kulis, 2004).

Exceptions do exist, and national organizations such as the Shriners operate health care institutions designed to provide specialty care for a specific population group. These services and all costs related to this care, including transportation, are provided to the eligible person free of charge. The only requirement for this care is sponsorship by a member of the supporting organization.

HEALTH INSURANCE PLANS

Historical Perspective

During the 1930s, in an effort to provide care and avoid bankruptcy, health care providers began to establish **health insurance plans.** One of the most recognizable of these plans is Blue Cross and Blue Shield. Those enrolled in the plan, called *enrollees,* paid a monthly fee for a guarantee of health care. Providers delivered services to the enrollees and collected payment from the health insurance plan. The insurance plan paid fees plus their administrative costs from money collected from the enrollees.

During World War II when prices and wages were frozen, industries began to offer health insurance as a fringe benefit. In 1953, as a further incentive to obtain health care coverage, money spent on health insurance was declared tax exempt. Over the years, workers' union groups began to negotiate for these benefits. With more available financial resources, the health care expenditures increased. Reimbursement based on operational costs represented a strong incentive for expansion (Higgins, 1997).

Types of Health Care Plans

This early Blue Cross and Blue Shield was an example of an **indemnity plan.** This plan paid all of the costs of covered services provided to the enrollee. The enrollee enjoyed free choice of the provider and services. Indemnity plans preserve the enrollee's right of choice and allow the person to manage his or her own health care. These plans lack incentives for cost containment. Although indemnity plans are still available, the monthly cost of enrollment has increased to exorbitant amounts, making these plans cost prohibitive. In an effort to infuse these incentives while preserving freedom of choice, mechanisms of cost sharing were introduced. These cost-sharing methods include **co-payment,** deductible amounts, and **co-insurance.** All of these represented efforts to have the enrollee share in the cost of medical care (Table 10-4).

As health care costs escalated, variations in health care insurance plans were developed. Industries, the major providers of insurance coverage, began to look for a more economical means of providing health care to their employees. In 1991, the cost of insurance was $15.40 per employee. In 2004, that cost had risen to $23.29. The largest increase was for industries that employed more than 500 workers; their costs increased 160% from 1991 to 2004 (NCHS, 2004). Large industrial giants, such as Kaiser Permanente, decided to assemble their own health care program. They built hospitals, hired physicians, and provided health care services to their employees. In an effort to market this concept, Dr. Paul Elwood coined the phrase **"health maintenance organization"** (HMO) (Higgins, 1997). HMOs were designed to provide a more comprehensive care. This type of program lacks enrollee freedom of choice. More preventive care is covered, but all care is restricted to the services rendered by the HMO. Health care providers are encouraged to reduce costs by providing only the most necessary services. This loss of choice led to a decrease in popularity of HMOs as a health care plan. The number of HMO plans declined from 643 in 1999 to 454 in 2003. Despite participants' dissatisfaction with the lack of choice and other health care provider complaints about the lack of competition, 25% of the U.S. population in 2003 was enrolled in HMOs (NCHS, 2004).

In an effort to compete with the HMO, physicians and hospitals organized the independent practice model (IPM). The IPM was a separate entity that provided services to enrollees of one insurance company. This model evolved into the **preferred provider organization** (PPO). These types of insurance plans negotiated with health care providers for services at a reduced rate in exchange for a guaranteed increase in consumers. A negotiated reimbursement rate allows the cost of the plan to be somewhat controlled. Plan enrollees are offered cost incentives for choosing health care from within the plan's network of health care providers. As they receive a specific amount of reimbursement, regardless of the rendered services, providers have an incentive to be cost-conscious in the services provided (Ginsburg, 2004).

Multistate networks or alliances are health insurance–purchasing cooperatives that establish purchasing pools responsible for negotiating health insurance arrangements for employers, employees, and state Medicaid recipients. These alliances use the sheer volume of health consumers that they represent as leverage to negotiate contracts for health care coverage. Provider membership into the alliance is voluntary but exclusive. If the provider is located in an area in which the alliance is the predominant insurance plan,

TABLE 10-4   Consumer Advantages and Disadvantages of Insurance Reimbursement Plans

TYPE	ADVANTAGES	DISADVANTAGES
Indemnity	No gatekeeper	High premiums
Fee for service	Unlimited choice of providers	Potential for overuse
	Full access to all services	No incentive for cost containment
Managed care	"Credentialed" providers promote quality assurance	
HMO	Comprehensive care	Restricted to plan provider
	Lower premium	Potential for lower quality care to maximized costs
	No deductibles or co-payment	
PPO	Greater selection of providers than with HMO	Gatekeeper
	Expedited provider reimbursement	Additional cost for out-of-plan provider
	Lower premiums	Potential for lower quality care to maximized costs
POS	More flexibility	Deductible
	Comprehensive services with plan	20%-50% co-payment for out-of-plan services
		Primary care provider referral needed for specialized care

HMO, Health maintenance organization; *POS*, point of service; *PPO*, preferred provider organization.

the provider is financially forced to join and accept the negotiated reimbursement.

Another means of providing the enrollee with choice, but at the same time allowing the plan to control prices, is a "cafeteria plan." Insurance providers may offer the enrollee or consumer a wide variety of choices. Employers may specify the amount of money that will be contributed toward health care. The consumers may then customize their health care coverage, depending on their needs and willingness to pay. By choosing the types of services they want covered and the provider of these services, consumers have some control over their own health care. Consumers assume financial responsibility for any costs that exceed the employer's contributing amount (Clark, 2003).

In 2002, 69% of those under the age of 65 years were covered by insurance, 95% of which is obtained through the workplace. Reasons for being uninsured are costs, change in employment, change in marital status, and death of spouse or parent (NCHS, 2004).

Reimbursement Mechanisms of Insurance Plans

The customary method of reimbursement has been a fee for the service rendered, or retrospective reimbursement. Calculation of the fee was based on the cost of providing the service. Included in this "umbrella" of costs were such things as salaries, supplies, equipment, building depreciation, utilities, and taxes. Cost-based reimbursement encouraged inflated prices and fraud. Physicians were encouraged to overtreat patients, and participants were encouraged to overuse the health care system. Soon, health care was costing Americans more than in any other industrialized country. The health care system needed to be reformed, but there was no clear consensus on how this was to be accomplished.

Prospective reimbursement, a concept derived from the HMO method of payment, seemed to be an effective financial alternative to cost-based reimbursement. Prospective reimbursement meant that care, no matter what the provider's cost, would be reimbursed according to a predetermined amount. The government introduced this method of reimbursement for Medicare in 1983, and an immediate savings was noted. For determination of the prospective amount, Medicare depended on the **diagnosis-related group** (DRG) to calculate the reimbursement. The amount to be paid to the provider was determined according to the client's primary and secondary diagnoses, age, gender, and complications. This amount was deemed sufficient cost for health care ascertained to be adequate for treatment. If the provider, at first limited to hospitals, could provide the treatment for less than this amount, a profit was made. If the required services cost more than this amount, then the provider took a loss (Rozzini, Sabatini, and Trabucchi, 2005).

This represented a reduction in Medicare costs but not the intended overall health care cost savings. Hospitals developed **cost shifting** as a means of supplementing the loss of Medicare funding. Private insurances reimbursement continued to be cost based. Therefore hospitals could include the loss from caring for Medicare patients to their cost. Private insurance companies were paying for the cost of providing care to their enrollees and Medicare patients. By 1985, Medicare paid $0.87 for each hospital dollar and the insurance provider paid $1.27 (Higgins, 1997).

It was not long before private health care plans followed the government's lead. In an effort to ensure appropriate reimbursement, more sophisticated methods of calculating the relative cost of health care were developed. **Actuarial classifications** ensured that adequate **premiums** were charged for the projected health care needs of those enrolled. Other means of cost control began to emerge. **Managed care groups** negotiated with health care providers to render care for a specified amount of reimbursement based on community ratings modified by group-specific demographics (Turner, 1999). Prospective reimbursement created incentives to control costs but also to undertreat and underuse the system. Soon, the public clamored for guarantees that the quality of care provided was being monitored as closely as the cost of care (Higgins, 1997) (see Table 10-4).

Covered Services

Insurance plans have always designated the types of services for which the plan would be financially responsible. When first developed, health insurance was meant to be a means of protecting an individual or family from economic catastrophe should a serious illness occur. Once an employee's fringe benefit included health insurance coverage, expanded benefit packages were developed. The scope of covered services began to increase to such things as physician's office visits, medication, and dental costs. Unions began to negotiate for these expanded covered medical services in lieu of additional wages. Health insurance began to represent a payer source for all health care needs.

When health care costs increased, the price of enrollment into the insurance plans increased. Industries began to balk at paying these higher premium rates. Workers became disgruntled when their employers passed the cost of increased rates to them. To curtail the escalating premium price, insurance companies began to limit the covered services and dictate the conditions under which these services would be covered. Sites of care delivery changed. Many treatments were required to be delivered outside the hospital, or in **ambulatory care** centers. The patient was held financially responsible for "uncovered" services. Providers were pressured to comply with these requirements. Providers began to modify the delivery of health care to accommodate for these changes (Clark, 2003). The rate of hospitalization declined, and the number of outpatient services increased. In 2002, 63% of all surgical operations in community hospitals were performed on an outpatient basis compared to 16% in 1980 (NCHS, 2004).

All of these changes resulted in conflicts among providers, patients, employers, and the insurance plans, particularly when services deemed necessary by the consumer and provider were denied insurance coverage. Disgruntled employees blamed the employer for their decrease in health care coverage. Employers looked to the insurance companies to provide health care services at a reasonable price. Insurance companies grabbled with ways to control costs. Providers searched for ways to provide needed care within the confines of the health care policy. To ensure quality control and guarantee provision of certain services, governmental involvement is required.

National Health Insurance

National health insurance is not a new concept. European countries began a social model of health insurance in the early 1900s. In 1916, President Theodore Roosevelt advocated enactment of a form of national medical coverage. President Franklin Roosevelt wanted national health insurance to be part of the Social Security Act of 1935 (Higgins, 1997). During the administration of President Lyndon Johnson, a modified form of national health insurance, Medicare and Medicaid, was instituted.

During the 1992 presidential campaign, Bill Clinton promised to reform America's health care system, ensure universal coverage, and reduce medical care costs without damaging the economy. At that time, it was felt that basic health care coverage for all individuals could be achieved over several years. The necessary changes required of the current health care system are as follows:

- Consumers will have to bear more of the costs for their own choices and accept treatment from nonphysician providers.
- Health care businesses will have to become more efficient.
- Physicians will have to practice in HMO-type organizations.
- Politicians will have to resist appeals to add benefits to the basic coverage.

Unfortunately, most Americans want a guarantee that all of the medical services that they and their families need, now and in the future, will be available no matter what the medical condition, age of the patient, job status, or ability to pay. The current system is a $1.5 trillion-per-year business, and the price tag for this type of universal coverage would be astronomical. Even with various cost containment measures, health care costs increased 7.1% in 2000, 8.5% in 2001, and 9.3% in 2002. These costs represent 14.9% of the gross national product compared to 13.2% in 1995 (NCHS, 2004).

ACCESS TO HEALTH CARE

Access to health care is a complex situation that is defined by the circumstances of the individual. The primary concern is inadequate access to health care, which leads to unnecessary illness. As stated previously, most Americans want to feel that the best possible health care will be available at any time regardless of their age, sex, race, or ability to pay. Anything that obstructs this pursuit can be considered a barrier to the access of health care.

Financial support for health care, either through private insurance coverage or participation in government programs, represents the "ticket" into the health care arena (Steinbrook, 2004). Lack of health care financing due to insurance coverage, preexisting conditions, unapproved care, or nonparticipating physicians represent the most frequent factors attributed to difficulty in obtaining care. According to the National Health Interview Survey in 2003, 20.2 million persons (7% of the population) delayed health care due to cost, and 15 million did not receive care due to cost. Adults aged 18 to 64 years old were more likely to delay or not receive care due to costs. Low levels of education and income, as well as lack of insurance were all reasons health care was delayed (NCHS, 2004).

Other impediments to health care access are physical barriers, including structural inaccessibility, lack of appropriate equipment, or inability to communicate. South Carolina State University developed a universal design for health care providers, which would render their services handicap accessible (Bailey, 2004). Some of these features include chairs for people who cannot sit, wheelchair scales, adjustable-height examination equipment, communication amplifiers, and the use of interpreter services (Ku and Flores, 2005).

Inequality in the distribution of health care services represents another type of physical barrier. Even those with insurance coverage may be unable to locate "participating" health care providers Transportation difficulty, conflict with work hours, and failure to provide services exemplify these types of physical barriers. Lack of transportation, either public or private, contributes to health care deprivation. Even when adequate transportation is available, the office hours tend to be the same as typical work hours. Opportunities to seek health care, especially preventive health care, during work hours is often discouraged by employers and sometimes forbidden. Rural areas and inner cities have been recognized as medically underserved for many years. Government incentives for increasing available medical services in these areas have not solved the problem.

Sociological barriers to health care access exist among poor and ethnic Americans. Research into the health care among the poor found that the major sociological risk factor for substandard care was lack of insurance (Steinbrook, 2004). Poor outpatient diagnosis and treatment, increased use of emergency rooms for primary care, and reluctance to hospitalize were possible explanations. Language and fear of reprisals have become important sociologic barriers. Hispanics now represent the fastest growing minority. Many of these are illegal aliens. Seeking medical attention, even during illnesses, may result in severe repercussions. Hispanics under the age of 65 are more than 1.5 times as likely as non-Hispanic persons to be uninsured. Ethnic Americans, although insured, are at risk for deprivation of services because guidelines and standards for determining the medical necessity of services are based on data derived from healthy European-American males. Application of restrictions derived from these data results in inadequate and unreliable health care for the poor and for ethnic Americans. Provision of ethnically sensitive health care is almost nonexistent (Ku and Flores, 2005).

Universal Coverage

The United States uses more of the gross national product (GNP) for health care than any other industrialized county, but it ranks only seventh in the world with regard to the health of the population. Among those younger than 65 years, 33.3% are uninsured. Hispanics are 3 times as likely to be uninsured as non-Hispanics. Those with a family income of less than $20,000 and those with less than a high school education are more likely to be uninsured compared to all other segments of the population. Of the children under 18 years of age, 12% had no health visit within the last 12 months, and 6% of these children had no usual source of health care (NCHS, 2004).

Medicare and the expanded eligibility of Medicaid have brought about national health insurance coverage for older adults, the disabled, and those, especially children, living below the poverty level. With this movement toward universal coverage, a new genre of uninsured has emerged (i.e., the working poor). Working males aged 18 to 64 years of age (21%) were nearly twice as likely as working females (11%) to have a usual source of health care. One of the main reasons for lack of insurance was cost (NCHS, 2004).

The current dilemma is how to provide affordable health care to the population at a level of care acceptable to the American public. Other countries provide their citizens with universal health care, but there are aspects of this care that are unpopular with U.S. society. Waiting several months for non-emergent treatment, lack of choice of treatment, and inaccessible or unavailable diagnostic and treatment modalities are not acceptable to most Americans. Currently, no successful solution to the problem of escalating health care costs exists.

COST CONTAINMENT

Costs have to be controlled to meet the public's demand for unlimited health care. This is known as **cost containment**. Numerous attempts to control costs have been made over the years, but none has been more than marginally successful. In 1960, health care expenditures represented 5.15% of the GNP. The federal government paid 3.3%, and the state paid 9.9% of these expenses. By 1995, health care expenses had risen to 13.4 % of the GNP, with the federal government paying 20.5% to the states' 14.9%. The rate of increase in health care cost had declined throughout the 1990s from 13.4% of the GNP in 1995 to 13.3% in 2000. Since the millennium, the rate has accelerated, with no indication of a slowdown (Centers for Medicare and Medicaid Services, 2004).

Assessment of the public perception of cost-containment strategies revealed that there is an overall lack of confidence in managed care. The general public does seem to be receptive to strategies that contain escalating health care costs. The challenge for those designing cost-containment strategies is to develop methods that balance restrictions with consumer control (Schur et al., 2004).

Historical Perspective of Cost Containment

By the late 1970s, the government realized its mistake. The political compromise necessary for passage of Medicare and Medicaid had resulted in a health care explosion. Hospitals were reimbursed at cost plus 2%, physicians received reimbursement for inflated fees, and private insurance companies were paid to process Medicare and Medicaid claims. All of these factors led to an unprecedented increase in use and escalation of health care costs (Higgins, 1997).

The first attempts at cost containment were directed at curtailing unnecessary proliferation of medical technology. Proposed health care projects had to demonstrate a community necessity or a certificate of need (CON) for additions to the current health care building or services. This information was then presented to a CON board, made up of those individuals with community and medical knowledge. Because these board members were closer to the communities, their judgment would ensure the community adequate, but not excessive, health care services. As these members were appointed, soon the political influences made them ineffective.

To further reduce use, hospital records were reviewed for the appropriateness of care provided. Admission and treatment

RESEARCH HIGHLIGHTS

The Cost of Home Care in the Prospective Payment System Based on Client Characteristics

There has been much speculation in the literature about the effect of the prospective payment system (PPS) on the home care industry but few reports of systematic investigation. The PPS was implemented in October 2000, in response to the passage of the Balanced Budget Act of 1997 in an effort to control Medicare home health expenditures. The PPS was developed to accurately predict the resource utilization (volume and type) of home health clients based on individual client characteristics identified in the admission assessment, thus encouraging the home health industry to provide more efficient, less costly care delivery. Client characteristics such as medical/nursing diagnoses, functional/clinical status, and demographics (age/sex/race/marital status) have been suggested as explanation for variations in resource utilization. A case-mix clinical model system was developed to predict variation of resource utilization based on client characteristics (clinical and functional) and intensity of service criteria. The system classifies Medicare home health clients into one of 80 mutually exclusive groups, referred to as home health resource groups.

Clearly, comprehension of client characteristics is essential for categorizing home care clients in the correct home health resource group, for allocating resources appropriately, and for implementing necessary organizational changes to accommodate clients who require variations in the amount of resources predicted by the PPS. The purpose of this study was to compare the characteristics of home health clients that resulted in a financial gain or a financial loss for one agency under the PPS with those of the interim payment system (IPS).

A secondary data analysis of 140 cases compiled by one not-for-profit, hospital-affiliated home care organization was completed. A general financial analysis of the entire 140-client sample was done using the PPS and the IPS. The PPS projections totaled $328,420, and the IPS reimbursement totaled $189,527, a projected gain of $48,893 under the PPS. If this trend continued, the agency would accumulate a gain of $586,718 over one fiscal year. The sample was then separated into cases projected to have a financial gain versus a financial loss for the agency. Of the 140 cases, 113 (80.7%) were projected to result in a gain that totaled $79,434 under the PPS when compared with the IPS. The remaining 27 cases (19.3%) were projected to result in a total loss of $30,541.

Clients for whom the agency projected a financial gain were likely to be initial certifications and were discharged within 60 days. Their home care length of stay was shorter, and they had fewer visits overall. Clients for whom the agency projected a financial loss were likely to be recertifications on admission and at the end of the 60-day episode. Their length of stay was about three weeks longer, with more visits, particularly from the skilled nursing discipline. Projected loss clients had more diagnoses associated with high-risk conditions, such as cardiovascular, orthopedic, wounds, and postoperative complications.

Prospective payment policies have the potential to alter the norms and practice patterns of home care. Home care agencies must be able to characterize accurately the clients they serve, predict the resources needed, and assign the correct home health resource group. When discrepancies exist between the projected and the actual resource utilization, investigation is necessary. Comprehension of client characteristics and the subsequent ability to adjust for the proper case mix is crucial if home care agencies are to remain financially viable under the PPS.

Livesay JL et al: Client characteristics and the cost of home care in the prospective payment system, *Public Health Nurs* 20(4):287-297, 2003.

ETHICAL Insights

Cost Containment: Whom Will You Deny?

You are the gatekeeper, meeting with others in your organization to determine what services to provide to clients. You have $400,000 to divide among four clients. Who will receive the required treatment? Who will not?
1. Child with broken leg, needs physical therapy (estimated cost: $10,000)
2. 55-year-old male requiring knee replacement surgery and physical therapy (estimated cost: $40,000)
3. 76-year-old requiring hip replacement (estimated cost: $40,000)
4. 32-year-old woman with leukemia, requiring a bone marrow transplant (estimated cost: $350,000)
What factors should be considered in the decision?
How much does the cost of treatment affect the decision?
How much does the age of the patient affect the decision?
Is social justice a factor in the decision?

was devoted to medical care. The only effective means of controlling costs seemed to be rate regulation or price control, both of which limited flexibility required to account for the patient's condition, age, or acuity adjustment. Prospective payment based on DRGs proved to be the effective compromise.

The cost reduction, as a result of prospective payment, gave rise to the managed care revolution. Unable to shift costs to another entity, and with a predetermined reimbursement rate, providers searched for the most cost-effective mechanism of care provision. Greater ability to predict the cost of care enabled health care plans to negotiate the best value for their premiums.

Current Trends in Cost Containment

The managed care form of health care financing changes economic incentives, which forces health care providers to rethink medical management decisions. Costs of the service rendered, rather than enhancement of revenue through service provision, must be considered. These economic or cost-containment incentives can be divided into the following broad categories: capitated reimbursement, access limitation, and rationing.

Capitated Reimbursement

The increasing visibility of HMOs and their associated success in cost containment through the use of prospective

of those hospitalized were reviewed by peer standard review organizations. Physicians and other medical personnel reviewed the hospital records and counseled the attending physician about unnecessary or excessively lengthy stays in the hospital as well as unwarranted services.

Both of these efforts proved ineffective. In 1970, medical care represented 7% of the GNP. By 1990, 14% of the GNP reimbursement to influence provider practice gave rise to various arrangements that link health care financing to service delivery or managed care. Managed care organizations create partnerships with health care providers using financial incentives to prevent overuse. Statistical norms, practice parameters, and population data determine the capitated, or maximum, payment for services. This is maximum reimbursement amount that the health care provider will receive for the provision of care. The actual cost of provision of care does not affect this the reimbursement. Health care providers must provide appropriate medical care while being cognizant of medical costs. As a reward for conservative medical practices, health care providers may receive a specified amount of money or a percentage of the agreed reimbursement if services are delivered below the limit set by the third-party payer. Providers whose services are inadequate or exceed this limit are excluded from the network.

Cost Containment Through Access Limitation

All third-party payers, or insurance plans, control access to health care through designation of covered services. **Managed care organizations** designate the type of covered services and specify the conditions under which the service is covered. Some services may only be accessed upon approval or referral from physicians who are used as **gatekeepers.** The enrollee must choose a **primary care provider** and consult this provider for a referral before seeking specialty services. Without this referral, the enrollee is financially responsible for the service. Even with the referral, choices may be limited to the providers who have contracted with the managed care plan. A study that compared gatekeeper-insured pediatric patients with "free choice" indemnity plans found that there was a 4% reduction in cost with the gatekeeper managed care plan (Pati et al., 2003).

Managed care plans may require that less costly health care modalities or medications be used. Exceptions to these modalities require justification. More technologically advanced and expensive treatment modalities may be accessed under the most stringent conditions. Preauthorization requirements determine the medical necessity of the service. The process is so complex that the client may not be aware that the service is not covered until the reimbursement for the service is denied.

Cost Containment Through Rationing

Rationing of health care is particularly distasteful to the public. Dr. David Eddy eloquently stated that health care deals with "the ultimate issues of human existence: life versus death, peace versus suffering and discomfort, function versus dysfunction" (Vermont Medical Roundtable, 1999). Every developing nation has various mechanisms in place that ensure inability to pay does not prevent receipt of health care. As the number of individuals older than 85 years of age grows, rationing will present greater ethical dilemmas.

Rationing is best described as determining the most appropriate use of health care or directing the health care where it can do the most good. The following case dramatizes the problem.

CLINICAL EXAMPLE

A middle-aged woman was diagnosed with ovarian cancer. After conventional and high-dose chemotherapy failed, her physician recommended an autologous bone marrow transplant, which was considered experimental at the time. The procedure was approved and performed. Medical costs exceeded $200,000, but the patient died 2 months later. ■

Was this a wise use of medical resources? Health care is not an exact science; too many variables exist. What appears to be the best course of action for one is not the best course of action for another. Making accurate treatment decisions is difficult, and the ramifications of a mistake are great. Health care providers and third-party payers, including the federal government, are currently investigating the **outcomes** of health care practices to determine what methods, if any, can be instituted to improve the accuracy of these choices. Ways to match the patient with the most effective treatment modalities are currently being investigated. Research into the area of treatment outcomes has brought about such treatment changes as laparoscopic surgery, genetically determined cancer treatment, and gender-specific interventions.

CARING FOR THE UNINSURED

More than 45 million Americans are uninsured; 28.2% of those between the ages of 18 and 24 are uninsured. Native Americans are 2.5 times as likely to be uninsured as white persons. Those with incomes at or below poverty level are 3.5 times more likely to be uninsured. Among Hispanic-origin population, those of Mexican origin are most likely to be uninsured. People younger than 65 years of age who are uninsured are 36.6% more likely to lack a usual source of health care and more than twice as likely to experience difficulty or delay in receiving needed medical care. Lack of insurance is the major factor associated with lack of access to medical care. Uninsured adults are more than 3 times as likely as insured adults to go without needed medical care (NCHS, 2004). By 2007, up to 54 million people or more may be uninsured.

Historical Perspective

Before the 1930s, most Americans were uninsured. Most health care providers considered it their duty to donate time and services to charity. Hospitals and clinics maintained charity wards. Society believed that those who could, and those who could not, should help themselves. The enactment of governmental entitlement programs, coupled with the availability of health care insurance as a benefit of occupation, helped change this belief. Quickly, the pervasive societal view was that those who could not help themselves should get government assistance, or go to work (Higgins, 1997).

Societal Perceptions

Social justice, or equal medical care for all, is a concept that the American public think they embrace. Most people state that health care should be one of those necessities available to all without cost. However, efforts to provide universal coverage through increased governmental involvement in health care have failed. Increase in taxes, no matter how humane the cause, is consistently unpopular. Managed care has curtailed escalating health care costs by diminishing and limiting use. The public, however, perceive this limitation as diminished quality of care. Compromise between societal perceptions and the reality of health care costs remains elusive.

Ethical Dilemmas

Most people in society view health care as a right for all rather than a commodity to be available only to those who can afford it. Economics and technological advances have presented health care providers with the ethical dilemma of allocation of health care. An ethical act is one that leads to the greatest benefit for the most people and increases the self-esteem of the person performing the act. Changes and shifts in the population have added a strain on the nation's limited health care resources (Weintraub and Shine, 2004).

Concern over possible changes in the basic goal of equal health care for all has prompted the creation of the Consumer Bill of Rights and Responsibilities of health care. Created by the President's Advisory Commission (1997), and supported by the American Nurses Association, the goals of this document are as follows:

* To strengthen consumer confidence by ensuring that the health care system is fair and responsive to consumer needs
* To reaffirm the importance of a strong relationship between patients and their health care providers
* To reaffirm the consumer's role in safeguarding his or her health

The idea is that patients should have the right to legal recourse against managed care insurers for damages in cases where their health had been seriously damaged due to withheld or delayed treatment. Patients, trial lawyers, and consumer advocates supported the legislation, whereas advocates of tort reform and the insurance industry opposed it. By 2000, the popular consensus favored a national version of patients' rights. Legislative compromise version was being readied for submission to the President. The terrorist events of September 11 eclipsed health care issues. The compromise became a victim to bipartisanism and special interest influence. The principle has remained popular enough that several states have enacted their own patients' bill of rights.

TRENDS IN HEALTH FINANCING

The public's demand for affordable health care has created a new environment for health care financing. Competition among health care providers and third-party payers has led to new and innovative health care. Outpatient services, patient education packages, electronic health records, and telehealth are just a few of these innovations. Increased competition has required insurance plans to be sensitive to the needs of the employee organizations and their enrollees. Individualized plans of covered services can be created.

Enrollees can choose the plan that provides them with the services they desire at a selected cost. Health care providers advertise to ensure that the consumer selects an insurance plan in which their services are included. Some providers, such as hospitals, campaign for provision into a plan.

Cost Sharing

Aware of the amount that the employer is willing to contribute for basic coverage, a third-party payer or insurance plan may propose several options, giving the employee freedom to choose services desired. Employees willing to pay may be able to increase the covered services not provided by the basic plan. Cost sharing may also require the consumer to pay an increased portion of the bill for covered services in return for lower premiums. Enrollees may opt to pay a higher premium for freedom to choose providers, or elimination of the gatekeeper. This can result in increased consumer control of health care.

Health Care Alliances

The creation of powerful regional or statewide insurance purchasing pools or health alliances is seen as one means of reform for the health care industry. The alliance would define basic benefits that all insurers would have to offer to everyone at the same price regardless of health status. These alliances would be chartered to not regulate insurance prices. Health alliances would collect premiums and help consumers choose among competing insurers and plans. The consumer's choice would be based on published, simple, standard information about benefits and outcomes of the different available plans. Plans would have to compete by offering better outcomes or less cost. Insurers would have to contract with providers that find ways of delivering cost-efficient care. Medicare is currently participating in health care alliance. Enrollees are given a choice between the traditional Medicare Parts A and B, or Medicare Advance (see Table 10-3).

Self-Insurance

Some organizations have used health care information collected by insurance plans to self-insure their employees. This has enabled industries and other types of organizations to reduce the administrative cost of insurance, which has been estimated to represent 12.5% of the cost of insurance. Unlike the large industrial HMOs, self-insured status organizations administer their own health care plan but purchase health care services from an established insurance plan.

Flexible Spending Accounts

Another source of funding for uncovered services is the **flexible spending account** (FSA). The employee determines how much he or she will have to spend for uncovered services and has this amount deducted from his or her paycheck. When these services are incurred, the employee can secure payment for these services from this account. The employee continues to pay into the account until the estimated amount is reached. If the employee overestimates the cost, the remaining amount is forfeited. If the cost of the services exceeds the estimate, only the amount estimated will be paid.

Health Promotion and Disease Prevention

Unfortunately, reimbursement for health promotion and disease prevention is limited. Most health insurances, both private and public, pay for screening procedures. However, funding or reimbursement for such treatment modalities such as support groups for smoking cessation, home safety evaluation, or relaxation techniques are not funded. These techniques, which have proven to help prevent some diseases and illness, are not funded. Obesity is one of this nation's most common health problems, yet weight loss programs are not reimbursed.

ROLES OF THE COMMUNITY HEALTH NURSE IN THE ECONOMICS OF HEALTH CARE

Researcher

Nurses need to be engaged in research into provision of efficient, cost-effective health care. Nurses are in a pivotal role to investigate culturally sensitive treatment modalities, health education, disease prevention, and factors to change behaviors. Health promotion and disease prevention are more cost effective than curative treatment modalities. Community Health nurse researchers need to investigate the effectiveness of health promotion and disease prevention. Research into health promotion intervention outcomes, program cost/benefit analysis, or health informatics are just a few of these areas.

Educator

Health education is the foundation of community health nursing practice. Community health nurses agree that knowledge empowers clients to actively participate in their health care. Funding for this education is provided primarily through public governmental plans. Educational plans for individuals are almost nonexistent. In the area of health care economics, the nurse needs to demonstrate the **effectiveness** and value of this education. Outcome measures for health education need to be established. Measuring these outcomes will provide evidence of the value of this education ("Health Illiteracy Leads to Billions in Avoidable Costs," 2004).

Provider of Care

Any service delivered by the nurse needs to be appropriate, necessary, and cost effective. Nurses, in all areas of practice, need to be cost conscious. Judicious application of the nursing process is imperative. An accurate assessment is foundation for an appropriate nursing diagnosis. Goals for care, jointly established between members of the community and the community health nurse, will guide the choice of interventions. Evaluation, using previously developed outcome measures, will provide appropriate modifications to the plan.

Nurses can serve as program service providers, health education providers, and health program participants. Nurses need to participate in the grant proposal process, program design, and evaluator of these programs. Nurses need to be familiar with and participate in the statistical information gathering process that serve as the basis for determining community health need.

Advocate

Nurses must become more involved in the economics of health care. Too often, nurses are cognizant of the effects of changes in health care economics, but feel powerless to act. Increasing knowledge of health care funding and policy making will empower nurses to advocate for the type of funding that provides appropriate care to obtain the greatest good. The large number of nurses provides our occupation with political clout. Nurses need to utilize this political power to influence health care funding. Nurses need to advocate for increase in health promotion/disease prevention funding from both the public and the private sector. Nurses need to plan programs, seek funding, evaluate program effectiveness through outcome measures. Nurses need to constantly seek sources of funding for health programs through any available sources.

SUMMARY

Health care economics is influencing health care practice at all levels. Nurses must become aware of the economics of health care to practice in this new era. Patient outcomes are quickly being seen as a measurement for health care financing. As the health care system evolves toward health promotion and disease prevention, nursing will play a pivotal role. Community health nurses, whose domain of practice has encompassed these areas, will be in the forefront of this change.

This chapter has presented the basics of health care economics. An understanding of these elements is essential for the practice of nursing. This is an ever-changing field with new innovations and changes coming every day. To be effective, the nurse must be attentive to these developments.

LEARNING ACTIVITIES

1. Create a health care system including services, eligible recipients, funding resources, and qualifying requirements for these services.
2. Evaluate a family's health care coverage. Investigate the type of coverage and the ability of this coverage type to meet the needs of the family. Is there another type of insurance coverage that would meet more of the family's needs? What prohibits their ability to obtain this coverage?
3. Investigate health care reform from the points of view of the consumer, health care provider, and third-party payer.

How would a change in the current health care system affect the concerns of each of these constituents?

4. Interview representatives from health care provider groups, insurance plans, and consumer groups regarding their suggestions for health care reform.

5. Interview public health nurses employed in a public health department regarding their perception of funding for health promotion/disease prevention.

REFERENCES

Alemayehu B, Warner K: The lifetime distribution of health care costs, *Health Serv Res* 39(3):627-642, Jun 2004.

Bailey L: Prices and healthcare, *South Carolina Nurse* 11(4):9, Oct-Dec 2004.

Centers for Medicare and Medicaid Services: *Health care directory for people with Medicare,* Baltimore, 2003, The Author, http://www.medicare.gov/Library/PDFNavigation/PDFInterim.asp?Language=English&Type=Pub&PubID=02231.

Centers for Medicare and Medicaid Services: *Medicare fraud: detection and prevention tips,* Baltimore, no date, The Author, http://www.medicare.gov/FraudAbuse/Tips.asp.

Centers for Medicare and Medicaid Service, http://www.cms.hhs.gov/.

Chattopadhyay S, Carande-Kulis V: Economics of prevention: the public health research agenda, *J Public Health Manag Pract* 10(5):467-471, 2004.

Clark K: Cost cure-all? Or unhealthy shift? Employers seek to pass on the workers more of the burden of soaring medical costs, *US News World Rep* 135(21):38-39, 2003.

Commonwealth of Kentucky Department of Revenue: *Tobacco taxes,* The Author, http://revenue.ky.gov/business/tobaccotax.htm.

Ginsburg P: Controlling health care costs, *New Engl J Med* 351(16):1591-1593, 2004.

Health illiteracy leads to billions in avoidable costs, *Oncol News Int* 13(6):53, 2004.

Higgins W: How did we get this way? *Health Care Econ* 11:35, 1997.

Ku L, Flores G: Pay now or pay later: providing interpreter services in health care, *Health Affairs* 24(2):435-444, 2005.

Livesay JL et al: Client characteristics and the cost of home care in the prospective payment system, *Public Health Nurs* 20(4):287-297, 2003.

National Center for Health Statistics: *Health: United States—2004,* Hyattsville, Md, 2004, The Author, http://www.cdc.gov/nchs/data/hus/hus04.pdf.

National Center for Health Statistics: *National Health Interview Survey,* Hyattsville, Md, 2003, The Author, http://www.cdc.gov/nchs/nhis.htm.

Pati S et al: Does gatekeeper control costs for privately insured children? *Pediatrics* 111(3):456-460, 2003.

President's Advisory Commission on Consumer Quality in the Health Care Industry: *Consumer bill of rights and responsibilities,* Washington, DC, 1997, US Government Printing Office.

Rozzini R, Sabatini T, Trabucchi M: Diagnosis related groups and hospital costs in elderly dependent patients, *J Am Geriatr Soc* 53(1):174-175, 2005.

Seshamani M, Gray A: *Time to death and health expenditure: an improved model for impact of demographic change on health care costs.*

University of Pennsylvania School of Medicine, Meensa.Seshamani @marshallscholoarship.org.

Schur CL, Berk ML, Yegian JM: Public perceptions of cost containment strategies: mixed signals for managed care, *Health Affairs Suppl* 2:W4-516-W4-525, 2004.

Sloan, T: Consumer-driven to nowhere: study throws cold water on recent efforts to beat health care cost inflation, *Mod Healthcare* 34(49):21, 2004.

Steinbrook R: The cost of admission: tiered co-payment for hospital use, *New Engl J Med* 350(25):2539-2542, 2004.

Turner SO: *The nurse's guide to managed care,* Gaithersburg, Md, 1999, Aspen.

US Department of Health and Human Services, Centers for Medicare and Medicaid Services: *Medicare overview,* 2004, Hyattsville, Md, 2004, The Author, http://www.cms.hhs.gov/review/supp/2003/overview.pdf.

Vermont Medical Roundtable: *Can we have it all? Balancing access, quality and cost in health care,* Montpelier, Vt, 1999, Vermont Business Roundtable: Healthcare Task Force.

Weintraub W, Shine K: Is a paradigm shift in US healthcare reimbursement inevitable? *Circulation* 109(12):1448-1455, 2004.

11

Policy, Politics, Legislation, and Community Health Nursing

Denise Snow ▪ MaryAnne Laffin

MEDIA RESOURCES

Additional Material for Study, Review, and Further Exploration

evolve Website at http://evolve.elsevier.com/Nies

❖ Quiz ❖ Case Studies ❖ Content Updates ❖ Glossary ❖ WebLinks

OBJECTIVES

Upon completion of this chapter, the reader will be able to do the following:

1. Describe the philosophical and historical foundations of government.
2. Identify the legislative process involved in establishing federal, state, or local health policy.
3. Identify the social and political processes that influence health policy development.
4. Discuss current health policy issues, including restructuring of the health care system, and the effective use of nurses.
5. Discuss nurses' roles in political activities.

KEY TERMS

Clara Barton	institutional policies	nursing policy	public health law
coalition	Lavinia Dock	organizational policies	public policies
Faye Wattleton	Lillian Wald	policy	Ruth Watson Lubic
Florence Nightingale	lobby	policy analysis	Sojourner Truth
government	lobbyist	political action committee	
health policy	Margaret Sanger	politics	

CHAPTER OUTLINE

NURSES WHO MADE A DIFFERENCE

INTRODUCTION TO HEALTH POLICY AND THE POLITICAL PROCESS
Definitions

HISTORICAL FOUNDATIONS OF HEALTH LEGISLATION AND POLICY

STRUCTURE OF THE GOVERNMENT OF THE UNITED STATES
Balance of Powers

THE LEGISLATIVE PROCESS
How a Bill Becomes a Law

OVERVIEW OF HEALTH POLICY
Government Authority for the Protection of the Public's Health
Health Policy and the Private Sector

PUBLIC POLICY: BLUEPRINT FOR GOVERNANCE
Policy Formulation: The Ideal
Policy Formulation: The Real World

Steps in Policy Formation
Policy Analysis

A MAJOR PARADIGM SHIFT
Shifts in Centers for Disease Control and Prevention Policy
Nursing's Involvement in Private Health Policy
Restructuring of the Health Care Industry
The Effective Use of Nurses

NURSES' ROLES IN POLITICAL ACTIVITIES
Nurses as Change Agents
Nurses as Lobbyists

PROFESSIONAL ASSOCIATIONS AND LOBBYING
Nurses and Political Action Committees
Nurses and Coalitions
Nurses in Public Office
Nurses and Health Policy Development
Nurses and Campaigning
Nurses and Voting Strength

INTERNET AND POLITICAL PROCESS

NURSES WHO MADE A DIFFERENCE

The significance of nurses' involvement in influencing health policy is not new. Many nurses in the past and present have been instrumental in working with legislation and politics. Information on a few exemplary nurse heroines who illustrate this point follows:

- **Florence Nightingale** was the first nurse to exert political pressure on a government (Hall-Long, 1995). She transformed military health and knew the value of data in influencing policy. She was a leader who knew how to use the support of followers, colleagues, and policy makers.
- **Sojourner Truth** became an ardent and eloquent advocate for abolishing slavery and supporting women's rights. Her work helped transform the racist and sexist policies that limited the health and well-being of African Americans and women. She fought for human rights and lobbied for federal funds to train nurses and physicians (Mason, Leavitt, and Chaffee, 2002).
- **Clara Barton** was responsible for organizing relief efforts during the U.S. Civil War. In 1882, she successfully persuaded Congress to ratify the Treaty of Geneva, which allowed the Red Cross to perform humanitarian efforts in times of peace. This organization has had a lasting influence on national and international policies (Hall-Long, 1995; Kalisch and Kalisch, 2004).
- **Lavinia Dock** was a prolific writer and political activist. She waged a campaign for legislation to allow nurses to control the nursing profession instead of physicians. In 1893, with the assistance of Isabel Hampton Robb and Mary Adelaide Nutting, she founded the politically active American Society of Superintendents of Training School for Nurses, which later became the National League for Nursing (Kalisch and Kalisch, 2004). She was also active in the suffrage movement, advocating that nurses support the woman's right to vote (Lewinson, 2002).
- **Lillian Wald's** political activism and vision were shaped by feminist values. Working in the early 1900s, she recognized the connections between health and social conditions. She was a driving force behind the federal government's development of the Children's Bureau in 1912. Wald appeared frequently at the White House to participate in the development of national and international policy (Mason et al., 2002).
- **Margaret Sanger,** who trained as a nurse, became an activist who transformed the nation's attitudes and approaches to family planning. Her actions and political voice spoke out for women and the need for birth control. Despite legal opposition and frequently intense criticism, in 1916 she opened the first birth control clinic in the United States in Brooklyn. She continued her crusade for decades, giving lectures and organizing meetings. In 1928, she founded the National Committee on Federal Legislation for Birth Control, which was a forerunner of Planned Parenthood (Kalisch and Kalisch, 2004; Mason et al., 2002).
- **Faye Wattleton,** who is a nurse-midwife, was president of Planned Parenthood Federation of America from 1978 to 1992. She was the first woman to be named to the presidency of this large reproductive health organization. Under Ms. Wattleton's guidance, Planned Parenthood grew to support family planning programs in dozens of developing nations. Today, Ms. Wattleton is the president of the Center for the Advancement of Women, a nonprofit research and education institution for women (Center for the Advancement of Women, 2005).
- **Dr. Ruth Watson Lubic** is a nurse-midwife who crusaded for free-standing birth centers in this country. After realizing the birth center model through the Maternity Center Association in New York City, Dr. Lubic expanded the model to Washington, DC, where the infant mortality rate was twice the national average. In 1993, Lubic was awarded the MacArthur Fellowship Grant, and in 2001, the Institute of Medicine's Lienhard Award (Institute of Medicine, 2001; Lyttle, 2000).

INTRODUCTION TO HEALTH POLICY AND THE POLITICAL PROCESS

The health care delivery system, including nursing practice, is profoundly influenced by policies set by government and private entities. Nurses must understand the system of health policy development and implementation to effectively interpret and influence policies that affect nursing practice and the health of individuals, families, groups, and communities.

The more an individual knows about the political process, the more he or she tends to become involved. Individual nurses may become politically active on a local, state, or national level, or they may work collectively within groups such as the American Nurses Association (ANA) or their state nurses association to lobby for health causes. All nurses assume an advocacy role; therefore, it follows that all nurses should be encouraged to become change agents and politically active. It is the hallmark of our system that citizens have the right to have a voice in the governance of the community. Nurses may communicate concerns about conditions and issues in health care for the profession of nursing and for issues confronting the health care needs of their community, especially the needs of those members of the community that may not be able to speak for themselves. As nurses gain experience in the political arena, they need to commit to mentorship of younger nurses. United, nurses can influence political leaders to make changes to the health care system that are beneficial to all.

Politics and legislation are processes through which health policies are instituted. Policy, politics, and legislation are the forces that determine the direction of health programs at every level of government. These programs are critical to the health and well-being of the nation and of every individual. This chapter addresses the interrelationships of these processes and outlines the importance of nurses' continual efforts to maintain and improve the health of individuals, groups, and communities.

TABLE 11-1 Terminology Example

TOPIC	EXAMPLE
Public policy	A local or regional effort to prevent the sale of tobacco or alcohol to minors. Public policy directs that the right to health of the majority must be preserved over individual freedoms and corporate interests.
Public health law (statute)	New York State Public Health Law §2164: "Every person in parental relation to a child in this state shall have administered to such child an adequate dose of an immunizing agent against poliomyelitis, mumps, measles, diphtheria, rubella, varicella, Haemophilus influenza type B, and hepatitis B…"
Common law	The Supreme Court decision in *Roe v. Wade,* making first-trimester abortion legal, is an example of how common law becomes enforceable.
Regulation	Health Insurance Portability and Accountability Act is a regulation enacted by a federal agency.
Treaties	Multilateral treaty: Treaty to Eliminate All Forms of Discrimination Against Women

Definitions

Policy denotes a course of action to be followed by a government or institution to obtain a desired end (Bonick, 2000). Policy reflects values and encompasses the choices that a society, segment of society, or organization makes regarding goals and priorities and the criteria used to allocate resources (Mason et al., 2002). Furthermore, policy involves the application of reason and evidence to problem solving in public and private settings (Helms, Anderson, and Hanson, 1996).

Politics, in contrast, is defined as the art of influencing others to accept a specific course of action (Bonick, 2000). It is a process by which an individual exerts control over situations and events (Mason et al., 2002). In general, politics constitutes a means, and policy is the end or outcome (Helms et al., 1996). All policies are shaped by politics and reflect social values, beliefs, and attitudes (Mason et al., 2002).

Public policies are principles and standards regarded by the legislature or by the courts as being of fundamental concern to the state and the whole of society (including the principle that a person should not be allowed to do anything that would tend to injure the public at large). Public policies are intended to serve the interests of the public as a whole. **Health policy** refers to public policies that pertain to, or influence, the pursuit of health, or a course of action to obtain a desired health outcome for an individual, family, group, community, or society (Bonick, 2000; Shi and Singh, 2004). **Nursing policy** can be viewed independently as its own policy sector or as a subset within the larger health policy arena. An example is included in Table 11-1.

Institutional policies govern work sites and identify the institution's goals, operation, and treatment of employees. **Organizational policies** are rules that govern organizations and their positions on issues with which the organization is concerned (Mason et al., 2002).

Administrative agencies are departments of the executive branch with the authority to implement or administer particular legislation.

Laws are rules of conduct or procedure; they result from a *combination* of legislation, judicial decisions, and administrative actions (the law of the land).

Public health law is a statute, ordinance, or code that prescribes sanitary standards and regulation for the purpose of promoting and preserving the community's health. Public health law consists of legislation, regulations, and court decisions enacted by governments at the federal, state, and local levels to protect the public's health (Brooke, 2005). An example is included in Table 11-1.

Common law is the body of law derived from judicial decisions rather than from statutes or constitutions. It may also be referred to as case law. An example is included in Table 11-1.

Statutes are any laws passed by a legislative body at the federal, state, or local level.

Regulations are the rules or orders that have legal force that are issued by an administrative agency. An example is included in Table 11-1.

Treaties are binding laws between nations. Treaties can be made between two or more countries. A treaty made among many countries is called a multilateral treaty. An example is included in Table 11-1.

Organizations are associations that set and enforce standards in a particular area. Some are recognized by the government as an accrediting body. For example, the not-for-profit Joint Commission on Accreditation of Healthcare Organizations confers Medicare and Medicaid certification on a health care facility.

Nongovernmental organizations are international organizations that use donations and grants to assist communities in need, with minimal support from, or influence of, a particular nation.

HISTORICAL FOUNDATIONS OF HEALTH LEGISLATION AND POLICY

In the United States, the government has been involved in efforts to improve or maintain the health of citizens since the late 1700s. As a result, over the past two centuries, federal, state, and local initiatives, laws, and organizations have fostered significant improvements in the health and life expectancy of Americans. However, the strength and focus of health policy efforts from the federal level were largely imparted during the latter part of the twentieth century (Box 11-1).

One of the earliest pieces of comprehensive health care legislation was the Hospital Survey and Construction Act, also known as the Hill-Burton Act, passed during the Truman administration in 1946 (Shi and Singh, 2004). The Hill-Burton Act provided grants to states for the construction of

---

BOX 11-1   History of Government-Funded Health Care

1965: The Social Security Act established both Medicare and Medicaid. Medicare was a responsibility of the Social Security Administration (SSA), whereas federal assistance to the state Medicaid programs was administered by the Social and Rehabilitation Service (SRS). SSA and SRS were agencies in the Department of Health, Education, and Welfare (HEW).

1977: The Health Care Financing Administration (HCFA) was created under HEW to effectively coordinate Medicare and Medicaid.

1980: HEW was divided into the Department of Education and the Department of Health and Human Services (HHS).

2001: HCFA was renamed the Centers for Medicare and Medicaid Services (CMS). CMS is the federal agency that administers the Medicare and Medicaid program.

---

new hospitals, targeting low-income and rural areas (Dowling, 2002). Two decades later, President Johnson's terms in office marked a time of dramatic growth in federal health policy, highlighted by the passage of Medicare and Medicaid in 1965. This landmark legislation strengthened the government's role in the health care system and dramatically shaped its rapid growth.

During the 1970s, the Nixon administration tried to shift emphasis in health policy issues to state and local agencies by combining local initiatives with policy input and national standards. During Nixon's presidency, two important pieces of health legislation were passed. In 1973, the Health Maintenance Organization Act was passed, which required employers to offer a health maintenance organization alternative to conventional health insurance. The National Health Planning and Resources Development Act of 1974 required states to obtain a certificate of need for new hospital construction and modernization projects, including technology, to procure federal funding (Shi and Singh, 2004). During this period, many of the federal responsibilities for a uniform, cooperative national public health system were removed, and individual states were expected to assume those responsibilities.

The federal government's involvement in public health services revived when Ronald Reagan took office in 1980. In response to the alarming inflation of health care costs under Reagan, new Medicare cost-control approaches for hospitals and health care providers (e.g., diagnosis-related groups) were created (Shi and Singh, 2004; Sultz and Young, 2001).

In the early 1990s, the public was anxious for reform, and President Clinton's administration worked diligently to set up a national health policy. This attempt to bring about national health insurance was the first since Truman's initiatives to provide nationally sponsored health coverage for all Americans in the late 1940s. However, like Truman's, Clinton's policy initiative was not successful.

As a result, health care insurance costs have escalated, and coverage has declined. The lack of coordinated government influence, coupled with the decline in insurance coverage, has increased the emphasis on managed care. Many observers view managed care as perhaps economically successful but popularly and practically problematic. Control of health decisions has moved from physician providers to managed care organizations (MCOs) and often leaves the patient as a helpless bystander.

The publication of *Healthy People 2000* by U.S. Surgeon General C. Everett Koop in 1990 led to a resurgence of interest by the federal government in the welfare of Americans. However, fiscal resources for public health interventions continued to decline, and only marginal progress was made in meeting the goals. In early 2000, *Healthy People 2010* (U.S. Department of Health and Human Services, 2000) marked the beginning of the new millennium and an enhanced focus on population-based health promotion strategies. Many *Healthy People 2010* objectives directly or indirectly involve health policy. Virtually all of the areas have multiple policy-related objectives, and the Healthy People table lists only a few of them. New objectives for the twenty-first century are to see a reduction in health disparities among groups and witness even greater improvements in the health of all Americans.

STRUCTURE OF THE GOVERNMENT OF THE UNITED STATES

Government is the structure of principles and rules determining how a state, country, or organization is regulated. Among its purposes are regulation of conditions beyond individual control and provision of individual protection through a population-wide focus. These tasks are accomplished through passage and enforcement of laws. Requirements of childhood immunizations for school attendance, vector control, and sewage treatment are examples of regulations to protect the health of the population.

Government can also be viewed as the sovereign power vested in a nation or state. Sovereign power is the independent and supreme authority of the nation or state. Historical documents describe the government's responsibility for health in the United States and the subsequent authority to enact laws (including health laws). These documents reflect the values of the country's founders. They give the government the authority to enact laws, but they also limit that power. The earliest of these statements was the Mayflower Compact, through which the Pilgrims committed themselves to making "just and equal laws" for the general good. The Declaration of Independence later established the doctrine of inalienable rights, life, liberty, and the pursuit of happiness. However, it was not until the Constitution of the United States was signed by the representatives of the individual states that the federal government realized its sovereign power. At the same time that power was realized, a limit to that power was placed on the federal government. The drafters of the Constitution sought to balance the need to empower the new federal government to "establish justice, insure domestic tranquility, provide for the common defence, promote the general welfare, and secure the Blessings of Liberty" for its people but with limits on that power. That balance is achieved in several important ways.

The federal government is a government of limited powers, which means that for a federal action to be legitimate, it must be authorized. Only those actions that are within the scope of

HEALTHY PEOPLE 2010 | Selected Objectives Related to Public Policy

Objective	Baseline	Goal
6-8: Eliminate disparities in employment rates between working-age adults with and without disabilities.	52%	82%
7-4: Increase the proportion of the nation's elementary, middle or junior, and senior high schools that have a nurse-to-student ratio of at least 1:750.	34%	50%
8-5: Increase the proportion of people served by a community water system who receive a supply of drinking water that meets the regulations of the Safe Drinking Water Act.	73%	95%
8-23: Reduce the proportion of occupied housing units that are substandard.	6.2%	3%
13-8: Increase the proportion of substance abuse treatment facilities that offer HIV and AIDS education, counseling, and support.	58%	70%
14-23: Maintain vaccination coverage levels for children in licensed day care facilities and children in kindergarten through first grade.	93% to 97%	95%
15-10: Increase the number of states and the District of Columbia with statewide emergency department surveillance systems that collect data on external cause of injury.	12 states	50 states and DC
15-22: Increase the number of states and the District of Columbia that have adopted a graduated driver licensing model law.	23 states	50 states and DC
15-24: Increase the number of states and the District of Columbia with laws requiring bicycle helmets for bicycle riders.	11 states	50 states and DC
16-20: Ensure appropriate newborn bloodspot screening, follow-up testing, and referral services.	NA	NA
21-9: Increase the proportion of the population served by community water systems with optimally fluoridated water.	11 states	50 states
25-13: Increase the proportion of STD programs that routinely offer hepatitis B vaccination to all STD clients.	5%	90%
26-24: Extend legal requirements for maximum blood alcohol concentration levels of 0.08% for motor vehicle drivers 21 years of age and older.	16 states	50 states and DC
26-26: Extend administrative license revocation laws or programs of equal effectiveness for people who drive under the influence of intoxicants.	41 states	50 states and DC
27-11: Increase smoke-free and tobacco-free environments in schools, including all school facilities, property, vehicles, and school events.	37%	100%
27-13: Establish laws on smoke-free indoor air that prohibit smoking or limit it to separately ventilated areas in public places and work sites.	13% work sites 3% restaurants 16% public transportation	51%
27-21: Increase the average federal and state tax on tobacco products.	$0.63 cigarettes $0.27 smokeless tobacco	$2.00
28-11: Increase the proportion of newborns who are screened for hearing loss by one month of age, have audiologist evaluation by three months of age, and are enrolled in appropriate intervention services by months of age.	NA	NA

From U.S. Department of Health and Human Services: *Healthy people 2010*, Conference edition, Washington, DC, 2000, The Author.

the Constitution, the supreme law of the land, are authorized. The Constitution separates governmental powers among the branches of government (Table 11-2).

Some examples of the separation of powers doctrine that are written into the U.S. Constitution include the following:

- The legislature is prohibited from interfering with the courts' final judgments.
- The Supreme Court cannot decide a "political question"; it must be an actual case or controversy.
- Congress must present a bill to the President before it can become law (Box 11-2).
- The President needs consent of the Senate to appoint Supreme Court Justices or to make treaties.

- The President and members of Congress are elected; the Judiciary is appointed.

The Constitution not only set forth the responsibilities of the federal government, but it also provided for the individual citizen's rights and freedoms. These are contained in the 10 amendments, which were added after the original Articles of the Constitution were ratified in 1787. These 10 amendments, added in 1791, are known as the Bill of Rights. The rights guaranteed in the Bill of Rights, such as the rights of free speech and freedom of religion, only applied to the laws and actions of the *federal* government. It would take another 72 years for these rights to be guaranteed within the states. "Liberty interests" and "privacy rights" have been found to

TABLE 11-2 Government Branches

BRANCH OF GOVERNMENT	INCLUDES
Executive branch	The president, the vice president, and the administrative agencies
Legislative branch	The Senate and the House of Representatives (Congress)
Judicial branch	At the federal level: district courts, circuit courts, and the Supreme Court
	At the state level: state and county courts

BOX 11-2 An Example of the President's Response to a Senate Bill (a President May or May Not Respond to a Bill)

STATEMENT OF ADMINISTRATION POLICY
S. 306—Genetic Information Nondiscrimination Act of 2005
(Senator Olympia J. Snowe [R-ME] and 19 co-sponsors)
The Administration favors enactment of legislation to prohibit the improper use of genetic information in health insurance and employment. The Administration supports Senate passage of S. 306 as reported, which would prohibit group health plans and health insurers from denying coverage to a healthy individual or charging that person higher premiums based solely on a genetic predisposition to developing a disease in the future. The legislation also would bar employers from using individuals' genetic information when making hiring, firing, job placement, or promotion decisions.

Administrative Agencies
One of the most dramatic changes in American government since the ratification of the Constitution is the growth of administrative agencies. Federal administrative agencies have broad power. They exercise all of the powers of government: executive, legislative, and judicial.

The Food and Drug Administration is one such administrative agency. Its power is in regulating the pharmaceutical industry as well as the food industry. ■

Decisions affecting the public's health are made not only at every level of government but also in each branch of government. The separation and balance of powers, referred to as checks and balances, is as important to health as it is to the economic or military status of the country.

The legislative branch (i.e., Congress at the federal level; legislature, general assembly, or general court at the state level) enacts the statutory laws that are the basis for governance. The executive branch administers and enforces the laws, which are broad in scope, through regulatory agencies. These agencies, in turn, define more specific implementation of the statutes through rules and regulations (i.e., regulatory or administrative law). The judiciary body provides protection against oppressive governance and against professional malpractice, fraud, and abuse. Its function, through the courts, both state and federal, is to determine the constitutionality of laws, interpret them, and decide on their legitimacy when they are challenged. Decisions of the U.S. Supreme Court are binding law for the nation. Decisions of the individual state's highest court are binding law within that state alone. The courts also have jurisdiction over specific infractions of laws and regulations.

exist by determinations by the Supreme Court and have become guiding principles in setting policy and enacting legislation. Note that these rights are *only* applicable to state or federal *government's* interaction with people. Violations of restrictions on rights such as free speech do not apply to nongovernmental entities, unless a specific law states otherwise.

Balance of Powers
Federalism is the relationship and distribution of power between the national and the state governments. This balance flows directly from the text of the Constitution: "The powers not delegated to the United States by the Constitution, nor prohibited by it to the States, are reserved to the States respectively, or to the *people.*"

States retain powers not delegated to the federal government; therefore much of public health law is under state jurisdiction and, as a result, varies considerably from state to state. These powers to enact laws for the public welfare are referred to as the states' "police powers." Additionally, states may delegate these powers to local governments. In the United States, legislative activities of the three levels of government (federal, state, and local) may vary greatly in their expectations, actions, and results. The state legislatures, for the most part, are directly involved in health care, yet the federal government influences health policy, directly and indirectly, through the financing of health care for many groups (e.g., Medicare), regulation activities (e.g., approval of drugs), and setting of standards (e.g., air quality).

THE LEGISLATIVE PROCESS
How a Bill Becomes a Law
As stated in the previous section, there is a balance of powers within the government at both state and federal levels. Along with a separation of powers of the three branches of government, there is an additional mechanism that balances the power of the Congress: bicameralism. Bicameralism ensures that the power to enact laws is shared between the House of Representatives and the Senate. The procedure through which legislation must pass to eventually become law is similar for all U.S. legislative bodies. Once a concept has been drafted into legislative language, it becomes a bill, is given a number, and moves through a series of steps. The

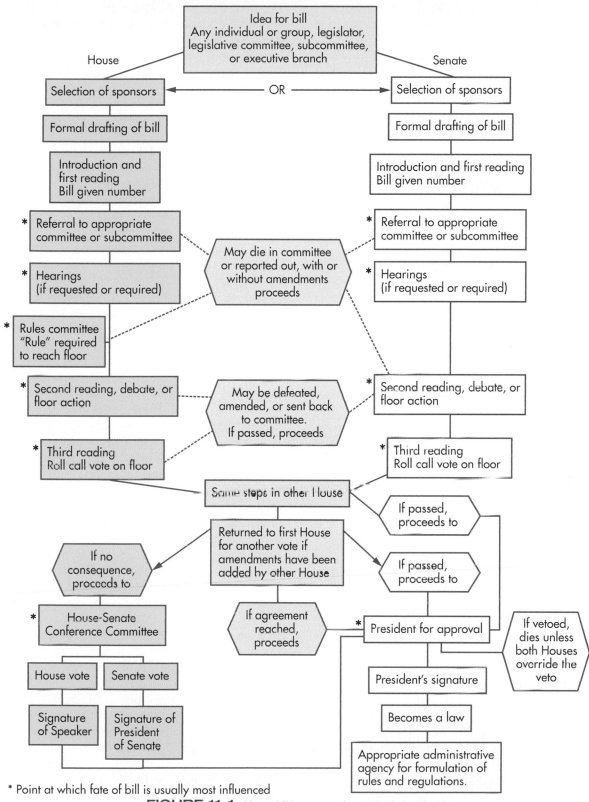

FIGURE 11-1   How a bill becomes a law at the federal level.

* Point at which fate of bill is usually most influenced

bill's passage is sometimes smooth, but, more often than not, the bill is extensively altered through amendments or even killed.

In Congress and in the 49 states that have a two-house legislature, a bill must succeed through the two legislative bodies, that is, the House of Representatives and the Senate (Figure 11-1). Nebraska, which has a single-house legislature, is the exception. A bill that has moved successfully through the legislative process has one final hurdle, which is the chief executive's approval. The approval may be a clear endorsement, in which case the governor or president signs it. If the executive neither signs nor vetoes it, the bill may become law by default. An explicit veto conclusively kills the bill, which then can be revived only by a substantial vote of the legislature to override the veto. This is another example of the checks and balances of the government process.

Issues that find their way into the legislative arena are commonly controversial, and proponents and opponents quickly align themselves. Defeating a bill is much easier than getting one passed; therefore the opposition always has the advantage. Health legislation, which usually requires preventive action (e.g., toxic waste management) or creates a new service (e.g., nursing center organizations for Medicare recipients), is at a disadvantage from several standpoints.

Few elected officials are knowledgeable about the health care field. Although health is readily recognized as a national resource, it is not easily quantified into the economic terms that make the issue easy to grasp. Other disadvantages are the backgrounds, biases, and ambitions of each legislator. The decision to run for public office is often made in keeping with personal goals that are likely to differ from health values aimed at the public good.

Despite these obstacles, good health laws can be passed when concerned nurses and other health care workers understand the legislative process and use it effectively. For nurses, this is yet another mode of intervention on behalf of clients. Legislation passed to reduce or prevent abuse for all children is as important as physical and emotional care of the abused child.

OVERVIEW OF HEALTH POLICY

As mentioned previously, *public policy* refers to decisions made by legislative, executive, or judicial branches of one of the three levels of government (i.e., local, state, or federal). These decisions are intended to direct or influence actions, behaviors, or decisions of others. When public policy addresses health issues, it is *health policy*. Health policies influence health care through the monitoring, production, provision, and financing of health care services. Virtually everyone, from providers (e.g., physicians, nurses, nurse practitioners, pharmacists, midwives, and dentists) to consumers, is affected by health policies. Likewise, health policy influences organizations, such as insurers, medical schools, health maintenance organizations, nursing homes, producers of medical equipment and technologies, and employers.

Health policies are developed, regulated, and enforced at all three levels of government. In addition to the public policy–making sector, health policies can also be made through the private sector. For example, an insurance company or employer will determine such matters as what illnesses will be covered by the insurance program, what drugs will be included in a formulary, and how much to charge for an insurance policy.

Government Authority for the Protection of the Public's Health

The authority for the protection of the public's health is largely vested with the states, and most state constitutions specifically delineate this responsibility. Municipal subdivisions of states, such as counties, cities, or towns, usually have the power of local control of the services conferred by the state legislature.

The responsibility of local, state, and federal governments for health services under varying conditions sometimes complicates attempts to determine the locus of political decision making. The supremacy of the state prevails in most situations; therefore the state is a critical arena for political action. An example is the state's authority to license health professionals, such as nurses and physicians, and health care institutions, such as hospitals, nursing homes, and day care centers.

Each state establishes policies or standards for goods or services that impact the health of its citizens. However, several factors may affect that authority. For example, the standards for pasteurization of milk sold within a state are determined by that state, but if the milk is sold in another state, it comes under the interstate commerce jurisdiction of the federal government. This could mean that a higher standard must be met, which negates the state standard. Alternatively, when public health authority is delegated to political subdivisions within the state, they too may impose a standard that is higher, and never lower, than that of the state.

The federal government also has a strong influence on health services. Constitutionally, this authority is derived from the federal role in regulation of interstate commerce (e.g., meat inspection) and through broad interpretation of the "general welfare" clause (e.g., Medicare). States vary considerably in resources allocated to provide health programs; therefore significant de facto authority derives from the promise of revenues or threats to remove funding (e.g., funds for interstate highway repair are often tied to air quality). Federal funds fully or partially fund many of the programs discussed in this and other chapters.

Compliance by states to federal program standards is voluntary, but the advantage of the revenue, which is withheld from the states if they do not comply, is seldom ignored. Programs such as control of sexually transmitted infections and the statistical reporting system are standardized across the country in response to the indirect but marked effect of federal funding.

Health Policy and the Private Sector

As described previously, the government has a profound role in setting and implementing health policy, but nurses must recognize that health policy is also made in the private sector. The private sector includes professional organizations (e.g., the American Medical Association and the American Hospital Association), non-profit health care organizations (e.g., Red Cross and the American Cancer Society) and for-profit corporations that deliver, insure, or fund health care services outside direct government control. Health insurance companies, and MCOs in particular, are increasingly setting policies that impact a large number of individuals (Pulcini et al., 2000).

In the private sector, health policy evolves differently than in the public sector. One difference is that private health policy is largely influenced by theories of economics and business management as opposed to the social and political theories that predominate in the public sector. In the private sector, economics is central, whereas in the public sector, economics is one of many factors. In the private sector, decisions can be swift and are often proactive, whereas in the public sector, decision making is more deliberate and tends to be reactive. Private sector change is dictated by consumer needs, economics, and market trends, whereas voting shifts and electoral realignments often delineate the need to change policy in the public sector. The private sector is managed by stockholders and boards of directors who are generally less accessible to the public than elected officials (Pulcini et al., 2000).

PUBLIC POLICY: BLUEPRINT FOR GOVERNANCE

Policy is directed by values. It articulates the guiding principles of collective endeavors, establishes direction, and sets goals. It influences and, in turn, is influenced by politics. Policy directives may become realized or obstructed at any stage in the political process.

Policy Formulation: The Ideal

In ideal circumstances, authorized authoritative bodies (e.g., state health departments, Occupational Safety and Health Agency, the Centers for Medicare and Medicaid Services) rationally determine actions to create, amend, implement, or rescind health care policy. These groups would decide what is right or best and then develop the political strategies to effect the desired outcomes. The question of whether a particular policy is advocated or adopted would depend on the degree that a group or the society as a whole may benefit without harm or detriment to subgroups. Of all the seemingly limitless factors that may influence policy formation, group need and group demand should be the strongest determinants. The premises supporting the goals of health policy should be equitable distribution of services and the guarantee that the appropriate care is given to the right people, at the right time, and at a reasonable cost.

Policy Formulation: The Real World

In the real world, policy for health care exemplifies both conflict and social change theories. Health policy is the product of continuous interactive processes in which interested professionals, citizens, institutions, industries, and other groups compete with one another for the attention of various branches of government. The most obvious and prominent among these is the legislative branch, although policy is also made through regulatory mechanisms and court decisions, as described previously. Health policy may also issue from

---

BOX 11-3   Balancing the Responsibilities of the Government With Individual Rights

Example of Statutory and Common Law
Jacobson v. Commonwealth of Massachusetts (1905)
- ➤ Massachusetts passes a statute requiring everyone to be vaccinated for smallpox.
- ➤ Jacobson refuses to be vaccinated, claiming the requirement of vaccination violated his liberty interests of bodily integrity and decisional privacy.
- ➤ The U.S. Supreme Court ruled that "a community has the right to protect itself against an epidemic of disease which threatens the safety of its members." Also, that individual liberty "does not import an absolute right in each person to be, at all times and in all circumstances, wholly freed from restraints. There are manifold restraints to which every person is necessarily subject for the common good."
- ➤ Result of the ruling: In this instance, the Supreme Court ruled that the Massachusetts law *was* constitutional. But when the Court rules against a statutory law, the Supreme Court's decision becomes the law.

U.S. Supreme Court, *Jacobson v. Commonwealth of Massachusetts*, 197 U.S. 11(1905).

BOX 11-4   Recommended Childhood and Adolescent Immunization Schedule: United States, 2005

Harmonized Childhood and Adolescent Immunization Schedule, 2005
The Advisory Committee on Immunization Practices (ACIP) periodically reviews the recommended childhood and adolescent immunization schedule to ensure that the schedule is current with changes in vaccine formulations and reflects revised recommendations for the use of licensed vaccines, including those newly licensed. Recommendations and format of the childhood and adolescent immunization schedule for July-December 2004 were approved by ACIP, the American Academy of Family Physicians, and the American Academy of Pediatrics and were published in April 2004. That schedule updated previous ones by adding the recommendation that, beginning in fall 2004, healthy children aged 6 to 23 months, as well as household contacts and out-of-home caregivers for healthy children aged 0 to 23 months, receive an annual influenza vaccine.

From Centers for Disease Control and Prevention: Recommended childhood and adolescent immunization schedule—United States, 2005, *MMWR Morb Mortal Wkly Rep* 53(51):Q1-Q3, 2005, http://www.cdc.gov/mmwr/preview/mmwrhtml/mm5351-Immunizationa1.htm.

---

the recommendations of fact-finding commissions established by the legislative or executive branch. This is illustrated in Box 11-3.

Health policy is rarely created through discrete, momentous determinations in relation to single problems or issues. It often evolves slowly and incrementally as an accumulation of many small decisions. It also changes slowly because changes in the social beliefs and values that underlie established policy develop within the context of actual service delivery. Once a direct health care service is offered, especially an official tax-funded service, it is often difficult to discontinue it. Existing programs create tradition by establishing vested interest and a sense of entitlement on the part of the public. This tradition also exerts political influence in a natural effort for self-preservation (see Box 11-4 for an example).

Steps in Policy Formulation

The tangible formulation of public policy begins with the most critical step, which is defining the issue and placing it on the agenda. The next step is the commitment of resources, most often, through the passage of legislation. A regulatory schedule for the implementation of the law into program is formulated. Then, an evaluation process is designed that satisfies regulatory and legislative remedies should they be needed.

Policy Analysis

Analysis of health policy is an objective process that identifies the sources and consequences of policy decisions in the context of the factors that influence them. Health **policy analysis** determines those who benefit and those who experience a loss as the result of a policy. These considerations are critical in order to develop health policies that are fair to all who are affected.

President Clinton's attempt to reform health care in the mid 1990s reflected ethical and practical considerations for a national health policy. The fundamental principle was access to health care for all Americans. Those benefiting would be the American public, as consumers of health care and payers for health care, through tax-supported insurance programs. The opposition consisted of those envisioning major financial losses from the proposed changes. Among these, the insurance industry was a dominant antagonist, with some provider groups joining the opposition forces. The public was confused by the complexity of the issues and wary of change. This effort to make an overdue change in health care policy eventually failed.

A MAJOR PARADIGM SHIFT

Policy is based on values, and the first step in forming policy is identification of the issue. Therefore, it would seem rational to define "health" as the starting point for any policy annexed to health care issues. Policy analysts can look to the experience of the international community and its recently altered view of health as one such definition. Historically, global concerns for health centered primarily on the spread of infectious disease. These concerns led to the formation of the World Health Organization (WHO). Defining health was central to the formation and mission of WHO. This definition was written as the preamble to its constitution: "Health is a state of complete physical, mental and social well-being and not merely the absence of disease or infirmity." Despite this broad definition, WHO directed most of its efforts in the past 50 years to disease containment. However, recent world events have led WHO back to its initial definition as it attempts to deal with, for example, environmental issues of nuclear contamination and industrial toxins and developed nations exporting carcinogenic commercial products, such as tobacco, and antibiotic resistant strains of bacteria. But it has been the emergence of the human immunodeficiency virus (HIV) that has changed the global health paradigm from the traditional notions of containment and treatment to a more comprehensive approach of social intervention and, in turn, has brought WHO back to its stated definition of health and the realization that health is a basic human right. The WHO's experience with the HIV pandemic has revealed that health problems are linked to government actions and, thus, affect human rights.

Human rights violations occur when governments fail to provide their people with the infrastructure, services, and information necessary to prevent and control disease. One example of how health is dramatically affected by human rights issues is the estimation that for every year of education a woman has, infant mortality decreases by 10%; yet education of women is not a global reality.

Shift in Centers for Disease Control and Prevention Policy

The existence of awareness of the health and human rights relationship is also seen nationally. In its 2004 annual report, the Centers for Disease Control and Prevention (CDC) describe health broadly and in terms similar to those used by WHO: "... health is more than the absence of threats of disease and disability ... it's a precious resource that helps us to create productive and satisfying lives for ourselves and our families" (CDC, 2004). A stated goal of the CDC is "All people, and especially those at greatest risk for health disparities, will achieve their optimal lifespan with the best possible quality of health in every stage of life." See Box 11-5 to follow the shifts in CDC philosophy.

However, a shift in the paradigm of health concepts would necessitate a substantial reallocation of resources since the vast majority of health spending (as much as 95% by some estimates) is directed toward medical care and biomedical research and, as such, reflects a viewpoint of health as a commodity. Indeed, it is not necessarily medical need but the ability to pay is what guides our system. Considering that more than 41 million Americans have no health insurance and more than 15% of children are uninsured (Feldstein, 2003; Shi & Singh, 2004), it becomes clear that the health and human rights relationship is not yet reflected in our health policies.

Nursing's Involvement in Private Health Policy

Nursing should incorporate private health policy into its policy agenda. Nurses can influence private health care organizations from internal and external positions. From an internal perspective, nurses can hold important management positions in MCOs. This would allow direct involvement in policy setting. Nurses can also support and use nursing research that demonstrates positive clinical and economic outcomes. This would serve to validate the importance of nursing within the health system (Pulcini et al., 2000).

External strategies that nurses can use to influence private health policy include participation in discussions regarding quality and managed care (Pulcini et al., 2000). Nurses should monitor the quality ratings of MCOs and suggest changes in providers accordingly. Nurses can also build entrepreneurial practices to provide lower-cost services for underserved groups and can encourage clients to call and write their managed care plan organization to request that

BOX 11-5 Shifts in Philosophy at the Centers for Disease Control and Prevention

FROM	TO
Disease orientation	Health protection focus
Designing and implementing sponsored programs	Informing and guiding health system actors
Allocating agency resources	Leveraging resources to steer larger health system
Emphasis on clinical prevention	Focus on prevention and health protection
Transaction-based relationships	Partnerships and strategic alliances
Program requirements	Incentives for participation/cooperation
Collecting and analyzing health data	Creating integrated health information systems
Issuing advisories and guidelines	Building decision-support system

Centers for Disease Control and Prevention. *State of the CDC: fiscal year 2004,* The Author.

nursing services be reimbursable. Nurses should work co-operatively with other health professions to influence MCOs to improve quality of care.

Restructuring of the Health Care Industry

Health care reform is a nursing issue, and few nurses will argue that reform is needed in the health system in the United States. In virtually every practice arena, nurses see the inequalities and inadequacies that diminish the nation's level of wellness. Identification of the problems is important to discussions of reform. Identification of politics and popular beliefs that create barriers to a comprehensive approach is also important for correction of the problems.

The economic structure of the United States is a market economy. There is a strong and prevailing political and popular belief in market-driven systems. Competition, which includes increasing quality and lowering costs, drives the market economy, thereby theoretically creating an even more robust economy with better goods and services. In the health care arena, efforts to lower costs have been aimed at decreasing payments to providers, hospitals, and pharmaceutical companies. Providers, in turn, avoid unprofitable patients. Competition between insurers exists less by increasing quality or lowering costs than by shifting costs. The business of health care generates huge administrative costs that, along with profits, divert resources from providing care to the demands of business.

Popular sentiments about governmental control over health care have mirrored attitudes concerning the governmental role in general. The politically viable range of cost-control measures available to public programs has been limited to cutbacks in payments to providers rather than limits on the demand for clinical services or limits on individual choice.

The failure of former President Clinton's Health Security Act, despite polls suggesting wide support for extension of insurance coverage, provides warnings to any politician who supports a proposal that may be characterized as a governmental takeover of individual decision-making authority. This was a particularly difficult disappointment for nurse advocates and is worth examining to prevent future policy

restructuring that nurses endorse. In the 1990s, Nursing's Agenda for Health Care Reform was developed through the collaborative efforts of the ANA and the National League for Nursing. Once completed, more than 75 nursing associations added their endorsements (de Vries and Vanderbilt, 1994). The agenda was a powerful tool to promote understanding of nursing and its special contributions to health care.

Armed with the plan set forth in the agenda, nurses were active participants in Clinton's efforts at health care reform. Soon after his inauguration, Clinton appointed a task force that included nursing association representatives and eventually designed a universal plan. Reducing barriers to practice for advanced nurse practitioners and redesigning personnel systems for use by nurses in a reformed system were two issues critical to nursing included in the plan (ANA, 1993).

The insurance industry and some provider groups opposed the unprecedented effort to redesign the health care system. The complexity of the plan and the issues involved confused the public. Despite general acknowledgment of the problems with the health care system, many were wary of the proposed changes. By the fall of 1994, efforts to support the plan waned, and it eventually died. Litman (1997) summarized the following reasons for the failure of Clinton's plan:

- Opposition forces were strong and well organized, whereas those in favor were disorganized and frequently at odds over the best way to attain reform.
- Ideological differences arose between the president and Congress.
- A lack of consensus existed between the majority party and the numerous House and Senate committees.
- The plan was too complex and bureaucratic.
- The plan's objectives were not easily understood and therefore were easily distorted.
- The administration took too long to introduce its plan, which allowed opponents to gather momentum.
- The plan's core reform was directed at a politically weak constituency and opposed by well-financed special interest groups.
- An improved economy and moderation in health insurance premium costs lessened the sense of urgency.

National Sample of Registered Nurses

The Division of Nursing, a component of the HRSA, helps direct policy through the National Sample Survey of Registered Nurses. This survey has been conducted seven times since 1977 and was done most recently in March 2000 and released in 2002 (HRSA, 2002). The national survey looks at trends in demographics, employment, education, and compensation among RNs. For example, Figure 11-2 shows a disturbing trend: For the last survey period, there were fewer nurses entering the workforce and more nurses leaving. Also, Figure 11-3 shows a comparison of the racial/ethnic and gender makeup of RNs and the general population.

Additional factors to consider from the data obtained in the 2000 survey include the following:

➤ In 1980, 25.1% of RNs were younger than age 30, but in 2000 only 9.1% were younger than age 30.

➤ The average age of an RN in the United States was 43.3 years.

➤ In 1980, the average annual salary of full-time RNs was $17,398. The 2000 average was $46,782, but that was only $23,369 in real dollars that reflect inflation and the cost of living.

➤ The expected need for RNs in the U.S. health care system is nearly three million by 2020, yet the projected available number of RNs is expected to remain at current levels of 2.7 million.

Data from Health Resources and Services Administration: *The registered nurse population: Findings from the national sample survey of registered nurses*, Washington, DC, 2002, The Author.

After the failed attempt at comprehensive reform, more intermediate reform steps have been proposed and taken, for example, enactment of the Medicare Prescription Drug Improvement and Modernization Act of 2003, which includes a long awaited prescription drug benefit. The U.S. Department of Health and Human Services (HHS) calls this act "the most significant expansion of Medicare since its enactment" (DHHS, 2004, para 6). However, many observers feel that the act falls far short of needed changes.

The Effective Use of Nurses

The Health Resources and Services Administration (HRSA) provides general resources and information to the public and for use in the development of policy by the government. The nursing workforce development programs administered by the HRSA through Title VIII provide federal support for nurse workforce development. This title includes the programs of the Nurse Reinvestment Act (NRA) of 2002.

The NRA significantly increased funding for nursing education and recruitment. It supports nursing programs through the educational scope of entry level to advanced degrees. Some of the ways this is done is through grants for mentoring, cultural competencies, and career ladders. It also promotes nursing through projects aimed at supporting advanced nursing education and increasing nursing workforce diversity. Additionally, it supports nursing education through loan repayment programs that provide incentives for nurses to work in facilities with critical shortages or in nurse faculty programs.

An issue that is vital to effective health care delivery relates to nurse staffing. Staffing has been a topic of concern of nurses for many years because inadequate and inappropriate staffing can threaten patients' safety, the nurses' health, and commit-

BOX 11-6 The Registered Nurse Staffing Act of 2005 (S. 71/H.R. 1372)

S. 71, the Registered Nurse Safe Staffing Act of 2005 allows for the development of staffing systems that require the input of direct care registered nurses (RNs) and provides for whistler-protection for RNs who speak out about patient care issues. S. 71, sponsored by Senator Daniel Inouye (D-HI) and H.R. 1372, sponsored by Representative Lois Capps (D-CA) and Representative Rob Simmons (R-CT) were developed and introduced at the urging of the ANA and its members in response to the current nursing crisis.

➤ A study published in the *Journal of the American Medical Association* (Aiken et al., 2002) found that RN staffing levels have a significant effect on preventable hospital deaths among surgical patients. According to researchers, the odds of patient mortality rose 7% for every additional patient added to the average nurse's workload.

➤ S. 71/H.R. 1372 requires the establishment of a staffing system that ensures a number of RNs on each shift and in each unit of the hospital to ensure appropriate staffing levels for patient care.

➤ The bills required public reporting of staffing information. Hospitals must post daily for each shift the number of licensed and unlicensed staff providing direct patient care, specifically noting the number of RNs.

➤ The staffing system must account for architecture and geography of the environment and available technology; reflect the level of preparedness and experience of those providing care; reflect staffing levels recommended by specialty nursing organizations; account for ancillary staff support; provide that an RN not be assigned in a particular unit without first having established the ability to provide professional care in such a unit; and be based on methods that ensure validity and reliability.

American Nurses Association: Registered Nurse Staffing Act of 2005, The Author, http://vocusgr.vocus.com/grconvert1/webpub/ana/ProfileIssue.asp?IssueID=3117%7CJOINT&XSL=ProfileIssue&hidLegislatorIDs=.

ment to the profession. Inappropriate staffing also contributes to pressure experienced by nurses because of increasing patient intensity, increasing complexity of care, and fatigue. The Registered Nurse Safe Staffing Act of 2005 (S. 71/H.R. 1372) was introduced in Congress to address these concerns. (See Box 11-6 for highlights of the Bill.) It was later referred to Committees in both the Senate and the House of Representatives.

NURSES' ROLES IN POLITICAL ACTIVITIES

A recent research study looked at facilitators and hindrances for political involvement among nurses. Factors identified that facilitated political involvement included being raised in a family that was politically active, positive role models (e.g., a politically involved nurse-mentor or national figure) who exemplified the importance of involvement in social issues, and education. Hindrances to political action included lack of resources (e.g., financial burdens of membership dues), the slow nature of the political process, time constraints, perceived lack of support from society and peers, gender issues, administrative structure, negative experiences, frustration, burnout, and apathy (Winter and Lockhart, 1997).

More effort needs to be given to educate nurses about the importance of being informed on health policy issues and to

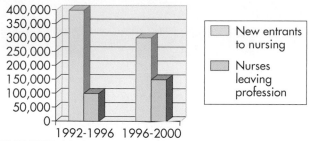

FIGURE 11-2 Comparison of registered nurses (RNs) entering and leaving the profession (1992-1996, 1996-2000). (HRSA, 2002.)

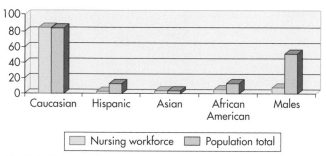

FIGURE 11-3 Race/ethnicity/gender comparison: registered nurses (RNs) and general population. (HRSA, 2002.)

encourage them to become politically active. Exposure to positive role models is particularly important. Nurses must obtain the tools to overcome factors that impede involvement. Nurses most often identify positive role models as the major influence that assisted them to become more politically involved in the profession. Mentorship is the most important aspect of involvement. Often, this occurred at the student level, but also can occur at any level, including the expert level of practice. But nurses often identify negative experiences that stimulated more awareness of policy within an institution and this occurred at the novice, skilled, and proficient levels of nursing practice. Negative influences appear to limit awareness of policy and politics to the institutional level, whereas positive influences have a much greater empowering capability. Responses to a survey asking what helped in developing awareness in the profession, policy, and politics illustrate this point in Box 11-7.

Nurses as Change Agents

Although nurses have historically been recognized as a necessary resource during wars and other emergencies, since the 1950s, all levels of government have begun to consider nurses as indispensable, even in ordinary times. The public now recognizes nurses as necessary and valued national resources. In their advocacy role, nurses are seen as professionals whose knowledge, skills, and concern are used to promote society's well-being. Nurses have a unique status in caring for patients, they are interpreters of the health care system to the public, and their professional activities are influenced by government-funded programs; therefore public health nurses must know how to participate in the political process. To do this effectively, they need a sound knowledge of community, state, and national government

BOX 11-7 Responses to Policy Activism Survey

Positive Influences and the Importance of Mentorship
"I became involved in policies through a relationship with a professor who felt strongly about an issue."
"I have found communication among peers to be informative and often inspiring. That has motivated my involvement in health care issues."
"I became aware of the potential role nurses could play related to policy as an undergrad. I had a few dynamic professors that were very inspiring by their involvement and passion related to various issues. At that point I didn't consider myself as someone to get involved but I think it ignited a spark for some day...."
"My exposure to professors that were actually involved in different 'causes' and not just teaching the course made a huge difference in my perspective of getting involved. The continual role model/mentor is also a huge inspiration."
"...nurses who take an interest in current events and enjoy discussing their opinions regarding public policies."
"I think if you don't get exposed to that 'spark' throughout your career it goes out. An inspiring speaker at a professional meeting will get me every time!"
"I was inspired by my professor who was past president for New York State Nursing Association."
"It would be great if one of the clinical nurse specialists at my hospital asked some nurses in a unit what they thought about something and how we could try to change or fix it. We just need that little nudge and some guidance to kindle that passion."

Negative Experiences Influencing Awareness
"I became more aware of the policies from my institution, from preceptors and when I had a problem. I was more aware as a novice because I was scared to do something that was going to get me into trouble."
"I became more involved at the institutional level after being 'wronged' by administration in regard to a policy, procedure, or benefit."
"I was usually unaware of a policy until it affected me directly, therefore the need to know became paramount."

organization and function and a clear understanding of how these bodies interact collectively to influence policy. Nurses must know how to influence the creation of health care legislation and how to contribute to the election and appointment of key officials.

Although there are more nurses than physicians, hospital administrators, or other health care professionals, nursing traditionally has not been seen as a major political influence because of a lack of public policy consensus within the nursing community. Unity within the professional organizations, coalitions, and lobby efforts has changed this perception. Policy is fundamental to governance; therefore nurses need to know about the formulation of public policy and the acts of government and its agencies. To assist in these activities, Table 11-3 presents sources for legislation information and Table 11-4 gives sources for information on electoral issues.

Nurses as Lobbyists

A **lobbyist** is a person who, voluntarily or for a fee, represents himself or herself, an individual, organization, or entity

TABLE 11-3   Sources for Legislative Information

GOVERNMENT LEVEL	INFORMATION AVAILABLE	LOCATION
Federal	Background of members of Congress	*Congressional Directory*
	Committee assignments	
	Terms of service	Government documents section of selected public or university libraries
	Congressional news	*Congressional Quarterly Weekly Report*
	Vote tabulations	Government documents section of selected public or university libraries
	Bills in process or legislated (bill number needed)	U.S representative or senator (may have local office)
	Health and nursing issues in U.S Congress	ANA
	ANA-PAC (*The American Nurse*)	600 Maryland Ave SW
		Suite 100
		Washington, DC 20024
		(202) 554-4444
	Public health issues in U.S Congress (*The Nation's Health*)	APHA
		1015 15th St NW
		Washington, DC 20005
		(202) 789-5600
State	Bills in process or legislated (bill number needed)	State representative or senator (may have local office)
	Health and nursing issues in state legislature, State PACs for nursing	SNA (for location, see April directory issue of the *American Journal of Nursing*)

ANA, American Nurses Association; *APHA*, American Public Health Association; *PAC*, political action committee; *SNA*, state nurses association.

TABLE 11-4   Sources for Electoral Information

GOVERNMENT LEVEL	INFORMATION AVAILABLE	LOCATION
State	State government operations	Secretary of (state capitol)
	Political subdivisions	Office of Lieutenant Governor (state capitol)
	Legislative information telephone number	
	State election laws and procedures	
	Campaign finance reports	
County or municipal	Similar to state as appropriate to local governmen	County clerk (county courthouse)
	Political jurisdictions for each household address	City clerk (city hall)
General	Government information	
	Political jurisdictions for each household address	League of Women Voters
	Names of current office holders in local jurisdictions	1730 M Street NW
		Washington, DC 20036
		(202) 429-1965
		Telephone directory
		(major cities)

before the legislature. The term derives from the fact that lobbyists usually stay in the areas (lobbies) next to the chambers of the Senate and the House, seeking either to talk with legislators as they walk to and from the chambers or await legislative action that might affect their interest.

To **lobby** is to try to influence legislators; it is an art of persuasion. A lobbyist is, by definition, a person who represents special interests (Loquist, 1999). Influencing lawmakers to pass effective health legislation requires the participation of individual nurses and nursing organizations. The initial step in this process involves request by telephone, e-mail, or letter to make an appointment with an elected official. Although exceptions exist, most officials are interested in meeting only with their own constituents (i.e., those registered to vote in their political jurisdiction) because the power of generating votes is the primary determinant of political influence.

Professional organizations are now making advocacy easier for members through the use of the Internet. Policy action centers are now part of many organizations' websites. E-mail alerts can be sent instantly to members residing in targeted districts to contact their legislators on a particular bill or issue. By entering one's zip code and a push of a button, a template letter can be signed and e-mailed to one's legislator.

The goal of the first contact with the official is to establish that the nurse is a concerned constituent and a credible source of information on health issues. The image of nurses as caring and helping people is a definite advantage at this point. In communities in which nurses have already established strong political credentials, their colleagues will be more readily accepted. An individual who establishes a reputation as a reliable and accurate resource as a lobbyist has substantial influence.

Legislators rely heavily on lobbyists to educate them on issues, and they usually want to hear from opposing sides before taking a position. The official must trust lobbyists to

Elizabeth Sacco, JD, and Tricia Asaro, JD, both of Greenberg Traurig, LLP, NYSALM's government affairs representative, with Nancy Kraus, midwife/quilter, in front of NYSALM quilt on display at 2005 Lobby Day, Albany, New York.

Tammy Farnham, CNM, and 2005 Lobby Day coordinator, with NYSALM President MaryAnne Laffin, CNM, NP, with "Proclaimation on Midwifery" signed by Governor George Pataki.

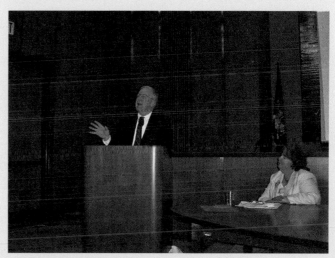

New York State Senator Hannon speaking to NYSALM members as they prepare to lobby.

Meeting together before the lobbying begins.

give accurate, though predictably biased, information. If a lobbyist does not have the information requested, he or she should obtain it and give it to the official quickly.

Each official represents a constituency with varied needs and interests, and each vote must be weighed within this context. The positions taken by legislators will not always be to an individual's liking, and evaluation of their performance should be based on their overall voting patterns, not on their votes on isolated issues. Many organizations (e.g., ANA, American Public Health Association, and Planned Parenthood) regularly tally and publish the records of each federal legislator on all issues related to the organization's priorities. This information can be helpful in evaluating elected officials. Internet addresses for these two organizations can be accessed through the WebLinks section of the Evolve website, http://evolve.elsevir.com/Nies/.

PROFESSIONAL ASSOCIATIONS AND LOBBYING

Collective action by nursing and health care organizations is critical to meeting their goals. Professional associations monitor legislative activity related to relevant health issues and link the process to their membership. This continual surveillance of the legislative environment is critical because even seemingly minor amendments can have profound effects on health services.

Thorough legislative surveillance requires the participation of people who are knowledgeable about nursing, health care, and the political intricacies of the legislative process. The ANA and American College of Nurse-Midwives have full-time staff lobbyists who work with Congress. State associations also work with state legislatures. State legislative contacts become the eyes, ears, and voices of their professional organizations. These associations can then provide comment and testimony on relevant issues to governing bodies. However, regardless of the effectiveness of association lobbyists in promoting the interests of nurses and society, they always need grassroots cooperation to truly influence decisions. In the final analysis, a sufficiently high number of communications from individual constituents, via letters, telephone calls, and e-mail messages has the greatest influence.

Lobbying is an ongoing activity for health policy issues influencing nursing and health care delivery. The ABC's of Lobbying provides an overview of the lobbying process (Box 11-8).

A State Organization: NYSALM

In New York State, more than 1,000 licensed midwives recognized a need for organized advocacy on the state level. The American College of Nurse-Midwives, which represents nearly 10,000 certified nurse-midwives and certified midwives nationally, did not have a mechanism in their structure (bylaws) to develop state organizations.

In 1999, the midwives of New York State formed the New York State Association of Licensed Midwives (NYSALM). NYSALM's organizational objectives include effecting legislation and regulations for their members.

BOX 11-8   ABCs of Lobbying

Before the Meeting

➤ Appointments will have been made with your legislator(s) for the Lobby Day. Tell the staff that you are a constituent and what issue(s) you would like to discuss with your representative. If your legislator is unavailable, you may have a scheduled appointment with a member of the legislative staff.

➤ If possible we will put together a delegation of midwives to attend the meeting. A number of individuals from the legislator's district who are concerned about the same issue will make a big impression. Take along students from their districts, as the legislators are impressed with their participation.

Preparing for the Meeting

➤ Establish your agenda and goals. Today we will focus on educating the legislators on the profession of midwifery, the legislation that we would like them to sponsor, our concerns about the malpractice insurance crisis and our interest in women's and children's health.

➤ Research your legislator's stance prior to the meeting. It is important that you know your official's position so that you can present your stance more effectively and have an intelligent discussion.

➤ Meet with the midwifery delegation that will participate in the lobbying. It is important that you review what each person will say during the meeting. Select someone as the group leader and make a list of points to be made and questions to be asked by each individual.

➤ Prepare materials. Review the packet of information you will leave with your legislator. It is important to include your name and phone number in the packet so that your legislator will have a contact person for more information. Leaving a business card would be appropriate.

During the Meeting

➤ Be on time for your meeting.

➤ Be concise and diplomatic. Keep your presentation short and to the point.

➤ Be a good listener. Look for indications of your legislator's views and watch for opportunities to provide useful information in order to strengthen or counter particular views.

➤ Stress why the issues concern you and others in your district.

➤ Don't be intimated. Your Legislator is in office to serve you. It is important to have a general knowledge of the issues, but you don't have to know every little detail. If he/she asks a question that you do not know the answer to, simply say that you do not know but are willing to find out. Find out the best way to get the information to him/her. (fax, e-mail, or a follow-up phone call).

After the Meeting

➤ Write a follow-up letter. After your visit, write a letter thanking your legislator for his/her time. Cards are included in your folder for you to mail prior to leaving the legislative building.

➤ Stay in contact with your legislator. Remember your goal is to strengthen midwifery relationships with your legislators.

From New York State Association of Licensed Midwives (NYSALM): *The Voice of Midwives* letter.

Each year, NYSALM brings midwives of the state together for a lobby day in the state capitol. In a few short years, their lobbying efforts have been successful in advancing their profession.

NYSALM reaches out to student midwives, encouraging their participation as advocates early in their professional career. ■

Nurses and Political Action Committees

Political action committees (PACs) have been important sources of collective political influence since the 1970s. These nonpartisan entities promote the election of candidates believed to be sympathetic to their interests. PACs are established by professional associations, business, and labor groups under federal and state laws that stipulate how they may contribute financially to campaigns. The advantage of a PAC is that small donations from many members, when added together, make an impressive addition to a campaign fund in the name of an organization. This gains the attention of the candidate and earns good will for the group.

Valid concern exists about the correlation of major PAC contributions and the legislator's votes on special interest legislation. However, as long as PACs are a reality of political life, nurses need to recognize their power and support those that are committed to electing candidates sympathetic to health care issues.

Most national associations of health care providers have PACs. Among the strongest are those representing hospitals, nursing homes, home health agencies, pharmaceutical interests, and insurance companies. A PAC that makes major political contributions is the American Medical Political Action Committee, sponsored by the American Medical Association. State medical associations also have strong PACs. This means that organized medicine has a powerful influence on national and state elections and on health care legislation at both levels.

The ANA and many other nursing organizations have PACs (Box 11-9). According to the information posted on their website, the ANA-PAC works "to ensure that nurses have the best representation possible in the United States Congress." Among other achievements, in 1998, the ANA-PAC helped procure funding increases for the Nurse Education Act and the National Institute of Nursing. In 2004, the ANA-PAC raised $785,000 (ANA, 2004b). Nurses made their mark on the 2004 elections with an unprecedented number of nurses coming together to support candidates in their commitment to advance nursing issues (ANA, 2004a) Box 11-9 lists priorities supported by the ANA-PAC.

Nurses and Coalitions

When two or more groups join to maximize resources, increasing their influence and improving their chances of success in achieving a common goal, it is called a **coalition.** Coalitions of health care providers often work together on issues such as family violence and fluoridation of water supplies. An outstanding example of such cooperative action is the establishment of rehabilitation programs for health professionals whose practice has been impaired by substance abuse or mental health problems.

Nursing and consumer groups often form coalitions to advance their shared interests in health promotion. In September 1999, the ANA joined 16 other organizations (e.g., American College of Nurse Practitioners, American Red Cross, Department of Veterans Affairs, and Sigma Theta

---

BOX 11-9   109th Congressional Legislative and Regulatory Priorities of the American Nurses Association

Nursing Shortage
Immigration and the nursing workforce
Funding for nursing workforce development programs

Appropriate Staffing
Adequate nursing facility staffing
Appropriate acute care staffing
Mandatory overtime

Workplace rights
Barriers to practice for advanced practice registered nurses
Fair Labor Standards Act: overtime regulations
Home health: plan of care designation
Medicaid coverage of advanced practice nursing
Safe Healthcare Reporting (SHARE) Act
Whistle-blowing/patient advocacy protections for nurses

Workplace Health and Safety
Health care worker safety
Safe patient handling and the Occupational Safety and Health Administration ergonomics standard

Patient Safety/Advocacy
Access to health care coverage
Association health plans
Medicaid cost containment
Medical errors
Medical malpractice liability/tort reform
Medicare reform/prescription drugs
Nursing research

From American Nurses Association: *Nursing's legislative and regulatory initiatives for the 109th Congress,* Silver Spring, Md, 2005b, The Author.

Tau) to form a coalition called Nurses for a Healthier Tomorrow. Responding to concerns about a potentially dangerous shortage of nurses, this coalition hopes to raise funds for a national advertising campaign designed to recruit new nurses and encourage existing ones to remain in the profession (Box 11-10). The coalition hopes to attract major health insurers, managed care companies, pharmaceutical firms, health care providers, nursing schools, and hospitals to support the campaign. The campaign focuses on the message that nurses are essential to the health care team and that they save health care dollars. The campaign shows that an increased demand exists for nurses, both in specialty areas and outside the hospital (ANA, 1999).

Nurses in Public Office

A profession derives its status from a contract with society to provide essential services under conditions of altruism and trust. Nurses are demonstrating this professionalism by serving the healthy and sick and by serving future generations through their influence in promoting wellness through public policy development. Although a few nurses are directly involved in health policy development, more are needed.

BOX 11-10   **Professional Organizations Joining Forces: Americans for Nursing Shortage Relief Alliance (ANSRA)**

ANSRA is a coalition of 37 nursing organizations that was founded in the early 2000s to influence policy and funding decisions related to nursing shortages. They do this through:
➤ Media attention to the nation's growing nursing shortage
➤ Advocacy for legislation that will reverse the nursing shortage
➤ Working with Congress to increase funding through the Nurse Reinvestment Act
➤ Promote nursing education, retention, and faculty development
➤ Develop funding initiatives for nursing education loans and scholarships
➤ Research into nursing workforce, staffing issues

In September 2004, ANSRA presented a briefing to Congress, titled "The Nursing Faculty Shortage: A National Perspective." In early 2005, ANSRA held a reception for members of Congress and their health legislative assistants to bring the nursing faculty shortage to the attention of federal policy makers.

Nurses and the public should be constantly attuned to opportunities to promote the appointment or election of nurses to policy-making positions.

Many women have become spokespeople for nursing and have a strong voice in politics. During the 2004 election cycle, nurses were very visible. The ANA endorsed some 250 candidates for the 109th Congress, with an 82% success rate (ANA, 2004c). The 109th Congress includes three nurses: Lois Capps, RN (D-CA), Carolyn McCarthy, LPN (D-NY), and Eddie Bernice Johnson, RN (D-TX). In addition, as of February 2000, a total of 97 nurses were serving as state legislators in 38 different states.

Nurse-legislators play a crucial role in interpreting health issues and influencing appropriate legislation. Nurses serve in county and city governments and on special governing bodies, such as school boards. Nurses also influence health policy through politically appointed positions. These appointments are based on individual qualifications for the position but may involve political connections.

Other women who have been active in the federal government are Carolyne Davis, who, in 2001, served as the administrator of the Health Care Financing Administration (renamed the Centers for Medicare and Medicaid Services), and Shirley Chater, who was Commissioner of the Social Service Administration. Virginia Trotter Betts, who served as the President of the ANA, was also the Senior Advisor on Nursing and Policy to the Secretary of the HHS in Washington, DC. Likewise, Dr. Beverly Malone resigned as President of the ANA in 1999 to assume the position of Deputy Assistant Secretary of the HHS. In this capacity, she advises the Assistant Secretary for the HHS, Dr. David Satcher, in program and political matters, policy and program development, and setting of legislative priorities. Denise H. Geolot, RN, PhD, FAAN, is Director of the Division of Nursing in the Bureau of Health Professions of the HRSA at HHS. Finally, nurses head 2 of the 10 regional offices of the HHS. Pat Monoya, MA, RN, is director for Region VI, headquartered in Dallas, and Pat Ford-Roegner, MS, RN, oversees Region IV, headquartered in Atlanta.

In the future, more nurses need to run for public office at all three levels of government. Whether serving as political appointees or career bureaucrats, nurses have much to offer. Young and beginning nurses should accept the challenge of helping advance the nursing practice and the nation's health.

Nurses and Health Policy Development

As the role of nurses in changing health care policy increases in importance, more nurses are needed who are equipped for this challenge. A strong cadre of nursing leaders who have the vision for change is essential to promoting nursing's policy agenda. National fellowships and internships are available for nurses who are interested in taking leadership roles (Sharp, 1999).

The Robert Wood Johnson Health Policy Fellowship is a 1-year career development program for mid career health professionals. The goal of this program is to help nurses gain an understanding of the health policy process and contribute to the formulation of new policies and programs. Robert Wood Johnson Health Policy fellows are selected from academic faculties from diverse disciplines, including medicine, dentistry, nursing, public health, health services administration, economics, and social services. After an extensive orientation on the legislative and executive branches of government, the fellows work with a member of Congress or on a congressional health committee (Sharp, 1999).

The President's Commission on White House Fellowships offers 20 fellowships each year to nurses early in their careers; the average age is 33. The White House fellows participate in an education program that involves working with government officials, scholars, journalists, and private-sector leaders to explore U.S. policy in action. Nurses who have been White House fellows may work at the Health Care Financing Administration and the Office of Science and Technology Policy, among others (Sharp, 1999). These fellowship programs are competitive, but strong leaders are desperately needed.

Nurses and Campaigning

Helping someone win an election is a sure way of gaining influence. All candidates are grateful for campaign assistance and usually remember to thank those who have helped. Although campaign contributions are commonly thought of as financial, they can also take the form of participation in campaign activities.

Nurses are frequently unable to contribute much money; therefore, they can provide these invaluable services. For the novice, veteran campaigners are eager to help him or her learn the necessary skills. Initially, a volunteer can address or stuff envelopes for mailings. The volunteer can also invite friends and neighbors for a social gathering to meet the candidate, thereby providing an opportunity to discuss issues of concern with constituents.

Telephone banks help a candidate identify supporters,

ETHICAL Insights

Nurses' Legislative Power

Nurses' interest in affecting health policies and legislation has expanded in recent years as nurses realize the influence they can have on their own practice and profession. As a body of more than 2.7 million, they can wield enormous power. This power of numbers is never more apparent than in the legislative process. A legislator carefully weighs the number of constituents supporting or opposing a bill before deciding how to vote. A sizable block of constituents on one side of an issue can significantly affect that vote. Representing the district is important to a legislator for ethical reasons and for political pragmatism.

opponents, and the critical undecided voter. These latter voters can make a difference on election day and are courted by all candidates. The telephone interviews are highly structured and easily handled by inexperienced campaign workers. Direct contact with potential voters may occur later in the form of house-to-house block walks or poll work on election day. The confidence that this requires comes with experience and a strong commitment to the candidate and the cause.

Hosting a social function to allow nurse colleagues to meet the candidate is a welcome contribution to the campaign. Nurses are substantial in number and their voting record is humanistic; therefore they are valued as a political force.

Government employees may be restricted by policies that limit or disallow political activism. Nurses employed at any level of government should be aware of such prohibitions.

Nurses and Voting Strength

With more than 2.7 million members, nurses make up the largest profession in health care (ANA, 2004a); one in 44 women voters is a registered nurse (RN) (Hadley, 1996). Therefore if every RN voted, their influence on health policy would be tremendous. If the nursing profession is to meet the challenges of the twenty-first century and work as a profession to positively influence the health of populations, political action is necessary, and an understanding of the factors that motivate or impede political action is needed (Winter and Lockhart, 1997).

INTERNET AND POLITICAL PROCESS

A 30-day window of opportunity is typical for public input into the development of regulations. Written comments about a political issue are made part of the public record. To facilitate correspondence, websites have been set up to promote contacting agencies, governmental organizations, and political figures. Nurses need to be aware of some of the important websites. Furthermore, many legislators may have their own web pages so that the nurse could easily access his or her office. Numerous websites related to health policy issues may be accessed through the WebLinks section of this book's website at http://evolve.elsevier.com/Nies/.

The Internet can provide almost unlimited access to information. However, access to information does not ensure the quality or credibility of the information. The user is responsible for evaluation of the information and separation of quality information from misinformation.

SUMMARY

Historically, nurses have been able to make significant differences in the quality of life experienced by the members of the communities in which they serve. By understanding how government works, how bills become law, and how legislators make decisions, nurses can influence policy decisions through individual efforts such as letter writing, participation in political campaigns, and selection of candidates who support policies conducive to improving the health and welfare of all citizens. When organized in lobbying groups, coalitions, and PACs, or when holding office, nurses can be a powerful force that brings about change in the delivery and quality of the health care of aggregates.

LEARNING ACTIVITIES

1. Develop an "insight" bulletin board, with each class member contributing cartoons, anecdotes, and clippings about issues affecting public health or nursing.
2. Look at a current public health issue that affects your community, including an understanding of the causes, effect on the public, and possible solutions. Influence its resolution through any of the following activities:
   a. Write a succinct letter to the editor of a local newspaper.
   b. Write a position paper and submit it to the "opinion page" of a local newspaper.
   c. Write to elected or appointed officials whose jurisdiction may be influential on the issue.
   d. Meet with an elected or appointed official to discuss the issue in groups of two or three.
   e. Call in to a radio talk show about the issue.
   f. Volunteer to speak on the issue to appropriate consumer or professional groups.
3. With a group of two or three, meet with an elected official for a 15-minute appointment to ask about the official's concerns and priorities. Remember to refer to the "ABC's of Lobbying" prior to meeting with the official.
4. Invite an elected official who is sympathetic to nurses to speak to the local chapter of the National Nursing Students Association to discuss the political process and health policy.
5. Invite an elected official to spend a day engaging in appropriate activities with a public health nurse or nursing student. Take black-and-white photos for press use.
6. Invite a medical reporter from the press, radio, or television to observe public health nursing activities that would appeal to the public.
7. Participate in a group organized around a public health issue (e.g., disposable diapers, toxic waste, or fluoride).
8. Serve as a volunteer in a campaign for a candidate who is supportive or potentially supportive of public health or nursing issues.
9. Serve as a volunteer for a political party.

REFERENCES

Aiken L, Clarke S, Sloane D, Sochalski J, Silber, J: Hospital nurse staffing and patient mortality, nurse burnout, and job dissatisfaction. *JAMA* 288(16):1987-1993, 2002

American Nurses Association: ANA advises on health care reform, *Capital Update* 11(8):1, 1993.

American Nurses Association: *ANA joins coalition formed to promote nursing* (press release), 1999, The Author, http://www.nursingworld.org/rnrealnews.

American Nurses Association: *Achieving access for all Americans: a proposal from the American Nurses Association for health coverage 2000,* 2000a, The Author, http://www.ana.org/readroom/rwjpaper.htm.

American Nurses Association: *American Nurses Association Political Action Committee: PAC FAQ,* 2000b, The Author, http://www.ana.org/gova/federal/anapac/gpacfaq.htmhttp://vocusgr.vocus.com/grconvert1/webpub/ana/Profile.asp?Entity=PRAsset&EntityID=760&XSL=Asset&PublishType=GR+Asset.

American Nurses Association: *ANA proposes universal Medicare program as solution to fragmented health care system* (press release), 2000c, The Author, http://www.nursingworld.org/rnrealnews.

American Nurses Association: ANA flexes its political muscle at the 2004 political conventions, *Am Nurse* 36(5):14, 2004a.

American Nurses Association: ANA-PAC needs you, *Am Nurse* 36(4):18, 2004b.

American Nurses Association: Saying goodbye to old friends, *Am Nurse* 36(6):12, 2004c.

American Association of Occupational Health Nursing: 2005 Key public policy issues, The Author, http://www.aaohn.org/public_policy/upload/2006%20Public%20Policy-2.pdf}.

American Nurses Association: *Nursing's legislative and regulatory initiatives for the 109th Congress,* Silver Spring, Md, 2005b, The Author.

Bonick J: Policy, politics and the law. In Stanhope M, Lancaster J, editors: *Community and public health nursing,* ed 5, St. Louis, 2000, Mosby.

Brooke PS: Legal context for community/public health nursing practice. In Maurer FA, Smith CM, editors: *Community/public health nursing practice: health for families and populations,* ed 3, Philadelphia, 2005, WB Saunders.

Center for the Advancement of Women: *Faye Wattleton Bio,* 2005, The Author, http://www.advancewomen.org/for-reporters/faye-wattleton-bio/.

Centers for Disease Control and Prevention: *Annual Report 2004,* http://www.cdc.gov.

Centers for Disease Control and Prevention: *State of the CDC: fiscal year 2004,* The Author, http//www.cdc.gov/about/stateofcdc/FY05/cd/SOCDC/SOCDC2004.pdf.

Centers for Disease Control and Prevention: Recommended childhood and adolescent immunization schedule—United States, 2005, *MMWR Morb Mortality Wkly Rep* 53(51):Q1-Q3, 2005, http://www.cdc.gov/mmwr/preview/mmwrhtml/mm5351-Immunizationa1.htm.

de Vries C, Vanderbilt M: Nurses gain ground during reform debate, *Am Nurse* 26(10):2-3, 1994.

Dowling WL: Hospitals and health systems. In Williams SJ, Torrens PR, editors: *Introduction to health services,* ed 6, Albany, NY, 2002, Delmar.

Feldstein PJ: *Health policy issues: An economic perspective,* ed 3, Chicago, 2003, Health Administration Press.

Hadley EH: Nursing in the political and economic marketplace: challenges for the 21st century, *Nurs Outlook* 44(1):6-10, 1996.

Hall-Long BA: Nursing's past, present, and future political experiences, *Nurs Health Care Perspect* 16(1):24-28, 1995.

Health Resources and Services Administration: *The registered nurse population: findings from the national sample survey of registered nurses,* Washington, DC, 2002, The Author.

Helms LB, Anderson MA, Hanson K: Doin' politics: linking policy and politics in nursing, *Nurs Admin Q* 20(3):32-41, 1996.

Institute of Medicine: *Biographical information: 2001 Lienhard Award Recipient Ruth Watson*

Lubic, 2001, The Author, http://www.iom.edu/subpage.asp?id=5046.

Kalisch PA, Kalisch BJ: *American nursing: a history,* ed 4, Philadelphia, 2004, Lippincott Williams & Wilkins.

Lewinson, SB: Pride in our past: nursing's political roots. In Mason DJ, Leavitt JK, Chaffee MW: *Policy and politics in nursing and health care,* ed 4, Philadelphia, 2002, WB Saunders.

Litman T: *Health, politics and policy,* ed 3, Albany, NY, 1997, Delmar.

Loquist RS: Regulation: parallel and powerful. In Milstead JA, editor: *Health policy and politics: a nurse's guide,* Gaithersburg, Md, 1999, Aspen.

Lyttle B: Humanizing childbirth, *Am J Nurs* 100(10):52-53, 2000.

Mason DJ, Leavitt JK, Chaffee MW: Policy and politics: a framework for action. In Mason DJ, Leavitt JK, Chaffee MW: *Policy and politics in nursing and health care,* ed 4, Philadelphia, 2002, WB Saunders.

Pulcini J et al: Health policy and the private sector: new vistas for nursing, *Nurs Health Care Perspect* 21(1):22-28, 2000.

Sharp N: Wanted: nurse leaders to craft health policy, *Nurse Pract* 24(10):85-86, 89, 1999.

Shi L, Singh DA: *Delivering health care in America: a systems approach,* ed 3, Sudbury, Mass, 2004, Jones and Bartlett.

Sultz HA, Young KM: *Health care USA: understanding its organization and delivery,* ed 3, Gaithersburg, Md, 2001, Aspen.

US Department of Health and Human Services: *Healthy People 2010,* Conference edition, Washington, DC, 2000, The Author.

US Department of Health and Human Services, Centers for Medicare and Medicaid Services, FY 2005 Budget in Brief, 2004, http://www.dhhs.gov/budget/05budget/centersformed.html#med.

Winter MK, Lockhart JS: From motivation to action: understanding nurses' political involvement, *Nurs Health Care Perspect* 18(5):244-250, 1997.

12

Cultural Diversity and Community Health Nursing

Margaret M. Andrews

MEDIA RESOURCES

Additional Material for Study, Review, and Further Exploration

evolve Website at http://evolve.elsevier.com/Nies

❖ Quiz ❖ Case Studies ❖ Content Updates ❖ Glossary ❖ WebLinks

OBJECTIVES

Upon completion of this chapter, the reader will be able to do the following:

1. Critically analyze racial and cultural diversity in the United States.
2. Analyze the influence of sociocultural, political, economic, ethical and religious factors that influence the health of culturally diverse individuals, groups, and communities.
3. Identify the cultural aspects of nursing care for culturally diverse individuals, groups, and communities.
4. Apply the principles of transcultural nursing to community health nursing practice.

KEY TERMS

biomedical	culture specific	universality	spirituality
cultural imposition	culture universal	magicoreligious	subculture
cultural negotiation	culturological assessment	naturalistic	transcultural nursing
cultural stereotyping	dominant value orientation	norms	value
culture	ethnocentrism	poverty	yin-yang theory
culture-bound syndrome	Leininger's theory of culture	religion	
culture shock	care diversity and	socioeconomic status (SES)	

CHAPTER OUTLINE

CULTURAL DIVERSITY

TRANSCULTURAL PERSPECTIVES ON COMMUNITY HEALTH NURSING

POPULATION TRENDS

CULTURAL PERSPECTIVES AND *HEALTHY PEOPLE 2010*
Addressing Racial and Ethnic Disparities in Health Care

TRANSCULTURAL NURSING

OVERVIEW OF CULTURE
Culture and the Formation of Values
Culture and the Family

CULTURE AND SOCIOECONOMIC FACTORS
Distribution of Resources
Education

CULTURE AND NUTRITION
Nutrition Assessment of Culturally Diverse Groups
Dietary Practices of Selected Cultural Groups
Religion and Diet

CULTURE AND RELIGION
Religion and Spirituality
Childhood and Spirituality

CULTURE AND AGING

CROSS-CULTURAL COMMUNICATION
Nurse-Client Relationship
Space, Distance, and Intimacy
Overcoming Communication Barriers
Nonverbal Communication
Language
Touch
Gender

HEALTH-RELATED BELIEFS AND PRACTICES
Health and Culture
Cross-Cultural Perspectives on Causes of Illness
Folk Healers ➤

Acknowledgment is given to Elda G. Ramirez for contributions to the chapter.

CULTURAL DIVERSITY

Cultural diversity is a multifaceted and complex concept that refers to the differences among people, especially those related to values, attitudes, beliefs, norms, behaviors, customs, and ways of living. The American Nurses Association's (ANA) position statement on cultural diversity in nursing practice (ANA, 1991) urges nurses to understand how cultural groups view life processes, how cultural groups define health and illness, how healers cure and care for members of their respective cultural groups, and how the cultural background of the nurse influences the way in which care is delivered. Nurses in community health settings also need to understand the diversity or differences that occur in families, groups, neighborhoods, communities, and public and community health care organizations.

TRANSCULTURAL PERSPECTIVES ON COMMUNITY HEALTH NURSING

Nurses' knowledge of culture and cultural concepts improves the health of the community by enhancing their ability to provide culturally competent care. Culturally competent community health nursing requires that nurses understand the lifestyle, value system, and health and illness behaviors of diverse individuals, families, groups, and communities. Nurses also should understand the culture of institutions that influence the health and well-being of communities. Nurses who have knowledge of, and an ability to work with, diverse cultures are able to devise effective interventions to reduce risks in a manner that is culturally congruent with community, group, and individual values.

In the United States, metaphors such as *melting pot, mosaic,* and *salad bowl* describe the cultural diversity that characterizes the population. Although there is a tendency to identify the federally defined racial and ethnic minority groups when referring to the cultural aspects of community health nursing, *all* individuals, families, groups, communities, and institutions, including nurses and the nursing profession, have

cultural characteristics that influence community health. When planning and implementing health care, community health nurses need to balance cultural diversity with the universal human experience and common needs of all people.

POPULATION TRENDS

The population of the United States is becoming increasingly diverse. In recent years, the populations within the federally defined minority groups have grown faster than the population as a whole. In 1970, minority groups accounted for 16% of the population. By 1999, this share increased to 30%. Assuming that current trends continue, the U.S. Census Bureau (2005) projects that by the mid twenty-first century, minorities will account for 51.1% of the total population. For the first time in U.S. history, minorities will make up a majority of the total population.

Furthermore, the numbers of certain minority groups are growing considerably faster than those of whites and other groups. Hispanics (of any race) accounted for almost 50% of the national population growth of 2.9 million between mid 2003 and mid 2004. The Hispanic growth rate of 3.6% over that 12-month period was more than three times that of the total population (1%). If current demographic trends continue, the United States will have the following population composition by the year 2080: Hispanic, 23.4%; black, 14.7%; and Asian and Pacific Islander, 12% (U.S. Census Bureau, 2004). At the same time, the Native-American and Alaska Native population is projected to remain at 0.7% or perhaps decrease slightly, due to intermarriage. Table 12-1 summarizes the current population composition by race, number, and percentage in 2001 and 2004.

Although the nursing profession has representatives from diverse groups, minorities are generally underrepresented. Currently about 13.4% of the nation's 2.3 million registered nurses come from racial and ethnic minority backgrounds. Estimates for each minority group are as follows: 4.9% black; 2.0% Hispanic; 3.7% Asian and Pacific Islander; and 0.5% Native-American and Alaska Native (Spratley et al., 2002). Additionally, each minority group is distributed differently

TABLE 12-1   Composition of United States Population, 2001 and 2004

POPULATION GROUP	2001 POPULATION	% OF POPULATION	2004 POPULATION	% OF POPULATION
Total	285,102,071	100	293,655,404	100
White (non-Hispanic)	196,320,116	68.9	197,840,821	67.4
Black (non-Hispanic)	34,812,941	12.2	35,963,702	12.2
Native American, Eskimo, and Aleut	2,129,624	0.7	2,206,748	0.7
Asian and Pacific Islander	11,243,028	3.9	12,466,585	4.2
Hispanic (any race)	37,060,356	13.0	41,322,070	14.1
Two or more races	3,536,006	1.2	3,855,478	1.3 .

From US Census Bureau: Annual estimates of population, 2001 & 2003, The Author, http://www.census.gov/popest/national/asrh/NC-EST2004/NC-EST2004-03.xls.

around the country. Black nurses are more likely to be found in the South, Hispanics in the West or South (i.e., especially states bordering Mexico), and Asian and Pacific Islanders in the West or Northeast. Native-American and Alaska Native nurses are predominantly in states with reservations.

The United States has grown and achieved its success largely through immigration. Since 1991, more than 13 million legal immigrants have come to United States (U.S. Department of Homeland Security, 2006). In 2003, the U.S. population included 33.5 million foreign-born individuals, or 11.7% of the total population. Among those foreign-born, 53.3% were born in Latin America, 25% in Asia, 13.7% in Europe, and the remaining 8% in other regions of the world (U.S. Census Bureau, 2004). The number of immigrants and refugees in the United States is projected to continue to increase.

In addition, people from other countries will continue to seek treatment in U.S. hospitals, particularly for cardiovascular, neurological, and cancer care, and U.S. nurses will to have the opportunity to travel abroad to work in a variety of health care settings in the international marketplace. In the course of a nursing career, it is possible to encounter foreign visitors, international university faculty members, international high school and university students, family members of foreign diplomats, immigrants, refugees, as well as members of more than 130 different ethnic groups, and Native Americans from more than 557 federally recognized tribes. A serious conceptual problem exists within nursing in that nurses are expected to know, understand, and meet the health needs of these culturally diverse individuals, groups, and communities.

Members of some cultural groups desire culturally relevant health care that incorporates their specific beliefs and practices. An increasing expectation exists among members of certain cultural groups that health care providers will respect their "cultural health rights," an expectation that frequently conflicts with the unicultural, Western biomedical worldview taught in most U.S. educational programs that prepare nurses and other health care providers.

Given the multicultural composition of the United States and the projected increase in the number of individuals from diverse cultural backgrounds, concern for cultural beliefs and practices of people in community health nursing is becoming increasingly important. Nursing is inherently a transcultural phenomenon, in that the context and process of helping people involves at least two people who often have different cultural orientations or intracultural lifestyles.

CULTURAL PERSPECTIVES AND *HEALTHY PEOPLE 2010*

Healthy People 2010, the prevention agenda for the nation, identifies priority areas and objectives. By developing a set of national health targets, which includes eliminating racial and ethnic disparities in health, U.S. health officials, together with state and local officials and members of the private sector, set goals to increase the quality and years of healthy life for all Americans (U.S. Department of Health and Human Services [USDHHS], 2000).

The *Healthy People 2010* objectives incorporate the government's Initiative to Eliminate Racial and Ethnic Disparities in Health and focus on ways to close the gaps in health outcomes. Particularly targeted are racial and ethnic disparities in areas including diabetes, acquired immunodeficiency syndrome (AIDS), heart disease, infant mortality rates, cancer screening and management, and immunizations. The objectives bring focus on disparities among racial and ethnic minorities, women, youth, older adults, people of low income and education, and people with disabilities (USDHHS, 2000). The Healthy People table lists selected objectives from *Healthy People 2010* specific to cultural health issues.

The aims of *Healthy People 2010* are the promotion of healthy behaviors, promotion of healthy and safe communities, improvement of systems for personal and public health, and prevention and reduction of diseases and disorders. The initiative is a tool for monitoring and tracking health status, health risks, and use of health services.

Addressing Racial and Ethnic Disparities in Health Care

As in many nations, people in the United States who come from various racial, ethnic, cultural and socioeconomic backgrounds often experience marked disparities in health care. A recent study by the Commonwealth Fund found that Hispanics and Asian Americans are the worst served by the U.S. health care system (Johnson et al., 2004). The study revealed that attention to three factors would enhance the health care of people from diverse cultures: (1) effective communication between client and health care provider, (2) overcoming cultural and linguistic barriers, and (3) access to affordable health insurance.

The occurrence of many diseases, injuries, and other public health problems is disproportionately higher in some

HEALTHY PEOPLE 2010 | Selected Objectives Related to Cultural Health

Objective	Baseline (1998)	Target
1-1: Increase the proportion of persons with health insurance.		
American-Indian or Alaska Native	79%	100%
Asian or Pacific Islander	83%	
Black	84%	
White	87%	
Hispanic	70%	
1-8 e-h: Increase nursing degrees awarded to underrepresented populations.		
e. American-Indian or Alaska Native	0.7%	1%
f. Asian or Pacific Islander	3.2%	4%
g. Black	6.9%	13%
h. Hispanic	3.4%	12%
3-1: Reduce the overall cancer death rate	201.4 per 100,000	158.7 per 100,000
American-Indian or Alaska Native	131.8	
Asian or Pacific Islander	127.2	
Black	262.1	
White	202.2	
Hispanic	125.5	
5-3: Reduce the overall rate of diabetes that is clinically diagnosed.	40 per 1000	25 per 1000
American-Indian or Alaska Native	NA	
Asian or Pacific Islander	NA	
African–American	74	
White	36	
Hispanic	61	
8-11: Eliminate elevated blood lead levels in children.	4.4% (one to five years of age)	0
American-Indian or Alaska Native	NA	
Asian or Pacific Islander	NA	
Black	11.5%	
White	2.6%	
Hispanic	4%	
9-7: Reduce pregnancies among adolescent females (overall).	72 per 1000	42 per 1000
American-Indian or Alaska Native	NA	
Asian or Pacific Islander	NA	
Black	133	
White	61	
Hispanic	110	
12-1: Reduce coronary heart disease deaths (overall).	208 per 100,000	166 per 100,000
American-Indian or Alaska Native	134	
Asian or Pacific Islander	125	
Black	257	
White	214	
Hispanic	151	
13-1: Reduce AIDS among adolescents and adults (overall).	19.5 new cases per 100, 000	1 new case per 100,000
American-Indian or Alaska Native	9.4	
Asian or Pacific Islander	4.3	
Black	82.9	
White	8.5	
Hispanic	33	
15-3: Reduce firearm-related deaths (overall).	11 per 100,000	4.9 per 100,000
American-Indian or Alaska Native	11.4	
Asian or Pacific Islander	5	
Black	23.7	
White	10	
Hispanic	10.7	
16-1 h: Reduce deaths from SIDS.	0.77 per 1000	0.3 per 1000
American-Indian or Alaska Native	1.56	
Asian or Pacific Islander	0.51	

HEALTHY PEOPLE **2010**	Selected Objectives Related to Cultural Health (cont'd)		
Objective	**Baseline (1998)**	**Target**	
Black	1.46		
White	0.71		
Hispanic	0.47		
18-1: Reduce the suicide rate (overall).	10.8 per 100,000	6 per 100,000	
American-Indian or Alaska Native	12.4		
Asian or Pacific Islander	7		
Black	6.5		
White	12.8		
Hispanic	6.4		
19-2: Reduce the proportion of adults who are obese (overall).	23%	15%	
American-Indian or Alaska Native	NA		
Asian or Pacific Islander	NA		
Black	30%		
White	21%		
Hispanic	29%		
26-1: Reduce deaths caused by alcohol-related motor vehicle crashes.	6.1 per 100,000	4 per 100,000	
American-Indian or Alaska Native	19.2		
Asian or Pacific Islander	2.4		
Black	6.4		
White	6		
Hispanic	NA		
27-1 a: Reduce cigarette smoking by adults (overall).	24%	12%	
American-Indian or Alaska Native	34%		
Asian or Pacific Islander	16%		
Black	26%		
White	25%		
Hispanic	20%		

From US Department of Health and Human Services: *Healthy people 2010*, Washington, DC, 2000, US Government Printing Office.
SIDS, Sudden infant death syndrome, *NA,* not available.

groups; access to health care may be more restricted, and the overall quality of health care is deemed inferior, for people from certain racial, ethnic, and cultural populations. Although the overall health of the U.S. population has improved during the past several decades, research reveals that all people have not shared equally in those improvements. For example, 17% of Hispanic adults and 16% of black adults report that they are in fair or poor health, compared with 10% of non-Hispanic whites (Agency for Healthcare Research and Quality, 2005). Primary care provides the foundation for the health care system, and research indicates that having a usual source of care increases the chance that people will receive adequate preventive care and other important health services. Data from the Agency for Health Care Research and Quality (2005) reveals the following facts:

- Cancer mortality rates are 35% higher in black Americans than in whites.
- Black Americans who are diabetic are seven times more likely to have amputations and develop renal failure than are white diabetics.
- 30% of Hispanics and 20% of black Americans lack a usual source of health care (compared with less than 16% of whites).

- Hispanic children are nearly three times as likely as non-Hispanic white children to have no usual source of health care.
- Black Americans (16%) and Hispanic Americans (13%) are more likely to rely on hospitals or clinics for health care than are whites (8%).

During the past two decades, health disparities have become the focus of numerous federal, state, and local government studies, and one of the major goals of *Healthy People 2010* is to eliminate health disparities. Therefore, it is essential to look at how to overcome these and other identified factors that contribute to poorer health among members of some minority groups.

TRANSCULTURAL NURSING

In 1959, Madeleine Leininger, a nurse-anthropologist, used the term **transcultural nursing** to define the philosophical and theoretical similarities between nursing and anthropology. In 1968, Leininger proposed her theory-generated model, and in 1970, she wrote the first book on transcultural nursing, *Nursing and Anthropology: Two Worlds to Blend* (Leininger, 1970). According to Leininger (1978), transcultural nursing is "a formal area of study and practice focused on a comparative analysis of different cultures and subcultures in the world with respect to cultural care, health and illness beliefs, values, and practices with the goal of using this knowledge to provide culture-specific and culture-universal nursing care to people" (p. 493). **Culture specific** refers to the "particularistic values, beliefs, and patterning of behavior that tend to be special, 'local,' or unique to a designated culture and which do not tend to be shared with members of other cultures" (Leininger, 1991, p. 491), whereas **culture universal** refers to the "commonalties of values, norms of behavior, and life patterns that are similarly held among cultures about human behavior and lifestyles and form the bases for formulating theories for developing cross-cultural laws of human behavior" (Leininger, 2001 p. 491).

Although many nurse-scholars have developed theories of nursing, **Leininger's theory of culture care diversity and universality** is the only one that gives precedence to understanding the cultural dimensions of human care and caring. Leininger's theory is concerned with describing, explaining, and projecting nursing similarities and differences focused primarily on human care and caring in human cultures. Leininger used worldview, social structure, language, ethnohistory, environmental context, and the generic or folk and professional systems to provide a comprehensive and holistic view of influences in cultural care and well-being. The following three models of nursing decisions and actions may be useful in providing culturally congruent and competent care (Andrews and Boyle, 2003; Leininger, 1978, 1991, 1995; Leininger and McFarland, 2002):

1. Culture care preservation and maintenance
2. Culture care accommodation and negotiation
3. Culture care repatterning and restructuring

Among the strengths of Leininger's theory is its flexibility for use with individuals, families, groups, communities, and institutions in diverse health systems. Leininger's Sunrise Model (Figure 12-1) depicts the theory of cultural care diversity and universality and provides a visual representation of the key components of the theory and the interrelationships among its components.

Although this text does not review all the recognized nursing theories from a transcultural perspective, the reader should critically evaluate the cultural relevance of a theory before using it in community health nursing. The nurse should examine the underlying assumptions of theories from a transcultural perspective. For example, those theories emphasizing self-care fail to recognize that many cultures and subcultures value group interdependence, cooperation, and responsibility for others. When clients' cultural values and expressions of care differ from those of the nurse, the nurse must exercise caution to ensure that mutual goals have been established.

The term *cross-cultural nursing* is sometimes used synonymously with *transcultural nursing*. The terms *intercultural nursing* and *multicultural nursing* and the phrase "ethnic people of color" are also used. Since Leininger's early work, many nurses have contributed significantly to the advancement of nursing care of culturally diverse clients, groups, and communities, and some of their contributions are mentioned in this chapter.

One of the major challenges that community health nurses face in working with clients from culturally diverse backgrounds is overcoming individual **ethnocentrism**, which is a person's tendency to view his or her own way of life as the most desirable, acceptable, or best and tendency to act in a superior manner toward individuals from another culture. Nurses also must beware of **cultural imposition**, which is a person's tendency to impose his or her own beliefs, values, and patterns of behavior on individuals from another culture.

OVERVIEW OF CULTURE

In 1871, the English anthropologist Sir Edward Tylor was the first to define the term *culture*. According to Tylor (1871), culture refers to the complex whole, including knowledge, beliefs, art, morals, law, customs, and any other capabilities and habits acquired by virtue of the fact that one is a member of a particular society. Culture represents a person's way of perceiving, evaluating, and behaving within his or her world, and it provides the blueprint for determining his or her values, beliefs, and practices. Culture has four basic characteristics:

1. It is learned from birth through the processes of language acquisition and socialization.
2. It is shared by all members of the same cultural group.
3. It is adapted to specific conditions related to environmental and technical factors and to the availability of natural resources.
4. It is dynamic.

Culture is an all-pervasive and universal phenomenon. However, the culture that develops in any given society is always specific and distinctive, encompassing all of the knowledge, beliefs, customs, and skills acquired by members of that society. Within cultures, groups of individuals share beliefs, values, and attitudes that are different from those of other groups within the same culture. Ethnicity, religion, education, occupation, age, sex, and individual preferences and variations bring differences. When such groups function within a large culture, they are termed *subcultural groups*.

The term **subculture** is used for fairly large aggregates of people who share characteristics that are not common to all members of the culture and which enable them to be a distinguishable subgroup. Ethnicity, religion, occupation, health-related characteristics, age, sex, and geographical location are frequently used to identify subcultural groups. Examples of U.S. subcultures based on ethnicity (e.g., subcultures with common traits such as physical characteristics, language, or ancestry) include blacks, Hispanics, Native Americans, and Chinese Americans. Subcultures based on religion include members of the more than 1200 recognized religions, such as Catholics, Jews, Mormons, Muslims, and Buddhists. Those based on occupation include health care professionals (e.g., nurses and physicians), career military personnel, and farmers. Those based on health-related characteristics include the blind, hearing impaired, and mentally retarded. Subcultures based on age include adolescents and older adults, and those based on sex or sexual preference include women, men, lesbians, and gay men. Those based on geographical location include Appalachians, Southerners, and New Yorkers.

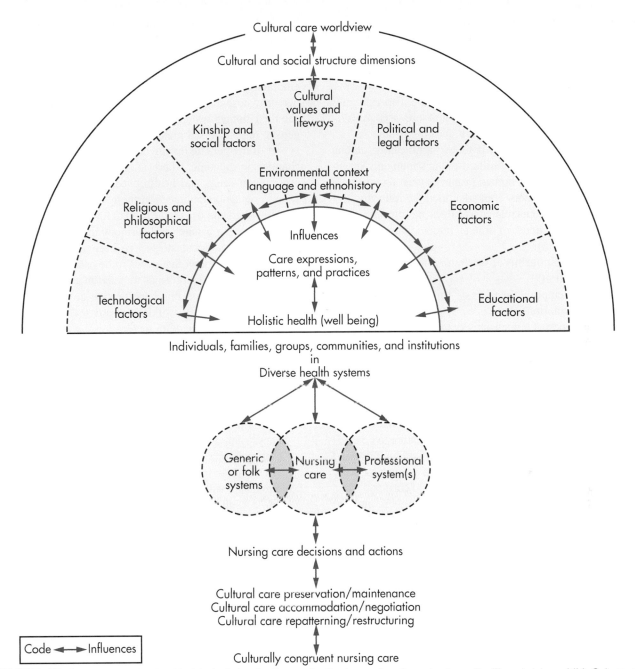

FIGURE 12-1   Leininger's Sunrise Model, depicting the theory of cultural care diversity and universality. (From Leininger MM: *Culture, care, diversity, and universality: a theory of nursing*, New York, 1991, National League of Nursing Press.)

Culture and the Formation of Values

According to Leininger (1995), **value** refers to a desirable or undesirable state of affairs. Values are a universal feature of all cultures, although the types and expressions of values differ widely. **Norms** are the rules by which human behavior is governed and result from the cultural values held by the group. All societies have rules or norms that specify appropriate and inappropriate behavior. Individuals are rewarded or punished as they conform to, or deviate from, the established norms. Values and norms, along with the acceptable and unacceptable behaviors associated with them, are learned in childhood.

Every society has a **dominant value orientation,** a basic value orientation that is shared by the majority of its members as a result of early common experiences. In the United States, the dominant value orientation is reflected in the dominant cultural group, which is made up of white, middle-class Protestants, typically those who came to the United States at least two generations ago from northern Europe. Many members of the dominant cultural group are of Anglo-Saxon descent; thus, they are sometimes referred to as white Anglo-Saxon Protestants (WASPs). In the United States, the dominant cultural group places emphasis on educational achievement, science, technology, individual expression, democracy, experimentation, and informality.

Although an assumption is sometimes made that the term *white* refers to a homogeneous group of Americans, a rich diversity of ethnic variation exists among the many groups that constitute the dominant majority. Countries of origin include those of eastern and western Europe (e.g., Ireland, Poland, Italy, France, Sweden, and Russia). The origins of people in Canada, Australia, New Zealand, and South Africa can ultimately be traced to western Europe. Appalachians, the Amish, Cajuns, and other subgroups are also examples of whites who have cultural roots that are recognizably different from those of the dominant cultural group.

Values and norms vary, sometimes significantly, among various cultural groups. According to Kluckhohn and Strodtbeck (1961), several basic human problems exist for which all people must find a solution. They identified the following five common human problems related to values and norms:

1. What is the character of innate human nature (human nature orientation)?
2. What is the relationship of the human to nature (person-nature orientation)?
3. What is the temporal focus (i.e., time sense) of human life (time orientation)?
4. What is the mode of human activity (activity orientation)?
5. What is the mode of human relationships (social orientation)?

Human Nature Orientation

Innate human nature may be good, evil, or a combination of good and evil. Some believe that life is a struggle to overcome a basically evil nature; they consider human nature to be unalterable or able to be perfected only through great discipline and effort. For others, human nature is perceived as fundamentally good, unalterable, and difficult or impossible to corrupt.

According to Kohls (1984), the dominant U.S. cultural group chooses to believe the best about a person until that person proves otherwise. Concern in the United States for prison reform, social rehabilitation, and the plight of less fortunate people around the world is a reflective perception of the belief in the fundamental goodness of human nature. Recent scientific advances, such as the advent of stem cell research and genome studies, have necessitated consideration of ethical quandaries regarding human nature. Questions emerge as to whether science can or should pursue activities that could alter the basic human orientation.

Person-Nature Orientation

The following three perspectives examine the ways in which the person-nature relationship is perceived:

1. Destiny, in which people are subjugated to nature in a fatalistic, inevitable manner
2. Harmony, in which people and nature exist together as a single entity
3. Mastery, in which people are intended to overcome natural forces and put them to use for the benefit of humankind

Most Americans consider humans and nature clearly separated; this is an incomprehensible perspective for many individuals of Asian heritage. The idea that a person can control his or her own destiny is alien to many individuals of culturally diverse backgrounds. Many cultures believe that people are driven and controlled by fate and can do very little, if anything, to influence it. Americans, by contrast, have an insatiable drive to subdue, dominate, and control their natural environment.

For example, the reader should consider three individuals who have been diagnosed with hypertension, where each embraces one of the values orientations described. The person whose values orientation is destiny may say, "Why should I bother watching my diet, taking medication, and getting regular blood pressure checks? High blood pressure is part of my genetic destiny and there is nothing I can do to change the outcome. There is no need to waste money on prescription drugs and health checkups." The person whose values orientation embraces harmony may say, "If I follow the diet described and use medication to lower my blood pressure, I can restore the balance and harmony that were upset by this illness. The emotional stress I've been feeling indicates an inner lack of harmony that needs to be balanced." The person whose values orientation leads to belief in active mastery may say, "I will overcome this hypertension no matter what. By eating the right foods, working toward stress reduction, and conquering the disease with medication, I will take charge of the situation and influence the course of my disease."

Time Orientation

People can perceive time in the following three ways:

1. *The focus may be on the past, with traditions and ancestors playing an important role in the client's life.* For example, many Asians, Native Americans, East Indians, and Africans hold particular beliefs about ancestors and tend to value long-standing traditions. In times of crisis, such as illness, individuals with a values orientation emphasizing the past may consult with ancestors or ask for their guidance or protection during the illness.
2. *The focus may be on the present, with little attention paid to the past or the future.* These individuals are concerned with the current situation, and they perceive the future as vague or unpredictable. Nurses may have difficulty encouraging these individuals to prepare for the future (e.g., to participate in primary prevention measures).
3. *The focus may be on the future, with progress and change highly valued.* These individuals may express discontent with the past and present. In terms of health care, these individuals may inquire about the "latest treatment" and the most advanced equipment available for a particular problem.

The dominant U.S. cultural group is characterized by a belief in progress and a future orientation. This implies a strong task or goal focus. This group has an optimistic faith in what the future will bring. Change is often equated with improvement, and a rapid rate of change is usually normal.

Activity Orientation

This values orientation concerns activity. Philosophers have suggested the following three perspectives:

1. *Being,* in which a spontaneous expression of impulses and desires is largely nondevelopmental in nature
2. *Growing,* in which the person is self-contained and has inner control, including the ability to self-actualize
3. *Doing,* in which the person actively strives to achieve and accomplish something that is regarded highly

The person often directs the doing toward achievement of an externally applied standard, such as a code of behavior from a religious or ethical perspective. The Ten Commandments, Pillars of Islam, Hippocratic oath, and Nightingale pledge are examples of externally applied standards.

The dominant cultural value is action oriented, with an emphasis on productivity and being busy. As a result of this action orientation, Americans have become proficient at problem solving and decision making. Even during leisure time and vacations, many Americans value activity.

Social Orientation

Variations in cultural values orientation are also related to the relationships that exist with others. Relationships may be categorized in the following three ways:

1. *Lineal relationships:* These exist by virtue of heredity and kinship ties. These relationships follow an ordered succession and have continuity through time.
2. *Collateral relationships:* The focus is primarily on group goals, and family orientation is important. For example, many Asian clients describe family honor and the importance of working together toward an achievement of the group versus a personal goal.
3. *Individual relationships:* These refer to personal autonomy and independence. Individual goals dominate, and group goals become secondary.

The social orientation among the dominant U.S. cultural group is toward the importance of the individual and the equality of all people. Friendly, informal, outgoing, and extroverted members of the dominant cultural group tend to scorn rank and authority. For example, nursing students may call faculty members by their first names, clients may call nurses by their first names, and employees may fraternize with their employers.

Members of the dominant culture have a strong sense of individuality. However, family ties are relatively weak, as demonstrated by the high rate of separation and divorce in the United States as well as the frequently widespread geographic separation of extended families. In many U.S. households, the family has been reduced to its smallest unit: the single-parent family.

When making health-related decisions, clients from culturally diverse backgrounds rely on relationships with others in various ways. If the cultural values orientation is lineal, the client may seek assistance from other members of the family and allow a relative (e.g., parent, grandparent, or elder brother) to make decisions about important health-related matters. If collateral relationships are valued, decisions about the client may be interrelated with the influence of illness on the entire family or group. For example, among the Amish, the entire community is affected by the illness of a member because the community pays for health care from a common fund. Members join together to meet the needs of the client and family for the duration of the illness, and the roles of many in the community are likely to be affected by the illness of a single member.

In another example, there are approximately five million illegal aliens in the United States (U.S. Census Bureau, 2005).

These individuals often create their own social groups in which they seek to protect themselves from being discovered by immigration authorities. These groups fear that attempting to access the health care system may lead to deportation, and they often have "underground" or private access to home remedies and pharmaceuticals for their health care. As a result, they often enter the formal health care system via emergency departments when their health status has declined considerably.

A values orientation that emphasizes the individual is predominant among the dominant cultural majority in the United States. Decision making about health and illness is often an individual matter, with the client being responsible, although members of the nuclear family may participate to varying degrees.

Culture and the Family

The family remains the basic social unit in the United States. Although various ways exist to categorize families, the following are commonly recognized types of constellations in which people live together in society:

- Nuclear (i.e., husband, wife, and child or children)
- Nuclear dyad (i.e., husband and wife alone, either childless or with no children living at home)
- Single parent (i.e., either mother or father and at least one child)
- Blended (i.e., husband, wife, and children from previous relationships)
- Extended (i.e., nuclear plus other blood relatives)
- Communal (i.e., group of men and women with or without children)
- Cohabitation (i.e., unmarried man and woman sharing a household with or without children)
- Gay (i.e., same-gender couples with or without children)

In addition to structural differences in families crossculturally, accompanying functional diversity may exist. For example, among extended families, kin residence sharing has long been recognized as a viable alternative to managing scarce resources, meeting child care needs, and caring for a handicapped or older family member. Sometimes the shared household is an adaptation for survival and protection. In general, families with a culturally diverse heritage include a large number of adults and a larger number of children.

The family constellations associated with teen parenting are unique and provide a special socialization context for infants. For example, Hispanic teen mothers receive more child care help from grandmothers and peers than do white teen mothers. Among blacks and Puerto Ricans, the presence of the maternal grandmother ameliorates the negative consequences of adolescent childbirth on the infant. In addition, grandmothers are more responsive and less punitive in their interactions with the infant than their daughters (Andrews and Boyle, 2003). Three-generational households can have an influence on the infant's development: by influencing the mother's knowledge about development and providing other more responsive social interactions with infants.

Families from diverse backgrounds are often characterized as being more conservative in terms of sex roles and parenting values and practices than white families. For example, tradi-

TABLE 12-2 Poverty Thresholds for 2004

SIZE OF FAMILY UNIT	RELATED CHILDREN UNDER 18 YEARS								
	NONE	ONE	TWO	THREE	FOUR	FIVE	SIX	SEVEN	EIGHT OR MORE
One person (unrelated individual)									
Under 65 years	9,827								
65 years and over	9,060								
Two persons									
Householder under 65 years	12,649	13,020							
Householder 65 years and over	11,418	12,971							
Three persons	14,776	15,205	15,219						
Four persons	19,484	19,803	19,157	19,223					
Five persons	23,497	23,838	23,108	22,543	22,199				
Six persons	27,025	27,133	26,573	26,037	25,241	24,768			
Seven persons	31,096	31,290	30,621	30,154	29,285	28,271	27,159		
Eight persons	34,778	35,086	34,454	33,901	33,115	32,119	31,082	30,818	
Nine persons or more	41,836	42,039	41,480	41,010	40,240	39,179	38,220	37,983	36,520

Data from US Census Bureau, Housing and Household Economic Statistics Division: *Poverty thresholds for 2004 by size of family and number of related children under 18 years,* The Author, http://www.census.gov/hhes/www/poverty/threshld/thresh04.html.

tional Japanese-American and Mexican-American families are family centered, enforce strict gender and age roles, and emphasize children's compliance with authority figures. Children of culturally diverse backgrounds are involved in family interactions that differ from those of children from the dominant U.S. cultural group. The values of children of immigrants typically evolve, depending on how far removed they are from the country of origin. These children may detach from their cultural traditions, becoming more individually focused or autonomous—often to the dismay of the elders in the family. Often the language of the ancestors is forgotten, or in certain subcultures, forbidden to be spoken, so that the children may assimilate to the dominant culture.

Relationships that may seem apparent sometimes warrant further exploration by nurses interacting with clients from culturally diverse backgrounds. For example, the dominant cultural group defines siblings as two people with the same mother, the same father, the same mother and father, or the same adoptive parents. In some Asian cultures, a sibling relationship is defined as involving infants who are breast-fed by the same woman. In other cultures, certain kinship patterns, such as maternal first cousins, are sibling relationships. In some African cultures, anyone from the same village or town may be called "brother" or "sister."

Certain subcultures, such as Roman Catholics, who may be further subdivided by ethnicity into those who are Italian, Polish, Spanish, Mexican, and so on, recognize relationships such as "godmother" and "godfather." The godmother/godfather is an individual who is not the biological parent but promises to assist with the moral and spiritual development of an infant and agrees to care for the child in the event of parental death. The godparent makes these promises during the religious ceremony of baptism.

When providing care for infants and children, the nurse must identify the primary provider of care because this individual may or may not be the biological parent. For example, among some Hispanic groups, female members of the nuclear or extended family (e.g., sisters or aunts) are sometimes the primary providers of care. In some black families, the grandmother may be the decision maker and primary caregiver of the children.

CULTURE AND SOCIOECONOMIC FACTORS

No single indicator can adequately capture all facets of economic status for entire populations, but measures such as median or average annual income, employment rate, poverty rate, and net worth are most often used. The economic status of most individuals, especially children, is better reflected by the pooled resources of family or household members than by their individual earnings or incomes. **Socioeconomic status** (SES) is a composite of the economic status of a family or unrelated individuals based on income, wealth, occupation, educational attainment, and power. It is a means of measuring inequalities based on economic differences and the manner in which families live as a result of their economic well-being. Most families with racially or ethnically diverse backgrounds have a lower SES than the population at large, with a few exceptions (e.g., Cuban Americans and subgroups of Asian Americans).

Poverty is another factor that dramatically influences health and well-being. National poverty data are calculated using the official U.S. Census Bureau definition of poverty, which has remained standard since it initial introduction in the mid 1960s. Under this definition, poverty is determined by comparing pretax cash income with the poverty threshold, which adjusts for family size and composition. Table 12-2 provides an overview of the poverty thresholds according to size of family and number of related children under age 18 residing in the home. The poverty guidelines are issued each year by the USDHHS. The guidelines are a simplification of the poverty threshold for administrative purposes, such as determining financial eligibility for federal

TABLE 12-3 Percentage of Minority Populations Living Below 100% Poverty Level: 2003

RACE	TOTAL (%)	CHILDREN YOUNGER THAN 18 YEARS OF AGE (%)	FEMALE HEAD OF HOUSEHOLD (%)
Total	12.5	17.6	30.0
Black	24.3	33.6	38.9
Hispanic	22.5	29.7	38.4
Asian and Pacific Islander	11.8	12.7	24.8
White (non-Hispanic)	10.6	14.4	25.8

From US Census Bureau: *Poverty: poverty by selected characteristics, 2003,* The Author, http://www.census.gov/hhes/poverty.

programs (e.g., Head Start, National School Lunch, Medicaid, Aid to Families with Dependent Children) (US Census Bureau, 2005).

As Table 12.3 shows, the U.S. Census Bureau (2005) reported that the poverty rate was 12.5%—up slightly from the previous year. The distribution of the poor varies considerably based on certain factors such as age, race or ethnicity, and marital status. For example, 30% of all female-headed household are poor (compared with 4.9% of families in which males are present), and that figure exceeds 38% among blacks and Hispanics. In addition, children under 6 years of age are particularly vulnerable to poverty, with 18.2% of all U.S. children in this age-group being poor.

Distribution of Resources

Status, power, and wealth in the United States are not distributed equally throughout society. Rather, a small percentage of the population enjoys most of the nation's resources, primarily through ownership of multibillion-dollar corporations, large pieces of real estate in prime locations, and similar assets. The U.S. population has traditionally been divided into the following three social classes: upper, middle, and lower. SES may be calculated by considering a variety of factors, but it is customarily determined by examining factors such as total family income, occupation, and educational level. In a less formalized examination of SES, factors such as age, sex, material possessions, health status, family name, location of residence, family composition, amount of land owned, religion, race, and ethnicity may also be considered.

A disproportionate number of individuals from the racially and ethnically diverse subgroups are members of the lower socioeconomic class, whereas a larger percentage of members of the dominant cultural group (i.e., WASPs) belong to the upper and middle socioeconomic classes (Council of Economic Advisers for the President's Initiative on Race, 1999). The United States has socioeconomic stratification; therefore, the idealization of America as the land of opportunity often applies more to members of the upper and middle classes than to those of the lower class. The outcome of social stratification is social inequality. For example, school systems, grocery stores, and recreational facilities vary significantly between the inner city, which has a high percentage of minority residents, and the suburbs, which are overwhelmingly WASP.

For many years, health care settings have been the subject of study and concern regarding distribution of resources, with members of racial and ethnic minority groups compellingly pointing out the inequalities. As the only industrialized Western nation in the world without a national health care delivery system, the United States provides the best health care to those with the highest SES and substantially inferior health care to those with low SES. In the United States, SES largely determines the quality of health care.

Education

One of the components considered in determining SES is educational level. Educational attainment is perhaps the single most important factor. In recent years, there has been an improvement in the level of education among those who have historically been less educated (e.g., elders, women, minorities). For example, women have a higher rate of high school completion than men. Also, graduation rates for both blacks and Hispanics are rising steadily (National Center for Educational Statistics, 2004).

Research suggests that differences between white and Mexican-American children's home educational development can be accounted for by differences in levels of formal schooling rather than by cultural differences or economic indices. According to a study by Garcia Coll (1990), mothers who had received more years of formal education inquired and praised their children more often than did mothers with less education. In contrast, the lower the mother's level of formal education, the more often she used modeling as a teaching strategy. Compared with white mothers, Hispanic mothers inquired and praised less often and used modeling, visual cues, directives, and negative physical control more often. However, these differences disappeared entirely when the mother's or father's educational level was controlled statistically. This study contributes to an understanding of the ways in which educational level attained by people from culturally diverse backgrounds affects the didactic aspects of the child-rearing environment.

CULTURE AND NUTRITION

Long after assimilation into U.S. culture has occurred, many members of various ethnic groups will continue to follow culturally based dietary practices and eat ethnic foods. When a new group of immigrants arrives in the United States, neighborhood food markets and ethnic restaurants are often established soon after arrival. The ethnic restaurant is often a place for members of the cultural group to meet and mingle,

TABLE 12-4   Dietary Practices of Selected Religious Groups

RELIGION	DIETARY PRACTICE
Hinduism	All meats are prohibited.
Islam	Pork and intoxicating beverages are prohibited.
Judaism	Pork, predatory fowl, shellfish, other water creatures (fish with scales are permissible), and blood by ingestion (e.g., blood sausage and raw meat) are prohibited. Blood by transfusion is acceptable. Foods should be kosher (meaning "properly preserved"). All animals must be ritually slaughtered by a shochet (i.e., quickly with the least pain possible) to be kosher. Mixing dairy and meat dishes at the same meal is prohibited.
Mormonism (Church of Jesus Christ of Latter-day Saints)	Alcohol, tobacco, and beverages containing caffeine (e.g., coffee, tea, colas, and select carbonated soft drinks) are prohibited.
Seventh-Day Adventism	Pork, certain seafood (including shellfish), and fermented beverages are prohibited. A vegetarian diet is encouraged.

and customers from the dominant cultural group may be of secondary interest. Food is an integral part of cultural identity that extends beyond dietary preferences.

Nutrition Assessment of Culturally Diverse Groups

Factors that must be considered in a nutrition assessment include the cultural definition of food, frequency and number of meals eaten away from home, form and content of ceremonial meals, amount and types of food eaten, and regularity of food consumption. Twenty-four-hour dietary recalls or three-day food records traditionally used for assessment may be inadequate when dealing with clients from culturally diverse backgrounds. Standard dietary handbooks may fail to provide culture-specific diet information because nutritional content and exchange tables are usually based on Western diets. Another source of error may originate from the cultural patterns of eating. For example, among low-income urban black families, elaborate weekend meals are frequent, whereas weekday dietary patterns are markedly more moderate.

Although community health nurses may assume that food is a culture-universal term, they may need to clarify its meaning with the client. For example, certain Latin-American groups do not consider greens, an important source of vitamins, to be food and fail to list intake of these vegetables on daily records. Among Vietnamese refugees, dietary intake of calcium may appear inadequate because low consumption rates of dairy products are common among members of this group. However, they commonly consume pork bones and shells, providing adequate quantities of calcium to meet daily requirements.

Food is only one part of eating. In some cultures, social contacts during meals are restricted to members of the immediate or extended family. For example, in some Middle Eastern cultures, men and women eat meals separately, or women are permitted to eat with their husbands but not with other males. Among some Hispanic groups, the male bread-winner is served first, then the women and children eat. Etiquette during meals, use of hands, type of eating utensils (e.g., chopsticks or special flatware), and protocols governing the order in which food is consumed during a meal all vary cross-culturally.

Dietary Practices of Selected Cultural Groups

Cultural stereotyping is the tendency to view individuals of common cultural backgrounds similarly and according to a preconceived notion of how they behave. However, not all Chinese like rice, not all Italians like spaghetti, and not all Mexicans like tortillas. Nevertheless, aggregate dietary preferences among people from certain cultural groups can be described (e.g., characteristic ethnic dishes and methods of food preparation, including use of cooking oils); the reader is referred to nutrition texts on the topic for detailed information about culture-specific diets and the nutritional value of ethnic foods.

Religion and Diet

Cultural food preferences are often interrelated with religious dietary beliefs and practices. As indicated in Table 12-4, many religions have proscriptive dietary practices and some use food as symbols in celebrations and rituals. Knowing the client's religious practice as it relates to food makes it possible to suggest improvements or modifications that will not conflict with religious dietary laws.

Fasting and other religious observations may limit a person's food or liquid intake during specified times. For example, many Catholics fast and abstain from meat on Ash Wednesday and each Friday of Lent, Muslims refrain from eating during the daytime hours for the month of Ramadan but are permitted to eat after sunset, and Mormons refrain from ingesting all solid foods and liquids on the first Sunday of each month.

CULTURE AND RELIGION

According to the *Yearbook of American and Canadian Churches* (National Council of Churches, 2005), in North America, more than 226 million people are affiliated with organized religion. A recent Gallup Poll (Gallup, 2005) found that 80% of Americans report that they are "convinced God exists" and an additional 8% state that God "probably exists, but have a little doubt." Further, about 66% note that they are members of a church, synagogue, or mosque. The largest religious groups are Protestant, 48%; "Christian/non-specific," 7%; Catholic, 25%; Jewish, 2%, and Mormon, 2%. The largest specific Protestant denominations are, in order, Baptist (other than Southern Baptist), Methodist, Southern Baptist, Lutheran, and Presbyterian.

Although the nurse cannot be an expert on each of the estimated 1200 religions practiced in the United States, knowledge of health-related beliefs and practices and general information about religious observances are important in providing culturally competent nursing care. For example, when planning home visits or scheduling clinic visits for members of a specific religious group, the nurse should consult the group's religious calendar and work around designated holy days. The nurse should also know the customary days of religious worship observed by members of the religion. Most Protestants worship on Sundays, whereas Muslims' holy day of worship extends from sunset on Thursday to sunset on Friday, and Jews and Seventh-Day Adventists' holy day extends from sunset on Friday to sunset on Saturday. Roman Catholics may worship in the late afternoon or evening of Saturday or all day Sunday. Some religions may meet more than once weekly.

In addition to regularly scheduled weekly religious services, most major religions also recognize special days of observance or celebration that last from one day (e.g., Christmas, Easter, Rosh Hashanah, and Janmashtami) to one month (e.g., Ramadan). Some days of commemoration or observation are based on a lunar calendar and some have rotating dates; the nurse may consult official information sources, such as religious leaders or religious calendars, to verify exact dates. The nurse should also ask clients what religious practices they follow, because individual activity within the religious organization may vary widely.

As an integral component of the individual's culture, religious beliefs may influence the client's explanation of the cause of illness, perception of its severity, and choice of healer. In times of crisis, such as serious illness and impending death, religion may be a source of consolation for the client and family and may influence the course of action believed to be appropriate.

Religion and Spirituality

Religious concerns evolve from, and respond to, the mysteries of life and death, good and evil, and pain and suffering. Nurses frequently encounter clients who find themselves searching for a spiritual meaning to help explain illness or disability. Some nurses find spiritual assessment difficult because the topic is abstract and personal, whereas others feel comfortable discussing spiritual matters. Comfort with personal spiritual beliefs is the foundation for effective assessment of spiritual needs in clients.

Although religions offer various interpretations of many of life's mysteries, most people seek a personal understanding and interpretation at some time in their lives. Ultimately, this personal search becomes a pursuit to discover a supreme being (e.g., Allah, God, Yahweh, or Jehovah) or some unifying truth that will render meaning, purpose, and integrity to existence.

An important distinction must be made between religion and spirituality. **Religion** refers to an organized system of beliefs concerning the cause, nature, and purpose of the

---

BOX 12-1 Methods of Assessing Spiritual Needs in Culturally Diverse Clients

Environment
- Does the client have religious objects in the environment?
- Does the client wear outer garments or undergarments that have religious significance?
- Are get-well greeting cards religious in nature or from a representative of the client's church?
- Does the client receive flowers or bulletins from a church or other religious institution?

Behavior
- Does the client appear to pray at certain times of the day or before meals?
- Does the client make special dietary requests (e.g., kosher diet; vegetarian diet; or diet free from caffeine, pork, shellfish, or other specific food items)?
- Does the client read religious magazines or books?

Verbalization
- Does the client mention a Supreme Being (e.g., God, Allah, Buddha, or Yahweh), prayer, faith, church, or religious topics?
- Does the client request a visit by a clergy member or other religious representative?
- Does the client express anxiety or fear about pain, suffering, or death?

Interpersonal Relationships
- Who visits the client? How does the client respond to visitors?
- Does a church representative visit?
- How does the client relate to nursing staff and roommates?
- Does the client prefer to interact with others or remain alone?

Data from Andrews MM, Boyle JS, editors: *Transcultural concepts in nursing care*, ed 4, Philadelphia, 2003, Lippincott Williams & Wilkins.

---

universe, especially belief in or the worship of a god or gods. More than 1200 religions are practiced in the United States. **Spirituality,** in contrast, is born out of the individual's unique life experience and personal effort to find purpose and meaning in life. Box 12-1 provides suggested guidelines for assessing the spiritual needs of culturally diverse clients.

Shared Beliefs Among Various Religions: The "Golden Rule"

Buddhism: "Hurt not others in ways that you yourself would find hurtful." (Udana-varga 5:18)

Christianity: "Whatsoever you would that men should do to you, do you even so to them." (Matthew 7:12)

Confucianism: "Do not do to others what you do not want them to do to you." (Analects 15:23)

Hinduism: "One should not behave towards others in a way which is disagreeable to oneself." (Mahabharata 5:1517; Mencius Vii.A.4)

Islam: "Not one of you is a believer until he loves for his brother what he loves for himself." (Number 13 of Al-Nawawi's Forty Hadiths)

Judasim: "Thou shalt love thy neighbor as thyself." (Leviticus 19:18).

Taoism: "Regard your neighbor's gain as your own gain and your neighbor's loss as your own loss." (T'ai Shang Kan Ying P'ien) ■

Religion may influence decisions regarding prolongation of life, euthanasia, autopsy, donation of a body for research, disposal of a body and body parts including fetus, and type of burial. The nurse should use discretion in asking clients and their families about these issues and gather data only when the clinical situation necessitates that the information be obtained. The nurse should encourage clients and families to discuss these issues with their religious representative when necessary. Before dealing with potentially sensitive issues, the nurse should establish rapport with the client and family by gaining their trust and confidence in less sensitive areas.

Childhood and Spirituality

Serious illness during childhood is especially difficult. Children have spiritual needs that vary according to the child's developmental level and the religious climate that exists in the family. Parental perceptions about the illness of their child may be partially influenced by religious beliefs. For example, some parents may believe that a transgression against a religious law is responsible for a congenital anomaly in their off-spring. Other parents may delay seeking medical care because they believe that prayer should be tried first. Certain types of treatment (e.g., administration of blood or medications containing caffeine, pork, or other prohibited substances and selected procedures) may be perceived as cultural taboos, which are to be avoided by children and adults.

CULTURE AND AGING

Values held by the dominant U.S. culture, such as emphasis on independence, self-reliance, and productivity, influence aging members of society. Americans define people 65 years and older as "old" and limit their work. In some other cultures, people are first recognized as being unable to work and then identified as being old. In some cultures the wisdom, not the productivity, of the older adult is valued; the diminishment of one's activity level and reduction of physical stamina associated with growing old are accepted more readily without loss of status among culture members. Retirement is also culturally defined, with some older adults working as long as physical health continues and others continuing to be active but assuming less physically demanding jobs.

The main task of older adults in the dominant culture is to achieve a sense of integrity in accepting responsibility for their own lives and having a sense of accomplishment. Individuals who achieve integrity consider aging a positive experience, make adjustments in their personal space and social relationships, maintain a sense of usefulness, and begin closure and life review. Not all cultures value accepting responsibility for an individual's own life. For example, among Hispanics, Asians, Arabs, and other groups, older adults are often cared for by family members who welcome them into their homes when they are no longer able to live alone. The concept of placing an older family member in an institutional setting to be cared for by strangers is perceived as an uncaring, impersonal, and culturally unacceptable practice by many cultural groups.

Older adults may develop their own means of coping with illness through self-care, assistance from family members, and social group support systems. Some cultures have developed attitudes and specific behaviors for older adults that include humanistic care and identification of family members as care providers. Older adults may have special family responsibilities (e.g., the older Amish adults provide hospitality to visitors, and older Filipinos adults spend considerable time teaching the youth skills learned during a lifetime of experience).

Older adult immigrants who have made major lifestyle adjustments in the move from their homeland to the United States or from a rural to an urban area, or vice versa, may need information about health care alternatives, preventive programs, health care benefits, and screening programs for which they are eligible. These individuals may also be in various stages of **culture shock,** the state of disorientation or inability to respond to the behavior of a different cultural group because it holds sudden strangeness, unfamiliarity, and incompatibility to the newcomer's perceptions and expectations (Leininger, 1995; Leininger & McFarland, 2002).

Several examples of how being an elderly immigrant influences health can be found in the nursing literature. Wilmoth and Chen (2003), for example, studied living arrangements and symptoms of depression among middle-aged and older immigrants and concluded that immigrants had significantly more depressive symptoms than non-immigrants. Further, immigrants who lived alone or with family had more depressive symptoms than those who lived with a spouse. In another example, Becker (2002) found that many older Cambodians wanted to return to their homeland to die.

CROSS-CULTURAL COMMUNICATION

Verbal and nonverbal communication are important in community health nursing and are influenced by the cultural background of the nurse and client. Cross-cultural, or intercultural, communication refers to the communication process between a nurse and a client with different cultural backgrounds as each attempts to understand the other's point of view from a cultural perspective.

Nurse-Client Relationship

From the introduction of the nurse to the client through termination of the relationship, communication is a continuous process for the community health nurse. First impressions are important in all human relationships; therefore cross-cultural considerations concerning introductions warrant a few brief remarks. To ensure a mutually respectful relationship, the nurse should introduce himself or herself and indicate how the client should refer to the nurse (i.e., by first name, last name, or title). Having done so, the nurse should ask the client to do the same. This enables the nurse to address the client in a manner that is culturally appropriate, thereby avoiding potential embarrassment. For example, some Asian and European cultures write the last name first; confusion can be avoided in an area of extreme sensitivity (i.e., the client's name).

TABLE 12-5 Functional Use of Space

ZONE	REMARKS
Intimate zone (0 to 1.5 feet)	Visual distortion occurs.
	Best for assessing breath and other body odors.
Personal distance (1.5 to 4 feet)	Perceived as an extension of the self, similar to a "bubble."
	Voice is moderate.
	Body odors are inapparent.
	Visual distortion does not occur.
	Much of the physical assessment will occur at this distance.
Social distance (4 to 12 feet)	Used for impersonal business transactions.
	Perceptual information is much less detailed.
	Much of the interview will occur at this distance.
Public distance (>12 feet)	Interaction with others is impersonal.
	Speaker's voice must be projected.
	Subtle facial expressions are imperceptible.

Data from Hall E: Proxemics: the study of man's spatial relations. In Galdston I, editor: *Man's image in medicine and anthropology,* New York, 1963, International Universities Press.

Space, Distance, and Intimacy

Sense of spatial distance is significant because culturally appropriate distance zones vary widely. For example, nurses may back away from clients of Hispanic, East Indian, or Middle Eastern origin who invade personal space with regularity in an attempt to bring the nurse closer into the space that is comfortable to them. Although nurses are uncomfortable with clients' close physical proximity, clients are perplexed by the nurse's distancing behaviors and may perceive the community health nurse as aloof and unfriendly. Table 12-5 summarizes the four distance zones identified for the functional use of space that are embraced by the dominant cultural group, including most nurses.

Interactions between clients and nurses may also depend on the client's desired degree of intimacy, which may range from formal interactions to close personal relationships. For example, some Southeast Asian clients expect those in authority (e.g., nurses) to be authoritarian, directive, and detached.

In contrast, Appalachian clients traditionally have close family interaction patterns that often lead them to expect close personal relationships with health care providers. The Appalachian client may evaluate the nurse's effectiveness on the basis of interpersonal skills rather than professional competency. Appalachian clients are likely to be uncomfortable with the impersonal, bureaucratic orientation of most health care institutions. Likewise, clients of Arab, Latin-American, or Mediterranean origin often expect an even higher degree of intimacy and may attempt to involve the nurse in their family system by expecting participation in personal activities and social functions. These individuals may come to expect personal favors that extend beyond the scope of professional nursing practice and may believe it is their privilege to contact the nurse at home at any time of the day or night for care.

Overcoming Communication Barriers

Nurses tend to have stereotypical expectations of the client's behavior. In general, nurses expect behavior to consist of undemanding compliance, an attitude of respect for the health care provider, and cooperation with requested behavior throughout the examination. Although clients may ask a few questions for clarification, slight deference to recognized authority figures (e.g., health care providers) is expected. However, individuals from culturally diverse backgrounds may have significantly different perceptions about the appropriate role of the individual and family when seeking health care. If nurses find themselves becoming annoyed that a client is asking too many questions, assuming a defensive posture, or otherwise feeling uncomfortable, they may pause for a moment to examine the source of the conflict from a cross-cultural perspective.

During illness, culturally acceptable "sick-role" behavior may range from aggressive, demanding behavior to silent passivity (Cockerham, 2001). Complaining, demanding behavior during illness is often rewarded with attention among Jewish and Italian-American clients, whereas Asian and Native-American clients are likely to be quiet and compliant during illness. Furthermore, during an interview, Asian clients may provide the nurse with the answers they think the nurse wants to hear, which is behavior consistent within their cultural value for harmonious relationships with others. The nurse should attempt to phrase questions or statements in a neutral manner that avoids foreshadowing an expected response. Appalachian clients may reject a community health nurse whom they perceive as prying or nosy because a cultural ethic of neutrality mandates that people mind their own business and avoid assertive or argumentative behavior.

Nonverbal Communication

Unless the nurse makes an effort to understand the client's nonverbal behavior, he or she may overlook important information such as that which is conveyed by facial expressions, silence, eye contact, touch, and other body language. Communication patterns vary widely cross-culturally, even for seemingly "innocent" behaviors such as smiling and handshaking. For example, among many Hispanic clients, smiling and handshaking are considered an integral part of sincere interaction and essential to establishing trust, whereas a Russian client may perceive the same behavior by the nurse as insolent and frivolous.

Gender issues also become significant. For example, among some groups of Middle Eastern origin, men and women do not shake hands or touch each other in any manner outside of the marital relationship. However, if the nurse and client are both female, a handshake is usually acceptable.

Wide cultural variation exists when interpreting silence. Some individuals find silence extremely uncomfortable and make every effort to fill conversational lags with words. In contrast, Native Americans consider silence essential to understanding and respecting the other person. A pause after a question signifies that what the speaker has asked is important enough to be given thoughtful consideration. In traditional Chinese and Japanese cultures, silence may mean that the speaker wishes the listener to consider the content of what has been said before continuing. The English and Arabs may use silence out of respect for another person's privacy, whereas the French, Spanish, and Russians may interpret it as a sign of agreement. Asian cultures often use silence to demonstrate respect for elders.

Eye contact is among the most culturally variable nonverbal behaviors. Although most nurses have been taught to maintain eye contact while talking with clients, individuals from culturally diverse backgrounds may misconstrue this behavior. Asian, Native-American, Indochinese, Arab, and Appalachian clients may consider direct eye contact impolite or aggressive, and they may avert their own eyes during the conversation. Native-American clients often stare at the floor when the nurse is talking. This culturally appropriate behavior indicates that the listener is paying close attention to the speaker.

In some cultures, including Arab, Hispanic, and some black groups, modesty for women is interrelated with eye contact. For Muslim women, modesty is achieved in part by avoiding eye contact with men, except for their husband, and keeping the eyes downcast when encountering members of the opposite sex in public situations. In many cultures, the only women who smile and establish eye contact with men in public are prostitutes. Hassidic Jewish men also have culturally based norms concerning eye contact with women. The male may avoid direct eye contact and turn his head in the opposite direction when walking past or speaking to a woman. The preceding examples are intended to be illustrative and are not exhaustive; nor do they represent values, actions, and beliefs of all members of the cultural groups described.

Language

To assess non–English-speaking clients, the nurse may need the help of an interpreter. Interviewing a non–English-speaking person requires a bilingual interpreter for full communication. Even the person from another culture or country who has a basic command of English may need an interpreter when faced with the anxiety-provoking situation of becoming ill, encountering a strange symptom, or discussing sensitive topics, such as birth control, gynecologic concerns, or urologic problems. The nurse may be tempted to ask a relative or friend of another client to interpret because this person is readily available and is anxious to help. However, this is disadvantageous because it violates confidentiality for the client, who may not want personal information shared with another. Furthermore, the friend or relative, although fluent in ordinary language, is likely to be unfamiliar with medical terminology, clinical procedures, and medical ethics.

Whenever possible, the nurse should use a bilingual team member or trained medical interpreter. This person knows interpreting techniques, has a health care background, and understands clients' rights. The trained interpreter is also knowledgeable about cultural beliefs and health practices, can help bridge the cultural gap, and can provide advice concerning the cultural appropriateness of recommendations.

Although the nurse is in charge of the client-nurse interaction, the interpreter is an important member of the health care team. Whenever feasible, the nurse should ask the

---

BOX 12-2 Overcoming Language Barriers: Use of an Interpreter

➤ Before locating an interpreter, the nurse should know what language the client speaks at home because it may be different from the language spoken publicly (e.g., French is sometimes spoken by aristocratic or well-educated people from certain Asian or Middle Eastern cultures).

➤ The nurse should avoid interpreters from a rival tribe, state, region, or nation (e.g., a Palestinian who knows Hebrew may not be the best interpreter for a Jewish client).

➤ The nurse should be aware of the gender difference between the interpreter and client to avoid violation of cultural mores related to modesty.

➤ The nurse should be aware of the age difference between the interpreter and client.

➤ The nurse should be aware of socioeconomic differences between the interpreter and client.

➤ The nurse should ask the interpreter to translate as closely to verbatim as possible.

➤ An interpreter who is not a relative may seek compensation for services rendered.

---

interpreter to meet the client before the visit to establish rapport and learn about the client's age, occupation, educational level, and attitude toward health care. This enables the interpreter to communicate on the client's level.

The nurse should allow more time for visits with culturally diverse clients who require an interpreter. With the third person repeating everything, it can take considerably longer than interviewing English-speaking clients. The nurse will need to focus on the major points and prioritize data.

Line-by-line and summarization are interpretation styles. Translation of line-by-line ensures accuracy, but it takes more time. The nurse and client should speak only a sentence or two and then allow the interpreter time to interpret. The nurse should use simple language, not medical jargon that the interpreter must simplify before translating. Summary translation is faster and useful for teaching relatively simple health techniques with which the interpreter is already familiar. The nurse should be alert for nonverbal cues as the client talks because they can give valuable data. A good interpreter will also note nonverbal messages and communicate those to the community health nurse. Box 12-2 summarizes suggestions for the selection and use of an interpreter.

Although use of an interpreter is ideal, the nurse may find himself or herself in a situation with a non–English-speaking client when no interpreter is available. Box 12-3 provides some suggestions for overcoming language barriers when an interpreter is not available.

Touch

Touching the client is a necessary component of a comprehensive assessment. Although benefits exist in establishing rapport with clients through touch, including the promotion of healing through therapeutic touch, physical contact with clients conveys various meanings cross-culturally. In many cultures (e.g., Arab and Hispanic), male health care providers

BOX 12-3 Overcoming Language Barriers When an Interpreter Is Not Available

- The nurse should be polite and formal.
- The nurse should greet the client using his or her last or complete name. The nurse should gesture to himself or herself and say his or her name. The nurse should offer a handshake or nod and smile.
- The nurse should proceed in an unhurried manner. The nurse should pay attention to efforts by the client or family to communicate.
- The nurse should speak in a low, moderate voice. The nurse should remember that he or she may have a tendency to raise the volume and pitch of his or her voice when the listener appears not to understand and the listener may perceive that the nurse is shouting or angry.
- The nurse should use words that he or she may know in the client's language. This indicates that the nurse is aware of and respects the client's culture.
- The nurse should use simple words, such as "pain" instead of "discomfort." The nurse should avoid medical jargon, idioms, and slang. He or she should avoid using contractions such as "don't," "can't," and "won't." The nurse should use nouns repeatedly instead of pronouns. For example, the nurse should say, "Do you take medicine?" instead of "You have been taking your medicine, haven't you?"
- The nurse should pantomime words and simple actions while verbalizing them.
- The nurse should give instructions in the proper sequence. For example, he or she should say, "First, wash the bottle. Second, rinse the bottle," instead of "Before you rinse the bottle, sterilize it."
- The nurse should discuss one topic at a time. He or she should avoid use of conjunctions. For example, the nurse should say, "Are you cold [while pantomiming]?" and "Are you in pain?" instead of, "Are you cold and in pain?"
- The nurse should determine if the client understands by having the client repeat instructions, demonstrate the procedure, or act out the meaning.
- The nurse should write out several short sentences in English and determine the client's ability to read them.
- The nurse should try a third language. Many Indo-Chinese speak French. Europeans often know three or four languages. The nurse should try Latin words or phrases.
- The nurse should ask who among the client's family and friends could serve as an interpreter.
- The nurse should obtain phrase books from a library or bookstore, make or purchase flash cards, contact hospitals for a list of interpreters, and use both formal and informal networking to locate a suitable interpreter.

may be prohibited from touching or examining all or certain parts of the female body. During pregnancy, the client may prefer female health care providers and may refuse to be examined by a man. The nurse should be aware that the client's significant other also might exert pressure on health care providers by enforcing these culturally meaningful norms in the health care setting.

Touching children may also have variable meanings cross-culturally. For example, Hispanic clients may believe in *mal ojo* (evil eye), in which an individual becomes ill as a result of excessive admiration by another. Many Asians believe that personal strength resides in the head and that touching the head is considered disrespectful. The nurse should approach palpation of the fontanelle of an infant of Southeast Asian descent with sensitivity. The nurse may need to rely on alternative sources of information (e.g., assessing for clinical manifestations of increased intracranial pressure or signs of premature fontanelle closure). Although it is the least desirable option, the nurse may need to omit this part of the assessment.

Gender

Violating norms related to appropriate male-female relationships among various cultures may jeopardize the therapeutic nurse-client relationship. Among Arab Americans, a man is never alone with a woman, except his wife, and is usually accompanied by one or more other men when interacting with women. This behavior is culturally significant, and failure to adhere to the cultural code (i.e., set of rules or norms of behavior used by a cultural group to guide their behavior and interpret situations) is viewed as a serious transgression, often one in which the lone male will be accused of sexual impropriety. The best way to ensure that cultural variables have been considered is to ask the client about culturally relevant aspects of male-female relationships, preferably at the beginning of the interaction before an opportunity arises to violate culturally based practices.

HEALTH-RELATED BELIEFS AND PRACTICES

One of the major aspects of a comprehensive cultural assessment concerns the collection of data related to culturally based beliefs and practices about health and illness. Before determining whether cultural practices are helpful, harmful, or neutral, the nurse must first understand the logic of the belief system underlying the practice and then be sure to grasp fully the nature and meaning of the practice from the client's cultural perspective.

Health and Culture

The first step in understanding the health care needs of clients is to understand personal culturally based values, beliefs, attitudes, and practices. Sometimes this requires considerable introspection and may necessitate that the nurse confront his or her own biases, preconceptions, and prejudices about specific racial, ethnic, religious, sexual, or socioeconomic groups. The next step is to identify the meaning of health to the client, remembering that concepts are derived, in part, from the way in which members of their cultural group define health.

Considerable research has been conducted on the various definitions of health that may be held by various groups. For example, Jamaicans define health as having a good appetite, feeling strong and energetic, performing activities of daily living without difficulty, and being sexually active and fertile. For traditional Italian women, health means the ability to interact socially and perform routine tasks such as cooking, cleaning, and caring for oneself and others. On the other hand, some individuals of Hispanic origin believe that coughing, sweating, and diarrhea are a normal part of living rather than symptoms of ill health, because the frequency of these problems in the clients' country of origin is high. Individuals may define themselves or others in their group as healthy even though the nurse identifies symptoms of disease.

Cross-Cultural Perspectives on Causes of Illness

For clients, symptom labeling and diagnosis depend on the degree of difference between the individual's behaviors and those the group define as normal. Other issues that the nurse should consider include the client's beliefs about the causation of illness, level of stigma attached to a particular set of symptoms, prevalence of the disease, and meaning of the illness to the individual and family.

Throughout history, humankind has attempted to understand the cause of illness and disease. Theories of causation have been formulated on the basis of religious beliefs, social circumstances, philosophical perspectives, and level of knowledge. Disease causation may be viewed from the following three major perspectives: biomedical (i.e., sometimes used synonymously with the term *scientific*), naturalistic (i.e., sometimes used synonymously with the term *holistic*), and magicoreligious.

Biomedical Perspective

The **biomedical** (i.e., scientific) theory of illness causation is based on the following:

1. All events in life have a cause and effect.
2. The human body functions more or less mechanically (i.e., the functioning of the human body is analogous to the functioning of an automobile).
3. All life can be reduced or divided into smaller parts (e.g., the human person can be reduced into body, mind, and spirit).
4. All of reality can be observed and measured (e.g., with intelligence tests and psychometric measures of behavior).

Among the biomedical explanations for disease is the germ theory, which posits that microscopic organisms such as bacteria and viruses are responsible for specific disease conditions. Most educational programs for nurses and other health care providers embrace biomedical, or scientific, theories that explain the causes of physical and psychological illnesses.

Naturalistic Perspective

Another way in which clients may explain the cause of illness is from the **naturalistic** (i.e., holistic) perspective. This viewpoint is found most frequently among Native Americans, Asians, and others who believe that human life is only one aspect of nature and a part of the general order of the cosmos. Individuals from these groups believe that the forces of nature must be kept in natural balance or harmony to maintain health and well-being.

Many Asians believe in the **yin-yang theory,** in which health is believed to exist when all aspects of the person are in perfect balance. Rooted in the ancient Chinese philosophy of Tao, the yin-yang theory states that all organisms and objects in the universe consist of yin or yang energy forces. The origin of the energy forces is within the autonomic nervous system, where balance between the opposing forces is maintained during health. Yin energy represents the female and negative forces (e.g., emptiness, darkness, and cold), whereas yang forces are male and positive, emitting warmth and fullness. Foods are classified as hot and cold in this theory and are transformed into yin and yang energy when metabolized by the body. Yin foods are cold, and yang foods are hot. Cold foods are eaten when one has a hot illness, and hot foods are eaten when one has a cold illness. The yin-yang theory is the basis for Eastern or Chinese medicine.

The naturalistic perspective posits that the laws of nature create imbalance, chaos, and disease. Individuals embracing the naturalistic view use metaphors such as the healing power of nature, and they may call the earth "Mother." For example, from the perspective of the Chinese, illness is not seen as an intruding agent but rather as a part of life's rhythmic course and an outward sign of the disharmony that exists within.

Many Hispanic, Arab, black, and Asian groups embrace a hot-cold theory of health and illness, an explanatory model with its origin in the ancient Greek humoral theory. Blood, phlegm, black bile, and yellow bile, the four humors of the body, regulate basic bodily functions and are described in terms of temperature, dryness, and moisture. The treatment of disease consists of adding or subtracting cold, heat, dryness, or wetness to restore the balance of the humors.

Beverages, foods, herbs, medicines, and diseases are classified as hot or cold according to their perceived effects on the body, not on their physical characteristics. Illnesses believed to be caused by cold entering the body include earache, chest cramps, paralysis, gastrointestinal discomfort, rheumatism, and tuberculosis. Illnesses believed to be caused by overheating include abscessed teeth, sore throats, rashes, and kidney disorders.

According to the hot-cold theory, the individual as a whole, rather than a specific ailment, is significant. Those who embrace the hot-cold theory maintain that health consists of a positive state of total well-being, including physical, psychological, spiritual, and social aspects of the person. Paradoxically, the language used to describe this artificial dissection of the body into parts is a reflection of the biomedical-scientific perspective, not a naturalistic or holistic one.

Magicoreligious Perspective

Another way in which people explain the causation of illness is from a **magicoreligious** perspective. The basic premise of this explanatory model is that the world is seen as an arena in which supernatural forces dominate. The fate of the world and those in it depend on the action of supernatural forces for good or evil. Examples of magical causes of illness include the belief in voodoo or witchcraft among some blacks and others from circum-Caribbean countries. Faith healing is based on religious beliefs and is most prevalent among selected Christian religions, including Christian Scientists. Various healing rituals may be found in many religions, such as Roman Catholicism, Mormonism (i.e., Church of Jesus Christ of Latter-day Saints), and others (Hanson and Andrews, 2003).

A combination of worldviews is possible, and many clients are likely to offer more than one explanation for the cause of their illness. As a profession, nursing largely embraces the biomedical-scientific worldview, but some aspects of holism have begun to gain popularity. These include a wide variety of techniques for management of chronic pain (e.g., hypnosis, therapeutic touch, and biofeedback). Many nurses hold a belief in spiritual power and readily credit supernatural forces with various unexplained phenomena related to clients' health and illness states.

Folk Healers

All cultures have their own recognized symptoms of ill health, acceptable sick-role behavior, and treatments. In addition to seeking help from the nurse as a biomedical-scientific health care provider, clients from many groups may also seek help from folk or religious healers.

Numerous types of folk healers exist, each with a unique scope of practice. Hispanic clients may turn to a *curandero* (male folk healer) or *curandera* (female folk healer), spiritualist, *yerbo* (herbalist), or *sabador* (healer who manipulates muscles and bones). In many instances, people from diverse cultures will combine folk healing and biomedicine. Among the main reasons for seeking care from folk healers is the perception that biomedical practitioners (e.g., physicians and nurses) fail to provide holistic care and use medicines that are not natural.

Some black clients may mention having received assistance from a *hougan* (voodoo priest or priestess), spiritualist, or "old lady" (an older woman who has successfully raised a family and specializes in child care and folk remedies). Likewise, Native-American clients may seek assistance from a shaman or a medicine man or woman. Clients of Asian descent may mention that they have visited herbalists, acupuncturists, or bone setters.

Each culture has its own healers, most of whom speak the native tongue of the client, make house calls, and cost significantly less than healers practicing in the biomedical-scientific health care system. In addition to relying on folk healers, many cultures rely on lay midwives (e.g., *parteras* for Hispanic women) or other health care providers to meet the needs of pregnant women.

In some religions, spiritual healers may be found among the ranks of the ordained or official religious hierarchy ranks and are called priest, bishop, elder, deacon, rabbi, brother, or sister. Other religions have a separate category of healer (e.g., Christian Science "nurses" [not licensed by states] or practitioners) (Hanson and Andrews, 2003).

A comprehensive discussion of the variety of healing beliefs and practices used by the numerous cultural groups is beyond the scope of this chapter. However, the nurse should be aware of alternative practices and folk healers that are used by the groups for which they care. The nurse should also be aware that most indigenous healing practices are innocuous, regardless of whether they are effective.

Cultural Expressions of Illness

A wide cultural variation exists in the manner in which certain symptoms and disease conditions are perceived, diagnosed, labeled, and treated. The disease that is grounds for social ostracism in one culture may be reason for increased status in another. For example, epilepsy is contagious and untreatable among Ugandans, a cause for family shame among Greeks, a reflection of a physical imbalance among Mexican Americans, and a sign of having gained favor by enduring a trial by God among the Hutterites.

Bodily symptoms are also perceived and reported in a variety of ways. For example, individuals of Mediterranean descent tend to report common physical symptoms more often than people of northern European or Asian heritage. The Chinese do not have a translation for the English word *sadness,* yet all people experience the feeling of sadness at some time in their life. To express emotion, Chinese clients sometimes somaticize their symptoms. For example, a client may complain of cardiac symptoms because the center of emotion in the Chinese culture is the heart. If the client has experienced a loss through death or divorce and is grieving, he or she may describe the loss in terms of a pain in the heart. Although some biomedical-scientific clinicians may refer to this as a psychosomatic illness, others will recognize it as a culturally acceptable somatic expression of emotional disharmony.

Cultural Expression of Pain

To illustrate the manner in which symptom expression may reflect the client's cultural background, pain, an extensively studied symptom, is used. Pain is a universally recognized phenomenon and an important aspect of assessment for clients of various ages. Pain is a private, subjective experience that is greatly influenced by cultural heritage. Expectations, manifestations, and pain management are all embedded in a cultural context. The definition of pain, like that of health or illness, is culturally determined.

The term *pain* is derived from the Greek word for penalty, which helps explain the long association between pain and punishment in Judeo-Christian thought. The meaning of painful stimuli for individuals, the way people define their situation, and the influence of personal experience combine to determine the experience of pain.

Much cross-cultural research has been conducted on pain (Ludwig-Beymer, 2003; Zborowski, 1969). Pain has been found to be a highly personal experience that depends on cultural learning, the meaning of the situation, and other factors unique to the individual. Health care professionals have identified silent suffering as the most valued response to pain. The majority of nurses have been socialized to believe that in virtually any situation, self-control is better than open displays of strong feelings.

Studies of nurses' attitudes toward pain reveal that the ethnic background of clients is relevant to the nurses' assessment of physical and psychological pain. Nurses view

TABLE 12-6 Selected Culture-Bound Syndromes

GROUP	DISORDER	REMARKS
Whites	Anorexia nervosa	Excessive preoccupation with thinness, self-imposed starvation
	Bulimia	Gross overeating, then vomiting or fasting
Blacks	Blackout	Collapse, dizziness, or inability to move
	Low blood	Not enough blood or weakness of the blood that is often treated with diet
	High blood	Blood that is too rich in certain components from ingesting too much red meat or rich foods
	Thin blood	In women, children, and the elderly; renders the individual more susceptible to illness in general
	Diseases of hex, witchcraft, or conjuring	Sense of being doomed by a spell, part of voodoo beliefs
Chinese or Southeast Asians	Koro	Intense anxiety that that penis is retracting into the body
Greeks	Hysteria	Bizarre complaints and behavior because the uterus leaves the pelvis and goes to another part of the body
Hispanics	Empacho	Food forms into a ball and clings to the stomach or intestines, causing pain and cramping
	Fatigue	Asthma-like symptoms
	Mal ojo (evil eye)	Fitful sleep, crying, and diarrhea in children caused by a stranger's attention; sudden onset
	Pasmo	Paralysis-like symptoms of face or limbs; prevented or relieved by massage
	Susto	Anxiety, trembling, and phobias from sudden fright
Native Americans	Ghost	Terror, hallucinations, and sense of danger
Japanese	Wagamama	Apathetic childish behavior with emotional outbursts

Jewish and Spanish clients as suffering the most and Anglo-Saxon Germanic clients as suffering the least. In addition, nurses who infer relatively greater client pain tended to report their own experiences as more painful. In general, nurses with an eastern or southern European or African background tend to infer greater suffering than do nurses of northern European background. Years of experience, current position, and area of clinical practice are unrelated to inferences of suffering (Ludwig-Beymer, 2003).

In addition to expecting variations in pain perception and tolerance, a nurse should expect variations in the expression of pain. Individuals turn to their social environments for validation and comparison. A first important comparison group is the family, which transmits cultural norms to its children.

Culture-Bound Syndromes

Clients may have a condition that is culturally defined, known as a **culture-bound syndrome.** Some of these conditions have no equal from a biomedical or scientific perspective, but others, such as anorexia nervosa and bulimia, are examples of health problems found primarily among members of the dominant U.S. cultural group. Table 12-6 presents selected examples from among more than 150 culture-bound syndromes that have been documented by medical anthropologists.

MANAGEMENT OF HEALTH PROBLEMS: A CULTURAL PERSPECTIVE

After a symptom is identified, the first effort at treatment is often self-care. In the United States, an estimated 70% to 90% of all illness episodes are treated first, or exclusively, through self-care, often with significant success. The avail-

ability of over-the-counter medications, a relatively high literacy level, and influence of the mass media in communicating health-related information to the general population have contributed to the high percentage of self-treatment. Home treatments are attractive because they are accessible compared with the inconvenience associated with traveling to a physician, nurse practitioner, and pharmacist, particularly for clients from rural or sparsely populated areas. Furthermore, home treatment may mobilize the client's social support network and provide the sick individual with a caring environment in which to convalesce.

However, the nurse should be aware that not all home remedies are inexpensive. For example, urban black populations in the Southeast sometimes use medicinal potions that cost much more than an equivalent treatment with a biomedical intervention.

Various nontraditional interventions are gaining the recognition of health care professionals in the biomedical-scientific health care system. Acupuncture, acupressure, therapeutic touch, massage, biofeedback, relaxation techniques, meditation, hypnosis, distraction, imagery, and herbal remedies are interventions that clients may use alone or in combination with other treatments.

Cultural Negotiation

Cultural negotiation refers to the process in which messages, instructions, and belief systems are manipulated, linked, or processed between the professional and lay models of health problems and preferred treatment. In each act, the nurse gives attention to eliciting the client's views regarding a health-related experience (e.g., pregnancy, complications of pregnancy, or illness of an infant).

Katon and Kleinman (1981) describe negotiation as a bilateral arrangement in which two principal parties attempt to work out a solution. The goal of negotiation is to reduce

conflict in a way that promotes cooperation. Cultural negotiation is used when conceptual differences exist between
the client and the nurse, a situation that may occur for one or
more of the following reasons:

- The nurse and client may be using the same words but
applying different meanings to them.
- The nurse and client may apply the same term to the
same phenomenon but have different notions of its causation.
- The nurse and client may have different memories or
emotions associated with the term and its use.

In cultural negotiation, the nurse provides scientific
information while acknowledging that the client may hold
different views. If the client's perspective indicates that
behaviors would be helpful, positive, adaptive, or neutral in
effect, the nurse should include these in the plan of care.
However, if the client's perspective would result in behaviors
that may be harmful, negative, or nonadaptive, the nurse
should attempt to shift the client's perspective to that of the
practitioner (Spector, 2004).

Pregnancy and childbirth are social, cultural, and physiological experiences; therefore, an approach to culturally sensitive nursing care of childbearing women and their families
must focus on the interaction between cultural meaning and
biological functions. Childbirth is a time of transition and
social celebration that is of central importance in any
society; it signals realignment of existing cultural roles and
responsibilities, psychological and biological states, and
social relationships. Child rearing is also a period during
which culturally bound values, attitudes, beliefs, and practices permeate virtually all aspects of life for the parents and
child (Andrews and Boyle, 2003). Careful assessment and
attention to culturally based practices are particularly important during these occasions.

MANAGEMENT OF HEALTH PROBLEMS IN CULTURALLY DIVERSE POPULATIONS

The factors responsible for the health disparity between
minority and white populations are complex and defy sim-
plistic solutions. Health status is influenced by the interaction
of physiological, cultural, psychological, and societal factors that are poorly understood for the general population
and even less so for minorities. Despite the shared characteristic of economic disadvantage among minorities, common
approaches for improving health are not possible. Rather,
solving problems among minorities necessitates activities,
programs, and data collection that are tailored to meet the
unique health care needs of many different subgroups. Solutions to health care problems among culturally diverse populations include the following:

- Providing health information and education
- Delivering and financing health services
- Developing health professionals from minority groups
- Enhancing cooperative efforts with the nonfederal sector
- Improving methods of data development
- Promoting a research agenda on minority health issues

Providing Health Information and Education

Minority populations tend to be less knowledgeable or less
aware of some specific health problems than whites. This is
demonstrated by the following (American Cancer Society,
2005; USDHHS, 2000):

- Blacks have the highest mortality rate for all cancers
combined and for most major cancers.
- Blacks receive less information about cancer and heart
disease than non-minority groups.
- Blacks tend to underestimate the prevalence of cancer, give
less credence to the warning signs, obtain fewer screening
tests, and are diagnosed at later stages of cancer than
whites.
- Many professionals and lay people, both minority and
white, do not know that heart disease is as common in black
men as in white men and that black women die from
coronary heart disease at a higher rate than white women.
- Among Mexican Americans, cultural attitudes regarding
obesity and diet are often barriers to achieving weight
control

Programs to increase public awareness about health problems have been well received in several areas. For example,
the Healthy Mothers and Healthy Babies Coalition, which
provides an education program in both English and Spanish,
has contributed to increased awareness of measures to improve
the health status of mothers and infants. In addition, increased
knowledge among blacks of hypertension as a serious health
problem is one of the accomplishments of the National High
Blood Pressure Education program. The success of these
efforts indicates that carefully planned programs have a
beneficial effect, but efforts must continue and expand to
reach even more of the target population and focus on
additional health problems.

Planning Health Information Campaigns

Sensitivity to cultural factors is often lacking in the health
care of minorities. Key concepts for the nurse to consider in
designing a health information campaign include meeting
the language and cultural needs of each identified minority
group, using minority-specific community resources to
tailor educational approaches, and developing materials and
methods of presentation that are commensurate with the
educational level of the target population. Furthermore, the
powerful influences of cultural factors over a lifetime in
shaping people's attitudes, values, beliefs, and practices
concerning health require health information programs to be
sustained over a long period. The following are examples of
ways in which the nurse can interweave these concepts into
health promotion efforts:

- The nurse should involve local community leaders who
are members of the targeted cultural group to promote
acceptance and reinforcement of the central themes of
health promotion messages.
- Health messages are more readily accepted if they do not
conflict with existing cultural beliefs and practices. Where
appropriate, messages should acknowledge existing cultural beliefs.

- The nurse should involve families, churches, employers, and community organizations as a support system to facilitate and sustain behavior change to a more healthful lifestyle. For example, although hypertension control in blacks depends on appropriate treatment (e.g., medication), blood pressure can be improved and maintained by family and community support of activities such as proper diet and exercise.
- Language barriers, cultural differences, and lack of adequate information on access to care complicate prenatal care for Hispanic and Asian women who have recently arrived in the United States. By using lay volunteers to organize community support networks, programs have been developed to disseminate culturally appropriate health information.

Health Education

Although printed materials and other audiovisual aids contribute to the educational process, client education is inherently interpersonal. The success of educational efforts is often determined by the credibility of the source and is highly dependent on the skill and sensitivity of the nurse in communicating information in a culturally appropriate manner. Education programs are particularly critical and necessary for several health problems with the greatest influence on minority health, such as hypertension, obesity, and diabetes. For example, if diabetics could improve their self-management skills through education, a significant number of complications (e.g., ketoacidosis, blindness, and amputations) could be avoided, saving human misery and health care dollars.

Delivering and Financing Health Services

Innovative models for delivering and financing health services for minority populations are needed. According to community health experts, models should increase flexibility of health care delivery, facilitate minorities' access to services, and improve efficiency of service and payment systems. One of the most commonly used indicators of adequacy of health services for a population is distribution of health care providers; however, this is an inadequate measurement. The following facts exemplify the problems associated with health services for minorities:

- The disparities in death rates between minorities and whites remain despite overall increases in health care access and use.
- Language problems hinder refugees and immigrants when they seek health care.
- Blacks with cancer postpone seeking diagnosis of their symptoms longer than whites and delay initiation of treatment once diagnosed (American Cancer Society, 2005).
- A smaller proportion of black women than white women begin prenatal care in the first trimester of pregnancy (USDHHS, 2000).

Models of Health Promotion

In most health models, SES is assumed to affect health status through environmental or behavioral factors. These models posit that poor families may not have the economic, social, or community resources needed to remain in good health. For example, poverty is thought to affect children's well-being by impacting health and nutrition, the home environment, caregiver interactions with children, caregiver mental health, and neighborhood conditions. The deficits associated with poverty may lead to an inadequate diet, which results in poor growth and delayed development. Likewise, poor housing results in increased risk for exposure that leads to other environmental hazards; overcrowding results in increased risk for infectious diseases such as tuberculosis, meningitis, influenza, and related conditions; and community violence threatens the safety and well-being of children. The combined effect of these stressors is thought to provide the foundation for a cycle of hopelessness and depression among family members, who, in turn, may engage in risky health behaviors (e.g., smoking, substance abuse, poor dietary habits resulting in obesity and high cholesterol levels, etc.) and unfavorable family interactions.

Although many Latino children live in poverty, they enjoy relatively good health compared to children in other low socioeconomic groups. This has been called an epidemiological paradox. It is believed that strong family-community support fosters optimum family health behaviors. The assumption is that if the family promotes beneficial health behaviors among its members, these behaviors will become integrated into the culture. Healthy lifestyle behaviors become an integral component of the family identity, traditions, and history.

Continuity of Care

Continuity of care is associated with improved health outcomes and is presumably greater when a client is able to establish an ongoing relationship with a care provider. Many of the leading causes of death among minorities (e.g., cancer, cardiovascular disease, and diabetes) are chronic rather than acute problems; therefore they require extended treatment regimens. Consider the following:

- Refugees are eligible for special refugee medical assistance during their first 18 months in the United States. However, after this period, refugees who cannot afford private health insurance and are ineligible for Medicaid or state medical assistance may become medically indigent.
- Many Native Americans and Alaska Natives live in areas where the availability of health care providers is half the national average.

Financing Problems

As mentioned previously, problems associated with financing health care tend to be more common in minority groups than in the dominant cultural group. Consider the following (National Center for Health Statistics, 2004):

- Economic inequalities cause members of minority groups to disproportionately rely on Medicaid for their health care needs.
- Older minority people are less likely than whites to supplement Medicare with additional private insurance.
- Proportionately, three times as many Native Americans, blacks, Hispanics, and certain Asian and Pacific Islander groups as whites live in poverty.

- In 2004, 27.8% of Hispanics lacked insurance coverage, compared with 10.5% of blacks and 6.3% of whites.

To better manage health problems and reduce the disparity in health indicators, these issues of financing must be addressed. Failure to do so will result not only in continued inequity in access to services but also in continued poor health among minority groups.

Developing Health Professionals From Minority Groups

The need to increase the number of health professionals from minority groups has been recognized for decades. With few exceptions, minorities are underrepresented as students and practitioners of the health professions. Although the number of minority nursing students has been steadily increasing, there still are proportionately more white nursing students.

Differences in the availability of health personnel resources in minority communities are apparent, regardless of the minority group being considered. Communities located in urban-metropolitan areas have significantly more professional resources. Among the factors that contribute to the imbalances in minority representation in health professions are the size of a minority population, number of cultural subgroups, and demographic features. Efforts to encourage more students from minority groups are ongoing, and government and private foundations offer grants, scholarships, and low-cost loans to recruit and retain students from underserved minority groups in nursing and other health care professions. Minority and non-minority health professional organizations, academic institutions, state governments, health departments, and other organizations from the public and private sectors should work together to develop strategies to improve the availability and accessibility of health care professionals to minority communities (Sullivan Commission, 2004).

Enhancing Cooperative Efforts With the Nonfederal Sector

Activities to improve minority health should involve participation of organizations at all levels (i.e., community, municipal, state, and national). Community involvement in developing health promotion activities can contribute to their success by providing credibility and visibility to the activities and facilitating their acceptance. Changes in health behavior frequently depend on personal initiative and are most likely to be triggered by efforts from locally based sources.

However, not all minority communities have the ability to identify their own health problems and initiate activities to address them. Support from the state and federal governments and private sector assistance is needed to assist with identifying and solving health-related problems afflicting the minority community. Assistance may be provided to minority communities in the following ways:

1. The use of technical assistance to identify high-risk groups
2. Assistance with planning, implementing, and evaluating programs to address identified needs
3. Specialized community services (e.g., federally funded projects for infants and frail older adults)
4. Programs supported by businesses and industries (e.g., health promotion programs organized by unions)

The private sector can also serve as an effective channel for programs targeted to minority health projects. National organizations concerned with minorities, such as the National Urban League and the Coalition of Hispanic Mental Health and Human Services Organizations, include health-related issues in their national agendas and are actively seeking effective ways to improve the health of minorities. Organizations such as these have a powerful potential for effecting change among their constituencies because they have strong community-level grassroots support.

Promoting a Research Agenda on Minority Health Issues

The National Center on Minority Health and Health Disparities (NCMHD) (http://ncmhd.nih.gov/) was developed in 2000 to assist in the investigation of factors affecting minority health. Its mission is to promote minority health and to ultimately eliminate health disparities. The NCMHD conducts and supports research that examines risk factor prevalence and treatment services. It also reviews health education interventions, preventive services interventions, and sociocultural factors that influence health and outcomes of care.

For further information on current research related to culture and community health nursing, the reader should search library databases for reports of completed studies (see Andrews, Burr, and Janetos, 2004). Electronic bulletin boards also may be valuable when searching for research in progress and for communicating with researchers studying a particular phenomenon of interest. An example of recent nursing research related to culturally competent care is discussed in "Research Highlights."

ROLE OF THE COMMUNITY HEALTH NURSE IN IMPROVING HEALTH FOR CULTURALLY DIVERSE PEOPLE

This chapter provides data detailing the health care problems of culturally diverse individuals, families, groups, and communities. Given the complexity of the problems and the wide variation in incidence and distribution of these problems within specific subgroups, no simple method exists for providing culturally sensitive community health nursing care to all clients. However, the following strategies may assist the community health nurse when working with culturally diverse clients:

- Conduct a "culturological" assessment.
- Conduct a cultural self-assessment.
- Seek knowledge about local cultures.
- Recognize the political issues of culturally diverse groups.
- Provide culturally competent care.
- Recognize culturally based health problems.

RESEARCH **HIGHLIGHTS**

Nutritional Patterns of Recent Immigrants

Edmonds (2005) examined the nutritional patterns of 23 recently immigrated women from Honduras to assist in understanding health-related nutritional issues in this Hispanic subgroup. She determined that the Honduran women had made both positive and negative changes in their diets since coming to the United States. Rice, beans, natural fruit juices, tortillas, bananas, beef, and eggs were reported as the typical foods eaten every day in Honduras. Positive changes in diets included eating a greater variety of fruits and vegetables, cooking with less grease, baking more frequently than frying, and using vegetable oil rather than lard. They also ate more meat and dairy products. Negative changes noted were more skipped meals and eating foods high in fat and calories (e.g., fast foods). Research suggests that classes be taught in WIC (Women, Infants, and Children) programs and other venues that would support the Hondurans' traditional diet and focus on how to eat nutritionally in fast food restaurants, eat a balance diet, plan meals and cook ahead, and read food labels.

Edmonds VM: The nutritional patterns of recently immigrated Honduran women, *J Transcult Nurs* 16(3):226-235, 2005.

Culturological Assessment

All nursing care is based on a systematic, comprehensive assessment of the client; therefore the community health nurse must gather cultural data on clients from racially and ethnically diverse backgrounds. A **culturological assessment** refers to a systematic appraisal or examination of individuals, groups, and communities regarding their cultural beliefs, values, and practices to determine explicit nursing needs and intervention practices within the cultural context of the people being evaluated (Leininger, 1995). The term *culturological* is a descriptive reference to cultural phenomena in their broadest sense.

Culturological assessments are as vital as physical and psychological assessments. Culturological assessments tend to be broad and comprehensive because they deal with cultural values, belief systems, and ways of living now and in the recent past. In conducting a culturological assessment, the community health nurse should be involved in determining and appraising the traits, characteristics, or smallest units of cultural behavior as a guide to nursing care. The following section summarizes major data categories pertaining to the culture of clients and offers suggested questions that the nurse may ask to elicit needed information.

Brief History of Ethnic and Racial Origins of the Cultural Group With Which the Client Identifies

- With what ethnic group or groups does the client report affiliation (e.g., Hispanic, Polish, Navajo, or a combination)? To what degree does the client identify with the cultural group (e.g., "we" concept of solidarity or a fringe member)?
- What is the client's reported racial affiliation (e.g., black, Native American, or Asian)?

- Where was the client born?
- Where has the client lived (i.e., country and city) and when (i.e., during what years)? If the client has recently relocated to the United States, knowledge of prevalent diseases in the country of origin may be helpful.

Values Orientation

- What are the client's attitudes, values, and beliefs about birth, death, health, illness, and health care providers?
- Does culture influence the manner in which the client relates to body image change resulting from illness or surgery (e.g., importance of appearance, beauty, strength, and roles in cultural group)?
- How does the client view work, leisure, and education?
- How does the client perceive change?
- How does the client value privacy, courtesy, touch, and relationships with individuals of different ages, of different social class, or caste, and of the opposite sex?
- How does the client view biomedical-scientific health care (e.g., suspiciously, fearfully, or acceptingly)? How does the client relate to people in a different cultural group (e.g., withdrawal, verbal or nonverbal expression, or negative or positive attitude)?

Cultural Sanctions and Restrictions

- How does the client's cultural group regard expression of emotion and feelings, spirituality, and religious beliefs? How are dying, death, and grieving expressed in a culturally appropriate manner?
- How is modesty expressed by men and women in the client's cultural group? Does the client's cultural group have culturally defined expectations about male-female relationships, including the nurse-client relationship?
- Does the client have restrictions related to sexuality, exposure of body parts, or certain types of surgery (e.g., amputation, vasectomy, or hysterectomy)?
- Does the client have restrictions against discussion of dead relatives or fears related to the unknown?

Communication

- What language does the client speak at home? What other language does the client speak or read? In what language would the client prefer to communicate with you?
- What is the written and spoken English fluency level of the client? Remember that the stress of illness may cause clients to use a more familiar language and temporarily forget some English.
- Does the client need an interpreter? If so, is a relative or friend available whom the client would like to have interpret? Is anyone available with whom the client would prefer not to interpret (e.g., member of the opposite sex, a person younger or older than the client, or a member of a rival tribe or nation)?
- What are the rules (i.e., linguistics) and modes (i.e., style) of communication?
- Is it necessary to vary the technique of communication during the interview and examination to accommodate the client's cultural background (e.g., tempo of conversation,

ETHICAL Insights

Disclosure of HIV/AIDS Status

Ortiz (2005) examined the experiences of disclosing they were living with HIV/AIDS of 19 Latinas. She described how the women decided to disclose their HIV status to partners, family members, friends, and employers. Four categories emerged: timing of the disclosure, the need to disclose, controlling disclosure, and supportive disclosing. These factors were influenced by the Latina's relationship with others, the perceived risks to the woman and others, the need to disclose, the wish to give support to themselves or others, and the desire to control who should know and when. It was concluded that nurses should be knowledgeable of the realities of Latinas' lives and to be able to incorporate that knowledge into comprehensive care plans that will help them maximize the utilization of appropriate resources.

Ortiz CE: Disclosing concerns of Latinas living with HIV/AIDS, *J Transcult Nurs* 16(3): 210-217, 2005.

eye contact, sensitivity to topical taboos, norms of confidentiality, and style of explanation)?

- How does the client's nonverbal communication compare with that of individuals from other cultural backgrounds? How does it affect the client's relationship with the nurse and with other members of the health care team?
- How does the client feel about health care providers who are not of the same cultural background (e.g., black, middle-class nurse, or Hispanic of a different social class)? Does the client prefer to receive care from a nurse of the same cultural background, sex, or age?
- What are the overall cultural characteristics of the client's language and communication processes?
- With which language or dialect is the client most comfortable?

Health-Related Beliefs and Practices

- To what cause(s) does the client attribute illness and disease (e.g., divine wrath, imbalance in hot-cold or yin-yang, punishment for moral transgressions, hex, or soul loss)?
- What does the client believe promotes health (e.g., eating certain foods, wearing amulets to bring good luck, exercise, prayer, ancestors, saints, or intermediate deities)?
- What is the client's religious affiliation (e.g., Judaism, Islam, Pentecostalism, West African voodooism, Seventh-Day Adventism, Catholicism, or Mormonism)?
- Does the client rely on cultural healers (e.g., curandero, shaman, spiritualist, priest, minister, or monk)? Who determines when the client is sick and when the client is healthy? Who determines the type of healer and treatment that should be sought?
- In what types of cultural healing practices does the client engage (e.g., herbal remedies, potions, massage, wearing talismans or charms to discourage evil spirits, healing rituals, incantations, or prayers)?
- How does the client perceive biomedical-scientific health care providers? How do the client and family perceive nurses? What are the expectations of nurses and nursing care?

- What comprises appropriate "sick-role" behavior? Who determines what symptoms constitute disease and illness? Who decides when the client is no longer sick? Who cares for the client at home?
- How does the client's cultural group view mental disorders? Do they show differences in acceptable behaviors for physical versus psychological illnesses?

Nutrition

- What nutritional factors are influenced by the client's cultural background?
- What meanings does the client attach to food and eating? With whom does the client usually eat? What types of foods does the client usually eat? What does the client define as food? What does the client believe comprises a "healthy" versus an "unhealthy" diet?
- How does the client prepare foods at home (e.g., type of food preparation; cooking oils used; length of time foods, especially vegetables, are cooked; amount and type of seasoning added to various foods during preparation)?
- Do religious beliefs and practices influence the client's diet (e.g., amount, type, preparation, or delineation of acceptable food combinations, such as kosher diets)? Does the client abstain from certain foods at regular intervals, on specific dates determined by the religious calendar, or at other times?
- If the client's religion mandates or encourages fasting, what does the term *fast* mean to the client (e.g., refraining from certain types or quantities of foods, eating only during certain times of the day)? For what period of time is the client expected to fast?
- During fasting, does the client refrain from liquids or beverages? Does the religion allow exemption from fasting during illness, and if so, is the client believed to have an exemption?

Socioeconomic Considerations

- Who constitutes the client's social network (i.e., family, peers, and healers)? How do they influence the client's health or illness status?
- How do members of the client's social support network define caring (e.g., being continuously present, doing things for the client, or looking after the client's family)? What are the roles of various family members during health and illness?
- How does the client's family participate in the client's nursing care (e.g., bathing, feeding, touching, and being present)?
- Does the cultural family structure influence the client's response to health or illness (e.g., beliefs, strengths, weaknesses, and social class)? Does a key family member have a role that is significant in health-related decisions (e.g., grandmother in many black families or eldest adult son in Asian families)?
- Who is the principal wage earner in the client's family? What is the total annual income? This is a potentially sensitive question that should be asked only if necessary. Does the family have more than one wage earner? Does

the family have other sources of financial support (e.g., extended family or investments)?

- What influence does economic status have on lifestyle, place of residence, living conditions, ability to obtain health care, and discharge planning?

Organizations Providing Cultural Support

- What influence do ethnic and cultural organizations have on the client's receiving health care (e.g., Organization of Migrant Workers, National Association for the Advancement of Colored People, Black Political Caucus, churches, schools, Urban League, and community-based health care programs and clinics)?

Educational Background

- What is the client's highest educational level obtained? Does the client's educational background affect the client's knowledge level concerning the health care delivery system, how to obtain the care needed, teaching and learning skills, and written material that is distributed in the health care setting (e.g., insurance forms, educational literature, information about diagnostic procedures and laboratory tests, and admissions forms)?
- Can the client read and write English, or does he or she prefer another language? If English is the client's second language, are materials available in the client's primary language?
- What learning style is most comfortable or familiar? Does the client prefer to learn through written materials, oral explanation, or demonstration?

Religious Affiliation

- How does the client's religious affiliation influence health and illness (e.g., death, chronic illness, body image alteration, and cause and effect of illness)?
- What is the role of the client's religious beliefs and practices during health and illness?
- Does the client believe in healing rituals or practices that can promote well-being or hasten recovery from illness? If so, who performs these?
- What is the role of significant religious representatives during health and illness? Does the client have recognized religious healers (e.g., Islamic imams, Christian Scientist practitioners or nurses, Catholic priests, Mormon elders, and Buddhist monks)?

Cultural Aspects of Disease Incidence

- Does the client have specific genetic or acquired conditions that are more prevalent in a specific cultural group (e.g., hypertension, sickle cell anemia, Tay-Sachs disease, or lactose intolerance)?
- Are any socioenvironmental diseases more prevalent among the client's specific cultural group (e.g., lead poisoning, alcoholism, AIDS, drug abuse, or ear infections)?
- Do diseases exist against which the client has an increased resistance (e.g., skin cancer in darkly pigmented individuals)?

Biocultural Variations

- Does the client have distinctive physical features that are characteristic of a particular racial group (e.g., skin color or hair texture)? Does the client have variations in anatomy that are characteristic of a particular racial or ethnic group (e.g., body structure, height, weight, facial shape and structure [nose, eye shape, and facial contour], or upper and lower extremity shape)?
- How do anatomical and racial variations affect the assessment?

Developmental Considerations

- Does the client have distinct growth and development characteristics that vary with his or her cultural background (e.g., bone density, psychomotor patterns of development, or fat folds)?
- What factors are significant in assessing children from the newborn period through adolescence (e.g., expected growth on standard grid, culturally acceptable age for toilet training, introduction of various types of foods, sex differences, discipline, and socialization to adult roles)?
- What is the cultural perception of aging (e.g., is youthfulness or the wisdom of old age more highly valued)?
- How are older people handled culturally (e.g., cared for in the home of adult children or placed in institutions for care)? What are culturally acceptable roles for older adults?
- Does the older adult expect family members to provide care, including nurturance and other humanistic aspects of care?
- Is the older adult isolated from culturally relevant supportive people or enmeshed in a caring network of relatives and friends?
- Has a culturally appropriate network replaced family members in performing some caring functions for older adults?

Cultural Self-Assessment

Community health nurses can engage in a cultural self-assessment. Through identification of health-related attitudes, values, beliefs, and practices that are part of the personal cultural meaning brought to the nurse-client interaction, the nurse can better understand the cultural aspects of health care from the perspective of the client, family, group, or community. Everyone has ethnocentric tendencies that must be brought to a level of conscious awareness so that efforts can be made to temper ethnocentrism and view reality from the perspective of the client.

Knowledge About Local Cultures

Community health nurses can learn about the cultural diversity characteristics of the subgroup or subgroups that are most prevalent within their communities. The nurse cannot know about all health-related beliefs and practices of the diverse groups served, but he or she can study select ones. The nurse can accomplish this cultural study by a review of nursing, anthropology, sociology, and related literature on culturally diverse groups; in-services held at community health agencies, educational institutions in the community, or organizations serving minority groups; enrollment in courses on transcultural or cross-cultural nursing and medical anthropology; and interviews with key members of the subgroups of interest, such as clergy members, nurses, physicians, and others, to obtain information about the influence of culture on health-related beliefs and practices.

Recognition of Political Issues of Culturally Diverse Groups

Awareness of the political aspects of health care for culturally diverse groups and communities can help community health nurses influence legislation and funding priorities aimed at improving health care for specific populations. Recognized for their leadership role in community health matters involving culturally diverse groups, community health nurses may be invited by political leaders to participate in political decision making affecting the health of a targeted subgroup. Community health nurses should also be active politically, both individually and collectively, to influence legislation affecting culturally diverse individuals, groups, and communities, and they should offer to serve on key community committees, boards, and advisory councils that impact the health of culturally diverse groups.

Providing Culturally Competent Care

When caring for individuals and families from culturally diverse backgrounds, the community health nurse can assess, diagnose, implement, and evaluate nursing care in a manner that is culturally congruent, competent, relevant, and appropriate. To provide this culturally appropriate nursing care, the nurse must create a relationship of mutual respect by becoming aware of the cultural similarities and differences between herself or himself and the client. A guideline for gathering cultural data has been presented, and the nurse may use this guideline or a similar one for identifying significant areas in which the nurse and client differ. Knowledge about biocultural variations in health and illness is particularly important when conducting cultural assessments.

Recognition of Culturally Based Health Practices

As discussed previously, the community health nurse should attempt to understand the nature and meaning of culturally based health practices of clients, groups, and communities. Once the practices are understood, the nurse can make a determination regarding their appropriateness in a particular context. Generally, the nurse should decide whether a cultural practice is useful, neutral, or harmful to the client, group, or community. The nurse should encourage or "tolerate" helpful and neutral practices, whereas he or she should discourage harmful practices.

The classification of some cultural healing practices is not so easily determined. For example, many Southeast Asians practice coining, which is the rubbing of a coin over body surfaces to expel "bad winds" that are believed to cause illness. Coining leaves abrasions on the skin. Community health nurses are faced with an ethical dilemma when coining is practiced on young children, because this practice may be construed by some members of the dominant cultural group as child abuse. This

practice is not useful, so the nurse must make the decision whether it is neutral or harmful. An argument for the practice being neutral is based on the facts that the abrasions usually heal quickly, no harm is done to the child as a result of the practice, and the practice is meaningful to parents who have much confidence in the healing powers associated with coining.

The argument can also be made that the practice is harmful. The red marks and skin abrasions caused by the coining place the child at increased risk for skin infection. Given that the child may require antibiotics or other medication for a respiratory disorder, encouragement of coining may prevent the child from receiving needed medical intervention and delay treatment.

As a solution, the community health nurse may suggest that parents combine traditional treatment with Western biomedicine (i.e., they can use coining in conjunction with a biomedical intervention). Therefore the healing will occur in a manner that has involved the use of both folk and professional health care systems.

RESOURCES FOR MINORITY HEALTH

Community health nurses will find federal resources for improving the health care of the federally defined minority populations through the Department of Health and Human Services (DHHS). Within the DHHS, the Office of Minority Health (OMH) and the Indian Health Service (INS) divisions relate to health promotion, disease prevention, service delivery, and research on minority groups.

Office of Minority Health

The OMH coordinates federal efforts to improve the health status of racial and ethnic minority populations (i.e., blacks, Hispanics, Native Americans and Alaska Natives, and Asians and Pacific Islanders). The OMH is directed by the deputy assistant secretary for minority health and was established by the Disadvantaged Minority Health Improvement Act of 1990 (PL 101-527), which was signed by President George H. W. Bush on November 6, 1990. Under the directives of the act, the OMH has the following responsibilities:

- Establish short- and long-range goals and objectives relating to disease prevention, health promotion, service delivery, and research on the health of minority people.
- Promote increased participation of disadvantaged people, including minorities, in health service and health promotion programs.
- Create a national minority health resource center.
- Support research, demonstrations, and evaluations of new and innovative models that increase understanding of disease risk factors and support better information dissemination, education, prevention, and service delivery to minority communities.
- Promote minority health–related activities in the corporate and voluntary sectors.

TABLE 12-7   Federally Sponsored Initiatives to Improve the Health of Minority Groups

INITIATIVE	DESCRIPTION
Health Resources and Services Administration Health Disparity Collaboratives (HDC)	HDC is a broad, multiyear plan to improve the health status of underserved populations. It seeks to ensure that clients receive evidence-based care, and it encourages clients to be active participants in their own care. For more information: http://bphc.hrsa.gov/quality/Collaboratives.htm
Racial and Ethnic Approaches to Community Health (REACH 2010)	This program was launched in 1999 to eliminate health disparities in six priority areas: cardiovascular diseases, immunizations, breast and cervical cancer screening and management, diabetes, HIV/AIDS, and infant mortality. REACH 2010 supports community coalitions in designing, implementing, and evaluating community-driven strategies to eliminate health disparities. For more information: http://www.cdc.gov/reach2010
National Breast and Cervical Cancer Early Detection Program (NBCCEDP)	NBCCEDP provides breast and cervical cancer screening, diagnosis and treatment to low-income, medically underserved, and uninsured women (emphasizing recruitment of minority women). For more information: http://www.cdc.gov/cancer/nbccedp
Ryan White Comprehensive AIDS Resources Emergency (CARE) Act B	Ryan White CARE Act provides services to persons living with HIV disease, primarily racial and ethnic minorities. For more information: http://hab.hrsa.gov/
National Center on Minority Health and Health Disparities (NCMHD)	NCMHD leads, coordinates, supports, and assesses the NIH research efforts to reduce and ultimately eliminate health disparities. For more information: http://ncmhd.nih.gov/

- Develop minority-focused health information and health promotion materials and teaching programs.
- Assist providers of primary care and preventive services in obtaining assistance of bilingual health professionals when appropriate.

As the focal point for minority health efforts, the OMH plays a key role in major initiatives launched by the USDHHS secretary. Table 12-7 lists some of the initiatives.

Indian Health Service

The IHS is responsible for providing federal health services to Native Americans and Alaska Natives. Federal Indian health services are based on the laws that Congress has passed pursuant to its authority to regulate commerce with the Indian Nations as specified in the Constitution and other documents.

The primary responsibility of the IHS is to elevate the health status of Native Americans and Alaska Natives to the highest level possible. The mission is to ensure quality, availability, and accessibility of a comprehensive, high-quality health care delivery system, providing maximum involvement of Native Americans and Alaska Natives in defining their health needs, setting health priorities for their local areas, and managing and controlling their health programs. The IHS also acts as the principal federal health advocate for Native Americans by ensuring that they have knowledge of, and access to, all federal, state, and local health programs to which they are entitled as American citizens. The IHS also works with these programs so Native Americans will be cognizant of their entitlements.

The IHS carried out its responsibilities through development and operation of a health services delivery system designed to provide a broad-spectrum program of preventive, curative, rehabilitative, and environmental services. This system integrates health services delivered directly through IHS facilities and staff with those purchased by IHS through contractual arrangements. Tribes are also actively involved in program implementation.

The 1975 Indian Self-Determination Act (PL 93-638), as amended, builds on IHS policy by giving tribes the option of staffing and managing IHS programs in their communities and provides funding for improvement of tribal capability to contract under the act. The 1976 Indian Health Care Improvement Act (PL 94-437), as amended, was intended to elevate the health care status of Native Americans and Alaska Natives to a level equal to that of the general population through a program of authorized, higher resource levels in the IHS budget. Appropriated resources were used to expand health services, build and renovate medical facilities, and step up the construction of safe drinking water and sanitary disposal facilities. It also establishes programs designed to increase the number of Native-American health professionals for Native-American needs and to improve health care access for Native Americans living in urban areas.

The operation of the IHS health care delivery system is managed through local administrative units called service units. A service unit is the basic health organization for a geographical area served by the IHS program, just as a county or city health department is the basic health organization in a state health department. These are defined areas usually centered around a single federal reservation in the continental United States or a population concentration in Alaska. The IHS serves approximately 50% of the total Native-American and Alaska Native population in the United States, primarily those residing on reservations.

SUMMARY

To provide community health nursing for individuals, groups, and communities representing the hundreds of different cultures and subcultures found in the United States, the nurse should include cultural considerations in nursing care. Guidelines for gathering data from clients of culturally diverse backgrounds have been suggested in this chapter and are interwoven throughout the text. Knowledge about culture-specific and culture-universal nursing care is foundational and is an integral component of community health nursing.

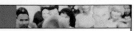

CASE STUDY | Application of the Nursing Process

Community health nurse Maria Gonzales visited the home of 5-year-old Nguyen Van Nghi, who was discharged from the hospital on the previous day. The pediatrician had diagnosed the child with pneumonia and "suspected failure to thrive" because the child's growth fell below the third percentile on a standard growth chart for height and weight and he performed poorly on a screening test used to identify developmental delays for a 5-year-old child.

Residing in the home were the child's parents, four siblings, grandmother, aunt, uncle, and three cousins. Although the child's father and uncle spoke some English, other members of the household communicated in a language unfamiliar to Maria, which "sounded like Chinese." When Maria approached the child, he did not look at her or speak to her, even when she called him Nguyen (pronounced "we'en").

ASSESSMENT

In a brief survey of the Nguyen's home, Maria noted that the home and furnishings were modest but very clean. The pantry held a considerable amount of food, including rice and dried noodles. The small refrigerator smelled of fish and contained some vegetables that Maria didn't recognize. She did not see any green vegetables, milk, or other dairy products.

During her initial assessment of Nghi, Maria observed multiple tender, ecchymotic areas with petechiae between the ribs on the front and back of the body, resembling strap marks. Suspecting child abuse, Maria told the family that she would return later in the day with an interpreter. She located an interpreter who spoke Mandarin Chinese and briefed him about her concerns with child abuse. When Maria and the interpreter returned to the client's home, she instructed the interpreter to ask the parents for an explanation of the bruises. The interpreter told Maria that the family was Vietnamese and could not understand his Chinese dialect. Both the interpreter and the child's father knew a little French and awkwardly managed to communicate.

The interpreter advised the nurse that, in the Vietnamese culture, the person's family name is given first, followed by the middle name and then the first name. Only a few different family names exist among the Vietnamese; therefore it is common practice to call people by their given first name. At this point, Maria also learned that the child was actually 4 years old, because the Vietnamese consider a newborn to be 1 year old at birth.

The interpreter explained that a Vietnamese healer performed *cao gio,* or coining, to exude the "bad wind" from Nghi. *Cao gio* is performed by applying a special menthol oil to the painful or symptomatic part of the body and then rubbing a coin over the area with firm, downward strokes. When Nghi's condition seemed to worsen after his hospital discharge, his grandmother convinced his parents that Western biomedicine had failed and that their son required the stronger power of folk healing.

DIAGNOSIS

- Maria must set priorities and focus on selected cultural data categories because they seem most relevant for the Nguyen family at present.

Individual

- High risk for Nghi's pneumonia to worsen
- Potential for child abuse/neglect
- Possible physical and/or developmental delay (low weight/height for age)

Family

- Increased risk for poor health outcomes related to distrust of Western health care practices
- Increased risk for nutritional deficits

Community

- Potential for poor health of area Vietnamese immigrants related to knowledge deficit of good nutritional practices and general health promotion

PLANNING

Individual
Short-term Goals

- Nghi's pneumonia will resolve.
- Nghi will show no more evidence of practice of "coining."

Long-Term Goal

- Nghi's height and weight will increase proportionally to at least 50th percentile for age.

Family
Short-Term Goals

- Family members will cease practice of "coining."
- Caregivers will recognize the importance of completing the antibiotics as prescribed.

Long-Term Goal

- A family nutritional assessment will be completed and adjustments will be made to their diet to provide needed nutrients.

Community
Long-Term Goal

- Leaders of the area's Vietnamese community will work with area health care providers to promote good nutritional practices.

INTERVENTION

Individual
Through the interpreter, Maria was able to communicate with the Nguyen family that it was vital for Nghi to complete the

Continued

CASE STUDY Application of the Nursing Process (cont'd)

prescribed antibiotics. She also attempted to convey the potentially harmful effect of the practice of coining and suggested that that procedure be stopped. She set a follow-up appointment for the following day.

Family

Maria was able to bring a Vietnamese interpreter for the follow-up appointment. So, in addition to reiteration of the importance of taking the medications, she was able to teach about basic nutritional principles and perform additional nutritional assessments. Although Nghi was not as small as initially thought, he was still below the 50th percentile for his age. Maria gave nutritional pamphlets written in Vietnamese to the parents and provided them with information on where to find low-cost foods in the neighborhood.

Community

Working with the health department's social worker, and the Vietnamese interpreter, Maria visited several area markets to gather information on diet and nutritional practices of Vietnamese immigrants. They decided that they would seek a small grant to develop more teaching materials on nutrition for this populations.

EVALUATION

Individual

By the third follow-up visit, Maria determined that although Nghi still had a residual cough, his chest was clearing. In addition, there was no evidence of coining. Further, Maria was shown that the family's refrigerator now contained whole milk and some leafy green vegetables. It was decided that she would return in 6 weeks for a follow-up visit to weigh and measure Nghi.

Family

The presence of the interpreter who spoke Vietnamese and who was familiar with the culture was vital. And, by the third visit, most of the family members appeared to be at ease with Maria. Mrs. Nguyn asked a number of questions about nutrition and other health issues and requested that Maria monitor the heights and weights of the other children.

Community

The health department's social worker was able to identify a small grant to develop and purchase teaching materials for the Vietnamese population. They applied for the funds and are eagerly waiting to hear the outcomes.

LEVELS OF PREVENTION

The following are examples of three levels of prevention as applied to the case study.

Primary

- Nutritional education for the Nguyn family.
- Health education targeted to developing comfort with the U.S. health care system and Western medicine.
- Education related to potentially harmful practices (e.g., coining).

Secondary

- Monitoring the height and weight of Nghi's and his siblings.

Tertiary

- Evaluation of resolution of pneumonia.

LEARNING ACTIVITIES

1. Examine the vital statistics of a community and compare differences in morbidity and mortality rates for whites and racial and ethnic subgroups. What data are available according to racial and ethnic heritage? What data are missing?
2. Visit an inner-city grocery store and compare quality, prices, customer services, and variety of products with those of a suburban grocery store.
3. Select a client from a racially or ethnically diverse background and conduct a cultural assessment.
4. Interview someone from racial or ethnic background different from your own to determine beliefs about illness causation, use of the lay and professional health care delivery systems, and culturally based treatments.
5. Dine at an ethnic restaurant. While dining, notice the type of cultural heritage in restaurant decor and information about the culture available from the menu, placemats, or elsewhere in the restaurant. Ask the owner or manager about the history of the restaurant.
6. Attend religious services at a church, temple, synagogue, or place of worship for a religion unfamiliar to you.
7. Interview an official representative (e.g., priest, elder, monk, or bishop) of a religion unfamiliar to you. Ask about health-related beliefs and practices, healing rituals, support network for the sick, and dietary practices.
8. Watch prime-time television and note the racial and ethnic diversity that is present during the commercials. During the program, note the role played by racially and ethnically diverse characters. Are they heroes or heroines or the "bad guys"? What are their occupations, SES, religions, and lifestyles?
9. Skim a popular magazine for references to racially and ethnically diverse subgroups. What is being written? Is the nature of the article favorable or unfavorable?

REFERENCES

Agency for Healthcare Research and Quality: *Addressing racial and ethnic disparities in health care: Fact sheet,* AHRQ 00-P041, Rockville, Md, Feb 2005, The Author.

American Cancer Society: *Cancer facts & figures for African Americans: 2005-2006.* Atlanta: American Cancer Society, 2005.

American Nurses Association: *Cultural diversity in nursing practice* (Position statement), Silver Spring, Md, 1991, The Author, http://www.ana.org/readroom/position/ethics/etcldv.htm.

Andrews M, Burr J, Janetos D: Electronic resources for transcultural nursing and health, *J Transcult Nurs* 15:242, 2004.

Andrews MM, Boyle JS, editors: *Transcultural concepts in nursing care,* ed 4, Philadelphia, 2003, Lippincott Williams & Wilkins.

Becker G: Dying away from home: quandaries of migration for elders in two ethnic groups. *J Gerontol B Psychol Sci Soc Sci* 57B(2):S79-S95, 2002.

Cockerham WC: *Medical sociology,* ed 8, Upper Saddle River, NJ, 2001, Prentice Hall.

Council of Economic Advisers for the President's Initiative on Race: *Changing America: indicators of social and economic well-being by race and Hispanic origin,* Washington, DC, 1999, The Author.

Edmonds VM: The nutritional patterns of recently immigrated Honduran women, *J Transcult Nurs* 16(3):226-235, 2005.

Gallup Poll News Service: *Religion,* Sept 2005, http://poll.gallup.com/content/default.aspx?ci=1690&VERSION=p.

Garcia Coll C: Developmental outcome of minority infants: a process-oriented look into our beginnings, *Child Dev* 61:270, 1990.

Hall E: Proxemics: the study of man's spatial relations. In Galdston I, editor: *Man's image in medicine and anthropology,* New York, 1963, International Universities Press.

Hanson PA, Andrews MM: Religion, culture and nursing. In Andrews MM, Boyle JS, editors: *Transcultural concepts in nursing care,* ed 4, Philadelphia, 2003, Lippincott Williams & Wilkins.

Indian Health Service: *Trends in Indian health,* Washington, DC, 1997, US Government Printing Office.

Johnson RL et al: Racial and ethnic differences in patient perceptions of bias and cultural competence in health care. *J Gen Intern Med* 19(2):101-110, 2004.

Katon W, Kleinman A: Doctor-patient negotiation and other social science strategies in patient care. In Eisenberg L, Kleinman A, editors: *The relevance of social science for medicine,* Boston, 1981, D. Reidel.

Kluckhohn F, Strodtbeck F: *Variations in value orientations,* Evanston, Ill, 1961, Row, Peterson.

Kohls LR: *Survival kit for overseas living,* Yarmouth, Me, 1984, Intercultural Press.

Leininger MM: *Nursing and anthropology: two worlds to blend,* New York, 1970, Wiley.

Leininger MM: *Transcultural nursing: concepts, theories, and practice,* New York, 1978, Wiley.

Leininger MM: *Culture, care, diversity, and universality: a theory of nursing,* New York, 1991, National League of Nursing Press.

Leininger MM: *Transcultural nursing: concepts, theories, research and practice,* ed 2, New York, 1995, McGraw-Hill.

Leininger MM, McFarland MR: *Transcultural nursing: concepts, theories, research and practice,* ed 3, New York, 2002, McGraw-Hill.

Ludwig-Beymer PA: Transcultural aspects of pain. In Andrews M, Boyle JS, editors: *Transcultural concepts in nursing care,* ed 4, Philadelphia, 2003, Lippincott Williams & Wilkins.

National Center for Educational Statistics, US Department of Education: *Digest of education statistics, 2004,* The Author, http://nces.ed.gov/programs/digest/d04/.

National Center for Health Statistics: *Trends in health insurance coverage by poverty status among persons under 65 years of age: United States, 1997-2002,* The Author, http://www.cdc.gov/nchs/products/pubs/pubd/hestats/healthinsur.htm.

National Council of Churches: *Yearbook of American and Canadian churches,* New York, 2005, Office of Minority Health.

Ortiz CE: Disclosing concerns of Latinas living with HIV/AIDS, *J Transcult Nurs* 16(3):210-217, 2005.

Spratley E et al: *The registered nurse population: March 2000: Findings from the National Sample Survey of Registered Nurses,* 2002, US Department of Health and Human Services, Health Resources and Services Administration, Bureau of Health Professions, Division of Nursing, http://bhpr.hrsa.gov/healthworkforce/reports/rnsurvey/rnss1.htm.

Sullivan Commission: *Missing persons: minorities in the health professions.* Report of the Sullivan Commission on diversity in the healthcare workforce, 2004, The Author, http://admissions.duhs.duke.edu/sullivancommission/documents/Sullivan_Final_Report.pdf.

Tylor EB: *Primitive culture,* London, 1871, Murray.

US Census Bureau: *Poverty: Poverty by selected characteristics: 2003,* Washington, DC, 2003, Government Printing Office, http://www.census.gov/hhes/poverty.

US Census Bureau: *Foreign-born populations in the United States: 2003,* Washington, DC, August 2004, US Government Printing Office.

US Census Bureau, Housing and Household Economic Statistics Division: *Poverty thresholds for 2004 by size of family and number of related children under 18 years,* The Author, http://www.census.gov/hhes/www/poverty/threshld/thresh04.html.

US Census Bureau, Population Division: *Poverty highlights, 2004.* The Author, http://www.census.gov/hhes/www/poverty/poverty04/pov04hi.html.

US Department of Health and Human Services: *Healthy People 2010,* Washington, DC, 2000, US Government Printing Office.

US Department of Homeland Security: *Yearbook of Immigration Statistics, 2004.* Washington DC, U.S. Department of Homeland Security, Office of Immigration Statistics, 2006.

Wilmoth JM, Chen PC: Immigrant status, living arrangements, and depressive symptoms among middle-aged and older adults. *J Gerontol B Psychol Sci Soc Sci* 58B(5):S305-S313, 2003.

Zborowski M: *People in pain,* San Francisco, 1969, Jossey-Bass.

Environmental Health

Joanne M. Hall ▪ Carolyn H. Robinson ▪ Tonya J. Broyles

MEDIA RESOURCES

Additional Material for Study, Review, and Further Exploration

evolve Website at http://evolve.elsevier.com/Nies

❖ Quiz ❖ Case Studies ❖ Content Updates ❖ Glossary ❖ WebLinks

OBJECTIVES

Upon completion of this chapter, the reader will be able to do the following:

1. Describe the broad areas of environmental health about which community health nurses must be informed and name environmental hazards in each area.
2. Recognize potential social, cultural, economic, and political factors affecting environmental health.
3. Apply the basic concepts of critical theory to environmental health nursing problems.
4. Identify aggregates at risk for particular environmental health problems.
5. Distinguish between environmental health approaches that focus on altering individual behaviors and those that aim to change health-damaging environments.
6. Formulate critical questions about environmental conditions that limit the survival and well-being of communities.
7. Understand the skills needed to facilitate community participation and partnership in identifying and solving environmental health problems.
8. Propose collective strategies in which community health nurses can participate to address the environmental health concerns of specific aggregates.

KEY TERMS

aggregate
atmospheric quality
critical theory
environment

environmental health
environmental justice
environmental racism
food quality

housing
living patterns
participatory action research
radiation risks

sick building syndrome
waste control
water quality
work risks

CHAPTER OUTLINE

A CRITICAL THEORY APPROACH TO ENVIRONMENTAL HEALTH
    Adults
    Children (Parents or Guardian)

AREAS OF ENVIRONMENTAL HEALTH
    Living Patterns
    Work Risks
    Atmospheric Quality
    Water Quality
    Housing
    Food Quality
    Waste Control
    Radiation Risks

EFFECTS OF ENVIRONMENTAL HAZARDS

EFFORTS TO CONTROL ENVIRONMENTAL HEALTH PROBLEMS

GLOBAL ENVIRONMENTAL HEALTH

EMERGING ILLNESSES RELATED TO THE ENVIRONMENT
    Other Emerging Threats
    Nursing Actions

APPROACHING ENVIRONMENTAL HEALTH AT THE AGGREGATE LEVEL

CRITICAL COMMUNITY HEALTH NURSING PRACTICE
    Taking a Stand: Advocating for Change
    Asking Critical Questions
    Facilitating Community Involvement
    Forming Coalitions
    Using Collective Strategies

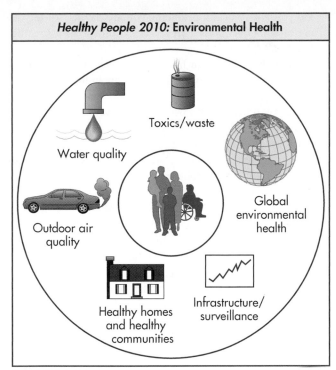

Healthy People 2010: Environmental Health

Toxics/waste

Water quality

Outdoor air quality

Global environmental health

Healthy homes and healthy communities

Infrastructure/ surveillance

FIGURE 13-1 *Healthy People 2010:* Elements of environmental health. (From US Department of Health and Human Services: *Healthy People 2010,* ed 2, Washington, DC, 2000, US Government Printing Office.)

The U.S. Department of Health and Human Services (2000) defines **environmental health** as

...those aspects of human health, disease, and injury that are determined or influenced by factors in the environment. This includes the study of both direct pathological effects of various chemical, physical, and biological agents, as well as the effects on health of the broad physical and social environment, which includes housing, urban development, land-use and transportation, industry and agriculture. (p. 8-3) (Figure 13-1)

Environmental health is of ever-increasing importance to community health nursing practice. Accumulated evidence shows that the environmental changes of the past few decades have profoundly influenced the status of public health. The safety, beauty, and life-sustaining capacity of the physical environment are unquestionably of global consequence. The ecological approach of the 1960s and 1970s tended to focus on clean water, clean air, and protected natural resources in specific locales. By the beginning of the twenty-first century, it is acutely apparent that the world must address urgent environmental difficulties, including extinction of some species, diminishment of tropical rain forests, proliferation of toxic waste dumps, effects of acid rain, progressive destruction of the ozone layer, shortage of landfill sites, consequences of global warming, development of deadly chemical and ballistic weapons, adulteration of food by pesticides and herbicides, oceanic contamination through toxic dumping and petroleum spills, overcrowding of urban areas, traffic congestion, and growing industrial hazards that pose health risks to workers.

This chapter uses critical theory to explore the health of communities in relation to the environment. Critical theory is particularly useful in examining environmental health, as it offers a framework for discussion and a basis for describing community health nursing practice (Bent, 2003; Clark, Barton, and Brown, 2002; Stevens and Hall, 1992). Applying critical theory is a way of thinking upstream (Chapter 3). **Critical theory** is an approach that raises questions about oppressive situations, involves community members in the definition and solution of problems, and facilitates interventions that liberate people from the health-damaging effects of environments. By applying the nursing process in a critical fashion, nurses can be dynamically involved in the design of interventions that alter the precursors of poor health.

Recognition of the gravity and pervasiveness of environmental hazards can be overwhelming. Looking beyond the individual to recognize the environmental determinants of illness and wellness can be complicated and threatening. Intervening to improve the quality of air, water, housing, food, and waste disposal and reducing the risks of occupational injury and radiation require basic social, economic, and political changes. Nurses must be aware of their ability to bring about changes in health-damaging environments.

For example, one nurse recently recognized this fact and challenged others to concern themselves with the health care industry's impact on the environment (Trossman, 2004). Fewer people will develop cancer associated with dioxin release into the environment when polyvinyl supplies, including IV bags, are no longer manufactured or incinerated. The elimination of products that contain mercury (sphygmomanometers, thermometers, and fluorescent lighting) could help prevent exposure of pregnant women and, in turn, neurologic defects in thousands of children annually. Money saved on disposing of these hazardous materials could be put to other uses.

Throughout this chapter, clinical examples illustrate how environmental health problems affect the everyday lives of aggregates. The term **aggregate** refers to a group that shares a common aspect, such as age, gender, race, economic status, cultural perspective, chronic illness, or area of residence. Aggregates may be a community in which the members know and interact with each other, such as a barrio neighborhood or a labor union. Aggregates may also be "theoretically defined" categories of individuals who may or may not interact regularly with others in the defined group, such as "crack cocaine users," "women with physical disabilities," or "men over the age of 65."

Two other terms used frequently throughout this chapter are environment and health. **Environment** is the accumulation of physical, social, cultural, economic, and political conditions that influence the lives of communities. The community's health depends on the integrity of the physical environment, the humaneness of the social relations in the environment, the availability of resources necessary to sustain life and manage illness, the equitable distribution of health risks, attainable employment and education, cultural preservation and tolerance of diversity among subgroups, access to historical heritage, and a sense of empowerment and hope.

A CRITICAL THEORY APPROACH TO ENVIRONMENTAL HEALTH

Critical theory suggests that community health nurses must be aware of environmental obstructions that affect the safety and well-being of particular aggregates or deprive them of access to resources necessary in the pursuit for health. Essentially, this is questioning what appears to be "given" in the environment and challenging "the way things have always been done." Public buildings, schools, workplaces, and mass transportation systems are environmental structures that are vital to people's everyday functioning. Ordinarily, society takes these systems and structures for granted, ignoring or overlooking potentially harmful environmental situations.

For example, the experiences of agricultural workers exposed to pesticides bring into question what society takes for granted about the environment. A recent study determined that farm workers and pesticide applicators who accumulate agricultural chemicals on their skin and clothing take these substances home with them, increasing their children's exposure to toxicants (Thompson et al., 2003). Nurses must provide answers to farm workers who ask questions such as What do I do if I'm exposed to a pesticide? How long should I wait until after a pesticide application to go back into the field? How do I find out how toxic a certain pesticide is? Where can I get information on a specific pesticide? In addition, nurses must advocate for pesticide legislation that will help protect the health of agricultural workers, as well as the safety of the food chain.

According to *Healthy People 2010* (U.S. Department of Health and Human Services [USDHHS], 2000), of the worldwide preventable illnesses, 25% are caused by poor environmental quality. Indeed, it is estimated that air pollution contributes to 50,000 premature deaths annually in the United States. The data suggest nurses need to ask critical questions about their clients' work and home environments to help discern the contributions of specific hazards to their health. This can be accomplished by taking an environmental health history. An environmental health history can benefit the client in the following ways:

- Increase awareness of environmental/occupational factors
- Improve timelines and accuracy of diagnosis
- Prevent disease and aggravation of conditions
- Identify potential work-related environmental hazards, and/or environmental hazards in and around clients' homes

Environmental health histories should be obtained on both adults and children, although the relationship between the environment and children's health is frequently overlooked (National Environmental Education & Training Foundation [NEETF], 2002). Also, although frequently overlooked, a parent's occupational exposures may put the child at risk for particular health problems.

The following are some suggestions for environmental health screenings (NEETF, 2002).

Adults

- What kind of work do you do? How long on the job? Types of work exposures?

- Do you notice health problems you are having while you are at work? At home? In the community? In a specific location?
- What is the age of your home? Characteristics of heating and ventilation? Do you live near an industrial site or landfill?
- Have you recently used pesticides, solvents, insecticides, or weed killers?
- What kinds of hobbies do you have?
- Has your workplace been treated recently for insects, weeds, or other pest problems?

Children (Parents or Guardian)

- Where does your child go to school, day care, playgrounds?
- Have any of these places been treated recently (e.g., sprayed) for insects, weeds, or other pest problems?
- Does your child help with gardening activities?
- What are sources of food, water (e.g., well water)? Is someone in the household breast-feeding an infant?
- Do parents have any occupational exposure to potential health threats (e.g., lead, pesticides, x-rays)?

According to Bent (2003), when looking at the community through a critical lens, nurses have the opportunity to promote "community-based" and "community-focused health." (p. 224). In identifying environmental sources of health problems, nurses must be involved with the affected communities. Rather than impose their views of the problem, nurses should share their ideas and dialogue with community members. For example, nurses should listen to what the community believes is problematic, help raise consciousness about environmental dangers, and help bring about change (Bent, 2003; Clark et al., 2002). If nurses become involved in conducting community assessments and analyses, they can learn how the community members perceive themselves, their health, and their environmental influences.

The ultimate goal of the critical practice of community health nursing is liberating people from health-damaging environmental conditions (Bent, 2003). From a critical standpoint, helping communities become more aware of the environmental effects on health and helping them make needed changes in their environment are legitimate nursing actions. Collective actions have been instrumental in accomplishing positive environmental changes since the 1980s. Some of the mechanisms have included strategic organization, litigation, public hearing testimony, letter-writing campaigns, legislative lobbying, and mass demonstrations. Currently, organizing, informing, and fund-raising for environmental causes is also done via the Internet. The immediate online donations from private individuals in the United States and elsewhere in response to the December 2004 Southeast Asia tsunami facilitated rapid availability of resources for minimizing loss of life and restoring basic necessities, such as clean water and shelter. Public response to "acute" environmental disasters needs to be extended to an ongoing, consistent pressure to ensure day-to-day environmental integrity; hence, "chronic" environmental problems need to be addressed more effectively.

A critical perspective can help nurses plan and implement aggregate-level interventions because it emphasizes collective

TABLE 13-1 Areas of Environmental Health

AREA	DEFINITION
Living patterns	Living patterns are the relationships among people, communities, and their surrounding environments that depend on habits, interpersonal ties, cultural values, and customs.
Work risks	Work risks include the quality of the employment environment and the potential for injury or illness posed by working conditions.
Atmospheric quality	Atmospheric quality refers to the protectiveness of the atmospheric layers, the risks of severe weather, and the purity of the air for breathing purposes.
Water quality	Water quality refers to the availability and volume of the water supply and the mineral content levels, pollution by toxic chemicals, and the presence of pathogenic microorganisms. Water quality consists of the balance between water contaminants and existing capabilities to purify water for human use and plant and wildlife sustenance.
Housing	Housing is an environmental health concern and refers to the availability, safety, structural strength, cleanliness, and location of shelter, including public facilities and family dwellings.
Food quality	Food quality refers to the availability, relative costs, variety, and safety of foods, and the health of animal and plant food sources.
Waste control	Waste control is the management of waste materials resulting from industrial and municipal processes, human consumption, and efforts to minimize waste production.
Radiation risks	Radiation risks are health dangers posed by the various forms of ionizing radiation relative to barriers preventing exposure of humans and other life forms.
Violence risks	The environmental risks of violence include the potential for victimization through the violence of particular individuals and the general level of aggression in psychosocial climates.

strategies for change. Acting collectively can empower nurses to impact environmental health. Assessing environmental health problems, planning and implementing interventions, and evaluating the effectiveness of community-based actions need to be based on a wide lens. Community health nurses should be familiar with physical surroundings and their mutual interaction with cultural realities, social relations, economic circumstances, and political conditions on communities, applying a critical perspective to community health.

AREAS OF ENVIRONMENTAL HEALTH

Environmental health hazards are ubiquitous in communities across the United States and place adults and children at risk for disease or injury. This chapter divides the vast field of environmental health into the following subcategories: living patterns, work risks, atmospheric quality, water quality, housing, food quality, waste control, and radiation risks (Alexander and Fairbridge, 1999; Kemp, 1998; Moore, 1999, USDHHS, 2000) (Table 13-1). The brief discussions of these areas are only introductions to environmental health and, as such, focus on basic problems and strategies to address them. The following sections define these eight areas of environmental health, provide clinical examples of problems relevant to each category, and describe the community health nursing responses to the environmental health concerns. Table 13-2 provides examples of health problems within each area.

It should be noted that a critical perspective does not separate the idea of a safe social environment from a safe physical environment. For example, interpersonal violence is a significant and growing risk, with consequences ranging from bodily injury to psychiatric aftereffects that may last for decades in some individuals. There are intergenerational patterns of abuse, hate crimes toward marginalized groups, sexual predators, and hazards of combat that might be considered from an environmental health perspective. There are also occupational hazards of sexual harassment, racial discrimination, and workplace distresses that have resulted

TABLE 13-2 Examples of Environmental Health Problems

AREA	PROBLEMS
Living patterns	Drunk driving
	Secondhand smoke
	Noise exposure
	Urban crowding
	Technological hazards
Work risks	Occupational toxic poisoning
	Machine-operating hazards
	Sexual harassment
	Repetitive motion injuries
	Carcinogenic worksites
Atmospheric quality	Gaseous pollutants
	Greenhouse effect
	Destruction of the ozone layer
	Aerial spraying of herbicides and pesticides
	Acid rain
Water quality	Contamination of drinking supply by human waste
	Oil spills in the world's waterways
	Pesticide or herbicide infiltration of groundwater
	Aquifer contamination by industrial pollutants
	Heavy metal poisoning of fish
Housing	Homelessness
	Rodent and insect infestation
	Poisoning from lead-based paint
	Sick building syndrome
	Unsafe neighborhoods
Food quality	Malnutrition
	Bacterial food poisoning
	Food adulteration
	Disrupted food chains by ecosystem destruction
	Carcinogenic chemical food additives
Waste control	Use of non-biodegradable plastics
	Poorly designed solid waste dumps
	Inadequate sewage systems
	Transport and storage of hazardous waste
	Illegal industrial dumping
Radiation risks	Nuclear facility emissions
	Radioactive hazardous wastes
	Radon gas seepage in homes and schools
	Nuclear testing
	Excessive exposure to x-rays

Examples of Environmental Health Issues Affecting Communities

Construction of new interstate bypass to relieve traffic congestion due to urban sprawl.

Motor vehicle emissions (primary mobile source of air pollutants).

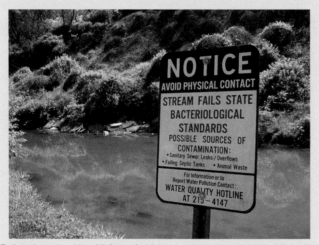

Polluted creek within 25 feet of children's urban playground in Knoxville, Tennessee.

Biological processing stage of wastewater treatment plant.

Land application of biosolids as part of a "sustainable" waste management program.

in shooting sprees. Issues of violence are discussed in more depth in Chapter 25.

Finally, we must be prepared for the public health effects of terrorism. Terrorism is a word that evokes many images and a range of reactions from rage to grief and loss. Acts of terrorism have drawn the public and political focus to establishing environmental security. Bioterrorism and homeland security are new areas where nurses will have an impact. A critical perspective is needed now more than ever, as security issues are linked to religious imperatives, moral stances, values, profit motives, health care systems and information, and cultural differences. These issues are also clearly in the scope of community health nursing and are discussed in more detail in Chapter 26.

Living Patterns

Living patterns are the relationships among people, communities, and their surrounding environments that depend on habits, interpersonal ties, cultural values, and customs. Most people live within areas that require almost daily contact with potential health risks and threats. These include intoxicated or impaired drivers, secondhand smoke, urban crowding, noise exposure, unabated traffic, and the stress of increased mechanization (Environmental Protection Agency [EPA], 2002; Frumkin, 2002; Harper and Lambert, 1994).

Urban sprawl is an emerging issue and an example of a living pattern that is of increasing concern. Urban sprawl has been defined as the conversion of land to non-agricultural or non-natural uses at a faster rate than the population growth (EPA, 2002). The sprawling development often occurs more rapidly than the expansion of the infrastructure (e.g., schools, sewer systems, water lines) needed for support. Typically, the desire to own one's vehicle, coupled with inadequate public mass transportation systems, contributes to a greater dependence on the automobile. This results in high volumes of traffic and a constant need to build more highways. Consequences of sprawl include air and water pollution, floods, infrastructure expenses, and a decrease in natural areas and forests (EPA, 2002; Frumkin, 2002) (see illustration depicting urban sprawl).

Living patterns reflect an individual's lifestyle choices (e.g., tobacco use, eating a diet rich in saturated fats, leading a sedentary lifestyle, becoming emotionally distressed while living with a substance abuser). Living patterns also contribute to population exposure to environmental conditions affected by mass culture, media, social policy, ethnic customs, and technology (Eckersley, 1992; Lawrence, 1999).

CLINICAL EXAMPLE

In an urban Chinese-American community, the economic aftershocks of a major earthquake caused the closure of a number of businesses. Some of these family businesses moved to parts of the city less characterized by the use of Chinese languages. These moves caused many elderly, non–English-speaking family members to experience depression, characterized by loss of appetite.

The community health nurses in the area began visiting these elders and brought interpreters with them. In their assessments, the nurses focused on psychiatric symptoms and suggested ventilation of emotions. They encouraged the Chinese elders to attend a local senior center staffed and attended mostly by European Americans. In some cases, they recommended psychiatric evaluations. In almost every instance, the elderly Chinese resisted these interventions.

The nurses failed to establish an alliance with the very strong Chinese family organizations before imposing their solutions. They also neglected to investigate Chinese cultural patterns before attempting to assist them with the life pattern ramifications of the earthquake. Generally, Chinese people do not readily talk about feelings with outsiders, and they do not conceptualize distress in psychiatric terms. They interpret the presence of fatigue and disturbances in eating and sleeping patterns as physical illness. They expect health care personnel to recognize and help them with these physical symptoms. The suggestion that socializing in centers populated by English speakers would cure their illness seemed quite incredulous to the families. ∎

One unfortunately common problem associated with living patterns relates to residing near hazardous facilities (e.g., waste incinerators, sewage treatment plants, landfills, refineries, and some correctional facilities). Discriminatory land use ensures that many impoverished and marginalized groups, especially people of color, live in close proximity to industrial contamination. This is called **environmental racism** (Northridge et al., 2003; Robinson, 2000; Williams and Collins, 2001). People who live near such environmental hazards are in danger of becoming victims of illness and injury related to violence, poisonings and exposures, fires, suicides, and malignant and non-malignant disease.

Many communities lack sufficient resources to respond when urban development and technological advances jeopardize the health and well-being of families in affected areas. The environmental movement of the 1960s and 1970s succeeded in building political power capable of passing monumental environmental reforms; however, charges that poor and minority communities are dumping grounds for environmental hazards have been substantiated by governmental agencies (EPA, 2005; Robinson, 2000).

Difficulties in alerting state and federal officials about environmental health dangers and difficulties in obtaining compensation for environmental toxin-causing disease and death often result in resident revictimization. Tightly knit social structures in the affected community and a lack of low-cost housing in other neighborhoods may hinder residents from leaving an area that poses potentially severe health risks from exposure to hazards. Residents may be unwilling to disrupt family ties and cultural roots to start over elsewhere, or they may be unable to afford a move. These residents may live with uncertainty and conflict. Long-term, community-wide effects of division, animosity, distrust, cynicism, and despair can abound in these situations.

In the 1990s, the central issues of equity and justice emerged in environmental health policy. In 1994, President Clinton signed Executive Order 12898, which required all federal agencies to develop comprehensive strategies for achieving **environmental justice.** Both the EPA and the National Institutes of Health responded with increased staffing and research funds to meet the needs of environmentally degraded communities (Northridge and Shepard, 1997). This legislation has served to increase public participation and

BOX 13-1 Landmark Federal Environmental Legislation

Year	Legislation
1970	Clean Air Act
	Poison Prevention Packaging Act
	Occupational Health and Safety Act
	Hazardous Materials Transportation Control
	National Environmental Policy Act
1971	Lead-Based Paint Poisoning Prevention Act
1972	Federal Water Pollution Control Act Amendments
	Noise Control Act
1976	Resource Conservation and Recovery Act
	Toxic Substances Control Act
1977	Clean Water Act
1980	Low Level Radiation Waste Policy Act
	Comprehensive Environmental Response, Compensation, and Liability Act (i.e., Superfund)

access to information, as well as provision of education about multiple risks and cumulative exposures (EPA, 2005) (Box 13-1). Much remains to be done, however, to attain environmental justice in the United States.

Work Risks

Work risks include poor employment environments and potential injury or illness due to working conditions. Environmental health problems posed by work risks include such issues as sexual harassment, occupational toxic poisoning, machine-operation hazards (e.g., falls, crushing injuries, burns), electrical hazards, repetitive motion injuries, carcinogenic particulate inhalation (e.g., of asbestos, coal dust), and heavy metal poisoning (Centers for Disease Control and Prevention [CDC], 2005d; Cralley, Cralley, and Cooper, 1990; Kaila, 2002; Le Moual, Kennedy, and Kauffmann, 2004). Prevention of work-related health problems requires integrated action to improve job safety and the working environment.

Worldwide, it is estimated that job-related accidents and illnesses claim more than 2 million lives annually, and this number appears to be rising because of industrialization in developing countries (World Health Organization [WHO], 2005b). In 2003, there were 4,365,200 recorded cases of non-fatal illnesses and injuries in the United States (US Department of Labor, Bureau of Labor Statistics, 2005). In that year, there were approximately 5,559 occupational fatalities; fishing, mining, construction, and agriculture have the highest rates of work-related deaths (CDC, 2005d).

These statistics do not reflect unreported health problems. For example, a clerical worker leaves the office every day with back strain and a headache because of ventilation problems in the building. After 5 years on a repetitive hand-movement job task, an employee develops carpal tunnel syndrome. An operating room nurse has a miscarriage and recalls that many of her coworkers have also been unable to carry their babies to term. A dry cleaner often leaves work feeling light-headed and dizzy from inhaling solvents at the shop, and one day she has a car accident on her way home. As a result,

collective problems related to employment or occupation are often perceived as individualized injuries, and no one "connects the dots."

CLINICAL EXAMPLE

Sanitation workers in an urban area experienced an increasing incidence of puncture injuries while transporting hazardous wastes from the public medical center; these puncture injuries caused several hepatitis cases. When the story became public, members of the city health commission contacted community health nurses and instructed them to politically support the interests of the city and the medical center "at all costs." Subsequently, the sanitation workers' union contacted the community health nursing office and requested information about procedures for safely packaging medical wastes. They also requested that a nurse speak to their membership about immediate measures for preventing further injuries on the job.

The nurses met to resolve the conflict. Most agreed that the union membership had pressing needs for education and support. Despite the city's demand for loyalty, they decided to "choose sides" with the workers and respond to their requests. They collectively drafted a letter to the city health commission and arranged a meeting with the commissioners to discuss their plan to assist the sanitation workers. The health commission held a press conference, which depicted the nurses' actions as mediational efforts that benefited the union and the city. Eventually, the nurses and the commission developed a new medical waste disposal plan, and injured workers received reasonable compensation through an out-of-court settlement. ■

Atmospheric Quality

Atmospheric quality refers to the amount of protection in the atmospheric layers, the risks of severe weather, and the purity of the air. Environmental dangers related to atmospheric quality include nitrogen dioxide, lead, particulate matter, and sulfur dioxide emitted from power plants, as well as motor vehicle emissions, by-products of industrial processes, and waste incinerators (Table 13-3). Tornadoes, electrical storms, smog, gaseous pollutants (e.g., carbon monoxide), excessive hydrocarbon levels, aerial herbicide spraying, and acid rain all contribute to air pollution. In addition, mercury, a potent neurotoxin released into the air from coal-fired power plants and waste incinerators, has resulted in fish consumption advisories in 45 states (EPA, 2003).

Two significant issues related to atmospheric quality are of global concern. First, the amount of protection in the atmospheric layers is diminishing (EPA, 2004; Last, 1993). Chemicals such as chlorofluorocarbons, halons, and carbon tetrachloride, which have been in widespread use for refrigeration, air conditioning, and aerosol propellants, remain in the atmosphere. These molecules cause depletion of the atmosphere's protective ozone layer. The resulting "holes" in the ozone layer allow excess ultraviolet radiation to penetrate, which cause harmful effects on many organisms. Long-term problems include increases in skin cancer and cataracts, suppression of immune response, and environmental damage.

Second, there is a disruption in the key processes that break down atmospheric carbon dioxide. The ongoing devegetation of the earth's surface, especially cutting the tropical rain forests, not only releases the carbon stored in the biomass,

TABLE 13-3 Major Air Pollutants

POLLUTANT	SOURCES	EFFECTS
Ozone: A colorless gas that is the major constituent of smog at the earth's surface.	Ozone is formed in the lower atmosphere as the result of chemical reactions between oxygen, volatile organic compounds, and nitrogen oxides in the presence of sunlight, particularly during hot weather. Sources of this harmful pollutant include vehicles, factories, landfills, lawn equipment, farm equipment, and industrial solvents.	Ozone can irritate the respiratory tract, produce impaired lung function, and cause throat irritation, chest pain, cough, and susceptibility to lung infection. Individuals with asthma and other existing respiratory conditions are particularly vulnerable. Ozone can also reduce agricultural yields and injure forests and other vegetation.
Carbon monoxide: A colorless and odorless gas that is emitted in the exhaust of motor vehicles and other kinds of engines during combustion of fossil fuels.	Carbon monoxide is emitted from cars, buses, trucks, and other small engines and from some industrial processes. High concentrations can be found in confined spaces (e.g., parking garages, poorly ventilated tunnels, or along roadsides during periods of heavy traffic).	Carbon monoxide reduces the ability of the blood to deliver oxygen to vital tissues, affecting primarily the cardiovascular and nervous systems. Lower concentrations have been shown to adversely affect individuals with heart disease and to affect exercise performance. Higher concentrations can cause symptoms such as dizziness, headaches, and fatigue.
Nitrogen dioxide: A light brown gas at lower concentrations; in higher concentrations, a significant component of brown urban haze.	Nitrogen dioxide forms from the burning of fuels in utilities, industrial boilers, cars, and trucks.	Nitrogen dioxide is a major component of smog and acid rain. When concentrations are high, it can harm cause increased respiratory illnesses (e.g., chest colds and coughing) in children. For asthmatics, it may cause increased breathing difficulty.
Sulfur dioxide: A colorless gas, odorless at low concentrations but pungent at very high concentrations.	Sulfur dioxide is emitted from industrial, institutional, utility, and apartment-house furnaces and boilers, as well as petroleum refineries, smelters, paper mills, and chemical plants.	Sulfur dioxide is one of the major components of smog. At high concentrations, it can harm humans; asthmatics are particularly vulnerable. It can also harm vegetation and metals and acidify lakes and streams
Particulate matter: Droplets from smoke, dust, ash, and condensing vapors that can be suspended in the air for long periods of time.	Particulates are emitted from industrial processes, vehicles, wood smoke, dust from paved and unpaved roads, construction, and agriculture.	Particulates can affect breathing and elicit respiratory symptoms, causing increased respiratory disease and lung damage. Children, elders, and people with heart or lung disease are especially at risk. They can also damage paint, soil, and clothing and reduce visibility.
Lead: A metal found in nature as well as a by-product of industry; can contaminate substances (e.g., soil, dust) that can be directly inhaled.	Metals processing is the major source of lead emissions into the air today. Lead is generally found near lead smelters, waste incinerators, utilities, and lead-acid battery manufacturers.	Lead can adversely affect mental development and performance, kidney function, and blood chemistry. Young children are particularly at risk to its effects.

From Environmental Protection Agency: *What are the six common air pollutants?* Last updated April 7, 2006, http://www.epa.gov/air/urbanair/6poll.html.

but it also eliminates sources of photosynthesis (i.e., the process by which plants absorb carbon and release oxygen) (Barnes et al., 1998; Bergstrom and Kirchmann, 1998). The loss of carbon dioxide–consuming resources increases carbon dioxide and traps part of the heat reemitted by the earth. As a result, the earth's surface temperature is increasing (i.e., the "greenhouse effect"), causing potentially catastrophic ecological consequences (Tchounwou, 1999). Scientists predict that by the year 2010, significant regional climate changes will have occurred, causing sea levels to rise and, in turn, causing serious coastal wetland loss (Patz and Khaliq, 2002; Raymo et al., 1998).

Severe weather conditions, another aspect of atmospheric quality that affects the public's health, can have dramatic results in the form of injury and loss of life, destruction of plants and wildlife, and property damage (Burns, 2002; Patz and Khaliq, 2002). Climatic changes associated with global warming may contribute to increasing the frequency and severity of the earth's weather extremes. Climatic disruption may be implicated in global geophysical destabilization, exemplified by earthquakes and tsunami effects.

Ground-level ozone, the primary component of smog, is the most common outdoor air pollutant in the United States (Physicians for Social Responsibility, 2001). Ozone is formed when nitrogen oxides (created by the burning of fossil fuels in power plants, automobiles, and industry) react with oxygen and sunlight (American Academy of Pediatrics, 2004). Ozone, along with other hazardous atmospheric pollutants cause and/or contribute to asthma, allergic reactions, bronchitis, lung cancer, chronic respiratory disease and death, and harms animal and plant species (Kleinman, 2000; National Toxic Inhalation Study Group, 1998). Further, sulfur dioxide, a by-product of burning coal and other fossil fuels, contributes to acid rain, which affects terrestrial ecosystems by increasing soil acidity, reducing nutrient availability, mobilizing toxic metals, leaching soil chemicals, and altering species composition (Foster, 1994).

CLINICAL EXAMPLE

A sudden increase occurred in the number of emergency calls from residents of a particular urban neighborhood to a medical hotline. These calls often involved elderly women who collapsed in their homes. In one case, an asthmatic child developed severe dyspnea.

The emergency calls continued, and two community health nurses noted that respiratory difficulties were often implicated. These nurses decided to visit the neighborhood and investigate. It was near rush hour and, within minutes, the traffic on the nearby freeway slowed to a crawl, apparently from road construction. Through their direct observations and critical assessment, these nurses determined that heavy car exhaust fumes seemed to stagnate around several residential buildings in the area. The nurses notified the Environmental Protection Agency and the city transportation department and recommended further investigation and resolution of the problem.

One week later, the nurses returned to the neighborhood and observed that the traffic moved more efficiently, although road construction continued. Within several weeks, the number of emergency medical calls decreased. ■

Water Quality

Water quality refers to the water supply's availability, volume, mineral content levels, toxic chemical pollution, and pathogenic microorganism levels. Water quality consists of the balance between water contaminants and the existing capabilities to purify water for human use and plant and wildlife sustenance. Water quality problems include experiencing droughts, dosing reservoirs with chemicals to reduce algae, contaminating aquifers with pesticides and fertilizers, leaching lead from water pipes, and oil spilling from transport tankers or leaking offshore wells. Other sources of water pollution are microbial contamination from poorly managed or maintained septic or sewage systems and animal feed lot wastes (Hamilton, Miller, and Myers, 2004; Schuurmann and Markert, 1998). Water pollution can be from point sources (a well-defined source, e.g., factory wastewater discharge) or non-point sources (urban runoff, domestic lawn care, and air-to-water transfer) (see illustration depicting water pollution).

Advances in water treatment technologies in industrialized countries have controlled many water-related diseases such as cholera, typhoid, dysentery, and hepatitis A. Despite this, disease outbreaks resulting from contamination by untreated groundwater and inadequate chlorination are increasing in both urban and rural areas (EPA, 2003; Gelberg et al., 1999). In addition, approximately 42 million Americans obtain their drinking water from private water supplies (e.g., wells) that have no treatment or monitoring guidelines (EPA, 2003).

Other potential water contaminants include accelerated soil erosion caused by construction, agriculture, and deforestation; these can contribute to high sediment levels in drinking water supplies. This necessitates higher levels of water treatment to remove heavy metals and chemicals. Heavy metal and toxic chemical pollution may also occur during the water treatment process or in the drinking water distribution system. In addition, the major disinfectant process, chlorination of water with high natural organic content (e.g., fulvic and humic acids emitted from decomposing animal and plant materials in the water) creates the formation of trihalomethane compounds that have been associated with a variety of adverse health effects. These include rectal and bladder cancer, shortened menstrual cycles, spontaneous abortion, small fetal size for gestational age, and birth defects (Bove, Shim, and Zeitz, 2002; Etzel, 2003; Hwang, Cash, and Zabik, 2002). Fortunately, the EPA has imposed regulations that limit the maximum allowable concentration of trihalomethanes in drinking water.

Pesticides, herbicides, and carcinogenic industrial waste infiltrate an increasing amount of groundwater, the underground source of half the U.S. population's drinking water (Sutherland, 1998). This is particularly tragic because groundwater is uniquely susceptible to long-term contamination. Unlike river or lake water, once groundwater becomes contaminated, it is impossible to cleanse.

CLINICAL EXAMPLE

In a midwestern farm community, there is growing concern about agricultural pesticide and herbicide seepage into groundwater. Families obtain water from their own wells rather than a central municipal source. The families recognized the long-range carcinogenic effects of the chemicals involved. Although family farmers decreased their use of these chemicals, the large-scale agribusiness companies continued to use excessive amounts of these chemicals.

County community health nurses lobbied local officials to begin a comprehensive program to monitor groundwater pollutants and enforce standards for herbicide and pesticide use; however, the powerful agribusiness companies pressured these officials to stand back. Together, some county farmers and nurses organized grassroots information and support groups among rural families. The families and nurses, in coalition with environmental activist groups in the state, established several participatory action research projects. These projects included collecting and testing samples from each family well, forming a local umbrella organization called "Water Watch" to coordinate actions and communications, involving a research project with a federal health agency to track the health problems of local residents who used these water sources on a long-term basis. The organization also disseminated an emergency plan for drinking water distribution if wells were found to have toxic levels of pesticides, herbicides, or other pollutants. ■

Housing

Housing is an environmental health concern and it refers to the availability, safety, cleanliness, and location of shelter, including public facilities and individual or family dwellings. According to *Healthy People 2010,* four of the major environmental health problems related to housing are elevated indoor allergen levels, radon poisoning, lead-based paint poisoning, and exposure to tobacco smoke (USDHHS, 2000).

Other environmental health problems related to housing include fire hazards; lack of access for disabled people; illnesses caused by overcrowding, dampness, and rodent or insect infestation; psychological effects of architectural design (e.g., low-cost, high-rise housing projects); injuries sustained from collapsed building structures; and exposure deaths from inadequate indoor heating or cooling.

Poor housing conditions can contribute to the spread infectious disease (EPA, 2003) and as well as cardiovascular and respiratory disorders, cancers, allergies, and mental illnesses (Lemus et al., 1998; Mariethoz et al., 1999). The term **sick building syndrome** describes a phenomenon in which public structures and homes cause occupants to experience a variety of symptoms, such as headache, fatigue, and exacerbation of allergies. This typically results from poor ventilation and building operations, hazardous building materials, furniture and carpeting substances, and cleaning agents (EPA, 2003).

Other problems may arise related to building structures, composition, and settings. For example, commercial buildings with offices near underground parking garages may cause workers to suffer carbon monoxide intoxication. Formaldehyde, asbestos, and volatile organic compounds which are common components of thermal insulation, cement, flooring, furnishings, and household consumer products—have carcinogenic properties. Additionally, "toxic mold" arising from chronically damp wood and improperly sealed areas in homes and offices has recently been recognized as contributing to respiratory irritation, allergies, and infections in susceptible individuals (Chapman et al., 2003).

Much controversy surrounds the economic hardship that industry, government, business, and multidwelling owners would face if they were forced to reduce concentrations of such toxic elements. Enforcement of mandatory toxic abatement, however, will ensure a safer future and exemplify community-level response to environmental health risks. For example, Massachusetts has a policy that requires lead paint abatement of children's homes and holds property owners liable for lead paint poisoning. This environmental management effort has been successful and has significantly reduced blood lead levels among the state's children (CDC, 2005b; Sargent et al., 1999).

CLINICAL EXAMPLE

In a large, northeastern U.S. city, an economic recession led to massive unemployment, rising housing costs, and drastically reduced housing subsidies. Simultaneously, funding was cut for several public health and mental health facilities. The result left approximately 4000 people "houseless." The local shelters housed a total of 500 people each night, but none of these shelters accepted women. Over a dozen people died from exposure to the elements during the winter.

Community health nurses met with local church groups who started a shelter for women. This coalition acquired a building in an area where many shelterless people congregated. They offered accommodations for 75 women. After 3 months, the city took over the women's shelter because the churches experienced difficulties filling the beds and maintaining the project's financial solvency. The city changed the shelter to a dwelling for 50 men and 25 women because women did not use it sufficiently.

In their evaluation, the nurses consulted with several shelterless women and workers from a popular soup kitchen. The answer was relatively simple. The women did not feel safe going to the shelter because the area had a high-crime reputation and lacked street lighting. Eventually, a new coalition formed, composed of community health nurses, several women who were or had been shelterless, a representative from the police force, and the church groups. A new women's shelter opened in a safer, well-lit neighborhood close to public transit lines. ■

Food Quality

Food quality refers to availability and relative cost of food, variety and safety of food, and the health of animal and plant food sources. Food quality problems include malnutrition, bacterial food poisoning, carcinogenic chemical additives

(e.g., nitrites, alar, and cyclamate), improper or fraudulent meat inspection or food labeling, microbial epidemics among livestock (e.g., cholera), food products from diseased animal sources, and disruption of vital natural food chains by ecosystem destruction. Further, increased mobility and globalized trade means that contaminants may rapidly be carried to distant destinations, through marketing, importing, and air travel.

Potential microbial contaminants of foods include bacteria (e.g., *Shigella coli, Salmonella, Escherichia coli [E. coli], Campylobacter*), parasites (e.g., *Balantidium coli, Cryptosporidium parvum, Entamoeba histolytica*), and viruses (e.g., Calicivirus, Rotavirus, hepatitis A virus, Enterovirus) (CDC, 2005c; Powell and Atwell, 1999). After increasing throughout the 1990s, the rates of food-borne illnesses are now declining. The biggest decline has been seen in *E. coli* 0157, most frequently identified in uncooked hamburger. The United States currently depends on the Foodborne Disease Active Surveillance Network (Foodnet) of CDC's Emerging Infections Program to collect data on diseases caused by enteric pathogens transmitted through food.

Agrichemicals, such as pesticides and fertilizers, materials from mechanical handling devices, detergents, and organic packaging materials can also contaminate food. Toxic chemicals from farming and ranching may be introduced into the food chain, increasing risk of reproductive and mutagenic effects in humans (EPA, 2004; Foster, 1994; Guillen, Sopelana, and Partearroyo, 1997). For instance, farmers spray dioxin-containing weed killers on rangeland. Beef cattle graze on the land, herbicide accumulates in their fatty tissue, and the contaminated meat is sold in markets. The complexity of transfer of these contaminants makes for difficulty in establishing causality and tracing accountability for these health risks.

Unsuitable handling, storage, processing, and transport techniques can damage food and make it unsuitable for consumption. Further, additives are often used to improve food properties. For example, vitamins and minerals are used to enhance nutritional content; salt, sugars, and monosodium glutamate are used to improve flavor; dyes are used to enhance color; leavening agents, gums, or thickening agents are used to improve consistency; and various preservatives are used to increase shelf life. Many of these additives are not nutritious, and some may be harmful. Additionally, residues from the overuse of antibiotics in animal husbandry remain in meat and milk products, causing consumers to develop resistance, thus rendering these antibiotics ineffective in treating human infections (Neu, 1992).

Another potential threat to food quality involves "genetically modified" (GM) or genetically engineered foods. Genetically modified foods have been in existence since the early 1970s and are created by a process in which scientists splice plant or animal genes with particular traits into the DNA of other organisms (Whitney, Maltby, and Carr, 2004). This technology has contributed to crops and livestock that grow faster, are more resistant to disease and insects, and produce higher yields and greater nutritive value; often GM crops require less water and fertilizer (Davies, 2003).

There is concern that genetic alteration of food is growing despite the fact that the long-term health effects of eating GM food are unknown. Some believe that allergies and other immunity problems may proliferate as unique antigens are present on GM proteins, and GM foods have unpredictable metabolic processes in animals, humans, and plants (Whitney et al., 2004). Indeed, animal studies suggest that developing infants and children may be particularly at risk for health problems caused by GM foods (Catani and Micera, 2001). Although the U.S. Department of Agriculture and the U.S. Food and Drug Administration set policy for foods produced from new plant varieties and breeding, a number of groups and organizations have called for increased public awareness on the dangers of genetically engineered foods and are working to require more stringent testing of them.

CLINICAL EXAMPLE

A southern U.S. town with a population of 10,000 has a large population of black farm workers and a smaller, but significant, number of white residents who work as textile workers. Located well off the interstate arteries, the town experienced very high food costs from shipping difficulties. Many families tapered their diets and ate mostly bread, rice, beans, and eggs. Health assessments of school-age children and toddlers indicated deficiencies of vitamins contained in fresh fruits and vegetables.

Local physicians, county health nurses, and the Parent-Teacher Association joined forces to improve the nutritional situation. The most popular proposed solution involved a community garden project. The groups leased land from the county, and the project began. Conflict arose when black community leaders realized that the mostly white textile workers formed their own garden project and competed with the original garden project for the town's support. Racial tensions intensified.

The nurses and parents originally involved in planning the project met to avert a crisis. They decided to focus on reaching church leaders and women in both black and white sectors of the town in the hope of supporting a dialogue and a just solution to the problem. Parents and church leaders spread the word in their respective communities. A community meeting was held at a convenient time for women in the town and at a neutral place that was acceptable to both groups.

Although tensions were strong enough to prevent the formation of a joint garden, the solution reached in the meeting caused each group to feel successful and to save face. On a per-capita basis, town funds were allocated to two gardening projects. The groups agreed that they would share vegetable and fruit yields equitably, depending on the yield from each site. In addition, the cooperative plan increased the total garden space allotted by 50% and began a gardening "tool library" so neither group had to purchase new tools. ■

Waste Control

Waste control is the management of waste materials resulting from industrial and municipal processes, human consumption, and efforts to minimize waste production. Environmental health problems related to waste control include non-biodegradable plastics, inefficient recycling programs, unlicensed waste dumps, inadequate sewage systems for increasing populations, unsafe dumping of industrial toxins, exportation of radioactive medical wastes, illicit dumping, and non-enforcement of environmental regulations.

American consumers' increasing trash production and the improper treatment, storage, transport, and disposal of waste are a significant concern (DeLong, 1993; National Research Council, 2002). Routinely, commercial and institutional wastes are dumped with household waste in the same municipal incinerator, landfill, or sewer system. These commercial enterprises are generally exempt from the strict waste regulation applied to industry, although they often generate the same hazardous materials. Small businesses such as dry cleaners, photography laboratories, pesticide formulators, construction sites, and car repair shops discard a variety of substances that can cause serious public health problems.

Traditionally, U.S. economic development has produced optimal wealth with the assumption that the environmental health consequences would be minor. This notion of sustainable development has proven inadequate, and cumulative hazardous episodes necessitate tough pollution control technologies. The sustainability paradigm has led to a shift from disposing to recycling of wastes reclaimed from sewage, called biosolids. Biosolids refer to sewage sludge that has been treated for pathogens to meet the regulatory requirements for land application. This has been a cost-effective practice, but more study needs to be conducted on human health risks of biosolid distribution in the ecosystem (see photo depicting waste disposal).

There are a number of potential health problems associated with waste management. For example, solid waste landfills accumulate methane gas, a by-product of decomposing organic wastes. Without proper venting, this volatile gas can move through soil and cause fires and explosions in nearby areas. Waste incineration is not the best solution because it causes particulate air pollution and is ineffective in the combustion of many materials. Improper design, operation, or waste site location causes hazardous substances to spread through air, soil, and water to poison humans, animals, and plant life. Alarmingly, only a percentage of hazardous waste actually reaches the designated waste sites; much is disposed of in open pits and in bodies of water, with dangerously uncertain long-term effects. New methods are only now being developed to estimate long-term rates of leaching of materials in various types of waste sites, based on probability principles (Sanchez and Kosson, 2005).

In 1980, Congress passed the Environmental Response Compensation and Liability Act, which established a revolving fund called the Superfund, to clean up several hundred of the worst abandoned chemical waste disposal sites. However, funds are insufficient, and improvements have been minor (Kilburn, 1999). One of the most notorious sites is the Love Canal in Niagara Falls, New York. For 40 years prior to the 1960s, more than 80 different types of chemicals including benzene, dioxin, trichloroethylene, toluene, and chloroform were dumped in an abandoned canal. Afterward, the covered area became the site for a school and several hundred homes. In the winters of 1976 and 1977, heavy snowfall and rain caused toxic wastes to reach the surface. Subsequently, the inhabitants experienced elevated miscarriage rates, blood and liver abnormalities, birth defects, and chromosome damage.

CLINICAL EXAMPLE

In a city on the Mississippi River, an outbreak of shigellosis was traced to a group of high school students who had been swimming in a particular area of the river. The local meat-packing plant was releasing waste material, including human and animal feces, directly into the river.

After intervening to contain the shigella outbreak, the local community health nurses began to assess the situation. Their research indicated that the meat-packing facility had been in violation of waste control laws for some time. City officials imposed fines, which the company paid, but the dumping continued. A sign at the riverside prohibited swimming. Frustrated by their attempts to negotiate with the city and the plant, the nurses wrote a letter to the state capital newspaper, which had a large state readership, and the local newspaper. In the letter, they voiced concern about the community's health and the river's ecological integrity. Both papers published their informative letter as a commentary, which prompted responses from two local environmental groups, several activist groups located downriver, and a national organization concerned with clean water. These groups provided legal support and brought a collective suit against the meat-packing company. Subsequently, the company improved its waste treatment process to avoid paying a large award in the civil suit. ■

Radiation Risks

Radiation risks are health dangers posed by various forms of ionizing radiation relative to barriers that prevent human exposure and other life form exposure. Radiation risks include nuclear power emissions, radioactive hazardous wastes, medical and dental radiographs, and wartime nuclear weapon dangers. According to WHO (2005c), the three primary sources and distribution of radiation exposure to the world's population are radon (43%), medical exposure (20%), and other non-natural sources (19%).

Manufactured sources of radiation contribute to humans' continuous exposure to ionizing radiation. Potential environmental radioactive pollution results from nuclear weapons testing, nuclear waste disposal, accidents at nuclear power plants, and the transportation, storage, loss, and misuse of radioactive sources (WHO, 2005c).

Nuclear industries can cause serious environmental problems. People and animals living near nuclear facilities such as power plants, waste storage sites, uranium-processing plants, nuclear weapons factories, and nuclear test sites have manifested increased rates of cancer, stroke, diabetes, cardiovascular and renal disease, immune system damage, premature aging, infertility, miscarriage, and birth defects (Harrison, Gustafson, and Dixon, 2003; International Physicians for the Prevention of Nuclear War, 1991). Further, there is the ever-present risk of nuclear accidents that release large amounts of radioactivity into surrounding areas.

In addition, nuclear wastes remain dangerously radioactive for thousands of years; a safe way to dispose of them does not exist. Interim collection centers currently stockpile much of the waste. There is a quandary not only about how, where, and when to dispose of newly generated nuclear wastes, but also about how to manage improperly disposed radioactive materials.

Millions of Americans are exposed to dangerous levels of radiation in the form of radon gas in their homes, schools, and workplaces (Platt, 1993). It is believed that radon contamination is the second leading cause of lung cancer mortality in the United States, contributing to an estimated 15,000 to 20,000 deaths from this disease each year (Alberg and Samet, 2003). Radon is a radioactive radium decay product that occurs naturally in certain kinds of phosphate- and uranium-containing rock, such as granite and black shale, and is associated with an increased risk of cancer. Radon may be present in building materials, drinking water, and soil. Radon gas diffuses into dwellings, mostly through soil, and is prevalent where uranium-bearing land is common. Radon seeps through basement walls, pipes, and cracks in the foundation and is trapped in buildings with inadequate ventilation.

Cumulative exposure to excessive or ill-performed radiographs can also cause radiation damage in the body (Alberg et al., 2003; Schleipman, 2005). People who work with medical sources of radiation, such as radium or radioactive iodine, are at increased risk for developing cancers and producing children with birth defects. Older x ray machines may emit excessive levels of radioactivity; all such equipment should undergo regular testing for leakage.

Finally, there is recent evidence of a new threat, as it has been noted that ammunition (bombs and bullets) made with depleted uranium was used in the Persian Gulf War (Salbu et al., 2005), and in Kosovo, and continues to be manufactured and used in Iraq and Afghanistan. Particulate contamination from the uranium has been discovered in Kosovo and Kuwait (Danesi et al., 2003). The long-term health consequences are purported to include teratogenic, immunological, and cancerous conditions, posing danger to both local populations and military personnel. Continued investigation is needed to identify long-term consequences of this practice.

CLINICAL EXAMPLE

During wartime, federal standards related to radioactive environmental contamination and the public's "right to know" are suspended for military projects. In the middle of the Persian Gulf War, information "leaked" about a military installation in the southwestern desert near Deserttown. The installation planned test explosions of several new nuclear bombs, which they called nuclear "devices."

Local townspeople expressed concern, but the military did not confirm or deny these plans. The possible dates for the tests were also unknown. Residents began to panic, and several families moved. Others built makeshift shelters and began stockpiling food. There was an increase in psychiatric hospitalization rates. The town reached a crisis when a spate of three related adolescent suicides occurred in 2 months. The entire community appeared disorganized, helpless, and hopeless.

Town officials organized town meetings. Public health nurses offered community education about the health effects of ionizing radiation and answered questions, but this did not raise resident morale. The nurses decided to contact other communities that faced similar threats to determine how they dealt with them.

When these communities received word about Deserttown, they organized a letter-writing campaign and a support demonstration. They converged on Deserttown for a weekend rally and celebration of solidarity. The youth of Deserttown extended this demonstration by performing weekly vigils at the military site. One year later, the community was more united and less depressed, and the adolescent suicide rate had decreased significantly. The nuclear threat remained. ■

EFFECTS OF ENVIRONMENTAL HAZARDS

Environmental hazards are ubiquitous, and their effect on the public's health is complex and generally interconnected (Jaga and Brosius, 1999; Lawrence, 1999). Nurses must understand the multiple and complex sequences leading to health disorders. For example, nuclear power plant emissions may contaminate water and air supplies, affecting water quality, atmospheric quality, and radiation risk. Overcrowded housing may exacerbate problems in managing human waste, which may taint foodstuffs and contribute to the spread of communicable disease.

Certain environmental exposures have been found to have a direct relationship to the development of some cancers, chronic diseases, and other health-related problems (Butterfield, 2002). For example, recent reports have shown that higher ozone levels exacerbate asthma attacks and link elevated ozone levels to increased hospital admissions and emergency room visits for asthma (Gent et al., 2003). Furthermore, oppressive environments may affect health directly. In one case, an American company dumped dangerous waste material in Mexico rather than pay for proper disposal (Schrieberg, 1991). Poor children who lived nearby and scavenged for food in the dump picked up and played with the shiny, brightly colored radioactive medical waste. The severe burns they suffered and the wine-colored spots on their skin were direct effects of the illegally dumped toxic waste.

Effects of environmental risks may also be indirect, such as in the case of global warming (Foster, 1994; Patz and Khaliq, 2002). It has been hypothesized that the sea level will eventually rise from the melting polar ice caps. The resulting coastal inundation and permanent flooding will threaten large areas of low-lying agricultural land and food supplies in many regions of the world. Rising global temperatures will enhance the quantity and distribution of parasites, insects, and other disease vectors, thus increasing the prevalence of a variety of infectious diseases.

Effects of environmental hazards may be general or specific. For example, the ramifications of massive unemployment, drought, and extensive smog cover affect the public generally, whereas the particular housing needs of elderly people who use walkers or canes, the occupational risks of electrical line repair workers, and the mentally incapacitating effects of elevated blood lead levels in children affect the public more specifically.

Environmental health effects can also be immediate, long term, or transgenerational. Burns, gunshot wounds, hurricane damage, and outbreaks of gastrointestinal distress among

ETHICAL Insights

Agent Orange

The controversial legacy of the Agent Orange defoliant (which contained dioxin) that was sprayed by the U.S. Army during the Vietnam War has caused pain for numerous citizens (past, present, and future). This toxic chemical killed many people in Vietnam, including civilians.

cafeteria customers are examples of immediate effects from health-damaging environments. Examples of long-term health effects include gradual occupational hearing loss, "black lung" in coal miners, and increased rates of cancer among farm workers who ingest pesticides from aerial spray (Jaga and Brosius, 1999). Transgenerational effects occur with female factory workers exposed to radiation at plutonium-processing plants. The radiation causes chromosomal anomalies, which results in birth defects.

Environmental exposures after the World Trade Center attack resulted in significant adverse health effects. The dust produced bronchial hyperactivity, persistent cough, and increased risk for asthma. Pregnant women who were inside or near the World Trade Center on September 11, 2001, bore small-for-gestational-age babies (likely related to exposures to polycyclic aromatic hydrocarbons and particulates). Further, scientists hypothesize that the future risk of mesothelioma may be increased, because of occupational exposure to asbestos (Landrigan et al., 2004).

Some negative environmental health effects may be reversible. Smokers who have quit demonstrate regeneration of cilia in the lungs after months to years, for example. Radiation damage to human cells and silicosis damage to lung capacity, however, are irreversible. Conversely, heavy metal exposure from many environmental hazards causes cumulative effects. Lead slowly collects in the long bones, and the lead can re-release into the body. This release may cause acute poisoning and additional damage over time (Needleman et al., 1992).

EFFORTS TO CONTROL ENVIRONMENTAL HEALTH PROBLEMS

The 1970s were the decade of environmental concern. Cynicism toward institutions grew during the years of U.S. involvement in Vietnam, and legislative activism for environmental preservation exploded (Burger, 1989). During the 1970s, Congress created new agencies to regulate environmental conditions on a national level, including the EPA, Occupational Safety and Health Administration, and the Nuclear Regulatory Commission. The EPA has enormous responsibilities for protecting the environment and minimizing risks to human health. Among its roles are health surveillance and monitoring; setting standards for air and water quality; evaluating environmental risks; acquiring information; screening new chemicals; performing basic research and training; and establishing, evaluating, and enforcing regulatory efforts.

The legislative activism of the 1970s was aimed toward a comprehensive national environmental policy. For example, stricter automobile fuel and emissions standards created improvements in air quality, which caused lead levels in urban air to decrease dramatically over the next decade (Bingham and Meader, 1990). The momentum to control environmental corruption in the United States slowed in the 1980s and 1990s with several policy reversals and the defunding of regulatory mechanisms. For instance, the Reagan administration's deregulation of industry weakened the Occupational Health and Safety Act. Through the 1990s, Congress was less attuned to environmental protection. Corporate industries launched publicity campaigns against stricter air-quality standards, regulated logging in old-world forests, and bans on marine dumping, claiming that environmentalists were a threat to local jobs and profits.

This trend has continued into the twenty-first century. For example, one piece of recent legislation regulating mercury pollution from power plants drew criticism from environmental advocates who noted that the rule was too weak. The Clean Air Mercury Rule is aimed at coal-fired power plants, which is the nation's largest remaining unregulated source of mercury emissions. According to the EPA, the rule will decrease mercury in two phases, eventually capping national mercury emissions at 15 tons by 2018 (down from about 48 tons). Environmental advocates argue that the EPA's mercury rule violates the 1900 Clean Air Act, ignores the science on mercury hazards, and allows industry to pollute beyond the 2018 deadline.

The EPA has limited some of its monitoring requirements, and this has resulted in compliance failures among some industries. For example, the widespread agricultural use of neurotoxic organophosphate pesticides continues even though they cause lasting central nervous system damage (Jaga and Brosius, 1999). Advocates for farm workers claim the EPA should ban pesticides registered in the highest toxicity category. Instead, the EPA requires that employers provide general pesticide safety information to all farm workers. The EPA also suggests regular blood tests to monitor toxin levels in those who apply the pesticides. Monitoring is required only for commercial applicators (i.e., companies that apply chemicals, not farm workers who apply pesticides in their job). Legislators and other policy makers have often made pesticide-use decisions based on economic impact on both chemical companies and large agricultural corporations.

Other laws and regulatory structures are weak or non-existent with regard to environmental health problems. For example, federal mandates for recycling do not exist, although local communities have made great strides in this area. Comprehensive groundwater legislation, similar to adopted measures to preserve marine and surface waters, also does not exist. In general, environmental laws have been too detailed or inflexible, causing problems in the articulation of federal and local regulatory efforts. Additionally, the EPA tends to set priorities for the reduction of environmental problems but does not allocate the resources necessary to accomplish these goals.

Most of the U.S. environmental health efforts have aimed for short-term results rather than anticipating future issues and problems. A crucial need exists in the development of human resources in the area of environmental health. Nurses in all areas of practice should be aware of the implications the environment has on their clients and their health. It is for this reason that nurses need to take and record an environmental health history on every client. The means of taking an environmental health history is discussed later in this chapter.

GLOBAL ENVIRONMENTAL HEALTH

Environmental health comprises those aspects of human health, including quality of life, that are determined by physical, chemical, biological, social, and psychosocial factors in the environment. It also refers to the theory and practice of assessing, correcting, controlling, and preventing those factors in the environment that can potentially affect adversely the health of present and future generations. (WHO, 2004)

Globalization and industrialization in the developing world have increased the number of health problems related to the environment. Urbanization has made it difficult to maintain clean air, clean water, and good sanitation practices. Consequently, humans are now exposed to serious amounts of environmental hazards (CDC, 2005d).

Large-scale hazards related to global environmental conditions include climate change, stratospheric ozone depletion, loss of biodiversity, degradation, stresses on food-producing systems, and changes in the hydrological systems and freshwater supplies. As corporations become global entities, many escape U.S. standards by moving operations to unregulated areas of the world. Global environmental health hazards cannot be fully outlined here, but it is incumbent on nursing as a profession to take a strong stance on global health at the international level.

EMERGING ILLNESSES RELATED TO THE ENVIRONMENT

The new science focusing on identifying and treating emerging illnesses recognizes the relationship between environmental change, human activities, disease, and public health. Emerging illness refers to newly identified diseases, as well as diseases that are establishing new niches in parts of the world where they previously were non-existent. Urban areas are susceptible to this phenomenon because they are densely populated and permit rapid entrance of microbes and contaminants from other countries due to the large number of seaports and airports (Center for Children's Health and the Environment, 2002).

For example, global climate change, along with international commerce and travel, contributed to the entry and propagation of the West Nile virus in the United States (Epstein, 2001). Increased air and water temperatures facilitate the spread of vector-borne diseases transmitted by mosquitoes (e.g., West Nile virus). As a result, in 2003, there were 9,862 reported cases of, and 264 related deaths from, West Nile virus in the United States (CDC, 2005a).

Similarly, a new coronavirus, severe acute respiratory syndrome (SARS), has recently been added to the list of environmental challenges for health professionals throughout

RESEARCH HIGHLIGHTS

I PREPARE: Development and Clinical Utility of an Environmental Exposure History Mnemonic

The I PREPARE environmental exposure history mnemonic is a quick reference tool created for primary care providers. A total of 159 health care providers, both students and professionals, were asked to evaluate a prototype mnemonic, to suggest new health history questions, and to propose the deletion of less relevant questions. The prototype was formatted as a pocket guide. The goal of this evaluation was to create a practical and clinically relevant mnemonic, rather than to obtain quantitative estimates of validity. This mnemonic serves as a mental cue to facilitate the collection and documentation of health information in a systematic manner.

I – Investigate Potential Exposures
P – Present Work
R – Residence
E – Environmental Concerns
P – Past Work

A – Activities
R – Referrals and Resources
E – Educate

Questions to ask are presented for each letter in the mnemonic, except for Referrals and Resources, which provides sources of additional information. A checklist of strategies to prevent or minimize exposures can be used by the health care provider to help clients identify potential exposures. The sequence of I PREPARE makes intuitive sense by cueing the provider to ask specific questions and provide educational materials to the client. The final version was reprinted on heavy laminated material. The I PREPARE mnemonic increases the repertoire of tools clinicians have available to elicit an appropriate health history. The national improvements in the quality of environmental exposure history are predicated, in part, on the creation of simple and convenient tools for use in clinical practice.

From Paranzino GK et al: I PREPARE: development and clinical utility of an environmental exposure history mnemonic, *AAOHN J* 53(1):37-42, 2005.

the world. This flulike disease swept through China and Southeast Asia before spreading to many parts of the world, including Canada and the United States, during the winter of 2002-2003 (Lovgren, 2003). International travel greatly contributed to the rapid spread of SARS, which epidemiologists have now identified as a global health threat.

Other Emerging Threats

It is a misconception that the United States is exempt from the environmental health hazards that less developed nations must endure. Within the past decade, we are beginning to recognize that our environmental public health infrastructure is quite weak and that the United States is susceptible to many of the same problems that burden the rest of the world. For example, the illegal use of pesticides, medical waste incineration, and the increased incidence of asthma related to air pollution are just a few of the challenges facing the United States today. The manufacturing of methamphetamine in home-based labs has risen dramatically in the past five years, and the "cooking process" emits dangerous levels of toxic chemicals into the air. Similarly, the abandoned labs also pose a threat.

Since September 11, 2001, U.S. citizens realize that our country is not safe from terrorist attack. Terrorist attacks can take many forms, some of which could include biological or chemical warfare or nuclear retaliation. Ongoing reports of actual attacks (e.g., the subway bombings in London during the summer of 2005) and threats of attacks promote recognition of personal vulnerability and the need to be aware and prepared.

There is also the threat of natural disasters that can disrupt and oftentimes overwhelm private and public health systems. Natural disasters, such as the tsunami that struck the coast of Indonesia in December 2004 and Hurricane Katrina in August, 2005, require mobilization of disaster relief units that offer substantial assistance and expertise. Natural disasters such as hurricanes, tornados, and earthquakes frequently receive notable publicity, but other, more insidious disasters such as droughts, floods, heat waves, and extreme cold also pose major public health concerns. The aforementioned threats can cause significant mortality and morbidity and, therefore, have the potential to burden the health care delivery system.

Nursing Actions

Nurses must work with the public to promote more stringent and actively enforced environmental legislation and regulations. In the twenty-first century, actions must include not only national but also worldwide environmental policies. Ozone depletion, global warming, fossil fuel burning, marine dumping, active land mine abandonment in war-torn areas, mass relocation of refugees across national borders, and destruction of tropical rain forests are among key global environmental health concerns.

In an era of globalization, nurses must support actions for biodiversity, including pushing back the deserts, replanting the forests, stabilizing the climate, and seeking alternative development pathways that do not destroy plant and animal species. The development of state-of-the-art methods for removing pollutants from the biosphere, managing ecosystems, handling hazardous wastes, and preserving oceans depends on the integration of scientific knowledge, complex sociopolitical processes, and values. In recognition of threats to the biosphere and exploitation of the world's ecosystems, environmental integrity will require international assistance, ameliorative actions, and an environmentally educated global public.

Environmental concerns for clean air, clean water, and freedom from noxious chemicals must become global nursing concerns. Community health nurses can be catalysts to neighborhood efforts to produce safe living environments. Community health nursing must expand its theory and practice to incorporate the fact that individual and community health ultimately depends on global environmental integrity. Countless organizations work to preserve and protect the environment and could benefit from the active involvement and support of nurses. Box 13-2 lists many of these organizations. Nursing must broaden its borders to include a global perspective. Global sustainability will be achieved through commitment to strong ethical principles and social justice and with initiatives for environmental responsibility in daily personal activity.

BOX 13-2 Environmental Organizations

- American Farmland Trust
- Animal Preservation League
- Citizens for a Better Environment
- Clean Water Action
- Earth Regeneration Society
- Forests Forever
- Greenpeace
- International Rivers Network
- National Environmental Law Center
- National Toxics Campaign
- Natural Resources Defense Council
- Ocean Alliance
- Pesticide Action Network
- Radioactive Wastes Campaign
- Rainforest Action Network
- Sierra Club
- Toxics Coordinating Project
- Trust for Public Land
- U.S. Public Interest Research Group
- Wilderness Society

Websites for these organizations can be accessed through the WebLinks section of the book's website at http://evolve.elsevier.com/Nies.

For further information, see the report by the Institute of Medicine Committee on Enhancing Environmental Health Content in Nursing Practice: *Nursing, health, and the environment*, Washington, DC, 1995, National Academies Press.

APPROACHING ENVIRONMENTAL HEALTH AT THE AGGREGATE LEVEL

In the United States, personal independence and individual responsibility for success and failure are valued. These values can lead nurses to overlook environmental hazards and instead blame individual clients for their health problems. By placing responsibility for the cause and cure of health problems exclusively on the individual, the belief is reinforced that all individuals are free to exert meaningful control over the quality and length of their lives. Such a perspective absolves society, government, industry, and business from accountability.

Research suggests that changing individual behaviors does not lead to significant reductions in overall morbidity and mortality in the absence of basic social, economic, and political changes (Milio, 1986). Emphasizing only interventions that address deleterious personal habits through exercise programs, weight-loss regimens, smoking-cessation classes, and stress-reduction tactics fails to take into account the broader environmental origins of disease, injury, and ecological destruction. An attempt to approach health at the aggregate level is the *Healthy People 2010* initiative (USDHHS, 2000). It focuses on health promotion and disease prevention in specific areas, such as environmental health. The *Healthy People* table lists selected *Health People 2010* environmental health objectives.

Nursing is not alone in its focus on individual health-promoting interventions. Most health agencies, health care institutions, and corporate workplaces, however, have principally addressed the idea of "controllable risk" in the individual,

with much less effort directed toward reducing risks in the environment. In addition, the government has also reduced its overall focus on environmental health. The effectiveness and power of agencies such as the EPA and the National Institute for Occupational Safety and Health have declined over the past 25 years. Therefore fewer studies of environmental health risks and enforcement regulatory policies have been conducted.

Interventions designed for individuals may overlook unhealthy environments. Further, although environmental hazards can be serious, the implication persists that little can alter the impact of technological and industrial growth. Therefore individuals are compelled to adjust to environments that might cause illness and injury.

Community health nurses who base their practices on the principles of critical theory are better prepared to respond to collective challenges (Bent, 2003; Clark et al., 2003). These nurses can facilitate community participation in identifying and solving environmental health problems and bring about changes that improve environments and eliminate hazards.

CRITICAL COMMUNITY HEALTH NURSING PRACTICE

Community health nurses who approach environmental health critically are action oriented (Ortner, 2004; Stevens and Hall, 1992). Several clinical examples throughout the chapter illustrate how nurses can focus their efforts by organizing groups of people, taking a stand, and acting as advocates for change. The nurses ask critical questions, stay engaged with the communities they serve, form coalitions, and use various collective strategies. In the interest of educating future practitioners about the critical practice of environmental community health nursing, the following sections discuss each of these interventions.

Taking a Stand: Advocating for Change

An old labor union folk song asks, "Whose side are you on?" Although a nurse may acknowledge that there are multiple sides to health and environmental issues, nurses cannot ultimately avoid taking a stand. Nurses must make individual and collective decisions about which interests they want to serve with their specialized knowledge and skills. To say that

HEALTHY PEOPLE 2010 | Selected Objectives for Environmental Health

Objective	Baseline	Target
8.1a: Reduce the proportion of persons exposed to air that does not meet the U.S. EPA's health-based standards for ozone.	43%	0%
8.6: Reduce waterborne disease outbreaks arising from water intended for drinking among persons served by community water systems.	6 outbreaks per year	2 outbreaks per year
8.11: Eliminate elevated blood lead levels in children.	4.4% of children aged 1-6	0%
8.15: Increase recycling of municipal solid waste.	27%	38%
8.18: Increase the proportion of persons who live in homes tested for radon concentrations.	17%	20%
10.2a: Reduce outbreaks of infections caused by *E. coli* 0157:H7.	22	11
16.15: Reduce the occurrence of spina bifida and other neural tube defects.	6 new cases per 10,000 births	3 new cases per 10,000 births
20.1e: Reduce deaths from work-related injuries—agriculture, forestry, and fishing.	24.1 deaths per 100,000 workers	16.9 deaths per 100,000 workers
24.3a: Reduce hospital emergency visits for asthma for children under age 5 years.	150 per 10,000	80 per 10,000
27.12: Increase the proportion of worksites with formal smoking policies that prohibit smoking or limit it to separately ventilated areas.	79%	100%

From US Department of Health and Human Services: *Healthy People 2010*, ed 2, Washington, DC, 2000, US Government Printing Office.

all must be served is certainly an ideal; however, people often experience consequences of hazardous environments inequitably. Vulnerable groups are exposed to more health-damaging effects than less vulnerable groups (EPA, 2005; Robinson, 2000). Nurses have the potential to increase or decrease these inequities through the decisions they make about the positions they accept and the interventions they undertake.

Environmental problems are clearly intertwined with social, political, and economic policies, resource barriers, and the interests of those in positions of control. Nurses need to connect the immediate and long-term health problems experienced by particular communities to this larger sphere of influence.

Asking Critical Questions

Community health nurses must also consider the relationships between non-health policies and health policies. They should ask how policies concerning ecological preservation, energy, housing, immigration, civil rights, crime, nutrition, minimum wage, occupational safety, and defense might affect the well-being of people. Addressing critical questions such as who has access to resources in this country, and whose interests are served in the existing system, provides a way to include social, political, and economic factors in environmental nursing assessments. Box 13-3 provides a sample set of questions that are useful in this endeavor. Nurses can ask these critical questions when approaching environmental health problems.

Dialogue resulting from critical questioning can frame the problem and assist in building collective strategies. Ideally, those directly affected by the problem should explore these questions collectively. However, even one individual involved in the situation can begin to explore a problem from this perspective and define an initial basis for action.

BOX 13-3   Critical Questions About Environmental Health Problems

- ➤ What is the problem?
- ➤ Who is defining the problem?
- ➤ In what terms is the problem described?
- ➤ How are others in the situation viewing the problem?
- ➤ What is the history of the problem?
- ➤ How did things get the way they are?
- ➤ What other situations does this problem directly affect?
- ➤ Who does the problem affect?
- ➤ Whose health is damaged because things are this way?
- ➤ Who benefits from the way things are?
- ➤ Whose interests do current solutions serve?
- ➤ What are the economic inequities in the situation?
- ➤ Who has political power in the situation?
- ➤ Who knows about the problem?
- ➤ Who needs to know or know more about the problem?
- ➤ How effective are current programs, strategies, and policies?
- ➤ What are the barriers to solving the problem?
- ➤ What strategies may alleviate the problem?
- ➤ How successful have these strategies been?
- ➤ What existing groups might deal with this problem?
- ➤ What resources are needed to solve the problem?
- ➤ How accessible are the resources?
- ➤ How can nurses evaluate potential solutions?

Facilitating Community Involvement

Approaching community health from a critical perspective requires working to improve health conditions and creating the context in which people can identify health-damaging problems in their environments. One important nursing goal is to help people learn from their own experiences and analyze the world with an intention to change it. It is essential that the affected people participate in the process of identifying and working to solve environmental problems. To foster active participation, nurses must be prepared to take leadership positions and join in mutual exchanges with community members that consider each person's experience. The nurse's role changes from presenting solutions and directing lifestyle changes to asking critical questions and helping groups reflect on the problematic environmental realities of their lives.

A second nursing role is to provide support, information, and expertise to groups to assist them in meeting the goals they set for environmental change. In each of these roles, nurses use the concept of solidarity, in which the relationship with the community and its individual members is maintained and nurtured despite disagreements that may occur over what is the best course of action. Rather than trying to compel people to behave in certain ways, nurses should assist aggregates in their collective search for effective change strategies. Actions dictated from those outside the situation are often culturally inappropriate and will most likely fail. Lasting rapport with aggregates depends on honesty, fairness, and mutuality in interactions over extended periods of time.

Using critical questions, community health nurses can help community members look beyond immediate environmental problems and explore social, cultural, economic, and political circumstances that contribute to them. Nurses can share their knowledge about the scientific basis for health problems, their insights about the historical origins of particular environmental hazards, their technical skills, and their expertise in communicating and organizing. Nursing expertise is not used to dominate a group but rather to develop a mutual plan of action to deal with the problems a group has collectively identified. By addressing people's everyday concerns and targeting the problems they identify, nurses situate their efforts in community struggles.

Forming Coalitions

Another very important nursing task that arises from approaching environmental health from a critical perspective involves forming coalitions to produce social change. By initiating dialogue and building a strong base of collective support, nurses join with communities to eliminate hazards and improve public health. Nurses can approach existing community organizations, churches, and family and friendship networks to help mobilize aggregate members who have not previously socialized or acted together. Nurses can then expose hazards, assess needs, plan actions, report abuses, and secure appropriate resources, personnel, funding, and legislative changes.

The environmental justice movement is an excellent example of coalition building wherein members of racial and ethnic minority groups have organized grassroots groups to address lead contamination, pesticide use, water and air pollution, native self-government, nuclear testing, and workplace safety. These groups focus on the disproportionate environmental challenges they face. Drawing insights from the civil rights movement and the environmental movement, environ-

mental justice groups have forged alliances with many conventional environmental and civil rights organizations to mount formal responses to environmental threats (EPA, 2004).

For example, the Mothers of East Los Angeles, one grassroots organization fighting for environmental justice, acquired the support of Greenpeace, Natural Resources Defense Council, Environmental Policy Institute, Citizens' Clearinghouse on Hazardous Waste, National Toxics Campaign, and Western Center on Law and Poverty to bring a lawsuit against state and federal agencies who granted a private corporation permission to build and operate a toxic waste incinerator in their urban neighborhood. Coalition allies provided the Mothers of East Los Angeles with valuable technical advice, expert testimony, lobbying, research, and legal assistance. The grassroots group spearheaded efforts in which hundreds of East Los Angeles residents placed intense political pressure on the state and federal agencies by attending every public hearing about the incinerator project. In the ensuing State Supreme Court battle, the decision prevented construction of the proposed facility.

Nurses can be instrumental in these efforts by helping community groups make connections with larger, more powerful organizations. Nurses can organize forums whereby community groups meet with scientific experts who can help them gather evidence about health threats, with businesses managers whose actions impinge on the economic life of the community, with industry leaders whose companies create ecological hazards, and with legislators who can bring community concerns to law-making bodies. Using available institutional resources, skills, and knowledge, nurses can also explore what is happening elsewhere. Making connections with groups in other locales who are struggling for similar environmental changes can enhance collective strength and solidarity. Press releases, media events, interviews, television spots, speeches, newsletters, and leaflets are important means of calling attention to a situation and raising awareness among communities.

Nurses usually find that establishing alliances with disenfranchised communities is a complex and often long-term process of building trust. Nurses must advocate for the fiscal, logistical, ideological, and labor support necessary to make community alliances possible. In many cases, this requires nurses to advocate for changes to develop resources and make the environment safer.

It is important to recognize that when nurses work to build coalitions for improving environmental conditions, each issue or problem requires appropriate strategic action based on its own merits. Allies in a current struggle may have been adversaries in a previous struggle. For example, although a bank refused to help farm families by granting farm loan extensions last month, it may be an ally this month when a superhighway development project threatens its location and an adjacent poor neighborhood. An ally need not be in complete agreement with the core group's philosophy, political agenda, or moral beliefs. Few individuals or factions can be completely discounted as an ally or remain untouched by environmental health issues. It is a good idea to brainstorm about all the possible groups in a locale that may have a stake in the outcome of an issue. A good coalition-building strategy is to consider the future and contemplate how one struggle, or one set of allies, can extend its network and subsequently form new coalitions for emerging issues.

Using Collective Strategies

Nurses can use a variety of strategies to intervene at the aggregate level and facilitate improvement in a community's health. Nurses can organize people to change health-damaging environments through combinations of strategies including coalition building; consciousness-raising groups; educational forums in neighborhoods, workplaces, schools, churches, and social clubs; seminars for health care providers, city officials, teachers, and employers; community needs assessments; dissemination of clinical research and policy analyses; use of mass media; canvassing; litigation; legislative lobbying; testimony at public hearings; demonstrations; and participatory research.

One collective strategy that is an effective aggregate-level community health nursing intervention is **participatory action research.** Participatory action research calls for nurses, community members, and other resource people to work together in identifying environmental health problems, designing the studies, collecting and analyzing the data, disseminating the results, and posing solutions to the problems (Garwick and Auger, 2003; Kelly, 2005). With the assistance of community health nurses, community members gather information on suspected environmental hazards, document their effects on health, educate their communities, persuade corporations to clean up, and lobby local, state, and federal governments for stricter regulations and improved enforcement. The goal of the research process is not merely the production of knowledge, but rather the generation of open discussion and debate that intensifies a community's consciousness of health-impairing environmental constraints. Box 13-4 presents an abstract of an article about illustrating a type of participatory action research related to environmental health.

Although nurses have not traditionally used all of these collective strategies to intervene in community health matters, environmental hazards are multiplying geometrically, pushing nurses to expand their skills repertoire. Pioneers such as Hollie Shaner, RN, have embraced that concept and are blazing the path to environmental awareness (Sattler, 2003). A decade ago, Shaner frequently left her home where she avidly separated and recycled, and arrived at the Vermont hospital where she worked, where none of the waste was recycled. Shaner was not comfortable throwing everything into a "red bag" and decided that there must be a way to change the environmental unfriendliness of her place of employment. She began voluntarily recycling the hospitals' cardboard and then began to recycle the newspapers, glass, and plastics. In addition, she received a grant from the state of Vermont to maximize her efforts in medical waste reduction. The efforts and savings did not go unnoticed by the hospital, as Shaner received a new job title of clinical waste reduction coordinator in which she saves the hospital $175,000 per year.

Shaner also authored a book for the American Hospital Association on medical waste management. She quickly

---

BOX 13-4 Participatory Action Research

Rates of overweight children and adolescents have nearly tripled over the past 30 years. Many barriers exist to healthy eating and physical activity for children and adolescents, including factors in the school and community environment. The Nutrition Friendly Schools and Communities (NFSC) model was developed to address these modifiable school environment factors with the intent of preventing the development of obesity among children and adolescents. The NFSC model was built upon the Coordinated School Health Program, the Baby Friendly Hospital Initiative, participatory research, and empowerment evaluation. The purpose of the NFSC environmental intervention is to actively engage the school community to prevent overweight in students through a multilevel, participative intervention that facilitates coordinated changes in the school environment in the following areas: health education, physical education, health services, food services, school policy, staff wellness, psychosocial services, and family/community involvement. The NFSC model is the basis by which school communities develop a plan and evaluation that lead to a healthy school environment and prevent the development of overweight in children.

Vecchiarelli S et al: Using participatory action research to develop a school-based environmental intervention to support healthy eating and physical activity, *Am J Health Educ* 36(1):35-42, 2005.

---

realized the negative impact the health care industry was having on the environmental health of the communities served. Mercury was being released into the streams from medical waste, and dioxins were being released into the air from medical waste incineration. From this realization, in 1996, Shaner and a small group of other health professionals launched a campaign to lead the health care industry toward environmental stewardship. This campaign, supported by the American Nurses Association, was named Health Care Without Harm. "The goal of the campaign was to reduce the environmental health risks that were being created by the health care industry" (Sattler, 2003, p. 8). The campaign still exists and is building momentum; today there are 433 participating organizations in 52 different countries (Health Care Without Harm, 2005).

If nurses do not possess these types of organizational skills, they can learn from experts in the community who have experience with conducting mass media campaigns, organizing demonstrations, canvassing neighborhoods, participating in class-action litigation, and testifying at public hearings. Nurses can also consult many available books about political action.

SUMMARY

This chapter provided a glimpse into the complex world of environmental health from a critical community health nursing perspective. The case study and clinical examples illustrate that nurses must evaluate the broader picture in assessing the environmental health status of communities and the vulnerable aggregates within communities. In preventing, minimizing, and resolving environmental health problems, nurses must recognize patterns, detect subtle changes, identify underlying issues, and work collaboratively with a variety of individuals

Text continued on p. 258

CASE STUDY — Application of the Nursing Process

In July 2001, the *Metro Pulse* newspaper reported an extensive air pollution problem in the city of Knoxville, Tennessee (Tarr, 2001). The American Lung Association had recently named Knoxville as the ninth most polluted city in the country, based on the ozone contamination in the air. The following case study expands upon some of the reported facts of the situation to construct hypothetical nursing interventions.

Knoxville's community health nurses and the public health department have long been involved with city residents and have been aware of high rates of asthma in particular neighborhoods. In the wake of alarming newspaper and research articles about the dangerous incidence of air pollution and related asthma, the nurses decided to make the health issues a priority. The community health nurses and several nursing students assigned to their department researched the topics and uncovered the following information.

Asthma has long been recognized as a condition in which an acute respiratory response may follow inhalation of a material to which a person is sensitized. Only recently, though, have scientists focused on agents that cause non-specific generalized inflammation, such as air pollution (Thurston and Bates, 2003).

A study conducted by the University of Southern California and funded by the California Environmental Protection Agency's Air Resources Board provides strong evidence that ozone can *cause*, as well as exacerbate, asthma (McConnell et al., 2002). The study found that days with higher ozone concentration resulted in significantly higher school absences due to respiratory illness, and children living in high ozone communities who actively participated in several sports were more likely to develop asthma than children in communities not participating in sports.

Indeed, the nation's leading group of pediatricians, the American Academy of Pediatrics (AAP, 2004) recently revised its policy statement on outdoor air pollution and the health hazards to children. The AAP's Committee on Environmental Health strengthened its warning of the dangers that air pollution poses to children because of the recent studies correlating air pollution with asthma and negative lung growth and function. Recent estimates are that more than 20 million Americans suffer from asthma (Asthma and Allergy Foundation, 2004).

An economically depressed neighborhood in Knoxville, hypothetically called Trent Park, is situated near numerous railways, freeways, and industrial yards. High numbers of African-American, Latino, and Southeast Asian residents live in the older homes that line the streets of Trent Park. Isolated by language and economic circumstances, many Trent Park residents do not know they are exposed to these environmental health hazards.

ASSESSMENT

Elena Garcia, an 8-year-old girl who lives in Trent Park, presented at the pediatric primary clinic at the health department at 8 AM on an early November morning, accompanied by her mother. Elena had been diagnosed with asthma 2 months previously and was now in mild respiratory distress. Elena explained to the nurse that she had gone trick-or-treating the night before in her neighborhood. It had turned cold that weekend, and she had also played outside in her neighborhood with friends the day before. In addition, Mrs. Garcia explained that Elena had contracted a respiratory virus a few days ago. The nurse realized that Elena and her mother both mentioned several factors such as her playing outside on a cold afternoon/evening in a polluted neighborhood with a respiratory virus that could have exacerbated her asthma.

At the clinic visit, the nurse assessed the following:
- Elena's heart rate and cardiovascular status
- Elena's pattern of breathing, which includes rate, rhythm, and effort
- Elena's asthma medication history
- Evidence of diaphoresis, papillary dilation, and fear, which are all features of the adrenergic response to hypoxia
- Elena's global central nervous system function, such as alertness, cooperation, and motor activity
- Elena's stress level and coping skills
- Mrs. Garcia's stress level and coping skills

DIAGNOSIS

Individual
- Ineffective airway clearance related to environmental exposure to air pollution
- Knowledge deficit related to precipitating factors that can cause/worsen an asthma attack
- Anxiety related to ongoing fear of daughter's illness

Family
- At risk for family crisis related to instability caused by the illness
- Knowledge deficit related to precipitating factors that can cause/worsen an asthma attack

Community
- At risk for increased incidence of asthma due to air pollution
- Inadequate programs for asthma screening

PLANNING

A plan of care is developed at the individual, family, and community levels. Mutual goal setting and contracting are essential if the outcome is to be optimal.

Individual
Long-Term Goals
- Client will not exercise outdoors on a day with high pollution levels.

Continued

- Client will reduce exposure to allergy triggers.
- Client will avoid tobacco smoke.
- Client will keep pets out of the bedroom.
- Client will experience successful maintenance of asthma.

Short-Term Goals
- Client will begin to keep an asthma diary and identify which allergy triggers are problematic.
- Client will remain free of acute asthma attacks.

Family
Long-Term Goals
- Family will follow the city's daily air quality index.
- Family will encourage child to stay indoors on days with high pollution levels.
- Family will remove as many allergy triggers from home as possible.
- Family will enforce the pets-out-of-the-bedroom policy.
- Family will cope effectively with daughter's asthma.

Short-Term Goals
- Family will provide encouragement for client to keep asthma diary to identify which allergy triggers are problematic.
- Family will express emotions regarding daughter's acute asthma attack.

Community
Long-Term Goals
- Citizens will be involved in decision-making process about proposed activities that could pose an environmental hazard.
- Citizens will encourage utility companies, government, and industries to reduce air pollution.
- Citizens will be encouraged to utilize mass transit and carpools to reduce vehicle emissions.
- Citizens will encourage officials to build new schools away from polluted areas.

Short-Term Goals
- Citizens will be alerted about the air pollution problem in the area.
- Citizens will be educated about the air quality index and its implications for outdoor activity.

INTERVENTION

The actions of the community health nurses in coalition with community members comprise interventions at the individual, family, and aggregate levels.

Individual
- Identify Trent Park children who are diagnosed and treated for asthma and plan follow-up home visits to provide education on basic pathophysiology, symptoms of distress, and environmental controls needed for successful asthma management.

- Redesign the community health agency's child health assessment protocol, adding several observations designed to detect symptoms of asthma and several questions that establish whether there are specific triggers for asthma in the home.
- Coordinate with school nurses to ensure they incorporate similar changes in their health assessment protocols.
- Establish an agreement with the state's TennCare Child Health Program that ensures they will screen for asthma if physicians, school nurses, or community health nurses recommend it.
- Prepare an educational pamphlet with members of Trent Park that details Trent Park residents' air pollution and asthma risks. The community health nurses mail the pamphlet to individual physicians and nurses who provide services to children in Trent Park.
- Prepare translations of the pamphlet in languages and reading levels appropriate for Trent Park residents and mail it to individual households.

Family
- Initiate a family-to-family program in which a core group of Trent Park community members attend educational meetings with the community health nurses. In these meetings, they share information about the environmental origins of air pollution and asthma and its prevention, diagnosis, and treatment. These specially trained community members then take charge of the program, sharing their knowledge with extended family members and neighboring families.
- Coordinate with school nurses to establish a health education program in Trent Park schools in which school-age children learn about air pollution and asthma. Encourage these children to take their knowledge home and teach younger preschool-age siblings about staying indoors on hot, sunny days when the ozone levels are apt to be the highest.
- Investigate how community health nurses might better assist Trent Park families by helping them apply for and obtain nutritional resources such as food stamps, food bank supplements, and school lunch programs. With improved nutritional status and immune system, symptoms of asthma may decrease.
- Facilitate the formation of a support group for families with children who have suffered asthma. The community health nurses volunteer their offices for evening meeting space and provide information about health care, social services, and government disability assistance.

Community
- Provide pamphlets with announcements about community health nurses' willingness to offer asthma education programs at churches, schools, hospitals, workplaces, medical association meetings, and nursing association meetings.
- Involve members of the Trent Park community at planning meetings and include African-American, Latino, and Southeast Asian community members.

CASE STUDY Application of the Nursing Process (cont'd)

- Contact neighborhood leaders, church leaders, ethnic clubs, the local Parent-Teacher Association, a senior citizen organization in the neighborhood, the Black Women's Health Project, and a local Latina women's political organization and organize planning meetings.
- Start multicultural grassroots effort by Citizens United to Combat Air Pollution (CUTCAP) that travels door to door educating Trent Park residents about the dangers of air pollution as it relates to asthma.
- Establish ties with local physicians, nurses, and health care institutions who allocate adequate funds and personnel to accomplish the coalition's goals.
- Establish a time frame for evaluating the Trent Park project.
- Encourage nursing students and community health nursing faculty from the local university and college programs to participate in the interventions.
- Lobby state legislatures, municipal officials, local medical associations, local hospitals, and city clinics regarding plan implementation.
- Form broader coalitions with Knoxville churches, local nurses association, several preschool and day care centers, and the Knoxville School Board to design a comprehensive, non-duplicative, cost-effective asthma screening program that will test all children in Knoxville on a regular basis.
- Contact researchers at a local university's environmental sciences program and request that they work with the coalition to conduct a house-to-house study of asthma triggers sources.
- Designate a CUTCAP committee to do daily reviews of the Environmental Protection Agency (EPA) index for air quality and provide monthly reports to Trent Park and surrounding communities.
- Contact state environmental groups for advice on local efforts and join in their fight for stricter regulation of air pollutants and toxic wastes.
- Contact local media (e.g., television, radio, and newspaper) about running a series of stories about Knoxville air pollutants and related asthma risks; supply information and contacts for interviews and photographs.

EVALUATION

Individual

- Evaluate the child and mother's understanding of asthma treatments at follow-up home visits.
- Facilitate the evaluation of ongoing interventions.
- Track the number of asthma screening tests Trent Park children receive and the rates of asthma to determine the effectiveness of their efforts in these areas.
- Keep close contact with the school nurses and organize an afterschool educational and screening program at schools that are understaffed.

- Ask school nurses to report on the educational sessions' success.

Family

- Document participation levels at educational programs and family training sessions.
- Document ongoing participation in referrals and support groups

Community

Although local officials supported their plan, CUTCAP's efforts at pushing for a comprehensive asthma screening program met a great deal of opposition from the state legislature. When repeated negotiations continued to fail, CUTCAP decided to align with environmental and civil rights groups who were suing the state of Tennessee for failure to provide federally mandated asthma screening tests for low-income children. The CUTCAP coalition became plaintiffs in the class-action suit. The community health nurses from Trent Park gave expert testimony in the case.

The court case proceeded, and some members of the state legislature began to show more interest in an asthma screening program; another vote was scheduled. The Trent Park Coalition participated in an Air Pollution and Asthma Awareness Day at the state capitol the week before the vote. They were active in the demonstration and gave speeches about their local experiences. They visited the offices of individual legislators, informing them of Trent Park's situation. Citing the tentative results from the environmental scientists' house-to-house research study and the community health nurses' asthma screening statistics proved very useful. This evidence strengthened the coalition members' arguments about the need for a comprehensive asthma screening program in the state. The coalition also shared these data with the national environmental groups with whom they worked. These groups used the data in testimony before federal legislators to secure federal funding for a new program to reduce emissions from automobiles and trucks by implementing an annual mandatory emissions test for all vehicles in the state.

LEVELS OF PREVENTION

Primary

Educating the community regarding air pollution and its relationship to asthma.

Secondary

Screening at-risk populations for asthma and testing blood levels for air pollutants.

Tertiary

Follow-up treatment for people with asthma and reducing air pollutants from the community environment.

and groups. In the past, environmental threats to health were usually suspected only when other possible causes of illness were ruled out. Nurses can expect this pattern to change dramatically in the twenty-first century as environmental health moves increasingly to the forefront of the public health agenda.

LEARNING ACTIVITIES

1. Identify a health-related problem associated with some aspect of the environment. It may be a problem in a nearby community, a problem publicized in the media, or a difficulty experienced by a family. Examine the problem using the sample series of critical questions listed in Box 13-3. Without sharing the results, present the problem to the group and ask them to discuss it by responding to the same questions. Were there differences or similarities in the initial results and the group's answers? On what points did everyone agree? Why? What questions caused the most disagreement? Why? Now repeat the entire activity by involving people other than nursing students in the group discussion. How did this discussion compare with the previous discussion and responses?

2. Attend meetings that hold environmental hazard discussions. If meetings or public forums are not available in the vicinity, write for information about the state's actions to fight environmental hazards. The reference librarians at colleges or public libraries can suggest ways of contacting sources and will supply addresses. Organizations that are likely to sponsor forums and provide information include those listed in Box 13-2, the EPA, the National Institute for Occupational Safety and Health, state and municipal agencies for environmental protection and occupational health, environmental caucuses of political parties, the American Public Health Association, the local public health department, farmers' organizations, and labor unions.

3. This chapter described how to use participatory research as an intervention in dealing with ecological hazards. In a group, brainstorm about possibilities for participatory action research projects in the area. Try to identify examples from a variety of environmental health areas. Be creative in planning. How might a nurse mobilize community support and participation in the research? What groups would be approachable? What critical questions might facilitate dialogue about the problem? What kinds of data could be collected and how could they be used? How could research results be publicized? What ramifications could the completed study have for community members, other communities in the state, and community health nurses in other locales?

4. Nurses may have to supplement their knowledge of collective strategies by reading books about political action and by learning from community members who are experienced in political organizing. Visit a college or public library to investigate books and journal articles outside the nursing literature. Compile a list of references related to one of these political strategies (e.g., grassroots organizing, legislative lobbying, community education, policy analysis, use of the media, coalition building, citizen surveys, public protest, letter-writing campaigns, or consciousness-raising groups). Exchange reference lists with peers to benefit from their efforts. Then choose one or two books of interest and read them.

REFERENCES

Alberg J, Samet JM: Epidemiology of lung cancer, *Chest* 123(1):21S-28S, 2003.

Alexander DE, Fairbridge RW: *Encyclopedia of environmental science,* Higham, Mass, 1999, Kluwer Academic Publishers.

American Academy of Pediatrics: *Air pollution: children more at risk than adults,* Press release, Dec 6, 2004, The Author, http://www.aap.org/advocacy/releases/decpollution.htm.

Asthma and Allergy Foundation: Asthma facts and figures, 2004, The Author, http://www.aafa.org/display.cfm?id=8&sub=42.

Barnes BV et al: *Forest ecology,* ed 4, New York, 1998, John Wiley and Sons.

Bent KN: Perspectives on critical and feminist theory in developing nursing praxis, *J Prof Nurs* 9(5):296-303, 2003.

Bergstrom L, Kirchmann H: *Carbon and nutrient dynamics in natural and agricultural tropical ecosystems,* New York, 1998, CAB International.

Bingham E, Meader WV: Governmental regulation of environmental hazards in the 1990s, *Annu Rev Public Health* 11:419-434, 1990.

Bove F, Shim Y, Zeitz P: Drinking water contaminants and adverse pregnancy outcomes: a review, *Environ Health Perspect* 110(suppl 1):61-74, 2002.

Burns WG: Climate change and human health: the critical policy agenda, *JAMA* 287(17): 2287, 2002.

Burger EJ: Human health: a surrogate for the environment: the evolution of environmental legislation and regulation during the 1970s, *Regul Toxicol Pharmacol* 9: 196-206, 1989.

Butterfield PG: Upstream reflections on environmental health: an abbreviated history and framework for action, *Adv Nurs Sci* 25(1):32-49, 2002.

Catani A, Micera M: Genetically modified foods and children potential health risks, *Eur Rev Med Pharmacol Sci* (5)1:25-29, 2001.

Center for Children's Health and the Environment: *Emerging illnesses in urban environments,* 2002, The Author, http://www.childenvironment.org/factsheets/emerging_illnesses.htm.

Centers for Disease Control and Prevention: *2003 West Nile virus activity in the United States,* The Author, http://www.cdc.gov/ncidod/dvbid/westnile/surv&controlCaseCount03_detailed.htm.

Centers for Disease Control and Prevention: Blood lead levels: United States—1999-2002, *MMWR Morb Mort Wkly Rep* 54(20):513-516, 2005b.

Centers for Disease Control and Prevention: Preliminary foodnet data on the incident of infection with pathogens transmitted commonly through food: 10 sites—United States, 2004, *MMWR Morb Mortality Wkly Rep Surveill Summ* 54(14):352-356, 2005c.

Centers for Disease Control and Prevention: *Worker health chartbook 2004,* NIOSH 2004-146, 2005, The Author, http://www2a.cdc.gov/NIOSH-Chartbook/, 2005d.

Chapman, JA et al: Toxic mold: phantom risk vs science. *Ann Allergy Asthma Immunol* 91(3): 222-232, 2003.

Clark, L, Barton JA, Brown NJ: Assessment of community contamination: a critical approach, *Public Health Nurs* 19(5):354-365, 2002.

Cralley LV, Cralley LJ, Cooper WC, editors: *Health and safety beyond the work place,* New York, 1990, John Wiley and Sons.

Cutter SL, Mitchell JT, Scott MS: Revealing the vulnerability of people and places: a case study of Georgetown Co, S.C., *Ann Assoc Am Geograph* 90(4):713-737, 2000.

Danesi PR et al: Isotopic composition and origin of uranium and plutonium in selected soil samples collected in Kosovo, *J Environ Radioact* 64(2-3):121-131, 2003.

Davies WP: An historical perspective from the green revolution to the gene revolution, *Nutr Rev* 61(6):S124-S134, 2003.

DeLong JV: Public policy toward municipal solid waste, *Annu Rev Public Health* 14: 137-157, 1993.

Eckersley R: *Environmentalism and political theory: toward an ecocentric approach,* Albany, NY, 1992, State University of New York Press.

Environmental Protection Agency: Urban sprawl modeling, air quality monitoring and risk communication: The Northeast Ohio Project. 2002, EPA/625/R-02/016. Washington, DC, 2002, The Author.

Environmental Protection Agency: *Indoors air facts No. 4 (revised): sick building syndrome (SBS),* 2003, The Author, http://www.epa.gov/iaq/pubs/sbs.html.

Environmental Protection Agency: *Why be concerned?* Nov 4, 2004, The Author, http://www.epa.gov/air/concerns.html.

Environmental Protection Agency: *Highlighting success: the region 9 environmental justice small grant program, fiscal years 1994-99,* EPA 909-R99-002, Washington, DC, 2005, The Author.

Environmental Protection Agency: *What are the six common air pollutants?* Last updated April 7, 2006, The Author, http://www.epa.gov/air/urbanair/6poll.html.

Environmental Protection Agency: *Ensuring risk reduction in communities with multiple stressors: environmental justice and cumulative risks/impacts.* Washington, DC, 2004, The Author.

Epstein PR: West Nile virus and the climate, *J Urban Health* 78:367-371, 2001.

Etzel R: How environmental exposures influence the development and exacerbation of asthma. *Pediatrics* 112, 233-239, 2003.

Foster HD: Health and the physical environment: the challenge of global change. In Hayes MV, Foster LT, Foster HD, editors: *The determinants of populations health: a critical assessment,* Victoria, BC, Canada, 1994, University of Victoria.

Frumkin H: Urban sprawl and public health, *Public Health Reports,* 117: 201-212, 2002.

Garwick AW, Auger S: Participatory action research: the Indian family stories project, *Nurs Outlook* 51:261-266, 2003.

Gelberg KH et al: Nitrate levels in drinking water in rural New York State, *Environ Res* 80(1): 34-40, 1999.

Gent JF et al: Association of low-level ozone and fine particles with respiratory symptoms in children with asthma, *JAMA* 290(14): 1859-1863, 2003.

Guillen MD, Sopelana P, Partearroyo MA: Food as a source of polycyclic aromatic carcinogens, *Rev Environ Health* 12(3): 133-146, 1997.

Hall JM, Stevens PE: A nursing view of the U.S.-Iraq war: psychosocial health consequences, *Nurs Outlook* 40:113-120, 1992.

Hamilton PA, Miller TL, Myers DN: *Water quality in the nation's streams and aquifers: overview of selected findings, 1991-2001,* US Geological Survey circular 1265, Reston, VA, 2004, US Geological Survey.

Harper AC, Lambert LJ: *The health of populations: an introduction,* ed 2, New York, 1994, Springer.

Harrison TW, Gustafson EM, Dixon JK: Radiologic emergency: protecting schoolchildren and the public, *Am J Nurs* 103(5):41-49, 2003.

Health Care Without Harm: *About us,* 2005, The Author, http://www.noharm.org/aboutUs/HCWHStory.

Hwang E, Cash JN, Zabik MJ: Chlorine and chlorine dioxide treatment to reduce or remove EBDCs and ETU residues in a solution, *J Agric Food Chem* 50(16):4734-4742, 2002.

Institute of Medicine Committee on Enhancing Environmental Health Content in Nursing Practice: *Nursing, health, and the environment,* Washington, DC, 1995, National Academies Press.

International Physicians for the Prevention of Nuclear War: *Radioactive heaven and earth: the health and environmental effects of nuclear weapons testing, in, on, and above the earth,* New York, 1991, Apex Press.

Jaga K, Brosius D: Pesticide exposure: human cancers on the horizon, *Rev Environ Health* 14(1):39-42, 1999.

Kaila HL: A review of the occupational health of women, *J Health Manage* 4(1):1-9, 2002.

Kelly PJ: Practical suggestions for community interventions using participatory action research, *Public Health Nurs* 22(1):65-73, 2005.

Kemp DD: *The environmental dictionary,* London, 1998, Routledge.

Kilburn KH: Neurotoxicity from airborne chemicals around a superfund site, *Environ Res* 81(2):92-99, 1999.

Kleinman M: *The health effect of our pollution on children,* Diamond Bar, Calif, Fall, 2000, South Coast Air Quality Management district, http://www.aqmd.gov/forstudents/health_effects_on_children.html.

Landrigan PJ et al: Health and environmental consequences of the World Trade Center Disaster, *Environ Health Perspect* 112(6):731-739, 2004.

Last JM: Global change: ozone depletion, greenhouse warming, and public health, *Annu Rev Public Health* 14:115-136, 1993.

Lawrence RJ: Urban health: an ecological perspective, *Rev Environ Health* 14(1):1-10, 1999.

Le Moual N, Kennedy SM, Kauffmann F: Occupational exposures and asthma in 14,000 adults from the general population, *Am J Epidemiol* 160(11):1108-1116, 2004.

Lemus R et al: Potential health risks from exposure to indoor formaldehyde, *Rev Environ Health* 13(1-2):91-98, 1998.

Lovgren S: The mystery of the SARS virus: how is it spread? *National Geographic News* April 9, 2003:1-4, http://news.nationalgeographic.com/news/2003/04/0409_030409_sars.html.

Mariethoz E et al: Allergy and the environment: a meeting report, *Rev Environ Health* 14(2): 63-78, 1999.

McConnell R et al: Asthma in exercising children exposed to ozone: a cohort study, *Lancet* 359.386-391, 2002.

Milio N: *Promoting health through public policy,* Ottawa, Ontario, 1986, Canadian Public Health Association.

Moore GS: *Living with the earth: concepts in environmental health science,* Boca Raton, Fla, 1999, Lewis Publications.

National Environmental Education & Training Foundation: *Pediatric environmental history initiative,* 2002, The Author, http://www.neetf.org/Health/screening.pdf.

National Research Council: *Biosolids applied to land: advancing standards and practice* Washington, DC, 2002, National Academies Press.

National Toxic Inhalation Study Group: Environmental pulmonary edema: an update, *Rev Environ Health* 13(1-2):27-58, 1998.

Needleman HL et al: The long-term effects of exposure to low doses of lead in children: an 11-year follow-up report, *N Engl J Med* 322:83-88, 1992.

Neu HC: The crisis in antibiotic resistance, *Science* 257:1064-1072, 1992.

Northridge ME, Shepard PM: Environmental racism and public health, *Am J Public Health* 87(5):730-732, 1997.

Northridge ME et al: Environmental equity and health: understanding completely and moving forward. *Am J Public Health* 93(2):209-213, 2003.

Ortner P. The nurse as change agent: an approach to environmental health advocacy, *Policy Polit Nurs Pract* 5(2):125-130, 2004.

Paranzino GK et al: I PREPARE: development and clinical utility of an environmental exposure history mnemonic, *AAOHN Journal* 53(1):37-42, 2005.

Patz JA, Khaliq M: Global climate change and health: challenges for future practitioners, *JAMA* 287(17):2283-2284, 2002.

Physicians for Social Responsibility: *Air pollution and health,* Washington, DC, 2001, The Author, http://www.psr.org/home.cfm?id=air_population.

Platt JR: Radon: its impact on the community and the role of the nurse, *AAOHN J* 41(11): 547-550, 1993.

Powell SC, Atwell R: The use of epidemiological data in the control of foodborne viruses, *Rev Environ Health* 14(1):31-38, 1999.

Raymo ME et al: Millennial-scale climate instability during the early Pleistocene epoch, *Nature* 392:699-702, 1998.

Robinson DM: Environmental racism: old wine in a new bottle, *ECHOES, World Council of Churches,* 2000, The Author, http://www.wcccoe.org/wcc/what/jpc/echoes/echoes-17-02.html.

Salbu C et al: Oxidation states of uranium in depleted uranium particles from Kuwait, *J Environ Radioact* 78(2):125-135, 2005.

Sanchez F, Kosson DS: Probabilistic approach for estimating the release of contaminants under field management scenarios, *Waste Manag* 25(4):463-472, 2005.

Sargent JD et al: The association between state housing policy and lead poisoning in children, *Am J Public Health* 89(11):1690-1695, 1999.

Sattler B: The greening of health care: environmental policy and advocacy in the health care industry, *Policy Polit Nurs Pract* 4(1): 6-13, 2003.

Schleipman AR: Occupational radiation exposure: population studies, *Radiol Technol* 76(3):185-192, 2005.

Schrieberg D: Death from a healing machine: radioactive waste goes on Mexican odyssey after sale of medical device, *San Francisco Examiner* June 23, 1991:1, 12.

Schuurmann G, Markert B, editors: *Ecotoxicology, ecological fundamentals, chemical exposure, and biological effects,* New York, 1998, John Wiley and Sons.

Stevens PE, Hall JM: Applying critical theories to nursing in communities, *Public Health Nurs* 9:2-9, 1992.

Sutherland WJ: *Conservation science and action,* Oxford, UK, 1998, Blackwell Science.

Tarr J: Knoxville's pollution rivals that of Los Angeles, Houston and Atlanta, but Green Power might help clear the air. *Metro Pulse* 11(18), May 3, 2001.

Tchounwou PB: Climate change and its potential impacts on the Gulf Coast region of the United States, *Rev Environ Health* 14(2): 91-102, 1999.

Thompson B et al: Pesticide take-home pathway among children of agricultural workers: study design, methods and baseline findings, *J Occup Environ Med* 45(1):42-53, 2003.

Thurston GD, Bates DV: Air pollution as an underappreciated cause of asthma symptoms, *JAMA* 290:1915-1917, 2003.

Trossman S: Catching the environmental health wave, *Am J Nurs* 104(3):73-74, 2004.

US Department of Health and Human Services: *Healthy People 2010,* ed 2, Washington, DC, 2000, US Government Printing Office.

US Department of Labor, Bureau of Labor Statistics: Current injury, illness, and fatality data, The Author, http://www.bls.gov/iif/home.htm.

Vecchiarelli S et al: Using participatory action research to develop a school-based environmental intervention to support healthy eating and physical activity, *Am J Health Educ* 36(1):35-42, 2005.

Whitney SL, Maltby HJ, Carr JM: "This food may contain . . ." What nurses should know about genetically engineered foods, *Nurs Outlook* 52, 262-266, 2004.

Williams DR, Collins C: Racial residential segregation: a fundamental cause of racial disparities in health, *Public Health Rep* 116(5): 404-417, 2001.

World Health Organization: *International travel and health,* Geneva, 2005a, The Author.

World Health Organization: *World day for safety and health at work 2005: a background paper,* Geneva, 2005b, International Labour Office.

World Health Organization: Ionizing radiation in our environment. 2005c, The Author, http://www.who.int/ionizing_radiation/env/en/.

World Health Organization: Protection of the human environment. 2004, The Author, http://www.who.int/phe/en/.

UNIT 4

Aggregates in the Community

Child and Adolescent Health

Susan Rumsey Givens ▪ Mary Brecht Carpenter

MEDIA RESOURCES

Additional Material for Study, Review, and Further Exploration

evolve Website at http://evolve.elsevier.com/Nies

❖ Quiz ❖ Case Studies ❖ Content Updates ❖ Glossary ❖ WebLinks

OBJECTIVES

Upon completion of this chapter, the reader will be able to do the following:

1. Identify major indicators of child and adolescent health status.
2. Describe how socioeconomic circumstances influence child and adolescent health.
3. Discuss the individual and societal costs of poor child health status.
4. Discuss public programs and prevention strategies targeted to children's health.
5. Apply knowledge of child and adolescent health needs in planning appropriate, comprehensive care at the individual, family, and community levels.

KEY TERMS

adolescent pregnancy
child abuse and neglect
childhood immunization
cultural competence
Early and Periodic
   Screening, Diagnosis,

and Treatment
   (EPSDT)
fetal alcohol syndrome (FAS)
Head Start
infant mortality
lead poisoning

Medicaid
preconceptional
   counseling
preterm birth
prenatal care

State Children's Health
   Insurance Program
   (SCHIP)
Women, Infants, and
   Children (WIC)

CHAPTER OUTLINE

ISSUES OF PREGNANCY AND INFANCY
   Infant Mortality
   Preterm Birth and Low Birth Weight
   Prenatal Care
   Prenatal Substance Use

CHILDHOOD HEALTH ISSUES
   Accidental Injuries
   Overweight
   Immunization
   Lead Poisoning
   Child Abuse and Neglect
   Children With Special Health Care Needs

ADOLESCENT HEALTH ISSUES
   Adolescent Pregnancy and Childbearing
   Violence
   Sexually Transmitted Diseases
   Substance Abuse

**FACTORS AFFECTING CHILD AND ADOLESCENT
HEALTH**
   Poverty
   Racial Disparities
   Single Parenting

   Parents' Educational Status
   Health Care Use
   Health Insurance Coverage

**STRATEGIES TO IMPROVE CHILD AND ADOLESCENT
HEALTH**
   Monitoring and Tracking
   Healthy People 2010: Child and Adolescent Health
   Health Promotion and Disease Prevention

**PUBLIC HEALTH PROGRAMS TARGETED TO CHILDREN
AND ADOLESCENTS**
   Health Care Coverage Programs
   Direct Health Care Delivery Programs

**SHARING RESPONSIBILITY FOR IMPROVING CHILD
AND ADOLESCENT HEALTH**
   Parents' Role
   Community's Role
   Employer's Role
   Government's Role
   Community Health Nurse's Role

**LEGAL AND ETHICAL ISSUES IN CHILD
AND ADOLESCENT HEALTH**
   Ethical Issues

A nation's destiny lies with the health, education, and well-being of its children. Children are the nation's youngest and most vulnerable population. The United States has made tremendous progress over the past century toward improving children's lives. Improvements in public health measures—such as sanitation, infectious disease control, environmental regulation, health screening, and education—and remarkable strides in medical care have all contributed to the good health status that most children enjoy. However, these improvements have not equally benefited children of all races and ethnic groups, children at all income levels, or children in all geographic areas of the country. For example, significant disparities persist in the health status of white children versus children of color. Children living in suburban areas and most outer urban areas experience superior access to health care services compared with children living in rural areas and inner cities, especially if they are poor.

Although most of the nation's children are healthy and succeed in school, many are not enjoying optimal health and well-being and are not reaching their full potential as contributing members of society. Despite improvements, the mortality and morbidity rates for children in all age-groups are unacceptably high. Consider:

- In 2003, over 28,000 infants died before reaching their first birthday.
- In that same year, over 323,000 babies were born with low birth weights (i.e., less than 5.5 lb). Many of these children will suffer long-term effects of low birth weight, including respiratory and vision problems, physical disabilities, and learning difficulties.
- An estimated 3 million children are victims of child abuse and neglect; most are under the age of 4.
- More than 420,000 adolescent girls give birth every year.
- In children aged 12 to 19, 33% use alcohol and over 11% use an illegal drug other than alcohol.
- Violence is the second leading cause of death among adolescents (Childstats, 2005).

The health of a child has long-term implications, and the health habits adopted by children and youth will profoundly influence their potential to lead a healthy, productive future. The physical and emotional health experienced by a child plays a pivotal role in his or her overall development and the well-being of the entire family. Children who go to school sick or hungry, who cannot see the chalkboard or hear the teacher, who have learning disabilities, who are troubled by abusive parents or disruptive living circumstances, or who fear for their safety at home or in school often do not perform on the level of their counterparts who are healthy, well-nourished, well cared for at home, and safe and secure in their world.

In 2002, there were 72.9 million children in the United States under age 18, forming about 25% of the country's population. The number of children is expected to increase to 80.3 million by the year 2020 (U.S. Department of Health and Human Services [USDHHS], 2003). The demographic composition of the nation is important to planners and policy makers because it influences how resources will be allocated. For example, a growing child population necessitates more resources for schools, child care, and health care.

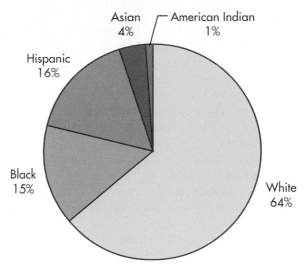

Figure 14-1 Percentage distribution of U.S. children by race/ethnicity, 2000 (estimate). (From Office of the Assistant Secretary for Planning and Evaluation: *Trends in the well-being of America's children and youth,* Washington, DC, 2003, The Author, http://aspe.hhs.gov/hsp/03trends/index.htm.)

The demographic composition of the United States' child and adolescent population (ethnic and racial diversity) is also changing. The percentage of non-Hispanic black children remained steady over the past two decades, but the Hispanic child population has increased from 9% to 16%, and the Asian and Pacific Islander child population has increased from 2% to 4% (Figure 14-1) (Childstats, 2005).

Children are a dependent population and rely primarily on parents or other adults to protect and promote their health and well-being. Community health nurses can learn more about this important population group and the positive and negative factors that influence their health. Nurses can use this information to help improve the chances that children will grow up to be healthy, contributing members of society.

This chapter focuses on the health status of children and adolescents; the medical, socioeconomic, environmental, educational, safety, and public health factors that nurses must address to improve child and adolescent health; and the community health nursing implications. This chapter also discusses indicators of child and adolescent health status, the individual and societal costs of poor child health, public programs targeted to children's health, and strategies to improve child and adolescent health at the individual, family, and community levels.

ISSUES OF PREGNANCY AND INFANCY

Genetic endowment, maternal health and behaviors, and intra-uterine and neonatal environments strongly influence early child health status. The conditions that surround a child's birth can shape his or her life. Protection and promotion of early child health can help ensure a healthy future for the child, whereas neglecting early child health may cause a number of problems.

- Children whose mothers have late or no prenatal care, or who smoked or used illegal drugs during pregnancy, are more likely to be born with low birth weights and serious health conditions (e.g., birth defects, mental retardation, and vision and hearing deficits).
- A fetus exposed to maternal conditions such as hypertension, poor nutrition, anemia, or infectious disease is more likely to suffer from chronic conditions that affect health and well-being.
- Similarly, children exposed to unsafe environmental conditions, such as secondhand smoke or lead-based paint, are more likely to suffer from chronic conditions throughout childhood and, in some cases, through adolescence and adulthood.
- Children who do not receive preventive health care and do not obtain all necessary immunizations by their second birthday are more likely to suffer from preventable diseases or chronic conditions that could have been prevented or minimized and controlled.

The first year of life is the most hazardous until the age of 65. Therefore, it is particularly important for pregnant women to receive prenatal care and adopt healthy lifestyle choices and for infants to receive primary health care to maintain health and prevent or minimize serious, long-lasting health problems.

Infant Mortality

Infant mortality, the death of an infant during the first year of life, is a critical gauge of children's health status. It is an important marker because it is related to several factors, including maternal health, medical care quality and access, socioeconomic conditions, and public health practices. Infant mortality reflects the health and welfare of an entire community and is used as an indicator of worldwide health status. In that regard, the United States ranks poorly, lagging behind many nations, including Japan, Sweden, Spain, Hong Kong, Italy, France, and Canada (Table 14-1).

In the past century, the infant mortality rate in the United States has declined substantially (Figure 14-2). The 2003 infant death rate of 6.9 deaths per 1000 live births (Hoyert, Kung, and Smith, 2005) was the lowest infant mortality rate ever recorded in this country. The incidence of infant mortality has decreased largely because of public health measures and improved standard of living (e.g., improved sanitation, a clean milk supply, immunizations against deadly childhood diseases, the increased availability of nutritious food, and enhanced access to maternal health care). Technological advances in neonatal care, for example, the introduction of synthetic lung surfactant, have also contributed to reductions in infant mortality.

The three leading causes of infant death in the United States are congenital malformations, deformations, and chromosomal abnormalities; disorders relating to short gestation and unspecified low birth weight; and sudden infant death syndrome (SIDS) (Hoyert et al., 2005). These three conditions account for 45% of all infant deaths.

Socioeconomic factors play an important role in infant mortality. Infant mortality rates are higher for children whose

TABLE 14-1	International Comparisons of Infant Mortality Rates* (2004)	
RANK	**COUNTRY**	**RATE**
1	Singapore	2.3
2	Sweden	2.8
3	Hong Kong	3.0
4	Japan	3.3
5	Finland	3.6
6	Norway	3.7
7	Czech Republic	4.0
8	Germany	4.2
9	France	4.3
10	Switzerland	4.4
11	Spain	4.5
12	Denmark	4.6
13	Austria	4.7
14	Australia	4.8
14	Belgium	4.8
14	Canada	4.8
17	Netherlands	5.1
17	Portugal	5.1
19	United Kingdom	5.2
20	Greece	5.6
21	New Zealand	6.0
22	Italy	6.1
23	Cuba	6.5
24	**United States**	**6.6**
25	Poland	7.4
26	Slovakia	7.6
27	Hungary	8.7
28	Chile	9.1
29	Puerto Rico	9.4
30	Costa Rica	10.3

*Infant mortality rate represents infant deaths per 1000 live births.
From U.S. Census Bureau: *Infant mortality rates and deaths and life expectancy at birth by sex.* International Data Base, Table 010, The Author, http://www.census.gov/ipc/www/idbagg.html.

mothers receive late or no prenatal care, who are adolescents, who did not complete high school, who are unmarried, or who smoked during pregnancy (Matthews, Menaker, and McDorman, 2004).

Infancy is defined as the first year of life. Infant mortality consists of two components: neonatal mortality (death in the first 28 days of life) and postneonatal mortality (death occurring after 28 days of life but within the first year). In the United States, most infant deaths occur during the first month of life (the neonatal period). These deaths are largely attributable to infant health problems or problems with the pregnancy itself, such as preterm birth or birth defects. The leading cause of postneonatal death is SIDS (Box 14-1). Other causes of postneonatal death are birth defects, diseases and infection, homicide, poor medical care access, and accidents.

Although the overall infant mortality rate in the United States has steadily declined since the 1960s, troubling disparities persist between racial and ethnic populations. For example, black infants continue to die at twice the rate of white infants (Figure 14-3). Higher rates of low birth weight among African-American babies help to account for this disparity. Infant mortality rates are lowest for Asian and Pacific Islanders (4.8), followed by whites (5.8), Native Americans (8.6), and blacks (13.8).

Infant mortality rates vary considerably among Hispanic subgroups. For example, the Puerto Rican infant mortality rate is 8.2, whereas the Cuban rate is 3.7 (Matthews et al., 2004). Identifying and remedying the causes of higher infant mortality rates among certain population subgroups remains a vexing societal problem (Box 14-2).

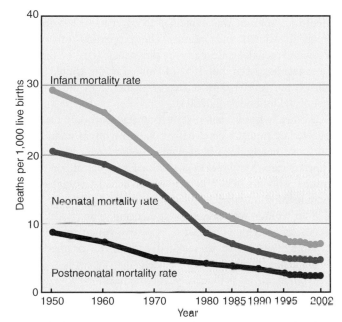

NOTES: Infant is defined as under 1 year of age, neonatal as under 28 days of age, and postneonatal as between 28 days and 1 year of age. See Data Table for data points graphed and additional notes.

SOURCE: Centers for Disease Control and Prevention, National Center for Health Statistics, National Vital Statistics System.

Figure 14-2 Infant mortality rates by decade from 1950 to 2000. (From Centers for Disease Control and Prevention, National Center for Health Statistics. National Vital Statistics System: *Infant mortality rates, fetal mortality rates, and perinatal mortality rates, according to race: United States, selected years 1950–99,* The Author, http://www.cdc.gov/nchs/data/hus/hus05.pdf.)

Preterm Birth and Low Birth Weight

Birth weight and length of gestation are the two most important predictors of an infant's health. About 1 in 8 infants born in the United States is born prematurely, and 1 in 13 is born at low birth weight (Hamilton, Martin, and Sutton, 2004). Alarmingly, both prematurity and low birth weight have been rising since the mid 1990s.

BOX 14-1 "Back to Sleep" Campaign

The rate of sudden infant death syndrome (SIDS) has dropped more than 40% since the advent of the 1992 public campaign "Back To Sleep" (American Academy of Pediatrics, 2000; Matthews et al., 2004; National Institute of Child Health and Human Development, 2005). This public education campaign, launched in 1994 by the National Institute of Child Health and Human Development, encourages caretakers of healthy infants, born full term, to place them on their backs for sleep and to learn other ways to prevent SIDS, including eliminating soft sleeping surfaces and loose bedding, overheating, and exposure to secondhand smoke. Despite dramatic reductions in the SIDS rate, there are still significant differences in the SIDS rates among racial and ethnic minorities. SIDS rates for non-Hispanic black and Native-American babies is over twice as high as for non-Hispanic white babies (Matthews et al., 2004). Reductions in the occurrence of SIDS, particularly among minority groups, would greatly lessen the overall infant mortality rate.

BOX 14-2 Sources of Vital Statistics Data for Children

Information concerning an infant's birth, including the mother's total prenatal care visits, the mother's name and father's name, and the infant's weight and birth date appear on a baby's birth certificate. Information concerning an infant's death, such as the cause(s), date, and other details appear on the death certificate. In each state, the vital statistics office in the state health department stores these certificates. This agency collects and regularly reports the aggregated data and forwards it to the National Center for Health Statistics. The National Center for Health Statistics collects, analyzes, and publishes numerous reports on the health and well-being of the nation's infants. These data sources are very important in tracking the health of infants and the health of other population groups; they help determine necessary interventions from various perspectives (e.g., clinical, public health, public policy, and environmental).

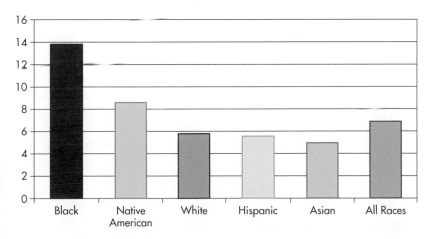

FIGURE 14-3 Infant mortality rates by race and Hispanic origin of mother, 2002. (From Matthews, TJ, Menaker F, McDorman MF: Infant mortality statistics from the 2002 period linked birth/infant death data set, *Natl Vital Stat Rep* 53(10), 2004, http://www.cdc.gov/nchs/pressroom/04facts/infant.htm.)

Infants born preterm (before 37 weeks' gestation) or at a low birth weight (less than 5.5 lb) have a far greater risk of death and physical and mental disabilities such as blindness, deafness, cerebral palsy, learning disabilities, and mental retardation than infants born at term with normal weight. Prematurity and low birth weight overlap. About half of preterm infants are born at low birth weight, but only two thirds of low-birth-weight babies are born prematurely. Babies born at term but at low birth weight are considered "growth-restricted."

Preterm birth is a complex disorder of pregnancy, the cause of which remains elusive despite many research efforts (Freda and Patterson, 2004). The most important risk factors are a history of preterm birth and having a multifetal gestation. A recent upswing in the rate of multiple births, stimulated in part by the rise in assistive reproductive technology (e.g., in vitro fertilization), has contributed to the rising preterm and low-birth-weight rates. Fewer than 1% of all live births result from assisted reproductive technology, yet this group accounts for one third of all twin births and 40% of all triplet and higher order births (Hogue, 2002).

Non-Hispanic black infants are disproportionately affected by preterm birth and low birth weight, and they are nearly twice as likely as white infants to be born at low birth weight (Hamilton et al., 2004). Factors associated with pre-term birth and low birth weight include the following:

- Minority status
- Maternal age of less than 17 years and over 35 years
- Chronic health problems such as diabetes mellitus, hypertension, and obesity
- Lack of prenatal care
- Low socioeconomic status
- Unhealthy maternal habits (e.g., poor nutrition, alcohol and drug use, and cigarette smoking)

The development of advanced life-support technologies for small infants has significantly improved the survival rate of low-birth-weight babies. Although technology can help to save tiny infants, preventing the occurrence of prematurity and low birth weight is a high priority for clinical and public health research and policy. Nurses can play important roles in preventing prematurity, through research, screening, counseling, education, referral, and implementation of interventions to reduce risk among target population groups (Freda and Patterson, 2004).

Prenatal Care

Obtaining early and regular **prenatal care** greatly enhances a woman's chance of delivering a healthy, full-term baby (Matthews et al., 2004). Prenatal care includes client education, risk identification, and monitoring and treatment of symptoms. It also includes referral to health, nutrition, and social service programs that can help a woman optimize her chances for a healthy pregnancy.

In addition to the important public health measures that improved the health of women and children early in the twentieth century, recent medical, public health, and public policy developments increased the availability of quality prenatal care. For example, in the past two decades, the

RESEARCH HIGHLIGHTS

Domestic Abuse and Infant Birth Weight

Medical records of almost 2000 women were reviewed to determine if domestic abuse and other factors during pregnancy affected infant birth weight. The researcher concluded that physical or psychological abuse had a small but significant effect on birth weight. Single marital status, smoking, less than 12 years of education, and low weight gain were also significantly associated with low birth weight of infants.

Kearney MH et al: Health behaviors as mediators for the effect of partner abuse on infant birth weight, *Nurs Res* 53(1):36-45, 2004.

Medicaid program was expanded to cover more low-income pregnant women and infants. The proportion of women receiving prenatal care early in pregnancy (i.e., in the first trimester) has risen, but 16% of women in the United States still do not receive prenatal care beginning in these first 3 months (Hamilton et al., 2004).

Women who do not receive prenatal care or those who receive late prenatal care, deliver babies with an infant mortality rate nearly 45% higher than mothers who receive first trimester care (Matthews et al., 2004). Examples of population groups who are less likely to receive early prenatal care include the following:

- Poor women who are under age 20 and unmarried
- African-American, Hispanic, or Native-American women
- Women who live in isolated rural areas or medically underserved urban areas
- Women with less than 12 years of education

Timely and comprehensive prenatal care increases the identification of specific and treatable causes of infant morbidity and mortality, such as maternal anemia, diabetes, hypertension, urinary tract infections, sexually transmitted diseases, and poor nutrition. Comprehensive prenatal care is particularly important for low-income women. It can help them obtain other services such as the Women, Infants, and Children (WIC) program, food stamps, smoking cessation, housing, child care, job training, substance abuse treatment, and domestic violence counseling.

Health education and counseling also are a part of comprehensive prenatal care and can provide women with the information they need to make lifestyle changes to help ensure a healthy pregnancy. Ideally, such counseling should begin before a woman becomes pregnant. This is known as **preconceptional counseling** (Box 14-3).

Prenatal Substance Use

Tobacco, alcohol, and illicit drug use are social factors that affect health. During pregnancy, substance use profoundly affects the neurological and physical development of the fetus. The use of these substances, in any combination, worsens infant health and development outcomes.

Smoking

The adverse health effects of tobacco use during pregnancy are well documented and include low birth weight, stillbirth, intrauterine growth retardation, preterm premature rupture

BOX 14-3 Preconceptional Counseling

Preconceptional counseling is a prevention strategy that helps women to identify potential risks to a fetus before pregnancy. Tiny developing fetal organ systems are highly vulnerable to the effects of maternal nutrition, drugs, alcohol, tobacco, chronic maternal diseases, environmental toxins, and other exposures. Preconception assessment encourages health and lifestyle modifications that can lead to healthier babies. Many pregnancies are unintended and the fetus can suffer damage before a woman knows she is pregnant; therefore all women capable of childbearing should have a source of regular medical care and adapt healthy lifestyles, for example consuming 0.4 mg of the B vitamin folic acid every day, even before conception, to decrease the likelihood of delivering a child with birth defects of the brain and spine, known as neural tube defects (Centers for Disease Control and Prevention, 1992). The Centers for Disease Control estimates that 50% to 70% of neural tube defects could be prevented if this recommendation were followed before and during early pregnancy.

of membranes, placenta previa, placental abruption, neuro-developmental impairment, and SIDS (Centers for Disease Control and Prevention [CDC], 2004a). The infant mortality rate for babies born to smokers is nearly 70% higher than the rate for nonsmokers (Matthews et al., 2004).

When a pregnant woman inhales cigarette smoke, the oxygen supply to her fetus is disrupted by nicotine and carbon monoxide (a lethal gas). Nicotine readily becomes concentrated in the breast milk of a smoking woman. During pregnancy, nicotine crosses the placenta and becomes concentrated in fetal blood and amniotic fluid. Nicotine concentrations in the fetus of a smoking woman can be as much as 15% higher than maternal levels. Secondhand smoke exposure also is dangerous to the fetus and newborn. It is linked to SIDS, decreased respiratory functioning, and childhood asthma (National Institute on Drug Abuse, 2001).

Eleven percent of women smoke during pregnancy (Hamilton et al., 2004). Smoking is far more common than alcohol and illicit drug use during pregnancy. Tobacco use varies by ethnic groups, ranging from 2.3% for Asian or Pacific Islanders to 18% for Native-American mothers.

The elimination of tobacco use among pregnant women would significantly reduce the percentage of low-birth-weight infants, preterm delivery, intrauterine growth restriction, and infant mortality. The need for widespread implementation of smoking cessation programs for women in the childbearing years is clear. Many smoking cessation programs have been developed and implemented by national, state, and local governments and organizations. *Treating Tobacco Use and Dependence* (Fiore et al., 2000) is an evidence-based, clinical practice guideline that helps clinicians counsel and advise clients about smoking cessation. Nurses can play a key role in reducing tobacco use in the United States.

Alcohol and Illicit Drug Use

The use of alcohol and illicit drugs is a major risk factor for poor infant outcomes. No level of alcohol intake has been determined to be safe during pregnancy. A fetus can be adversely affected by maternal alcohol consumption before its mother even knows she is pregnant. In 2005, the U.S. Surgeon General urged all women who are pregnant or who may become pregnant to abstain from alcohol (USDHHS, 2005c).

Alcohol use during pregnancy can lead to spontaneous abortion, low birth weight, and a cluster of congenital defects, including the nervous system dysfunction called **fetal alcohol syndrome (FAS)**. The spectrum of FAS ranges from mild subtle learning disabilities to severe learning disabilities, and may manifest with physical abnormalities, growth deficiencies, and central nervous system disorders.

An estimated 9% of pregnant women use alcohol during pregnancy; 3% of pregnant women report frequent or binge drinking (five or more drinks on the same occasion) (Office of Applied Studies, 2004b).

Like alcohol, illicit drugs can also cause permanent harm to an unborn baby. Approximately 3% of pregnant women aged 15 to 44 years used an illicit drug in the past month, according to the 2002 National Survey on Drug Use and Health. This compares to 9% of nonpregnant women in this age-group. Marijuana was the most commonly used illicit drug in both groups (Office of Applied Studies, 2004b).

Substance use is often a sign of more complex psychosocial problems such as depression, poverty, abuse, and violence. Because of serious potential risks to the developing fetus, women who are pregnant, or who could become pregnant (most pregnancies are not planned), should be counseled to abstain from alcohol and the use of illicit drugs. For those women who already use alcohol and drugs, a comprehensive and long-lasting approach to treatment is required.

CHILDHOOD HEALTH ISSUES

At all ages, appropriate and timely medical care plays an important role in children's health status. However, other factors, including parental influences, nutrition, environmental hazards, community safety, and the overall quality of home life, exert stronger influences over a child's well-being. Childhood is generally a healthy time of life, as evidenced by the improvement in many indicators of child health status over the past century. For example, the incidence of childhood disease has decreased because the majority of children receive a full complement of immunizations during infancy and toddlerhood.

The causes of childhood death vary with age. Parents and the community have important responsibilities in promoting healthy lifestyles, creating safe environments, and ensuring access to medical care. They must take steps to protect children from the leading threats to children's health (i.e., accidental injury and exposure to environmental toxins, abuse, and violence).

Accidental Injuries

After the first year of life, accidental injury (e.g., motor vehicle accidents, drowning, burning, and suffocation) is the leading cause of death in children. Motor vehicle accidents are the greatest danger to their life and health. Many injuries occur because adults fail to secure children in car seats or insist that older children buckle up. The most important step

This clinic provides services through the Early Periodic Screening Diagnostic Treatment (EPSDT) Program, which was developed to provide health care for children in low-income families.

Unfortunately, clinic schedules are often crowded and clients may not be able to get appointments for several weeks.

The nurse has an opportunity to observe the client and the family as they register and wait for their appointment. The parent registers the 5-year-old daughter for a school entry health physical. Medicaid insurance is verified for the physical examination.

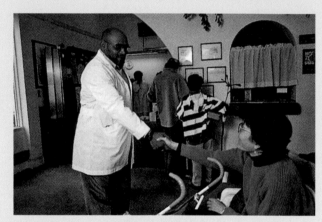

Introduction of the nurse to the client should include your name and role with the agency. It is important to address clients by their proper names and titles—Mr., Mrs., Ms.

The nurse understands the importance of developing a comfortable atmosphere by beginning with social talk and general questions about the client and family.

Trust can be established in a short period of time. The nurse can begin by explaining the steps in the clinic process so that the client knows what is expected. Always listen to the client attentively, and allow enough time for the client to reflect and respond to questions.

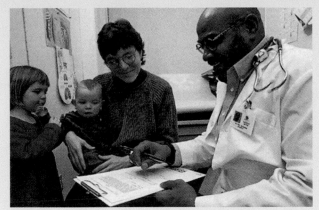

Asking an introductory question, such as "What brought you here today?", provides an open range of responses from the client. The parent's signature is required on a consent form in order for a physical examination and laboratory tests to be performed. The nurse explains the consent form to the parent.

The nurse interacts with the child to include her in the interview process. This provides an opportunity for the nurse to develop a clearer picture of the relationship between the child and parent. It will promote a smoother transition through the examination process.

As you move from one part of the history to another, it is helpful to orient the client with brief transitional phrases such as, "Now I would like to ask you some questions about…"

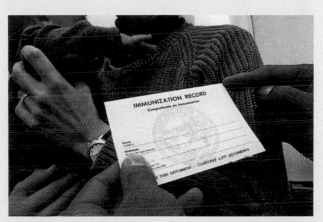

Reviewing immunization records is an important primary prevention role for the community health nurse. This is a teachable opportunity for the nurse to stress the importance of maintaining immunizations for the child. In California parents are provided with a yellow state immunization record for the child, which they should use for recording all immunizations and showing proof of immunizations when needed.

The child requires booster immunizations. The immunization consent forms are given to the parent for a signature. The nurse goes over the consent form with the parent and obtains a signature.

The clinic staff often take vital signs on clients, which include height and weight.

Blood pressure is taken for children 3 years and older.

A vision screen is first attempted on a 4-year-old child. If the child is younger, a verbal report is taken from the parent.

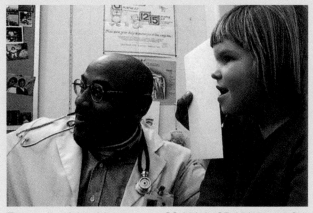

The results of the vision test are: OS:20/40; OD:20/50; and OU: 20/50.

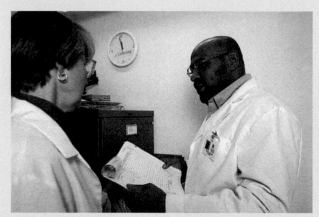

The nurse discusses any concerns about the client with the practitioner prior to the examination. The nurse reports the vision test results to the practitioner, as well as any other concerns the nurse may have about the family.

The practitioner performs the physical examination on the child with the help of the parent. The practitioner discusses the result of the vision test with the parent and the need for a follow-up appointment with ophthalmologist. The child has not had a lead level done and requires booster immunizations. The practitioner orders laboratory tests, immunizations, and a referral to an ophthalmologist.

The clinic staff perform the laboratory work: hematocrit, urinary analysis, and lead level. The immunization consent forms have been signed by the parent. The nurse administers the immunizations and takes this opportunity to reinforce the importance of immunizations for both children.

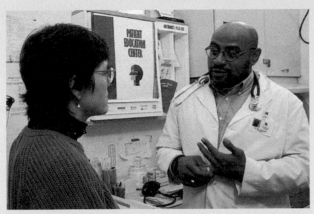

The nurse also offers suggestions to relieve the common side effects of immunizations.

The exit interview provides an opportunity for the nurse to review any issues the parent has raised about the child. The nurse may ask, "Is there anything else I can assist you with?"

The parent asks about an ophthalmologist who takes Medicaid and about day care facilities in the area for the younger child. The parent also asks about family planning services in the community.

The family agrees to maintain immunizations on the children and to follow-up with appointments with an ophthalmologist and a family planning clinic. The nurse returns the immunization record to the parent documenting today's immunization as well as when the next immunizations are due. The nurse will call with a referral for an ophthalmologist, a family planning clinic, and a day care facility.

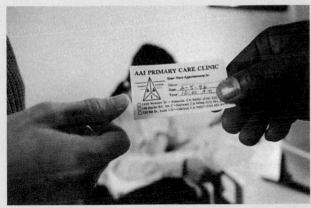

The nurse gives the parent a business card with the nurse's name and agency's address and phone number. The CHN advises the parent to call the nurse if there is anything else that the family may need.

The nurse charts accurately, clearly, and concisely after the clinic visit.

The nurse searches for resources for an ophthalmologist and a family planning clinic that accept Medicaid and a resource for day care providers. The nurse obtains phone numbers for a couple of ophthalmologists, a family planning clinic, and a day care consortium service.

The nurse calls the day care consortium and finds out that there is a list of day care providers available.

The nurse calls the family with the referrals for an ophthalmologist and a phone number to obtain a list of day care providers.

Story by Leonard Kaku, RN, MSN. Photography by George Draper.

that a parent can take to ensure a child's safety in a motor vehicle is to correctly secure them into car seats, or seat belts when they are older, for each ride. Restraint use by infants approaches 99%, but only 83% of 4- to 7-year-olds are properly restrained (Glassbrenner, 2003).

Head injury from cycling and other wheeled sports, such as skateboarding and inline skating, is another leading cause of child death and disability. Without proper head protection, a fall from as little as 2 feet can cause traumatic brain injury. Although the use of helmets can substantially reduce the risk of head injuries in biking accidents, a recent study revealed that only 41% of children regularly wear helmets. One third of those children wear helmets improperly, with helmets tilted or unsecured (Glassbrenner, 2003).

Other leading causes of accidental injury in children include pedestrian accidents, drowning, and burns. Box 14-4 discusses how toys can be another threat to small children.

Overweight

One in every seven children in America is overweight. The percentage of children who are overweight has increased more than threefold since the 1960s (USDHHS, 2003). Minority groups, those with less income, and those with lower education levels are more likely to be overweight (Strauss and Pollack, 2001).

Overweight in children is calculated based on growth charts, physical development, gender, and age. To avoid stigma, the terms *at-risk* and *overweight* are used rather than the term *obese* when referring to children and youth.

Being overweight in childhood can lead to type 2 diabetes and cardiovascular disease. Further, overweight adolescents are more likely to become overweight adults. Obesity in adulthood can lead to a number of health problems, including hypertension, coronary disease, diabetes, and gallbladder disease (USDHHS, 2003). Further, overweight children often

BOX 14-4   Toy-Related Injuries

Although most toys are safe, children are at risk from toy-related injuries and death. In 2002, an estimated 165,200 children under the age of 14 were treated in hospital emergency rooms for toy-related injuries (National Safe Kids Campaign, 2004). Although the majority of toy-related injuries are minor, permanent disability can occur. The leading cause of toy-related death is riding toys, both powered and unpowered.

Laws and regulations have been put into place to protect children from toy injuries. Examples include the Federal Hazardous Substances Act, which bans children's toys that contain any hazardous substance such as lead. The Child Safety Protection Act (PL 103-267, 1994) was designed to reduce toy-related choking and requires manufacturers to place choking hazard warning labels on balloons, marbles, small balls, and games with small parts intended for use only by children aged 3 and older. The Act also requires manufacturers, importers, distributors, and retailers to report choking incidents involving such products to the Consumer Product Safety Commission. The U.S. Department of Commerce requires toy guns to be distinguished from real guns. In addition, the toy industry has established voluntary safety standards to minimize risk of injury.

Although regulations and laws are helpful, parents and caretakers must also provide adequate supervision of children and adopt strategies recommended to prevent toy-related injuries. These include the following: use only age-appropriate toys; use Mylar balloons instead of latex (which can cause children to choke or suffocate); purchase a "small parts tester" to determine whether small toys pose choking hazards; check the Web site of the U.S. Consumer Product Safety Commission (www.cpsc.gov) to obtain information on toy recalls; never allow young children to play with toys with strings, straps, or cords longer than seven inches; follow age and safety recommendations on toy labels; and ensure that toys are used in a safe and proper environment.

Data from *National Safe Kids Campaign toy injury fact sheet*, Washington DC, 2004, http://www.safekidscharmeck.org/Safe%20Kids/Library/ToyFactSheet.pdf#search ='national%20safe%20kids%20campaign%20toy%20injury%20fact%20sheet'.

face social discrimination, which may lead to poor self-esteem and depression.

A number of factors have contributed to the increase of overweight in children. Two of the leading causes of overweight are a lack of physical activity and poor nutrition. Modern technologies such as electronic games, television, and readily accessible transportation have contributed to more sedentary lifestyles. The typical American diet, which is high in fat and calories and low in nutrients, has also led to an increase in overweight. Widely available fast food, increasing portion sizes, vending machines in schools, and fewer meals eaten at home have also contributed to the trend.

Nurses can play a leading role in generating public awareness, designing and implementing food and physical activities policies and standards in schools, and challenging policy makers and industry leaders such as fast food restaurants to mobilize resources for good nutrition and fitness.

Immunization

Childhood immunization is a benchmark of child health. Maintaining appropriate immunization protects all members of the community, especially immunocompromised individuals and pregnant women who are particularly vulnerable to certain infectious diseases. Adequate immunization pro-

tects children against several diseases that killed or disabled many children in the past. Polio, a crippling disease of the past, was eliminated in the United States thanks to the public health effort that made the polio vaccine accessible and affordable. Since this effort 50 years ago, children can now be protected from more than 14 vaccine-preventable diseases.

The national health objective for 2010 is to sustain at least 95% vaccination coverage among children kindergarten through first grade. It is estimated that coverage is approximately 90% overall, except for hepatitis B and varicella (CDC, 2004b). State laws requiring proof of vaccination before entry to school or child care has helped ensure high vaccination levels.

Despite positive overall vaccination rates, only one in three children is *age-appropriately* vaccinated. Factors associated with delay in vaccinations include having a mother who is unmarried or who does not have a college degree, living in a household with two or more children, being non-Hispanic black, and using public vaccination providers (Luman et al., 2005). Minimizing the time children are undervaccinated will help to prevent disease outbreaks.

The following vaccines are recommended for children and adolescents (CDC, 2005):

- Diphtheria
- Tetanus
- Pertussis
- Inactivated poliovirus
- Measles
- Mumps
- Rubella
- Hepatitis B
- Varicella
- Haemophilus influenzae type B (Hib)
- Influenza (for selected populations)
- Pneumococcal (for selected populations)
- Hepatitis A (for selected populations)
- Meningococcal (for selected populations)

Lead Poisoning

Lead poisoning is a preventable cause of childhood death, mental retardation, cognitive and behavioral problems, decreased growth, and neurological disabilities. The reduction of lead levels in both children and adults is among the greatest public health stories of the latter half of the twentieth century. Over the past three decades, lead has been removed from the manufacture of gasoline, household paint, food and drink cans, and plumbing systems. Public health, legislative, and commercial measures tremendously reduced the problem of lead poisoning in the United States (Meyer et al., 2003).

Unfortunately, lead is still a threat. The neurotoxic properties of lead have been apparent for at least a century, but the nature and extent of subtle long-term effects are newly realized. Unlike the obvious signs of measles or polio, it is difficult to recognize low-level lead poisoning in children. Lead poisoning affects virtually every system in the body and rarely yields distinctive symptoms.

Before 1950, lead-based paint was quite common, but the 1972 Lead Paint Poisoning Prevention Act limited the manufacture of lead-based paint. However, many millions of housing units in the United States still contain lead-based paint. Most of these units are located in poor, inner-city neighborhoods. Contamination can result from contact with paint dust or chips (e.g., raising and lowering windows) and from exposure to contaminated soil. Despite dramatic declines in blood lead levels for most U.S. populations, levels remain high among children in low-income families who live in older housing with lead-based paint. Black and Hispanic children are at greatest risk (Meyer et al., 2003).

Treatment for children with elevated lead levels is long, difficult, and carries risks. Better prevention, more efficient tracking, and reporting of children who receive public assistance are essential to further reduce the menace of lead poisoning.

Child Abuse and Neglect

Child abuse and neglect rates are other indicators of children's physical and emotional health status. *Neglect* is the failure to provide basic needs for children, such as food, shelter, education, medical care, and supervision. *Abuse* is the intentional injuring of a child. This includes hitting, punching, kicking, burning, or shaking a child so as to cause marks, bruising, or even death. Failure to provide affection, warmth, understanding, and supervision adequate for healthy development is *emotional abuse*. *Sexual abuse* refers to any sexual act with a child by an adult or older child.

Each week, child protective services agencies throughout the United States receive more than 55,000 reports of suspected child abuse or neglect. An estimated 900,000 children each year are victims of abuse or neglect (Children's Bureau, 2004). The majority of reports are from community professionals, illustrating the important role nurses play in protecting children's safety. The individuals most likely to report child abuse are professionals such as nurses, social service workers, and teachers. Many professionals, including nurses, are required by law to report child abuse.

Child abuse affects children of all races, ages, and ethnicities. Girls are slightly more likely to be victimized than boys, and children from birth to age 3 have the highest rate of victimization at 16.4 per 1000 children. Likewise, younger children (under age 4) account for three quarters of those killed (Children's Bureau, 2004).

Most often, the perpetrators of abuse and neglect are parents (Children's Bureau, 2004). The two dominant characteristics of abusive parents are a history of substance abuse and abuse from their own parents. Often, caretakers do not intend to hurt their children. They may be stressed by poverty, illness, or disability, and they may lack social support systems or coping skills. Young and inexperienced parents may not understand the physical, emotional, and behavioral needs of their children.

There are many long-term effects of abuse and neglect. The effects may be physical, such as brain damage in shaken baby syndrome; emotional, such as depression and low self-esteem; and behavioral, such as delinquency, poor academic achievement, and drug abuse. Community organizations must become more involved in preventing child abuse and creating a climate that supports families and provides alternatives to abusive behavior. Tragically, such services are in short supply in most communities.

Children With Special Health Care Needs

Children and youth with special health care needs are those who have a chronic physical, developmental, behavioral, or emotional condition that requires health and related services beyond those required by children generally. All children receiving special education and all children with mental disorders are included in this group. An estimated 13% of the U.S. population of children and youth have special health care needs (USDHHS, Health Resources and Services Administration, Maternal and Child Health Bureau, 2004).

Children with special health care needs frequently have multiple service needs, including public health, physical and mental health care, specialized diagnostic services, social services, and educational, vocational, and sometimes corrective services. Families trying to obtain care for children with special needs face challenges in trying to deal with differing eligibility criteria, duplication and gaps in services, inflexible funding sources, geographic cultural and financial barriers, and poor coordination of care.

Children with special needs can benefit from a coordinated, comprehensive, integrated system of care—often called a "medical home." A medical home is not a place, but rather an approach to providing care. Having a medical home strengthens the ability of children with multiple service needs to receive comprehensive care for complex conditions (Box 14-5).

ADOLESCENT HEALTH ISSUES

Adolescence is a time of generally good health. It is a period when adolescents form lifelong health habits, including dietary and exercise habits and emotional health skills such as problem-solving and coping strategies. Typically, adolescents do not use health services unless they have an underlying

---

BOX 14-5 The Medical Home

The American Academy of Pediatrics has long endorsed the concept of a "medical home." This ideal suggests that each child should have "accessible, continuous, comprehensive, family-centered, coordinated, and compassionate" health care (American Academy of Pediatrics, 2002). A medical home has the following characteristics: the provision of preventive care, the assurance of ambulatory and inpatient care 24 hours a day, strategies and mechanisms to ensure continuity of care from infancy through adolescence, and appropriate use of subspecialty consultation and referrals.

Experts recommend that a health care provider should consistently examine children eight times during their first year, three times during their second year, and once a year until age 6. This allows children and parents to build trusting relationships with their health care providers and enables providers to monitor growth and development.

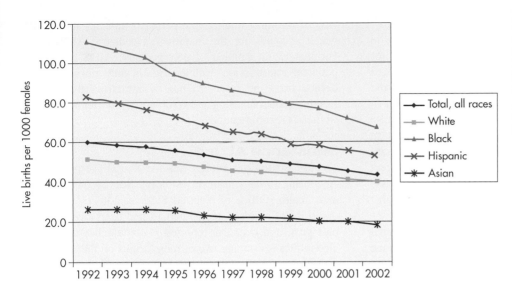

FIGURE 14-4 Adolescent births ages 15-19, by race and Hispanic origin of mother, 1992-2002. (From Federal Interagency Forum on Child and Family Statistics: *Adolescent births: birth rates by mother's age, race, and Hispanic origin*, Childstats Table HEALTH9, http://www.childstats.gov/ac2004/tables/Health9.asp.)

chronic condition or an acute illness. They rarely use preventive health services.

In their struggle to gain independence and with their sense of immortality, many adolescents engage in risk-taking behaviors that threaten their health, including alcohol and drug abuse, early and unprotected sexual activity, unsafe driving, and participation in delinquent and violent activities. The leading cause of death for those aged 15 to 24 years is unintentional injury. For every ethnic and racial group except non-Hispanic blacks, the leading cause of unintentional injury is motor vehicles. Among non-Hispanic blacks, the leading cause of unintentional injury is firearms (Childstats, 2004).

The health threats that adolescents face at the beginning of the twenty-first century are very different from those that threatened the health of this age-group only a generation or two ago. The community health nurse can help parents and communities understand the nonmedical, public health nature of these morbidities and assist in developing community-wide strategies to effectively deal with them.

Adolescent Pregnancy and Childbearing

Giving birth at an early age can have negative consequences for both teenagers and their babies. Fortunately, the teen birth rate has shown a steady decline for the past decade; however, **adolescent pregnancy** is a persistent and troubling problem (Figure 14-4). In the United States, nearly a quarter of a million girls and women under age 20 become pregnant each year. Latinas and black Americans have higher teen pregnancy rates than their white counterparts (Hamilton et al., 2004).

One of the many risk-taking adolescent behaviors is sexual intercourse among unmarried teenagers. Adolescent sexual activity is often unprotected and can result in pregnancy and sexually transmitted diseases (STDs). Several factors predispose a child to engage in sexual activity in the teen years. Twenty-nine percent of teens aged 15 to 17 report feeling pressure to have sex, and nearly 10% of 9th- through 12th-

grade students report having been physically forced into having sexual intercourse against their wishes (Kaiser Family Foundation, 2003). Many teens have limited access to reproductive health care counseling. This may be influenced by insurance coverage, transportation issues, and the ability to seek certain services without parental consent in certain states (Huck-Long et al., 2003).

The consequences of early childbearing are significant. Teen childbearing poses serious health risks to the infant, including death, prematurity, low birth weight, abuse, and neglect. Researchers disagree on the causes of poor pregnancy outcomes among teenagers, but most agree on the importance of socioeconomic factors associated with young age, such as lack of education, low income, and inadequate prenatal care, than biological factors.

Adolescent childbearing and parenting often have long-term, negative consequences for both child and mother. Children born to teenage parents are more likely to have poor health, are less likely to complete high school, and are more likely to end up on welfare (Annie E. Casey Foundation, 2000).

The causes and effects of teen pregnancy are complex, and the solutions are multifaceted. Primary prevention models are most successful when tailored to the community's individual needs. Components of such programs can include the following:

- Abstinence promotion
- Education about contraception and its availability
- Sexual education
- Character development
- Problem-solving skill development
- Strategies for ensuring teenagers' school success
- Job training

Such efforts benefit from partnerships between parents, adolescents, and agencies for health, education, religion, social service, and government. Nurses working within such organizations can play leadership roles in developing community programs for adolescent pregnancy prevention.

Violence

A decline in the level of violence affecting adolescents in recent years is a positive public health trend. However, for too many of the nation's youth, violence is a way of life, a way of coping with challenging and difficult situations, and a significant public health problem. Nearly 13 children in America die each day from gunfire (Children's Defense Fund, 2000). Although violence is most predominant in inner cities, adolescents in suburbs and rural areas are increasingly faced with violence and its direct and indirect impact on the entire community. African-American youths are at the greatest risk for homicides, suicides, and firearm accidents (Bureau of Justice Statistics, 2002).

Violence among youth is a multifaceted problem. Social factors, such as unemployment and poverty, strongly influence the risk of violent behavior exposure. Violence in the home, in the media, and in the community; gun ownership; and child abuse, violence, or severe corporal punishment may socialize youth to viewing violence as an expected and unavoidable part of life.

Handguns are readily accessible to America's youth. Federal law prohibits anyone under age 21 from purchasing a handgun from a licensed dealer, but it does not prohibit anyone under age 21 from purchasing a handgun from a non-licensed dealer. Teen violence does not have simple remedies. Solutions require community and neighborhood efforts to help young people diffuse anger and frustrations before they escalate; help parents, religious organizations, and schools assist their youth in managing anger and resolving conflicts; and work with children and teenagers to assure them that they are loved, appreciated, and accepted for who they are and that help is available. Reducing children's unsupervised exposure to guns, engaging communities in strengthening law enforcement, modifying the design of guns, and limiting the flow of illegal guns to youth are also strategies to reduce youth gun violence (Reich, 2002).

Sexually Transmitted Diseases

Sexually transmitted diseases (STDs) include AIDS, hepatitis B, chlamydia, gonorrhea, syphilis, genital herpes, genital warts, vaginal trichomoniasis, and other vaginal infections. Compared to adults, teenagers are more likely to acquire STDs. For some infections, for example, chlamydia trachomatis, this may be due to a physiological susceptibility. Barriers to health care such as lack of transportation, concerns about confidentiality, and lack of access to preventive health services also contribute to a higher prevalence of STDs among teens (CDC, 2003).

Although most STDs are treatable with antibiotics, they can have long-term health consequences. For women, untreated STDs can lead to pelvic inflammatory disease, ectopic pregnancy, cervical cancer, and infertility. Young men infected with STDs do not suffer the same health consequences as women because male symptoms typically appear earlier than female symptoms; thus men can obtain early treatment.

Not only is a woman's health affected, especially if the infections go untreated, but infants born to women with STDs are at risk of infection and can suffer long-term consequences.

One of the most tragic is the perinatal transmission of HIV, which accounts for the majority of pediatric AIDS cases. Fortunately, the number of new pediatric AIDS cases from perinatal transmission declined significantly during the last decade from the increased use of antiretroviral treatment. Routine HIV counseling and voluntary testing for all pregnant women is recommended.

Substance Abuse

Alcohol is the drug adolescents use and abuse most often. According to data from the National Survey on Drug Use and Health (Office of Applied Studies, 2004a), more than one third of children aged 12 to 17 had used alcohol in the past year, and over 2% reported *heavy* alcohol use. Heavy alcohol use is drinking five or more drinks on the same occasion on each of 5 or more days in the past 30 days. Children reporting heavy alcohol use were more likely to have engaged in delinquent behaviors, such as getting into a serious fight, attacking someone with the intent to seriously hurt them, trying to steal more than $50, selling illegal drugs, or carrying a handgun. Teenage alcohol use is strongly associated with a number of health risks, including early and unprotected sex, tobacco use, violence, and traffic fatalities (Ellickson, Tucker, and Klein, 2003).

Likewise, *tobacco* use is a prevalent and dangerous problem among adolescents. Smoking can lead to lung disease and cancer. About 25% of high school seniors report smoking within the past 30 days (O'Malley, Bachman, and Schulenberg, 2005). Smoking rates among teens have declined since peaking in the mid 1990s, but the rate of decline has decelerated sharply in recent years.

Illicit drug use by youths has also declined in recent years, but concerns remain, particularly about an upswing in the use of painkillers and inhalants. Illicit drugs include marijuana/hashish, cocaine (including crack), heroin, hallucinogens (including LSD and PCP), inhalants, or any prescription-type psychotherapeutic used non-medically. Among youths aged 12 to 17, an estimated 11.2% are current illicit drug users. The most commonly used drug is marijuana (Office of Applied Studies, 2004a). Participation in some community activities (e.g., team sports) is associated with a lower risk of illicit drug use (Office of Applied Studies, 2002). Participation in school-based, community-based, and church or faith-based activities lowers the risk of alcohol, tobacco, and illicit drug use (Office of Applied Studies, 2004a).

FACTORS AFFECTING CHILD AND ADOLESCENT HEALTH

Like all age-groups, social, non-medical factors largely determine children's health. Children are dependent on their families or caregivers for health and well-being; therefore the following factors significantly impact children's physical and mental health and overall well-being:

- Parents' or caregivers' education, income, and stability
- Security and safety of the home
- Nutritional and environmental issues
- Health care use

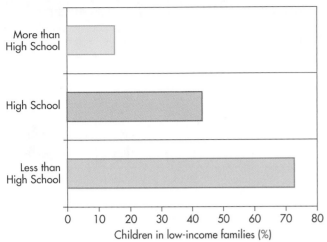

Figure 14-5 Effect of parental education on income (2004). (From National Center for Children in Poverty: *The effects of parental education on income,* New York, 2004, Columbia University, Mailman School of Public Health, http://www.nccp.org/pub_pei04.html.)

Poverty

Poverty is the greatest threat to child health. Child poverty in the United States is higher than in most other industrialized countries, including Canada and most western European countries (Children's Defense Fund, 2004). Nearly 13 million of the nation's children, more than one in six, live below the poverty threshold (i.e., the federal poverty level), which was $19,350 for a family of four in 2005 (USDHHS, 2005a). Research suggests that even to meet basic needs, families need an income equal to about two times the federal poverty level (Bernstein, Brocht, and Spade-Aguilar, 2000).

Children are far more likely than adults to live in poverty. Young children are more likely than older children to live in low-income families. Children who are poor are most likely to be white, non-Hispanic, to live in suburban or rural areas, and to live in a household where someone worked full- or part-time at least part of the year (Children's Defense Fund, 2004).

Parental education plays a key role in child poverty (Figure 14-5). Eighty-two percent of children whose parents do not have a high school education live in low-income families. Even if parents have full-time employment, low education levels make their children susceptible to poverty (National Center for Children in Poverty, 2004).

Poverty alone does not always place a child at risk; children in higher income groups can also suffer similar health and related problems. However, poor children face the following health and socioeconomic risks that can compound the burdensome influence of poverty (Center for the Future of Children, 1997):

- Children in poverty have less access to nutritious food, shelter, and health care.
- Poor children are often deprived of advantages such as good schools, libraries, and other community resources.
- Deaths from unintended injuries, child abuse, homicide, STDs, and infectious diseases (including AIDS) are more common among poor children.

- Many poor children live in substandard housing, have stressful home lives, may live surrounded by drugs and crime, and lack positive and nurturing adult role models.
- Poor children may feel hopeless about the future.
- Poor children often suffer from low birth weight, asthma, dental decay, elevated blood lead levels, learning disabilities, and teenage unmarried childbearing.
- Poor children are more likely to move frequently. Residential instability and extreme living conditions of poor children who are homeless or migrants usually compound their health problems.

These social and economic burdens can be overwhelming to parents or caregivers and may cause them to neglect other matters, such as providing a nutritious breakfast before school, taking a child for a well-child appointment, or getting his or her immunizations completed on schedule. They can create a sense of despair and hopelessness among parents and children, which greatly hinders healthy behavior. These factors clearly increase a child's physical and emotional health risks.

Racial Disparities

Although children in the United States are healthier now than in any other time in our nation's history, overall improvements in health mask the poor health of some racial and ethnic subgroups. For example, the infant mortality rate has plunged over the past century, yet babies born to black mothers are twice as likely as babies born to white mothers to die in the first year of life and to be born prematurely. Native Americans and African Americans account for a disproportionate share of deaths due to FAS. African-American and Hispanic mothers are less likely than white mothers to enter prenatal care early or to breast-feed their babies. African-American youth are at high risk for gun violence. Disparities also exist *within* ethnic groups. For example, U.S.-born women of Mexican decent have a higher risk of poor pregnancy outcomes than do immigrant Mexican women (Cervantes, Keith, and Wyshak, 1999).

Eliminating health disparities is an important national health priority. *Healthy People 2010* targets persistent differences in health among children of varying racial and ethnic groups and calls for the elimination of social disparities in health. The root causes underlying these disparities are complex, but several factors appear to contribute to the problem. These include systemic inequities in the health care system, for example, lack of health insurance and access to quality care, poverty, and lack of education (Egerter et al., 2004; Smedley, Stith, and Nelson, 2002). A recent study showed, for example, that the race/ethnicity of children significantly influenced their wait time in emergency departments. Hispanic white children waited 18% longer than did non-Hispanic white children. Non-Hispanic black children waited 6% longer than non-Hispanic white children (James, Bourgeois, and Shannon, 2005).

Cultural and linguistic barriers also pose challenges. For example, African Americans, Asian Americans, and Hispanics are more likely than whites to experience difficulty communicating with their physician and to feel like they are treated with disrespect (Collins et al., 2002). Bias, stereotyping, and prejudice contribute to disparities in health care (Smedley et al., 2002).

Providing health care services that are culturally competent will help make care more acceptable to all races and cultures (Beach, Price, and Gary, 2005). **Cultural competence** requires that services and assistance are provided in a manner that demonstrates respect for individual dignity, personal preferences, and cultural differences. Nurses can develop the skills needed to provide culturally competent care by learning how to perform cultural assessments, cultural interpretation, culturally appropriate interventions, and cross-cultural communication (Moore and Moos, 2003). Many resources are available to help nurses understand the perspectives of various cultures, including the March of Dimes module, *Cultural Competence in the Care of Childbearing Families* (Moore and Moos, 2003), and the USDHHS's *The Provider's Guide to Quality and Culture* (Bureau of Primary Health Care, 2002).

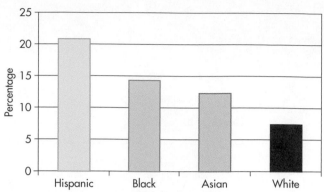

Figure 14-6   Children lacking health insurance by race and origin of mother, 2003. (From DeNavas-Walt C, Proctor BD, Mills RJ: *Income, poverty, and health insurance coverage in the United States: 2003,* Current Population Reports P60-226, August 2004, US Bureau of the Census, http://www.census.gov/prod/2004pubs/p60-226.pdf.)

Single Parenting

Family structure is associated with child well-being. Generally speaking, children living in households with two married parents fare better economically, socially, and academically (Biblarz and Rafferty, 1999). The number of children living in households headed by single parents has increased since 1975. Approximately 32% of children do not live with two, married parents (Mills and Bhandari, 2003). Children in households headed by a single parent (usually the mother) are far more likely to live in poverty.

Parents' Educational Status

Children's health is also tied closely to their parents' education level. About 15% of U.S. children have a parent who has not received a high school diploma (Childstats, 2005). Low birth weight and infant mortality are more common in the children of less educated mothers. Women with higher education are more likely to obtain prenatal care, delay childbearing until after adolescence, and breast-feed their babies. Women with less than 12 years of education are almost 10 times more likely to smoke during pregnancy than mothers with 16 years of education.

Health Care Use

Children grow and develop rapidly between infancy and adolescence; therefore they are extremely vulnerable to the effects of illness and environmental factors that influence physical and emotional health. Preventive health and dental care offers children and parents a chance to periodically meet with a health care provider to do the following:

- Discuss the child's physical and emotional growth and development.
- Learn about good nutrition.
- Address safety issues, such as the use of car seats.
- Receive immunizations and vision and hearing screening.
- Learn about potential environmental threats to the child's health.
- Begin prompt treatment for a condition discovered during the examination.
- Ask other questions or obtain a referral if necessary.

Access to a regular health care source can facilitate prompt attention to acute medical problems, which can help prevent chronic, disabling conditions. For example, untreated ear infections can lead to hearing loss, which can lead to learning disabilities, school problems, and even school dropout. Resulting low self-esteem can increase the likelihood of depression, behavior problems, early sexual activity, STDs, and unplanned pregnancy. Comprehensive, regular health care helps all children achieve their potential (Box 14-5).

Health Insurance Coverage

Approximately 11% of American children under the age of 18 do not have health insurance. Hispanic children are far more likely than children of other races to be uninsured (Mills and Bhandari, 2003) (Figure 14-6). Children who do not have health insurance are more likely to lack a source of health care, to have unmet health needs, and to experience worse health outcomes than children with insurance (Kaiser Family Foundation, 2002). Although most children are insured as dependents through their parent's workplace, an increasing number of children are losing this coverage. The cost of health insurance has risen over the years, and an increasing number of employers are no longer offering coverage for employees or their dependents. This is a more prevalent problem in small businesses and in businesses with mostly low-wage earners.

Medicaid (Title XIX of the Social Security Act) is a health insurance program for poor and low-income people. It is a federal/state entitlement program that plays an important role in providing health insurance for low-income women and children. Initiated in 1965, it is the largest source of funding for medical and health-related services for America's poor. It covers more than one in four children (U.S. Census Bureau, 2004) and pays for nearly 40% of all births in the United States (Cornell, 2003).

Within broad national guidelines, each state establishes eligibility standards, determines the type and scope of services, and administers its own Medicaid program. States have some discretion in determining which population groups their program will cover. A pregnant woman or child who is eligible for the program in one state may not be eligible in another. Under federal guidelines, however, states must cover pregnancy-related services to pregnant women whose family income is at or below 133% of the federal poverty level and health coverage to children under the age of 6 whose family income is at or below 133% of poverty.

Families who earn too much to qualify for Medicaid may be able to qualify for the **State Children's Health Insurance Program (SCHIP),** a publicly subsidized health insurance program for children. This program was formed in 1997 to help close the gap between higher income and lower income families whose children need insurance.

Expansions in public health care insurance programs have helped many children achieve insurance coverage, but many children still lack insurance or other health care coverage like Medicaid or SCHIP for many reasons. Some of these include the following:

- It is too expensive.
- Medicaid has a welfare stigma, and parents do not want to be associated with it.
- Medicaid application forms and processes are complex, burdensome, and can intrude upon a family's privacy.
- Parents may be concerned that their illegal immigration status may be revealed.
- Parents may not consider the importance of health insurance.
- Parents may not know their child is eligible for programs such as Medicaid or SCHIP.
- Applications and other information may not be available in the family's language.

Although insurance gives a child financial access to health care, some children may not obtain the health care they need. Numerous health care or family barriers can still stand in the way. These may include the following:

- Lack of transportation
- Language barriers
- Misunderstanding or denial of the child's health problem
- Clinic or office hours that conflict with work or school schedules
- Overcrowded clinics with long delays in securing an appointment
- Long delays in the waiting room (and parents often have more than one child in tow)
- Competing family or personal priorities that reduce the importance of obtaining care
- Some doctors' unwillingness to see Medicaid or low-income clients
- Parents' concerns that care providers are either unresponsive to their medical needs or interpersonally disrespectful
- Cost of deductibles or co-payments

To successfully meet the health needs of children and adolescents, especially those with known risk factors, the community health nurse must be cognizant of health care access issues, family and neighborhood influences, and other social concerns in a child's life. The nurse must be

prepared to help the family solve problems, be their health care system advocate, and address the child's health needs in a culturally competent manner.

RESOURCES: Monitoring the Health and Well-Being of Children

Centers for Disease Control and Prevention (CDC). Monitors many health and disease prevention efforts, including the Youth Risk Behavior Surveillance System, which monitors youth tobacco, alcohol, and drug use; dietary behaviors; and sexual behaviors contributing to unintended pregnancy and sexually transmitted infections. http://www.cdc.gov.

Federal Interagency Forum on Child and Family Statistics. On an annual basis, produces *America's Children: Key National Indicators of Well-Being*, a report that includes detailed information on a set of key indicators of child well-being. http://www.childstats.gov.

National Center for Education Statistics (NCES). The primary federal agency for collecting and analyzing data related to education in the United States. http://www.nces.ed.gov.

National Center for Health Statistics (NCHS). Provides birth and death data, including birth certificate information. http://www.cdc.gov/nchs.

U.S. Bureau of Justice. Collects information about juvenile offenders. http://www.ojp.usdoj.gov/bjs.

U.S. Bureau of Labor Statistics. Provides a variety of employment data. http://www.bls.gov

U.S. Census Bureau. Provides current census figures and analysis. http://www.census.gov

U.S. Department of Health and Human Services (USDHHS). *Healthy People 2010* provides a framework of goals and objectives for the nation's health. http://www.healthypeople.gov.

U.S. Department of Health and Human Services (USDHHS). *Trends in the Well-Being of America's Children and Youth* monitors trends in the well-being of the nation's children on a yearly basis. http://aspe.hhs.gov/search/hsp/03trends.

STRATEGIES TO IMPROVE CHILD AND ADOLESCENT HEALTH

One of the most important ways to ensure the success and well-being of future generations is for each child to start life healthy and maintain their physical and emotional health status throughout childhood and adolescence. Since the beginning of the twentieth century, the nation has made remarkable progress in many areas of child and adolescent health, but the results are mixed. Fortunately, scientific, medical, environmental, parenting, and other knowledge can lessen or eliminate many of the problems. It is a matter of making these concerns a priority and taking the necessary steps to elicit change.

Monitoring and Tracking

The federal, state, and local governments and many national organizations collect and analyze data tracking the well-being of children. For example, the USDHHS (2003) generates a yearly report on more than 80 indicators of the well-being of America's children and youth. Such data are readily accessible online to citizens, health professionals, policy makers, and the

HEALTHY PEOPLE 2010 | Objectives for Child and Adolescent Health

Objective	Baseline (1998)	% Target
1-4b: Increase the proportion of children and youth aged 17 years and under who have a specific source of ongoing care.	93%	96%
8-11: Eliminate elevated blood lead levels in children.	4.5% of children aged one to five years	0
9-7: Reduce pregnancies among adolescent females.	72 per 1000 females aged 15 to 17 years	46 per 1000 females aged 15 to 17 years
9-8a: Increase the proportion of adolescent females who have never engaged in sexual intercourse before age 15 years.	81%	88%
13-17: Reduce new case of perinatally acquired HIV infection.	NA	NA
14-4: Reduce bacterial meningitis in young children.	13.0 per 100,000	8.6 per 100,000
14-22a: Achieve and maintain effective vaccination coverage levels for universally recommended vaccines among young children (i.e., four doses of Dtap vaccine)	84%	90%
15-20: Increase use of children restraints.	92%	100%
15-39: Reduce weapon carrying by adolescent on school property.	8.5%	6%
16-1a: Reduce fetal and infant deaths during perinatal period (i.e., 28 weeks of gestation to seven days or more after birth).	7.5 per 1000	4.5 per 1000
16-15: Reduce the occurrence of spina bifida and other NTDs.	6 per 10,000 live births	3 per 10,000 live births
18-2: Reduce the rate of suicide attempts by adolescents.	2.6% per year	1% per year
19-3a: Reduce the proportion of children aged 6 to 11 years who are overweight or obese.	11%	5%
21-1b: Reduce the proportion of children with dental caries experienced either in their primary or permanent teeth.	52%	42%
22-11: Increase the proportion of children and adolescents who view television two or fewer hours per day.	60%	75%
24-2a: Reduce hospitalizations for asthma in children under age five years.	60.9 per 10,000	825 per 10,000
26-10: Reduce past-month use illicit substances by adolescents aged 12 to 17.	77%	89%
27-2a: Reduce tobacco use by adolescents in grades 9 to 12.	43%	21%
28-12: Reduce otitis media in children and adolescents.	344.7 visits per 1000	294 visits per 1000

From US Department of Health and Human Services: *Healthy people 2010: conference edition*, Washington, DC, 2000, USDHHS.

media. A number of key indicators are tracked on a regular basis by the federal statistical system so that trends are revealed. State and local data also are used to track the well-being of children.

Healthy People 2010: Child and Adolescent Health

Many professions establish goals and set measurable objectives. Educators use these techniques to organize their teaching materials, measure their students' progress, and evaluate the effectiveness of their teaching strategies and plans. Health care professionals use them for similar purposes in client care. The individual community health nurse uses them in working with a family to ensure the nurse and family are organized and guided by common purposes. Goals and objectives help the nurse and family evaluate progress and make necessary mid-course corrections.

These strategies are also important at the macro level and the programmatic level, where multiple players must col-laborate to address complicated statewide or nationwide problems. In 1979, the Surgeon General of the United States embarked on an ambitious task of convening hundreds of public health experts, health care researchers, health professional organizations, and others to develop the first health goals and objectives for the nation. At each of the intervening decades, these groups have developed a new set of goals and objectives to help bring clear focus to the health concerns of the nation and to set measurable and attainable goals for different age-groups and issues across the country.

Healthy People 2010 (USDHHS, 2000) sets broad national health goals for the first decade of the twenty-first century. This initiative, like its predecessors, helps define the nation's health agenda and guide policy development. *Healthy People 2010* addresses many challenges facing the country and will help the public and private sectors understand the nation's leading health problems, develop strategic plans for addressing them, and collaborate to reach common goals. The *Healthy People* table lists selected objectives from *Healthy People 2010* related to child and adolescent health.

Since the inception of the *Healthy People* initiative in 1979, child and adolescent health has improved. For instance, there have been improvements in infant, child, and adolescent mortality, use of prenatal care, adolescent smoking, pregnancy, and violence.

Health Promotion and Disease Prevention

Health promotion and disease prevention are more significant and cost effective for children than for any other age-group. Primary health care and early intervention for children and families can help prevent costly problems, suffering, and lost human potential. The following examples illustrate this need:

- The average hospital charge for a healthy newborn is $1500. For newborns with the primary diagnosis of prematurity, the average cost is $79,000 (March of Dimes Perinatal Data Center, 2002). The costs do not end there. Infants who are born prematurely are more likely than healthy full-term infants to need specialized services for chronic conditions such as cerebral palsy, blindness, and learning disabilities (Hack et al., 2002). Children born prematurely tend to have lower test scores and more behavioral problems than their full-term counterparts (Bhutta et al., 2002).
- Preventing pregnancy among teenagers can reduce the dropout rate, welfare dependency, low birth weight, and infant mortality. It has been estimated that teen child-bearing costs taxpayers at least $7 billion every year in expenses associated with health and foster care, criminal justice, and public assistance (National Campaign to Prevent Teen Pregnancy, 2001).

Health promotion and disease prevention strategies for improving child and adolescent health come in many forms and originate in research institutions, public agencies, private businesses, and community-based organizations. They can include the following:

- Clinical interventions
- Public health efforts that identify trends and develop population-based, community-wide, or individual strategies to affect these trends
- Philanthropic endeavors that fund initiatives at the community, state, and regional levels for the purpose of testing a strategy or establishing an initiative
- Public policy initiatives that create or improve public programs or provide incentives for non-governmental entities to address identified problems

PUBLIC HEALTH PROGRAMS TARGETED TO CHILDREN AND ADOLESCENTS

A number of public programs address the health needs of children, and many help medically underserved or low-income individuals specifically. In addition, local and state public health and social service agencies aim to protect the health of an entire community or state through programs such as water fluoridation, sanitation, and infectious disease control. Furthermore, broad-based strategies such as lead-based paint elimination, mandatory child safety seats in automobiles, bicycle helmet laws, teen pregnancy prevention programs, comprehensive school health clinics, and drug and violence prevention programs serve to improve the health of children through community-wide approaches.

Health Care Coverage Programs
Medicaid

The ability to pay for health care greatly influences whether a parent takes a child to see a health care provider. This is especially true for preventive care. Access to health care services has significantly improved since the introduction of Medicaid and the **Early and Periodic Screening, Diagnosis, and Treatment (EPSDT)** program in the mid 1960s. State and federal governments jointly finance Medicaid. Medicaid pays for health care services delivered to eligible individuals (i.e., primarily those receiving welfare payments) under the age of 21. In the late 1980s, Congress and states passed legislation that expanded Medicaid eligibility for pregnant women, infants, and children in higher income groups in an effort to improve the nation's infant mortality rate and children's health status.

Over the years, Medicaid has become a primary payer for prenatal care and deliveries. Across the states, Medicaid now pays for 40% of all births (Cornell, 2003) and covers close to 25% of all children under age 18 (U.S. Census Bureau, 2004).

Through the EPSDT program, a child covered by Medicaid can receive a range of health and health-related services beginning in infancy. The program is designed to assure availability and accessibility of health care resources and to help Medicaid recipients and their parents effectively use these resources. The program's services far exceed those usually covered by private insurance and include the following:

- Health, developmental, and nutritional screening
- Physical examinations
- Immunizations
- Vision and hearing screening
- Certain laboratory tests
- Dental services

Not all Medicaid-eligible children are enrolled in the program. The families, the Medicaid application and enrollment process, or the health care system present many barriers. These barriers are similar to those discussed earlier concerning insurance coverage.

State Children's Health Insurance Program SCHIP

Again, Medicaid does not cover all poor children, nor does it cover children in the "gap group," (i.e., children whose family income is above Medicaid limits but whose families do not receive health insurance through the parents' employment). This population group is often called the working poor. How to insure the uninsured has been a perplexing public policy issue for years. However, in August 1997, Congress passed the State Children's Health Insurance Program (SCHIP) into law with the support of the President, states, countless organizations, advocacy groups, individuals, and others in an effort to solve this problem for children in working poor families. This program is the single largest public investment in children's health since the creation of the Medicaid program. SCHIP gives each state permission to offer health insurance to children up to the age of 19 who are not already insured. Each state sets its own guidelines regarding services and eligibility.

Direct Health Care Delivery Programs

Although Medicaid and SCHIP finance health care for their enrollees like private insurance, several other public programs deliver health care services directly to underserved populations. Most underserved aggregates live in inner cities or rural areas with few health care providers and facilities. Some have Medicaid, SCHIP, or insurance coverage, but many are uninsured.

Maternal and Child Health Block Grant

The Maternal and Child Health Block Grant (also called Title V, because it is the fifth section, or title, of the Social Security Act) provides funds to the states for maternal and child health care. The Maternal and Child Health Block Grant program allocates federal funds to the states, and the states must contribute their own funds. It is administered by the Maternal and Child Health Bureau as a part of the Health Resources and Services Administration, U.S. Department of Health and Human Services.

The Block Grant Program has three components: Formula Block Grants to States and Other Jurisdictions, Special Projects of Regional and National Significance, and Community Integrated Service Systems Grants. In most states, these resources are combined with local funding to help ensure the delivery of basic health care to pregnant women and children and help deliver additional services to children with special health care needs. Title V agencies in state health departments also monitor the health status of mothers and children throughout their respective states and work with other state agencies to develop programs to improve the health of this population.

Healthy Start Initiative

The Healthy Start Initiative is a series of demonstration programs initiated in 1991 by the Health Resources and Services Administration of the U.S. Public Health Service. The goal was to improve maternal and infant health (especially in high-risk populations) and to reduce infant mortality by 50%. It is administered by the Maternal and Child Health Bureau.

Grantees are awarded funding based on their assessment of local needs, efforts to increase public awareness, implementation of an infant mortality review, community involvement, design of innovative health and social services programs, and evaluation methods. Grantees are usually city, county, or state health departments. Ninety-six programs are currently funded. Promising results from this initiative have been reported—for example, improved adequacy of prenatal care and decreased low–birth weight rates (Devaney, 2000).

Community and Migrant Health Centers Programs

The Community and Migrant Health Centers Programs began in 1965 and were two of the early programs of the U.S. Office of Economic Opportunity. Through a network of approximately 700 centers that operate more than 3000 service delivery sites, these health centers provide comprehensive primary and preventive health care to nearly 7 million low-income people. Nearly 4 million of these people are uninsured (Bureau of Primary Health Care, 2001). Health centers are located in medically underserved areas, which are mostly rural and inner-city areas. Health centers also obtain funds from sources such as local governments, foundations, corporations, and clients.

National Health Service Corps

The National Health Service Corps is another federal program that helps children receive primary health care services. The National Health Service Corps sends physicians, nurses, and other health care providers to underserved areas of the country. The program assists students with medical, nursing, and other training through scholarships and loan repayment plans if they agree to provide a certain number of service years in a rural or urban underserved area. Currently, about 2700 health care professionals serve in the National Health Services Corps (NHSC, 2006).

School-Based and School-Linked Health Services

Adolescents are the least likely aggregate to use health care services, especially preventive services. Their adolescent health care needs are different from their childhood needs, and they may be uncomfortable seeing a pediatrician or their childhood provider. Furthermore, they may or may not be able to discuss sensitive topics such as puberty, contraception, and peer relationships with their parents. Some may not want their parents to know they have a health problem; therefore they may not want to see the family's health care provider out of concern for privacy and confidentiality. This can cause their health care needs to go unmet.

The school-based health movement began in the 1970s in a St. Paul, Minnesota, high school. Since then, school-based health clinics have grown in both numbers and variety of available services. Although centers are more common in high schools, they are spreading to elementary and middle schools. More conservative areas of the country are somewhat reluctant to allow adolescent health care at or near schools.

State dollars, mostly from general funds and the Maternal and Child Health Block Grant, are the primary sources of funding for school-based health care. An increasing number of health centers participate in the Medicaid and SCHIP programs, and some provide services within a managed care network.

Special Supplemental Nutrition program for Women, Infants, and Children

Although it is not a health program exclusively, **Women, Infants, and Children (WIC)** provides highly nutritious foods, nutrition education and counseling, and screening and referral to nearly 8 million low-income pregnant and breast-feeding mothers, their infants, and their children under age 5 each year (Food and Nutrition Service, 2004). To be eligible, women and children must meet income guidelines established by each state, and a health professional must determine they are at "nutritional risk." Women and children who participate in Medicaid, the Food Stamp program, or the Temporary Assistance for Needy Families program are automatically income eligible for WIC.

WIC clinics operate in a number of sites including health clinics, hospitals, schools, public housing sites, and mobile clinics. Women participating in the program are encouraged to obtain prenatal care if they are pregnant. They also are encouraged to maintain healthy diets and obtain preventive health care for themselves and their children, including childhood immunizations. WIC participants receive checks or vouchers to purchase specific, nutritious foods. Most grocery stores and supermarkets participate in WIC and carry the foods designated by the program.

Established in 1972, WIC is one of the most successful, popular, and cost-effective public health programs. Some of the many benefits attributed to WIC include the following:
- Improved birth outcomes and health care cost savings
- Improved infant feeding practices, improved low–birth weight rate, more regular primary care
- Improved cognitive development (Food and Nutrition Service, 1999; Kowaleski-Jones and Duncan, 2002)

Head Start

Formed in 1965, **Head Start** is a comprehensive, federally funded early childhood program for low-income children aged 3 to 5 years. In 1994, Congress also created Early Head Start, which serves children from birth to 3 years. Together, these programs are comprehensive child-development programs that aim to increase the school readiness of young children in low-income families. They provide educational opportunities and medical, dental, mental health, nutritional, and social services. They strongly emphasize parental involvement on a voluntary or paid-staff basis.

The Head Start Bureau in the USDHHS administers Head Start and Early Head Start. The Bureau awards grants to local public agencies, private nonprofit organizations, Native-American groups, and school systems. The grantee organizations provide a range of services in the following areas:
- Education and early childhood development
- Medical, dental, and mental health
- Nutrition
- Parental involvement

Head Start has served more than 22 million children since its inception in 1965. About 13% of participants are children with disabilities (Administration on Children and Families, 2004). Although it is a successful program, it does not reach all eligible children. Congress has steadily increased the funding level in an attempt to reach the goal of full enrollment for both Head Start and Early Head Start.

SHARING RESPONSIBILITY FOR IMPROVING CHILD AND ADOLESCENT HEALTH

Most children in the United States are born healthy and remain healthy throughout childhood. However, the protective factors operating in the lives of healthy children and the interventions they receive are not available to all children. Although public sector programs have attempted to provide a "safety net" for children, these interventions cannot address all needs of the children. For example, the health care system may provide emergency care to a 9-year-old child injured by gunfire in a drive-by shooting, but it cannot address the community conditions that perpetuate violence.

Child health is affected by many factors; therefore, the responsibility for improving children's health rests with the entire community. This responsibility begins with parents and includes health care professionals, community groups, businesses, and the public sector. When a child gets older, he or she can be responsible for practicing healthy behaviors and obtaining proper health care.

Parents' Role

Even before conception, a mother is responsible for ensuring the health of her fetus. Preconception care can help a woman learn about specific actions she can take to increase her chances for having a healthy baby, for example, achieving optimal weight and taking folic acid before she becomes pregnant. During pregnancy, she should develop healthy behaviors, including proper nutrition and avoidance of tobacco, alcohol, drugs, and other behaviors that could harm her developing baby. This is particularly important in the early stages of gestation when fetal organ systems are developing. It is also important for the mother to receive prenatal care early in pregnancy.

Starting with breast-feeding, parents must give their children nutritious food and ensure that they are immunized, receive needed health care services, and acquire healthful lifestyles. Breast-feeding provides many health benefits for mothers and their children (Box 14-6).

Another important task for parents is to ensure their children have a safe environment at home, in the neighborhood, and at school. They must protect their children from injury, violence, abuse, and neglect. Parents must learn how to nurture, guide, and protect their children effectively through the developmental stages of childhood.

Community's Role

Families need support from their community and society to fulfill their roles and responsibilities. This is particularly true for families who live in poverty and for parents who are isolated and disenfranchised. Ensuring access to health care is an important community role, but communities also are responsible for promoting well-being, which goes far beyond the provision of traditional medical care.

Communities should work to create safe neighborhoods and support the development of community-based, compre-

---

BOX 14-6 Breast-feeding: The Feeding Method of Choice

Breast-feeding is uniquely superior for infant feeding. The practice imparts many health benefits for mothers and babies. Benefits for children include the following:

➤ Decreased incidence and severity of a wide range of infectious diseases
➤ Decreased infant mortality
➤ Decreased risk of SIDS
➤ Reduction in the incidence of diabetes, asthma, and some cancers
➤ Lower risk of overweight
➤ Enhanced cognitive development

Benefits for mothers who breast-feed include the following:

➤ Decreased postpartum bleeding
➤ Earlier return to pre-pregnancy weight
➤ Decreased risk of breast and ovarian cancer

The American Academy of Pediatrics and many other health organizations recommend exclusive breast-feeding for the first 6 months of life (American Academy of Pediatrics, 2005).

---

hensive health, education, and social service programs. Also, communities can promote community health education campaigns concerning prenatal care, smoking, nutrition, teenage pregnancy, drug and violence prevention, and other health topics. Communities and community organizations can sponsor health fairs, immunization drives, car safety seat checks, bicycle safety helmet campaigns, crime prevention and reduction programs, and other projects that help families develop healthy lifestyles and gain access to needed health services.

Communities are well situated to facilitate the integration of health, education, and social services; to eliminate fragmentation and duplication of services; to provide culturally competent care; and to better organize more comprehensive and streamlined systems of care. Although many health and social service programs exist, they can be poorly coordinated with each other with little collaboration among the professional disciplines. Through public awareness campaigns, communities can facilitate the integration and coordination of services. For example, these initiatives can alert parents about the importance of immunizations, a safer environment, prenatal care, and other services and can inform families about how and where to obtain these services.

The media are part of the community at large and should be involved in promoting child and adolescent health. The media significantly influence children's lives, their perceptions of the world, and their self-images. From developing informational campaigns about prenatal care and immunizations to discouraging violence and explicit sex in advertising and popular television programs, the media can have a profound effect on improving children's health and well-being.

Employer's Role

Business and industry have an enormous stake in the health of the nation's children. A strong, productive workforce is ensured only when the health, social, and educational needs of the next generation of workers are met. Furthermore, health risks cost employers in lost productivity and increased health care costs.

The private sector can play a role in improving the health of individual children or the community in general. An employer can make health care more accessible to families with children by offering affordable health insurance that covers employees and dependents. The provision of insurance plans that offer full pregnancy and well-child health care benefits is essential to employee health promotion.

Maintaining a workplace that allows flexible leave for prenatal and pediatric health care and allows time off to care for newborn and sick children can also contribute to child health improvements. In 1993, the Family and Medical Leave Act mandated that employers with 50 or more employees must allow a total of 12 work weeks of unpaid leave during any 12-month period for the birth or adoption of a child or for the care of a sick family member.

In addition, employers can sponsor education opportunities for employees about healthy diets, healthy pregnancies, substance abuse, and stress management. Businesses can also offer on-site child care and can work with community leaders and public officials to initiate community-wide health promotion projects targeted to children. Finally, employers can be catalysts for linking health, education, and social services for children.

Government's Role

In the United States, government's role in promoting or ensuring children's health is more limited than in many other countries. Other countries often have defined policies on children's health; the United States does not. Not only do such policies indicate that children are a priority of the citizenry, but they also help shape the operation of programs and their funding.

As discussed earlier, U.S. state and federal governments have several public health programs that provide assistance to children, especially to those at risk from poverty or other disadvantages. Monitoring the health of children is also a governmental role. Although these programs are not a substitute for a family's or caregiver's care and concern, they are important in protecting and promoting health and delivering services to those who would otherwise go without. Although programs with significant funding exist, many children with health problems do not receive the services they need.

Managers and front-line workers (e.g., community health nurses, social workers, physicians, and caseworkers) in effective community programs should be encouraged to collaborate and thereby assist children with problems that adversely impact their health. "One-stop shopping" (i.e., user-friendly, accessible services for children and families) is an important concept for public programs to embrace to ensure that children easily receive needed services, especially preventive health and social services, before a problem becomes a crisis. Outreach efforts should be an integral part of health initiatives to provide children in need with the services they require. Community health nurses are often an essential part of these outreach efforts.

Community Health Nurse's Role

Public health nurses have always played pivotal roles in improving the health status of pregnant women and children. Within the community, the community health nurse is often most aware of children's health status, any barriers that prevent children from receiving necessary care, and other factors that may adversely affect their health. Armed with this information and knowledge about available health resources in the community, the community health nurse is as follows:

* An advocate for improved individual and community responses to children's needs
* A participant in publicly funded programs
* A promoter of social interventions that enhance the living situations of high-risk families
* A partner with other professionals to improve service collaboration and coordination

Many resources are available to help the community health nurse advocate for children within the community. Internet-based resources such as the March of Dimes, Peristats, can also help nurses to construct maps, charts, and graphs reflecting local child health trends.

One important role of the community health nurse is to help link local health and social services with the school system. Children must be healthy to learn; however, children often come to school with vision, hearing, and other health problems that appropriate education, screening, and treatment could have prevented or alleviated. When children pass the preschool years, the school health nurse is sometimes their only connection to the health care system. School health nurses can be an important source of primary health care and health information for students and their families.

Community health nurses can alert the health professional community, business leaders, religious groups, and voluntary organizations to children's needs and the strategies that can improve their health. Community health nurses, both individually and in groups, can influence the planning and implementation of necessary changes in the health care system to ensure improved children's health and to achieve the national health goals for the year 2010. Also, they can promote commitment within their own institutions for comprehensive, culturally competent care.

LEGAL AND ETHICAL ISSUES IN CHILD AND ADOLESCENT HEALTH

Every day, community health nurses are involved in making decisions. In each encounter with a client, the nurse's decisions or the family's choices have the potential to influence the health and well-being of the family or the community at large for better or for worse.

People often assume that health care professionals, particularly nurses, are by nature attuned to the ethical implications of their decisions. In addition, the community trusts that nurses are aware of the legal ramifications of their actions and decisions, of their client's decisions, and of the health care and legal systems' decisions. In reality, the ever-changing pressures of serving the community's health care needs leave little time to

---

> ### ETHICAL Insights
>
> #### Ethical Issues Related to Child and Adolescent Health
>
> ➤ *Allocation decisions:* Given limited time and resources, what level of care should a nurse offer a child and his or her family?
>
> ➤ *Maternal-fetal conflict:* Sometimes there are opposing ethical concerns for the pregnant woman and her fetus, for example, whether the benefits of prolonging a pregnancy justifies the risk of complications for a pregnant woman or whether court-ordered treatment for a substance-abusing pregnant woman overrides the right to autonomy for a pregnant woman.
>
> ➤ *Client autonomy:* In each specific case, who should make health care decisions for a young client, especially when opposing opinions arise? The client? The parents or guardian? The nurse or other health care professional? At what age does a child become mature enough to participate in such decision making? What laws does any given state have that affect adolescent client autonomy? What should the community health nurse do if he or she believes the client's or parent's decisions are not in the best interest of the client?
>
> ➤ *Privacy and confidentiality:* Is an intervention appropriate if the community health nurse identifies gross noncompliance, neglect, or abuse? Is it appropriate if the nurse must break confidentiality? When and how should the nurse take action?
>
> ➤ *"Gaming the system":* When the health care system's rules appear to impede the nurse's ability to serve the client's best interest, is it acceptable to circumvent the system? If so, what are the moral and legal costs?
>
> ➤ *Cultural competence:* The United States will continue to experience huge demographic changes and increased diversity; nurses will face different cultural definitions of what is and what is not acceptable or ethical. How should the community health nurse respond to a client or population group that does not share the same cultural outlook on health? What is the nurse's legal justification, if any, for responding in a certain way?

---

reflect on the ethical and moral implications of a given situation. In some cases, it may seem easier to avoid tough decisions. An ethical approach to decision making allows the community health nurse to evaluate a client's needs or a population's needs more honestly and completely and take appropriate action. Understanding the legal environment will help the nurse make informed decisions and assist clients with their decision-making processes more effectively.

Ethical Issues

The complex nature of public health and health care delivery environments often sets the stage for conflicts of interest and values. Meanwhile, nurses and other health professionals must work within the system to improve child and adolescent health in a country of great differences. Such differences exist between races and cultures, and there are great dichotomies, such as the affluence of some and the poverty of many others. For the perinatal nurse, ethical dilemmas may arise because she is an advocate for two clients: the pregnant woman and her fetus. This dilemma is further complicated because the law does not recognize the fetus as an autonomous individual. Regardless of the law, some consider the fetus to be a vulnerable individual who needs protection (Langa and

Text continued on p. 288

CASE STUDY   Application of the Nursing Process

By applying the principles of the nursing process to the individual, family, and community, the community health nurse can provide services to children and adolescents more systematically and effectively. Most communities offer a range of preventive services and other important programs that children need. The community health nurse must thoroughly understand the needs of the individual child and family and must be aware of available community resources to help meet the child's health needs.

Maria Martinez, a community health nurse working for the county health department, received a call from the high school nurse informing her that a 16-year-old high school student named Tara Parkhurst would come in that afternoon for a pregnancy test. Tara had already missed three menstrual periods and was afraid to talk about it with her family. She had a long discussion with the school nurse and asked her boyfriend to take her to the health department clinic after school for the pregnancy test.

ASSESSMENT

Tara's pregnancy test was positive, and she was an estimated 3 months pregnant. She was upset and would not speak with Maria at the health department. Maria arranged to make a home visit the next afternoon.

The school nurse told Maria that Tara wanted to keep her baby and that Tara's family struggled financially. Knowing that she needed to address a number of issues at the first home visit, Maria prepared by developing a list of possible assessment areas that covered individual, family, and community concerns. Her list included the following:

Individual
- Medical risk factors
- Emotional well-being, including concerns about domestic violence and sexual abuse
- Cultural beliefs and attitudes toward pregnancy and medical care
- Barriers to communication with providers, such as language, hearing, or sight
- Understanding and acceptance of pregnancy
- Health-promoting and risk-taking behaviors
- Understanding the importance of obtaining preventive care services
- Health insurance status
- Access to transportation

Family
- Adequacy of housing structure
- Safety of neighborhood
- Ability of family members to provide emotional support
- Ability of family to provide financial support

Community
- Availability of affordable and local prenatal and pediatric care
- Health and social services coordination
- Availability of culturally sensitive health care
- Emotional guidance and counseling
- Educational opportunities for pregnant and parenting teenagers
- Job training
- Nutrition services such as WIC and food stamps
- Pregnancy and parenting education
- Child care availability

ASSESSMENT DATA

Individual
- Tara was already in the early second trimester of pregnancy and had not received prenatal care. She also engaged in risk-taking behaviors (i.e., smoking, alcohol use, unprotected sex, and poor eating habits) potentially detrimental to her baby.
- During the interview, Tara seemed quiet and reserved. She said she was excited to have a baby, but she feared labor and delivery. Her boyfriend wanted her to keep the baby.
- She said she did not think about prenatal care much, but would probably visit a health clinic sometime before her delivery. Her family did not have health insurance, and she said they could not afford prenatal care.
- She wanted to keep the baby and remain in school, yet she did not have a realistic understanding of parental responsibilities.

Family
- When Tara told her parents she was pregnant, they expressed disappointment. Her mother voiced a willingness to provide emotional support, but her seemingly emotionally distant father expressed anger.
- Both parents expressed concern about how the family would manage financially.
- After a brief review of the family's financial situation, it appeared that Tara was eligible for Medicaid and WIC.

Community
- Maria determined that prenatal services were available, but only during school hours. Although the only clinic that accepted Medicaid clients was on the other side of town, a nearby obstetrical practice with a certified nurse-midwife on staff accepted clients with Medicaid coverage. However, their primary clientele was middle-class, married women.
- Applying for Medicaid and the WIC program required Tara to go to the welfare office and apply during school hours. However, the hospital outpatient department could make a preliminary Medicaid eligibility determination, which might be more convenient.

- Although Medicaid would pay for some prenatal classes, those nearby were geared to older, married couples.
- Tara's school encouraged her to remain in regular classes until her delivery date and participate in home study for a limited time thereafter.
- No parenting classes geared toward adolescents were available.
- Child care was not available at the high school, which made returning to school more difficult for Tara.
- Although the community has a lay home visitor program that matches mentors with pregnant and parenting teens and provides health information and encouragement, the project does not serve Tara's neighborhood.

DIAGNOSIS

Individual

- Altered health maintenance related to the lack of prenatal care and the effect of poor nutrition, smoking, and alcohol use on fetal development
- Altered parenting potential related to unrealistic expectations about parenting responsibilities
- Knowledge deficit of infant and child safety issues such as the use of child safety seats, prevention of lead poisoning, advantages of breast-feeding, and use of preventive health care, including immunization

Family

- Altered family processes related to anger and disappointment over daughter's pregnancy
- Altered financial status resulting from the addition of another dependent to the family

Community

- Lack of coordinated, culturally sensitive, accessible prenatal and parenting services for adolescents
- Existing lay home visitor program not available

PLANNING

To ensure the action plan is complete, realistic, and successfully implemented, Maria must thoroughly identify the factors affecting Tara's health and well-being. In addition, Tara, her family, and Maria must set mutual goals.

Individual
Long-Term Goals
- Pregnancy outcome will be healthy for mother and infant.
- Tara will demonstrate successful parenting behaviors.
- Tara will complete high school.

Short-Term Goals
- Tara will obtain prenatal care.
- Tara will understand the reasons to change nutrition and substance use habits.
- Tara and the nurse will plan actions to change poor health habits.

- Tara will remain in school throughout her pregnancy and will use the home study program until she returns to school after her baby is born.
- Tara will enroll in parenting class. If classes are not available, she will use age-appropriate reading materials, films, videotapes, opportunities for group discussion with other teens, or visits with experienced parents.
- Tara will breast-feed her baby.
- Tara will speak with the community health educator to determine methods to protect the health and safety of her newborn.

Family
Long-Term Goal
- The family's ability to handle crises will improve with their ability to discuss problems and engage in mutual problem solving.

Short-Term Goal
- Tara's parents will display supportive behaviors, such as accompanying her to prenatal care appointments, helping her engage in healthy behaviors, and helping her arrange child care to remain in school.

Community
Long-Term Goal
- Accessible, comprehensive, culturally sensitive prenatal and other health care services will be established, including home visiting and parenting classes targeted to adolescents.

Short-Term Goals
- The health department clinic will extend evening hours to accommodate students and working families.
- A child care facility will open in or near the high school.

INTERVENTION

The nurse, family, and individual must address their immediate, mutual goals to help Tara achieve a healthy birth outcome and begin successful parenting. Interdisciplinary planning between Tara's school health nurse, caseworker, community health nurse, primary pregnancy care provider, child birth educator, and family planning nurse is critical. In addition, the nurse must be an advocate for community-wide change to ensure that the community is meeting individuals' needs.

Individual

Maria worked with the school nurse and other health professionals to help Tara obtain Medicaid and WIC; she was referred to an obstetrician who saw her regularly. Tara's pregnancy was also monitored by the school nurse who had her come to the clinic on a weekly basis to check her weight and blood pressure and to talk with her about pregnancy-related issues.

Continued

CASE STUDY   Application of the Nursing Process (cont'd)

Working with the school nurse, Maria provided Tara with information on child birth classes and nutrition as well as booklets detailing how to promote a healthy pregnancy. She was counseled to avoid tobacco, alcohol and all drugs. Near the end of the pregnancy, Tara was encouraged to attend parenting classes with her boyfriend.

Family

Maria and the social worker referred Tara's parents to other social service agencies that might be able to help financially. In particular, they focused on providers who could assist with utilities, job placement and child care. The family was also referred to a family counselor who specialized in working with families with adolescent children.

Community

Maria worked with the Maternal Child Health Division of the County Health Department to help facilitate offering parenting classes at an area high school, targeting the learning needs of pregnant teens. She and the school nurse also met with school district officials and community leaders to stimulate dialogue about the consequences of dropping out of high school and facilitate action in policies such as child care for parenting teenagers to help them remain in school.

EVALUATION

Evaluation strategies must involve both process and outcome measures on the individual, family, and community levels.

Individual

The school nurse was able to monitor Tara throughout her pregnancy and was aware that she finished classes for the term. Tara's pregnancy was unremarkable and she delivered a healthy boy. Their health care expenses were covered by Medicaid and the baby was determined to also be eligible for SCHIP. A home-based teacher was assigned to work with her for 1 month after delivery to ensure that she was able to keep up with her coursework. With the assistance of the social worker, Tara was able to place the baby in a subsidized day care facility, allowing her to finish school.

Family

Family counseling helped the family resolve some of their issues. Maria observed that Tara's parents were proud of their grandson and eager to help with his care.

Community

With the help of the school nurse and other interested parties, Maria was able to initiate a collaborative program in which health department nurses and developmental specialists offered parenting classes in high schools on a regular basis. They were also planning on writing for a Maternal Child Block grant to implement a school-based clinic focusing on the needs of pregnant teens and their infants.

LEVELS OF PREVENTION

Primary

- Primary prevention depends largely on the child's age. For the youngest children, strategies include preconceptional counseling and the practice of healthy behaviors by mothers before pregnancy.
- Primary prevention also includes the prevention of unwanted pregnancy, which is especially important for adolescents.

Secondary

- Once pregnant, the woman must receive early and adequate prenatal care, practice healthy behaviors, obtain necessary social and supportive services, and prepare herself for becoming a parent.
- It is incumbent on the community to ensure that adequate preventive health services, such as prenatal care, nutrition and dietary counseling, pregnancy and parent education, and social services, are available.

Tertiary

- Initiate programs and services that prevent future unwanted pregnancy among teenagers and help the parenting teenager provide the best possible care to the child.
- Establish programs such as parenting classes; support services to help adolescents complete their education; coordination of health and social services for the mother and her child; and well-child care, immunizations, and nutrition services.

Duderstadt, 2003). The scope of ethical and legal dilemmas is broad. See Ethical Insights for specific ethical issues related to child and adolescent health.

These issues invariably involve value judgments and challenge a nurse's bounds of professional and personal duty. They also require the community health nurse to stay abreast of legislative changes at the local, state, and national levels and participate in professional activities that can help him or her

stay current in these important matters. By recognizing the ethical implications of the care and advice they give or the actions they take, nurses can embrace their duty to promote the health and well-being of individual clients and the community more completely, protect their clients from harm, and strive for health care fairness and justice for all clients.

Recognizing the value of engaging in a shared dialogue with colleagues regarding ethical decision-making issues and understanding the possible legal implications of their decisions are equally important. The choices can be complex; therefore receiving the guidance of an ethics board or gaining a second opinion can be critical to making the right choices. On a broader scale, a community health nurse's ethical perspective can enhance any discussion about individual client care and overall community health, and it also can affect the direction of the country's public health policy.

SUMMARY

Child and adolescent health status remains an important indicator of the nation's health. The health of a child sets the foundation for school readiness and future success. Child and adolescent health problems are a reflection of rapidly changing social conditions, not isolated events. Despite generally improving trends in health for most children, community health nurses must address discrepancies that exist between racial and ethnic groups. Poverty is the basis for many continuing health problems among children in this country, and nurses must recognize and treat it as such.

The best way to ensure the success and well-being of future generations is for each child to begin life healthy and maintain that health status throughout childhood. Any health problem (e.g., hunger and poor nutrition, increased lead blood levels, asthma, poor vision or hearing, anemia, dental caries, illicit drug use, or teen pregnancy) can interfere with school attendance, academic success, normal growth and development, learning ability, and life success.

The prevention of health problems is most significant and cost effective for children. Each dollar spent on the prevention of physical and emotional problems in children is a sound investment. Primary health care and early intervention for children and families can help prevent costly problems, suffering, and lost human potential.

Community health nurses can use their experience and "inside knowledge" of barriers to child health to educate others. Rather than limiting their approach to caring for the individual and family only, community health nurses can maximize their roles to collaborate and forge necessary alliances to solve children's health problems. Nurses are

authority figures in the least expected places. Working on health care's front line is a powerful and very real position to members of Congress, state legislators, mayors, and others. By creatively using this kind of power, community health nurses can contribute greatly to improving the health and well-being of all children.

LEARNING ACTIVITIES

1. Examine infant mortality statistics in the community and compare the rates with state and national averages. Is infant mortality higher for any particular racial or ethnic group within the community?
2. Determine how a non–English-speaking immigrant without finances or available transportation would obtain prenatal care.
3. Accompany a pregnant woman to a local department of social services and observe as she tries to establish Medicaid eligibility for herself and her unborn child.
4. Develop strategies to inform parents whose children are uninsured about the availability of SCHIP.
5. Spend a day with a school health nurse and analyze what could help prevent the health problems and issues he or she encountered throughout the day.
6. Survey businesses in the community to determine whether they offer maternity health insurance benefits, paid or unpaid maternity or paternity leave for new parents, and leave for prenatal care appointments. Is there a location within the worksite where women can pump breast milk? Use this information to develop a strategy to encourage family-friendly policies and practices in the business community.
7. If the community has a lay home visitor program, meet with a home visitor and, if possible, accompany him or her during home visits.
8. Communicate with those in policy-making positions by writing letters or holding meetings about children's needs.
9. Identify the public health and advocacy organizations in the community that are working to address children's health needs and identify their strategies for promoting child health within the community.

REFERENCES

Administration on Children and Families: *Head Start program fact sheet: 2004,* The Author, http://www.acf.hhs.gov/programs/hsb/research/factsheets.htm.

American Academy of Pediatrics, Task Force on Infant Sleep Position and Sudden Infant Death Syndrome: Changing concepts of sudden infant death syndrome: implications for infant sleeping environment and sleep position, *Pediatrics* 105:650-657, 2000.

American Academy of Pediatrics: The medical home, *Pediatrics* 110(1):184-186, 2002.

American Academy of Pediatrics: Breastfeeding and the use of human milk, *Pediatrics* 115(2):496-506, 2005.

Annie E. Casey Foundation: *When teens have sex: Issues and trends,* 2000, The Author, http://www.aecf.org/kidscount/teen/index.htm.

Beach MC, Price EG, Gary TL: Cultural competence: A systemic review of health care provider educational interventions, *Med Care* 43(4):356-373, 2005.

Bernstein J, Brocht C, Spade-Aguilar M: *How much is enough? Basic family budgets for working families,* Washington, DC, 2000, Economic Policy Institute.

Bhutta AT et al: Cognitive and behavioral outcomes of school-aged children who were born preterm, *JAMA* 288(6):728-737, 2002.

Biblarz, TJ, Raferty AE: Family structure, educational attainment, and socioeconomic success:

rethinking the pathology of matriarchy, *Am J Sociol* 105(2):321-365, 1999.

Bureau of Justice Statistics: *Teens experience the highest rates of violence crime,* Washington, DC, 2002, The Author, http://www.ojp.usdoj.gov/bjs/glance/vage.htm.

Bureau of Primary Health Care: *Experts with experience: community and migrant health centers highlighting a decade of service 1990-2000,* Rockville, Md, Sept 2001, Health Resources and Services Administration, US Department of Health and Human Services, http://bphc.hrsa.gov/chc.

Bureau of Primary Health Care: *The provider's guide to quality and culture,* Rockville, Md, 2002, The Author, Management Sciences for

Health, and USDHHS, http://erc.msh.org/mainpage.cfm?file=1.0.htm&module=provider&language=English.

Center for the Future of Children: *Children and Poverty,* 7(2), Los Altos, Calif, Summer/Fall 1997, The David and Lucille Packard Foundation.

Centers for Disease Control and Prevention: Recommendations for the use of folic acid to reduce the number of cases of spina bifida and other neural tube defects, *Morb Mortal Wkly Rep* 41(RR-14):1-7, 1992.

Centers for Disease Control and Prevention: *STDs in adolescents and young adults 2003,* STD Surveillance Report, Washington, DC, 2003, US Department of Health and Human Services, http://www.cdc.gov/nchstp/dstd/Stats_Trends/Stats_and_Trends.htm.

Centers for Disease Control and Prevention: *The health consequences of smoking: a report of the surgeon general,* Washington DC, 2004a, USDHHS, National Center for Chronic Disease Prevention and Health Promotion, Office on Smoking and Health.

Centers for Disease Control and Prevention: Vaccination coverage among children entering school—United States, 2003-04 school year, *Morb Mortal Wkly Rep* (53)44:1041-1044, 2004b.

Centers for Disease Control and Prevention: Recommended childhood and adolescent immunization schedule: United States, 2005, *Morb Mortal Wkly Rep* 53(51-52):Q1-Q3, 2005.

Centers for Disease Control and Prevention, National Center for Health Statistics. National Vital Statistics System. *Infant mortality rates, fetal mortality rates, and perinatal mortality rates, according to race: United States, selected years 1950–99,* The Author, http://www.cdc.gov/nchs/data/hus/hus01.pdf.

Cervantes A, Keith L, Wyshak G: Adverse birth outcomes among native-born and immigrant women: replicating national evidence regarding Mexicans at the local level, *Matern Child Health J* 3(2):99-110, 1999.

Children's Bureau: *Child maltreatment 2002,* Washington, DC, 2004, US Government Printing Office.

Children's Defense Fund: *Yearbook 2000: The state of America's children,* Washington, DC, 2000, The Author.

Children's Defense Fund: *2003 Facts on Child Poverty,* Washington, DC, 2004, The Author, www.childrensdefense.org/familyincome/childpoverty.

Childstats 2004: *Death rates among adolescents. Adolescent Mortality Table 8*, Health Resources and Services Administration, www.childstats.gov.

Childstats 2005: *Population and family characteristics*, Health Resources and Services Administration, http://www.childstats.gov/americaschildren/pop.asp.

Collins KS et al: *Diverse communities, common concerns: assessing health care quality for minority Americans,* New York, 2002, The Commonwealth Fund.

Cornell EV: MCH update 2002: states' health coverage for low-income pregnant women, children, and parents, June 2003, *Nat Gov Assoc Issue Brief,* National Governor's Association, http://www.nga.org/center/divisions/1,1188,C_ISSUE_BRIEF^D_5568,00.html.

DeNavas-Walt C, Proctor BD, Mills RJ: *Income, poverty, and health insurance coverage in the United States: 2003,* Current Population Reports P60-226, August 2004, US Census Bureau, http://www.census.gov/prod/2004-pubs/p60-226.pdf.

Devaney B et al: *Reducing infant mortality: Lessons learned from Healthy Start,* Final report, Princeton, NJ, July 2000, Mathematica Policy Research, Inc.

Egerter S et al: *Disparities in maternal and infant health: are we making progress? Lessons from California,* KFF 7157, Menlo Park, Calif, 2004, The Henry J. Kaiser Foundation, www.kkf www.kff.org/womenshealth/upload/ Disparities-in-Maternal-and-Infant-Health-Are-We-Making-Progress-Lessons-From-California-Issue-Brief.pdf.

Ellickson PL, Tucker JS, Klein DJ: Ten-year prospective study of public health problems associated with early drinking, *Pediatrics* 111:949-955, 2003.

Federal Interagency Forum on Child and Family Statistics: *Adolescent births: birth rates by mother's age, race, and Hispanic origin,* Childstats Table HEALTH9, http://www.childstats.gov/ac2004/tables/Health9.asp.

Fiore MC et al: *Treating tobacco use and dependence,* Clinical practice guideline, Rockville, Md: June 2000, US Department of Health and Human Services, Public Health Service.

Food and Nutrition Service: *About WIC: how WIC helps,* Alexandria, VA, 1999, The Author, http://www.fns.usda.gov/wic/aboutwic/howwichelps.htm#birth%20outcomes.

Food and Nutrition Service: *WIC program: total participation,* 2004, The Author, http://www.fns.usda.gov/pd/wifypart.htm.

Freda MC, Patterson ET: *Preterm labor: prevention and nursing management,* ed 3, 2004, White Plains, NY: March of Dimes Birth Defects Foundation.

Glassbrenner D: *The use of child restraints in 2002,* Washington, DC, 2003, United States Department of Transportation, National Highway Traffic Safety Administration, www.nhtsa.gov/CPS/ChildRestraints/ChildRestraints.html.

Hack M et al: Outcomes in young adulthood for very-low-birth-weight infants, *Obstet Gynecol Surv* 57(6):342-344, 2002.

Hamilton BE, Martin JA, Sutton PD: Births: preliminary data for 2003, *Natl Vital Stat Rep* 53(9), 2004, http://www.cdc.gov/nchs/pressroom/04facts/birthrates.htm.

Hock-Long L et al: Access to adolescent reproductive health services: financial and structural barriers to care, *Perspect Sex Reprod Health* 35(3):144-147, 2003.

Hogue CJ: Successful assisted reproductive technology: the beauty of one, *Obstet Gynecol* 100:1017-1019, 2002.

Hoyert DL, Kung H-C, Smith BS: Deaths: preliminary data for 2003, *Natl Vital Stat Rep* 53(15), 2005, http://www.cdc.gov/nchs/data/nvsr/nvsr53/nvsr53_15.pdf.

James CA, Bourgeois FT, Shannon MW. Association of race/ethnicity with emergency department wait times, *Pediatrics* 115(3): e310-e315, 2005.

Kowaleski-Jones L, Duncan GJ: Effects of participation in the WIC program on birthweight: evidence from the national longitudinal survey of youth, *Am J Public Health* 92(5):799-804, 2002.

Kaiser Family Foundation: *Children's health: why health insurance matters,* May 2002, http://www.kff.org/uninsured/loader.cfm?url=/commonspot/security/getfile.cfm&PageID=14132.

Kaiser Family Foundation: *National survey of adolescents and young adults sexual health knowledge, attitudes, and behaviors,* May 2003, The Author, http://ww.kff.org/youth-hivstds.

Kearney MH et al: Health behaviors as mediators for the effect of partner abuse on infant birth weight, *Nurs Res* 53(1):36-45, 2004.

Larsen LJ: *The foreign-born population in the United States: 2003,* Current Population Reports P20-551, August 2004, US Census Bureau, http://www.census.gov/prod/2004-pubs/p20-551.pdf.

Lagana K, Duderstadt K: *Perinatal and neonatal ethics: facing contemporary challenges,* White Plains, NY, 2003, March of Dimes Birth Defects Foundation.

Luman ET et al: Timeliness of childhood vaccinations in the United States, *JAMA* 293(10):1204-1211, 2005.

March of Dimes Perinatal Data Center: *The big picture: hospital costs,* 2002, March of Dimes Birth Defects Foundation, http://www.marchofdimes.com/prematurity/15341_10734.asp.

Matthews, TJ, Menaker F, McDorman MF: Infant mortality statistics from the 2002 period linked birth/infant death data set, *Natl Vital Stat Rep* 53(10), 2004, http://www.cdc.gov/nchs/pressroom/04facts/infant.htm.

Meyer PA et al: Surveillance for elevated blood lead levels among children: United States, 1997–2001, *Morbid Mortal Wkly Rep* 52(SS10):1-21, 2003, http://www.cdc.gov/mmwr/preview/mmwrhtml/ss5210a1.htm.

Mills RJ, Bhandari S: *Health insurance coverage in the United States 2002,* Current Population Reports P60-223, Sept 2003, US Census Bureau, http://www.census.gov/prod/2003-pubs/p60-223.pdf.

Moore ML, Moos MK: *Cultural competence in the care of childbearing families,* White Plains NY, 2003, March of Dimes Birth Defects Foundation.

National Health Service Corps (NHSC): *About the NHSC,* 2003, The Author, http://nhsc.bhpr.hrsa.gov/about/.

National Campaign to Prevent Teen Pregnancy: *Halfway there: a prescription for continued progress in preventing teen pregnancy,* Washington, DC, 2001, The Author.

National Center for Children in Poverty: *The effects of parental education on income,* New York, 2004, Columbia University, Mailman School of Public Health, http://www.nccp.org/pub_pei04.html.

National Institute of Child Health and Human Development: *SIDS: Back to Sleep Campaign,* Rockville, Md, 2005, The Author, http://www.nichd.nih.gov/sids.

National Institute on Drug Abuse: Smoking and pregnancy: what are the risks? *Research Report Series: Nicotine addiction,* NIH 01-4342, 2001, National Clearinghouse on Drug Information, http://www.drugabuse.gov/researchreports/nicotine.

Office of Applied Studies: *Team sports participation and substance use among youths,* National Survey on Drug Use and Health report, Feb 8, 2002, Substance Abuse and Mental Health Services Administration, http://www.oas.samhsa.gov/2k2/athletes/athletes_DrugUse.htm.

Office of Applied Studies: *Participation in youth activities and substance use among youths,* National Survey on Drug Use and Health report, Rockville, Md, 2004a, Substance Abuse and Mental Health Services Administration, http://www.oas.samhsa.gov/2k4/activities/activities.cfm.

Office of Applied Studies: *Pregnancy and substance abuse,* National Survey on Drug Use and Health report, Rockville, Md, 2004b, Substance Abuse and Mental Health Services Administration, http://www.oas.samhsa.gov/2k3/pregnancy.

Office of Applied Studies: *Alcohol use and delinquent behaviors among youths,* National Survey on Drug Use and Health report, Rockville, Md, 2005, Substance Abuse and Mental Health Services Administration, http://www.oas.samhsa.gov/2k5/alcDelinquent/alcDelinquent.cfm.

Office of the Assistant Secretary for Planning and Evaluation: *Trends in the well-being of America's children and youth,* Washington, DC, 2003, The Author, http://aspe.hhs.gov/hsp/03trends/index.htm.

O'Malley LD, Bachman JG, Schulenberg JE: *Monitoring the Future. national results on adolescent drug use—overview of key findings, 2004,* Bethesda, Md, 2005, National Institute on Drug Abuse.

Reich K, editor: Children, youth, and gun violence, *Future Child* 12(2), 2002, The David and Lucile Packard Foundation, http://www.futureofchildren.org/pubs-info2825/pubs-info_show.htm?doc_id=154414.

Smedley B, Stith A, Nelson A, editors: *Unequal treatment: confronting racial and ethnic disparities in health care,* Washington, DC, 2002, National Academies Press.

Strauss RS, Pollack, IIA. Epidemic increase in childhood overweight, 1986-1998, *JAMA* (286):2845-2848, 2001.

US Census Bureau. *America's families and living arrangements: 2003,* Current Population Reports P20-553, Annual Social and Economic Supplement, Washington, DC, 2004, The Author, http://www.census.gov/prod/2004pubs/p20-553.pdf.

US Census Bureau: *Infant mortality rates and deaths and life expectancy at birth by sex,* International Data Base, Table 010, http://www.census.gov/ipc/www/idbagg.html.

US Department of Health and Human Services: *Healthy People 2010*: conference edition, Washington, DC, 2000, US Government Printing Office.

US Department of Health and Human Services: *Overweight prevalence, 2003: trends in the well-being of America's children and youth,* 2003, The Author, http://aspe.hhs.gov/search/hsp/03trendss/HC2.pdf.

US Department of Health and Human Services, Health Resources and Services Administration, Maternal and Child Health Bureau: *The national survey of children with special health care needs chartbook 2001,* Rockville, Md, 2004, The Author, http://mchb.hrsa.gov/chscn/pages/prevalence.htm.

US Department of Health and Human Services: 2005 poverty guidelines, *Fed Reg* 70(33): 8373-8375, Feb 18, 2005a.

US Department of Health and Human Services: *U.S. surgeon general releases advisory on alcohol use in pregnancy,* News release, Feb 21, 2005c, The Author, http://www.surgeongeneral.gov/pressreleases/sg02222005.html.

Women's Health

Lisa Jensen

OBJECTIVES

Upon completion of this chapter, the reader will be able to do the following:

1. Identify the major indicators of women's health.
2. Examine prominent health problems among women of all age-groups (i.e., from adolescence to old age).
3. Identify barriers to adequate health care for women.
4. Discuss issues related to reproductive health.
5. Explain the influence of public policy on women's health.
6. Discuss issues and needs for increased research efforts focused on women's health.
7. Apply the nursing process to women's health concerns across all levels of prevention.

KEY TERMS

Civil Rights Act
domestic violence
ectopic pregnancy
Family and Medical Leave Act (FMLA)
family planning
hypertension

life expectancy
maternal mortality
multiple family configurations
osteoporosis
pelvic inflammatory disease (PID)
sexual harassment

CHAPTER OUTLINE

MAJOR INDICATORS OF HEALTH
Life Expectancy
Mortality Rate
Morbidity Rate

SOCIAL FACTORS AFFECTING WOMEN'S HEALTH
Health Care Access
Education and Work
Employment and Wages
Working Women and Home Life
Family Configuration and Marital Status

HEALTH PROMOTION STRATEGIES FOR WOMEN
Acute Illness
Chronic Illness
Reproductive Health
Other Issues in Women's Health

MAJOR LEGISLATION AFFECTING WOMEN'S HEALTH
Public Health Service Act
Civil Rights Act

Social Security Act
Occupational Safety and Health Act
Family and Medical Leave Act

HEALTH AND SOCIAL SERVICES TO PROMOTE THE HEALTH OF WOMEN
Women's Health Services
Other Community Voluntary Services

LEVELS OF PREVENTION AND WOMEN'S HEALTH
Primary Prevention
Secondary Prevention
Tertiary Prevention

ROLES OF THE COMMUNITY HEALTH NURSE
Direct Care
Educator
Counselor

RESEARCH IN WOMEN'S HEALTH

HEALTHY PEOPLE 2010	Selected Objectives for Women's Health	
Objective	**Baseline**	**Target**
3-3: Reduce breast cancer death rate.	27.9 deaths per 100,000	22.3 deaths per 100,000
3-4: Reduce death rate from cervical cancer.	3 deaths per 100,000	2 deaths per 100,000
3-11b: Increase the proportion of women 18 years of age and older who have received a PAP test within the preceding three years.	79%	90%
3-13: Increase the proportion of women 40 years of age and older who have received a mammogram within the preceding two years.	67%	70%
16-4: Reduce maternal deaths.	7.1 deaths per 100,000 live births	3.3 deaths per 100,000 live births
16-5a: Reduce maternal complications during labor and delivery.	31.2 per 100 deliveries	24 per 100 deliveries
16-6a: Increase the proportion of pregnant women who receive early and adequate prenatal care beginning in the first trimester.	83%	90%
16-15: Reduce the occurrence of neural tube defects.	6 cases per 10,000 live births	3 cases per 10,000 live births
25-1a: Reduce the proportion of females 15 to 24 years of age attending STD clinics with chlamydia infections.	12.2%	3%
25-6: Reduce the proportion of females who have required treatment for PID.	8%	5%

From U.S. Department of Health and Human Services: *Healthy People 2010,* ed 2, Washington, DC, 2000a, The Author.

To achieve "health for all" in the twenty-first century, health care services must be affordable and available to all. Although adequate health care for women is a key to realizing this goal, a significant number of women and their families face tremendous barriers in gaining access to health care. Additionally, knowledge deficits related to health promotion and disease prevention activities prevent women of all educational and socioeconomic levels from assuming responsibility for their own health and well-being.

Beginning in the 1970s, the women's movement called for the reform of systems affecting women's health. Women were encouraged to become involved as consumers of health services and as establishers of health policy. More women entered health professions in which they were previously underrepresented, and those in traditionally female-dominated professions, such as nursing and teaching, became more assertive in their demands to gain recognition for their contributions to society.

In "Preamble to a New Paradigm for Women's Health," Choi (1985) declared that collaboration and an interdisciplinary approach are necessary to meet the health care needs of women. She further stated, "essential to the development of health care for women are the concepts of health promotion, disease and accident prevention, education for self-care and responsibility, health risk identification and coordination for illness care when needed" (p. 14). To realize this paradigm, community health nurses must work with other health care professionals to formulate upstream strategies that modify the factors affecting women's health. Many *Healthy People 2010* objectives address health problems pertaining to women and include specific objectives and strategies to improve the health of this aggregate. The *Healthy People 2010* tables above and on p. 304 present a small selection of these objectives. This chapter examines the health of women from adolescence to old age. It explores the major indicators of

health, including specific health problems and the socioeconomic, sociocultural, and health policy issues surrounding women's health. This chapter also discusses identification of current and future research aimed at improving the health of women. An understanding of these points will enable community health nurses to appropriately apply expertise in a community setting to help improve women's health.

MAJOR INDICATORS OF HEALTH

In the United States, data collected on major causes of death and illness appraise the health status of aggregates. These data are typically presented in terms of gender, age, or ethnicity and can help us interpret the levels of health in different groups. The primary indicators of health this chapter covers are life expectancy, mortality (i.e., death) rate, and morbidity (i.e., acute and chronic illness) rate.

Many factors that lead to death and illness among women are preventable or avoidable. If certain conditions receive early detection and treatment, a significant positive influence on longevity and the quality of life could ensue. Recognition of patterns demonstrated by these indicators can address problems preventatively. This section presents an overview of these major indicators of health among women.

Life Expectancy

Except in a few countries, such as Bangladesh, Malawi, Niger, Pakistan, Qatar, and Zimbabwe, women typically experience greater longevity than their male counterparts (World Health Organization, 2004a). For example, females born in the 1970s in the United States had an average life expectancy of 74.7 years, or 7.6 years longer than males born in the same year.

Life expectancy for Americans is at an all-time high, but the discrepancy between males and females has remained. Males born in 2003 have a life expectancy of 72.3 years

TABLE 15-1 Five Leading Causes of Death Among American Women for All Races by Age-Groups in 2001

AGE-GROUP (YEARS)	CAUSE OF DEATH (IN RANK ORDER)
15 to 24	Unintentional injury or accidents
	Malignant neoplasm
	Homicide
	Suicide
	Heart disease
25 to 44	Malignant neoplasm
	Unintentional injury or accidents
	Heart disease
	Suicide
	HIV infection
45 to 64	Malignant neoplasm
	Heart disease
	Chronic obstructive pulmonary disease
	Cerebrovascular disease
	Diabetes mellitus
65 to 74	Malignant neoplasm
	Heart disease
	Chronic obstructive pulmonary disease
	Cerebrovascular disease
	Diabetes

Modified from U.S. Census Bureau: *Statistical abstract of the United States: 2004-2005,* Washington, DC, 2005, U.S. Government Printing Office, http://www.census.gov/prod/2004pubs/04statab/pop.pdf.

compared with 79 years for females. This suggests a trend toward narrowing the gap between male and female life expectancy (Centers for Disease Control and Prevention [CDC], 2005).

Ethnic/racial disparities in life expectancy unfortunately continued into the twenty-first century, as there is considerable variation between races. For example, black females gained an additional 6.7 years, rising from 69.4 years for those born in 1970 to 76.1 years in 2003. Although that is a significant gain, it falls behind the 80.5 years of life expectancy of white females born in that year (U.S. Census Bureau, 2005).

Mortality Rate

Table 15-1 lists the five major causes of death among American women in 2001 by age-group. As this table shows, before age 75, the most common causes of death are accidents and cancer. Overall, however, cardiovascular disease (CVD) continues to be the number one killer of women even though the number of deaths due to CVD decreased dramatically from 424.2 per 100,000 in 1950 to 273 per 100,000 in 2003. Further, CVD caused more deaths among females (493,623, or 53.2%) than among males (433,825, or 46.8%) (American Heart Association [AHA], 2005). Nevertheless, disparities continue related to prevention, diagnosis, and management of heart disease in women. Some investigators believe this phenomenon exists because women display different symptoms of heart disease and are managed differently than men (Chang et al., 2003; Martin et al., 2004; Schulman et al., 1999; Wexler et al., 2005). For example, women with heart disease may not

RESEARCH HIGHLIGHTS

Nurse Researchers Study the Inclusion of Women in Research

A group of nurse researchers examined more than 1000 articles published in nursing journals between 1995 and 2001 to determine if women had been included in research studies focusing on the leading causes of mortality. They found that 87% of the studies did include women participants. They also noted that there appeared to be a slight increase in inclusion of women from the earlier years to the later years.

Crane PB et al: Inclusion of women in nursing research: 1995-2001, *Nurs Res* 53(4): 237-242, 2004.

respond positively to exercise tests; therefore, they are not treated the same way as men (e.g., with cardiac catheterization or heart surgery).

Maternal Mortality

According to the Safe Motherhood Organization (2005), statistics around the world are as follows:

- Complications of pregnancy and childbirth are the leading cause of disability and death among women between the ages of 14 and 49.
- At least 40% of women experience complications during pregnancy, childbirth, and the postpartum period; 15% develop potentially life-threatening problems.
- Each day, about 55,000 unsafe abortions take place; 10% to 50% will need additional medical care for complications.

Maternal mortality is the death of a woman while pregnant or within 42 days after termination of pregnancy, irrespective of the duration and the site of the pregnancy, from any cause related to or aggravated by the pregnancy or its management, but not from accidental or incidental causes. The World Health Organization (WHO) has acknowledged that the 42-day limit is somewhat arbitrary and has introduced a new category, late maternal death, which is defined as death of a woman from direct or indirect obstetric causes more than 42 days but less than 1 year after termination of pregnancy (WHO, 2004a).

It is important for community health nurses to be aware of the global situation surrounding maternal mortality. Wide gaps continue to exist in the availability and quality of reproductive health care services globally. This results in uneven rates in maternal mortality. Indeed, for each woman who dies in the developed world, 99 will die in the developing world (WHO, 2000).

The United States ranks 17th in maternal mortality among all nations (WHO, 2000). Reduction of maternal mortality is one of the *Healthy People 2010* objectives for the United States.

Beginning in the 1950s, maternal mortality rates began to decline in the United States. The decline is largely attributed to the use of blood transfusions, antimicrobial drugs, and the maintenance of fluid and electrolyte balance during serious complications of pregnancy and birth. The development of obstetric training programs and obstetric anesthesia programs was also important.

TABLE 15-2 Maternal Mortality Rate per 100,000 Live Births—Selected Years

YEAR	TOTAL	WHITES	BLACKS	OTHER (NONWHITE)
1985	7.8	5.2	20.4	18.1
1992	7.8	5.0	20.8	18.2
1995	7.1	4.2	22.1	18.5
2002	8.9	6.0	24.9	NA

Centers for Disease Control and Prevention: Pregnancy related mortality surveillance: United States, 1991-1999, *MMWR Morb Mortality Wkly Rep* 52(SS2), 2003.

Racial discrepancy persists, however, in maternal mortality rates as in life expectancy. Table 15-2 illustrates how non-white women have a significantly higher incidence of death during pregnancy than whites. The gap in maternal mortality rates between black and white women has widened over the past several decades. Early in the twentieth century, black women were two times more likely to die of pregnancy-related complications than white women. Currently, black women are three times more likely to die as white women (CDC, 2003). Major risk factors for maternal death include lack of antepartal care and family planning services, inadequate health education, and poor nutrition. An additional risk factor, regardless of race, is advancing age. Women aged 40 and older have nearly four times the risk of dying from a pregnancy-related cause as women aged 30 to 34 years and twice the risk for women aged 35 to 39 years (CDC, 2003). Intrinsic maternal factors, such as increasing frequency of hypertension and a greater likelihood of uterine hemorrhage, help explain this increase in the mortality rate among older mothers.

In decreasing order of occurrence, the leading cause of maternal death is pulmonary embolism (17%), followed by pregnancy-induced hypertension, ectopic pregnancy, hemorrhage, stroke, and anesthesia (Cunningham et al., 2005). Death associated with legal surgical abortion is rare in the United States. Complications that result in death from legal abortion relate to the woman's age, the type of procedure, the gestational age of the fetus, and general health problems at the time of the abortion (Cates, Ellertson, and Stewart, 2004).

Since 1988, a medical method of abortion using mifepristone (i.e., RU-486), an antiprogestin medication, together with prostaglandins has been used in European countries and China. Although this method is as effective as surgical abortion, public pressure in the United States caused a delay in the testing, licensing, and manufacturing of RU-486 until the mid 1990s when it became available for clinical trials. In September 2000, the Food and Drug Administration (FDA) approved the use of RU-486, yet news reports suggest that physicians may be reluctant to provide this method of abortion for fear of being targeted as an "abortion doctor."

In time, as clinicians gain experience with this medical method of abortion, protocols may be adapted for women to use it at home. Additional research is needed to examine the acceptability of the newer medical methods of abortion among American women, the relationship between the medical method of abortion and a woman's cultural beliefs, and her decision-making process to choose between a medical method or surgical abortion.

Abortion is a controversial issue for providers and for the women in their care. An upstream intervention would certainly be the best strategy; however, until that time, nurses must continue to keep abreast of all available pregnancy prevention and termination options to provide the best counsel. ∎

According to the CDC (1999), **ectopic pregnancy** is the leading cause of maternal death in the first trimester, accounting for 13% of maternal deaths. Since the 1980s, the incidence of ectopic pregnancy has increased fourfold to 11.3 per 1000 pregnancies among women 15 to 44 years of age. Racial discrepancy is evident and yields a rate of 14.7 per 1000 among non-whites compared with 10.3 per 1000 among whites. This disparity continues to increase throughout the reproductive years of non-white women, possibly because sexually transmitted diseases (STDs) are more frequently diagnosed among non-white women, and these clients have less access to health care.

The most significant risk for ectopic pregnancy is previous pelvic inflammatory disease (PID) or salpingitis; therefore women at risk for acquiring STDs must learn to protect themselves from these diseases. Additional risk factors for ectopic pregnancy include tubal pathology, previous ectopic pregnancy, tubal surgery, and the use of intrauterine contraceptive devices. Prevention interventions are critical in reducing a woman's risk for an ectopic pregnancy because early diagnosis and treatment greatly reduce the mortality rate. An important task of health care providers is to assist women and men to reduce personal health risk-taking behaviors related to sexuality.

Cancer

Cancer is the second leading cause of death in the United States, as 1 in every 4 Americans dies from some form. Further, cancer is expected to become the overall leading cause of death in the next decade (CDC, 2004).

Cancer rates appear to be increasing for a number of reasons including lifestyle choices (smoking, diet, sun exposure), increasing exposure to environmental carcinogens, and probably most importantly, age. To illustrate, death rates from cancer among women have increased from 136 per 100,000 women in 1960 to 167.3 per 100,000 women in 2000 (CDC, 2004). The American Cancer Society (ACS) estimates that 275,000 deaths will occur among women as a result of cancer in 2005 (ACS, 2005).

In 1987, lung cancer surpassed breast cancer as the leading cause of cancer deaths in women, and death rates increased sharply until about 1990; since then, lung cancer deaths have leveled off. In 2004, 27% of cancer deaths in American women were attributed to lung cancer; in comparison, breast cancer resulted in 15% of all cancer deaths (ACS, 2005). Colorectal cancer, the third most frequent cause of cancer deaths, accounts for 10% of all cancer deaths, and claims the lives of some 28,000 women annually.

Other female-specific cancers include uterine cancer (fourth most common cancer), ovarian cancer (seventh most common cancer), and cervical cancer (fourteenth most common cancer). Cervical cancer, in particular, has received considerable attention of late as it has been determined that 100% of women with cervical cancer have evidence of cervical infection with human papillomavirus (HPV) (ACS, 2005). In June, 2006, the FDA licensed Gardasil (Merck & Co, Inc), the first vaccine to prevent HPV infection (CDC, 2006; MedScape Today, 2006). Gardasil has been shown to be highly effective in preventing the most common types of HPV infection and was approved for use in females between 9 and 26 years of age. For additional information on the availability and recommended use of this vaccine, consult the CDC's website (http://www.cdc.gov/nip/acip/).

The good news is that healthy lifestyle changes and early detection and intervention have contributed to the decrease in mortality rates from some cancers. For example, the death rate for colorectal cancer has been decreasing for the past 15 years due to early detection and treatment (ACS, 2005).

Five-year survival rates vary according to the type of cancer and stage at diagnosis. For instance, the 5-year survival rate for all clients with lung cancer is only 15%. For localized breast cancer, it is 98%, but it is only 26% when diagnosed with distant metastases. Of cancers related to the reproductive tract, ovarian cancer has the lowest survival rate, as only around 44% of women survive for 5 years. When diagnosed at an early stage, 5-year survival rate for women with colon cancer is 90%, and for those with rectal cancer it is 87% (ACS, 2005).

Early diagnosis and prompt treatment are major factors in surviving many types of cancer. In addition, certain health choices may reduce an individual's risk of cancer. All women need to avoid health-deteriorating practices and replace them with health-promoting behaviors that foster a health-protecting lifestyle. If providers and clients applied everything known about cancer prevention, approximately two thirds of cancer cases would not occur. For example, women could reduce their risk for cancer by never smoking or by quitting if they already use tobacco products. Eating a nutritious diet can decrease a woman's risk of both heart disease and cancer. Also, physical activity helps protect against heart disease and some cancers by achieving or maintaining a healthy body weight. Obesity has been associated with an increased risk for cancers such as colon and rectum, endometrium, and breast (i.e., among postmenopausal women) (ACS, 2005).

Community health nurses play a major role in providing cancer control services that should be culturally sensitive and appropriate to the targeted aggregate. Community health nurses must encourage all females (i.e., from childhood to old age) to avoid tobacco in any form, maintain a healthy weight, stay physically active, and eat a low-fat, high-fiber diet filled with needed nutrients and calories (Rhodes, 2002; Vogel,

2003). The nurse should also recommend limiting alcohol and the consumption of salt-cured, smoked, and nitrite-cured foods and to practice safe sex (ACS, 2004).

For women, cancer is not just another chronic disease. It evokes more fear than heart disease, which is the number one killer. In addition, cancer's relevance for women changes across the lifespan.

Cardiovascular Disease

CVD accounts for about 38% of all deaths in the United States, or about 1 out of every 2.6. Each day, more than 2600 Americans die from CVD. About one in four Americans has one or more forms of CVD (e.g., high blood pressure, coronary heart disease, stroke, congenital defects, and rheumatic heart disease). One in ten women under age 60 has some form of CVD; the ratio increases to one in three after age 65. Black women are more likely to die from CVDs than white women. In 2002, the CVD death rate among white females was 265.5 per 100,000, compared with 368.1 per 100,000 for black females. Black women are also more likely to die from stroke than white women (39.2 per 100,000 and 22.9 per 100,000, respectively, or 71% higher) (AHA, 2005).

Rates of CVD among women can decline further when individuals become more aware of risk factors and accept responsibility for managing their own health and well-being (Kuehn, McMahon, and Creekmore, 1999). Concerned and motivated providers must encourage women to practice heart-healthy behaviors.

Diabetes

Diabetes mellitus is another disease that causes the premature death of many women and overall ranks sixth in mortality among that group. Furthermore, diabetes ranks fourth as the cause of death among several aggregates, including Native-American, black, and Asian, and is fifth among Hispanics (National Center for Health Statistics, 2004). The incidence of non–insulin-dependent diabetes (NIDDM) increases with age and is slightly higher for women than for men (i.e., except among those aged 65 to 74 years). The highest prevalence of NIDDM is found among the Pima Indians (35%), which is significantly higher than among the entire Native-American population (15%). Blacks have a prevalence rate of 11.4%, which is almost twice that of the general population (6.3%); likewise, about 8% of Hispanics are diabetics, significantly higher than the population as a whole (CDC, 2003).

In addition to being a serious illness in itself, diabetes is a risk factor for the development of CVD; furthermore, it dramatically influences the severity and course of the CVD. When diabetic clients suffer heart attacks, their overall in-hospital mortality rate is much higher than that of non-diabetic clients. The prognosis for diabetic women after a myocardial infarction is particularly grave: the overall in-hospital mortality rate is 37% for women, compared with 19% for men. Among the aggregates at highest risk of death are obese, diabetic women. An upstream approach to this problem includes helping women maintain a desirable weight throughout life in an effort to avoid nutrition-related causes of death, such as diabetes and CVD.

Morbidity Rate
Hospitalizations

The 1999 National Hospital Discharge Survey (CDC, 2001) reported that more women than men are hospitalized each year in the United States. However, the average length of hospitalization for males (5.4 days) exceeds that for females (4.7 days) until after age 65. Pneumonia resulted in an average hospital stay of 6 days, which occurred most frequently among women aged 65 or older. Fractures accounted for an average of 5.5 days, malignant neoplasms for an average 7 days, and diseases of the heart for an average 4.7 days.

The prospective payment system for hospitalization resulted in an increased demand for skilled nursing services in the home. After hospitalization for several of these conditions, community health nurses may provide ongoing nursing care in the home by referral. Nurses practicing in home environments must be prepared to deliver high-tech and high-touch services. Chapter 31 discusses home health care in detail.

Chronic Conditions and Limitations

Women are more likely than men to be disabled from chronic conditions. Arthritis and rheumatism, hypertension, and impairment of the back or spine decrease women's activity level more often than they affect their male counterparts. In fact, almost twice as many women (25.9%) as men (16.8%) are limited in activity from arthritis and rheumatism. Women are more likely than men to have difficulty performing activities such as walking, bathing or showering, preparing meals, and doing housework (CDC, 2005).

Functional limitations may require home health care that community health nurses supervise and deliver. Nurses plan and implement interventions based on functional assessments. The care plan facilitates optimal resumption of the individual's independence in personal care activities.

Surgery

Hysterectomy is the second most frequently performed major surgical procedure among women of reproductive age; approximately 600,000 hysterectomies are performed each year (CDC, 2002). Hysterectomy rates for black women are slightly higher than those for white women (6.2 and 5.3 per 1000 women, respectively).

The most common reason for hysterectomy is uterine fibroids or leiomyoma, which contributes to more than one third of all such surgeries, but considerably more for blacks (68%) than for whites (33%) (CDC, 2005). White women are more often diagnosed with endometriosis and uterine prolapse, which are the second and third most common reasons for hysterectomy. Hysterectomy rates are the highest in women aged 40 to 44 years (CDC, 2002).

New procedures and options have become available to women over the past few years. Myomectomy, or removing only the tumors with repair of the uterus and the use of gonadotropin-releasing hormone to shrink the tumors can decrease the need for hysterectomy; women may not know about these alternatives. Community health nurses function as advocates for women and can provide health education programs related to alternatives to hysterectomy, indications for hysterectomy and oophorectomy (i.e., removal of ovaries), and information regarding the type of surgical approach and the purpose of a second opinion. Second opinions and higher levels of education tend to decrease the rate of hysterectomies (Finkel and Finkel, 1990).

Birth by cesarean delivery is the most prevalent surgical procedure experienced by women in the United States and accounts for 1 out of every 4 births. Several factors contribute to the high rates of cesarean delivery, including physicians' fear of malpractice suits, physicians not performing vaginal breech deliveries and mid-pelvic floor forceps deliveries, and progress in technology that facilitates fetal monitoring. As part of the childbirth curriculum, childbirth educators offer information related to the cesarean birth experience. Some hospitals or groups, such as Cesarean Support, Education, and Concern, hold classes in preparation for a repeat cesarean birth or for couples desiring vaginal birth after cesarean (Olds, London, and Ladewig, 2004).

Mental Health

The most frequently occurring interruption in women's mental health relates to depression. Well-controlled epidemiological studies consistently demonstrate that women experience depression at two to three times the rate of men (American Psychological Association, 2005). Symptoms of depression range from depressed mood to apathy, anxiety, irritability, and thoughts of death and suicide (Evans et al., 1999). Women with socioeconomic barriers such as lower income and lower educational levels, racial/ethnic discrimination, unemployment, poor health, single parenthood, and high-stress jobs are at greater risk for depression than women with higher educational levels or higher economic status. Those lacking adequate financial or emotional support often express a sense of frustration and futility.

Nurses practicing in community health settings should be aware of the signs and symptoms of depression and identify referral sources for professional help within the community. The nurse needs to also be aware of the impact a mother's depression may have on her child's development and family functioning. A woman experiencing depression may display some signs and symptoms listed in Box 15-1.

SOCIAL FACTORS AFFECTING WOMEN'S HEALTH

Health Care Access

An estimated 15.6% of the population, or 45 million U.S. citizens lacked health insurance coverage in 2003, up from 43.6 million people in 2002 (U.S. Census Bureau, 2004). Owing to the nature of their employment, women frequently lack health insurance but may not be eligible for Medicaid benefits because their income is too high. Young adults (i.e., those between ages 16 and 24 years) make up approximately 50% of individuals without health insurance. Lacking economic means for meeting the costs of health care, these women are not likely to seek health care until they or a

BOX 15-1 Signs and Symptoms of Depression

➤ Mood disturbance and emotional distress
➤ Sad, blue, and gloomy feelings
➤ Feelings of helplessness, hopelessness, inadequacy, and worthlessness
➤ Loss of interest in work, friends, family, and sex
➤ Sleep pattern disturbances
➤ Loss of appetite or voracious appetite
➤ Feelings of heaviness in head or chest
➤ Tendency to cry easily and sigh often
➤ Complaints of headaches, backaches, and constipation
➤ Difficulty in concentrating and making decisions
➤ Flat to hectic gaiety
➤ Everything drooping (i.e., mouth, eyes, posture, and body language)

family member is in acute distress. Others may rely on home remedies, over-the-counter drugs, or folk healers for health care. Older adults, who are usually covered by Medicare, may also delay seeking health care. Older women on fixed incomes may have difficulty meeting copayments required by Medicare and paying for prescription medications. Many senior citizens have paid hospitalization insurance premiums for policies that fail to meet the gap.

Education and Work

In the workplace, women predominate as librarians, teachers, social workers, and nurses, which accounted for 65% of working women in 1990 (Pollard and Tordella, 1993). However, in the 1980s, more women began to enter professions traditionally held by men (e.g., lawyers, physicians, and dentists), and by 1990, more than half (57%) of young professionals were women. According to Pollard and Tordella, this is a revolutionary development and the likely trend of the future.

Academic statistics show a significant rise in the achievements of women. In 1970, 55.4% of all women aged 25 or older were high school graduates compared with 81.6% in 1995 and 85% in 2003. Of this same age-group, 25.7% had completed college in 2003, which was more than three times the 1970 rate of 8.1% (U.S. Census Bureau, 2004). An increasing number of women earned degrees in traditionally male-dominated professions. Table 15-3 reflects recent changes occurring in percentages of women receiving degrees in medicine, dentistry, law, and theology.

Employment and Wages

In 2005, more than 60% of women of working age (ages 18 to 64 years) were employed (i.e., compared to 73% of men). In addition, more than half (62%) of women with young children (younger than 6 years) were working outside the home (U.S. Department of Labor, 2005). In 1950, only 12% of women were combining these roles (Chadwick and Heaton, 1992).

Several questions concern women's health and well-being related to employment issues. A review of female-dominated versus male-dominated jobs discloses inequalities in wage and salary scales; despite the diminishing gap between

TABLE 15-3 Percentages of Degrees Received by Women

DEGREE	1970	1980	1988	1996	2002
Medicine (MD)	8.4	23.4	33.3	40.9	44.4
Dentistry (DDS or DMD)	0.9	13.3	26.7	35.8	38.5
Law (LLB or JD)	5.4	30.2	40.8	43.4	48.0
Theology (BD, MDiv, or MHL)	2.3	13.8	19.3	23.3	33.2

From US Department of Education: *Digest of education statistics*, Washington, DC, 2003, The Author.

TABLE 15-4 Median Annual Earnings by Type of Household: 1969, 1979, 1989, 1999, and 2003

HOUSEHOLD TYPE	1969	1979	1989	1999	2003
Married couple with children	41,453	47,793	50,613	56,827	62,405
Female householder with children	16,327	18,468	17,651	26,164	29,307
Male householder with children	33,749	36,619	34,646	41,830	41,959

From US Census Bureau: *Income, poverty, and health insurance coverage in the United States: 2003*, Current Population Reports P60-226, 2004, The Author, http://www.census.gov/prod/2004pubs/p60-226.pdf.

women's and men's incomes, there is still much room for improvement. Table 15-4 depicts median weekly earnings income by sex and ethnicity for both men and women (U.S. Census Bureau, 2004). Disparities in income, based on sex and ethnicity, are clear.

Women heads of households and their children are the poorest aggregate in the United States. This phenomenon is labeled "the feminization of poverty." The nurse working with impoverished families should be aware of social services, child care programs, emergency services, and other resources for families in need. The community health nurse often needs to act as case manager and advocate for families with social service agencies and other public entities.

Working Women and Home Life

Added to inequalities outside the home are inequalities within the home. A working woman is less likely to have a spouse or partner help with the home and children. Even when a spouse or partner is present, the burdens of housework and child care usually fall more heavily on women, regardless of ethnicity. Mothers generally spend more time than fathers preparing meals and training and disciplining their children. These multiple-role demands and conflicting expectations contribute to stress (American Academy of Pediatrics, 2005; Matthews and Power, 2002).

However, changes are occurring as younger and older men now report spending more time in family activities compared with middle-aged men. Blacks and Hispanics tend to spend a

TABLE 15-5   Characteristics of Black, White, and Hispanic Female-Headed Households: 2004

CHARACTERISTIC	BLACK	WHITE	HISPANIC
Never married	49.9	25.7	39.5
Married and spouse absent	15.3	14.1	24.1
Widowed	11.1	18.1	10.5
Divorced	23.5	41.4	25.8
Number of children per female-headed household	1.92	1.58	1.90

Modified from U.S. Census Bureau: *Statistical abstract of the United States: 2004–2005*, http://www.census.gov/prod/2004pubs/04statab/pop.pdf.

little more time working at family tasks than white men. Increasingly, books and articles encourage wives and husbands to make their needs known. As a result, many couples emphasize increased communication between partners. Marriage enrichment programs, often offered through churches and synagogues, teach couples how to communicate more effectively with each other. Such efforts should foster equality between partners.

Family Configuration and Marital Status

Women are members of **multiple family configurations** (e.g., nuclear families, extended family units, single-parent units, families of group marriages, blended family units, adoptive family units, non-legal heterosexual unions, lesbian family units, and others). This diversity causes changes in women's roles within families. Whether or not they function in a traditional role, most women do whatever is necessary to maintain the integrity of their families. Early assessment of the strengths of family units by the community health nurse provides a database for positive nursing interventions established on upstream strategies to enhance each family's level of health and well-being.

Many women are delaying marriage, and an increasing number are not marrying. Overall marriage rates have remained stable perhaps because the increasing number of remarriages balances the declining rate of first marriages. When a relationship ends in divorce or separation, more women than men have the responsibility of providing for themselves and their children. According to the U.S. Census Bureau (2004), single-parent households in 2000 represented 58.6% of all households with children. Single mothers are most often the head of a single-parent family. Percentages of female single-parent households with children under the age of 18 years are as follows: African American, 19.3%, Hispanic or Latina, 13.6%, white, 5.2% (U.S. Census Bureau, 2004) (Table 15-5). Even in the face of changing lifestyles, divorce, and increased mobility, which leads to long-distance relationships, most Americans report they remain connected to their extended families through parents, grandparents, siblings, aunts, and uncles.

One contemporary family configuration involves single women with one or more adopted children. Single-parent adoptions are legal, and an increasing number of single women are becoming adoptive parents. An often-ignored family structure is one headed by a lesbian parent. Lesbians who become parents have needs similar to those of all mothers. Many cities have lesbian-gay parent groups that provide support, anticipatory guidance, and strategies for coping in society. However, lesbian women often neglect their own health. This self-neglect may be traced to hostile and rejecting attitudes of health care providers (Zeidenstein, 2004). However, the parents or guardians must remain healthy to ensure the child's well-being. A delay in health-seeking services may have devastating consequences for both parent and child.

HEALTH PROMOTION STRATEGIES FOR WOMEN

A woman's ability to carry out her important roles can affect her entire family; therefore women should receive services that promote health and detect disease at an early stage. Early detection and improved treatments for disease allow women to return to work or remain working throughout the course of an illness. Although work is essential to the economic and social well-being of many women's families, the workplace itself creates physical and social stress. As more women enter the workforce and face many of the same risks and stressors as men, it is not surprising that their formerly favorable mortality and morbidity rates have been declining.

Many women seek information that will allow them to be in control of their own health. Since the early 1970s, women have met in self-help groups to develop a better understanding of their own health needs. Some of the health behaviors that women learn in self-help groups are the importance of nutrition and exercise, breast self-examination (BSE), pregnancy testing, and contraceptive awareness; recognition of the early signs of vaginal infections and STDs; and awareness of the variations in female anatomy and physiology.

For women who desire to become more knowledgeable about their own health, there are books available in bookstores, public libraries, and among the holdings of traditional women's groups such as sororities, federated women's clubs, and others. An excellent resource for women is the *FDA Consumer*, the official magazine of the FDA. The *FDA Consumer* reports on FDA studies that cover a variety of women's health issues, such as mammography standards, menopause, treatment for STDs, eating disorders, infertility, cosmetic safety, silicone breast implants, and osteoporosis. The *FDA Consumer* magazine can be found online at http://www.fda.gov/fdac/.

Pender's Health Promotion Model synthesizes the literature on health promotion and wellness. Pender notes that health-promoting behaviors are directed toward sustaining or increasing the level of well-being, self-actualization, and fulfillment of a given individual or group (Pender, Murdaugh, and Parsons, 2006). The community health nurse can use this model in teaching health behaviors that lead to general health promotion among women. However, because many models were developed for the middle class, they may not be useful to community health nurses working with low-income families. Health promotion for low-income, underserved women may differ from that for their middle-class counterparts.

Knowledge deficits related to body awareness prevail among all women, regardless of socioeconomic or educational level. Regardless of whether a group comprises college-educated professional women or blue-collar working women, many of the questions they pose are the same. For example, a woman may ask if she will menstruate after hysterectomy, whether she should perform a BSE, or what she can do to prevent recurrent episodes of vaginitis. Nurses can play an instrumental role in helping women develop a greater sense of self-awareness. Furthermore, community health nurses can remove the mystery surrounding the woman's body and encourage clients to ask previously unmentionable questions.

Acute Illness

Females report a greater incidence of acute conditions than males. This section describes several of the most common.

Urinary Tract Infection and Dysuria

By age 32, half of all women report a history of at least one UTI. Peak incidence in women is ages 20 to 24 (Foxman and Brown, 2003). In every age-group, adult women have a higher incidence of UTI than men, with an annual incidence of 12.6% compared with 3% among men. The higher incidence among women is attributed to differences in anatomy, which enhance the exposure to potential uropathogens and enhance the ability of these pathogens to colonize the urinary tract.

Women often experience dysuria, the sensation of pain, burning, or discomfort on urination. Dysuria accounts for 5% to 15% of visits to family physicians; approximately 25% of American women report acute dysuria every year. The symptom is most prevalent in women 25 to 54 years of age and in those who are sexually active. Although many physicians equate dysuria with urinary tract infection (UTI), it is actually a symptom that has many potential causes, infection being only one. Treatment with antibiotics may be inappropriate, except in carefully selected clients (Bremnor and Sadovsky, 2002). Risk factors for both UTI and dysuria are female gender, advancing age, sexual activity, vaginitis, renal stone, and a history of sexual abuse, which can result in psychogenic dysuria (Bremnor and Sadovsky, 2002).

Diseases of the Reproductive Tract

Acute illnesses specific to the reproductive tract include conditions such as vulvovaginitis, pelvic inflammatory disease, and toxic shock syndrome.

Vulvovaginitis

Vulvovaginitis may start in girls before puberty and is more common than in women of reproductive age. The labia of young girls lack fat and the vaginal mucosa is thin and friable. Vaginitis continues to be a frequent and often acute painful problem for which thousands of women seek relief annually. Women often report an increase in vaginal discharge, itching, burning, dysuria, and dyspareunia. The physical examination may reveal vaginal and/or vulvar edema and erythema and a discharge that varies in color, odor, and consistency (Mou, 1999). The reader is referred to a women's health text to learn more about the etiology of these conditions, their treatment, and comfort measures.

Pelvic Inflammatory Disease

Pelvic inflammatory disease (PID) refers to acute infection of the upper genital tract structures in women, involving any or all of the uterus, fallopian tubes, and ovaries. It is estimated that more than one million women experience an episode of acute PID each year (Epperly and Viera, 2005). PID most commonly affects young, sexually active women. Risk factors include multiple sexual partners, non-barrier contraceptive use, instrumentation of the cervix, and smoking. PID is considered a community-acquired infection initiated by a sexually transmitted agent; the most common is *Chlamydia trachomatis. Neisseria gonorrhea* is the second most common cause and may be concurrent with chlamydial infection. Women with PID often have atypical or no symptoms. If symptomatic, a woman may experience lower abdominal or pelvic pain, malodorous or new-onset vaginal discharge, abnormal uterine/vaginal bleeding, dyspareunia, dysuria, nausea, vomiting, and fever.

The diagnosis of PID is often based on imprecise clinical findings. Diagnosis is critical because even mild to moderate forms of the disease have serious reproductive sequelae, including ectopic pregnancy and infertility. The causative organism is usually unknown at the time of initial therapy, and treatment includes antimicrobial coverage against the broadest possible range of pathogens. The CDC (2002) has developed criteria for the diagnosis and treatment of PID. All clients with PID must return for evaluation after initiation of therapy, usually in 2 to 3 days and again in 4 days after completion of therapy. In addition, the woman's sex partner(s) needs evaluation and treatment. The woman and her partner or partners are advised to avoid sexual activity until they are treated/cured. As with other STDs, counseling for women diagnosed with PID must include individualized behavioral messages aimed at risk reduction.

Toxic Shock Syndrome

Toxic shock syndrome (TSS) is a rare but serious disorder caused by toxins released by some strains of *Staphylococcus aureus.* TSS came to public attention in 1980 based on a series of menstrually associated cases (Davis et al., 1980). The number of cases of menstrual TSS has declined from 9 out of 100,000 women in 1980 to 1 out of 100,000 women since 1986 (CDC, 1990). It is most associated with tampon use during menses; non-menstrual TSS risk is increased for women who use vaginal barrier methods for birth control (Cates and Stewart, 2004). The incidence of TSS has declined over the years owing to product changes and media warnings about tampon use (Farley, 1994). Although rare, TSS is a serious disorder to women's health, and providers must make women aware of this acute illness and its potential consequences, encourage them to report symptoms early, and exercise caution when using tampons and vaginal family planning methods (Cates and Stewart, 2004). Although TSS occurs most often in women of reproductive age who are menstruating, it has also occurred in children and men (Creehan, 1995).

Chronic Illness

Included among chronic diseases that may affect a woman during her life span are arteriosclerotic heart disease (ASHD), hypertension, diabetes, arthritis, osteoporosis, and cancer.

Arteriosclerotic Heart Disease

According to clinical evidence, ASHD may have its beginnings in the second and third decades of a woman's life. Changing lifestyles are altering these statistics, but some risk factors such as race or family history of ASHD are non-modifiable. As discussed earlier, black women are more vulnerable to ASHD than white women and experience congestive heart failure and angina pectoris after myocardial infarction more frequently (AHA, 2005). Among the modifiable risk factors are the following:

- Cigarette smoking
- Obesity
- Diet high in calories, total fats, cholesterol, refined carbohydrates, and sodium
- Hypertension
- Glucose intolerance
- Elevated serum lipid levels
- Personality type
- Sedentary lifestyle
- Stress

Women should reduce their risk for ASHD by controlling as many of these factors as possible.

Hypertension

The latest report of the Joint National Committee on Prevention, Detection, Evaluation, and Treatment of High Blood Pressure defines **hypertension** as blood pressure of 140/90 mm Hg or greater. The guidelines have included a new category, "prehypertensive," which refers to systolic pressure of 120 to 139 and/or diastolic pressure of 80 to 89. Clients with prehypertension are at increased risk for progression to hypertension and require lifestyle modifications to prevent CVD (Chobanian et al., 2003).

Essential hypertension is the most common type of chronic hypertensive disorder in women of childbearing age, accounting for 85% of such cases. It is also responsible for approximately one third of all hypertension cases during pregnancy. Hypertension is more common in women than in men and affects more blacks than whites. Additional factors associated with primary hypertension are age (older than 35 years), family history of hypertension, obesity, cigarette smoking, and diabetes mellitus (AHA, 2005). Hypertension usually starts with an asymptomatic phase; therefore, every woman should be screened on an average of every 2 years beginning in her teenage years. Diagnosis is crucial to prevent or modify possible complications of this disease.

Diabetes

According to the American Diabetes Association (2002), 18.2 million people (6.3% of the population) have diabetes in the United States. Furthermore, although an estimated 13 million have been diagnosed, some 5.2 million people are not aware they have the disease. In previous years, community health nurses have worked to educate women to assume responsibility in their management of diabetes mellitus. More recently, community health nurses have been actively involved in education and screening programs for groups at high risk. Included in these groups are individuals who have a family history of diabetes, those who are obese, and older adults. Nurses who design education programs need to be aware of the ethnic differences in the prevalence of diabetes. African American are 1.6 times more likely to have diabetes than non-Latino whites, and 1 in 4 African-American women over 55 years of age has diabetes. Latinos have an increased prevalence of 1.5 times higher than non-Latino whites (American Diabetes Association, 2002).

According to Cunningham and colleagues (2005), pregnancy is potentially diabetogenic. Pregnancy may aggravate the condition, and clinical diabetes may appear in some women only during pregnancy. Consequently, considerable attention has been given to screening for diabetes in pregnancy.

Controversy surrounds the most effective method of screening for diabetes, but regardless of the selected method, the nurse is involved in explaining the purpose of the screening and how to prepare for the tests. In most public health settings, the nurse is responsible for explaining the results.

Arthritis

In 2005, 66 million people in the United States, nearly 1 in 3 adults, were afflicted with arthritis. The incidence of osteoarthritis is higher in women than in men: approximately 41.0 million women have the condition compared with 28.9 million men (Arthritis Foundation, 2005). The cause of arthritis is not known; however, recurring multiple factors in the development of arthritis include diet, environment, and stress.

Rheumatoid arthritis (RA) can affect anyone, but 70% of people with RA are women. Onset usually occurs between 30 and 50 years of age. Interestingly, RA often goes into remission in pregnant women, although symptoms tend to increase in intensity after the baby is born, and RA develops more often than expected the year after giving birth. Although women are two to three times more likely to get RA than men, men tend to be more severely affected when they do get it (Arthritis Foundation, 2005). Nursing interventions focus on prevention of joint deformity and lifestyle modification if necessary.

Osteoporosis

Osteoporosis is a major disorder affecting women. Estimates of its occurrence range from 25% to 50% of postmenopausal women. Although men may experience osteoporosis, it is four times more common among women. The National Osteoporosis Foundation (2005) estimates that of the 10 million Americans who have osteoporosis, 8 million are women and 2 million are men. An additional 34 million Americans have osteopenia. Half of all non-Hispanic white women in the United States will sustain an osteoporosis-related fracture during their lifetime. The most serious complication of osteoporosis is hip fracture. Indeed, some 280,000 Americans experience hip fractures each year; approximately 24% die within a year from complications from the injury (U.S. Department of Health and Human Services [USDHHS], 2000b).

Postmenopausal white women are at highest risk for osteoporosis. In women, loss of bone begins at an earlier age and proceeds twice as rapidly as in men. The recent guidelines issued by the National Osteoporosis Foundation recommend bone mineral density tests for selected post-menopausal women and the use of oral bisphosphonates as the first-line pharmacological treatment of osteoporosis. In light of the results of the women's health initiative study showing that non-estrogen therapies fail or cause intolerance to side effects, hormone replacement therapy is currently considered second-line therapy (Wei et al., 2003). Osteoporosis has no cure; therefore prevention is especially important early in life. Prevention involves an awareness of dietary practices such as maintaining a correct balance of calcium, vitamin D, and protein throughout life, in addition to regular weight-bearing, muscle-strengthening, and aerobic exercise.

Nurses in ambulatory health practices should encourage women to become more knowledgeable of the strategies to prevent osteoporosis. For women diagnosed with osteoporosis, nurses can assist in various aspects of management (e.g., education regarding prescribed medication, follow-up care, avoidance of complications, and dietary modifications as needed).

Breast Cancer

The incidence of breast cancer has been increasing since the 1950s. Presently, 1 of every 7 women will acquire breast cancer sometime in her life. The chance of dying from breast cancer is about 1 in 33. The ACS estimates that 213,000 women in the United States will be found to have invasive breast cancer in 2006. Risk factors include aging, personal or family history (especially mother or sister) of breast cancer, early age at menarche, late age at menopause, never having children, or having a first child after age 30. Female gender and aging are the most significant risk factors for breast cancer (ACS, 2006).

According to the results of a randomized trial of women employed in Shanghai textile factories from October 1989 through July 2000, the mortality rate from breast cancer in women who practiced BSE was no lower than in women who did not practice BSE. In the group that practiced BSE, there was a higher rate of breast biopsy that did not reveal breast cancer. The current position of the U.S. Preventive Health Services Task Force is that there is insufficient evidence to recommend for or against the teaching of BSE (Thomas et al., 2002).

The ACS (2005) makes the following recommendations related to BSE for early detection of breast cancer:

- BSE should be performed monthly beginning at age 20. But BSE is only one part of a three-part early detection program, which should include mammography and clinical breast examination (examination preformed by a medical professional).

- Mammography and clinical breast examination have the greatest impact on reducing breast cancer mortality. BSE's role in early detection is a supporting but important one.
- BSE contributes to awareness, helping women be alert to changes in their breasts and identify changes earlier. However, for women 40 and older, the greatest potential to save lives from breast cancer is through early detection with mammography (ACS, 2005).

When a palpable lump or an abnormality is found on mammography, health care providers use specific algorithms to evaluate the lump and determine a course of action (Love et al., 1996). All nurses must be familiar with resources that may assist women in the diagnostic process (Facione, 1999). Breast health centers are excellent resources for women, and many centers accept self-referrals.

Lung Cancer

Although breast cancer is the most common cancer among women (i.e., excluding skin cancer), cancer of the lung and bronchus is responsible for more cancer deaths. Lung cancer is responsible for 20,000 more deaths yearly in U.S. women than breast cancer. In fact, lung cancer kills more women annually than breast, ovarian, and uterine cancers combined (Patel, 2005). Between 1990 and 2003, there was a 60% increase in the number of new cases of lung cancer in American women, whereas the number of men diagnosed with lung cancer remained stable (Patel, 2005). The increase in the incidence of lung cancer in women is due primarily to an increase in their tobacco use: 85% to 90% of all clients who develop lung cancer have a history of cigarette smoking. Yet, only 20% of cigarette smokers develop lung cancer, suggesting that the cause of lung cancer is multifactorial.

Widely accepted risk factors for lung cancer include exposure to environmental tobacco smoke, certain occupational exposures (especially asbestos), genetic predisposition, sex, gender, diet, chronic lung disease, and a history of tobacco-related cancer (Rivera and Stover, 2004). Studies have shown that the risks for development of lung cancer are different in women compared with men and that lung cancer appears to be a biologically different disease in women. Women smokers are more likely than men to develop adenocarcinoma of the lung, and women who have never smoked are more likely to develop lung cancer than men who have never smoked. These differences are due to hormonal, genetic, and metabolic differences between the sexes (Patel, 2005).

Although medical treatment may be similar for men and women, the symptom distress, quality of life, and demands of illness experienced by women may be different than they are for men because the competing household, child care, and other role-related demands take a toll on many women (Sarna and McCorkle, 1996). Further, women with advanced lung cancer report more psychological symptoms than men (Hopwood and Stephens, 1995).

Lung cancer is often a fatal illness because it is difficult to obtain early detection and effective treatment for advanced disease. Lung cancer at diagnosis is most commonly at an advanced stage. Women appear to have a slight survival advantage over men: the 5-year survival rate for women who have lung cancer is 15.6% compared with 12.4% for men (Patel, 2005)

The primary factor in preventing lung cancer is for individuals to never start smoking or to quit smoking. Nurses must work with other health care providers to reverse the morbidity and mortality rates related to this disease. The Agency for Healthcare Research and Quality has developed a useful guideline for health care professionals to assist women and their families in smoking cessation efforts. The Agency for Healthcare Research and Quality has summaries of more than 400 guidelines on a wide variety of topics, which can be found on their website (http://www.ahrq.gov).

Gynecological Cancers

About 20% of all malignant diseases in women occur in the genital tract. Carcinoma of the cervix is the most common and accounts for 21% of all new genital tract malignancies. The cervix is accessible to cytologic study; therefore the mortality rate related to cervical cancer has decreased. Risk factors for cervical cancer include coitus at an early age, multiple sexual partners, history of sexually transmitted infections with certain types of HPV, cigarette smoking, and low socioeconomic status (ACS, 2006).

The incidence of invasive cervical cancer has declined dramatically as a result of regular Pap tests that allow for identification of a precancerous condition (i.e., cervical carcinoma in situ). However, the ACS (2006) estimated that 3700 women would die from the disease in 2006.

RESEARCH HIGHLIGHTS

Cancer Screening Study

Surveys from 209 Vietnamese women residing in Houston, Texas, describing their beliefs and actions related to breast and cervical screening were analyzed in this study. The researchers found that 68% of the women had never had a Pap test. Also, 27% reported they performed breast self-examination (BSE) monthly, 45% had a yearly breast examination by a health provider, and 45% had had a mammogram in their lifetime. Only 15%, however, had had a mammogram during the current year. The main predictors of Pap test were educational level (higher), marital status (married), and lack of barriers. Predictors of regular BSE and mammography include lack of barriers, education level (higher), family history of breast cancer, and age (older).

Ho V, Yamal JM, Atkinson EN, Basen-Engquist K, Tortolero-Luna G, Follen M: Predictors of breast and cervical screening in Vietnamese women in Harris County, Houston, Texas, *Cancer Nurs* 28(2):119-131, 2005.

In recent years, a debate has arisen regarding how often a woman should have a Pap smear. Current guidelines recommend screening to begin approximately 3 years after a woman begins having vaginal intercourse, but no later than 21 years of age. Screening should be done every year with regular Pap tests or every 2 years using liquid-based tests. At or after age 30, women who have had three normal test results in a row may get screened every 2 to 3 years. However, doctors may suggest a woman get screened more frequently if she has certain risk factors, such as HIV infection or a weakened immune system. Women age 70 and older who have had three or more consecutive Pap tests in the past 10 years may choose to stop cervical cancer screening (ACS, 2004).

A self-collected tissue sample that detects HPV may become an effective alternative to the Pap smear (Wright, 2000). This test is especially important for use with populations at risk for HPV infection and for poor regions of the world (see Cancer Prevention Study).

The incidence of carcinoma of the endometrium has increased significantly during the past three decades, being commonly found in women during their sixth and seventh decades of life (i.e., 80% of women with this condition are postmenopausal). Approximately 7350 women in the United States will die from endometrial cancer in 2006 (ACS, 2006). Factors related to its occurrence are obesity, low parity, diabetes mellitus, and conditions in which high circulating estrogen levels are not countered by adequate progesterone levels. The most common sign of endometrial cancer, occurring in 90% of women, is abnormal vaginal bleeding. Postmenopausal women experiencing vaginal bleeding should seek immediate gynecological evaluation.

Cancer of the ovary causes more deaths than any other pelvic malignancy. In the United States, ovarian cancer's annual incidence usually ranges between 5 and 15 cases per 100,000 women. Approximately 1 out of 70 women will acquire ovarian cancer, a rate that increases fairly rapidly after age 40. Risk factors include increasing age, nulliparity, a history of breast cancer, and a family history of breast and ovarian cancer (ACS, 2006). Early-stage detection of

HEALTHY PEOPLE 2010 | Selected Objectives for Family Planning

Objective	Baseline	Target
9-1: Increase the proportion of pregnancies that are intended.	51%	70%
9-7: Reduce pregnancies among adolescent females.	68 pregnancies per 1000 females 15 to 17 years of age	43 pregnancies per 1000 females 15 to 17 years of age
9-11: Increase the proportion of young adults who have received formal instruction before turning 18 years of age on reproductive health issues.	64%	90%
9-12: Reduce the proportion of married couples whose ability to conceive or maintain a pregnancy is impaired.	13%	10%

From U.S. Department of Health and Human Services: *Healthy People 2010,* ed 2, Washington, DC, 2000a, The Author.

ovarian cancer is difficult; therefore it has usually reached an advanced stage once discovered. The health professional should be alert to ovarian enlargement with suspicion that ovarian malignancy may be present. This is especially true in postmenopausal women.

The most common sign a woman experiences is abdominal enlargement. She may complain that her skirts and slacks are getting tighter in the waist. This is a silent cancer; therefore any woman older than age 40 who experiences vague digestive complaints that persist and are not explained by another cause must have a thorough evaluation for ovarian cancer. According to the ACS (2006), transvaginal ultrasound and a blood test for tumor marker CA-125 may assist in the diagnosis of ovarian cancer; however, these are not recommended for routine screening of all women.

Mental Disorders and Stress

Various circumstances and conditions influence the mental health of women. Women face stressful decisions about career and family, and many express anxieties with these decisions. A woman may feel pressured to make decisions regarding childbearing before she has fulfilled her career goals. Deciding to focus on a career may mean decreased authority and the suffering of stress in the workplace. Women combining motherhood and a career have additional decisions such as working during pregnancy and choice of child care. More women are occupying middle-management positions, which are known for creating stress-related illness associated with high demands and little or no power.

A woman's emotional state is influenced by ovarian function from the onset of menstruation to the cessation of menstrual periods. Depression may be triggered or worsened by hormonal changes premenstrually. Women with a history of depression are also at increased risk for a recurrent episode of depression during the postpartum period, and they also are at risk for depression during the perimenopausal transition (Blehar, 2003). Depression is more prevalent among women than among men. In all age-groups from adolescents through the elderly, approximately two thirds of those affected are women. According to Bhatia and Bhatia (1999), the higher prevalence of depression in women is most likely due to a combination of gender-related differences in cognitive styles,

certain biological factors, and a higher incidence of psycho-social and economic stressors.

Mental disorders often go undiagnosed and untreated or undertreated despite the availability of effective treatments. Women may fail to recognize or correctly identify their symptoms, and even when they do, they may be reluctant to seek care because of stigma associated with mental illness (Blehar, 2003). Community health nurses are in a good position to assess women's moods in diverse aggregates and to assist in seeking and maintaining continuity of care (see Box 15-1).

Reproductive Health

Community health nurses provide a variety of services in the area of women's reproductive health from menarche through the postmenopausal phase. Nurses, in collaboration with other health care professionals, have identified a persistent group of preventable and correctable problems related to maternal-child health. *Healthy People 2010* (USDHHS, 2000b) provides numerous recommendations for improving maternal and infant health, including reduction of cigarette smoking, reduction of alcohol and other drug use, better nutrition, better socioeconomic opportunities (including education), and a decrease in environmental hazards.

For the *Healthy People 2000* initiative, family planning objectives witnessed progress. For example, the number of unintended pregnancies decreased from 56% to 49% between 1988 and 1995, yet the objective to reduce the rate of adolescent pregnancy still remains distant. With *Healthy People 2010* family planning objectives, the focus is on the positive that "all pregnancies should be intended." Examples of *Healthy People 2010* objectives related to family planning are shown above.

Nutrition

One of the most important factors in a woman's reproductive health is her total life nutritional experience from infancy through childhood and adolescence. Obesity has become a major public health concern. The community health nurse is in an advantageous position to provide nutritional counseling. The U.S. Department of Agriculture updates the dietary recommendations every 5 years based on current scientific information, and the 2005 Food Guide Pyramid stresses a personalized approach to healthy eating and physical activity. The new dietary pyramid includes the addition of the variable of activity, focusing on the importance of moderation, proportionality, and variety. It also depicts the five food groups and oils, and advocates personalization and gradual improvement. The updated guidelines encourage most Americans to eat fewer calories, be more active, and make wiser food choices (USDHHS, 2005).

Pregnancy may provide a motivational factor for developing an awareness of proper nutrition. During the nutritional assessment of a prenatal client, the community health nurse can take the opportunity to determine dietary habits and initiate a referral to the Special Supplemental Food Program for Women, Infants, and Children (WIC) when necessary. Women, Infants, and Children provides food vouchers for pregnant or breast-feeding women, infants, and children who are at nutritional risk.

Good nutrition must include factors other than kinds and amounts of foods. Other elements to consider include age, lifestyle, economic status, and culture. For example, when counseling a pregnant adolescent, the nurse can include the primary person responsible for meal preparation. The nurse should not ignore the adolescent in the planning of her diet, but should ask her to identify foods that she likes from those recommended. The nurse should to make the adolescent aware of the influence of her nutrition on fetal growth and development. This information must be balanced with the young woman's individual needs.

Family Planning

The community health nurse has many opportunities to provide counseling in the area of **family planning.** Although the phrase "family planning" has come to imply planned limitation of pregnancies, another important aspect of family planning concerns couples attempting to increase their chances of conception. This is because infertility occurs in a surprising number of otherwise healthy adults. Indeed, approximately 10% to 15% of couples in the United States are unintentionally childless (Nelson and Marshall, 2004).

Community health nurses are in a strategic position to provide support and guidance for women in the area of fertility control. Numerous factors contribute to the decision of whether to use family planning methods and what methods to use. When counseling women on this matter, the nurse should use a holistic approach. The nurse must consider factors such as age, sexual activity, cost, health care access, and the woman's and her partner's values and beliefs. After a discussion with the nurse about benefits and risks, indications and contraindications, and advantages and disadvantages of the various contraception methods, the client selects a method that she believes is safe, effective, and comfortable.

Health care professionals often neglect to mention natural family planning as a method of contraception. Although many consider this approach to be synonymous with the rhythm method, proponents of natural family planning are describing this method as *natural reproductive technology,* a term that is broader in scope and

---

ETHICAL Insights

Working With Women's Health

Community health nurses working in the field of women's health will be exposed to ethical dilemmas during their career. Due to this, nurses must have a working knowledge of the principles of health care ethics. The commonly accepted principles include the following:

➤ Respect for autonomy
➤ Beneficence
➤ Non-maleficence
➤ Justice

Nursing care revolves around moral values such as compassion, empathy, honesty, trust, and respect. Most encounters will be non-problematic. Occasionally, nurses may be exposed to clinical situations that challenge their values and beliefs. Clients and family members may, at times, also disagree with the nurse's professional advice/plan. It is important for the nurse to keep his or her personal philosophy, politics, religion, and moral values out of their clinical work with individuals and families.

Examples of potential ethical dilemmas related to women's health care are emergency contraception, abortion, assisted reproductive technology, and end-of-life issues.

---

encompasses the health of a woman's reproductive system. Such knowledge allows feelings of empowerment and a sense of control over fertility. Women experience self-knowledge and thereby gain autonomy in relation to fertility. Family and community health care professionals need to have up-to-date information concerning natural family planning. ∎

Women who decide that their families are large enough and do not wish to be concerned with temporary methods of fertility control may select voluntary surgical contraception (VSC) or contraceptive sterilization by tubal ligation. Vasectomy as a VSC continues to be a simpler, safer, and less expensive procedure than tubal ligation. The VSC is one of the most effective, safest, and cost-effective methods of family planning, and developed and developing countries use it widely (Pollack, Carignan, and Jacobstein, 2004). The client's decision must be based on clear, complete information for sterilization more than any other phase of family planning. The reversibility of sterilization procedures is not dependable; if a woman has doubts about her future childbearing, the nurse should encourage her to use other methods of fertility control.

Nurses worldwide have a major role to play if the health of women and their families is to improve. Besides being knowledgeable about family planning methods and services, all nurses must work for universally accessible maternal and child health care and seek to protect the rights of couples and individuals to receive good information about family planning. In addition, nurses must be involved in shaping policy that affects every woman's reproductive health. Research in the area of family planning will hopefully provide several safe options designed to meet the individual needs of all women.

Sexually Transmitted Diseases and Human Immunodeficiency Virus

STDs are commonly found among U.S. women. Community health nurses and other health providers, including physicians, NPs, nurse midwives, and social workers, must be prepared to provide age-appropriate STD prevention, education, and counseling.

Sexually Transmitted Diseases

Genital chlamydia infection is now the most commonly reported infectious disease in the United States; an estimated 3 million new cases occur annually. Furthermore, more than 650,000 cases of gonorrhea are reported every year, making it the second most commonly reported communicable disease in the United States (Cates, 2004). Further, the actual numbers are estimated to be about double, owing to underreporting.

A woman may acquire chlamydia infection simultaneously with gonorrhea; therefore she should be treated presumptively with a regimen effective against both organisms. As mentioned earlier, complications resulting from STDs include tubal occlusion, leading to infertility and ectopic pregnancy; pregnancy loss and neonatal injury caused by transmission of organism to fetus; genital cancers; and epidemiological synergy with HIV transmission (Cates, 2004). Other commonly occurring STDs are HPV, herpes, trichomoniasis, and syphilis. Chapter 23 contains detailed information on these diseases, their incidence, symptoms, and treatment.

Human Immunodeficiency Virus and Acquired Immunodeficiency Syndrome

Today, the HIV/AIDS epidemic represents a growing and persistent health threat to women in the United States, especially young women and women of color. In 2001, HIV infection was the leading cause of death for African-American women aged 25 to 34 years and was among the four leading causes of death for African-American women aged 20 to 24 and 35 to 44 years, as well as Hispanic women aged 35 to 44 years (CDC/NCHS, 2005). In 1992, women accounted for estimated 14% of adults and adolescents living with AIDS. By the end of 2003, this had grown to 22%. Rate of AIDS diagnoses for African-American women was approximately 25 times the rate for white women and 4 times the rate for Hispanic women (CDC/NCHS, 2005). Worldwide, AIDS is a leading cause of death among young women (WHO, 2004c).

According to the CDC (2005), risk factors and barriers to prevention for women include the following:

- Young age
- Lack of recognition of partner's risk
- Sexual inequality in relationships
- Biologic vulnerability and sexual transmitted infections
- Substance abuse
- Socioeconomic and other societal factors
- Working in the sex trade
- Participants in unprotected sex

In April 2005, the USDHHS released the updated *Guidelines for the Use of Antiretroviral Agents in HIV-1 Infected Adults and Adolescents* (USDHHS, 2005). Treatment guidelines continually evolve with new research and experience. It is imperative that the community health nurse working with this population stays abreast of the current trends for both counseling and treatment options.

Other Issues in Women's Health

Unintentional Injury or Accidents

Although unintentional injury affects women less commonly than it does men, several areas of concern still exist for women. For example, older women are at increased risk for accidents such as falls. Falls account for the majority of serious unintentional injuries and lead to 40% of all deaths from injury in people older than 75 years of age. Factors that may be responsible for this major cause of injury among older adults are an unsteady gait, reduced vision, or a hazardous environment. Older women experience an increasing number of falls; therefore the nurse must identify the preventable factors. Nurses, whether working with older adults in the home or in institutional settings, must be knowledgeable of hazards that may be corrected to decrease the incidence of falls.

Domestic violence is the single largest cause of injury to women between the ages of 15 and 44 in the United States—more than muggings, car accidents, and rapes combined. Each year between 2 million and 4 million women are battered, and 2,000 of these battered women will die of their injuries (American College of Emergency Physicians, 2003).

Abuse in women is often explained as accidental injury. Approximately 6% of visits made by women to emergency rooms are for injuries that result from physical battering by their husbands, former husbands, boyfriends, or lovers. Domestic violence includes physical, sexual, and psychological attacks and economic coercion (Warshaw, Ganley, and Salber, 1995).

All women should be questioned directly about abuse. However, according to Blair (1999), barriers can interfere with such screening, including frustration when clients fail to leave the abusive situation after intensive intervention or counseling. Also, many nurses are past or current victims of abuse; assessing abuse with clients can evoke painful emotions that the nurse may not be ready to confront.

Nurses employed in community health settings need to know how to make assessments, provide support, and make referrals to agencies dealing with domestic violence. In addition, nurses and other health care professionals must know the state laws related to reporting known or suspected domestic violence. Chapter 25 contains additional information about domestic violence.

Disability

More women than men have disabilities resulting from acute conditions, but women experience fewer disabilities resulting from chronic conditions because they report their symptoms earlier and receive necessary treatment. According to the U.S. Census Bureau (2000), of the population aged 16 to 64 years living with a disability, 19.6% are men and 17.6% are women. Women report proportionately more days of restricted activity than men. Women average 16.1 days of disability per year compared with 12.7 days for men (U.S. Census Bureau, 2000).

A frequently encountered disabling condition is dysmenorrhea, which is most often associated with ovulatory cycles and is one of the most common concerns of women. Dysmenorrhea affects approximately 50% to 80% of the female population between ages 15 and 24 years but continues to plague women throughout the reproductive years (Nelson, 2004). At least 10% to 20% of women with dysmenorrhea are incapacitated for 1 to 3 days each month. Dysmenorrhea is the greatest single cause of absenteeism from school and work among young women and causes the loss of approximately 140 million working hours annually; therefore the economic influence of this condition is significant.

Disabling conditions limit the physical functional abilities of many women, but the health care delivery system has often overlooked the unique needs of this aggregate. In planning care for disabled women, community health nurses should focus attention on enabling women to strengthen their capabilities. In addition, nurses should be sensitive to barriers in the clinical setting that affect the access of disabled women to health care services. Chapter 19 discusses the needs of disabled people in greater detail.

MAJOR LEGISLATION AFFECTING WOMEN'S HEALTH

Several legislative acts have a direct or indirect influence on the health of women. Many changes have been made in the past two decades that have the potential for improving the health and welfare of all women.

Public Health Service Act

The Public Health Service (PHS) Act, passed in 1982, provides biomedical and health services research, information dissemination, resource development, technical assistance, and service delivery. In the area of women's health, the PHS Act supports activities related to general health issues, reproductive health, social and behavioral issues, and mental health. Aggregates of women targeted by the PHS Act include those disabled by specific diseases, victims of sexual abuse and domestic violence, recent immigrants, and occupational groups.

The Family Planning Assistance Program, which is one component of the PHS Act, helps millions of women obtain family planning services each year. The need for subsidized family planning remains significant, and generous federal funds should be made available to meet documented needs. With regard to the particular relationship of family planning and low birth weight, both young teenage status and poverty are major risk factors for delivering infants with low birth weight. The program is an important part of the public effort to prevent low birth weight.

Civil Rights Act

Title VII of the **Civil Rights Act** of 1964 prohibits discrimination based on sex, race, color, religion, or national origin in determining employment eligibility or termination, wages, and fringe benefits. The Act was amended to prohibit discrimination against pregnant women or conditions involving childbirth or pregnancy. This landmark legislation makes it unlawful for employers to refuse to hire, employ, or promote a woman because she is pregnant. In addition, employee benefit plans that continue health insurance, income maintenance during disability or illness, or any other income support program for disabled workers must include disabilities resulting from pregnancy, childbirth, and other related conditions. If employers allow disabled employees to assume lighter or medically restricted assignments, the same considerations must extend to pregnant women.

The amendment does not require employers to pay health insurance benefits for abortions or abortion-related care unless the mother's life is endangered or she has medical complications after an abortion. Employers are prohibited from firing or refusing to hire a woman because she had an abortion.

Sexual harassment is a violation of the Civil Rights Act. Sexual harassment is "conduct of a sexual nature . . . unwelcome by the target . . . severe or pervasive enough to create an intimidating work environment" (Women Employed Institute, 1994). Female and male workers may face unwelcome sexual advances or requests for sexual favors or other verbal or physical conduct of a sexual nature. Awareness of sexual harassment in the workplace has increased dramatically over the past decade, but sexual harassment has not been eliminated.

Social Security Act

The Social Security Act provides monthly retirement and disability benefits to workers and survivor benefits to families of workers covered by Social Security. Full retirement benefits are available to workers after 10 years of covered employment.

The Social Security Act permits a divorced person to receive benefits based on a former spouse's earning record when that spouse retires, becomes disabled, or dies if the marriage lasted at least 10 years. Since January 1985, a woman who has been divorced for at least two years can receive spousal benefits at age 62, if her former husband is eligible for benefits, regardless of whether he is actually receiving them.

Medicare and Medicaid also resulted from the Social Security Act. Medicare is the insurance plan that covers the majority of the health care expenses of older adults, including payments for hospital care, physicians, home health care, and other services and supplies after co-payments and deductibles. Medicaid covers health care for indigent and eligible children and includes family planning, obstetric care, and preventive cancer screening for women, such as mammography and PAP smears. Chapters 9 and 10 describe Medicare and Medicaid in detail.

Occupational Safety and Health Act

The Occupational Safety and Health Act, enacted in 1970, helps ensure safe and healthful working conditions for workers throughout the United States. Although there is an increasing emphasis in the study of the health of women

TABLE 15-6 Hazardous Occupations in Which Women Are Employed

OCCUPATION	HEALTH HAZARD
Clerical workers	Organic solvents in stencil machines, correction fluids, rubber cement, and ozone from copying machines
Textile and apparel workers	Cotton dust, skin irritants, and chemicals
Hairdressers and beauticians	Hair, nail, and skin beauty preparations
Launderers and dry cleaners	Heat, heavy lifting, and chemicals
Electronics workers	Solvents and acids
Hospital and other health care workers	Infectious diseases, heavy lifting, radiation, skin disorders, and anesthetic gases
Laboratory workers	Biological agents; flammable explosive, toxic, or carcinogenic substances; exposure to radiation; and bites from and allergic reactions to research animals

workers, gaps in knowledge exist. For example, little is known about women who work in cottage industries, as domestic workers, as prostitutes, in agriculture, and in the garment industry. In addition, the work of some women is classified as "women's work" and includes such things as housework, child care, caregiver of the sick, and farming (Misner, Beauchamp-Hewitt, and Fox-Levin, 1995). These women experience physical demands and hazards, yet government economic reports have not recognized these individuals as workers. Investigations of factors that influence the health of these women workers are needed. Table 15-6 lists specific positions in which a large number of women are employed and the potential for health hazards within these positions.

Community health nurses, occupational health nurses, and nurse practitioners (NPs) need to be cognizant of environmental hazards wherever they find women at work. In taking health histories, the nurse should collect data regarding the client's occupational environment to assess the potential risk to emotional, general, and reproductive health. In addition, nurses must work individually and as an aggregate with their legislatures to maintain strong worker health and safety programs to protect the health of all women.

Family and Medical Leave Act

Enacted in 1993, the **Family and Medical Leave Act (FMLA)** allows an employee a minimum provision of 12 weeks unpaid leave each year for family and medical reasons such as personal illness; an ill child, parent, or spouse; or the birth or adoption of a child. This act guarantees the employee the same or equivalent job with the same pay and benefits upon the employee's return to work. In addition, health benefits must continue throughout the leave. Approximately 20% of the U.S. workforce needed some form of FMLA-covered leave after the law was enacted (Gilinson, 1999).

The FMLA is particularly important to female workers because they are more likely to use leave to care for seriously ill family members, whereas male workers more often use leave for personal illness (Gilinson, 1999). It has been observed that employees who must be away from work for family and medical reasons lose income. However, the loss is most severe for those without job-protected leave. The FMLA is an important step toward equitable leave policies, but more change is needed.

HEALTH AND SOCIAL SERVICES TO PROMOTE THE HEALTH OF WOMEN

Medicaid is a health insurance program that was instituted in 1965 for the poor. Medicaid is funded jointly by the federal and state governments but is administered by individual states. Medicaid is the largest source of funding for medical and health-related services for people with limited income, regardless of age eligibility. Medicaid is classified into five broad coverage groups: children, pregnant women, adults in families with dependent children, individuals with disabilities, and individuals 65 years or older.

Many of the pregnant women who are eligible for Medicaid are at high risk for poor pregnancy outcome, including low birth weight. Ideally, a maternity care provider should examine women with high maternal risk immediately after conception. However, too often these women seek prenatal care late in the pregnancy or arrive at the emergency department when delivery is imminent without having previously received prenatal care. This case is not unusual. Barriers limit access to prenatal care among those most in need. Medicaid allows some access to care. Greater public awareness of facilities and maternity care providers who accept Medicaid is necessary. Recent changes in payment plans that allow billing for care at higher rates have increased the number of providers who accept Medicaid clients.

CLINICAL EXAMPLE

Anita Rogers, a 16-year-old unemployed single woman, arrived at the Family Services Health Center seeking initial prenatal care at 36 weeks' gestation. She stated that for a few days she noted some brown discharge from her vagina. She told the nurse she knew she should have begun prenatal care earlier, but when she called several physicians' offices, the receptionist told her she should bring $1000 for her first visit. She said that neither she nor her parents had that much money. Her father was unemployed, and her mother worked at a cafe as a waitress. She also had difficulty with transportation. Anita was sent to the hospital immediately for an ultrasound examination. The sonogram revealed triplets, but two of them had died in utero. Anita was hospitalized and began to hemorrhage. She delivered a 3-lb infant. ■

Women's Health Services

Since the mid 1970s, women have sought health services beyond the conventional mode of care delivery. Many self-help groups have emerged, and new approaches to women's health services have been accepted. Women have demanded a participatory role and have become more assertive; therefore, health care facilities, including physicians' offices, are more responsive to women's perceptions of their health needs. A complete revolution in maternity care has occurred with the emergence of freestanding and hospital-based birth centers and family- and sibling-attended births. The health care needs of women go beyond their reproductive status and include their primary health care needs. The health care needs of women must be addressed more effectively and should include services for the following (Star, Lommel, and Shannon, 2004):

1. Eating disorders
2. All forms of abuse
3. Disease prevention, including smoking cessation
4. Health promotion focusing on nutrition, exercise, and stress management

The National Women's Health Network has been a strong advocate for women's concerns and has provided testimony before congressional hearings dealing with women's issues. This organization is concerned with women's rights, environmental safety, reproductive rights, warnings regarding the effects of alcohol and drugs on the developing fetus, and safety in relation to medical devices. For example, the network was instrumental in the worldwide recall of the Dalkon Shield intrauterine device.

Another concern of the National Women's Health Network is drug safety, especially concerning drugs that may have teratogenic or carcinogenic effects. For example, the network has attempted to identify women who may have been exposed to diethylstilbestrol in utero.

Women's health consumers are requesting more emphasis in the area of well-women's health care (i.e., health care aimed at well-being, health promotion, and disease prevention). Several nurses throughout the United States have established collaborative practices with other health professionals to meet this demand for nonconventional services.

Other Community Voluntary Services

Networking has been one of the major movements during the past two decades. Networking is a system of interconnected or cooperating individuals. It is the means by which women seek to advance their careers, improve their lifestyles, and increase their income while helping other women become successful. Networks in business, professional support, politics and labor, arts, sports, and health have been established throughout the United States. These multiple networks have enabled women to develop new identities and become empowered to achieve mutual goals.

Many private voluntary organizations spend money, time, and energy in attempting to increase health awareness among its members and provide direct services to the public. Most urban areas have crisis hotline services in which women volunteer to provide counseling to battered women, battering parents, rape victims, those considering suicide, and those with multiple needs. One of the most effective, low-cost, voluntary efforts to assist abused women involves shelters and safe houses scattered throughout the United States. Many women needing shelter are often denied emergency housing. One of the goals of *Healthy People 2010* relates to this problem.

Women's organizations have a long history of voluntary involvement with the community. An increasing number have added activities to their agenda to improve pregnancy outcomes, prevent teen pregnancy, and support older women's rights. Organizations such as the Older Women's League, United Methodist Women, other religious denomination women's groups, Urban League, sororities, Junior League, YWCA, National Association of Colored Women's Clubs, and many others have made women's health a major item on their agenda.

LEVELS OF PREVENTION AND WOMEN'S HEALTH

Primary Prevention

The focus of primary prevention is preventing the disease from occurring. The author became involved in primary prevention with other community health-nursing faculty as members of an ACS committee called Stop Cancer Among Minorities (SCAM). The SCAM committee members represented several ethnic groups from churches, schools, and health care agencies. The committee assessed the needs of a community that revealed a lack of knowledge of health promotion practices necessary to decrease the risk of cancer.

The committee planned a health fair to promote cancer awareness in the community. The state chapter of the ACS and a local community health center sponsored it. Nursing students and undergraduate faculty members from the local nursing college joined the committee to plan and implement the program.

Nursing students offered nutritious snacks (i.e., low in fat and high in fiber and complex carbohydrates) and discussed the relationship of diet to cancer risk reduction. They also taught breast self-examinations and testicular self-examinations. Other students shared the risks of smoking and the benefits of quitting. Seven booths located at the fair were associated with the seven danger signals of cancer.

Secondary Prevention

The focus of secondary prevention is detecting the disease once it has begun but before it appears clinically. Examples of this level of prevention would be routine screening for cervical cancer through Pap smears, chlamydial infections through nucleic acid amplification tests either by urine or cervical specimen, and clinical breast examination and mammogram.

Tertiary Prevention

Tertiary prevention seeks to stop further complications after a disease has become clinically evident. For example, Sandra Smith, a 55-year-old Native American, has had diabetes mellitus for the past 3 years. She attended an urban clinic for monitoring her diabetes. After the physician examined her, he suggested that she have her annual pelvic examination. She was overdue for this and agreed to be seen by the women's health care NP. Ms. Smith described symptoms of a yeast infection (e.g., increase in vaginal discharge and itching) to the nurse. Her examination and a wet mount confirmed the diagnosis of *Candida albicans* infection, a common problem among diabetic women. The woman

CASE STUDY   Application of the Nursing Process

John Lawrence, an educator at the state women's correctional center, contacted Donna Williams, a women's health care nurse practitioner and faculty member at the College of Nursing, and expressed concern for the health of an inmate, Lela Marvin. According to Mr. Lawrence, Lela, a 19-year-old pregnant primigravida, was being seen at the state-supported hospital for antepartal care; however, she was not permitted to attend perinatal education classes. He stated that other pregnant women in the facility could benefit from perinatal education. In fact, approximately 6.1% of female state prison inmates are pregnant when admitted to prison and could benefit from perinatal education (Snell, 1994).

Lawrence's call was followed by a call from Herman Martin, an RN who also expressed concern for the other women's needs for information regarding their personal hygiene. Although an RN, Mr. Martin was not knowledgeable of women's health because his primary clinical focus was emergency and trauma care. He indicated that many of the women were overweight, cared little about themselves, and lacked a general knowledge of how to maintain their health.

ASSESSMENT

After gaining clearance by the prison officials, Ms. Williams made an assessment of health care information needs and started offering classes for the inmates. The immediate need was for perinatal education for women in the last weeks of pregnancy. Lela said she wanted to learn about labor because she had heard only horror stories from other women. Donna noted that three other women were close to term and they also seemed eager to learn. Donna knew that students' readiness to learn was key to the course's success. Success of this course would be crucial to future course offerings.

The traditional perinatal education course was designed to promote healthy birth outcomes and an emotionally satisfying birth experience. These goals are also important to pregnant women in a correctional facility; however, perinatal education should be modified to meet this group's special needs. For example, information on newborn care is not appropriate because the infant is usually placed with the mother's family or in foster care.

Assessment of nonpregnant women provided opportunities for other health education classes. The next spring and each spring thereafter, junior nursing students under the guidance of Ms. Williams were assigned to develop and carry out a 1-hour weekly health education and awareness session at the correctional facility. Although each student expressed some initial anxiety toward the experience, each evaluated it as being worthwhile.

DIAGNOSIS

After assessment, the community health nurse developed community and aggregate diagnoses, which served as the basis for the care plan.

Individual
- Inadequate preparation for childbirth related to lack of resources in prison (Lela)
- Lack of family support related to separation secondary to incarceration (Lela)
- Potential for feelings of loss related to separation from infant after birth (Lela)

Family
- Lela's family visits were rare; therefore she looked for others to provide support during her pregnancy. Lela told Ms. Williams that her cellmate, Julieanna, offered to be her labor support person.
- Lack of knowledge of her role as a labor support person (Julieanna)

Community
- Knowledge deficit of adequate health-seeking behaviors of women in the correctional facility (i.e., pregnant and nonpregnant women)
- Lack of programs to promote health and prevent diseases among women prisoners

PLANNING

After validating the nursing diagnosis with the individual, family, or community, the plan of care is developed. Examples of long- and short-term goals follow.

Individual
Long-Term Goal
- Individual family members will have a positive birth experience (Lela).

Short-Term Goal
- Family member or friends will help Lela use relaxation techniques to cope with discomforts of labor.

Family
Long-Term Goal
- The family members will be strengthened through their newly acquired knowledge and skills.

Short-Term Goal
- The family members will demonstrate increased ability to perform role as labor support people.

Community
Long-Term Goal
- The health and well-being of incarcerated women (i.e., pregnant and nonpregnant) will improve.

Short-Term Goal
- Health education programs will be instituted to individuals, families, and aggregates in the correctional facility.

CASE STUDY Application of the Nursing Process (cont'd)

INTERVENTION

The community health nurse works with the individual, family, or community to achieve mutually established goals. Intervention is aimed at empowering individuals and groups to take responsibility for themselves and form links with others to accomplish goals.

Individual

Providing a perinatal education program for Lela is Ms. Williams' first priority. In addition, counseling related to feelings of loss after birth may be appropriate. Referral to a counselor may be necessary, and Ms. Williams must become familiar with available resources.

Family

Teaching the family the roles and responsibilities of a labor support person is an important intervention. In the correctional facility, interventions must ensure that Lela has a labor support person to practice her relaxation techniques and be available. In this case, Lela's cellmate, Julieanna, was willing to act in this role, and the nurse must negotiate with prison officials to allow this arrangement.

Community

Specific interventions with a group of pregnant women in the correctional facility are based on the specific needs of the group. The community health nurse must identify prison officials who are supportive of health education programs and request input as to which women should be targeted for such programs. Then the nurse meets with targeted women to assess level of knowledge and skills regarding women's health. For example, the nurse should survey what the woman perceives as learning needs (e.g., well-women's care, women's anatomy and physiology, self-care in health promotion, health protection, and disease prevention). Then the nurse tailors an intervention that is compatible with the community. Ms. Williams asked each nursing student to select a topic based on the survey and develop a teaching plan for presentation to female prisoners (i.e., pregnant and nonpregnant) at least once during the spring semester.

EVALUATION

The community health nurse compares the actual and predicted outcomes to determine the efficacy of the plan of care and make revisions.

Individual

For example, Lela learned necessary relaxation techniques that were useful to her in labor and assisted in making the birth experience positive. Follow-up of Lela's psychosocial concerns in postpartum was also important.

Family

Evaluation of this nontraditional family would include their level of satisfaction with their role in the birth experience. Evaluation would also include learning how this interaction between family members (i.e., Lela and Julieanna) prepared them for other situations.

Community

The aggregate evaluation focuses on the community. For example, in health education programs designed for pregnant and nonpregnant women in the correctional facility, it is important to do the following:
- Maintain attendance records.
- Seek feedback from women, the referring nurse-educator, and prison officials regarding changes in self-care behavior regarding health.
- Obtain student response to learning experience.
- Make changes in health education programs based on evaluation.

LEVELS OF PREVENTION

The following are examples of the three levels of prevention as applied to the individual, family, and community.

Primary
- Assessment and teaching perinatal education course to pregnant inmates
- Assessment and teaching health education classes to nonpregnant inmates
- Teaching the family the roles and responsibilities of a labor support person

Secondary
- Screening at the community level (correctional facility) of what is perceived as learning needs
- Educating the family and community of the signs of postpartum depression

Tertiary
- Educating HIV-positive pregnant inmates on the need of antiviral treatment and delivery by cesarean
- Educating family members and foster parents about the need of neonatal follow-up with regard to HIV status
- Assessing available community resources for counseling and treatment of postpartum depression

Continued

learned about the nature, predisposing factors, and treatment of the infection.

ROLES OF THE COMMUNITY HEALTH NURSE

Direct Care

The community health nurse provides direct care in a variety of settings. Often, this is considered the "hands-on" nursing care given to a client in the home or a clinic.

Educator

The nurse encounters many opportunities for teaching. To be successful with health education, the nurse must attempt to gain trust and be sensitive to any cultural issues present. The nurse must also be aware of the emotional and physical state of the client. If the client is anxious or in pain, teaching may be ineffective.

Counselor

The counseling role of the nurse occurs in almost every interaction in the area of women's health. Before beginning counseling in the area of reproductive health, it is essential for effective intervention that the nurse becomes aware of his or her value system, including how biases and beliefs about human sexual behavior affect the counseling role.

RESEARCH IN WOMEN'S HEALTH

Women have long been the major users of the health care system. However, until recently, little research involving women provided information enabling prediction, explanation, or description of phenomena affecting health. In many cases, medical treatment for women is based on research with male subjects exclusively. This is also true in conditions that cause more deaths in women. Fortunately, increased effort includes women in studies related to cardiovascular health and lung and colon cancer. This emphasis came after a federal mandate that research must include women and minorities. If women are not included, a rationale must be given for their exclusion.

The National Institutes of Health established the Office of Research on Women's Health in 1990. Through a special task force, recommendations were made for the research agenda for women's health for the next two decades. In addition, nurse researchers are encouraged to test interventions and question rituals in nursing by conducting ritual-busting research. The following are some of the areas for exploration and research among women:

- Health promotion
- Barriers to care
- Disease prevention
- Health education at various literacy levels
- Wellness across the life cycle
- Differences among women experiencing menopausal symptoms

- Dysmenorrhea
- Safe and effective contraception
- Promotion of breast feeding
- Infertility
- Coping with chronic illness, such as systemic lupus erythematosus or arthritis
- Discomforts of pregnancy, including morning sickness
- Strengths of single, female heads of households
- Adolescent sexuality
- Multiple-role adaptation
- Menstrual cycle variations
- Control of obesity
- Substance abuse and its effect on pregnancy
- HIV infection and pregnancy
- Influence of diet on osteoporosis
- Effect of socialization on role
- Domestic violence

More recently, research on the financing and delivery of health services for women has been supported. This research will address the changing health care environment; the unmet need for primary and preventive health services; the historic lack of research on women's health; and the importance of social, cultural, legal, economic, and behavioral factors influencing women's health care (Hinshaw, 2000).

With the increased emphasis on community health, community health nurses can make significant contributions toward the improvement of women's health through scholarly research, either as principal investigators or through data gathering. Furthermore, they can become consumers of research and develop nursing interventions based on sound research and recommendations.

SUMMARY

Women's health care has multiple facets. Many areas for community health nursing intervention exist. Nurses are advocates and activists for women's health through their involvement in health policy making as a profession. Along with other multidisciplinary and consumer groups, professional nurses are in the forefront of making changes in the health care delivery system that will promote an overall quality and research-based health plan for women. Women are at the center of the health of the United States; therefore, if better models are developed for improving the health of women, the health of the entire nation will benefit.

LEARNING ACTIVITIES

1. Identify examples from everyday life that support or encourage violence against women (e.g., magazines, books, and television advertisements). Share findings with classmates.
2. Survey lay magazine advertisements and estimate the percentage of total pages that use a woman's image, including aging, menopause, overweight and obesity, and sexuality to sell products. Share these with classmates.
3. Discuss the need for cancer screening with female relatives; refer to the ACS guidelines.

4. Discuss with female relatives the need for a heart-healthy nutritional plan based on AHA guidelines.
5. Identify resources for mammograms and PAP smears for low-income women.
6. Visit with a women's group in the community (e.g., business, church, sorority, and Parents Without Partners) to discuss members' health care needs and concerns. From these data, develop research questions.
7. Call a family planning clinic and determine the population served (i.e., eligibility), available services, and costs.
8. Review county or state health department statistics for leading causes of death among women of varying ethnic or racial groups.

REFERENCES

American Academy of Pediatrics: *Family pediatrics: report of the task force on the family,* Elk Grove Village, Ill, 2005, The Author.

American Cancer Society: *Cancer facts and figures 2006,* Atlanta, 2006, The Author, http://www.cancer.org.

American College of Emergency Physicians: Domestic violence, The Author, 2003, The Author, http://www.acep.org.

American Diabetes Association: *National diabetes facts,* 2002, The Author, http://www.diabetes.org/diabetes-statistics/national.

American Heart Association: *Heart disease and stroke statistics, 2005 update,* Dallas, Texas, 2005, The Author, http://www.americanheart.org.

American Psychological Association: Women and depression, 2005, http://www.apa.org.ppo/issues/pwomenanddepress.html.

Arthritis Foundation: *Disease center,* 2005, The Author, http://www.arthritis.org/conditions.asp.

Bhatia SC, Bhatia SK: Depression in women: diagnostic and treatment considerations, *Am Fam Physician* 60(1):225, 1999

Blair T: Domestic abuse: What is the ob/gyn nurse's role? *Ob Gyn Nurse Forum* 7(2):1, 1999.

Blehar M: Public health context of women's mental health research, *Psychiatr Clin North Am* 26:781-799, 2003.

Bremnor JD, Sadovsky R: Evaluation of dysuria in adults, *Am Fam Physician* 65(8):1589-1596, 2002.

Cates W: Reproductive tract infections. In Hatcher RA et al: *Contraceptive technology,* ed 18, New York, 2004, Ardent Media.

Cates W, Ellertson C, Stewart F: Abortion. In Hatcher RA et al: *Contraceptive technology,* ed 18, New York, 2004, Ardent Media.

Centers for Disease Control and Prevention: APV vaccine questions and answers, The Author, http://www.cdc.gov/std/hpv/STDFact-HPV-vaccine.htm#vaccine.

Centers for Disease Control and Prevention: Racial/ethnic differences in prevalence and impact of arthritis: U.S. 2002. *MMWR Morb Mortality Wkly Rep* 54(5):119-123, 2005.

Centers for Disease Control and Prevention: Reduced incidence of menstrual toxic-shock syndrome, United States 1980-1990. *MMWR Morb Mortality Wkly Rep* 39:421-424, 1990.

Centers for Disease Control and Prevention: Achievements in public health, 1900-1999: healthier mothers and babies, *MMWR Morb Mortality Wkly Rep* 48(38):849, 1999.

Centers for Disease Control and Prevention: Hysterectomy surveillance, United States, 1994-1999, *MMWR Morb Mortality Wkly Rep* 51(SS03), 2002, http://www.cdc.gov/mmwr/preview/mmwrhtml/ss5105al.htm.

Centers for Disease Control and Prevention: Pregnancy related mortality surveillance: United States—1991-1999, *MMWR Morb Mortality Wkly Rep* 52(SS2), 2003.

Centers for Disease Control and Prevention: *National diabetes fact sheet, United States, 2003,* rev ed, Atlanta, 2004, The Author, http://www.cdc.gov/diabetes/pubs/pdf/ndfs_2003.pdf.

Centers for Disease Control and Prevention, National Center for Health Statistics: *1999 National hospital discharge survey,* Atlanta, 2001, The Author.

Centers for Disease Control and Prevention: Sexually transmitted disease treatment guide: 2002. *MMWR Morb Mortality Wkly Rep* 51(RR-6) 2002.

Centers for Disease Control and Prevention, National Center for Health Statistics: *Health: United States—2005.* Hyattsville, Md, 2005, The Author.

Chadwick BA, Heaton TB, editors: *Statistical handbook on the American family,* Phoenix, 1992, Oryx Press.

Chang WC et al: Impact of sex on long-term mortality from acute myocardial infarction vs. unstable angina, *Arch Intern Med* 163:2476-2484, 2003.

Chobanian AV et al: The seventh report of the joint national committee on prevention, detection, evaluation, and treatment of high blood pressure, *JAMA* 289(19), 2003.

Choi M: Preamble to a new paradigm for women's health, *Image* 17:14, 1985.

Clark RA: Infections during the postpartum period, *J Obstet Gynecol Neonatal Nurs* 24(6):542-548, 1995.

Crane PB et al: Inclusion of women in nursing research: 1995-2001, *Nurs Res* 53(4):237-242, 2004.

Creehan PA: Toxic shock syndrome: an opportunity for nursing intervention, *J Obstet Gynecol Neonatal Nurs* 24(6):557-561, 1995.

Cunningham FG et al: *Williams' obstetrics,* ed 21, Norwalk, Conn, 2005, Appleton & Lange.

Davis JP et al: Toxic-shock syndrome: epidemiologic features, recurrence, risk factors, and prevention, *N Engl J Med* 303(25):1429-1435, 1980.

Donaldson K, Briggs J, McMaster D: RU 486: an alternative to surgical abortion, *J Obstet Gynecol Neonatal Nurs* 23(7):555-559, 1995.

Epperly AT, Viera AJ: Pelvic inflammatory disease, *Clin Fam Pract* 7(1):67-78, 2005.

Evans DL et al: Depression in the medical setting: biopsychological interactions and treatment considerations, *J Clin Psychiatry* 60(suppl 4):40, 1999.

Facione NC: Breast cancer screening in relation to access to health services, *Oncol Nurs Forum* 26(4):689, 1999.

Farley D: Preventing TSS: tampon labeling allows women to compare absorbencies. In USDHHS: *FDA consumer special report: current issues in women's health,* ed 2, Rockville, Md, 1994, The Author.

Finkel ML, Finkel DJ: The effect of a second opinion program on hysterectomy performance, *Med Care* 28:776, 1990.

Foxman B: Epidemiology of urinary tract infections: incidence, morbidity, and economic costs, *Am J Med* 113(suppl 1A):5S-13S, 2002.

Foxman B, Brown P: Epidemiology of urinary tract infections transmission and risk factors, incidence, and costs, *Infect Dis Clin North Am,* 17:227-241, 2003.

Fishwick NJ: Assessment of women for partner abuse, *J Obstet Gynecol Neonatal Nurs* 27(6):661, 1998.

Guest F: Education and counseling. In Hatcher RA et al: *Contraceptive technology,* ed 18, New York, 2004a, Ardent Media.

Hinshaw AS: Nursing knowledge for the 21st century: opportunities and challenges, *J Nurs Sch* 32(2):117-123, 2000.

Hopwood P, Stephens RJ, Medical Research Council (MRC) Lung Cancer Working Party: Symptoms at presentation for treatment in patients with lung cancer: implications for the evaluation of palliative treatment, *Br J Cancer* 71:633, 1995.

Karlson EW et al: A retrospective cohort study of cigarette smoking and risk of rheumatoid arthritis in female health professionals, *Arthritis Rheum* 42(5):910, 1999.

Kuehn J, McMahon P, Creekmore S: Stopping a silent killer: preventing heart disease in women, *AWHONN Lifelines* 3(2):31, 1999.

Love S et al: Practice guidelines for breast cancer, *Cancer J Sci Am* 2(3A):S7, 1996.

Martin R et al: Gender disparities in common sense models of illness among myocardial infarction victims, *Health Psychol* 23:345-353, 2004.

Matthews S, Power C: Socio-economic gradients in psychological distress: A focus on women, social roles and work-home characteristics, *Soc Sci Med* 54:799-810, 2002.

Medscape Today: Merck's HPV vaccine wins U.S. approval, http://www.medscape.com/viewarticle/535729.

Misner ST, Beauchamp-Hewitt JB, Fox-Levin P: Occupational issues in women's health. In McElmurry BJ, Parker RS, editors: *Annual review of women's health,* vol 11, New York, 1995, NLN.

Mou SM: Gynecologic infections. In Seltzer VL, Pearse WH, editors: *Women's primary health care,* ed 2, New York, 1999, McGraw-Hill.

National Center for Health Statistics: *Health, United States, 2004, with chartbook on trends in the health of Americans,* Hyattsville, Md, 2004, The Author.

National Osteoporosis Foundation: Fast facts on osteoporosis, 2005, The Author, http://www.nof.org/osteoporosis/diseasefacts.htm.

Nelson AL: Menstrual problems and common gynecologic concerns. In Hatcher RA et al, editor: *Contraceptive technology,* ed 18, New York, 2004, Ardent Media.

Nelson AL, Marshall JR: Impaired fertility. In Hatcher RA et al: *Contraceptive technology,* ed 18, New York, 2004, Ardent Media.

Olds S, London M, Ladewig P: *Maternal-newborn nursing,* ed 7, Menlo Park, Calif, 2004, Addison-Wesley.

Patel JD: Lung cancer in women, *J Clin Oncol* 23(14):3212-3218, 2005.

Pender NJ, Murdaugh CL, Parsons MA: *Health promotion in nursing practice,* ed 4, Upper Saddle River, NJ, 2006, Prentice Hall.

Pollack AE, Carignan CS, Jacobstein R: Female and male sterilization. In Hatcher RA et al: *Contraceptive technology,* ed 18, New York, 2004, Ardent Media.

Pollard K, Tordella S: Women making gains among professionals, *Population Today* 21:1, 1993.

Rhodes, DJ: Identifying and counseling women at increased risk for breast cancer. *Mayo Clinic Proc* 77:355-361, 2002.

Rivera MP, Stover DE: Gender and lung cancer, *Clin Chest Med* 25(2):391-400, 2004.

Safe Motherhood Organization: Safe Motherhood Initiative, 2005, http://www.safemotherhood.org/resources/pdf/e_facts.pdf

Sarna L, McCorkle R: Burden of care and lung cancer, *Cancer Pract* 4:245, 1996.

Schulman KA et al: The effect of race and sex on physicians' recommendations for cardiac catheterization, *N Engl J Med* 340(8):618-626, 1999.

Snell T: *Survey of state prison inmates: 1991—women in prison,* US Department of Justice, Bureau of Justice Statistics, Washington, DC, 1994, US Government Printing Office.

Thomas B et al. Randomized trial of breast self-examination in Shanghai: final results, *J Natl Cancer Inst* 94(19), Oct 2002.

Government Printing Office, 1990.

US Census Bureau: *Income, poverty, and health insurance coverage in the United States: 2003,* Current Population Reports P60-226, 2004, The Author, http://www.census.gov/prod/2004pubs/p60-226.pdf.

US Census Bureau: *Disability status by sex: 2000.* http://factfinder.census.gov/servlet/QTTable?_bm=y&-geo_id=01000US&qr_name=DEC_2000_SF3_U_QTP21&ds_name=DEC_2000_SF3_U&redoLog=false.

US Census Bureau: *Statistical abstract of the United States: 2004-2005,* Washington, DC, 2005, US Government Printing Office, 2005, http://www.census.gov/prod/2004pubs/04statab/pop.pdf.

US Department of Education: *Digest of education statistics,* Washington, DC, 2003, The Author.

US Department of Health and Human Services: *Healthy People 2010,* ed 2, Washington, DC, 2000a, US Government Printing Office.

US Department of Health and Human Services, Public Health Service: *Healthy People 2010: national health promotion and disease prevention objectives,* Washington, DC, 2000b, US Government Printing Office.

US Department of Health and Human Services: *Guidelines for the use of antiretroviral agents in HIV-1 infected adults and adolescents,* 2005b, http://www.aidsinfo.nih.gov/guidelines.

US Department of Labor: *Women in the labor force: a databook,* Washington, DC, 2005, The Author.

Vogel WH: The advance practice nursing role in a high-risk breast cancer clinic, *Oncol Nurs Forum* 30:115-122, 2003.

Warshaw C, Ganley AL, Salber PR: *Improving the health care response to domestic violence: a resource manual for health care providers,* San Francisco, 1995, Family Violence Prevention Fund.

Wei G et al: Osteoporosis management in the new millennium, *Prim Care* 30(4):711-741, 2003.

Wexler DJ et al: Sex disparities in treatment of cardiac risk factors in patients with type 2 diabetes, *Diabetes Care* 28:514-520, 2005.

Women Employed Institute: *Sexual harassment: the problem that isn't going away,* Chicago, 1994, The Author.

World Health Organization, Department of Reproductive Health and Research: *Maternal mortality in 2000,* Geneva, 2004a, The Author, http://www.WHO.int/reproductivehealth/publications/maternal_mortality2000/.

World Health Organization: *World Health Report: 2004,* Geneva, 2004b, The Author, http://www.who.int/whr/2004/en/index.html.

World Health Organization: Joint United Nations Programme on HIV/AIDS, 2004c, The Author, http://www.who.org.

Wright TC: Patient-collected tissue samples may offer effective option to Pap smear, *JAMA* 283:81, 2000.

Zeidenstein L: Health issues of lesbian and bisexual women. In Varney H, editor: *Varney's midwifery,* ed 4, Sudbury, Mass, 2004, Jones and Bartlett.

Men's Health

Carrie Morgan

MEDIA RESOURCES

Additional Material for Study, Review, and Further Exploration

evolve Website at http://evolve.elsevier.com/Nies

❖ Quiz ❖ Case Studies ❖ Content Updates ❖ Glossary ❖ WebLinks

OBJECTIVES

Upon completion of this chapter, the reader will be able to do the following:

1. Identify the major indicators of men's health status.
2. Describe physiological and psychological factors that have an impact on men's health status.
3. Discuss barriers to improving men's health.
4. Discuss factors that promote men's health.
5. Describe men's health needs.
6. Apply knowledge of men's health needs in planning gender-appropriate nursing care for men at the individual, family, and community levels.

KEY TERMS

acute condition
androgen
chronic condition

illness orientation
life expectancy

medical care
morbidity

mortality
prevention orientation

CHAPTER OUTLINE

MEN'S HEALTH STATUS
Longevity and Mortality in Men
Morbidity

USE OF MEDICAL CARE
Use of Ambulatory Care
Use of Hospital Care
Use of Preventive Care
Use of Other Health Services

THEORIES THAT EXPLAIN MEN'S HEALTH
Biological Factors
Socialization
Orientation Toward Illness and Prevention
Reporting of Health Behavior
Discussion of the Theories of Men's Health

FACTORS THAT IMPEDE MEN'S HEALTH
Medical Care Patterns
Access to Care
Lack of Health Promotion

MEN'S HEALTH CARE NEEDS

PRIMARY PREVENTIVE MEASURES
Health Education
Interest Groups for Men and Men's Health
Men's Increasing Interest in Physical Fitness and Lifestyle
Policy Related to Men's Health

SECONDARY PREVENTIVE MEASURES
Health Services for Men
Screening Services for Men

TERTIARY PREVENTIVE MEASURES
Sex-Role and Lifestyle Rehabilitation
New Concepts of Community Care

It is common knowledge that women live longer than men and that health care use is greater among women than men. Death rates for men are higher than for women in the major causes of death. Although the overall interest in health promotion and illness prevention has increased, men's health issues remain largely unaddressed. Women's health has become a specialty practice with courses and programs available in many colleges of nursing. A specialty in men's health has not been established.

This chapter focuses on exploring the health needs of men and the implications for community health nursing. Specific areas that are discussed include the current health status of men, physiological and psychological theories that attempt to explain men's health, factors that impede men's health, factors that promote men's health, men's health needs, meeting men's health needs, and planning gender-appropriate care for men at the individual, family, and community levels.

MEN'S HEALTH STATUS

Traditional indicators of health include rates of longevity, mortality, and morbidity. Reviewing these rates provides nursing students with a better understanding of this community aggregate.

Longevity and Mortality in Men

Major gender differences in longevity and mortality rates reveal that men remain disadvantaged despite advances in technology. Although women are more likely to use health services and experience higher morbidity rates, mortality rates for men remain higher. Gender differences are generally associated with both physiological and behavioral factors, which place men at greater risk of death. These behavioral factors, together with men's reluctance to seek preventive and health services, have marked implications for community health nursing.

Standardized Terminology

In the fields of demography and sociology, the following terms are standardized:

People of all ages: Males and females

Children younger than 18 years of age: Boys and girls

Adults 18 years of age or older: Men and women

Sex: The biological distinction between males and females

Gender: The attitudes and behavior of men and women that are shaped by socialization and have a potential to be changed

Role: The part one plays in society ■

Modified from Skelton R: Man's role in society and its effect on health, Nursing 26:953, 1988; Verbrugge LM, Wingard DL: Sex differentials in health and mortality, Women Health 12:103, 1987.

Longevity

Rates of longevity are increasing for both men and women. People can now expect to live more than 20 years longer than their forefathers and foremothers lived at the turn of the nineteenth century. Infants born in the United States in 1996 can expect to live 76 years, whereas those born in 1900 lived an average of 47.3 years when the death rate was highest. **Life expectancy** for both males and females has increased; however, since the 1970s this gender gap in longevity has decreased. Between 1990 and 2001, men gained two years of longevity while females gained one year of longevity (National Center for Health Statistics [NCHS], 2004). This change in male longevity may be attributed to the advances in treatment of heart disease and cancer, which have been the major causes of death in U.S. males.

Factors that influence the incongruencies between males and females are race or ethnic origin, social economic status, and education. Reported by race, gender mortality rates show that less advantaged populations in the United States, especially minorities, live significantly fewer years. African American males live 6.3 years less than white males (NCHS, 2004). Native Americans live an average of 4 years less than white males, and black males live approximately 8 years less than white males. Hispanics have a life expectancy comparable with their white counterparts.

The United States lags behind several other countries in mortality rates for males. In 1999, the United States ranked 23rd in life expectancy for men and women (Table 16-1) (NCHS, 2004).

Mortality

In the United States, as in most industrialized countries, males lead females in **mortality** rates in each leading cause of death. Although males were the primary source of medical data before the 1970s, and most of the treatment advances have been developed from this data, gender-related disparity in death rates continue. Other factors account for this mortality gender gap (Table 16-2).

The gender disparity for disease-related deaths has narrowed. Heart disease remains the leading cause of death, but the ratio of male to female deaths decreased by .38 between 1992 and 2002. Since the 1990s, female, cancer-related deaths have declined at a slower rate than men. The death rate for chronic lower respiratory disease among females increased 150% between 1980 and 2002, whereas death rates for males increased 7% (NCHS, 2004). Unintentional injury deaths due to accidents, suicide, or homicide for the whole population have increased. Males continue to be at risk for death due to unintentional injury. Males aged 15 to 64 are 2 to 3 times more likely to die as a result of unintentional injury than females of the same age. Men are 6 times more likely to commit suicide. Males over age 85 are 11 times more likely to die as a result of suicide.

Race and ethnic background also are factors to be considered when evaluating male mortality rates. Black men between ages 45 and 64 are more than 10 times as likely to die from HIV infection than white males. Among males ages 15 to 24, African-American males are twice as likely to die from vehicle accidents, and 7 times more likely to die from homicide (NCHS, 2004). Hispanic males fare somewhat better but are twice as likely to die as a result of homicide as white males.

TABLE 16-1   Life Expectancy at Birth According to Sex and Race, United States, 1900 to 2002

	ALL RACES			WHITE			BLACK		
YEAR	BOTH SEXES	MALE	FEMALE	BOTH SEXES	MALE	FEMALE	BOTH SEXES	MALE	FEMALE
1900	47.3	46.3	48.3	47.6	46.6	48.7	33.0	32.5	33.5
1960	69.7	66.6	73.1	70.6	67.4	74.1	63.2	60.7	65.9
1992	75.8	72.3	79.1	76.5	73.2	79.8	69.6	65.0	73.9
1990	75.4	71.8	78.8	76.1	72.7	79.4	69.6	64.5	73.6
2002	77.3	74.5	79.9	77.7	75.5	80.3	72.3	68.8	75.6

Data from National Center for Health Statistics: *Health, United States: 2004*, Hyattsville, Md, 2004, US Public Health Service.

TABLE 16-2   Ratio of Age-Adjusted Death Rates for 12 Leading Causes of Death for the Total Population by Sex and Race: United States, 2002

RANK ORDER	CAUSE OF DEATH (NINTH REVISION, INTERNATIONAL CLASSIFICATION OF DISEASES, 1975)	RATIO MALE TO FEMALE	RATIO BLACK TO WHITE
—	All causes	1.72 (1.03)	1.61 (1.69)
1	Diseases of the heart	1.88 (1.50)	1.48 (1:81)
2	Malignant neoplasms	1.45 (1.46)	1.3 (1.71)
3	Cerebrovascular diseases	1.18 (1.02)	1.86 (1:69)
4	Chronic obstructive pulmonary disease (COPD) and allied conditions	1.70 (1.43)	0.81 (1.13)
5	Accidents and adverse effects	2.63 (2.19)	1.27 (1.76)
—	Motor vehicle accidents	2.35 (2.30)	1.03 (1.08)
6	Pneumonia and influenza	1.69 (1.36)	1.44 (1:90)
7	Diabetes mellitus	1.14 (1.24)	2.41 (1:53)
8	HIV infection	6.97 (2.96)	3.69 (10:1)
9	Suicide	4.28 (4.38)	0.58 (0.49)
10	Homicide and legal intervention	3.98 (3.36)	6.46 (6.86)
11	Chronic liver disease and cirrhosis	2.42 (2.05)	1.48 (1.33)
12	Nephritis, nephrotic syndrome, and nephrosis	1.53 (1.44)	2.70 (2.46)

Data from Kochanek MA, Hudson DL. Advance report of final mortality statistics, 1992, *Mon Vital Stat Rep* 43(6 suppl):152, 1995.
Modified from National Center for Health Statistics: *Health, United States, 2004*, Hyattsville, Md, 2004, US Public Health Service.

Morbidity

Despite the differences in mortality rates, men tend to perceive themselves to be in better health than women. In the National Health Interview Survey of 2003 (NCHS, 2004), which asked people to rate their health status, men were more likely to rate their health as excellent or very good as opposed to fair or poor. **Morbidity** rates, or rates of illness, are difficult to obtain and have been available usually only in Western industrialized countries. For example, in the United States, reports of analyses of morbidity rates by gender lag several years behind analyses of mortality rates by gender. Gender differences in morbidity rates reflect the latest available reports. The following are common indicators of morbidity rate:

- Incidence of acute illness
- Prevalence of chronic conditions
- Use of medical care

Although variations exist, women are more likely to be ill, whereas men are at greater risk for death.

Acute Illness

According to the National Health Interview Survey, an **acute condition** is a type of illness or injury that usually lasted less than 3 months and either resulted in restricted activity (e.g., causing a person to limit daily activities for at least half a day) or caused the patient to receive medical care. The incidence rate for acute infective and parasitic disease, digestive system conditions, and respiratory conditions is higher for women than for men (Benson and Marano, 1994). The only exception is for injuries, which were 12% greater for men in 1993. In addition, the severity of these injuries is reported to be greater in men than in women. When conditions associated with childbearing are excluded from the list of acute illnesses, the incidence rate for women remains 18% greater than men.

Women reported that they slowed their activities and rested more often than men. The number of restricted-activity days associated with acute conditions per 100 people is 33% greater for women than for men; similarly, the number of bed days associated with acute conditions per 100 people is 38% greater for women than for men (Benson and Marano, 1994).

Chronic Conditions

A **chronic condition** is a condition that persists for at least 3 months or belongs to a group of conditions classified as chronic regardless of time of onset, such as tuberculosis, neoplasm, or arthritis. In general, women have higher morbidity rates than men. Women are more likely than men to have a higher prevalence of chronic diseases that cause disability and limitation of activities but do not lead to death. However, men have higher morbidity and mortality rates for conditions that are the leading causes of death.

Sources of Data

Health, United States: Submitted by the Secretary of the Department of Health and Human Services, Health, United States is a report of the health status of the nation. The data are compiled by the National Center for Health Statistics and the Centers for Disease Control and Prevention. The National Committee on Health and Vital Statistics reviews the report. (http://www.cdc.gov/nchs/data/hus/hus04.pdf)

National Center for Health Statistics (NCHS): Through the National Vital Statistics System, the NCHS collects data from each state, New York City, the District of Columbia, the U.S. Virgin Islands, Guam, and Puerto Rico on births, deaths, marriages, and divorces in the United States. (http://www.cdc.gov/nchs/Default.htm)

National Health Interview Survey: Directed by the National Center for Health Statistics of the Centers for Disease Control and Prevention, the National Health Interview Survey is a continuing, nationwide sample survey in which data are collected by personal interviews about household members' illnesses, injuries, chronic conditions, disabilities, and use of health services. (http://www.cdc.gov/nchs/nhis.htm) ■

USE OF MEDICAL CARE

Medical care, the use of ambulatory care, hospital care, preventive care, or other health services, also illustrates the different gender patterns.

Use of Ambulatory Care

Men seek ambulatory care less often than women. According to the 2003 National Health Interview Survey (NCHS, 2004), the physician's office is the primary setting for ambulatory care for both men and women. In this report, males visited physician offices, outpatient departments, or emergency rooms less often than women in all age-groups, with the exception of males over age 75. Physicians see men more frequently than women for the chronic diseases that are more prevalent among them. Males are twice as likely to visits specialists other than obstetricians and gynecologists. Injury-related visits to hospital emergency department are higher for males that females. Males aged 18 to 24 are twice as likely to visit hospital emergency departments for unintentional injuries than females in the same age range. Even though gender differences in ambulatory care utilization are lessening, males continue to delay medical treatment, resulting in men being sicker when they do seek health care. Because they are sicker, they require more intensive medical care.

Use of Hospital Care

The literature indicates that hospitalization rates also vary by sex. In 2003, rates of discharges from short-stay hospitals were lower for males (102 per 1000) than for females (133 per 1000), even when discharges for deliveries were excluded. However, males had a longer length of stay in the hospital than females (4.3 vs. 3.8 days). Discharge rates increase for both men and women after 45 years of age; however, rates for men increase more rapidly. After 65 years of age, men's discharge rates continue to be higher than women's rates (NCHS, 2004).

Use of Preventive Care

Preventive examinations are necessary for early diagnosis of health problems. Most men do not have routine checkups. National health surveys indicate that women are more likely than men to receive physical examinations (NCHS, 2004). Men are twice as likely to report no usual source of care. Men may not perceive the need for a regular source of care and often feel exercise is sufficient to compensate for unhealthy behaviors.

Use of Other Health Services

Admission for serious mental disease accounts for the largest number of hospital admissions for men aged 45 to 74. Women of the same age are more likely to be admitted for disease of the heart. Women are also more likely to reside in nursing homes because they have longer life expectancy. Men are more likely than women to be admitted for psychiatric services in state and county mental hospitals (NCHS, 2004).

THEORIES THAT EXPLAIN MEN'S HEALTH

As discussed previously, a gender gap exists in health. The data reviewed raise many questions for community health nurses to explore, regarding gender differences in health and illness. Although men have shorter life expectancy and higher rates of mortality for all leading causes of death, women have higher rates of morbidity, including rates of acute illness and chronic disease and use of medical and preventive care services. Verbrugge and Wingard (1987) asked why "females are sicker, but males die sooner" (p. 135). Several explanations exist for this paradox.

Nurses traditionally use developmental theories to explain individual behavior. Erickson's model was not gender specific (Erickson, 1963). Levinson focused somewhat on male development (Levinson, 1978). There remains a need for literature detailing the factors and combinations of factors that influence gender differences in the health and illness of populations.

The following explanations proposed by Waldron (1995a, 1995b, 1995c, 1995d, 1995e) and Verbrugge and Wingard (1987) attempt to account for gender differences in this important area:

- Biological factors, including genetics, effects of sex hormones, and physiological differences, which may be influenced by genetics, hormones, and environment
- Socialization

- Orientations toward illness and prevention
- Data collection of health behavior

Biological Factors

Several biological factors influence sex differences in mortality and morbidity rates, including genetics, effects of sex hormones, and physiological differences, which may be influenced by genetics, hormones, and environmental factors (Waldron, 1995a, 1995b, 1995c, 1995d, 1995e). The embryo is unisexual until the seventh week of gestation. **Androgen,** a hormone from the Y-chromosome coupled with the maternal androgen source, results in the development of the male sex. Male embryos outnumber female embryos 115 to 100. Higher rates of miscarriage and stillbirths in males reduce this gender difference to 105 to 100. More male births occur than female births, but a higher number of male infant deaths during the first 6 months reduces this ratio (Legato, 1997). Sex ratios at birth appear to be lower for births to older fathers, black fathers, higher-order births (i.e., second, third, or fourth births), and births after induced ovulation.

Whether sex ratios at birth are influenced by sex ratios at conception or sex differentials in mortality rates before birth is unknown. Current evidence suggests that more than two out of three prenatal deaths occur before clinical recognition of the pregnancy. Sex differences in late fetal mortality rates, once favoring males in developed countries, have decreased since the early and mid twentieth century; currently, because of improved medical care and maternal health, no differences in late fetal mortality rates exist (Waldron, 1995d). These factors also have decreased deaths resulting from difficult labor, injuries at birth, and maternal diseases and accidents.

In 2002, the U.S. infant mortality rates increased for the first time in more than 40 years. Analysis of the data is incomplete, but it is known that two thirds of all infant deaths occur in the neonatal (less than 28 days) period (NCHS, 2004). Infant mortality rate for males is higher than for females. Males' experience of higher mortality rates for perinatal conditions are attributed to biological disadvantages such as males' greater risk of premature birth, higher rates of respiratory distress syndrome, and infectious disease in infancy resulting from the influence of male hormones on the developing lungs, brain, and possibly the immune system of the male fetus (Waldron, 1995d). Sex chromosome–linked diseases, such as hemophilia and certain types of muscular dystrophy, are more common among males than females (Waldron, 1995d).

Biological advantages for females may also exist later in life because the mechanism produced by estrogen protects against heart disease; studies must be interpreted cautiously, however (Waldron, 1995b). Some evidence supports the hypothesis that men's higher testosterone levels contribute to men's lower HDL levels. Body fat distribution, specifically the tendency for men in Western countries to accumulate abdominal body fat versus the tendency for women to accumulate fat on the buttocks and thighs, may also contribute to sex differences in ischemic heart disease risk (Waldron, 1995b). Men's higher levels of stored iron also may contribute to risk for ischemic heart disease. Some additional physiological gender differences are the following (Tanne 1997):

- During the process of aging, men's brain cells die faster than women's brain cells. This may explain why men are more often hospitalized for serious mental disease.
- Male immune systems are weaker than women's

Socialization

A second theory for explaining sex differences in health is socialization. U.S. society emphasizes assertiveness, restricted emotional display, concern for power, and reckless behavior in males. Pursuit of these attributes results in increased risks in work, leisure, and lifestyle. Gender-role socialization may influence these differences. Men enculturate their sons to believe that risking personal injury demonstrates masculinity.

According to the NOSH Workers health chartbook (2004), 54.2% of U.S. workers are males. Male workers account for 66.1% of the reported occupational injuries and 92% of work-related fatalities. Men's higher exposure to carcinogens at the work site is associated with high rates of mesothelioma and coal worker's pneumoconiosis. In the United States, men score higher than women on measures of hostility and lack of trust of others, which may place them at higher risk of ischemic heart disease (Matthews et al., 1992). Although occupational hazards to women's health are being identified, evidence indicates that, unlike men, employment of U.S. women outside the home has a positive effect on their health (Waldron, 1995c).

Traits and characteristics of the traditional male gender role are combative and competitive, physically active, strong, coarse, and independent. Modern men must cope with the expectations of the traditional role coupled with the expectation that their relationships with women should include emotional intimacy, tenderness, and companionship (Harrison and Dignan, 1999).

Popular male leisure, sports, and play activities place men at high risk for injury. Males between the ages of 18 and 24 are twice as likely than women to visit a hospital emergency department due to motor vehicular accidents, stabs, or intentional injury than other males (NCHS, 2004). Statistics show that men drive faster than women, receive more traffic violations, and are less likely to wear seat belts, all of which contribute to a greater number of motor vehicle fatalities (Waldron, 1995a). Although prevalence of smoking is decreasing, 25.5% of males smoke (NCHS, 2004); 68% of men consume alcohol and are five times more likely than women to drink heavily. Male have a greater use of illegal psychoactive substances and are three times more likely to be involved in criminal activity (NCHS, 2004).

Men are more likely to be involved in violent crimes, and violence is a typical precursor to homicide. Men are victims in four out of five homicides. Black males are involved in a homicide seven times more often than European-American males (NCHS, 2003).

Four Dimensions of Stereotyped Male Gender-Role Behavior

No Sissy Stuff: The need to be different from women

   The Big Wheel: The need to be superior to others

   The Sturdy Oak: The need to be independent and self-reliant

   Give 'em Hell: The need to be more powerful than others, through violence if necessary ■

Modified from David DS, Brannon R: The male sex role: our culture's blueprint of manhood, and what it's done for us lately. In David DS, Brannon R, editors: The forty-nine percent majority: the male sex role, Reading, Mass, 1976, Addison-Wesley.

Orientation Toward Illness and Prevention

Illness orientation, or the ability to note symptoms and take appropriate action, also may differ between the sexes. Most diseases, injuries, and deaths prevalent among men are preventable. However, the stereotypical view of men as strong and invulnerable is incongruent health promotion. Boys are socialized to ignore symptoms and "toughen up." Women are more likely to cut down their activities when ill, seek health care, and report more details to health care providers (Waldron, 1995a). Surveys done by *Men's Health* reveal that 9 million men have not seen a health care provider in 5 years. Men may be aware of being ill, but they make a conscious decision not to seek health care to avoid being labeled as "sick."

Prevention orientation, or the ability to take action to prevent disease or injury, also may vary between the sexes. Perhaps as a result of the contraceptive developments of the 1970s, women have a higher likelihood to seek preventive examinations. Routine reproductive health screening (i.e., the Pap test and breast examination) has been expanded to include some general screening, such as testing blood pressure and urine and blood for chronic problems. Men do not have routine reproductive health checkups that include screening, which would detect other health problems at an early stage. Specific national health objectives have only recently addressed the health care needs of this aggregate. Uniformly recognized preventive screening programs for males have only recently been developed. With the advent of managed care, men who are eligible for coverage will have access to these routine health screenings. However, it is undetermined whether men will take advantage of these programs. Box 16-1 discusses matters related to men's reproductive health needs.

Actual gender differences in preventive health behavior are variable and must be viewed with caution for the following reasons: Little research has been completed and the efficacy of many behaviors is still in question (Waldron, 1995a). In addition, existing research shows decreasing gender differences for some health behaviors and increasing gender differences for others.

Among respondents to the National Health Interview Survey of Health Promotion and Disease Prevention, more women than men reported wearing seat belts, receiving blood pressure checks, having their blood cholesterol checked, and seeking help for an emotional or personal problem in the past year (NHISH, 2002a). Men reported spending more time in leisure activities than women, including playing sports regularly. The rapid growth of gymnasiums and health spas

indicates a growing interest in maintaining physical fitness. Only 4.9% of male respondents and 5.5% of female respondents reported knowing that exercise periods of 20 minutes per session three times per week are necessary to strengthen the heart and lungs.

The survey results also revealed that in other areas of preventive health behaviors, men are less likely than women to visit a dentist, and 26.1% of males over age 65 have no natural teeth. Males tend to participate in exercise, but 68% of men over 20 years of age are overweight. Men consume more fatty foods and are less likely than women to change their eating habits.

Reporting of Health Behavior

Data regarding health behaviors are collected from a variety of sources, such as interviews, surveys, questionnaires, or reports. Data from these sources may not be accurate because males are less likely than females to participate in the data collection process. Men may be less willing to talk, may not recall health problems, and may lack a health vocabulary. Men may be more hesitant to talk about their illness. Not only do women participate in the data collection process but they also are often solicited in health surveys to report the health behavior of men. In this manner, women are proxies, and proxies have a tendency to underreport behavior. The accuracy of the data does increase with male participation, but men may not want to participate in the socialization of sickness and will make light of health problems. Males with an extreme conception of masculinity are less likely to express their health problems and may conceal or suppress pain in an effort to appear strong (Helgasend, 1995). Males are far less likely than women to seek counseling. Socialization to suppress expressiveness may represent the explanation for gender differences in reporting health behaviors.

Discussion of the Theories of Men's Health

Interpreting the Data

Verbrugge and Wingard (1987) cautioned that all four theories (i.e., biology, socialization, illness and prevention orientations, and health-reporting behavior) must be considered when interpreting data. When only diagnostic data from examinations or laboratory tests are considered (i.e., a highly medical perspective), gender differentials are most likely the result of inherited and acquired risks. However, when data have the potential to be affected by social factors, such as gender differences in illness and prevention orientations and health-reporting behavior, these factors should not be ignored. Verbrugge and Wingard (1987) stated, "A sex differential in emphysema partly reflects risks men and women incur, but also whether they are aware of the condition or feel like reporting it" (p. 134). Health interview data such as those from the National Health Interview Survey and the National Survey of Health Promotion and Disease Prevention are the most common types available concerning a population's health. Verbrugge and Wingard (1987) cautioned that the social factors of gender differences in illness and prevention

BOX 16-1 Men's Reproductive Health Needs

Reproductive health needs are beginning to be recognized as important to men's health and to women's health. Usually the term *reproductive health* is applied to women of childbearing age. Used here, the term applies to the health of reproductive organs, which develop in utero and with which a person is born, in both males and females, regardless of whether a person has sex or reproduces. Males may have reproductive health needs whether child or adult, straight or gay, or virgin or sexually experienced.

Many STDs are at epidemic proportions in the United States and are a major health hazard for many men and women. AIDS in the United States is twice as likely to occur in males than in females. In 2002, death due to HIV in African-American males was 49.9 per 100,000, and African-American females deaths due to HIV was 25.9. Less well known, perhaps, is that many STDs are considered intrinsically "sexist" because clinical evidence, more overt in men, is more likely to facilitate a correct diagnosis in men than in women. These STDs are easier to detect in men because men are more likely to be symptomatic, laboratory tests are more reliable in men, efficiency of transmission is greater from male to female, and men are more likely to seek care for STDs that are symptomatic. For example, incidence rates for chlamydia in 2003 for males was 134.6 per 100,000; for females, the rate was 468.1 per 100,000. The rate of gonorrhea was slightly lower among men (113.3 per 100,000 population) than among women (119 per 100,000 population). Only syphilis was more common in men than in women (4.2 per 100,000 males; 0.8 per 100,000 females (Centers for Disease Control and Prevention, 2003).

Testicular cancer represents only 1% of cancers in males and is the most common cancer to affect young men between ages 15 and 35 years. Cancer of the prostate is a leading cause of death from cancer in men and was estimated to account for 171 per 100,000 population in 2002 and remains twice as common in African-American males as white males. The increase in the incidence of prostate cancer has been attributed to factors such as improved methods of detection and increased exposure to environmental carcinogens.

Mortality rates for all cancers remain high, especially in males over 75 years of age. Men over age 85 are twice as likely to die from cancer than those ages 75 to 84.

Many occupational and environmental agents associated with adverse sexual and reproductive outcomes in men have been identified, including pesticides, anesthetic gases in the operating room and dental office, inorganic lead from smelters, paint, printing materials, carbon disulfide from vulcanization of rubber, inorganic mercury manufacturing and dental work, and ionizing radiation from x-rays (Cohen, 1986; McDiarmid et al., 1991; Whorton, 1984). Nonchemical agents have also been identified as hazardous in men; for example, hyperthermia experienced by firefighters has been linked to male infertility.

Many pharmacological agents, including prescription, over-the-counter, and recreational drugs, have been found to affect the reproductive outcomes or sexual functioning of men. Examples include drugs from the following categories: antihypertensives, antipsychotics, antidepressants, hormones, sedatives, hypnotics, stimulants, chemotherapy agents used in cancer treatment, amphetamines, opiates, alcohol, marijuana, cocaine, barbiturates, and lysergic acid diethylamide (LSD). Erectile dysfunction has become a "socially acceptable" topic of discussion since many high profile men, such as Senator Bob Dole, former National Football League coach Mike Ditka, and retired General Norman Schwarzkopf have openly discussed their problem. Pharmaceutical companies market their products for treatment of this disorder via mass media. Controversy has arisen as to the use of public funding for these products.

A focus on homosexual men's health has come about largely through the advent of AIDS. Today, homosexuality encompasses not only the male but also the entire family. The community health nurse should develop nonjudgmental assessment skills that foster honest and open expression for all members of the community. Nurses may need specialized skills to work with these individuals.

---

orientations, as well as health-reporting behavior, are critical in interpreting health interview data.

Community health nurses should be aware of this gender disparity when collecting and interpreting data. To avoid bias, the community health nurse should consider the following things:

- Gender-specific interview techniques may be necessary to obtain the most accurate health history. Men respond better to direct questioning rather than open-ended questions.
- How do data obtained by male nurses differ from those obtained by female nurses? Is there personal gender bias in data collection?
- The accuracy of secondary sources of information is skewed toward the interpretation of the source. How does the data provided by women about male health behavior compare with the data collected from males regarding these same behaviors?
- Men are not enculturated to be caregivers. Men need assistance to learn how to provide support to the caregiver or to develop a caregiver role.

In response to the question of why "females are sicker, but males die sooner," several reasons can be provided. Conditions that affect morbidity rates (e.g., arthritis and gout) do not significantly affect mortality rates. Conditions that affect mortality rates may not significantly affect day-to-day activity until the condition is advanced. Men tend to delay seeking health care until their condition is advanced. Although mortality rates are, in large part, the outcome of inherited or acquired risks, gender differences in illness and prevention orientations and the reporting of health behaviors suggest that social and psychological factors also affect morbidity rates. Although males have a higher prevalence and death rates for "killer" chronic diseases, injuries, and accidents, females have higher prevalence rates for a greater number of nonfatal chronic conditions. In addition, adult women report higher rates of morbidity from acute conditions than adult men. Verbrugge and Wingard (1987) stated that "females' greater willingness and ability to take care of themselves when ill, to seek preventive help, and to talk about health all boost their morbidity rate" (p. 136).

Gender-Linked Behavior

The largest gender differences in mortality rates occur for causes of death associated with gender-linked behavior and suggest that gender-linked behavior, which is more prevalent and encouraged in men, correlates with the following major categories of death (Harrison, 1984):

Doctors and Patients: Gender Interaction in the Consultation

Much research on gender differences in medicine has centered on women as better communicators, more egalitarian, more patient-centered, and more involved with psychosocial problems, preventive care, and female-specific problems. Little research has examined the interaction between a health care provider and the patient's gender. Anecdotal evidence says that women prefer to see women doctors. Research indicates that men as well as women are more satisfied with the care given by a woman doctor. This leads to the question of why this is.

Research indicates that women doctors demonstrate more "humanitarian" and "patient-care values." They conduct longer consultations and manage more problems of a psychosocial nature. Women doctors tend to use a conversational style of communication that is egalitarian and encourages participation, whereas men doctors tend to be more dominant and directive. Clearly, men and women have different styles of consultation. Does this imply that consultation outcomes are influenced by a doctor's gender? Does the patient's gender influence the doctor's management? In other words, do men and women doctors treat men and women patients equally?

A study was planned that tested a cohort of medical students to see if their gender interacted with that of their patients, influencing the outcome of the consultation. The study examined the perceptions of medical students and the comfort levels of patients during consultation. This cross-sectional study used a self-administered questionnaire to survey 132 final-year medical students at one school in 1999. It tested students' patient-centeredness, "patient-care" values, and degree of comfort in performing certain intimate physical examinations.

The study showed that women medical students were more patient-centered than were men medical students. Both genders were more attuned to the concerns of patients of their own gender, were more comfortable with personal rather than sexual issues, and were more uncomfortable with performing more intimate examinations upon the opposite gender. Using comparable case studies, it was also shown that the female student–female patient dyad had significantly greater "patient care" values than did the male student–male patient dyad.

The study showed that medical students did not behave in a gender-neutral way in the consultation. There is a powerful interaction between a health provider's gender and a patient's gender.

Zaharias G, Piterman L, Liddell M: Doctors and patients: gender interaction in the consultation, *Acad Med* 79(2):148-155, 2004.

- *Tobacco use:* Lung cancer, bronchitis, emphysema, and asthma
- *Substance abuse:* Cirrhosis, accidents, and homicide
- *Poor preventive health habits and stress:* Heart disease
- *Lack of other emotional channels:* Cirrhosis, suicide, homicide, and accidents

Physical conditions can be seriously affected by social and environmental conditions, such as occupational hazards (e.g., carcinogens and stress), unemployment, and massive advertising campaigns that use gender and gender roles to sell alcohol and tobacco. These lifestyle factors are compounded by men's lack of willingness to seek preventive care such as screening and to seek health care when a symptom arises. To counter these types of factors, research is needed to determine gender-specific methods of data collection, education, and practice that are aimed at health promotion, illness prevention, and political processes for males.

FACTORS THAT IMPEDE MEN'S HEALTH

Many factors present as barriers to men's health, including their risk taking behavior and infrequent use of the health care system. In addition, gaps in preventive health behavior and differences in illness and health orientations and reporting health behavior all contribute to a diminished health status for men. Several other barriers have been proposed, including the patterns of medical care provided in the United States, access to care, and lack of health promotion.

Medical Care Patterns

DeHoff and Forrest (1984) stated, "The usual pattern of medical care in this country—'the system'—has contributed indirectly to men's health problems" (p. 5). Although the data that serve as a foundation for medical treatment were collected from males, the concept of a health care provider that specializes in men's health is a relatively recent phenomenon. Many health professionals provide care for men with complex health needs in a wide variety of settings. A specialist to which a male could go to for care that "feels right" for them has not been developed. Little effort has been made to create a male-specific health care climate. Urologists, who may see men for genital abnormalities or diseases of the prostate, became the proxy "male health specialist." The medical specialty andrology, which originated in Europe to treat problems of fertility and sterility, is considered too narrow in focus to treat "the whole man." Without a primary care specialty that focuses specifically on men's needs and gender-role influences on health and lifestyle, the gender disparity will continue. Currently, male health concerns are addressed by specialists and generalists who have not received gender-specific training that would enable them to focus on men's health needs. In the current era of managed care, men will still be left without a gender-specific primary care provider with training focused specifically on men's needs.

Access to Care
Mission Orientation
Historically, society's interest in men's health has focused on efforts necessary to maintain an effective workforce (DeHoff and Forrest, 1984). Men are socialized to view health as a commodity or resource that enables the body to work (Harrison and Dignan, 1999). Mission-oriented health care is a priority for large industries and organized sports. Industries provide workers with preventive health care to maintain workplace productivity. Mission-oriented health care in the sports arena has given birth to the specialty of sports medicine. Insurance programs such as health maintenance organizations (HMOs) may provide more comprehensive health care to men. Perhaps the most complete care is currently offered by the military; however, marked deficiencies exist in the lack of a focus on prevention and health promotion at the individual

BOX 16-2   Precursors of Death

The following precursors of death are frequently unaddressed by the present health care system:

- Heart disease and stroke
- Hypercholesterolemia
- Hypertension
- Diabetes mellitus
- Obesity
- Type A personality
- Family history
- Lack of exercise
- Cigarette smoking

- Cancer
- Sunlight
- Radiation
- Occupational hazards
- Water pollution
- Air pollution
- Dietary patterns
- Alcohol
- Heredity
- Certain medical conditions

and aggregate levels and inattention to policy regarding environmental hazards.

Financial Considerations

Another barrier to health care for men is financial ability. A man may receive an annual physical examination if he belongs to an HMO or if he is an executive or an airline pilot, but many private insurance companies will reimburse more fully for a diagnosed condition (e.g., for pathology) and less fully for preventive care. A man is more likely insured for acute or chronic illness conditions than for health education, counseling, or other types of preventive health care. Women have annual gynecological examinations that include screening for other conditions and allow a woman to express other physical or psychological needs; however, men have lacked entrée to the health care system for a physical examination on a routine basis. With the advent of managed care and societal interest in preventative health focus, gender differences in routine physical examinations for preventive reasons have narrowed. However, socialization has a marked influence on behavior, and current trends may prevail despite attitudinal changes in health care delivery. Men must become advocates for programs that meet their own health care needs.

Time Factors

Historically, medical care could be accessed between the hours of 9:00 AM and 5:00 PM Monday through Friday. Men were reluctant to take time from work for a medical visit, especially for reasons other than illness. Fear of loss of income or the stigmatization of being "weak," "ill," or "less of a man" inhibited medical care access for males. Variety in the times and locations of care delivery clinics should increase male access. More walk-in primary care clinics that provide evening and weekend appointments have appeared. These clinics may be housed in occupational settings, malls, and even grocery stores. Data need to be collected regarding male utilization of these additional health care sites.

Lack of Health Promotion

Limiting the concept of health as merely absence of disease eliminates health promotion. Using traditional mortality and morbidity rates as reflective of the state of "health" of a population represents only a biological basis of health. To provide the community health nurse with a clearer picture of male health, the presence of behavioral risk factors such as smoking, alcohol consumption, obesity, and sedentary lifestyle should be considered. When asked, men describe "healthy" people as those with proportional body weight and height who do not engage excessively in behaviors detrimental to health. Physical recovery after impairment, illness, or injury is also considered a factor in men's definition of "healthy." Disease prevention and health promotion are not often reflected in a man's perception of health. Addressing and limiting the precursors of death is a recent health care phenomenon (Box 16-2). Interventions by many disciplines are needed to prevent current health problems. Nursing can play a pivotal role in the contribution to practice and research in this area of concern.

The continued focus on disease cure in the present health care system reinforces men's perception of health. Coronary heart disease, cancer, and stroke are three conditions that account for two thirds of all deaths and require the greatest use of health care resources. The increase in life expectancy exhibits the effect these medical advances have had on mortality rates from these diseases. These advances have resulted in an increase in years of disability, which may account for the increase in suicide among males over the age of 65 (NCHS, 2004). An increase in health care costs has also resulted.

Social Demography and Social Epidemiology

Epidemiology is the method of research used to determine the nature and distribution of a health problem in a community. Social demographers and social epidemiologists study social and psychological factors that affect the distribution of health problems in a community. Factors associated with the occurrence of the problems can be identified, and resources can be focused on prevention. Social epidemiologists have identified men as a population at risk for premature death. Concentrated efforts can improve men's health. ■

Financial resources are invested in traditional disease curative care rather than health promotion action. An inordinate amount of funding is poured into the health care system each year, with only minimal amounts allotted to public health promotion, as discussed in earlier chapters. In 2002, total

Social Justice Versus Market Justice Ethics

Community health nurses should be involved in political activities that develop health policies that will make a difference in the health of males and the entire population. Such activities are congruent with the philosophy of public health as "health for all" and a commitment to a social justice ethic of health care rather than a market justice ethic of health care. Examining men's health gives the community health nurse an opportunity to observe the market justice ethic of health care's influence on men's health in the United States from men's traditional roles in the family, the health of women, family, and community. The community health nurse can play a vital role in contributing to a social justice ethic of health care, particularly in relation to promoting men's health. Nurses must focus on health promotion and prevention at the aggregate and population levels rather than focus on treatment and cure.

health expenditures accounted for 14.1% of the gross domestic product. Of every dollar spent on health care in 2002, more than half went to hospital care and physician services, which are, in large part, curative in focus. The current health care system is making limited advances in addressing the precursors of death. It is questionable whether medical care, or another medical specialty, is the answer to men's health needs when social, occupational, environmental, and lifestyle factors continue to place men at risk.

Milio (1983) asserted that healthy lifestyles are not a matter of free choice but rather a result of opportunities that are not always equally available to people. Although available, prevention and health promotion are not uniformly applied at the aggregate and population levels. Health policies shape these opportunities for a healthy lifestyle for individuals and aggregates. Policies related to environmental and occupational changes beyond an individual's control are required to significantly impact the health of the population.

MEN'S HEALTH CARE NEEDS

DeHoff and Forrest (1984) delineated men's health care needs that draw from the biological and the psychosocial causes of men's distinctive health situation. According to these authors, men need the following:

- Permission to have concerns about health and talk openly to others about their concerns
- Support for the consideration of gender-role and lifestyle influences on their physical and mental health
- Attention from professionals regarding factors that may result in illness or influence a man's expression of illness, including such things as occupational factors, leisure patterns, and interpersonal relationships
- Information about how their bodies function, what is normal, what is abnormal, what action to take, and the contributions of proper nutrition and exercise
- Self-care instruction, including testicular and genital self-examination

- Physical examination and history taking that include sexual and reproductive health and illness across the lifespan
- Treatment for problems of couples, including interpersonal problems, infertility, family planning, sexual concerns, and sexually transmitted diseases (STDs)
- Help with fathering (i.e., being included as a parent in child care)
- Help with fathering as a single parent, in particular with a child of the opposite sex, in addressing the child's sexual development and concerns
- Recognition that feelings of confusion and uncertainty in a time of rapid social change are normal and that they may mark the onset of healthy adaptation to change
- Adjustment of the health care system to men's occupational constraints regarding time and location of health care sources
- Financial ways to obtain these goals

Additional health care needs of men are for primary prevention, and for secondary and tertiary prevention at the individual, family, and community levels, to address the precursors of death that influence males so greatly. Men are less likely to be consumers in the health care system than are women; therefore alternative approaches must be developed that address their health needs. The most significant approaches in the future will be those that reach men in the community, schools, the workplace, and public settings. These approaches call for political processes that set policy, for health marketing techniques, and for advocacy.

Community Health Nursing Services for Men

A male can be seen by a community health nurse in a well-baby clinic, by a school nurse, by an occupational health nurse, and by a community health nurse or home health nurse on a home visit for follow-up of a chronic disease. However, men are less likely than women to be seen by a community health nurse. Not only is maternal and child health a major focus of many health departments, but neither a medical nor a nursing specialty within a health department routinely exists to specifically address men's health. Preventive reproductive health care (i.e., family planning, prenatal care, and cancer screening) and associated general screening are not routinely available for men. The hours of services offered by health departments usually do not provide convenient access for men. The community health nurse's commitment to health for all requires an increased awareness of men's health issues in their social and cultural context and individual and group action that will improve men's physical, psychological, and social well-being.

Meeting men's health care needs can be viewed in a traditional public fashion. By viewing the problem from a primary, secondary, and tertiary intervention method, the nurse can look at the problem in a holistic manner. Factors that promote men's health are in the community, including interest groups in men and men's health, men's increasing interest in physical fitness and lifestyle, policy related to men's health, and health services for men. ∎

Gaining Skills Necessary to Address Men's Health Needs

Assessment skills necessary to carry out screening activities with men to detect reproductive health needs may be lacking in nursing education. One community health nurse who worked in a rural health department felt unable to respond to male partners' requests for genital examinations when couples came to seek family planning services. This community health nurse requested to work for specified periods of time with a urologist and in an STD clinic in a large urban area to gain the necessary skills. On return to the rural health department, she felt comfortable with male patients and taught the skills she had learned to nurse colleagues. ■

PRIMARY PREVENTIVE MEASURES

Health Education

Health care professionals, including the community health nurse, find that health education is the cornerstone of prevention. Although criticized by some as too narrow, health education can be a means of empowerment that assists individuals to make behavioral changes. Education about male health issues should begin early. At school, boys should learn the anatomical and physiological aspects of their bodies and the social aspects of taking responsibility for their health. Coeducational discussion classes that cover a variety of social and personal topics can be a venue to encourage boys to talk about their bodies and their feelings. This may lead to a less self-conscious attitude toward health seeking when boys reach adulthood.

Access to health education should follow males into the workplace. Many employers have experienced benefits such as lower health care costs when their employees receive health education programs coupled with health screening. Government and private insurance incentives given to employers who provide such programs would provide further impetus. Men who are not in the workplace can access health education in other areas, such as shopping malls, barbershops, and local senior centers. Some health care professionals are concerned about this informal dispersion of health literature, citing concern about the literacy level of the population. Government benefits programs can be a medium for health education by including such in their benefit mailing. More control over the readability and the information included can be exerted over this material. Educational material should be written in the context of male interests.

Interest Groups for Men and Men's Health

Unlike the consumer movement that occurred on behalf of women's health in the 1960s and early 1970s, a consumer movement has not taken place advocating men's health. However, a viable men's consumer movement is forming. The National Organization for Changing Men is interested in redefining the male role, particularly those aspects of the male role that are detrimental to health and growth. The American Assembly for Men in Nursing sponsors annual meetings that address issues such as men's health, men's work environments, research on men's health, and networking and support among male nurses. Researchers are beginning to define and study men's health beyond men's occupational role (e.g., reproductive health). Marketing has changed to include male health promotion public service announcements.

Men's Increasing Interest in Physical Fitness and Lifestyle

Although cardiovascular diseases (CVDs) are a major health hazard for men, research on the validity and usefulness of preventive and treatment modalities is an issue of considerable debate (Waldron, 1995b). Men's interest in altering behavior that places them at risk for cardiovascular and other major diseases is increasing. For example, men's smoking behavior has changed dramatically. In 1965, over 50% of males smoked compared to 25% in 2002. Today, 59.4% of men report exercising three times a week or more, compared to 52.1% of females (NCHS, 2004).

However, those health behaviors that have reported the greatest change in a positive direction have been those most influenced by legislative action (e.g., seat belt use, use of smoke detectors, and drunk driving) (Piani and Schoenborn, 1993). Even with these legislative actions, males remain three times less likely to use a seatbelt as females of the same age. In the Southeast, pickup truck usage of seat belts was 25% compared to greater than 75% for other vehicles. The states of Alabama, Florida, Georgia, Kentucky, Mississippi, North Carolina, South Carolina, and Tennessee have begun a campaign called "Buckle Up Your Pickup Truck." The campaign's centerpiece is the use of targeted television and radio advertisements to encourage seat belt use. Intensive enforcement mobilizations in the form of Selective Traffic Enforcement Programs (STEPs), like Click It or Ticket, will immediately follow the periods of pickup truck advertisements.

The Southeast's Buckle Up in Your Truck campaign is a 16-month campaign, whereby program processes and outcomes will be measured and documented. Progress will be measured using a number of data collection methods (Preusser Research Group, 2003).

Policy Related to Men's Health

Policies related to any group of people should include the opinions and perceptions of those directly affected. Policy related to men's health should include the male perception of health. Community health nurses can encourage and assist males to be advocates for policies regarding their health care. Male nurses can be extremely instrumental in this endeavor. Liaisons between male consumers and policy planners should be formed.

SECONDARY PREVENTIVE MEASURES

Health Services for Men

Fewer health care clinics are tailored to men's special needs than women's special needs. The "well-man clinics" set up in the 1980s were designed to identify lifestyle risk factors, not to provide screening clinics like the women's clinics. Once identified, a method or resolution for these lifestyle risk factors is formulated. These clinics still exist, with emphasis placed on CVDs (Sadler, 1979). Male screening methods typically have been limited to detecting high blood cholesterol levels and cancers such as prostate cancer, skin cancer, and testicular lumps. Although many well-man clinics exist in the United Kingdom, male usage of these clinics is far below female usage of women's clinics (Roberts and Gerber, 2003). This era of managed care may not encourage the concept of gender-specific care, as men and women receive primary care from the same health services.

Screening Services for Men

The U.S. Preventive Services Task Force (2004) outlines the kinds of screening tests the population should receive. According to the Task Force, healthy men under age 50 should have the following:

- Dental examination: Yearly
- Eye examination: Every 3 to 5 years
- Blood pressure check: Every 2 years
- Blood cholesterol check for men aged 53 years and older every year
- Prostate examination: Every year after age 50; blacks every year after age 40
- Colorectal screening: Every 3 to 5 years
- Tobacco use and cessation information every year
- One-time screening for abdominal aortic aneurysm for men 65 years old if the male has smoked

Community health nurses should be familiar with these recommended screening test frequencies and should take every opportunity to encourage men to have these screenings. Through the institution of male health care fairs and other organized screenings, nurses are able to work with other health care providers to ensure these routine screenings are performed.

TERTIARY PREVENTIVE MEASURES

Sex-Role and Lifestyle Rehabilitation

Traditional health services for males are available in both private and governmental arenas. The emphasis of these services is on diagnosis and treatment. The traditional male role may change dramatically from treatment modalities. Rehabilitation services for males must include counseling on lifestyle, role changes, and job retraining. Men must be given permission to express their emotions, such as fear and anxiety, over the resultant change.

Goal setting and possible methods for achievement must be acceptable to the man. For example, after a heart attack, a man may be told to stop smoking and begin an exercise program. To be successful, the male must be an active partner in the formation of the plan. He may be able to exercise, for example, by walking to the nearest automotive shop to talk with friends rather than spending time on a stationary bicycle at a local gym.

Time away from work due to occupational injuries should be kept to a minimum. Males should be encouraged to return to work in an altered capacity rather than remaining away from work until the injury is completely healed. Occupational accommodation for treatment regiment will help ensure compliance. Provision of medical care, supportive physical and occupational therapies, and "light-duty" jobs at the worksite help preserve the masculine persona.

Door Openers: Ways to Address Men About Health Concerns

Strategies to address men about health concerns include the following:

- Ask a man to talk about the last time he had a physical examination, what was done, why it was done, where it was done, and what the recommendations were.
- Ask a man how he feels about his health insurance coverage. If he lacks health insurance, ask about the resources he used to obtain medical care for himself and for his family.
- Ask a man about how he spends his leisure time, what he is doing to take care of himself, and what his usual physical activities are.
- Observe a man for signs of stress such as moist palms, nail biting, posture, and nervous movements. If signs of stress are present, ask about how he is coping with an identified health problem, family problem, or being unemployed.
- Observe a man for difficulty clearing airway (e.g., from smoking) and flushing of the face (e.g., from alcohol). Inquire as to habits of smoking and drinking and whether these habits have increased since the occurrence of the particular health or social problem.
- Involve men in decision making about health care to instill a sense of control over events. ■

New Concepts of Community Care

Specific services for men within health departments continue to be lacking in the United States. With the exception of STD clinics and selected family planning service models, male health concerns remain unaddressed. Two male health visitors (the British term for public health nurses) from the National Health Service (NHS) started an innovative public health nursing program directed at men in Glasgow, Scotland (Sadler, 1979). Health visitors Bill Deans and Bob Hoskins established a nurse-run well-man clinic with the help of the NHS and the Scottish Council for Health Education. During home visits with mothers and infants, Deans and Hoskins observed that fathers excused themselves and went to the local pub when they arrived.

Noting characteristics of the male population in their community (e.g., overweight, heavy smoking, drinking, and high unemployment), Deans and Hoskins decided to modify their practice to serve their clients' needs. One afternoon per week, the clinic, which is based on a nursing model rather than a medical model, offers health screening, health education, and primary prevention to men. Marketing is important, and men are referred from general practitioners' and specialists' practices and recruited through newspaper advertisements. Clients with clinical signs and symptoms are referred back to their physicians. Lifestyle counseling and education are offered in areas such as fat and fiber content in diet, smoking, alcohol use, and exercise.

Text continues on p. 330

CASE STUDY   Application of the Nursing Process

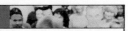

Community health nurses are in an ideal position to address the health needs of men at the individual, family, and community levels. The community health nurse may promote self-care in male members of the family, facilitate men's health by addressing needed changes at the family level, buttress women's roles as caregivers of the family's health, and bring about change that influences policies that affect men at the community level.

Planning gender-appropriate care for males is outlined in the following case study, which is an application of the nursing process at the individual, family, and aggregate levels initiated in a home visit and applies the previous discussions about the levels of prevention, roles of the community health nurse, research, and men's health.

Application of the nursing process to aggregates is facilitated by the use of systems theory, in which the nurse identifies the system and subsystems involved. The nurse may use a deductive or an inductive approach. A deductive approach would involve carrying out a community assessment and identifying an area or areas, such as a program needed by the community. Planning, implementation, and evaluation of the program would be carried out at the family or group level. An inductive approach would involve entering the community system through a person or client via a referral about a problem or concern. Assessment of the individual would be followed by identification of those groups to which the client belongs, such as family and community, and assessment of those groups.

Beth Lockwood, a community health nursing student at a health department, received a referral from the high school nurse to visit the Connors family to assess Richard Connors' mental health status. Richard was a 16-year-old sophomore whose academic work in school had declined rapidly after the premature death of his 46-year-old father. He died from a myocardial infarction, which he suffered while cleaning the garage with Richard one evening after school. Richard and the neighbors failed to revive Mr. Connors and Richard carries feelings of guilt. Household members include Mrs. Connors, age 44, and Richard's sister Yvonne, age 12.

ASSESSMENT

The referral to assess the Connors family called for an inductive approach to assessment. Beth used a deductive approach later, when her experience with the Connors family piqued her concern about the status of men's health in her community. Beth assessed Richard, his mother, and his sister as household members of the family. However, she could not stop with the immediate family; she had to continue to identify the other groups within the community to which each individual family member belonged. Viewing the community as a system and focusing on systems and subsystems helped Beth organize the data she collected during assessment. Knowing that "the whole is greater than the sum of its parts," Beth prepared for her visit by reviewing adolescent theories of development and family theory. Beyond individual assessment, she noted factors related to the development of sex-role–related behavior that may influence health. Examples of assessment areas include the following:

Family configuration, traditional or nontraditional

- Sex-role–related behavior of parents, including work patterns in and out of the home, division of household labor, and decision-making patterns
- Patterns of parenting: mothering, fathering, and substitute father figure(s)
- Ability of male children to disclose feelings to family members and others
- Degree of assertiveness in female children
- Ability of family members to give emotional and physical support during crises and noncrises
- Ability of family members to trade off role-related behavior during crises and noncrises
- Risk-taking health behaviors
- Processing stress and grief
- Communal lifestyle patterns that place the individual or family at risk (e.g., lack of exercise, poor diet, smoking, and drinking)
- Family history of death and illness
- Healthcare–taking patterns of family members
- Preventive health behaviors
- Leisure activities

Assessment of other groups includes neighborhood and other peer groups, school environments, sports, and church and civic activities.

DIAGNOSIS

Through induction, the nurse makes a diagnosis for each individual and each system component, including family and the community. The following are examples of diagnoses.

Individual

- Loss of interest or involvement in an activity, related to conflicting stages of grief process secondary to premature death of father (Richard)
- Expressed dissatisfaction with parenting role, related to feelings of helplessness and hopelessness secondary to premature death of husband (Mrs. Connors)
- Risk of interpersonal conflict, resulting from prolonged, unrelieved family stress secondary to premature death of father (Yvonne)

Family

- Decreased ability to communicate, related to family stress secondary to premature death of father
- Risk of family crisis, related to disequilibrium

Community

- Inadequate systematic programs for linking families in crisis to community resources

Continued

- Inadequate systematic programs for populations at risk of premature death, related to inadequate planning among community systems

PLANNING

Planning involves contracting and mutual goal setting and is an outcome of mutually derived assessment and diagnosis. A contract with the family alone is shortsighted and may provide little community benefit over time. The following are examples of other aggregates with which a contract may be established:

- The school subsystem that does not provide ongoing counseling, but will meet periodically to evaluate pupil progression with family members
- The school subsystem that provides physical education in football, basketball, and baseball (i.e., nonaerobic, non-lifetime sports), but offers extramural aerobic, lifetime sports such as swimming and track after school hours
- The American Red Cross, which does not offer cardiovascular pulmonary resuscitation (CPR) courses on evenings or weekends, but offers to consider doing so for a defined minimum-size community.

Mutual goal setting requires collaboration regarding long- and short-term goals. Again, mutually defined needs and diagnoses are important to this process. Regardless of the diagnosis, each individual in the family and the subsystem must participate in developing a care plan. The following are examples of goals.

Individual
Long-Term Goal
- Individual family members will be able to trade off role-related behavior.

Short-Term Goal
- Individual family members will express feelings related to abandonment and loss.

Family
Long-Term Goal
- The family will exhibit an increased ability to handle crisis, as evidenced by ability to discuss roles and interdependencies.

Short-Term Goal
- The family will identify specific ways to recognize and use support services.

Community
Long-Term Goal
- Systematic programs, with ongoing program evaluation, will be established for populations at risk of premature death from coronary heart disease, as evidenced by local planning bodies.

Short-Term Goals
- Dissemination is provided to individuals, families, groups, and planning bodies in the community about the incidence of coronary heart disease.
- Existing programs are identified that address coronary heart disease.
- Existing programs are coordinated to bridge gaps and avoid duplication of effort.

INTERVENTION

The nurse, family, and other aggregates carry out interventions contracted during the planning phase to meet the mutually derived goals. Most important, the nurse empowers the family and community to develop the networks and linkages necessary to care for themselves.

Individual

Individual counseling regarding loss and grief may be beneficial to each family member, but options may need to be explored and referrals may need to be reevaluated for members of the rural family. Education regarding preventive measures that combat risk factors for heart disease include those aimed at individual family members and address areas such as diet, exercise, smoking, alcohol use, and stress management.

Family

Examples of interventions with the family include counseling, education, and referral aimed at family self-care promotion. For example, Beth's interventions with the Connors family were dependent on the family's ability to solve problems, investigate community resources, and create linkages between the family and resources. Periodic family conferences at school and more inclusive family therapy may enable the family to work through the death of Mr. Connors; this results in the development of new roles and the communication necessary to maintain family equilibrium. Education regarding preventive measures to combat risk factors for heart disease may need discussion at the family and individual levels (e.g., diet, exercise, smoking, alcohol use, and stress management).

Community

The nurse must also carry out interventions with other aggregates. These may involve activities such as educating, facilitating program expansion, or tailoring programs to meet community needs. Intervention at the aggregate level calls for group and community work. The nurse carries out interventions at this level in several ways (e.g., by communicating community statistics from a community analysis, relating anecdotes from families served, or linking family experience to program need by acting as an advocate and bringing family members to board meetings or hearings on community health issues).

CASE STUDY Application of the Nursing Process (cont'd)

Education regarding preventive measures to combat risk factors for heart disease also includes those interventions aimed at the community. A rationale for the development of lifetime aerobic sports is needed not only by Richard, but also by school districts. Exploration of options with the school nurse and review of the school district health education curriculum would be beneficial. A community assessment of heart disease awareness, including determination of the availability of resources such as emergency response and CPR courses, is an aggregate intervention. Taking the outcome of the assessment in the form of statistics and the anonymous anecdotal story of the Connors family to planning bodies in the community is also intervention at the aggregate level. Creative programs other communities used (e.g., teaching CPR within the school system) should be investigated and proposed.

EVALUATION

Evaluation is multidimensional and ongoing. Using a systems approach to evaluation, the nurse evaluates each component of the system, from individual family member to family and community, in terms of goal achievement. Evaluation includes noting degrees of equilibrium established, degree of change, how the system handles change, whether the system is open or closed, and patterns of networking. Ongoing evaluation includes noting referrals and follow-up of the individual, the family, and other aggregates in resource use.

Individual

Use of resources such as support groups by the individual family member may be noted. These resources may include a teen support group, a women's support group, support groups for those experiencing the loss of a spouse or other family member, reentry programs for women at a local junior college or university, and parents without partners.

Family

Evaluation of the Connors family would include follow-up of their use of support services specifically for the family, such as counseling options for the family as a unit. Evaluation would also focus on the family's ability to handle crises in the future.

Community

Aggregate evaluation would focus on the community. For example, to what extent do school programs encourage sports options that promote lifetime aerobic activities and prevent premature death from heart disease? Are programs systematically planned in the community for populations that are at risk of premature death from heart disease?

LEVELS OF PREVENTION

Society's expectations of men and women are in transition. Application of levels of prevention by the community health nurse must take into account men's health status, men's socialization, men's use of health care services, men's primary needs for prevention and health promotion, and the role of women as caregivers in family health.

Primary

Men are more likely to engage in risk-taking behavior than women and are less likely to engage in preventive behaviors; therefore, primary prevention must be marketed specifically to men. Examples of primary prevention for the Connors family are applied at the following individual, family, and community levels:

Individual
- Assessment, teaching, and referral related to diet and exercise behaviors

Family
- Assessment and teaching related to food selection and preparation at home and fast-food restaurant food selection
- Teaching and role modeling gender roles that allow male members of the family to use alternative expressions of emotion

Community
- Provision of CPR courses for members of the community; consultation with schools regarding need for aerobic activities in physical education and sports programs

The nurse must pull men from the family, workplace, or other aggregates into involvement with family planning, education, antepartum and postpartum care, parenting, dental prophylaxis, and accident prevention. In addition, assessment of need for immunizations and classes (e.g., retirement preparation) is considered action aimed at primary prevention.

Secondary

Men have higher mortality, morbidity, and health care use rates for many of the leading causes of death, but they are second to women in overall use of health care services, including preventive physical examinations and screening; therefore, early diagnosis and prompt intervention must also meet men's needs. Examples of secondary prevention regarding the Connors family include the following:

Individual
- Screen for risk factors related to CVD in the individual, such as how the individual handles stress.

Family
- Screen for risk factors related to CVD in the family, such as how the family processes stress.

Community
- Organize screening programs for the community, such as health fairs.

Continued

The nurse must screen individuals and aggregates of men according to lifestyle risk factors, mortality rates at different age levels, morbidity rates, and occupational health risks.

Tertiary

Activities that rehabilitate individuals and aggregates and restore them to their highest level of functioning are aimed at tertiary prevention. The nurse in the community is ideally situated to locate people in need of rehabilitation services. The nurse may provide evaluation and physical, mental, and social restoration services. Men in need of rehabilitation may have special needs because their disability influences them, their families, and ultimately their communities. Financial assistance and vocational counseling, training, and placement may be priorities for the well-being of the family. Socialization causes men to have difficulty admitting they need help. Community health nurses who teach men with chronic disease to rest at specified periods during the day or continue with medical regimens or speech or occupational

therapy are providing tertiary prevention. Working with couples as a unit is also important because caregiving patterns may shift as a result of chronic disease and disability. Encouraging men to express their concerns about their health, families, and jobs and frustration with themselves is important. The following are examples of tertiary prevention with the Connors family.

Individual

- Assist individual family members in dealing with grief from the loss of the father and husband.

Family

- Assist family in dealing with grief and assuming alternate roles.

Community

- Assist the community in dealing with loss of a fully functioning family by providing grief support services that include males or target males and females.

Deans and Hoskins consider the clinic a way to extend the health visitor's role in the NHS's efforts in health education with an aim to "nip potential diseases in the bud" (Sadler, 1979, p. 18). Deans and Hoskins are concerned that the NHS does not provide male services and are clear that "the unemployed chain-smoking husband needs as much care and health education from the health visitor as do his wife and baby" (Sadler, 1979, p. 18). The well-man clinic and the well-woman clinic models can now be found in several communities throughout Great Britain and have been expanded to serve inmates in prison (Fareed, 1994; Woodland and Hunt, 1994). After 10 years in existence, the well-man clinics in Great Britain are only sporadically used by males. Even when the services were expanded to the home, nurses found that men were purposely absent at the appointment time. Usage was highest with informal evening clinics directed by male nurses (Roberts and Gerber, 2003).

Public health nurses working in the Benton County Health Department in Corvallis, Oregon, responded to the challenge of teen pregnancy in the 1970s by launching a community-wide effort that included developing a men's health clinic and marketing reproductive health services directly to teenage boys and men. An early effort established an advisory committee that included people from churches, schools, and health care facilities. A public health nurse health educator launched an extensive education program in the high school, which focused on decision-making processes and services available in the community. Later efforts involved the establishment of a clinic for men. Teenage boys were members of a consumer advisory committee established by the nurses that recommended the wording and format for advertisements about the clinic that ran in the high school newspaper. The advisory committee also recommended a flyer format that would be attractive to males. Specifically, they requested a

card with information about the clinic and how to use condoms that would discreetly fit into their wallets and be available to share with peers.

The nurses have expanded their focus to create inclusive service environments in which teenage girls and boys and adult men and women will feel accepted and comfortable. Particular attention is given to the clinic decor and advertising, reading materials, and posters to transmit a message that includes offering health care for males and females. Clinic staff will see males or females at any time; however, a room in which staff members see men has decor geared toward men (e.g., no gynecological stirrups on the examining table) and pamphlets available for men on topics such as testicular cancer and chewing tobacco. Integrated services exist in the areas of family planning, STDs, and HIV counseling and testing.

LEARNING ACTIVITIES

1. Examine the vital statistics in the community and compare the gender-specific differences in mortality rates.
2. During a one-week period, determine the frequency of newspaper articles in the local major newspaper that identify the top 12 causes of death for men.
3. Survey the billboards in the community and determine the frequency of those that depict gender-linked behavior of men associated with risk-taking behavior.
4. Survey local businesses and industries in the community to determine what health promotion and prevention programs are available and used by men and women.
5. Select a family that has a man in the household who is accessible. Select two "door openers" appropriate to initiate discussion of health concerns with this man. Devise a gender-appropriate nursing care plan that includes primary, secondary, and tertiary prevention for this man as an individual, for his family, and for his community.

6. Select a family that has a man in the household who is not readily accessible. Interview the female caregiver in the household and obtain information by proxy about the man's health. If possible, arrange to meet the man for lunch, at work, or after work and obtain information about his health.

Compare the information obtained by proxy with that obtained from the client.

7. Review major nursing texts (e.g., medical-surgical); examine the tables of contents and the indexes for content on men's health versus women's health.

REFERENCES

Benson V, Marano MA: *Current estimates from the National Health Interview Survey, 2001-2002,* http://www.cdc.gov/nchs/data/10_190_1.pdf.

Centers for Disease Control and Prevention, National Center for Health Statistics: *Men's health 2002,* Hyattsville, Md, 2002, The Author, http://www.cdc.gov/nchs/fastats/mens-health.htm.

Cohen FL: Paternal contributions to birth defects, *Nurs Clin North Am* 21:49, 1986.

David DS, Brannon R: The male sex role: our culture's blueprint of manhood, and what it's done for us lately. In David DS, Brannon R, editors: *The forty-nine percent majority: the male sex role,* Reading, Mass, 1976, Addison-Wesley.

DeHoff JB, Forrest K: Men's health. In Swanson J, Forrest K, editors: *Men's reproductive health,* New York, 1984, Springer.

Erikson E: *Childhood and society,* New York, 1963, WW Norton.

Fareed A: Equal rights for men, *Nurs Times* 90:26, 1994.

Gotch KE et al: Surveillance for fatal and nonfatal firearm-related injuries –1990-2000, *MMWR Morb Mortality Wkly Rep*

Harrison JB: Warning: the male sex role may be dangerous to your health. In Swanson J, Forrest K, editors: *Men's reproductive health,* New York, 1984, Springer.

Harrison T, Dignan K: *The state of man 1999: a special report,* New York, 1999, Churchill Livingstone.

Helgeson VS: Masculinity, men's roles and coronary heart disease. In Sabo D, Gordon DF, editors: *Men's health and illness: gender, power and the body,* Thousand Oaks, Calif, 1995, Sage, pp. 68-104.

Kochanek MA, Hudson BL: Advance report of final mortality statistics, 1992, *Mon Vital Stat Rep* 43(6 suppl):152, 1995.

Legato M: *Gender-specific aspects of human biology for the practicing physician,* Armonk, NY, 1997, Futura.

Levinson D: *The seasons of a man's life,* New York, 1978, Alfred A. Knopf.

Matthews KA et al: Influence of age, sex, and family on type A and hostile attitudes and behaviors, *Health Psychol* 11:317, 1992.

McDiarmid MA et al: Reproductive hazards of fire fighting: II. Chemical hazards, *Am J Ind Med* 19:447, 1991.

Milio N: *Primary care and the public's health,* Lexington, Mass, 1983, Lexington Books.

Montiero L: *Monitoring health status and medical care,* Cambridge, Mass, 1976, Ballinger.

National Center for Health Statistics: 2004a, The Author, http://www.cdc.gov/nchs/fastats/mens_health.htm

National Center for Health Statistics: *Health, United States, 2004,* Hyattsville, Md, 2004b, US Public Health Service.

National Health Interview Survey: 2002a, The Author, http://www.cdc.gov/nchs/nhis.htm.

National Health Interview Survey, 2002b, The Author, http://www.cdc.gov/nchs/data/series/sr_10_222.pdf.

National Institute for Occupational Safety and Health: *NIOSH workers health chartbook* NIOSH publ 2004-146, 2004, The Author, //www.cdc.gov/niosh/doc./chartbook.

Preusser Research Group: 2003, The Author, http://www.pickupsafetybelt.com/index.php.

Roberts A, Gerber L: *Nursing perspective on public health programming in Nunavat,* Iqaluit, Nunavat, Dec 2003, Department of Health and Social Services, http://www.gov.nu.ca/hsssite/Report%20on%20Nursing%20Perspectives%20on%20Public%20Heatlh%20Programming%20in%20Nunavut.pdf.

Skelton R: Man's role in society and its effect on health, *Nursing* 26:953, 1988.

Sadler C: DIY male maintenance, *Nurs Mirror* 160:16, 1979.

Simon HB: Men's health: a conversation with an expert, *Harv Health Lett* 28(3):6, Jan 2003.

Tanne JH: Medicine's new motto: One sex does not fit all. A*me Health Women* 16(5):54-58, 1997.

Verbrugge LM, Wingard DL: Sex differentials in health and mortality, *Women Health* 12:103, 1987.

Waldron I: Changing gender roles and gender differences in health behavior. In Gochman DS, editor: *Handbook of health behavior research,* New York, 1995a, Plenum.

Waldron I: Contributions of changing gender differences in behavior and social roles to changing gender differences in mortality. In Sabo D, Gordon DF, *Men's health and illness: gender, power and the body,* London, Sage Publication, 1995b.

Waldron I: Contributions of biological and behavioral factors in changing sex differences in ischaemic heart disease mortality. In Lopez A, Caselli G, Valkonen T, editors: *Adult mortality in developed countries: from description to explanation,* New York, 1995c, Oxford University Press.

Waldron I: Contributions of changing gender differences in behavior and social roles to changing gender differences in mortality. In Sabo D, Gordon D, editors: *Men's health and illness: gender, power, and the body,* Thousand Oaks, Calif, 1995d, Sage.

Waldron I: Factors determining the sex ratio at birth. In United Nations, editors: *Sex differentials in infant and child mortality,* New York, 1995e, United Nations.

Waldron I: Sex differences in infant and early child mortality: major causes of death and possible biological causes. In United Nations, editors: *Sex differentials in infant and child mortality,* New York, 1995f, United Nations.

Whorton MD: Environmental and occupational reproductive hazards. In Swanson J, Forrest K, editors: *Men's reproductive health,* New York, 1984, Springer.

Woodland A, Hunt C: Healthy convictions . . . well-man clinic for the inmates of Lindholme prison, *Nurs Times* 90:32, 1994.

Zaharias G, Piterman L, Liddell M: Doctors and patients: gender interaction in the consultation, *Acad Med* 79(2):148-155, 2004.

Senior Health

Mary Ellen Trail Ross ▪ Edith Summerlin

MEDIA RESOURCES

Additional Material for Study, Review, and Further Exploration

evolve Website at http://evolve.elsevier.com/Nies

❖ Quiz ❖ Case Studies ❖ Content Updates ❖ Glossary ❖ WebLinks

OBJECTIVES

Upon completion of this chapter, the reader will be able to do the following:

1. Discuss the aging process.
2. Discuss the demographic characteristics of elders.
3. Describe psychosocial issues related to aging.
4. Describe physiological changes due to aging.
5. Recognize *Healthy People 2010* wellness goals and objectives for older adults.
6. Describe health/illness concerns common to the elderly.
7. Identify nursing actions that address the needs of elders.
8. Identify resources available to seniors.

KEY TERMS

advance directives
aging
alternative housing options
Alzheimer's disease

anxiety disorders
crime
depression
elder abuse

falls
glaucoma
guardianship
macular degeneration

Medicaid
Medicare
Social Security
suicide

CHAPTER OUTLINE

CONCEPT OF AGING

THEORIES OF AGING

DEMOGRAPHIC CHARACTERISTICS
    Population
    Racial and Ethnic Composition
    Geographic Location
    Gender
    Marital Status
    Education
    Living Arrangements
    Sources of Income
    Poverty and Health Education

PSYCHOSOCIAL ISSUES

PHYSIOLOGICAL CHANGES

WELLNESS AND HEALTH PROMOTION
    Healthy People 2010
    Recommended Health Care Screenings
     and Examinations
    Physical Activity and Fitness
    Nutrition

COMMON HEALTH CONCERNS
    Chronic Illness
    Medication Use by Elders

ADDITIONAL HEALTH CONCERNS
    Vision Impairment
    Hearing Loss
    Dental Concerns
    Incontinence

ELDER SAFETY AND SECURITY NEEDS
    Falls
    Driver Safety
    Residential Fire-Related Injuries
    Cold and Heat Stress
    Elder Abuse
    Crime

PSYCHOSOCIAL DISORDERS
    Anxiety Disorders
    Depression
    Substance Abuse
    Suicide
    Alzheimer's Disease

END-OF-LIFE ISSUES
    Advance Directives
    The Nurse's Role and End-of-Life Issues

In America, individuals age 65 or older are an important and growing segment of the population. Life expectancy is increasing, thus, larger numbers of people are reaching 65 years of age and older. In view of the increasing number of seniors who potentially will remain living in the community, the role of the community health nurse becomes very important in helping these seniors to continue to live independently and to increase their years of healthy life. For community health nurses to assist older adults, they must be familiar with the characteristics of seniors, their socioeconomic situations, their health behaviors, health status, health risks, and available community resources. This chapter discusses these issues and gives suggestions as to how community health nurses might address them.

CONCEPT OF AGING

Aging is a natural process that affects all living organisms. The concept of aging is most often defined chronologically. Chronologic age refers to the number of years a person has lived. In the United States, an older adult is generally defined as one who is 65 years of age or older. However, it is important to remember that older adults cannot be grouped collectively as just one segment of the population. The older adult population is a heterogeneous group. The young-old (ages 65 to 74), the middle-old (ages 75 to 84), the old-old (ages 85 to 99), and the elite-old (more than 100 years old) are four distinct cohort groups (Lueckenotte, 2000).

Functional age, on the other hand, refers to functioning and the ability to perform activities of daily living (ADLs), such as bathing and grooming, and instrumental activities of daily living (IADLs), such as cooking and shopping. This definition of aging is a better measure of age than chronologic age. After all, most older adults are more concerned with their functional ability than their chronologic age. Assisting older adults to remain independent and functional is a major focus of nursing care.

THEORIES OF AGING

Since early times, scientists have attempted to explain why humans age. There are many biologic and psychosocial theories on aging. Biologic theories of aging answer questions such as How do cells age? and What triggers the actual aging process? (Miller, 2004). The biologic theories can be subdivided into two main divisions: stochastic and nonstochastic. Stochastic theories explain aging as events that occur randomly and accumulate over time, whereas nonstochastic theories view aging as predetermined. Some of the popular biologic theories are included in Box 17-1.

The three classic psychosocial theories of aging are behavioristic and examine how humans experience late life. The disengagement theory, proposed by Cumming and Henry (1961), states that aging is an inevitable, mutual withdrawal or disengagement, resulting in decreased interaction between the aging person and others. The activity theory posits that activity is necessary to maintain life satisfaction and a positive self-

---

BOX 17-1   Biologic Theories of Aging

Stochastic Theories

Error Theory

The error theory proposes that an accumulation of errors in protein synthesis occurs over time, resulting in impaired cellular function. Defective cells are produced, which eventually interfere with biologic function (Orgel, 1963).

Somatic Mutation Theory

This theory is similar to the error theory but also suggests that when cells are exposed to x-ray radiation or chemicals, alteration of DNA occurs, increasing the incidence of chromosomal abnormalities and decreasing cellular and organ function. The deleterious effects appear in later life (Morley, 1995).

Free Radial Theory

Free radicals are highly reactive molecules that possess an extra electric charge (free electron) that can damage protein membranes, enzymes, and DNA. The body produces antioxidants that scavenge the free radicals (Hayflick, 1996).

Cross Link Theory

This theory posits that aging causes body chemicals (proteins, lipids, nucleic acid, and carbohydrates) to become cross-linked. This causes abnormal metabolic activity and waste products to accumulate in the cells. The result is poor functioning of body tissues and structures (Hayflick, 1996).

Wear and Tear Theory

This theory describes a human as similar to a machine in that the human body eventually wears out due to decline in cellular function, death of cells, and mechanical injury and use (Hayflick, 1996).

Nonstochastic Theories

Programmed Theory

This theory postulates that normal cells divide a specific number of times. The number of cell divisions is proportional to the life span of the species. Human cells double 40 to 60 times before the ability to replicate is lost and cellular death occurs (Hayflick, 1996).

Immunologic Theory

There is alteration of the B and T cells, which causes a loss of a self-regulatory pattern between the body and the cell. Autoaggression occurs when cells normal to the body are misidentified as alien and are attacked by the body's immune system (Miller, 1996).

---

concept (Lemon, Bengston, and Peterson, 1972; Maddox, 1963). The continuity theory suggests that a person continues through life in a similar fashion as in previous years (Havighurst, Neugarten, and Tobin, 1968).

Concepts gleaned from the various theories are useful to nurses as they care for older adults. For example, knowledge that the immune system is affected by aging implies the need for nurses to be vigilant about preventing infections (Miller, 2004). Psychosocial theories of aging point out the uniqueness of older individuals as they age and make life adjustments. Knowledge of these theories may help nurses to dispel common myths of aging.

DEMOGRAPHIC CHARACTERISTICS

Population

Americans are living longer than ever before, and it is expected that the older population will continue to grow. Presently, people who survive to age 65 can expect to live an average of nearly 18 more years. The life expectancy of people who survive to age 85 today is about 7 more years for women and 6 more years for men. Life expectancy varies by race, but the difference decreases with age. In 1900, people age 65 and older made up 4% of the population. In 2003, nearly 36 million people age 65 and over lived in the United States, accounting for just over 12% of the total population. The oldest-old population (those 85 years and older) grew from just over 100,000 in 1900 to 4.2 million in 2000 (Federal Interagency Forum on Aging-Related Statistics, 2004). There are about 40,000 centenarians in the United States (Boston University, 2002).

The baby boomers (individuals born between 1946 and 1964) will start turning 65 in 2011, and the number of older adults will increase dramatically. By 2030, the number of Americans age 65 years and older is expected to be twice as large as their counterparts in 2000, growing from 35 million to 71.5 million, and will represent nearly 20% of the total U.S. population. The greatest growth will occur in the population age 85 and older, whose numbers are projected to grow from 4.2 million in 2000 to nearly 21 million by 2050 (Horiuchi, 2000; Oeppen and Vaupel 2002; Tuljapurkar, Nan, and Boe, 2000).

Racial and Ethnic Composition

In addition to growing larger, the older population is becoming more diverse, as is the rest of the population. In 2003, non-Hispanic whites accounted for nearly 83% of the U.S. older population. Blacks made up just over 8%, Asians made up nearly 3%, and Hispanics (of any race) accounted for nearly 6% of the older population. The older population will grow among all racial and ethnic groups; however, the older Hispanic population is projected to grow the fastest.

Geographic Location

The proportion of the population age 65 and over varies by state. In 2002, Florida had the highest proportion (17%) of people age 65 and over. Pennsylvania and West Virginia also had high proportions, each slightly over 15% (Federal Interagency Forum on Aging-Related Statistics, 2004). The nine states with the largest number of elderly individuals (1 million or more) are California, Florida, New York, Texas, Pennsylvania, Ohio, Illinois, Michigan, and New Jersey (Administration on Aging, 2001).

Gender

Older women outnumber older men in the United States. In 2003, women accounted for 58% of the population age 65 and over and 69% of the population age 85 and over (Federal Interagency Forum on Aging-Related Statistics, 2004). The ratio between the two sexes narrows with increasing age.

Marital Status

Older men are more likely than older women to be married. In 2003, over three quarters (78%) of men ages 65 to 74 were married, compared with over half (56%) of women in the same age-group. The proportion married is lower at older ages: 36% of women ages 75 to 84 and 14% of women age 85 and over were married. Widowhood is more common among older women than older men. Women age 65 and over were three times as likely as men of the same age to be widowed: 44% compared with 14%. In 2003, 78% of women age 85 and over were widowed, compared with 35% of men. Relatively small proportions of older men (7%) and women (9%) were divorced in 2003. A small proportion of the older population had never married (Federal Interagency Forum on Aging-Related Statistics, 2004).

Education

Educational attainment has increased among older adults. In 2003, 72% of older adults were high school graduates (compared to 17% in 1950). Older blacks and Hispanics age 65 and older completed high school at lower rates than their white and Asian counterparts (52% and 36%, compared to 76% and 70%). In 2003, 17% of older adults had a bachelor's degree or higher (compared to 3% in 1950). Older Asians had the highest proportion with a bachelor's degree or higher (29%), compared to 20% for non-Hispanic whites, 10% for blacks, and 6% for Hispanics. Older men attained a bachelor's degree more often than older women (23%, compared with 13%); however, the gender gap in completion of a college education is narrowing (Federal Interagency Forum on Aging-Related Statistics, 2004).

Living Arrangements

As age increases and widowhood rates rise, the percentage of the population living alone increases accordingly. In 2003, 73% of older men lived with their spouse, whereas only half (50%) of older women did. In contrast, older women were twice as likely as older men to live alone (40% and 19%, respectively). Older Asian women were far more likely than women of other races to live with relatives other than a spouse. Older white and black women were more likely than others to live alone (approximately 40% each, compared with about 20% for Asian and Hispanic women). Older Asian men were more likely (31%) than men of other races and ethnicities to live with relatives other than a spouse (Federal Interagency Forum on Aging-Related Statistics, 2004).

Housing and Residential Services

Older adults typically prefer to "age in place" or live in their own home for as long as possible. In 2002, 93% of Medicare enrollees age 65 and over resided in traditional community settings. Two percent of the Medicare population age 65 and over resided in community housing with at least one service available, such as meal preparation, housekeeping, laundry, and assistance with medication. Approximately 5% resided in long-term care facilities. The percentage of people residing in community housing with services and in long-term care facilities was higher for the older age-groups. For example, among older adults age 85 and older, 74% resided in traditional housing, whereas, 7% resided in community housing with services, and 19% resided in long-term care facilities (Federal Interagency Forum on Aging-Related Statistics, 2004).

Alternative Housing Options for Seniors

The significant majority (93%) of older adults age 65 and older reside in the traditional, single-family home; however, some choose to downsize to smaller housing, such as townhouses or condominiums, where maintenance needs are eliminated or minimized. In 2002, only 2% of elders age 65 and over resided in community housing with at least one service available. The types of **alternative housing options** included retirement communities or apartments, continuing care retirement facilities, assisted living facilities, and board and care facilities/homes. Services at these facilities include meal preparation, housekeeping, laundry, and medication administration. Approximately 5% of older adults reside in long-term care facilities that provide 24-hour personal and/or skilled care, seven days a week. The percentage of people residing in community housing with services and in long-term care facilities is higher for individuals age 85 and older. These older adults generally have more functional limitations (Federal Interagency Forum on Aging-Related Statistics, 2004). It is important to note that many older adults who would like to change current living arrangements find that organized senior housing is too expensive for middle-class and lower-middle-class citizens. On the other hand, these individuals often have too many assets to qualify for subsidized housing.

Although not considered a housing option, adult day care provides a safe and supportive environment during the day for adults who cannot or choose not to stay alone. This service is often needed for caregivers who work during regular hours or need respite. Socialization, recreational activities, medication supervision, and meals are provided on-site. Often transportation to and from the facility is provided.

Sources of Income

In 2002, the median household income of older adults was $23,152. Aggregate income for the population age 65 and over came largely from four sources: **Social Security** provided 39%, earnings accounted for 25%, pensions provided 19%, and asset income accounted for 14%. Among older Americans in the lowest fifth of the income distribution, Social Security accounts for 83% of aggregate income, and public assistance accounts for another 9%. For those whose income is in the highest income category, Social Security, pensions, and asset income each account for about one fifth of aggregate income, and earnings account for the remaining two fifths (Federal Interagency Forum on Aging-Related Statistics, 2004).

With aging, a good percentage of income is spent on health care. Most older adults have **Medicare,** which provides health insurance for those who are 65 years of age or older, disabled, or have end-stage renal disease. Medicare is funded, in part, by Social Security contributions from employers, employees, and

the self-employed. Medicare Part A is a hospital insurance plan that covers acute care, short-term rehabilitative care, and some costs associated with hospice and home health care. For 2005, the copayment for acute care is $912 for the first 60 days of a hospital stay per benefit period. This amount increases for longer hospital stays. Rehabilitative care generally provided in skilled nursing facilities is only covered if it occurs after a 3-day hospital stay and requires "skilled care" provided by a licensed nurse or by a physical or occupational therapist. Medicare Part A will pay 100% of the first 20 days of a nursing home stay, with a daily co-pay for days 21 to 100 and no coverage after that (U.S. Department of Health and Human Services [USDHHS]/Centers for Medicare and Medicaid Services [CMS], 2006).

Medicare Part B covers the costs for physician and nurse practitioner services; outpatient services, such as diagnostic procedures (e.g., laboratory and x-ray); qualified physical, speech, and occupational therapy; ambulance services; durable medical equipment; and some home health care services. Charges are paid by Medicare at a rate of 80% of what Medicare considers an "allowable charge." The client is responsible for the remaining 20% of the charge. In addition, the client is responsible for an annual Part B deductible of $110.00 and a monthly premium of $78.20 (2005). This amount is generally deducted directly from the monthly Social Security check. Most individuals purchase Medigap policies, which cover the deductibles and co-pays. Another option is to join a Medicare Advantage Plan, which often provides more choices and benefits such as extra days in the hospital. To join a Medicare Advantage Plan, an older adult must have Medicare Part A and Part B. In addition to the Part B premium, there may be an additional monthly premium for the extra benefits provided (USDHHS/CMS, 2006).

The newest component of Medicare is the new prescription drug coverage that was implemented in January 2006. The prescription drug plan will help lower prescription drug costs. The individual chooses the drug plan and pays a monthly premium (about $37/month) and an annual deductible ($250 in 2006—this may increase in subsequent years). After the plan participant meets the deductible, he or she is responsible for 25% co-pay up to $2250. The individual is responsible for 100% of the next $2850, or a total out-of-pocket cost of $3600. At that point, the plan will pay 95% of prescription drug costs (USDHHS/CMS, 2006).

For older adults with low incomes, **Medicaid** may be available to offset the Medicare deductibles and co-pays and to provide additional health benefits. Each state establishes its own eligibility criteria within the broad guidelines established by the federal government. Medicaid generally covers more services than Medicare, including custodial care in nursing homes, without deductibles or co-pays.

Poverty and Health Education

To determine who is considered poor, the U.S. Census Bureau compares family income (or an unrelated individual's income) with a set of poverty thresholds that vary by family size and composition and are updated annually for inflation. By 2002, the proportion of the older population living in poverty had decreased dramatically to 10%. Older women (12%) were more likely than older men (8%) to live in poverty in 2002. Older people who live alone have higher rates of poverty than those who are married. Race and ethnicity are also related to poverty among the older population. In 2002, older whites were far less likely than older blacks and Hispanics to be living in poverty (about 8% compared with 24% and 21%, respectively) (Federal Interagency Forum on Aging-Related Statistics, 2004).

Community nurses will be increasingly called upon to care for older adults of diverse backgrounds who reside in various living arrangements. Although educational attainment has increased among the elderly population, many older adults have less than a high school education; therefore nurses must be sensitive and creative when providing instruction and teaching. Nurses cannot assume that an older adult has had a formal education. In addition, instructions may need to be given at a slower pace. It may also be imperative to include family or significant others when providing instruction. Also, written information may be sent home for further reference.

On the other hand, increased educational levels of current and future elders also provide a challenge for the community health nurse. These elders are, and will be, more informed and will make greater demands for current and scientifically based information, thus requiring the community health nurse to be knowledgeable about the latest developments in health care. Lastly, nurses must be aware of community programs and services that address the needs of a diverse older population. Many of these resources are discussed in this chapter.

PSYCHOSOCIAL ISSUES

In addition to adjusting to physiological changes related to aging and health concerns (discussed later in this chapter), older adults must cope with psychosocial and role changes such as retirement, relocation, widowhood, loss of family and friends, and possibly raising their grandchildren. Retirement may be a happy occasion when voluntary; however, the opposite may be true if it is involuntary. When older adults retire, they inevitably must cope with a change in social status and possibly income level; this may be especially difficult for people whose self-concept is related to job status. For retirees who are married, the spouse must also adjust to the changes related to retirement. Indeed, the adjustment may be more difficult for the spouse than the retiree as the retiree's leisure time will be increased. For elders who have no hobbies or interests, this extra leisure time may be a source of boredom. Nurses should encourage older retirees to pursue old hobbies and interests or establish new ones.

Relocation is another psychosocial issue that many older adults must manage. Often, relocation occurs as a result of health and functional impairment, lack of ability to maintain one's home, unsafe neighborhoods, and lack of assistance with ADLs or IADLs. The relocation may be prompted by the older adult's desire to be closer to family or medical care, or interest in moving to a new location or more supportive

---

RESEARCH HIGHLIGHTS

Recognizing the Needs of the Elderly

Tsai (2005) recently examined factors that predicted distress and depression among elders with arthritis. Performing secondary analysis of data from 234 people aged 65 and older (mean age 74.1 years), she determined that elders with higher levels of disability, more financial hardship, less social support, and younger age were more likely to have higher levels of distress than those who did not share these characteristics. Furthermore, distress, along with pain and disability, significantly predicted depression. She concluded that nurses should recognize the needs of elders with arthritis, considering a number of both physical (e.g., pain, level of disability) and psychosocial (e.g., social support, financial hardship) factors that might lead to depression, and intervene where appropriate and feasible.

From Tsai P: Predictors of distress and depression in elders with arthritic pain, *J Adv Nurs* 51(2):158-165, 2005.

housing (as discussed in the section Alternative Housing Options for Seniors).

Widowhood is an event experienced by most older adults, especially elderly women. According to Miller (2004), common consequences of widowhood are loss of one's sexual partner, loss of companionship and intimacy, feelings of grief, loneliness and emptiness, increased responsibilities and dependency on others, loss of income and less efficient financial management, and changes in relationships with children, married friends, and other family members. Widowhood may be especially traumatic for elders who have been married for many decades. In addition to the loss of a spouse, older adults must also cope with loss of family (sometimes their own children) and friends.

On the other hand, many older adults are faced with the responsibility of raising their grandchildren. Substantial increases have occurred in the number of children under age 18 living in households maintained by grandparents, often without the presence of the grandchildren's parents. Antecedents to children being raised by grandparents include neglect related to parental substance abuse, abandonment, emotional and physical abuse, parental death, mental and physical illness, incarceration, teen pregnancy, and grandparent's assisting adult children who work or attend school. Ross and Aday (2006) investigated the degree of stress in 50 African-American grandparents and found that 94% of the grandparents reported a "clinically significant" level of stress. Use of professional counseling, special school programs, and length of caregiving greater than 5 years were associated with less stress. Coping strategies that were significantly correlated with less stress included accepting responsibility, confrontive coping, self-control, positive reappraisal, planful problem solving, and distancing.

The role of the community health nurse is to identify, support, and assist older adults experiencing various psychosocial changes and role adjustments. In addition, the nurse should provide information about various community resources and make referrals to agencies that might be helpful.

HEALTHY PEOPLE 2010	Selected Objectives for Older Adults		
Objective		**Baseline (1994-2002)**	**Target**
1-15: Increase the proportion of persons with long-term care needs who have access to the continuum of long-term care services.		—	—
2-9: Reduce the proportion of adults with osteoporosis.		10%	8%
3-12a: Increase the proportion of adults 65 years of age and older who have received a fecal occult blood test within the preceding 2 years.		33%	50%
7-12: Increase the proportion of older adults who have participated during the preceding year in at least one organized health promotion activity.		12%	90%
12-6b: Reduce hospitalizations of adults between 75 and 84 years of age with heart failure as the principal diagnosis.		27.1 per 1000	13.5 per 1000
14-5b: Reduce invasive pneumococcal infections in adults 65 years of age and older.		51 per 100,000	42 per 100,000
14-29a: Increase the proportion of adults aged 65 years and older who are vaccinated annually against influenza.		66%	90%
15-27: Reduce deaths from falls. 65-84 years old (not age adjusted)		22.1	—
85 years and older (not age adjusted)		130.4 per 100,000	—
15-28a: Reduce hip fractures among females 65 years of age and older.		1029.2 per 100,000	416 per 100,000
17-3: Increase the proportion of primary care providers, pharmacists, and other health care professionals who routinely review with their patients aged 65 years and older and patients with chronic illnesses or disabilities all new prescribed and over-the-counter medicines.		—	—
21-4: Reduce the proportion of older adults aged 65-74 years who have experienced complete tooth loss.		24%	20%
24-2c: Reduce hospitalizations for asthma among adults aged 65 years and older.		11.8 per 10,000	7.7 per 10,000
28-15: Increase the number of persons who are referred by their primary care physician for hearing evaluation and treatment.		—	—

From US Department of Health and Human Services: *Healthy People 2010: national health promotion and disease prevention objectives,* Washington, DC, 2000, US Government Printing Office, http://www.health.gov/healthypeople.
—, Data not available.

PHYSIOLOGICAL CHANGES

Normal physiological aging changes occur in all body systems. However, it is important to note that the rate and degree of these changes are highly individualized. These changes are influenced by genetic factors, diet, exercise, the environment, health status, stress, lifestyle choices, and many other elements. Table 17-1 depicts common physiological changes that occur with aging.

WELLNESS AND HEALTH PROMOTION

Health promotion and illness prevention interventions for older adults may be beneficial in reducing death and disability and improving quality of life. These are goals of *Healthy People 2010.* To address these goals, health care professionals must inform and educate elders about the benefits of health care screenings and examinations, physical activity and fitness, and good nutrition.

Healthy People 2010

A primary goal of *Healthy People 2010* is to increase the quality and years of healthy life. Although people are living longer, many older adults have chronic illnesses that interfere with the quality of their lives. To address this issue, *Healthy People 2010* includes specific objectives related to increasing health promotion programs and decreasing morbidity and mortality in older adults.

Recommended Health Care Screenings and Examinations

Many organizations such as the American Cancer Society, the American Heart Association, and the USDHHS Preventive Services Task Force have established recommendations for health promotion screenings and examinations. Box 17-2 depicts some of the more widely agreed-on screenings and exams for older adults. These established recommendations might be very useful to community nurses when educating older adults about the benefits of screening and early detection of disease. Frequently, earlier detection of disease allows better treatment, lower health care costs, and the possibility of cure.

Physical Activity and Fitness

Physical activity is beneficial for the health of people of all ages, including older adults. Although there are various types of exercises, walking is one of the best forms of exercise and

TABLE 17-1   Normal Physiological Changes Associated With Aging

PHYSIOLOGICAL CHANGES	NURSING INTERVENTIONS
Sensory Changes	
Vision	
Decreased visual acuity	Use large print for teaching
Decreased visual accommodation	Encourage adequate lighting (e.g., nightlights)
Increased opacities	Encourage use of corrective lenses as prescribed
Increased sensitivity to glare	Decrease glare
Decreased ability to discriminate within blue-green color range caused by yellowing of the lens	Advise to use caution with blue-green color range (e.g., when taking medications and selecting clothing)
	Advise use of contrasting colors, reds, and yellows
Hearing	
Decreased ability to hear—presbycusis	Decrease extraneous sounds
Decreased ability to hear consonants with high-frequency sounds	Use concise sentences and speak slowly and distinctly in low-pitched voice
	Face person when talking; use gestures
	Encourage hearing examination (see Hearing Loss section)
	Encourage use of hearing aid if needed
Taste	
Diminished taste sensation	Encourage well-balanced meals
Decreased saliva production	Advise to drink plenty of fluids
Increased sensitivity to bitterness	Observe for overconsumption of sweets and salts
Decreased sensitivity to sweetness and salt	Give options for seasoning other than salt
	Teach about good oral hygiene
Smell	
Decreased smell acuity	Advise to use other senses and other people to assist with monitoring the environment for safety (e.g., spoiled food and gas fumes)
Touch	
Decreased sensitivity to touch	Provide a safe environment
	Monitor for extreme temperature changes in the environment (e.g., water temperature)
	Maintain adequate room temperature
	Ensure adequate clothing is worn for body warmth
Nervous System	
Decreased brain weight	Assess neurological status
Slower autonomic and voluntary reflexes	Assess for pain
Increased pain threshold	
Increased amount of senile plaque and neurofibrillary tangles	
Reduction in functioning neurons	
Cognitive Changes	
Slower reaction time	Teach fall precautions (see Falls section)
Slower learning time	Break instructions into small units
Memory: long-term memory better than short-term memory	Use shorter teaching sessions
Intelligence: little change	Use cues and gestures
Personality consistent with earlier years	Relate education to prior experience
	Allow adequate time for completing tasks
Sleep	
Decrease in Stages 3 and 4 sleep pattern	Avoid interruptions at night
Increase in arousals during the night	Allow naps as needed
Total sleep time is slightly reduced	
	Avoid sleep medication use if possible
	Provide quiet environment for sleep
	Avoid stimulants and caffeine
	Assess quantity and quality of sleep
Cardiovascular System	
Decrease in tone and elasticity of aorta and great vessels	Pace activities
Thicker and stiffer heart valves	Allow rest periods
Slowing down of heart's conduction system	Encourage use of ambulation aids when appropriate
Myocardium slower to recover its contractility and irritability	Monitor for activity intolerance
Decreased cardiac reserve	Prevent or eliminate stressors
Decreased cardiac output	Monitor heart rate and blood pressure
Decreased ability to increase heart rate when stress occurs	Encourage regular exercise program
Increased peripheral resistance and pulse pressure	
Increased systolic blood pressure	

Continued

TABLE 17-1 Normal Physiological Changes Associated With Aging (cont'd)

PHYSIOLOGICAL CHANGES	NURSING INTERVENTIONS
Respiratory System Reduced size of lungs, lung expansion, activity, and recoil Increased rigidity of lungs and thoracic cage Decreased cough response Decreased vital capacity Decreased number of alveoli and gas exchange Increased anterior:posterior chest diameter	Encourage influenza and pneumovax vaccinations (see recommended scheduling, Box 17-2) Encourage regular exercise Auscultate lung sounds Encourage adequate fluid intake Monitor oxygen administration
Musculoskeletal System Atrophy and decrease in muscle fibers Decreased muscle mass and strength Reduced bone minerals and mass, causing porous and brittle bones Shortening vertebra, causing shrinkage in height Kyphosis more common	Prevent immobility Encourage regular exercise program Teach safety precautions to prevent falls (see Falls section) Encourage adequate calcium intake
Gastrointestinal System Teeth become more brittle Decreased esophageal peristalsis and emptying Decreased stomach motility Decreased production of saliva, HCl, and digestive enzymes Decreased absorption of fat and vitamins B_1 and B_{12} Decrease in thirst response	Encourage good dental health (see Dental Concerns section) Encourage diet that is well balanced and has adequate protein and vitamins Encourage adequate fluids Encourage fiber in the diet Advise to eat slowly and assess for indigestion Monitor diet for deficiencies Encourage toileting schedule and monitor frequency of bowel movements
Renal Decreased weight of kidneys Decrease in number of nephrons Reduced renal blood flow and tubular function Decrease in glomerular filtration rate Decreased ability to concentrate urine	Monitor drugs—smaller doses may be needed Monitor electrolytes Prevent dehydration
Genitourinary System Weakening of bladder muscle, causing increased urinary frequency, urgency, and nocturia Decreased bladder capacity Increased retention Increased nocturia	Assess bladder function and assist with frequent toileting Encourage bladder training program, exercises, and medication when needed Observe for signs of urinary tract infection
Women Atrophy of vulva and flattening of labia Vaginal drying Atrophy of cervix and ovaries Shrinkage of uterus Ovulation ceases Decreased amount and elasticity of breast tissue	Differentiate between changes due to normal aging, disease, and medications Advise about use of lubricants for comfort during intercourse Provide education in normal reproductive changes Recommend breast examinations and mammograms
Men Decreased elasticity of scrotal skin Decrease in size and firmness of testes Takes 2-3 times longer to achieve an erection, but able to maintain a long erection without ejaculation Venous and arterial sclerosis of the corpus spongiosum Prostatic enlargement	Differentiate between changes due to normal aging, disease, and medications Recommend prostate examination
Endocrine System Increased fibrosis and nodularity of thyroid gland Shrinkage of thymus and pituitary glands Decline in natural antibodies Decrease in adrenal gland secretion of glucocorticoid Decreased levels of aldosterone Delayed insulin release Reduced peripheral sensitivity to insulin Reduced ability to metabolize glucose Decrease in testosterone, estrogen, and progesterone	Recommend pneumococcal, influenza, and tetanus vaccinations (see recommended scheduling, Box 17-2) Monitor electrolytes and glucose Prevent infection Observe for hypoglycemia or hyperglycemia
Integumentary System Decreased skin elasticity Generalized thinning Loss of subcutaneous fat Atrophy of sweat glands	Encourage frequent position changes and inspect skin Be careful of skin tears, bruising, and pressure ulcers Recognize need for less frequent bathing; avoid harsh soaps; use lotion Advise to eat a good diet, exercise, and limit exposure to harmful radiation

Continued

TABLE 17-1 Normal Physiological Changes Associated With Aging (cont'd)

PHYSIOLOGICAL CHANGES	NURSING INTERVENTIONS
Atrophy of sweat glands Variation in pigmentation (age spots) Hair thins and grays on head and becomes thicker in nose, ears, and eyebrows (men) Increased facial hair on women Fingernails are fragile and brittle and grow more slowly	Advise to eat a good diet, exercise, and limit exposure to harmful radiation

From Eliopoulos C: *Gerontological nursing,* ed 6, Philadelphia, 2005, Lippincott Williams & Wilkins.

BOX 17-2 Recommended Examinations for Health Promotion and Disease Prevention in Older Adults

Examinations/Tests for All Older Adults

Complete physical: Annually
Blood pressure: Annually, more frequently if hypertensive or at risk
Serum cholesterol: Every 5 years; more frequently if high risk
Fecal occult blood test: Annually
Sigmoidoscopy: Every 3-5 years after age 50
Visual acuity and glaucoma screening: Annually
Dental examination: Annually for those with teeth; cleaning every 6 months, every 2 years for denture wearers
Hearing test: Every 2 to 5 years

Women

Breast self-examination: Monthly
Clinical breast examination: Annually
Pelvic examination and Pap smear: Not needed if age 65 or older and not otherwise at risk
Digital rectal examination: Annually with pelvic examination
Mammogram: Every 1-2 years if age 40 or older

Men

Digital rectal examination and prostate examination: Annually
Prostate specific antigen (PSA) blood test: Annually

Immunizations for All Older Adults

Tetanus-diphtheria: Every 10 years
Influenza/flu vaccine: Annually
Pneumonia vaccine: Once after age 65 years; ask physician about booster
Hepatitis B and C: For those at risk

From US Preventive Services Task Force, 1996, 2002; Zoorob et al., 2001.

it's free. Many older adults engage in walking, swimming, dancing, yoga, and tai chi for exercise. Regular exercise preserves muscle strength, enhances bone density, improves balance, neuromuscular coordination, joint function and endurance, reduces blood pressure, improves mood, relieves depression, and help prevent falls (Beers and Berkow, 2000). Yet, more than two thirds of older adults in the United States do not get enough physical activity (National Institute on Aging, 2002c). In 2001 to 2002, men age 65 and over were more likely than women in the same age-group to report engaging in regular leisure time physical activity (26% vs.

18%) (Federal Interagency Forum on Aging-Related Statistics, 2004).

Barriers to exercising that have been identified in older adults include impaired health, fear of injury, unpleasant sensations associated with exercise, lack of access to appropriate facilities, and lack of knowledge about the benefits of exercise (Resnick, 2002). Other concerns are safety of the neighborhood (e.g., fear of criminal activity or dogs running freely) and weather conditions. Health-related barriers identified as interfering with physical activity in older adults include pain, fatigue, and sensory and mobility impairments (Cooper et al., 2001).

Objective 22-2 of *Healthy People 2010* recommends that health care providers work to "increase the proportion of adults who engage regularly, preferably daily, in moderate physical activity for at least 30 minutes per day" (USDHHS, 2000). Nurses may help older adults accomplish this goal by assessing their understanding of the beneficial effects of exercise. Nurses should also educate, encourage, and assist older adults with exercise. When applicable, antiinflammatory medications may be administered before physical activity to address accompanying pain.

Nutrition

In *Healthy People 2010,* nutrition was identified as a priority area of health promotion for people of all ages. Poor nutrition in the elderly population is common. An inappropriate diet is related to constipation, dental disease, physical inactivity, and depression. Normal physiological changes related to aging affect nutritional status. Fewer calories taken in may result in a decreased intake of essential nutrients. A diminished sense of smell may reduce the enjoyment of eating. Gastrointestinal changes can interfere with absorption of vitamin B_{12} and folic acid, leading to anemia. A diminished thirst sensation may lead to dehydration. Other factors that can affect the nutritional status of the elderly are income, functional status, taking multiple medications, social isolation, lack of transportation, and dependence on others for grocery shopping and cooking. The nutrition checklist presented in Table 17-2 lists warning signs and risk factors of poor nutritional health described by the mnemonic DETERMINE.

The new U.S. Department of Agriculture's (USDA's) food pyramid, known as MyPramid, is a personalized approach to healthy eating and physical activity (Figure 17-1). Each person can find the amounts of food they should eat daily by going to

TABLE 17-2   Nutrition Checklist for Older Adults: Warning Signs of Poor Nutritional Health

POSSIBLE PROBLEM	QUESTION TO ANSWER	SCORE FOR "YES" ANSWER (CIRCLE IF "YES")
Disease	Do you have an illness or condition that makes you change the kind and/or amount of food you eat?	2
Eating poorly	Do you eat fewer than two meals per day?	3
	Do you eat few fruits, vegetables, or milk products?	2
	Do you have three or more drinks of beer, liquor or wine almost every day?	2
Tooth loss/mouth pain	Do you have tooth or mouth problems that make it hard for you to eat?	2
Economic hardship	Do you sometimes have trouble affording the food you need?	4
Reduced social contact	Do you eat alone most of the time?	1
Multiple medications	Do you take three or more prescribed or over-the-counter drugs a day?	1
Involuntary weight loss/gain	Have you lost or gained 10 lb in the last 6 months without trying?	2
Needs assistance in self-care	Are you sometimes physically not able to shop, cook, or feed yourself?	1
Elder years >80 yr	Are you over 80 years old?	1
	TOTAL	

Scoring:
- *0-2:* Good!
  Recheck your nutritional score in 6 months.
- *3-5:* You are at moderate nutritional risk.
  See what can be done to improve your eating habits and lifestyle. Your office on aging, senior nutrition program (e.g., Meals on Wheels), senior center, or health department can help. Recheck your nutritional score in 3 months.
- *6 or more:* You are at high nutritional risk.
  Bring this checklist the next time you see your physician/nurse practitioner, dietitian, or other qualified health or social service professional. Talk with them about any problems you may have. Ask for help to improve your nutritional health.

From American Academy of Family Physicians, American Dietetic Association, National Council on Aging: *Nutrition screening initiative*, Washington, DC, 1992, The Authors, http://www.acsu.buffalo.edu/~drstall/nutrition.html.

http://www.MyPyramid.gov. Variety of food is symbolized by the six color bands of the pyramid representing the five food groups (grains, vegetables, fruits, milk, and meat and beans). Physical activity is emphasized by the picture of a person walking up steps. Figure 17-2 depicts a sample food plan for a 70-year-old female who engages in 30 to 60 minutes of physical activity per day. Tips are provided on how to incorporate foods from each food group.

The USDA's key dietary recommendations relate to adequate nutrients within calorie needs, weight management, physical activity, food groups to encourage, fats, carbohydrates, sodium and potassium, alcoholic beverages, and food safety. Available at the MyPyramid.gov website are lists of what foods are found in each of the food groups, oils, moderate and vigorous physical activities, and a discussion about discretionary calories.

Many elderly have chronic diseases such as osteoporosis, chronic lung disease, cardiac disease, and diabetes; nutritional interventions can help these people. Unless indicated by a medical condition, overly restrictive diets in the elderly are not advised. Small, easy steps in following the new guidelines can add up to short- and long-term health benefits. Recipes for success suggested by the http://www. Mealtime.org website are plan ahead for healthful eating, fit more in, choose your "carbs" by the company they keep, make calories count, get the power of Omega-3s, watch the sodium, boost the potassium, refresh with less, keep it clean, chilled and properly cooked, and, finally, move it to be fit. Food choices need to be nutrient-dense for the prevention of deficiencies.

The community health nurse should use a nutrition checklist to evaluate the nutritional status and needs of the elderly. A copy of a personalized food pyramid can be obtained and then used to assess the current eating pattern of the elderly, and from that, recommendations for dietary changes can be made. The physical and mental status of the individual must be taken into account when making recommendations. Also, the social factors influencing nutritional choices need to be considered. The benefits of good nutrition are an important factor in helping to maintain independence and quality of life.

In 2002, the World Health Organization, in collaboration with the Tufts University School of Nutrition and Policy, established recommendations for improving the health and nutritional status of older persons. Their recommendations for nutrients can be found in the pamphlet *Keep Fit for Life: Meeting the Nutritional Needs of Older Persons* (available at http://whqlibdoc.who.int/publications/9241562102.pdf). It is unknown whether these recommendations are in keeping with the new USDA pyramid recommendations, but they serve as a basis for the specific vitamin and mineral levels recommended in 2002.

COMMON HEALTH CONCERNS

Chronic Illness

The prevalence of chronic diseases increases with aging. Most older adults have at least one chronic disease, but more often they have several chronic illnesses. The 10 leading chronic conditions affecting the population age 65 and older

MyPyramid
STEPS TO A HEALTHIER YOU
MyPyramid.gov

GRAINS	VEGETABLES	FRUITS	MILK	MEAT & BEANS
GRAINS Make half your grains whole	**VEGETABLES** Vary your veggies	**FRUITS** Focus on fruits	**MILK** Get your calcium-rich foods	**MEAT & BEANS** Go lean with protein
Eat at least 3 oz. of whole-grain cereals, breads, crackers, rice, or pasta every day 1 oz. is about 1 slice of bread, about 1 cup of breakfast cereal, or ½ cup of cooked rice, cereal, or pasta	Eat more dark-green veggies like broccoli, spinach, and other dark leafy greens Eat more orange vegetables like carrots and sweetpotatoes Eat more dry beans and peas like pinto beans, kidney beans, and lentils	Eat a variety of fruit Choose fresh, frozen, canned, or dried fruit Go easy on fruit juices	Go low-fat or fat-free when you choose milk, yogurt, and other milk products If you don't or can't consume milk, choose lactose-free products or other calcium sources such as fortified foods and beverages	Choose low-fat or lean meats and poultry Bake it, broil it, or grill it Vary your protein routine — choose more fish, beans, peas, nuts, and seeds

For a 2,000-calorie diet, you need the amounts below from each food group. To find the amounts that are right for you, go to MyPyramid.gov.

Eat 6 oz. every day	Eat 2½ cups every day	Eat 2 cups every day	Get 3 cups every day; for kids aged 2 to 8, it's 2	Eat 5½ oz. every day

Find your balance between food and physical activity
- Be sure to stay within your daily calorie needs.
- Be physically active for at least 30 minutes most days of the week.
- About 60 minutes a day of physical activity may be needed to prevent weight gain.
- For sustaining weight loss, at least 60 to 90 minutes a day of physical activity may be required.
- Children and teenagers should be physically active for 60 minutes every day, or most days.

Know the limits on fats, sugars, and salt (sodium)
- Make most of your fat sources from fish, nuts, and vegetable oils.
- Limit solid fats like butter, stick margarine, shortening, and lard, as well as foods that contain these.
- Check the Nutrition Facts label to keep saturated fats, *trans* fats, and sodium low.
- Choose food and beverages low in added sugars. Added sugars contribute calories with few, if any, nutrients.

MyPyramid.gov
STEPS TO A HEALTHIER YOU

U.S. Department of Agriculture
Center for Nutrition Policy and Promotion
April 2005
CNPP-15

USDA

USDA is an equal opportunity provider and employer.

FIGURE 17-1 USDA Food Pyramid. (US Department of Agriculture: *My pyramid,* 2005, The Author, http://www.mypyramid.gov.)

My Pyramid Plan*

▶ Grains¹	6 ounces	tips
▶ Vegetables²	2.5 cups	tips
▶ Fruits	1.5 cups	tips
▶ Milk	3 cups	tips
▶ Meat & Beans	5 ounces	tips

FIGURE 17-2   Sample food plan for 70-year-old woman. (From U.S. Department of Agriculture: MyPyramid, 2005, The Author, http://www.mypyramid.gov.)

TABLE 17-3   Leading Causes of Death for Persons 65 Years of Age and Older

CAUSE OF DEATH	NUMBER OF DEATHS
All causes	1,753,220
Heart disease	605,673
Malignant neoplasms (cancer)	384,186
Cerebrovascular (stroke)	139,144
Chronic obstructive pulmonary disease	97,896
Pneumonia and influenza	82,989
Diabetes	48,974
Accidents	32,975
Alzheimer's disease	22,416
Nephritis, nephritic syndrome, nephrosis	22,640
Septicemia	19,012

US Department of Commerce: *Statistical abstract of the United States*, ed 121, Washington, DC, 2001, US Census Bureau, p. 82.

are: arthritis, hypertension, heart conditions, diabetes, hearing and vision impairment, orthopedic impairments, chronic sinusitis, hay fever/allergic rhinitis (without asthma), and varicose veins (U.S. National Center for Health Statistics, 2003).

Chronic illness may cause limitations with ADLs and IADLs. Chronic illnesses are a major cause of disability and are also the leading causes of death. Table 17-3 displays the 10 leading cause of death for those age 65 and older.

Medication Use by Elders

The high prevalence of chronic diseases in the elderly population causes this group to use a large number of medications. According to the Center for Medicare Education (2002), older adults consume slightly more than one third of all prescription drugs and spend billions annually on medications. Older adults also consume many over-the-counter medications, as well as "folk" or herbal remedies.

The elderly are vulnerable to the effects of drugs because of normal aging changes (see Table 17-1) and age-related differences in pharmacokinetics and pharmacodynamics. Polypharmacy may also make older adults vulnerable to drug interactions and dangerous adverse reactions. During a 12-month period (1999 to 2000), Gurwitz et al. (2003) studied Medicare enrollees (30,397 person-years of observation) cared for by a multispecialty group practice. The researchers found 1,523 identified adverse drug events, of which 27.6% (421)

were considered preventable. Of the adverse drug events, 578 (38%) were categorized as serious, life-threatening, or fatal; 244 (42.2%) of these more severe events were deemed preventable, compared with 177 (18.7%) of the 945 significant adverse drug events. Errors associated with preventable adverse drug events occurred most often at the stages of prescribing and monitoring. Errors involving client adherence also were common. The most common medication categories associated with preventable adverse drug events were cardiovascular medications (24.5%), followed by diuretics (22.1%), nonopioid analgesics (15.4%), hypoglycemics (10.9%), and anticoagulants (10.2%). The most common types of preventable adverse drug events were electrolyte/renal (26.6%), gastrointestinal tract (21.1%), hemorrhagic (15.9%), metabolic/endocrine (13.8%), and neuropsychiatric (8.6%). The researchers concluded that prevention strategies should target the prescribing and monitoring stages of pharmaceutical care and that interventions should focus on improving client adherence to prescribed regimens.

One of the roles of community health nurses is to closely monitor medication use in the home to ensure safety. An easy-to-use pill organizer may be helpful to older adults. In addition, older adults should be educated about potential adverse reactions, as well as drug-drug and drug-food interactions.

ADDITIONAL HEALTH CONCERNS

Vision Impairment

Visual acuity and accommodation normally decrease with age. Presbyopia, loss of elasticity of the lens of the eye causing difficulty with near vision, generally occurs in people in their 40s. Nearly 95% of adults older than 65 years of age wear glasses (Burke and Laramie, 2000), and 18% also use a magnifying glass for reading and close-up work (Desai et al., 2001). Among older adults, the three most common pathologic eye conditions are cataracts, macular degeneration, and glaucoma. In 2002, among people age 65 and older who reported trouble seeing, 44% reported having had cataracts in the past 12 months, 16% reported having macular degeneration, and 16% reported having glaucoma (Federal Interagency Forum on Aging-Related Statistics, 2004).

Cataracts

Cataracts are the leading cause, as well as the most reversible cause, of visual impairment in older adults. A cataract is a clouding of the normally clear lens of the eye. It's like trying to see through a frosted or fogged-up window. Most cataracts develop slowly, are painless, and do not disturb a person's eyesight early on. However, as the clouding progresses, the cataract eventually interferes with vision. Signs and symptoms of a cataract include clouded, blurred or dim vision, increasing difficulty with vision at night, sensitivity to light and glare (e.g., sunlight, lamps, or oncoming headlights), halos around lights, the need for brighter light for reading and other activities, frequent changes in eyeglass or contact lens prescription, fading or yellowing of colors, and double vision in a single eye (Mayo Clinic Staff, 2004a).

Age is the single greatest risk factor for cataracts. By age 65, half of all Americans have developed some degree of lens clouding, although it may not impair vision. Other risk factors that increase a person's risk of cataracts include diabetes, family history of cataracts, previous eye injury or inflammation, previous eye surgery, prolonged use of corticosteroids, excessive exposure to sunlight, and smoking. Older adults should have annual eye examinations with an eye specialist (US Preventive Services Task Force, 2002). This examination will allow early detection and tracking of cataract development. The only effective treatment for a cataract is surgical removal of the clouded lens and replacement with a clear lens implant (Mayo Clinic Staff, 2004a).

Macular Degeneration

Macular degeneration causes severe loss of vision in older adults in the United States and other developed countries. Macular degeneration is a chronic eye disease that occurs when tissue in the macula, the part of the retina responsible for central vision, deteriorates. The retina is the layer of tissue on the inside back wall of the eyeball. Degeneration of the macula causes blurred central vision or a blind spot in the center of the visual field.

The first sign of macular degeneration may be a need for more light when doing close-up work. Fine newsprint may become harder to read and street signs more difficult to recognize. Eventually, one may notice that when looking at a grid, some of the straight lines appear distorted or crooked. Gray or blank spots may mask the center of the visual field. The condition usually develops gradually but sometimes progresses rapidly, leading to severe vision loss in one or both eyes. Other signs and symptoms of macular degeneration include the need for increasingly bright illumination when reading or doing close-up work, increasing difficulty adapting to low levels of illumination (such as when entering a dimly lit restaurant), printed words that appear increasingly blurry, colors that appear less bright, difficulty recognizing faces, gradual increase in the haziness of overall vision, blurred or blind spot in the center of the visual field combined with a profound drop in central vision acuity, a need to scan all around an object to provide a more complete image, visual distortions (such as straight lines appearing wavy or crooked), a doorway or street sign that seems out of alignment, objects appearing smaller or farther away than they should, decrease in or loss of central vision, and a central blurry spot (Mayo Clinic Staff, 2004c).

In the United States, macular degeneration is the leading cause of vision loss in people age 60 and older. Although researchers have not identified the exact causes of macular degeneration, they have identified some contributing factors. In addition to age, the risk factors include family history of macular degeneration, race (more common in whites than in other groups, especially after age 75), gender (women are more likely to develop macular degeneration), obesity (severe overweight increases the severity of the disease), light-colored eyes, long-term exposure to ultraviolet light, low levels of nutrients (including minerals such as zinc and antioxidants such as vitamins A, C, and E), cigarette smoking, and cardiovascular diseases (Mayo Clinic Staff, 2004c).

Annual eye examinations can detect early signs of macular degeneration before the disease leads to vision loss. Any change to central vision or in the ability to see colors and fine detail should be reported to one's eye care specialist. An Amsler grid is a simple test that may be used to detect changes in vision. Treatment options depend on the location and the extent of the abnormal blood vessels. Damage already caused by macular degeneration cannot be reversed (Mayo Clinic Staff, 2004c).

Glaucoma

Glaucoma is sometimes referred to as the silent thief because it can slowly diminish vision before one realizes anything is wrong. The common feature of this disease is damage to the optic nerve, usually accompanied by an abnormally high pressure inside the eyeball. The most common form of glaucoma, primary or chronic open-angle glaucoma, develops gradually without warning and progresses with few or no symptoms until the condition reaches an advanced stage. The drainage angle formed by the cornea and the iris remains open; however, the aqueous humor drains too slowly. This leads to fluid backup and a gradual buildup of pressure within the eye. Increased eye pressure continues to damage the optic nerve, and more and more peripheral vision is lost. If left untreated, tunnel vision develops, followed by total vision loss (Mayo Clinic Staff, 2004b).

Acute or closed-angle glaucoma is less common but develops suddenly. The disease occurs when the drainage angle formed by the cornea and the iris closes or becomes blocked, resulting in a rapid rise in eye pressure. Permanent vision loss can occur within hours of the attack; therefore it requires immediate medical attention. Signs and symptoms of glaucoma include blurred vision, halos around lights, reddening of the eye, severe eye pain, and nausea and vomiting. Increasing age is a significant risk factor. Other risk factors include family history, race (African Americans and other minorities have a higher risk), medical conditions (including diabetes, history of hypertension or heart disease, retinal detachment, eye tumors, and eye inflammations), physical injuries or severe trauma (such as being hit in the eye), nearsightedness, and prolonged corticosteroid use. Regular eye examinations (every 2 to 4 years after age 40 and every 1 to 2 years after age 65) are essential for detecting glaucoma early enough for successful treatment. Glaucoma cannot be cured, and damage caused by the disease cannot be reversed; however, glaucoma can be controlled by the use of eye drops, oral medication, or surgery (Mayo Clinic Staff, 2004b).

Nurses should educate clients about recommended vision screening. To determine the influence of visual impairment, the nurse should inquire about activity limitations associated with poor vision. Determining whether the client is using visual assistive devices such as glasses, contact lenses, magnifying lenses or large print books can be beneficial in recognizing the degree of adaptation. The community health nurse should be knowledgeable about resources to assist older adults with eye care and assistive devices. Organizations that provide information include the National Eye Institute, the American Foundation for the Blind, the Lighthouse National Center for Vision and Aging, Lighthouse for the Blind and Visually Impaired, and the National Society to Prevent Blindness.

Hearing Loss

In 2002, 37% of elders age 65 and over reported having trouble with hearing. This number increases to 60% in elders who are age 85 and over. Elderly men are more likely than women to be hearing impaired. Nineteen percent of all older men and 10% of all older women reported having ever worn a hearing aid. Whites report hearing loss more frequently than blacks. Consequences of hearing loss may include withdrawal, isolation, and depression (Federal Interagency Forum on Aging-Related Statistics, 2004).

According to Miller (2004), the following are the most common types and characteristics of hearing loss: presbycusis, conductive hearing loss, and sensorineural hearing loss. Presbycusis is caused by age-related changes of the inner ear structures. An early functional consequence of presbycusis is the loss of ability to hear high-frequency sounds. Conductive hearing loss results from abnormalities of the external and middle ear that impair the sound-conduction mechanism. Sensorineural hearing loss results from abnormalities of the inner ear that interfere with the sensory and neural structures. Sensorineural hearing loss is often age related or noise induced. Tinnitus, a persistent ringing or buzzing in the ear unrelated to the external environment, is a common pathologic condition in older adults that is often associated with both conductive and sensorineural hearing loss, ototoxic medications, and with Meniere's disease.

Nurses should assess older adults for hearing loss by using a tuning fork to detect hearing impairments and to differentiate between conductive and sensorineural loss. An otoscopic examination also should be done to examine the external ear canal and the tympanic membrane. If there is an abnormal accumulation of cerumen, it may need to be removed. The nurse may also need to refer the client for further assessment by an audiologist or otolaryngologist, who might recommend use of hearing aids. In general, Medicare and Medicaid do not cover the costs of hearing aids. Box 17-3 contains tips for health care providers who work with older adults with hearing difficulties.

Dental Concerns

The dental health of elderly individuals is often neglected with advanced age due to inadequate dental care, limited mobility and transportation, poor nutrition, the myth that it is natural for older adults to become edentulous, and lack of finances and reimbursement (Medicare and some states' Medicaid programs do not provide adequate reimbursement for dental needs). These risk factors predispose older adults to periodontal disease and tooth loss.

Serious dental problems are related to both age and income. For example, the prevalence of edentulism (having no natural teeth) was higher for people age 85 and over (38%)

BOX 17-3   Working With Older Adults With Hearing Difficulties

Face the person and speak clearly.
Stand where there is good lighting and low background noise.
Speak clearly, naturally, and at a reasonable speed.
Do not hide or cover mouth, eat, or chew gum.
Use facial expressions or gestures to give useful clues.
Reword statements if needed.
Be patient and stay positive and relaxed.
Ask if there are ways to help the listener.
Include the hearing-impaired person in all discussions to prevent feelings of isolation.
Use pencil and paper if necessary.

From National Institute on Aging: *Age page: hearing loss,* Sept 2002a, The Author, http://www.niapublications.org/agepages/hearing.asp.http://www.niapublications.org/agepages/hearing.asp.

than for people ages 65 to 74 (24%). Forty-six percent of older people with family income below the poverty line reported no natural teeth, compared with 27% of people above the poverty threshold (Federal Interagency Forum on Aging-Related Statistics, 2004).

Nurses should routinely assess their clients' oral and dental health. Gums should be inspected for color and palpated for lesions and swelling. If the client wears dentures, proper fit should be assessed, as well as excessive wear and rough spots. The teeth should be inspected for looseness, caries, and lost fillings. The tongue and mucous membranes should also be inspected for color, swelling, lesions, and moistness (Ebersole, Hess, and Luggen, 2004). The nurse should teach the client or their caregiver proper dental care, including brushing at least twice a day and flossing once a day. The nurse may also be helpful in providing referrals to dentists and periodontists.

Incontinence

Aging does not cause incontinence; however, at least 1 in 10 people age 65 or older has this problem (National Institute on Aging, 2002b). Incontinency is a symptom of underlying problems. Urinary incontinence can occur for many reasons. Urinary tract infections, vaginal infection or irritation, constipation, and certain medicines can cause short-term bladder control problems. Weak bladder muscles, overactive bladder muscles, blockage from an enlarged prostate, or damage to nerves that control the bladder may cause longer-lasting incontinence. However, in most cases, urinary incontinence can be treated or controlled, if not cured.

The choice of treatment depends on the type of bladder control problem. Types of urinary incontinence are stress incontinence, urge incontinence, and overflow incontinence or functional incontinence. One of the treatments that health care providers may suggest is Kegel exercises. These exercises make the muscles that are used to stop urination stronger.

An individual may also experience fecal incontinence. Loss of control of the bowels leads to stool leakage from the large intestine. Medical evaluation to determine the cause should be recommended. Treatment varies, depending on the cause. Self-treatment is rarely successful (American Academy of Family Physicians, 2005).

ELDER SAFETY AND SECURITY NEEDS

Injuries and violence are serious threats to seniors. According to the National Center for Injury Prevention and Control (2005), the injuries and violence that pose the greatest threat to seniors are elder abuse and maltreatment, falls, driving, residential fire-related injuries, suicide, and traumatic brain injury. Older adults are at higher risk for injuries that can lead to death or disability. The leading cause of death due to unintentional injuries for seniors is fall-related injuries. Seniors who experience a hip fracture are likely to die in the first year following that injury.

Falls

Many of the physiological changes that normally occur with aging, as well as a variety of chronic illnesses, can affect balance and make **falls** more likely. Medications such as blood pressure pills, heart medicines, diuretics, and tranquilizers may increase the risk of falling. Osteoporosis, a disease that causes a gradual loss of bone tissue or bone density, makes bones more susceptible to breaking. There is a link between osteoporosis and broken bones from falls. A person who falls and sustains a fracture may become afraid of falling again and thus will limit his or her activities. Seniors living independently before a fall may be institutionalized for as long as a year after their fracture. Loss of footing and loss of traction are factors that can lead to a fall. Uneven surfaces such as sidewalks, curbs, or floor elevations, wet or slippery ground, and climbing up on household items not intended for climbing can result in loss of footing or loss of traction. In addition, drinking alcoholic beverages increases the risk of falling because alcohol slows reflexes and response time; causes dizziness, sleepiness, or lightheadedness; and alters balance.

Steps can be taken to reduce the chance of falls. The community health nurse can educate seniors regarding measures they can take to lessen the risk of falls. Adequate amounts of calcium and vitamin D, exercising several times a week, obtaining a bone density test and taking medications that are available for slowing bone loss are activities that can help. Nowak (2003) reported on a study of 1500 women that found that vitamin D deficiency increased the risk of falls. Simple exercises that strengthen muscle and exercises that can improve balance are recommended (Box 17-4). Seniors can also improve their environment in order to reduce their risk of falling by checking floor surfaces, curb heights, identifying weather related problems before venturing outside, wearing supportive, low-heeled shoes, making sure that rooms are well lit, and ensuring that safety equipment is installed in bathrooms and stairwells. In the event of a fall, if the senior remembers to fall forward or backward or to land on their hands to break a fall, it will lessen the risk of hip fracture. Another factor older adults should consider is having a cellular phone with them at all times to call for help

---

BOX 17-4 Improving Balance

Focus on the following areas
Muscle strengthening exercises.
Obtain maximum vision correction.
When using bi-trifocal glasses, practice looking straight ahead and lowering the head.
Practice balance exercises daily.

Balance Exercises
While holding on to a stable item like a chair or counter, practice standing on one leg at a time for a minute.
Gradually increase time, try balancing with eyes closed, and try balancing without holding on to anything.
Practice standing on toes, then rock back to balance on heels.
Hold for count of 10.
Hold on to stable item with both hands, then make a big circle to the left with hips.
Repeat to the right.
Do not move shoulders or feet.
Repeat five times.

From National Institutes of Health Osteoporosis and Related Bone Diseases, National Resource Center: *Preventing falls and related fractures,* Bethesda, Md, 2005, The Author, http://www.osteo.org/newfile.asp?doc=r613i&doctitle-falls+and+Related+Fractures&3A.

---

directly. Telephone systems providing personal emergency response services, may be available on a subscription basis thus allowing seniors to be monitored. If no answer is received, then help can be sent.

Traumatic Brain Injury

Traumatic brain injury (TBI), also called acquired brain injury or simply head injury, occurs when a sudden trauma causes damage to the brain. TBI can result when the head is suddenly and violently hit, or when an object pierces the skull and enters brain tissue (National Institute of Neurological Disorders and Stroke, 2005). TBI results in a number of deaths and cases of permanent disability. Men have consistently composed about three quarters of the number of TBI cases. Motor vehicle crashes account for 48.3%, and falls, the next most common cause of TBI, account for 18.5% (Millis and Wood, 2005). Mosenthal (2002) found that the mortality rate from TBI is higher in the geriatric population at all levels. Prevention of TBI is directly related to measures taken to prevent falls and driving accidents.

TBI symptoms may be mild, moderate, or severe. Symptoms of mild TBI include headache, confusion, lightheadedness, dizziness, blurred vision or tired eyes, ringing in the ears, bad taste in the mouth, fatigue or lethargy, and a change in sleep patterns or thinking. Moderate or severe TBI may demonstrate the same symptoms as mild TBI plus a headache that gets worse or does not go away, repeated vomiting or nausea, convulsions or seizures, an inability to awaken from sleep, dilation of one or both pupils of the eyes, slurred speech, weakness or numbness in the extremities, loss of coordination, and increased confusion, restlessness, or agitation (National Institute of Neurological Disorders and Stroke, 2005). Medical attention should be sought for monitoring and treatment of symptoms. Nothing can be done to correct damage of brain cells. Referral for rehabilitation may be required for persons with disabilities resulting from TBI.

Driver Safety

One of the quality-of-life factors that is important to the senior is the ability to drive. Older drivers depend on driving in order to maintain independence and personal mobility. Seniors overwhelmingly prefer to drive as their means of transportation, with being a passenger their second preferred option. Over the next 30 years, the number of drivers over the age of 85 is expected to be four to five times greater than it is today. Seniors are generally safe drivers. Unfortunately, they are more likely than other age-groups to be injured or killed in an accident (Tucker, 2004).

Age alone should not be the determining factor of whether or not a senior can drive safely. Driving skills vary from one elderly person to another. However, there are certain functional capabilities that are essential for safe driving. The functional capabilities needed are body strength, range of motion, and coordination (Russo-Meek, 2004). In addition, hearing and vision are essential for responding safely to the driving environment. Most older drivers monitor their own driving ability and gradually limit or stop driving; others risk personal injury rather than give up their driver's license. Aging-related physiological and psychological changes and medical, physical, and mental illnesses are factors that may interfere with an individual's ability to drive safely.

The community health nurse should be alert to signs of driving impairment in older clients and offer practical advice so that the driver may either continue to drive safely or be encouraged to find alternative transportation. The nurse can discuss issues with the senior driver, family, or friends and refer them to multiple resources available for identifying the warning signs of when someone should begin to limit driving or to stop altogether.

The American Association of Retired Persons (AARP) provides a list of 15 warning signs to help identify unsafe older drivers (Box 17-5). These drivers can be encouraged to take a driver safety program or be educated to make changes in their behavior that might help them to continue driving safely.

Some interventions older adults could implement are limiting their driving to daylight hours, planning their trips to avoid rush hour, not listening to the radio, or avoiding talking with passengers, and there are more measures that might be taken to assure their safe driving. The driver should also be encouraged to find other methods of transportation such as family and friends, or public transportation, taxis, or other private transportation options available in the community. A helpful booklet that offers many suggestions as to what the individual can do to prolong the ability to drive safely is "Driving Safely While Aging Gracefully" (National Highway Safety Administration, 2005). When the question of driving safely becomes personal, elderly drivers might get very defensive. Therefore it is important that the elderly person, if at all possible, be involved in the decision-making process of identifying their ability and deciding what should be done. However, if the individual is

---

BOX 17-5   Warning Signs for Driving Cessation

Feeling less comfortable and more nervous or fearful while driving

Difficulty staying in the lane of travel

More frequent close calls (i.e., almost crashing)

More frequent dents, scrapes on the car or on fences, mailboxes, garage, doors, curbs, etc.

Trouble judging gaps in traffic at intersections and on highway entrance and exit ramps

Other drivers honking at you more often; more instances when you are angry at other drivers

Friends or relatives not wanting to ride with you.

Getting lost more often

Difficulty seeing the sides of the road when looking straight ahead (i.e., cars or people seem to come "out of nowhere" more frequently)

Trouble paying attention to or violating signals, road signs and pavement markings

Slower response to unexpected situations; trouble moving foot from gas to brake pedal or confusing the two pedals

Easily distracted or hard to concentrate while driving

Hard to turn around to check over shoulder while backing up or changing lanes

Medical conditions or medications that may be increasingly affecting your ability to handle the car safely

More traffic tickets or "warnings" by traffic or law enforcement officers in the last year or two

From American Association of Retired Persons: *Keeping safe: when to stop driving,* Washington, DC, 2004, The Author, http://www.aarp.org/life/drive/safetyissues/Articles/a2004-06-21whentostop.html.

---

greatly impaired and, therefore, is dangerous to themselves and others, it may be necessary to involve the family, family physician, or department of motor vehicles in determining whether to suspend or revoke an older person's license. In addition, it may be necessary to take the keys, disable the car, or move it to a location beyond the individual's control in order to protect the senior and others from injury or accidents.

Residential Fire-Related Injuries

In the United States, more than 1000 older adults aged 65 years and older die each year in home fires and more than 2000 are injured. In addition, older adults are 2 times more likely to die in a residential fire than the rest of the population. This risk may be attributed to reduced sensory abilities such as smell, touch, vision, and hearing, diminished mental faculties, slower reaction time, increased disabilities, and economic and social concerns which may prevent necessary home improvements that could reduce fire risk. The predominant cause of fires which result in injuries to older adults are cooking, open flames, smoking, and heating (National Fire Data Center, 2006). Community health nurses making home visits can assess their elderly client's for fire risk and teach fire safety including the importance of home smoke detectors and fire extinguishers. In many communities, the fire department will install free smoke detectors for older adults. In addition to the U.S. Fire Administration's public information campaign, A Fire Safety Campaign for People 50-Plus, organizations like the National Fire

Protection Association and the American Burn Association have active fire prevention and education programs for older adults.

Cold and Heat Stress
Cold Stress Disorders

Hypothermia is the most serious of the cold stress–related disorders and is the one elderly individuals might experience in the home due to failure of their heating system or lack of financial resources to pay for sufficient heat. Factors that contribute to the development of hypothermia are age, health, nutrition, exhaustion, exposure and duration of exposure, wind, temperature, wetness, and medications that may decrease heat production or increase heat loss or interfere with thermo stability.

Hypothermia is a body temperature–related disorder. Hypothermia is defined as a core temperature of less than 35° Celsius. At this temperature, the body is unable to produce sufficient heat to efficiently maintain functioning. Normal functioning requires a body temperature of 37° Celsius (98.6° Fahrenheit). The body can self-compensate for small upward or downward variations in temperature through vasoconstriction. The response to an upward variation in body temperature is the initiation of perspiration that moves moisture from body tissues to the body surface. When moisture reaches the skin, it evaporates. The response to a downward variation in body temperature is shivering, which generates heat. Shivering is an involuntary contraction and expansion of muscles on a large scale. This muscle action creates heat through friction (Search and Rescue Society of British Columbia, 1995).

The stages of hypothermia are impending, mild, moderate, and severe. In the impending stage, the skin will become pale, numb, and waxy. Muscles tense and shivering may begin. Fatigue and signs of weakness begin. In mild hypothermia, uncontrolled intense shivering begins. The individual is still alert and able to help himself, but movement becomes less coordinated and some pain and discomfort may be present. In moderate hypothermia, muscles begin to stiffen and mental confusion and apathy occurs. Speech becomes slow, vague, and slurred; breathing becomes slower; and sleep drowsiness and strange behavior may develop. In severe hypothermia, the skin is cold, may be a bluish color, and pupils may be dilated. The individual is very weak, demonstrates a marked lack of coordination, slurs his or her speech, appears exhausted, and may appear drunk. There is a gradual loss of consciousness, with little or no breathing, that progresses to death.

Initial management is to prevent further loss of heat. Rewarming of the core temperature at a safe, slow rate is important in order to avoid lethal side effects. The reason for rewarming the core first is to prevent vasodilatation that would place the individual in ventricular fibrillation. Measures that can be taken are (1) remove the individual from the cold area as soon as possible; (2) add more clothing, especially to the head (e.g., use a hat or scarf); (3) provide a warm sweetened drink (no coffee or tea); and (4) apply mild heat to the head, neck, chest, and groin areas using hot water bottles or warm moist towels. Medical help is imperative, and hospitalization may be needed depending on the stage of hypothermia. Other cold stress disorders are frostbite and trench foot, which occur from long exposure to extremely cold temperatures.

Heat Stress Disorders

The heat stress disorders are heatstroke, heat syncope, heat exhaustion, and heat cramps. As the environment becomes warmer, all methods of heat elimination become less effective. These conditions should be taken seriously and require immediate medical attention; heatstroke is life threatening. Heat cramps are painful spasms of muscles of the arms, legs, or abdomen that occur during or after work. Heat exhaustion signs and symptoms are fatigue, nausea, headache, and giddiness. The skin is clammy and moist, and the complexion may be pale, or flushed. The individual may faint on standing with a rapid, thready pulse and low blood pressure. Heatstroke signs and symptoms are hot dry skin, which is usually red, mottled, or cyanotic. Confusion, loss of consciousness, or convulsions might occur. All of these may occur in the home without fans or air conditioning, or from being in the sun for prolonged periods of time, either in recreation or working in extremely hot temperatures and humidity. In all instances, the individual should be moved to a cooler environment and made to lie down and rest. With heat stroke, immediate and rapid cooling with chilled water or by wrapping in a wet sheet, as well as removing to a cooler area, should be done while seeking immediate medical attention.

Elder Abuse

Elder abuse is a serious problem throughout the United States. It is important to remember that abuse is not only a health concern but also a legal problem. States have laws defining abuse and identifying who is required to report abuse to Adult Protective Services. Abuse is generally defined as the willful infliction of pain, injury, or debilitating mental anguish; unreasonable confinement; or deprivation by a caretaker of services that are necessary to maintain mental and physical health. The categories of abuse are domestic, institutional, or self-neglect. Domestic abuse is that which occurs in the home. Institutional abuse is that which occurs in a nursing home or other residential care facility. Self-neglect is that which occurs when a person living alone threatens his or her own health or safety.

There are four common types of elder abuse. One is physical abuse, which includes slapping, pushing, pinching, and beating; physical restraint that results in broken bones, sprains, dislocations, bruises, black eyes, cuts, and rope marks; or sexual assault. Second is psychological or emotional abuse, which includes humiliation, intimidation, threats, and destruction of belongings (e.g., broken glasses). Behaviors displayed by the elder might be agitation, withdrawal, or unusual behavior such as rocking, biting, or sucking. The third type of abuse is financial or material exploitation, which refers to the improper or illegal use of the resources of an older person without consent (e.g., use of ATM card). The final type is neglect. Signs of neglect might include dehydration, malnutrition, untreated health problems, bedsores, unclean or inappropriate clothing, and weight loss.

Elder abuse affects approximately 2 million elderly each year; an accurate number is unknown because it is estimated that for every case reported, five go unreported. This problem will steadily increase as more and more elderly are living longer and remaining in their homes. Abuse of the elderly is underreported for a number of reasons, including denial, fear of further abuse, no other place to go, love of the abuser and not wanting the abuser locked up, dependence on an abuser, and shame and embarrassment that someone they love could act in an abusive manner. Another reason is that elder abuse is often not recognized by health care providers (Meeks-Sjostrom, 2004).

Diagnosis is very difficult because many of the signs and symptoms may truly be the result of normal physiological aging. Ways to tell the difference include conflicting stories about how physical injuries were obtained, "physician shopping", clusters of signs and symptoms, increasing depression of the elder, new poverty, poor personal care, malnutrition, unresponsiveness, hostility, anxiety, confusion, new health problems, improper medication, dehydration, and longing for death.

The abuser is frequently the spouse, sibling, child, friend, or other caregiver. The family member profile of an abuser is an individual who is middle age or older, a daughter or son of the elder, someone with low self-esteem and impaired impulse control. Caregiver behavior to look for is aggression, defensive or increasingly resentful attitude toward the elder, blames the victim for an injury, and treats the elder like a child; or, if the caregiver shows new affluence while withholding food or medication from the elder. Factors that lead to abuse are a lack of knowledge about normal aging, caregiver exhaustion, anger and frustration with the elder, financial problems, and drug and alcohol use of the caregiver. Elders who are most vulnerable are older females who are widows, single, and over 75; those dependent on a caregiver for their shelter and food; those with incontinence; individuals who are frail or who have illness or mental disability.

Prevention activities include professional training of health care personnel, public education about elder abuse and its seriousness, and development of reliable assessment tools for the detection of abuse appropriate for the categories of abuse. Nurses should report suspected abuse to Adult Protective Services through their state's hotline. Suggestions the community health nurse can give to the elder are to stay sociable, maintain friendships, and participate in senior citizen activities; have pension and Social Security checks deposited directly into bank accounts and obtain durable power of attorney when no longer able to manage property and assets; consider co-guardians so more than one person knows and can act on the elder's behalf; ask for help if needed, keep records, property, and a will in order; and plan ahead for possible disability. Community health nurses also should advise elders to avoid leaving cash, jewelry, and other valuables lying around visible; refuse to sign a document unless someone the elder trusts reviews it first; and resist letting anyone isolate them from others (Iowa State University, 1994). Additional resources that can be used for further information are the Administration on Aging (http://www.aoa.dhhs.gov)

and the National Center on Elder Abuse (http://www.elderabusecenter.org).

Crime

Older adults are less likely to be victims of **crime** than are teenagers and young adults; however, if an older person becomes a victim of a crime, the result is that the individual is more likely to be seriously hurt than someone who is younger. Crime against the elderly occurs in the form of robbery, purse snatching, pocket picking, car theft, and home repair scams (National Institute on Aging, 2003). Elder abuse is not only a health concern but also a legal one. According to the National Crime Victimization Survey, serious violent crimes of the elderly include rape and sexual assault, robbery, and aggravated assault (Perkins, 1997).

The key for crime prevention for the senior is to be careful and alert to what is going on in the environment and to the types of crimes to which elders are vulnerable. Measures can be taken to lessen the risk of crime happening to the elderly person. In the home, safety measures include making sure that door and window locks are strong. Bars on doors and windows need to be installed with caution, because they may increase the risk of harm in the event public officials need to access the home due to fire or need to gain access to assist the elderly who may be injured from a fall or is ill. The use of a safe deposit box should be recommended to store a list and pictures of expensive belongings and other important documents, such as a copy of the individual's will. Installation of a monitored alarm system with its accompanying outdoor security sign would also help deter criminals. Caution should always be used before answering the door. The elder should note who is at the door before opening the door and, if it is a stranger, have them show identification. Nurses should remind elders that if they are uneasy about the visitor, they should not answer the door.

When out in the community, measures that should be observed are to stay away from unsafe places, keep car doors locked and windows up at all times, and park in well-lit areas. Don't open the car door or roll down the window for strangers. Use inside pockets of clothing for valuables such as a wallet, money, or credit cards. A purse should be carried close to the body and kept closed. Credit cards and money should be kept separately so that if a thief steals a purse, the credit card signature cannot be used to forge a signature for illicit use of checks. Only carry what is needed at the time. In addition, the elderly person should be advised not to resist the thief, but to hand over immediately what the person is requesting.

Fraud is the crime that frequently is mentioned in the media as happening to elders. Older people are subject to con games, insurance scams, home repair, and telephone scams. Types of Internet fraud include auction fraud, non-delivery of products ordered, securities fraud, credit card fraud, identity theft, bogus business opportunities, and unnecessary professional services. According to the Federal Bureau of Investigation, senior citizens are targeted at a rate of 34% of individuals in fraud schemes (Perkins, 1997). One strategy to recommend to seniors to prevent fraud from happening to them is to hang up the phone on telephone salespeople. Today, the elder can get caller ID service for the telephone; if no number or individual is identified, the elder may choose not to answer the call. No personal or financial information should be given over the phone unless the elder made the phone call. When in doubt about an inquiry or opportunity, the elder should be encouraged to say no and in this way protect himself or herself. The elder should check the references of anyone seeking to do home repairs and be sure to get, in writing, the details of the work to be completed as well as the cost. A job should never be paid for in advance.

Identity theft is on the increase, and elderly individuals are particularly vulnerable. To avoid this problem, Social Security and monthly pension checks should be deposited directly into a bank account. Any information that is sent to the home with credit card offers, personal information, and so forth should be shredded so that the information cannot be used illegally. All cancelled and new checks should be kept in a safe place. The elder should check carefully the bank statement and credit card account statements for any discrepancies and report them immediately to the respective business. Caution should be used in using the Internet for buying products or paying bills, due to websites without security.

PSYCHOSOCIAL DISORDERS

Psychosocial disorders account for a significant number of suicides, especially among older men. Depression is likely to lead to suicides. Alzheimer's disease more commonly affects the old than the young. Alcohol and drug abuse are less common in older individuals; however, this is still a concern. Depression and abuse of drugs and alcohol can coexist with one or more anxiety disorders. These conditions are discussed in the following section.

Anxiety Disorders

Anxiety is a normal human emotion that everyone experiences at one time or another. For elderly individuals, normal age-related worries experienced are financial concerns, health problems, and reduced social interactions due to loss of friends because of death and relocation, but these do not mean that the individual has an anxiety disorder. An **anxiety disorder** is diagnosed only if symptoms are excessive, uncontrollable, create significant distress, or interfere with normal activities (Grayson, 2005).

However, anxiety disorders are a very real and relatively common problem among older adults. Some older adults with anxiety disorders may have had the problem for a long time, whereas others may experience anxiety problems only later in life. Studies have shown that among older adults, anxiety disorders occur anywhere from two to seven times more often than depression problems. It is possible that depression and abuse of drugs or alcohol can coexist with one or more anxiety disorders. Generalized anxiety disorder, social phobia, and agoraphobia seem to be the most common types of anxiety in the elderly; obsessive-compulsive disorder, panic disorder, and posttraumatic stress disorder also occur in the

elderly but at a lower rate. Approximately 5 to 6 out of every 100 elders is coping with at least one anxiety disorder (Stanley and Beck, 2000).

Generalized anxiety disorder is characterized by excessive, exaggerated anxiety and worry about everyday events and is accompanied by physiological problems, including headaches, muscle tension, nausea, trembling, and frequent trips to the bathroom (Grayson, 2005). The worry is often unrealistic or out of proportion to the real situation because anxiety dominates the individual's thinking to such a point that it interferes with daily activities. Social phobia involves overwhelming worry and self-consciousness about everyday social activities. Worry centers on fear of being judged by others or fear of behaving in a way that might cause embarrassment. Agoraphobia is a fear of leaving the familiar setting of home that is so invasive that the individual avoids social situations or enters into life situations reluctantly. Symptoms vary depending on the type of anxiety; as noted earlier, an anxiety disorder is diagnosed only if the symptoms are excessive, uncontrollable, create significant distress, or interfere with daily living.

Anxiety disorders cannot be prevented. Some things that can be suggested to control or lessen symptoms are stop or reduce consumption of caffeine, check over-the-counter medicines or herbal remedies for any chemicals that can increase anxiety symptoms, exercise daily and eat an adequate nutrient-based diet, and seek counseling and support after experiencing a traumatic or disturbing event (Haines, 2005). All anxiety disorders are serious medical conditions, and elderly clients should be referred to their physician for evaluation and treatment. The nurse can help elders realize that what they are experiencing does not need to interfere with their lives if they seek medical help.

Depression

Everyone has times when they are unhappy with their lives. Feelings of sadness are not a weakness or a character flaw. These feelings can happen at any time and to anyone, and they are not necessarily related to an unhappy event. **Depression** can affect people of all ages, backgrounds, and ethnic groups.

Many myths exist concerning depression. Depression may last for days, weeks, months, or even years without treatment. Treatment is not just for those who are threatening suicide but also for anyone with symptoms that last more than 2 weeks. Depression is a serious condition that lasts longer and increases the risk of death in the elderly population. For example, depression is likely to lead to suicide. Elderly white men are at greatest risk. Suicide rates in people ages 80 to 84 are more than twice that of the general population. Also, depression is associated with increased risk of death following a heart attack. In addition, depression may coexist with other medical illnesses and disabilities such as diabetes, stroke, heart disease, cancer, chronic lung disease, Alzheimer's disease, Parkinson's disease, and arthritis. Health care providers may miss the diagnosis of depression associated with one of these diagnoses as well as depression in general (Healthy Place.com, 2000-2004).

Depression refers to a lasting (2 weeks or longer) sad mood or loss of interest or pleasure in most activities. People may experience several or all of the following symptoms: changes in appetite or weight, changes in sleep patterns, restlessness, loss of energy, feelings of worthlessness or guilt, and repeated thoughts of death or suicide. If any of these symptoms exist, the client should be referred to their physician for diagnosis. A physician can only make a diagnosis of clinical depression, which calls for the presence of five or more of the symptoms mentioned above. Clinical depression usually interferes with a person's work, social life, or daily life. Seniors with depression usually do not complain of depressed mood or a loss of interest in previous areas of activity; family or friends usually observe these symptoms. Elders who are no longer able to live independently are at great risk for suicide (Scanlon, 2006).

Treatment is available and is helpful. The physician and the individual determine which treatment would be used. There is medication alone or medication with psychotherapy. How long depression lasts depends a great deal on identifying the condition early and seeking treatment early. Depression is undiagnosed or underdiagnosed. Delay in treatment in the elderly can be very dangerous as noted before.

Thus, the community health nurse can play an important part in recognizing individuals who may be experiencing depression and who need to be referred for medical diagnosis and supervision. There are a number of checklists, including the Geriatric Depression Scale short form (Healthy Place.com, 2000-2006), which can be used to help the nurse recognize those at risk.

Substance Abuse

Data from the Substance Abuse and Mental Health Services Administration's (SAMHSA) National Survey on Drug Use and Health conducted from 2002 to 2003 revealed that 13.7 million (17.1%) of persons age 50 or older smoked cigarettes and 36 million (45.5%) drank alcohol during the month prior to responding to the survey. Approximately 12.2% of older adults reported binge alcohol use, and 3.2% reported heavy alcohol use. A binge drinker is defined as a person who drinks five or more drinks on the same occasion on at least one day in the past 30 days. Among older adults, 1.4 million (1.8%) used an illicit drug during the past month. Marijuana was the most commonly used illicit drug, followed by prescription-type drugs used non-medically and cocaine (SAMHSA, 2005).

Older males were more likely to report substance use than females in this age-group. However, the rate of nonmedical use of prescription drugs tended to be greater among older females than older males, although not statistically significant. Past-month cigarette use by older adults was significantly greater among non-Hispanic blacks (22.6%) than among non-Hispanic whites (17%) and Hispanics (13.8%). Past-month alcohol use by older adults was greater among non-Hispanic whites (48.3%) than among non-Hispanic blacks (30.2%) and Hispanics (33.6%). For older adults, overall illicit drug use in the past month did not differ significantly by race/ethnicity, but marijuana use was greater among non-Hispanic whites (1.2%)

and non-Hispanic blacks (0.9%) than among Hispanics (0.2%). Lastly, there were no significant differences in the rates of binge alcohol use or heavy alcohol use across these racial/ethnic groups (SAMHSA, 2005).

Although alcohol and illicit drug use is lowest among the elderly population compared to other adult cohorts, alcohol-related problems are a significant cause of acute-care hospitalizations in this group (Rigler, 2000). The number of illicit drug users among older adults is expected to increase due to the aging of the "baby boom" generation. Elderly adults consume more over-the-counter and prescription drugs than any other age-group and are more likely to consume psychoactive drugs with a potential for misuse, abuse, and addiction (Levin and Kruger, 2000).

Although the statistics discussed above are helpful in estimating the number of elderly substance abusers, it is difficult to adequately determine rates of use and abuse due to isolation, retirement, and lack of report (Benshoff, Harrawood, and Koch, 2003). In addition, the symptoms of alcohol and drug abuse are often mistaken for health problems associated with aging, such as dementia or depression (Levin and Kruger, 2000).

Elderly substance abusers may be categorized as early or late onset abusers (also referred to as chronic or situational). Early-onset abusers began drinking or drugging behavior before the age of 65. Rigler (2000) reported that about two thirds of elderly individuals with alcoholism problems are early-onset drinkers. Those individuals who survive the rigors of alcoholism problems in earlier life often have significant mental and physical health complications. Late-onset abusers began their substance abuse (usually alcohol vs. illicit drug abuse) after age 65, typically in response to a negative life situation or event, such as retirement, death of a spouse, or disability.

As a result of normal physiological changes (discussed earlier in this chapter), older adults generally experience increased sensitivity and decreased tolerance to alcohol and drugs. Because of loss of body mass, decreased absorption rate in the gastrointestinal system, slower kidney function, and slower metabolism, drugs and alcohol remain in the body longer and at higher rates of concentration, thus prolonging and increasing their effects. The problem is compounded when alcohol and illicit drugs interact with prescribed or over-the-counter drugs.

Careful screening must include a thorough review of factors that may be directly affecting substance use and abuse. Several instruments have been utilized with the population of elderly individuals including the CAGE, the Michigan Alcohol Screening Test—Generic Version (MAST-G), and the Alcohol Use Disorders Identification Test (AUDIT). The CAGE is an easy-to-use, four-question interview. The MAST-G (23 questions) and AUDIT (10 items) are screening instruments that provide more detailed description of alcohol use. All three of these instruments rely on client self-report. According to Menninger (2002), research has demonstrated that the MAST-G and the CAGE have comparable sensitivity for identifying alcoholism in elderly individuals, whereas the AUDIT is somewhat less sensitive.

However, Rigler (2000) cautioned that the MAST-G and CAGE fail to distinguish between current and past drinking behaviors.

There are several levels of care for substance abusers. These levels of care include outpatient care, where individuals may receive 1 to 3 hours of group and individual counseling per week; intensive outpatient counseling, where consumers may receive 9 to 20 hours of individual and group counseling per week; residential care with medical monitoring, consisting of 24-hour supervision by substance abuse professionals and access to medical and psychiatric treatment; and medically managed care, where services may be provided in a medical setting such as a psychiatric hospital (Benshoff et al., 2003). Alcoholics Anonymous (AA) is a community peer self-help group that may be very beneficial; however, elderly individuals may believe that they do not fit into the group or have differing concerns from younger members. In addition, they may have age-related mobility or hearing problems that prevent participation in peer self-help groups.

It is important that nurses recognize, assess, and screen for substance abuse in older adults so that they can refer these individuals to appropriate community resources. Nurses are involved in assisting elderly substance abusers at every level of care discussed in this section. Lastly, nurses are in a prime position to educate clients about the dangers of substance abuse.

Suicide

Suicide, the act of intentionally taking ones own life, is a serious health concern related to the elderly, who account for 19% of all suicides. Elder suicide may be underreported (40% or more). Omitted are "silent suicides," for example, deaths from medical noncompliance or overdoses, self-starvation or dehydration, and "accidents." Elders at highest risk are white males over the age of 85; second highest are American-Indian and Native-Alaskan men (Centers for Disease Control and Prevention [CDC], 2004). Elderly individuals have a high success rate for suicide because they use firearms, hanging, and drowning. "Double suicides" involving spouses or partners occur frequently among the aged.

Elder suicide is associated with depression, chronic illness, physical impairment, unrelieved pain, financial stress, loss and grief, social isolation, and alcoholism. Depression is tied to low serotonin levels. Serotonin is a neurotransmitter that limits self-destructive behavior. Serotonin levels decrease with age.

Warning signs to watch for in the elderly are loss of interest in things or activities that are usually found enjoyable, cutting back from social interactions, self-care, and grooming activities, not following medical regimens (e.g., going off diets, not taking prescriptions), experiencing or expecting a significant personal loss (e.g., spouse or friend), feeling hopeless or worthless, putting affairs in order, giving things away, making changes in will, and stock-piling medications or obtaining other lethal means for committing suicide. The most significant warning sign is any expression of intent. Risk factors that should also be considered in determining if an elder

might be at risk are previous suicide attempts, history of mental disorders, alcohol and substance abuse, family history of suicide, and local epidemics of suicide.

Prevention activities include dispelling any myths that exist relating to suicide. Many think that winter holidays are linked to suicide, but, in fact, suicide rates in the United States are lowest in the winter and highest in the spring (CDC, 2004). Other myths that need to be discussed and banished are those who kill themselves must be crazy, asking someone about suicide can lead to suicide, pain goes along with aging so nothing can be done, those who talk about suicide rarely actually do it, and if someone is determined to kill themselves, no one can stop them. Other prevention concepts are promote awareness, develop broad-based support, reduce stigma associated with aging and being a consumer of mental health, urge use of substance abuse and suicide prevention services, develop community-based suicide prevention programs if none exist, reduce access to lethal means of self-harm, promote participation in education programs related to recognition of at-risk behaviors, and lastly promote and support research.

Alzheimer's Disease

Alzheimer's disease is a slowly progressive brain disorder that begins with mild memory loss and progresses through stages to total incapacitation and eventually death. Diagnosing whether an individual has Alzheimer's disease is very difficult because it mimics other conditions such as depression and other types of dementia. Usually, a tentative diagnosis is reached after all other conditions have been ruled out. The only sure way to diagnose Alzheimer's disease is by autopsy. There is no cure, and limited treatment options are available.

The estimate of Americans who have the disorder is 3 to 4 million; however, the exact number is unknown due to difficulty in diagnosing dementia of the Alzheimer's type. The numbers are expected to increase to 7 million as people are living longer. As age increases, so does the risk of Alzheimer's disease. The percentage of individuals with the disease doubles every 5-year period beyond 65 (Alzheimer's Disease Education & Referral Center, 2005). Many of these individuals live in their homes and are taken care of by family members or friends.

Wolf-Klein et al. (1989) studied 312 active outpatient geriatric clients to measure the validity of the clock drawing test in screening individuals with probable Alzheimer's disease. They found that clients with Alzheimer's disease were unable to draw a normal clock and demonstrated five characteristically abnormal patterns. As a test for Alzheimer's disease, clock drawing had a sensitivity of 86.7% and a specificity of 92.7%. There was correct identification in 97.2% of normals. The researchers reported that the findings indicate that the clock drawing test, an easily administered, low-cost screening tool, can be useful to health care professionals in characterizing cognitive loss in a general geriatric clinic population. Research also is being conducted on developing a diagnosis test that could help individuals in the early stages so that the drugs and therapies that are available can be initiated. The Food and Drug Administration has approved four drugs for people in the mild to moderate stages of the disease. They are Cognex (tacrine), Aricept (donepezil), Exelon (rivastigmine), and Reminyl (galantamine) (Alzheimer's Disease Education and Referral Center, 2005). These drugs appear to slow down some of the symptoms, but they do not stop the progression of the disease. Research continues related to diagnosis, causes and risk factors, and treatment and care issues.

The behavioral and physical changes create many challenges for caregivers, family, and friends. If the individual is living alone and develops short-term memory loss, problems such as fires from leaving the stove on, having the electricity turned off because bills have not been paid, or leaving to go to the store and forgetting how to get home are just some of the problems that might occur. Some of the behavioral symptoms are agitation, aggression, wandering, and sleep disturbances.

Management strategies for caring for the individual with Alzheimer's disease should be elicited from the Alzheimer's Association's many publications, experts, and local chapter programs. Medical supervision of the physical condition and medications (if clinically indicated) is essential. In addition, Alzheimer disease centers throughout the country offer diagnosis and treatment, provide information about the disease, services and resources, and provide volunteers an opportunity to participate in drug trials and other research projects. Any number of resources is available for respite for the caregiver, support groups for both client and family, and day care facilities for the client. These resources can be found by contacting the local chapter of the Alzheimer's Association. If wandering is a problem, the local police should be informed of the potential problem, current pictures of the individual should be available, and safety measures such as locks, bells on the doors, or other means to ensure safety should be installed.

END-OF-LIFE ISSUES

Advance Directives
Decision making at the end of life is complex. Older adults often experience multiple chronic illnesses, some life threatening. An older person who is approaching death may not be able to make end-of-life decisions. In this case, confusion as to how to provide appropriate care may develop.

The Patient Self-Determination Act is a federal law that requires health care facilities that receive Medicare and Medicaid funds to inform patients in writing of their rights to execute **advance directives** concerning end-of-life care. In the absence of written advance directives, oral advance directives may be challenged legally if family members are not in agreement about the person's wishes (Hooyman and Kiyak, 2005).

The most common type of advance directive is a living will. Living wills are legal documents whose purpose is to allow individuals to specify what type of medical treatment they would or would not want if they became incapacitated or had an irreversible terminal illness.

Living wills can direct physicians to withhold life-sustaining procedures and can assist family members in

ETHICAL Insights

Making End-of-Life Decisions When the Client Cannot

The Terri Schiavo case, which riveted the nation for weeks in 2005, demonstrated a worst-case scenario in an end-of-life situation. The case involved a brain-damaged client without a written advance directive and a family bitterly divided on what to do. In the end, the court ruled in favor of Schiavo's husband, who won the right to have her feeding tube removed over her parents' objections.

Similar situations occur with regularity in caring for elders who are near the end of their lives. According to Erlen (2005), family members sometimes don't agree with specific wishes of their family member regarding continuation of treatment and/or providing comfort through palliative care. Even though health care providers want to respect their clients' wishes, this is not always easy. Factors to consider are whether the client has provided written advance directives, the vulnerability of the client, whose interests and wishes should prevail, and quality of life.

making decisions when they are unable to consult a comatose or medically incompetent relative. An individual must be competent to initiate a living will, and he or she can revoke or change it at any time (Miller, 2004).

A durable power of attorney is another type of advance directive that authorizes someone to act on an individual's behalf with regard to property and financial matters. A durable power of attorney for health care is an advance directive that allows an individual to designate a health care proxy or surrogate to make decisions about medical care if the person is unable to make them for himself or herself. When an individual has no advance directive, is incompetent, or unable to handle his or her affairs adequately, a guardian may be appointed by the court to direct the individual's medical treatment, housing, personal needs, finances, and property. Because the guardian manages all the individual's affairs and assumes legal rights, a **guardianship** is generally considered a last resort (Hooyman and Kiyak, 2005).

Lastly, a do-not-resuscitate (DNR) order is another kind of advance directive. A DNR order is a request not to have cardiopulmonary resuscitation (CPR) if an individual's heart stops or if the person stops breathing. Persons should place their request on an advance directive form or tell their physician. Afterward, a DNR order is placed in the medical chart by the physician.

Advance directives not only makes a person's wishes known, but they may also decrease the stress of decision making experienced by family members at the end of a loved one's life. State-specific advance directives can be ordered from the national organization, Caring Connections, or downloaded from their website (http://www.partnershipforcaring.org).

The Nurse's Role and End-of-Life Issues
The nurse is encouraged to discuss and educate clients about end-of-life issues. These include advance directives and pre-funeral considerations when death is imminent. When a client enters a health care facility with an advance directive,

Text continued on p. 356

CASE STUDY Application of the Nursing Process

Mrs. Darren, a 75-year-old widow, was referred to the community health nurse by her physician, who did not believe she could care for herself sufficiently. Her diagnoses were hypertension, mild congestive heart failure, arthritis, and occasional confusion after transient ischemic attacks.

During the initial home visit, the nurse observed that Mrs. Darren lived in a run-down house in an inner-city neighborhood. The roof leaked, and the house had no functioning heat unit. A rat was scrambling in the garbage. Mrs. Darren told the nurse that she did not have children and her only relative was a sister who lived with her family in another state. She was used to the neighborhood and knew her neighbors, but she was frightened of the teenagers who lingered when she took the bus to the supermarket to cash her Social Security check.

Mrs. Darren received Supplemental Security Income, Medicare, Medicaid, and food stamps. She ate mostly bread and butter and drank coffee, but she enjoyed fried chicken and oranges after going to the supermarket. Constipation was sometimes a problem and she took a laxative every night. She said she did not always remember whether she took her medication and held out a small bottle containing an assortment of pills of different colors, shapes, and sizes.

ASSESSMENT

With Mrs. Darren as the system, or central planning focus, the nurse identified her biopsychosocial subsystem strengths and weaknesses and looked for actual or potential connections to her family and community suprasystems. Considering aging theories, the nurse believed Mrs. Darren was undergoing disengagement from her physical and social circumstances and decided that this might reverse if her health could be maintained and her links to the community strengthened. On a practical level, the nurse also checked with Mrs. Darren's physician regarding the prescriptions and identified the assortment of pills by taking them to the pharmacist who filled the prescriptions.

The nurse used a problem-solving approach to data gathering and identified Mrs. Darren's assets as the following:
- Being basically able to care for herself
- Receiving medical treatment
- Receiving income from various sources
- Being accustomed to the neighborhood and knowing her neighbors
  Her liabilities were more extensive, as follows:
- Inadequate nutrition
- Confusion with medications and improper use of laxatives
- Condition of the house, which was not supportive of health
- Threat of violence in neighborhood and possibility of attack for her Social Security money
- Physical impairment resulting from age and illness
- No children or other family living nearby
- Probable progression of confusion
- Possibility of a major stroke at home while unattended

DIAGNOSES

Diagnoses and related short- and long-term goals address Mrs. Darren's situation. The nurse wrote plans at the three levels of prevention for the diagnoses and included suggestions for intervention with families.

Individual
- Altered nutrition of less than body requirements, which was related to difficulty or inability to procure food
- Potential for injury related to inadequate housing, possibility of robbery for Social Security money, aging, and progression of disease

Family
- Potential for injury to family unit related to unanticipated loss of interaction with Mrs. Darren because her health is declining and her residence is distant

Community
- Knowledge deficit of nutritional services, related to lack of publicity of available nutritional programs for older adults
- Lack of support programs for medication consistency related to unrecognized need
- Lack of programs and resources for older adult residents of limited income related to cost of services and competition for limited funds

PLANNING

Individual
Long-Term Goals
- Mrs. Darren will maintain a nutritionally adequate diet through self-care and use of community programs as evidenced by a steady weight and normal tests for nutritional status during physical examinations.
- Mrs. Darren will avoid inconsistency in her medication regimen related to forgetfulness and mild confusion.
- Mrs. Darren will continue to take medications as ordered, as evidenced by stabilization of disease processes and intermittent demonstration to a nurse.
- Mrs. Darren will explore sheltered housing for older adults and continue contact with a community health nurse and neighborhood friends.

Short-Term Goals
- Mrs. Darren will improve her diet to include a recommended daily allowance of nutrients, including fiber and fluids, as evidenced by diet recall, and she will report regular bowel habits without use of laxatives.
- Mrs. Darren will utilize memory aids for consistent medication regimen.
- Mrs. Darren will identify medications and know when to take them, as evidenced by demonstration to a nurse.

CASE STUDY | Application of the Nursing Process (cont'd)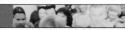

- Mrs. Darren will improve her home to allow healthy habitation, avoid robbery by varying her routine and using banking services, expand her social network, and maintain health care appointments.

Family
Long-Term Goal
- Mrs. Darren will maintain family contact by mail, telephone, or possible visits.

Short-Term Goal
- The family's addresses are included in Mrs. Darren's record to facilitate emergency contact.

Community
Long-Term Goals
- Promote publicity campaign to advertise nutritional services for older adults in the community.
- Support community pharmacists in the campaign to increase public awareness of the need to take medications as prescribed.
- Identify and support programs that will assist with provision of prescribed medications for people who have difficulty obtaining prescriptions because of a lack of insurance, money, transportation, or other problems.
- Community groups work together to maximize use of resources.

Short-Term Goal
- Identify existing programs for older adults in the community.

INTERVENTION

Individual
When the nurse discussed the nursing diagnoses and plans with Mrs. Darren, Mrs. Darren agreed with the short-term goals, but she was not sure that she wanted to leave her home for other housing or meet other people through community activities. She agreed, however, to try. During the course of the next few visits, the nurse explained basic nutritional principles and helped make a shopping list and menus for one week. Together, they developed a plan to assist with medication scheduling.

The nurse encouraged Mrs. Darren to talk about her earlier life during the nurse's visits. She had been widowed soon after her marriage when her husband was killed serving the army overseas, and she had never remarried. She lived in the neighborhood where she grew up, although it had deteriorated over the years. She had worked as a secretary until her retirement and had no pension plan.

Family
Because Mrs. Darren's family did not live close by, the nurse designed a plan to increase Mrs. Darren's social contacts by introducing her to a group that met frequently and offered several activities she might enjoy. If she were unexpectedly absent, the group would check on her. A neighbor invited her to a senior center, where she became involved in a domino-playing group. Mrs. Darren allowed her name to be put on the waiting list for an apartment for older adults. With the other changes, the apartment was no longer a priority, and Mrs. Darren could make a decision when an apartment became available.

Community
Referrals initiated by the nurse resulted in a greatly improved living situation. A financial advisor from the city's Supportive Services to the Elderly program encouraged Mrs. Darren to open a bank account for the direct deposit of her checks and showed her how to use it. A home health aide from the same program came for half a day each week to assist with shopping and cleaning. The sanitation department of the health district exterminated the rats, the local Area Agency on Aging fixed the roof, and a church-sponsored group painted the house and cleaned the yard. A small heater was purchased from the Salvation Army store, and application was made to the utility company for help with bills during the winter months.

EVALUATION

Individual
With the nurse as intermediary and coordinator of community services, Mrs. Darren easily accepted help with the problems related to security and survival. When her home improvements were completed, Mrs. Darren was able to maintain herself more comfortably with the help of the weekly visit from the home health aide.

Family
In the absence of family support, the establishment of an orderly routine, the companionship at the nutrition site, and safer financial arrangements increased Mrs. Darren's feelings of belonging and self-esteem. The nurse reduced her home visits but maintained contact with Mrs. Darren during her visits to the health clinic for blood pressure checks and preventive health care to supplement her medical care.

Community
Discussion with the home health aide informed the nurse of proposed funding cuts to the city's Supportive Services to the Elderly program, which would result in reduced services. The nurse spoke to the president of the district branch of the professional nurse's association, who notified the state level of the association to monitor funding on the state level. The association also assisted the nurse in working with other local agencies for older adults to establish a publicity campaign against proposed funding cuts through writing letters to the editors of local newspapers, speaking at public hearings on the city budget, and speaking at city council meetings. Although funds were reduced, the cuts were much less severe than they would have been without the campaign, and most services were able to continue, although with increased waiting time for admission of new clients.

Continued

CASE STUDY   Application of the Nursing Process (cont'd)

LEVELS OF PREVENTION

Primary

Goal: Promote good nutrition.

Individual
- Instruct about nutritional needs.
- Plan a shopping list and menus incorporating a prescribed diet for health problems.

Family
- Instruct about nutritional needs of family members by age, sex, or special needs.

Community
- Increase nutrition information where food is sold.

Goal: Promote safety and prevention of injury.

Individual
- Provide immunizations as appropriate.
- Provide community services for assistance to maintain property and prevent deterioration.
- Encourage a network of friends and family members.

Family
- Provide services of community health nurse or case manager.
- Provide counseling.
- Provide respite care.

Community
- Provide community education programs for older adults.
- Be aware of potential hazards for older adult residents and provide intervention as needed.

Secondary

Goal: Assess and treat nutrition-related disorders.

Individual
- Provide referral for assessment of possible nutrition-related disorders.
- Provide hospitalization or prescribed nutritional supplements for illness resulting from inadequate nutrition.

Family
- Provide referral for nutritional assessment and counseling.

Community
- Encourage emergency food supplies.

Goal: Diagnose and treat medication-related injuries.

Individual
- Provide referral for apparent overmedication or undermedication symptoms.
- Diagnose and treat drug or food reactions.

Family
- Reassess the client's understanding of medications.

Community
- Provide a 24-hour poison hotline.
- Provide an emergency department with 24-hour response.
- Provide medical services.

Tertiary

Goal: Maintain improved nutrition.

Individual
- Encourage use of community services.

Family
- Encourage exchange of family recipes.
- Encourage attendance of home economics classes.

Community
- Provide campaigns for nutritional awareness and healthy eating.
- Encourage the eating of healthy snacks in food machines.
- Encourage use of funding of community food services for aggregates or emergencies.
- Encourage use of services providing access to food (e.g., food banks, Meals on Wheels, and food stamps).
- Encourage use of transportation to grocery stores or nutrition services.

Goal: Be consistent with prescribed medications and prevent medication error.

Individual
- When medications are dispensed, provide written and oral instructions at the level of understanding and in the language of the client.
- Have the client repeat instructions to the health care provider.

Family
- Have the client repeat instructions to family members.

Community
- Provide a community education program about understanding medications.

---

nurses should ensure that it is current and reflects the client's wishes. The nurse should inform other members of the health care team and make sure that the document is visible and accessible in the client's chart. Nurses should also

encourage clients to discuss with their family their wishes regarding decisions in these documents. Clients should provide copies of advance directives such as living wills for their family members in case of emergency. Furthermore, clients should discuss the living will with their physician so that this document is made a part of their medical record. A copy of advance directives should also be kept in the individual's automobile.

SUMMARY

Increasing life expectancy, coupled with aging baby boomers, will cause a dramatic and continual rise in the number of older adults. In addition to longevity, older adults desire to function independently for as long as possible. This chapter has described aging, demographic characteristics, normal aging changes, health promotion and illness prevention interventions, common health and psychosocial concerns, end-of-life issues, and various resources that may assist older adults. Community health nurses should be aware of and address these issues and concerns so that they can help elders have a better quality of life.

LEARNING ACTIVITIES

1. Interview an elderly person you know to assess his or her physical activity level and nutritional status using the nutrition checklist and food pyramid. Review the results with the person and help the person plan a nutritious menu for one day. What factors hindered or enhanced interaction with this person?
2. Find the names, addresses, and phone numbers of local resources for someone interested in, for example, exercise programs for the elderly, smoking cessation programs, and so forth.
3. Devise a nursing care plan for an elder with a visual disturbance (i.e., cataracts, glaucoma, or macular degeneration).
4. You are asked to lead a 1-hour discussion (see topics below) for a group of 10 seniors at a senior citizens center. What would be your goal? What physiological aspects would you include? What psychosocial aspects would you consider?
   - Issues related to urine control
   - Fall prevention
   - Prevention of influenza and pneumonia
   - Medications and aging
   - Normal aging changes
5. Speak with police officers in a local community about elder abuse and crimes against elders. Identify community strengths and weaknesses. Discuss needs and solutions.
6. The family of your elderly client is considering taking the keys from him. They asked you how to decide if their loved one should stop driving. How would you respond?
7. Your 80-year-old client has become very frail and needs assistance with several activities of daily living. There are no family members who are able or willing to take care of him full time. The family has asked you for advice. What information would you share with them about alternative housing options?
8. Your elderly client has a terminal illness. You note that she does not have an advance directive. What issues surrounding this topic would you discuss with her?

REFERENCES

Administration on Aging: *Geographic distribution: a profile of older Americans,* Washington, DC, 2001, The Author, http://www.aoa.gov/aoa/stats/profile/2001/6.html.

Administration on Aging: *Elder rights & resources: elder abuse,* Washington, DC, 2004, The Author, http://www.aoa.gov/eldfam/Elder_Rights/Elder_Abuse/Elder_Abuse.asp.html.

Alzheimer's Disease Education and Referral Center: *Alzheimer's disease fact sheet,* Silver Spring, Md, 2005, The Author, http://www.alzheimers.org/pubs/adfact.html.

American Academy of Family Physicians: *Fecal incontinence,* 2005, The Author, http://familydoctor.org/ 067.xml?printxml.

American Academy of Family Physicians, American Dietetic Association, National Council on Aging: *Nutrition screening initiative,* Washington, DC, 1992, The Author, http://www.acsu.buffalo.edu/~drstall/nutrition.html.

American Association of Retired Persons: *Keeping safe: when to stop driving,* Washington, DC, 2004, The Author, http://www.aarp.org/life/drive/safetyissues/Articles/a2004-06-21-whentostop.html.

Beers M, Berkow R: *Merck manual of geriatrics,* ed 3, Whitehouse Station, NJ, 2000, Merck Research Laboratories.

Benshoff J, Harrawood L, Koch D: Substance abuse and the elderly: unique issues and concerns, *J Rehabil* 69(2):43-48, 2003.

Boston University: *The New England Centenarian Study: a look at centenarians,* 2002, The Author, http://www.bumc.bu.edu/Dept/Content.aspx?DepartmentID=361&PageID=5749.

Burke MM, Laramie JA: *Primary care of the older adult: a multidisciplinary approach,* St. Louis, 2000, Mosby.

Center for Medicare Education: Prescription drug coverage for people with Medicare: issue brief, *Center Medicare Educ* 3(9):1, 2002.

Cooper K et al: Health barriers to walking for exercise in elderly primary care, *Geriatr Nurs* 22:258-262, 2001.

Cumming E, Henry W: *Growing old,* New York, 1961, Basic Books.

Desai M et al: Trends in vision and hearing among older Americans, *Aging Trends,* No. 2, Hyattsville, Md, 2001, National Center for Health Statistics.

Ebersole P, Hess P, Luggen A: *Toward healthy aging: human needs and nursing response,* ed 6, St. Louis, 2004, Mosby.

Eliopoulos C: *Gerontological nursing,* ed 6, Philadelphia, 2005, Lippincott Williams & Wilkins.

Erlen JA: When patients and families disagree, *Orthop Nurs* 24(45):279-282, 2005.

Federal Interagency Forum on Aging-Related Statistics: *Older Americans 2004: key indicators of well-being,* Washington, DC, Nov 2004, US Government Printing Office, http://www.agingstats.gov.

Grayson CE: Mental health: anxiety disorders, *WebMD,* April 2005, http://my.webmd.com/content/article/60/67142.htm.

Gurwitz J et al: Incidence and preventability of adverse drug events among older persons in the ambulatory setting, *JAMA,* 289(9):1107-1116, 2003.

Haines C: Mental health: generalized anxiety disorder, *WebMD,* July 2005, http://my.webmd.com/content/article/60/67148.htm.

Havighurst RL, Neugarten BL, Tobin SS: Disengagement and patterns of aging. In Neugarten BL, editor: *Middle age and aging,* Chicago, 1968, University of Chicago Press.

Hayflick L: *How and why we age,* New York, 1996, Ballantine Books.

Healthy Place.com, Depression Community: *Geriatric depression scale (GDS) short form,* 2000-2004, The Author, http://www.healthyplace.com/communities/depression/elderly_2a.asp.

Hooyman NR, Kiyak HA: *Social gerontology: a multidisciplinary perspective,* ed 7, Boston, 2005, Allyn and Bacon.

Horiuchi S: Greater lifetime expectation, *Nature* 405:744-745, 2000.

Iowa State University: *Understanding abuse: elder abuse,* Ames, Iowa, 1994, The Author.

Lemon BW, Bengston VL, Peterson JA: An exploration of the activity theory of aging: activity types and life satisfaction among in movers to a retirement community, *J Gerontol* 27:511, 1972.

Levin SM, Kruger J: *Substance abuse among older adults: a guide for social service providers,* Rockville, Md, 2000, Substance Abuse and Mental Health Services Administration.

Lueckenotte AG: *Gerontological nursing,* ed 2, St. Louis, 2000, Mosby.

Mayo Clinic Staff: *Cataracts,* 2004a, The Author, http://www.mayoclinic.com/health/cataracts/DS00050.

Mayo Clinic Staff: *Glaucoma,* 2004b, The Author, http://www.mayoclinic.com/health/glaucoma/DS00283.

Mayo Clinic Staff: *Macular degeneration,* 2004c, The Author, http://www.mayoclinic.com/health/macular-degeneration/DS00284.

Meeks-Sjostrom D: A comparison of three measures of elder abuse, *J Nurs Scholarsh* 36(3):247-250, 2004.

Menninger JA: Assessment and treatment of alcoholism and substance-related disorders in the elderly, *Bull Menninger Clin* 66(2):166-184, 2002.

Millis S, Wood K: *Database update,* TBI National Data Center, http://www.tbindc.org.

Miller CA: *Nursing for wellness in older adults: theory and practice,* ed 4, Philadelphia, 2004, Lippincott Williams & Wilkins.

Miller RA: The aging immune system: primer and prospectus, *Science* 273:70, 1996.

Morley A: The somatic mutation theory of aging, *Mutat Res 338*(1-6):19-23, 1995.

National Center on Elder Abuse: *Frequently asked questions,* The Author, http://www.elderabusecenter.org/default.cfm?p-faqs.cfm.

National Center for Injury Prevention and Control: *Injuries among older adults, 2006,* The Author, http://www.cdc.gov/ncipc/olderadults.htm.

National Fire Data Center: *Fire and the older adult, 2006,* The Author, http://www.usfa.fema.gov/downloads/pdf/publications/fa-300.pdf.

National Highway Safety Administration: *Driving safely while aging gracefully.* The Author, http://www.nhtsa.dot.gov/people/injury/olddrive/Driving%20%Safely%20Aging%20Web/.

National Hospice and Palliative Care Organization: *Caring connections.* The Author, http://www.partnershipforcaring.org.

National Institutes of Health, Osteoporosis and Related Bone Diseases—National Resource Center: *Preventing falls and related fractures,* Bethesda, Md, 2005, The Author, htttp://www.osteo.org/newfile.asp?doc=r613i&doctitle-falls+and+Related+Fractures&3A.

National Institute of Neurological Disorders and Stroke: *NINDS Traumatic brain injury information page,* The Author, http://www.ninds.nih.gov/disorders/tbi/tbi.htm.

National Institute on Aging: *Age page: hearing loss,* Sept 2002a, The Author, http://www.niapublications.org/agepages/hearing.asp.

National Institute on Aging: *Age page: urinary incontinence,* Aug 2002b, The Author, http://www.niapublications.org/engagepages/urinary.asp.

National Institute on Aging: *It's never too late to start,* 2002c, The Author, http://www.nia.nih.gov/news/pr/2002.

National Institute on Aging: *Age page: crime and older people,* 2003, The Author, http://www.niapublications.org/engagepages/crime.asp.

Nowak R: *Elderly falls linked to vitamin deficiency,* 2003, The Author, http://www.newscientist.com/article.ns?id=dn4433.

Oeppen J, Vaupel J: Broken limits to life expectancy, *Science* 296:1029-1031, 2002.

Orgel LE: The maintenance of the accuracy of protein synthesis and its relevance to aging, *Proc Natl Acad Sci* 49:517-521, 1963.

Perkins C: *Age patterns of victims of serious violent crime,* Bureau of Justice Statistics special report, Washington, DC, 1997, US Department of Justice.

Resnick B: Testing the effect of the WALC intervention on exercise adherence in older adults, *J Gerontol Nurs* 28(6):40-49, 2002.

Rigler SK: Alcoholism in the elderly, *Am Fam Physician* 61:1710-1716, 2000.

Ross MET, Aday L: Stress and coping in African-American grandparents who are raising their grandchildren, *J Fam Issues* 27(7):912-932, 2006.

Russo-Meek PA: Nurses can help older drivers steer clear of trouble, *NurseWeek* Nov 15, 2004, http://www.nurseweek.com.

Scanlon B: *Recognizing depression in later years,* 2006, The Author, http://healthyplace.healthology.com/printer_friendlyAR.asp?b=healthyplace&f=healthyaging&c=aging_depression.

Search and Rescue Society of British Columbia: *Hypothermia-physiology, signs, symptoms, and treatment considerations,* 1995, The Author, http://www.sarbc.org/hypo1.html.

Stanley MA, Beck JG: Anxiety disorders, *Clin Psychol Rev* 20:731-754, 2000.

Substance Abuse and Mental Health Association: *Substance use among older adults: 2002 and 2003 update,* National Survey on Drug Use and Health report, April 22, 2005, The Author, http://www.oas.samhsa.gov/2k5/olderadults/olderadults.htm.

Tsai P: Predictors of distress and depression in elders with arthritic pain, *J Adv Nurs* 51(2):158-165, 2005.

Tucker LE: *Community based approach to promoting older driver safety,* 2004, National Association of Area Agencies on Aging, http://www.n4a.org.

Tuljapurkar S, Nan L, Boe C: A universal pattern of mortality decline in the G8 countries, *Nature* 405:789-792, 2000.

US Department of Agriculture: *My pyramid,* 2005, The Author, http://www.mypyramid.gov.

US Department of Commerce: *Statistical abstract of the United States,* ed 121, Washington, DC, 2001, US Census Bureau.

US Department of Health and Human Services: *Healthy People 2010: national health promotion and disease prevention objectives,* Washington, DC, 2000, US Government Printing Office, http://www.health.gov/healthypeople.

US Department of Health and Human Services/Centers for Medicare and Medicaid Services (USDHHS/CMS): *Medicare and you,* Baltimore, Md, 2006, The Author, http://www.medicare.gov/publications/pubs/pdf/10050.pdf.

US National Center for Health Statistics: *Vital and health statistics,* 2003, The Author, http://www.cdc.gov/nchs/data/hus/tables/2002.

US Preventive Services Task Force: *Guide to clinical prevention services,* ed 2, Baltimore, Md, 1996, Williams & Wilkins.

US Preventative Services Task Force: Screening for colorectal cancer: recommendations and rationale, *Am Fam Physician* 66(12):2287, 2002.

Wolf-Klein G et al: Screening for Alzheimer's disease by clock drawing. *Am Geriatr Soc* 37:730-734, 1989.

World Health Organization, Tufts University School of Nutrition and Policy: *Keep fit for life: meeting the nutritional needs of older people,* Geneva, 2002, World Health Organization, http://whqlibdoc.who.int/publications/9241562102.pdf.

Zoorob R et al: Cancer screening guidelines, *Am Fam Physician* 63(6):1101-1112, 2001.

Family Health

Beverly Cook Siegrist

MEDIA RESOURCES

Additional Material for Study, Review, and Further Exploration

evolve Website at http://evolve.elsevier.com/Nies

❖ Quiz ❖ Case Studies ❖ Content Updates ❖ Glossary ❖ WebLinks ❖ Resource Tools
18A Family Health Assessment Form

OBJECTIVES

Upon completion of this chapter, the reader will be able to do the following:

1. State a definition of *family.*
2. Identify characteristics of the family that have implications for community health nursing practice.
3. Describe strategies for moving from intervention at the individual level to intervention at the family level.
4. Describe strategies for moving from intervention at the family level to intervention at the aggregate level.
5. Discuss a model of care for families.
6. Apply the steps of the nursing process to individuals within the family, the family as a whole, and the family's aggregate.

KEY TERMS

cohabitation
contracting
culture of poverty
ecological framework
ecomap

expressive functioning
external structure
family
Family Health Assessment
family health tree

family interviewing
gay or lesbian family
general systems theory
genogram
instrumental functioning

internal structure
network therapy
nuclear family
transactional model

CHAPTER OUTLINE

UNDERSTANDING FAMILY NURSING

THE CHANGING FAMILY
    Definition of Family
    Characteristics of the Changing Family

APPROACHES TO MEETING THE HEALTH NEEDS
OF FAMILIES
    Moving From Individual to Family
    Moving From Family to Community

APPROACHES TO FAMILY HEALTH
    Family Theory
    Systems Theory
    Structural-Functional Conceptual Framework
    Developmental Theory

ASSESSMENT TOOLS
    Genogram

    Family Health Tree
    Ecomap

FAMILY HEALTH ASSESSMENT
    Social and Structural Constraints

EXTENDING FAMILY HEALTH INTERVENTION
TO LARGER AGGREGATES AND SOCIAL ACTION
    Institutional Context of Family Therapists
    Models of Social Class and Health Services
    Models of Care for Communities

APPLYING THE NURSING PROCESS
    Home Visit

The four families described below depict broad contemporary definitions of family and are examples of families carried in caseloads by undergraduate community health nursing students. Assessments made by students during home, office, and hospital visits with these families triggered interventions that linked the families to resources provided by the community and, in turn, triggered questions about health needs of groups of families or larger aggregates living in the same communities.

CLINICAL EXAMPLE 1

Rebecca Martin is a 72-year-old widow of 10 years who lives in a rural town in Tennessee. She resides in the home that she and her husband purchased before his death. Her primary source of income is her deceased husband's Social Security benefits, and she also receives a small income from providing child care for infants at her church. Medicare benefits are her only source of payment for health care. Her only child, a daughter from whom she has been estranged for many years, recently died. The daughter was a never-married, single mother of an 8-year-old, medically fragile child with asthma. As the only surviving relative, Rebecca has become the custodial parent for her granddaughter. ■

CLINICAL EXAMPLE 2

Joe Hudson is a 74-year-old alcoholic who is being treated at an outpatient department in a large medical center. He lives in a hotel room in downtown Salt Lake City, Utah. He has one living relative, a 76-year-old brother. Mr. Hudson states, "I had a falling out with my brother 20 years ago. I never hear from him. I reckon he's still in Boston, if he's alive at all." Mr. Hudson frequently falls out of bed, dislodging the telephone that the desk clerk has placed precariously close to the bed, which signals the desk clerk that something is amiss. The clerk then goes to Mr. Hudson's room and puts him back in bed. Mr. Hudson's source of income is a check sent to him the first day of each month by a minister who lives in a town 75 miles away. The desk clerk cashes Mr. Hudson's check and assists him in paying his bill from the hotel, which provides congregate dining facilities. ■

CLINICAL EXAMPLE 3

Lai Chan is a refugee from Vietnam who moved with her family to San Francisco 3 months ago. Mrs. Chan is a single parent; Mr. Chan died in an automobile accident shortly after arriving in the United States. Mrs. Chan has two children, an 11-year-old son and a 5-year-old daughter. The family resides in a one-room efficiency apartment in the Tenderloin district in downtown San Francisco. ■

CLINICAL EXAMPLE 4

Jaime Gutierrez, a 72-year-old Mexican-American man, lives with his 36-year-old son, Roberto; his 34-year-old daughter-in-law, Patricia; and his three grandchildren who are 14, 13, and 12 years of age. Mr. Gutierrez was in good health until he fell from a tree while helping his son make roof repairs on the house in 1995. He suffered a concussion, right hemothorax, and fracture of vertebra T-11 and T-12. Confined to bed, he is receiving home health care. He requires intermittent catheterization but feels uncomfortable when the nurse suggests that his daughter-in-law is willing to carry out this procedure for him. Therefore Roberto quit work to provide this personal care to his father. Consequently, the family of six lives on Mr. Gutierrez's retirement income, which consists of $239 from Social Security and $244 from a pension plan per month. Roberto would like to increase his job skills while at home. He has finished the fourth grade and has failed the Graduate Equivalency Degree examination twice. Patricia also would like to return to school and pursue job training. Although agreeable to Patricia's interests, Roberto is hesitant to support active steps taken by Patricia to initiate her plan. ■

Families have major health care needs that are not usually addressed by the health care system. Instead, the health care system most frequently addresses the individual. This holds true for nursing interventions within the health care system. The majority of nurses work in hospitals where interventions traditionally occur at the individual client level. However, nurses are on the forefront of a trend toward intervention at the family level.

UNDERSTANDING FAMILY NURSING

Family nursing is not a new concept and has been taught in schools of nursing since Nightingale's "district nursing" concept (Cook, 1913) and Lillian Wald's (1904) principles on how to nurse families in the home. The National League for Nursing (NLN) has emphasized the importance of family nursing in standard curriculum guides for schools of nursing since 1917 (Beard, 1999; NLN, 1937). Early NLN publications directed nurses in "household science" and later required that 10 to 15 hours of study should be directed toward understanding the "modern family," in which the nurse must consider the family as a unit (NLN, 1937). Modern nurse theorists such as Newman, King, Orem, Roy, and others extensively discuss the family and its importance to individuals and society. Previously, nurses defined the family conceptually in the following ways: as the environment affecting individual clients; as small to large groups of interacting people; as a single unit of care with definable boundaries; or as a unit of care within a specific environment of a community or society. Current family theorists recognize the diversity of American families. Hanson (2001) defines family as "two or more individuals who depend on one another for emotional, physical, and economical support. The members of the family are self-defined" (p. 6). Wright and Leahey (2000) stated, "the family is who they say they are" (p. 70). These later definitions are perhaps more useful to the nurse and allow the focus on the needs of the family. Family nursing care may be focused on the individual family member, within the context of the family, or the family unit. Regardless of the identified client, the nurse establishes a relationship with each family member within the unit and understands the influence of the unit on the individual and society (Box 18-1).

The family is composed of many subsystems and, in turn, is tied to many formal and informal systems outside the family. The family is embedded in social systems that have an influence on health (e.g., education, employment, and housing). Many disciplines are interested in the study of families; interdisciplinary perspectives and strategies are necessary to understand the influence of the family on health and the influence of the broader social system on the

---

BOX 18-1   Nursing an Individual Client Versus Nursing a Family as Client

Ross and Helmer discuss the similarities and differences between nursing an individual as client versus nursing a family as client. Using the Neuman Systems Model as a guide, these present factors that contribute to the decision to use one approach versus the other. These factors include the following:

➤ The perception of the client as to the need for nursing
➤ The nature of the stressors as affecting only one member of the family or other family members
➤ The risk of instability to the family as a whole posed by the health status of an individual member
➤ The feasibility of the family-nurse collaboration (i.e., the availability of family members and the availability of nursing time to meet with family members)
➤ The knowledge and skill of the nurse

Using a case study, the authors then make comparisons between an individual approach and a family approach by applying the nursing process to an individual client and to the family client.

Data from Ross MM, Helmer H: A comparative analysis of Neuman's model using the individual and family as the units of care, *Public Health Nurs* 5:30, 1988.

---

family. Traditionally, nursing, and even community health nursing, has relied heavily, if not solely, on theoretical frameworks for intervention with families from the disciplines of psychology or social psychology, which target individuals (Cody, 2000; Duvall, 1977; Erikson, 1963; Maslow, 1970). Dreher (1982) questioned the usefulness of these frameworks for the public health nurse "who is ministering to the health of socially and economically diverse populations. . . . Such psychological themes often draw our attention away from broader social issues that are the essence of public health nursing" (p. 505).

Intended for clinical rather than public health use, these models do not address why some social and economically advantaged populations are successful as family units and others are not. Dreher (1982) stated that improvement must come about by addressing the socioeconomic conditions that make some families more dysfunctional than others and to alter the system itself that produces such inequities. Dreher cautioned that socioeconomic causes cannot be interpreted as psychological symptoms. Social and policy changes are necessary to alter the conditions under which families function. This chapter addresses how community health nurses work with families within communities to bring about healthy conditions for families at the family, social, and policy levels. This chapter focuses on the following five areas:

1. The changing family
2. Approaches to meeting the health needs of families
3. Family theory approach to meeting the health needs of families
4. Extending family health intervention to larger aggregates and social action
5. An example of the nursing process applied to a family

THE CHANGING FAMILY

Definition of Family

Many definitions of *family* exist. The nurse's definition of *family* is influenced by personal involvement with his or her own family and clinical experiences. Vaughan-Cole and colleagues (1998) suggest that traditional definitions of *family* are based on the following myths: the typical family as the nuclear family consisting of parents and children and the commonality of the extended family of several generations working toward a common family goal. The examples presented at the beginning of this chapter describe the variations found in today's families.

The term family as used in this chapter is defined as an aggregate made up of a body of units, the individuals that represent the whole, or the family. Definitions of *family* vary by professional discipline and type of family described. For example, psychologists may define *family* in terms of personal development and intrapersonal dynamics; the sociologist has used a classic definition of *family* in terms of a "social unit interacting with the larger society" (Johnson, 2000). Other professionals have classically defined *family* in terms of kinship, marriage, and choice: "a family is characterized by people together because of birth, marriage, adoption, or choice (Allen, Fine, and Demo, 2000, p. 7). Friedman, Bowden, and Jones (2003) incorporate the idea of many nontraditional definitions: "a family is two or more persons who are joined together by bonds of sharing and emotional closeness and who identify themselves as being part of the family" (p. 10). Again, this definition supports the idea of letting the family define their composition and relationships (Wright and Leahey, 2000).

In the past, the dominant American definition focused on the intact **nuclear family**. African American families focus on a wide network of kin and community. The "nuclear" family does not exist for Italians. To them, *family* means a strong, tightly knit three- or four-generational family, which includes godparents and old friends. The Chinese go beyond this and include in their definition of *family* all their ancestors and all their descendants (Patterson, 1999).

The community health nurse interacts with communities made up of many types of families. When faced with great diversity in the community, the community health nurse must formulate a personal definition of *family* and be aware of the changing definition of *family* held by other disciplines, professionals, and family groups. The community health nurse who interacts with Mr. Hudson, the alcoholic who lives in a hotel, must have a broad conceptualization of the family. Both the surveillance activity of the hotel manager and the financial support of the minister could be accounted for in Jordheim's (1982) definition of *family* as a "relationship community of two or more persons" (p. 61), whether from the same or different kinship groups.

Regardless of the definition of *family* accepted, what is evident is the importance of the family unit to society. The family fulfills two important purposes. The first is to meet the needs of society, and the second is to meet the needs of individual family members (Friedman et al., 2003). The family meets the needs of society through procreation and socialization of family members. "The basic unit (family) so strongly influences the development of an individual that it may determine the success or failure of that person's life" (p. 4). The family is the "buffer" between individuals and society. The family meets individual needs through provision of basic needs (food, shelter, clothing, affection). The family supports spouses or partners by meeting affective, sexual, and socioeconomic needs. For children, the family is the "first teacher," instructing the children in societal rules and providing values needed for growth and development.

Characteristics of the Changing Family

The characteristics of the U.S. family continue to change. The typical family, the nuclear family, has traditionally been defined as "the family of marriage, parenthood, or procreation; it is composed of a husband, wife, and their immediate children—natural, adopted or both" (Friedman et al., 2003, p. 10). The stereotypical view of this family as father, mother, and non-adult children is eroding. For example, in 1970, 85% of children younger than 18 years of age were living with two parents (Saluter, 1994), defined as "mother and father." In 2002, 74% of children younger than 18 years of age were living with two parents, defined as two adults including grandparents, same sex partners, and other adults as parents (Annie E. Casey Foundation, 2004). The percentage of black children living with both parents decreased from 58.5% in 1970 to 50% in 2003 (U.S. Census Bureau, 2005). About 44% of white children lived with both parents in 2003, whereas 65% of children of Hispanic origin lived with both parents (U.S. Census Bureau, 2005).

Cohabitation, which is defined as "two unrelated adults of the opposite sex (one of whom is the householder) who share a housing unit with or without the presence of children under 15 years old," has also increased over time (Saluter, 1994, p. vii). The number of cohabiting unmarried people increased from 523,000 in 1970 to 105,480,101 in 2000 (U.S. Census Bureau, 2005). In 2000, more than one third of the cohabiting-couple households included children. Cohen (1999) reported that differences in family income and education are significant in cohabiting families when compared with married couples, especially for white males. White cohabiting males tend to earn less income and have lower educational levels than their married counterparts.

Single parenting has also increased over time. In 1970, 12% of children lived with one parent (Saluter, 1994); in 2000, 28% of children were found in single-parent homes (with 84% of these homes headed by women) (U.S. Census Bureau, 2005). The increase in the teenage birth rate among this group raises concern. During the years 1980 to 2000, the birth rate for unmarried women 15 to 17 years of age increased from 21 to 32 per 1000 in the United States. The majority of teen parents raise the children alone. Of the children living with one parent, 38% live with a divorced parent, 19% live with a separated parent, 35% with a never-married parent, 19% with a separated parent, 4% with a widowed parent, and 4% with a spouse who lives some other place (U.S. Census Bureau, 2003).

The proportion of children younger than 18 years of age who are living with their grandparents is also growing. In 1970, only 3% of children lived with their grandparents. This has increased 30% since 1990. AARP (2005) statistics note that currently 4.5 million children under the age of 18 years of age live in grandparent-headed families with the majority of the grandparents between the ages of 55 and 64 years of age. There are eight times more children in grandparent-headed families than in foster homes (AARP, 2005).

A **gay or lesbian family** is made up of a cohabiting couple of the same sex who have a sexual relationship. The homosexual family may or may not have children. Estimates of the number of children who live in lesbian- or gay-parented families, including children conceived in heterosexual marriages, range from 6% to 11% of children (Parke, 2004; Women's Educational Media, 2005). Between one and five million lesbian mothers and between one and three million gay fathers live in the United States (Patterson, 2002). These numbers are estimates because the U.S. Census Bureau does not count the number of lesbians and gay men.

Single parenting is associated with greater risk associated with lesser social, emotional, and financial resources, which affects the general well-being of children and families. In 2003, 28% of all U.S. children lived in single-parent homes. Single parenting is a key indicator of well-being in children. Numbers of single-parent families vary among ethnic groups (Figure 18-1) (Annie E. Casey Foundation, 2005).

The number of unmarried teen mothers (ages 16-19) remain fairly constant at about 23 births per 1,000 females. There is a significant difference between and among teen birth rates from various ethic groups as illustrated in Figure 18-2 (Annie E. Casey Foundation, 2005).

APPROACHES TO MEETING THE HEALTH NEEDS OF FAMILIES

Community health nursing has long viewed the family as an important unit of health care, with awareness that the individual can be best understood within the social context of the family. Observing and inquiring about family interaction enables the nurse in the community to assess the influence of family members on each other. However, direct intervention at the family rather than the individual client level is a new frontier for many nursing students, most of whom have experience in acute care settings before the community setting. A family model, largely a community health nursing or psychiatric–mental health intervention model, is now expanding into the areas of birthing and parent-child interventions, adult day care, chronic illness, and home care. However, nursing assessment and intervention must not stop with the immediate social context of the family, but it must also consider the broader social context of the community and society. Friedman et al. (2003, pp. 5-6) suggest reasons why it is important for nurses to work with families:

- "The family is a critical resource." The importance of the family in providing care for its members has already been

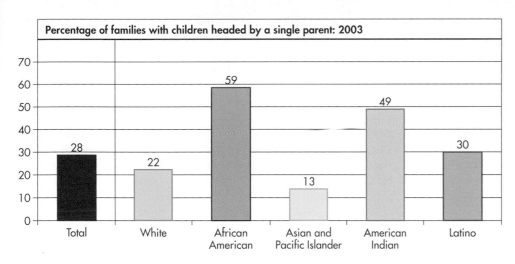

FIGURE 18-1 Percentage of families with children headed by a single parent: 2003. (From Annie E. Casey Foundation: *10 key indicators of child well-being, by race and ethnicity,* KIDS COUNT 2004 Data Book Online, http://www.aecf.org/kidscount/databook/indicators.htm.)

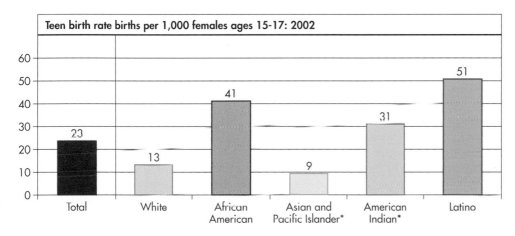

FIGURE 18-2 Teen birth rate: 2002. (From Annie E. Casey Foundation: *10 key indicators of child well-being, by race and ethnicity,* KIDS COUNT 2004 Data Book Online, http://www.aecf.org/kidscount/databook/indicators.htm.)

established. In this caregiver role, the family can also improve individual members' health through health promotion and wellness activities.

- "In a family unit any dysfunction (illness, injury, separation) that affects one or more family members will affect the members and unit as a whole." Also referred to as the "ripple effect," changes in one member causes changes in the entire family unit. The nurse must assess each individual and the family unit.

- "Casefinding" is another reason to work with families. As the nurse assesses an individual and family, he or she may identify a health problem that necessitates identifying risks for the entire family.

- "Improving nursing care." The nurse can provide better and more holistic care by understanding the family and its members.

Moving From Individual to Family

Community health and home care nurses have traditionally focused on the family as the unit of service. With the move to managed care throughout the United States, most of these nurses continue to focus their practice on individuals residing in the home. As a result of the current era of cost containment, constraints on the community health nurse and on nurses working within hospitals and in other settings will increase. For example, reimbursement, which is almost entirely calculated

for services rendered to the individual, is a major constraint toward moving toward planning care for the family as a unit. Various creative approaches to meeting the health needs of families are needed, reflecting interventions appropriate to the needs of the population as a whole.

Family Interviewing

Approaches to the care of families are needed and must be creative, flexible, and transferable from one setting to another. Community health nurses are generalists who bring previous preparation in communication concepts and interviewing to the family arena. Wright and Leahey (2000) proposed the realm of **family interviewing** rather than family therapy as an appropriate model. In this model, the community health nurse uses general systems and communication concepts to conceptualize the health needs of families and a family assessment model to assess families' responses to "normative" events such as birth or retirement or to "paranormative" events such as chronic illness or divorce. Intervention is straightforward, as in helping parents educate prepubescent teenage family members about sex by providing appropriate educational materials or making a referral to another health professional, if the level of intervention is beyond the preparation of the nurse. For the purposes of this text, the model is extended to include intervention at the level of the larger aggregate. For example, the index of suspicion based on the health needs of a particular family would prompt the community health nurse to assess the need for similar information and the resources for intervention with other families in the community, schools, churches, or other institutions. Family interviewing requires thinking "interactionally," not only in terms of the family system but also in terms of larger social systems.

Wright and Leahey (2000) identify the following critical components of the family interview: manners, therapeutic conservation and questions, family genogram (and ecomap when indicated), and commendations. With experience, they believe that the family interview can be accomplished in 15 minutes.

Manners

Manners are common social behaviors that set the tone for the interview and begin the development of a therapeutic relationship. Wright and Leahey (2000) believe that erosion of these social skills prevents the family nurse from collecting essential data. Many nurses argue that too much formality establishes artificial barriers to communication; however, studies identify that the essentials of a therapeutic relationship begin with manners. The nurse introduces himself or herself by name and title, always addresses the client (and family members) by name (i.e., Mr., Mrs., or Ms., unless otherwise directed by client), keeps appointments, explains the reason for the interview or visit, and brings a positive attitude. Other behaviors (manners) that invite rapport include being honest with the client and checking attitude (the nurses) before each client encounter.

Therapeutic Conversations

The second key element in the interview is the therapeutic conversation. This type of conservation is focused, planned, and engages the family. The nurse must listen and remember that even one sentence has the potential to heal or help a family member. The nurse encourages questions, engages the family in the interview and assessment process, and commends the family when strengths are identified. Every encounter, whether brief or extended, has what Wright and Leahey (2000) call "healing potential." Therapeutic conversation may initiate further discussion that brings the family together on issues.

Genogram and Ecomap

The genogram and ecomap constitute the third element and are described in detail later in this chapter. These tools provide essential information on family structure and are an efficient way to gather information, such as family composition, background, and basic health status, in a way that engages the family in the interview process.

Therapeutic Questions

Therapeutic questions are key questions that the nurse uses to facilitate the interview. The questions are specific for the context or family situation but have the following basic themes (Wright and Leahey, 2000): family expectations of the interview or home visit; challenges, concerns, and problems encountered by the family at the time of the interview; and sharing information (e.g., who will relate the family history or information).

Commending Family or Individual Strengths

The fifth element of the family interview is commending the family or individual strengths. Wright and Leahey (2000) suggest identifying at least two strength areas and, during each family interview, sharing them with the family or individual. Sharing strengths reinforces immediate and long-term positive relationships between the nurse and family. Interviews that identify and build upon family strengths tend to progress toward more open and trusting relationships and often allow the family to reframe problems, thereby increasing problem solving and healing (Wright and Leahey, 2000).

Issues in Family Interviewing

Creative family interviewing requires interviewing families in many types of settings. The prediction of decreased hospitalization, supplemented by a wide variety of health care settings ranging from acute to ambulatory to community centers, calls for flexible, transferable approaches. Clinical settings for family interviewing are reviewed by Wright and Leahey (2000) and include inpatient and outpatient ambulatory care and clinical settings in maternity, pediatrics, medicine, surgery, critical care, and mental health. According to Wright and Leahey, community health nurses have many opportunities besides the traditional home visit to engage the family in a family interview. Community health nurses are employed in ambulatory care centers, occupational health and school sites, housing complexes, day care programs, residential treatment and substance abuse programs, and other official and nonofficial agencies. At each of these sites, community health nurses meet families and can assess and intervene at the family and community levels.

The community health nurse can implement preventive programs for family units. The family is particularly appropriate because it experiences similar risk factors (i.e., physiological, behavioral, and environmental). For example, in a classic study conducted by Manley and Graber (1977) in a community hospital, family members of patients with coronary heart disease were invited to attend preventive screening and educational programs. Family members were evaluated for hypertension, smoking, and triglycerides. Findings were similar to those in large epidemiological studies. For example, 25% had lipid abnormalities, 44% were overweight, 12% smoked, and 15.5% had previously undetected hypertension. Later studies (Allen and Blumenthal, 1998; Yarnell et al., 2003) also found similar results. A study by Conger et al. (2003) documented how the family of origin influenced antisocial or aggressive behaviors among family members. Such programs can occur in community health settings and demonstrate the need to go beyond intervention with the individual family to groups of families, serving the population as a whole.

Another example would be a Mexican-American family in which a family member has diabetes; the nurse could implement a family health promotion plan based on the needs of the individual within an at-risk family. The family plan for diabetes prevention is based on the nurse's understanding that Mexican Americans have three times the rate of diabetes as compared with white, non-Hispanic Americans (Klever, 2004).

Involving family members in newborn assessments can aid the community health nurse in determining the family's adjustment to the newborn and parenthood. The nurse can do this in the home, clinic, or other health care center. Family members should be involved during the first contact or visit, and if they do not attend, a telephone call explaining the nurse's interest in them should take place (Wright and Leahey, 2000).

More husbands and family members are becoming involved in the pregnancy and delivery phases of childbirth. The community health nurse in the well-baby clinic may often see parents for whom a family interview or home visit may be valuable. A general statement may introduce the commonality of hurdles faced by new parents. For example, "many new parents face similar problems, which usually last only a short period of time. We find that bringing all of the family members together is important because the entire family is affected when a new baby comes into the home."

The community health nurse working with single-parent families may face particular challenges. Mothers in single-parent families report a higher incidence of children's academic and behavioral problems than do mothers in two-parent families. For example, Teachman, Tedrow, and Crowder (2001) found that single-parent family children are two to three times more likely to have behavior and emotional problems than children in two-parent families and are more likely to drop out of school or become teenage parents. Children in these families need a chance to express their concerns; the family interview is important and may provide the nurse with necessary information needed to care for these families.

School Nurse

The school nurse has a unique opportunity to compare the child in the school system with the child in the family system. The school nurse is becoming increasingly involved in planning special programs in the schools. Astute assessment of children's needs within the context of their families in interviews at school or in the home can lead to innovative interventions such as support groups for children with chronic illness. Other areas of assessment and intervention that benefit from a family approach include learning or behavioral problems and absenteeism (Wright and Leahey, 2000).

Occupational Health Nurse

The nurse in the occupational health setting also can use a family approach to care to improve the health of the worker and contribute to overall productivity. For example, alcohol and chemical abuse account for much absenteeism in the workplace. Effective intervention with these families has been demonstrated. Assessment of occupational hazards may involve conducting reproductive histories in an effort to determine the effects of a chemical or agent on the reproductive capacity of the couple. Toxic agents can also transfer to family members from the workplace via clothes and equipment.

An awareness and a high degree of suspicion about the risks of occupational hazards in community industry are necessary. Obtaining an occupational history from all family members who have entered the workplace and obtaining referrals for family members' screening and health education will contribute to unraveling occupational hazards and effects in the future. In addition, the community health nurse should be aware of the many family-related work issues that may trigger stress-related illness, such as job promotion, job loss, or shift work.

Intervention in Cases of Chronic Illness

Perhaps as many as 80% of families are dealing with chronic illness in a family member (Hopia, Paavilainen, and Astedt-Kurki, 2004). Also significant is the fact that resources such as third-party reimbursement cause most of these families to learn to manage the chronic problems with limited or infrequent intervention by health professionals. The community health nurse working with families coping with chronic illness in a child, adult, or older adult is aided by the family interview. As Glaser and Strauss (1975) stated, chronic illness interjects change into various areas of family life:

> Sex and intimacy can be affected. Everyday mood and interpersonal relations can be affected. Visiting friends and engaging in other leisure time activities can be affected. Conflicts can be engendered by increased expenses stemming from unemployment and the medical treatment . . . different illnesses may have different kinds of impact on such areas of family life, just as they probably will call for different kinds of helpful agents (p. 67).

Changes in family patterns, fears, emotional responses, and expectations of individual family members can be assessed in the family interview. Special needs of the primary caretaker (i.e., often the spouse, daughter, or daughter-in-law) can be assessed. The community health nurse making family visits to older adults and the terminally ill is able to assess intergenerational conflict and stress and influence family interaction positively (Wright and Leahey, 2000).

Moving From Family to Community

The health of families can affect the health of society as a whole, in both positive and negative ways. The health of communities is measured by the well-being of its people and families (Hanson, 2001). Circumstances such as low-birth-weight infants, lack of health insurance, homelessness, violence, poverty, and low employment rates provide a description of families and nations. Community health nurses provide family nursing to improve individual and family health; however, the potential result is that of improving the health of society. The care of entire populations is the major focus, as stated by Freeman in her classic work (1963).

> The selection of those to be served . . . must rest on the comparative impact on community health rather than solely on the needs of the individual or family being served. . . . The public health nurse cannot elect to care for a small number of people intensely while ignoring the needs of many others. She must be concerned with the population as a whole, with those in her caseload, with the

---

HEALTHY PEOPLE 2010 | Access to Health Care

In relation to improving family health, all of the leading health indicators listed as priority in *Healthy People 2010* can serve as a guide for family nursing interventions. Access to quality health care affects every aspect of family nursing. The objectives for measurement of this goal are:

➤ Increase the proportion of persons with health insurance.

➤ Increase the proportion of persons who have a specific ongoing care.

➤ Increase the proportion of pregnant women who begin prenatal care in the first trimester of pregnancy.

  In this chapter, we have discussed the disparities that exist among families and populations with regard to health care access. The community nurse should use political skills, advocacy, and education to influence policy that will result in increased access to health care. The nurse can educate families about available resources and help communities develop resources to improve health care access.

From US Department of Health and Human Services: *Healthy People 2010*, Washington, DC, 2000, US Government Printing Office, http://www.health.gov/healthypeople.

---

need of a particular family as compared to the needs of others in the community (p. 35).

The challenge to the community health nurse is to provide care to communities and populations and not to focus only on the levels of the individual and family. The community health nurse, who traditionally carries a caseload of families, extends his or her practice to the community. To do so, an aggregate, community, and population focus must serve as a backdrop to the entire practice.

For example, families must be viewed as components of communities. The community health nurse must know the community. As stated in previous chapters, a thorough community assessment is necessary to practice in the community. By way of review, the nurse must remember that communities must be compared not only in terms of different health needs but also in terms of different resources to effect interventions that influence policies and redistribute resources to ensure that community and family health needs are met.

Community health nurses must then compare city data with county data and then county data, state data, and national data. In addition, they may need to compare local census tract data and areas of a city or county with other areas of the city or county.

For example, community health nursing students in San Antonio, Texas, who were planning home visits to families of pregnant adolescents attending a special high school, compared local, state, and national statistics on infant mortality rates as a part of a community assessment. They found higher rates of infant mortality in San Antonio in census tracts on the south side of the city in which the population was predominantly Mexican-American. They also found the population to be younger, to have a higher rate of functional illiteracy among adults, to be less educated, to be more likely to drop out of high school, to have higher fertility rates, to have higher birth rates among adolescents, and to be more likely to be unemployed. They found that specific health needs varied among census tracts. Common major health needs of this subpopulation were identified from the community assessment, which assisted the students in planning care for these families. For example, their goals were broadened from carrying out interventions at the individual level to interventions at the family and community levels. In addition to targeting good perinatal outcomes for the individual teenage parent, nursing students planned to include assessments of

functional literacy at the individual and family levels and arranged for group sessions in clinic waiting rooms that informed and referred individuals and family members to alternative resources to enable teenage parents to complete school, take classes in English as a second language, and use resources for family planning and employment at the community level.

In addition to the cross-comparison of communities, the community health nurse also cross-compares the needs of the families within the communities and sets priorities. The nurse in the community finds that specific health needs vary among families. The nurse must account for time spent with families and choose those families on the basis of their needs compared with the needs of others in the community.

Delegation of Scarce Resources

Although the community health nurse serves the community or population as a whole, fiscal constraints hold the nurse accountable for the best delegation of scarce resources. Time spent on home visits has traditionally allowed the community health nurse to assess the environmental, social, and biological determinants of health status among the population and the resources available to them. Fiscal accountability, nevertheless, means setting priorities. In 1985, Anderson, O'Grady, and Anderson listed the factors that influence public health nursing practice, especially home visits, as "the need to justify personnel costs in a time of fiscal constraint, the increasing number of medically indigent who turn to local public health services for primary care, and the change in reimbursement mechanisms by the federal government and some states" (p. 146). Anderson's observations still hold true. In 2000, more than 40,000 Americans lacked health insurance (Hanson, 2001). Many of these individuals are Americans working in low-paying jobs and their families. The Children's Health Insurance Program (CHIP) of 1997 has greatly increased access to health care for many low-income children. When the CHIP program was initiated, there were 10 million children in the United States and 14% were uninsured; by December 2001, 3.5 million (7%) children were enrolled in state CHIP plans (Families USA, 2002). The majority of these children lived in families with working, low-income parents. It is predicted, by legislators, that fiscal budget cuts will result in 900,000 children being dropped from CHIP programs by 2006.

Double Standard in Public Health

A double standard is tolerated in public health. Although the government is responsible for the maintenance of health, a minimal amount of health care is guaranteed to each person because public resources are limited.

A minimum is established for all; however, as demonstrated with Medicare and Medicaid unequal care exists as a result of differences in income (i.e., Medicare) and geographical location (i.e., Medicaid). In a market system, the wealthy can purchase all the health care services they desire and the poor cannot afford these services. The few supplemental resources provided by the government to ensure a minimum for all vary among communities, states, administrations, and counties.

In a period of cost containment, the focus of community health nurses on prevention and health maintenance, which are difficult areas to justify, must carefully legitimate home visiting services by identifying aggregates in need of care.

Prioritizing groups at highest risk and using home visits in conjunction with planning for larger aggregates' needs are necessary. Working for social and policy changes to alter the conditions that place these families at high risk goes hand-in-hand with this activity. More research needs to be done that documents the importance of family nursing through home visits or community-based programs.

Nursing education programs need to educate students in the roles and skills needed to promote family health. Murray (2004) describes the family nursing curriculum based on the 2000 World Health Organization (WHO) document, *The Family Nurse: Context, Conceptual Framework and Curriculum*. In this curriculum, nursing students provide care to families throughout the nursing program, expanding acute care skills to include caring for families through the roles of care provider, decision maker, communicator, leader, and manager.

Many populations at high risk benefit from family nursing through home visits. WHO (1998) describes the benefits of nurses providing family health:

> Help individuals and families to cope with illness and chronic disability or during times of stress, by spending a large part of their time working in patients' homes and with their families. Such nurses give advice on lifestyle and behavioral risks, as well as assisting families with matters concerning health. Through prompt detection, they can ensure that the health problems of families are treated at an early stage. With their knowledge of public health and social issues and other social agencies, they can identify the effects of socio-economic factors on a family's health and refer them to the appropriate agency. They can facilitate the early discharge of people from hospital by providing nursing care at home, and they can act as the lynchpin between the family and the physician, meeting identified needs relevant to nursing expertise.

APPROACHES TO FAMILY HEALTH

Many schools of thought regarding the approaches to meeting family health needs exist among community health, community mental health, and public health nursing professionals.

Dreher (1982) stated that the traditional basis for community health nursing intervention has a focus that has long endorsed psychological and social-psychological theories to explain variations in health and patterns of health care, such as those set forth by Erikson (1963), Maslow (1970), and Duvall (1977). Dreher (1982) stated that what is needed are "more encompassing theories which explain the relationship between society and health [and] the policies which will be most effective in assuring health and health care" (p. 508). To help bridge this gap, four frameworks are presented (i.e., meeting family health needs through the application of family theory, systems framework, structural-functional conceptual framework, and developmental theory).

CLINICAL EXAMPLE

Ten-year-old Jean Wilkie was referred by her teacher to the school nurse. She was withdrawn, had no school friends, and was dropping behind in her schoolwork. The school nurse talked to Jean in her office. Jean said that she had no friends because the other girls stayed overnight with one another "all the time" and that she did not want to bring her friends home because her father "drank all the time." The school nurse decided that Jean's problems needed assessment within the context of the family and arranged to visit the family at home. The father refused to participate in the family interview, but Jean's mother, her 13-year-old brother Peter, and Jean expressed concerns that the father had changed jobs several times in the past year, was frequently absent from work, and had been in two recent car accidents while "drinking." The school nurse was able to verify the family context as the basis of Jean's "problems," continue her family assessment, and plan for intervention at the family level. In addition, she was prompted to assess the community's preventive efforts directed toward drinking and the ability to provide ongoing care for families of alcoholics. ∎

Family Theory

Many reasons exist for why the community health nurse should work with families. Friedman (1998) listed the following six reasons:

1. Any "dysfunction" (e.g., separation, disease, or injury) that affects one or more family members probably affects other family members and the family as a whole.
2. The wellness of the family is highly dependent upon the role of the family in every aspect of health care, from prevention to rehabilitation.
3. The level of wellness of the whole family can be raised through care that reduces lifestyle and environmental risks by emphasizing "health promotion, 'self-care,' health education, and family counseling" (p. 5).
4. Commonalities in risk factors and diseases shared by family members can lead to case finding within the family.
5. A clear understanding of the functioning of the individual can be gained only when the individual is assessed within the larger context of the family.
6. The family as a vital support system to the individual member needs to be incorporated into treatment plans.

Nurses have relied heavily on the social and behavioral sciences for approaches to working with families. These approaches include psychoanalytical, anthropological, sys-

TABLE 18-1 Major Definitions From Systems Theory

TERM	DEFINITION
System	"A goal-directed unit made up of interdependent, interacting parts which endure over a period of time" (Friedman, 1992, p. 115). A family system is not concrete. It is made up of suprasystems and subsystems and must be viewed in a hierarchy of systems. The system under study at any given time is called the focal, target, or system. In this chapter, the family system is the focal system.
Suprasystem	The larger system of which the family is a part, such as the larger environment or the community (e.g., churches, schools, clubs, businesses, neighborhood organizations, and gangs).
Subsystem	Smaller unit within the family, such as the relationship between spouses, parent and child, sibling and sibling, or extended family.
Hierarchy of systems	The levels of units within the system and its environment, which, in their totality, make up the universe. Higher level units are composed of lower level units (e.g., the biosphere is made up of communities, which are made up of families). Families are made up of family subsystems and, in turn, family subsystems are made up of individuals, who are made up of organs, which are made of cells, which are made of atoms.
Boundary	An imaginary definitive line that forms a circle around each system and delineates the system from its environment. Auger (1976) conceptualized the boundary of a system as a "filter" that permits the constant exchange of elements, information, or energy between the system and its environments. . . . The more porous the filter, the greater the degree of interaction possible between the system and its environment" (p. 24). Families with rigid boundaries may lack necessary information and resources pertinent to maintaining family health or wellness.
Open system	A system that interacts with its surrounding environment and gives outputs and gets inputs necessary to survival. An exchange of energy occurs. All living systems are open systems. However, if a boundary is too permeable, the system may be too open to input new ideas from the outside and may be unable to make decisions on its own (Wright and Leahey, 1994).
Closed system	A system that theoretically does not interact with the environment. This is a self-sufficient system; no energy exchange occurs. Although no system has been found that exists in a totally closed state, if a family's boundaries are impermeable (i.e., less open as a system), needed input or interaction cannot occur. An example is a refugee family from Vietnam living in San Francisco; they may remain a closed family for some time because they have differences in culture and language.
Input	Information, matter, or energy that the open system receives from its environment that is necessary for survival.
Output	Information, matter, or energy dispensed into the environment as a result of receiving and processing the input.
Flow and transformation	The system's use of input may occur in two forms. Some input may be used in its original state, and some input may have to be transformed before it is used. Both original and transformed input must be processed and flow through the system before being released as output (Friedman, 1992).
Feedback	"The process by which a system monitors the internal and environmental responses to its behavior (i.e., output) and accommodates or adjusts itself" (Friedman, 1992, p. 117). The system controls and modifies inputs and outputs by "receiving and responding to the return of its own output" (Friedman, 1992, p. 117). Internally, the system adjusts by making changes in its subsystems. Externally, the system adjusts by making boundary changes.
Equilibrium	A state of balance or steady state that results from self-regulation or adaptation. As with the concept of a system as a mobile in the wind, balance is dynamic and, with change, is always reestablishing itself.
Differentiation	The tendency for a system to actively grow and "advance to a higher order of complexity and organization" (Friedman, 1992, p. 117). Energy inputs into the system make this growth possible.
Energy	Energy is needed to meet a system's demands. Open systems will require more input through porous boundaries to meet high energy levels needed to maintain high levels of activity.

tems or cybernetic, structural-functional, developmental, and interactional frameworks (for reviews, see Friedman, 1998; Whall and Fawcett, 1991; Wright and Leahey, 2000). The use of a framework for assessing families is useful to help the nurse understand the health potential for the family. Three conceptual frameworks (systems, structural-functional, and developmental), often used by nurses in providing health care to families, are described. These models help the nurse empower the family in the process of family health promotion.

Systems Theory

The systems approach has been used in such diverse areas as education, computer science, engineering, and communication. **General systems theory** (Minuchin 2002; Sameroff, 1994; von Bertalanffy, 1968, 1972, 1974) has been applied to the study of families. General systems theory is a way to explain how the family as a unit interacts with larger units outside the family and with smaller units inside the family (Friedman, 1998). The family may be affected by any disrupting force acting on a system outside the family (i.e., suprasystem) or on a system within the family (i.e., subsystem).

Parke (2004) stated that there are three subsystems of the family that are most important: parent-child subsystem, marital subsystem, and sibling-sibling subsystem. Allmond, Buckman, and Gofman (1979) compared the family as a system to a piece of a mobile suspended from the air that is in constant movement with the other pieces of the mobile. At any time, the family, like any piece of the mobile, may be caught by a gust of air and become unbalanced, moving "chaotically" for a time; however, eventually, the stabilizing force of the other parts of the mobile will reestablish balance. Table 18-1 presents the major definitions from the systems approach.

Characteristics of Healthy Families

Otto (1973) and Pratt (1976) characterized healthy families as "energized families" and provided descriptions of healthy families to guide in assessing strengths and coping. Curran (1983) and Montalvo (2004) helped to identify healthy families. These authors suggest the following traits of a healthy family:

- Members interact with each other; they communicate and listen repeatedly in many contexts.

BOX 18-2 Summary of Family Functional Assessment

Summary of Family Functional Assessment

I. Instrumental functioning (i.e., activities of daily living)
II. Expressive functioning
   a. Emotional communication
   b. Verbal communication
   c. Nonverbal communication
   d. Circular communication
   e. Problem solving
   f. Roles
   g. Influence
   h. Beliefs
   i. Alliances and coalitions

Data from Wright LM, Leahey M: *Nurses and families: a guide to family assessment and intervention,* ed 2, Philadelphia, 1994, FA Davis.

- Healthy families can establish priorities. Members understand that family needs are priority.
- Healthy families affirm, support, and respect each other.
- The members engage in flexible role relationships, share power, respond to change, support the growth and autonomy of others, and engage in decision making that affects them.
- The family teaches family and societal values and beliefs and shares a religious core.
- Healthy families foster responsibility and value service to others.
- Healthy families have a sense of play and humor and share leisure time.
- Healthy families grow from problems and know when to seek help from professionals.

Structural-Functional Conceptual Framework

With the structural-functional conceptual framework approach to the family, the family is viewed according to its structure, or the parts of the system, and according to its functions, or how the family fulfills its roles.

Structural

Wright and Leahey (2000) stated that three aspects of family structure can be examined (internal structure, external structure, and context). **Internal structure** of the family refers to the following five categories:

1. Family composition, the family members, and changes in family constellation
2. Gender
3. Rank order, or positions of family members by age and sex
4. Subsystem or labeling of the subgroups or dyads (e.g., spouse, parental, and interest) through which the family carries out its functions
5. Boundary, or who participates in the family system and how they participate (e.g., a single-parent mother who does not allow her 17-year-old son to have his girlfriend spend the night in their home)

External structure refers to the extended family and larger systems (Wright and Leahey, 2000). It includes the following two categories:

1. Extended family, including family of origin and family of procreation
2. Larger systems, including work, health, and welfare

Context refers to the background or situation relevant to an event or personality in which the family system is nested (Wright and Leahey, 2000). It includes the following five categories:

1. Ethnicity
2. Race
3. Social class
4. Religion
5. Environment

CLINICAL EXAMPLE: ROLE RELATIONSHIPS

When Edna Smith, a 64-year-old client with severe arthritis, was diagnosed with diabetes, her longtime friend, Frank Gardens, a widower of several years, moved in with her and assumed a caregiver role. The community health nurse assessed the dietary habits of Mr. Gardens and Mrs. Smith and found that Mr. Gardens did the shopping and the cooking because Mrs. Smith's mobility was severely restricted from her arthritis. Mr. Gardens did the cooking; therefore he purchased canned fruits and vegetables rather than fresh or frozen. Mr. Gardens perceived cooking, which was a new role for him, as demanding. After several visits, he disclosed to the nurse that his resistance to preparing fresh or frozen fruits and vegetables came from "the time it takes to clean the darn things, cook 'em, store 'em, and clean up the fridge when they go bad on ya." He stated unequivocally that it was stressful caring for Mrs. Smith and that he wanted to do it, but it was "much easier" to just "open a can" and "heat it in a pan" than to take the time and energy that preparation of fresh or frozen foods would require. The shift in roles that is often required of couples when one is diagnosed with a chronic illness can have an influence on the health of the family. Miller (2000) provides additional reading about how couples manage with chronic illness. ■

Functional

Wright and Leahey (2000) also dichotomized family functional assessment, or how family members behave toward one another, into two categories (instrumental functioning and expressive functioning). **Instrumental functioning** refers to activities of daily living (e.g., elimination, sleeping, eating, or giving insulin injections) (Box 18-2). This area takes on important meaning for the family when one member of the family becomes ill or disabled and is unable to carry out daily functions and must rely on other members of the family for assistance. For example, an older adult may need assistance getting into the bathtub, or a child may need to have medications measured and administered.

The second type of family functional assessment is **expressive functioning**, or affective or emotional aspects. This aspect has nine categories, which follow:

1. Emotional communication: Is the family able to express a range of emotions, including happiness, sadness, and anger?

2. Verbal communication focuses on the meaning of words. Do messages have clear meanings rather than distorted meanings? Wright and Leahey (2000) gave the example of masked criticism when a father states to his child, "Children who cry when they get needles are babies."

3. Nonverbal communication, which includes sounds, gestures, eye contact, touch, or inaction. An example is when a husband remains silent and stares out the window when his wife is talking to him.

4. Circular communication is commonly observed between dyads in families. A common example is the blaming, nagging wife and the guilty, withdrawn husband.

5. Problem solving refers to how the family solves problems. Who identifies problems? Someone inside or outside the family? What kinds of problems are solved? What patterns are used to solve and evaluate tried solutions?

6. Roles refer to established patterns of behavior for family members (Wright and Leahey, 2000). Roles may be developed, delegated, negotiated, and renegotiated within the family. It takes other family members to keep a person in a particular role. Traditional roles are being challenged and are changing with economic and feminist changes; many women are entering the workforce outside the home. Formal roles, with which the larger community agrees, may come into conflict with roles set by family members and influenced by religious, cultural, and other belief systems.

7. Influence refers to methods used to affect the behavior of another. Instrumental influence refers to the use of reinforcement via objects or privileges (e.g., money or watching television). Psychological influence refers to the influence of behavior through the use of communication or feelings. Corporal control refers to use of body contact (e.g., hugging and spanking).

8. Beliefs refer to assumptions, ideas, and opinions that are held by family members and families as a whole. Beliefs shape the way families react to chronic or life-threatening illness. For example, if a family of a person with colon cancer believes in alternative treatments, then acupuncture may be a viable option.

9. Alliances and coalitions are important within the family. What dyads or triads appear to occur repeatedly in the family? Who starts arguments between dyads? Who stops arguments or fighting between dyads? Is there evidence of mother and father against child? When does this change to parent and child against the other parent? The balance and intensity of relationships between subsystems within the family are important. Questions may be asked regarding the permeability of the boundary. Does it cross generations?

Developmental Theory

Nurses are familiar with developmental states of individuals from prenatal through adult. Duvall (Duvall and Miller, 1985), a noted sociologist, is the forerunner of a focus on family development. In her classic work, she identified eight stages that normal families traverse from marriage to death (Box 18-3).

To assess the family, the community health nurse must

BOX 18-3 Family Life Cycle

1. Beginning family (marriage)
2. Early childbearing family (eldest child is in infancy through 30 months of age)
3. Preschool children (eldest child is 2.5 to 5 years of age)
4. School-age children (eldest child is 6 to 12 years of age)
5. Teenage children (eldest child is 13 to 20 years of age)
6. Launching family (youngest child leaves home)
7. Middle-age family (remaining marital dyad to retirement)
8. Aging family (from retirement to death of both spouses)

Data from Duvall EM, Miller BC: *Marriage and family development,* ed 6, New York, 1985, Harper and Row.

BOX 18-4 Stages and Tasks of Middle-Class North American Family Life Cycle

I. Launching: single young adult leaves home
  a. Coming to terms with the family of origin
  b. Development of intimate relationships with peers
  c. Establishment of self: career and finances
II. Marriage: joining of families
  a. Formation of identity as a couple
  b. Inclusion of spouse in realignment of relationships with extended families
  c. Parenthood: making decisions
III. Families with young children
  a. Integration of children into family unit
  b. Adjustment of tasks: childrearing, financial, and household
  c. Accommodation of new parenting and grandparenting roles
IV. Families with adolescents
  a. Development of increasing autonomy for adolescents
  b. Midlife reexamination of marital and career issues
  c. Initial shift toward concern for the older generation
V. Families as launching centers
  a. Establishment of independent identities for parents and grown children
  b. Renegotiation of marital relationship
  c. Readjustment of relationships to include in-laws and grandchildren
  d. Dealing with disabilities and death of older generation
VI. Aging families
  a. Maintenance of couple and individual functioning while adapting to the aging process
  b. Support role of middle generation
  c. Support and autonomy of older generation
  d. Preparation for own death and dealing with the loss of spouse and/or siblings and other peers

Data from Wright LM, Leahey M: *Nurses and families: a guide to family assessment and intervention,* ed 2, Philadelphia, 1994, FA Davis.

---

comprehend these phases and the struggles that families experience while going through them. Wright and Leahey (2000) called attention to the need to distinguish between "family development" and "family life cycle." They stated that the former is the individual, unique path that a family goes through, whereas the latter is the typical path many families go through.

The developmental categories listed in Box 18-4 outline the six stages of the middle-class North American family life cycle

Adolescent Mothers: Resilience, Family Health Work, and Health-Promoting Practices

The dominant perspective of adolescent mothering is that it is an immense social problem. The complexities of adolescent development combined with parenting challenges are thought to place adolescent mothers and their children at high risk for poor health and developmental outcomes. However, findings of some qualitative studies suggest that, although some adolescent mothers struggle as parents, others embrace their parenting responsibilities with optimism and determination. Given that relatively little is known about the successes of these young women in caring for themselves and their children, the purpose of this study was to examine how an adolescent mother's strengths affect her health promotion efforts.

The study was conducted with a convenience sample of 41 adolescent mothers recruited through a variety of strategies. Mothers were asked to provide verbal responses to items on three study instruments: the Resilience Scale, the Health Options Scale, and the Health Promoting Lifestyle Profile. This study examined the relationships among the mother's resilience, family health promotion, and the mother's health-promoting lifestyle practices in single-parent families led by adolescent mothers by testing hypotheses derived from the Developmental Model of Health and Nursing.

The Developmental Model of Health and Nursing (DMHN) gives a perspective from which to understand health promotion in families led by adolescent mothers. The DMHN focuses on process and emphasizes family strengths. Health is seen as a characteristic of the family—a way of living that develops over time within the context of everyday family life. In the DMHN, family health is a composite of four distinct but interrelated concepts: health work, health potential, competence in health behavior, and health status. Health work, the central concept of the theory, is a process of active involvement through which families learn ways of coping with health challenges and of using strengths and resources to achieve goals for individual and family development.

Study findings support the premise that resilience is a critical source for single adolescent mothers. Both mother's resilience and health work predicted health-promoting lifestyle practices, suggesting that both of these variables play an important role in creating a family context in which health is nurtured. Adolescent mothers have been found to be at increased risk for a variety of social, psychological, and physiological problems, including poverty, domestic violence, abuse, and low educational attainment. Giving that resilience is an internal strength that develops in the context of adversity, it is not surprising that levels of resilience were relatively high since half of the participants reported some type of past abuse. The results raise issues for nurses working with adolescent mothers and provide a basis for developing their nursing practice.

From Black C, Ford-Gilboe M: Adolescent mothers: resilience, family health work and health-promoting practices, *J Adv Nurs* 48(4):351-360, 2004.

(Carter and McGoldrick, 1988; Wright and Leahey, 2000) and the tasks necessary for the family's resolution of each stage. Nurses may use the stages to delineate family strengths and weaknesses.

The profiles of families living in North America and in many other parts of the world are changing dramatically from what they have been in the recent past, both in structure and form (Wright and Leahey, 1994, 2000). Language used in reference to the family should be inclusive of many kinds of "families," including those headed by dual-career parents, single parents, unmarried couples, gay or lesbian couples, or remarried couples. The nurse should no longer use terms such as *working mother, children of divorce,* or *fatherless home* when speaking of the family.

Alterations in Family Development: Divorce and Remarriage

Alterations to the life cycle occur, as seen in previously reviewed statistics of separation, divorce, single-parent families, and remarriage. Carter and McGoldrick (1988) and Wright and Leahey (2000) identified phases involved in the processes of divorce, post divorce, and remarriage (Tables 18-2 and 18-3). The family must engage in emotional work as a result of divorce, a process that may occur suddenly or may be long and drawn out. In her classic study, Stern (1982b) interviewed stepfather families in their homes and conceptualized the integration of the blended family, once remarriage occurs, as the integration of two distinct family cultures. In addition, Stern (1982a) identified a set of affiliating strategies that families can learn to establish stepfather-child friendship.

ASSESSMENT TOOLS

Many tools exist for the community health nurse to use in assessing the family (Friedman, 2003; Wright and Leahey, 2000). Reviewed here are the genogram, family health tree, and ecomap.

Genogram

The **genogram** is a tool that helps the nurse outline the family's structure. It is a way to diagram the family (Figure 18-3, p. 373). Generally, three generations of family members are included in a family tree, with symbols (Figure 18-4, p. 374) denoting genealogy. Children are pictured from left to right, beginning with the oldest child.

The community health nurse may use the genogram during an early family interview, starting with a blank sheet of paper and drawing a circle or a square for the person initially interviewed. The nurse tells the family that he or she will ask several background questions to gain a general picture of the family. The nurse may draw circles around family members living in separate households.

For example, as depicted in the case study (Figure 18-5, p. 375) family order across generations can be illustrated and specific personal characterics can be noted in the drawing. Mr. and Mrs. Garcia are non–English speaking, a factor that will be of importance to the nurse as he or she plans nursing interventions. At times the usefulness of the Genogram is limited by how freely the family member relates significant information such as divorces and remarriages, or family health concerns. Other families may be

TABLE 18-2 Dislocations of the Family Life Cycle Requiring Additional Steps to Restabilize and Proceed Developmentally

PHASE	EMOTIONAL PROCESS OF TRANSITION; PREREQUISITE ATTITUDE	DEVELOPMENTAL ISSUES
DIVORCE		
1. Decision to divorce	Acceptance of inability to resolve marital tensions sufficiently to continue relationship	Accepting own part in the failure of the marriage
2. Planning of the breakup of the system	Support of viable arrangements for all parts of the system	a. Working cooperatively on problems of custody, visitation, and finances b. Dealing with extended family about the divorce
3. Separation	a. Willingness to continue cooperative coparental relationship b. Work on resolution of attachment to spouse	a. Mourning loss of intact family b. Restructuring marital and parent-child relationships: adaptation to living apart c. Realigning relationships with extended family; staying connected with spouse's extended family
4. Divorce	More work on emotional divorce: overcoming of hurt, anger, and guilt	a. Mourning the loss of intact family: giving up fantasies of reunion b. Retrieving hopes, dreams, and expectations from the marriage c. Staying connected with extended families
POSTDIVORCE FAMILY		
1. Single-parent family	Willingness to maintain parental contact with ex-spouse and support contact of children and ex-spouse and ex-spouse's family	a. Making flexible visitation arrangements with ex-spouse and ex-spouse's family b. Rebuilding own social network
2. Single-parent (i.e., noncustodial)	Willingness to maintain parental contact with ex-spouse and support custodial parent's relationship with children	a. Finding ways to continue effective parenting relationship with children b. Rebuilding own social network

From Wright LM, Leahey M: *Nurses and families: a guide to family assessment and intervention,* Philadelphia, 1984, F.A. Davis, as adapted from Carter E, McGoldrick M: The family life cycle and family therapy: an overview. In Carter E, McGoldrick M: *The family life cycle: a framework for family therapy,* New York, 1980, Gardner Press.

TABLE 18-3 Remarried Family Formation: A Developmental Outline

STEPS	PREREQUISITE ATTITUDE	DEVELOPMENTAL ISSUES
1. Entering the new relationship	Recovery from loss of first marriage (i.e., adequate "emotional divorce")	Recommitment to marriage and to forming a family with readiness to deal with the complexity and ambiguity
2. Conceptualizing and planning new marriage and family	a. Acceptance of own fears and those of new spouse and children about remarriage and formation of a stepfamily b. Acceptance of need for time and patience for adjustment to complexity and ambiguity of the following: • Multiple new roles • Boundaries: space, time, membership, and authority • Affective issues: guilt, loyalty conflicts, desire for mutuality, and unresolvable past hurts	a. Work on openness in the new relationships to avoid pseudomutuality b. Plan for maintenance of cooperative coparental relationships with ex-spouse(s) c. Plan to help children deal with fears, loyalty conflicts, and membership in two systems d. Realignment of relationships with extended family to include new spouse and children e. Plan of maintenance of connections for children with extended family of ex-spouse(s)
3. Getting remarried and reconstituting family	Final solution of attachment to previous spouse and ideal of "intact" family: acceptance of a different model of family with permeable boundaries	a. Restructure of family boundaries to allow for inclusion of new spouse-stepparent b. Realignment of relationships throughout subsystems to permit interweaving of several systems c. Room for relationships of all children with biological (i.e., noncustodial) parents, grandparents, and other extended family d. Sharing of memories and histories to enhance stepfamily integration

From Wright LM, Leahey M: *Nurses and families: a guide to family assessment and intervention,* Philadelphia, 1984, F.A. Davis, as adapted from Carter E, McGoldrick M: The family life cycle and family therapy: an overview. In Carter E, McGoldrick M: *The family life cycle: a framework for family therapy,* New York, 1980, Gardner Press.

sensitive to the sharing of such information, particularly when it is shown to recur with each generation. For example a family history of alcohol or substance abuse or depression may be a sensitive issue. For other families, the development of the Genogram is an excellent opening to the discussion of family history, herediatary health problems, or highlights the need for health education and promotion.

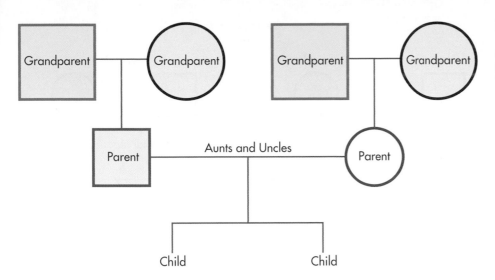

FIGURE 18-3 Genogram. (Redrawn from Wright LM, Leahey M: *Nurses and families: a guide to family assessment and intervention,* Philadelphia, 1984, FA Davis.)

Family Health Tree

The **family health tree** is another tool that is helpful to the community health nurse. Based on the genogram, the family health tree provides a mechanism for recording the family's medical and health histories (Diekelmann, 1977; Friedman, 1992; U.S. Health and Human Services, 2005). The nurse should note the following on the family health tree:

- Causes of death of deceased family members
- Genetically linked diseases, including heart disease, cancer, diabetes, hypertension, sickle cell anemia, allergies, asthma, and mental retardation
- Environmental and occupational diseases
- Psychosocial problems, such as mental illness and obesity
- Infectious diseases
- Familial risk factors from health problems
- Risk factors associated with the family's methods of illness prevention, such as having periodic physical examinations, PAP smears, and immunizations
- Lifestyle-related risk factors (i.e., by asking what family members do to "handle stress" and "keep in shape")

The family health tree can be used in planning positive familial influences on risk factors, such as diet, exercise, coping with stress, or pressure to have a physical examination. Recently, the U.S. Department of Health and Human Services (2005), under the direction of U.S. Surgeon General Richard Carmona, launched the "Family History Initiative." Included in this initiative is an online interactive tool "My Family Health Portrait" to help families learn about their risk for disease (www.hhs.gov/familyhistory). Included are questions to ask family members about common diseases, questions that suggest health promotion activities and goals as established in *Healthy People 2010.* When completed, the "family tree" can be printed. This tool could be incorporated into the family assessment and utilized by the nurse to plan family interventions to improve health.

Ecomap

The **ecomap** (Figure 18-6) is another classic tool that is used to depict a family's linkages to their suprasystems (Hartman, 1979; Wright and Leahey, 2000). As originally stated by Hartman (1978):

The eco-map portrays an overview of the family in their situation; it depicts the important nurturant or conflict-laden connections between the family and the world. It demonstrates the flow of resources, or the lacks and deprivations. This mapping procedure highlights the nature of the interfaces and points to conflicts to be mediated, bridges to be built, and resources to be sought and mobilized (p. 467).

As with the genogram, the nurse can fill out the ecomap during an early family interview, noting people, institutions, and agencies significant to the family. The nurse can use symbols used in attachment diagrams (see Figure 18-4) to denote the nature of the ties that exist. For example, in Figure 18-7, which presents a sample ecomap of the Garcia family, the ecomap suggests that few contacts occur between the family and the suprasystems. The community health nursing student was able to use the ecomap to discuss with the Garcia family the types of resources in the community and the types of relationships they wanted to establish with them.

The nurse can use these tools for family assessment with families in every health care setting. They help increase the nurse's awareness of the family within the community and help guide the nurse and the family in the assessment and planning phases of care.

FAMILY HEALTH ASSESSMENT

Many agencies in the community have developed guidelines for assessment of the family that help practitioners identify the health status of individual members of the family and aspects of family composition, function, and process. Often included in family health assessment guidelines is information about the environment, or community context, and information about the family. A **Family Health Assessment** form can be used as a guide to assist the nurse in data collection and organization of the data collected from families over time. (See **Resource Tool 18A,** Family Health Assessment Form on the book's evolve site.)

The nurse can obtain information for the Family Health Assessment through interviews with one or more family members individually, interviews of subsystems within the family (e.g., dyads of mother-child, parent-parent, and sibling-

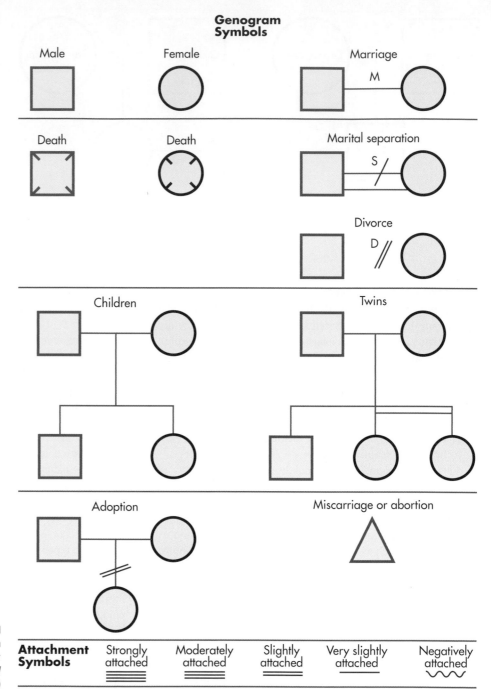

Genogram Symbols

Male	Female	Marriage
Death	Death	Marital separation
		Divorce
Children		Twins
Adoption		Miscarriage or abortion

| Attachment Symbols | Strongly attached | Moderately attached | Slightly attached | Very slightly attached | Negatively attached |

FIGURE 18-4 Genogram and attachment symbols. (Redrawn from Wright LM, Leahey M: *Nurses and families: a guide to family assessment and intervention,* Philadelphia, 1984, FA Davis.)

sibling), or group interviews with more than two members of the family. The nurse can also obtain information through observation of individual family members, dyads, and the entire family and observation of the environment in which the family lives, including housing, the neighborhood, and the larger community.

Family assessment tools have been developed by nurses and other professionals, such as sociologists, social workers, and psychologists working with families, to assess a range of dimensions of the family, such as marital satisfaction, parental coping abilities, and family dysfunction.

The Family Health Assessment addresses family characteristics, including structure and process and family environment (i.e., residence, neighborhood, and community). Not all dimensions on the Family Health Assessment will be appro-

priate for every family; therefore the nurse should modify content of the assessment guideline and adapt it as necessary to fit the individual family. The guidelines should serve as a guide only, as a means to record pertinent information about the family that will assist the nurse in working with the family. The nurse should gather information in the assessment spontaneously over several contacts with the family and various members and dyads within the family. It should also include multiple forays into the community, neighborhood, and home in which the family resides. Several contacts with the family will be required to complete the Family Health Assessment.

Social and Structural Constraints

In addition to the tools just reviewed, an important aspect of family assessment and planning for intervention is the need to

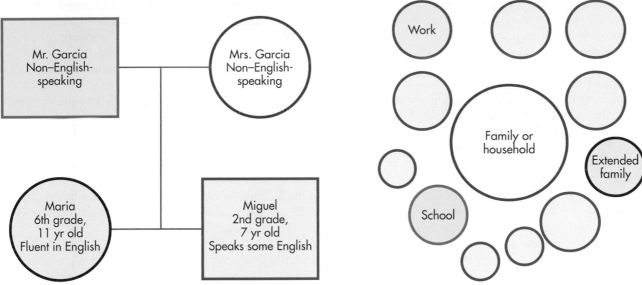

FIGURE 18-5   Sample genogram of the Garcia family.

FIGURE 18-6   Ecomap. (Redrawn from Hartman A: Diagrammatic assessment of family relationships, *Soc Casework* 59:496, 1978.)

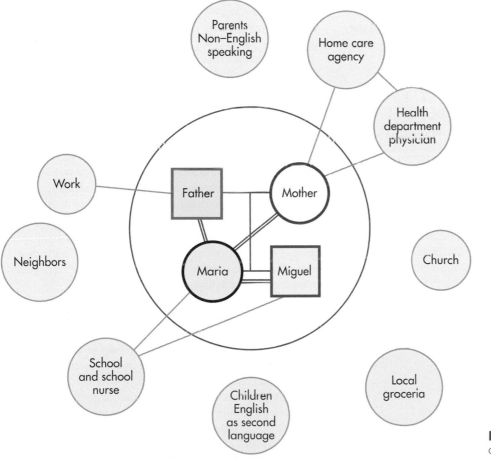

FIGURE 18-7   Sample ecomap of the Garcia family.

make note of the social and structural constraints that prevent families from receiving needed health care or achieving a state of health. These constraints explain why some families differ in mortality rates, ability to achieve "integrity" rather than "despair," or ability to "self-actualize." Social and structural constraints are usually based in social and economic causes, which affect a wide range of conditions (e.g., literacy, education, and employment) associated with major health indicators (i.e., mortality and morbidity rates). Families most frequently served by the community health nurse are disadvantaged in that they are unable to buy health care from the private sector. However, constraints to obtaining needed health and social services are well documented and may come from characteristics of health and social services rather than individual family limitations. The nurse can note these constraints on the ecomap because they influence each family's ability to interact with a specific agency. For example, in addition to noting the strength of the relationship between family and agency or institution, the nurse should note those constraints that prevent use or full use of the resource. Constraints include hours of service, distance and transportation, availability of interpreters, and criteria for receiving services (e.g., age, sex, and income barriers). Specific examples include the different guidelines posed by each state for Medicaid and by each community for home-delivered meals to the homebound.

Helping families understand constraints and linking them to accessible resources is necessary, but intervention at the family level is not sufficient. The common basic human needs of families in a community add up, and the community health nurse must tally structural constraints faced repeatedly by families and compare them with families in other communities. The nurse can then plan and implement interventions at the aggregate level. The following section is an overview of how community health nurses can extend intervention at the family level to larger aggregates and social action.

EXTENDING FAMILY HEALTH INTERVENTION TO LARGER AGGREGATES AND SOCIAL ACTION

Institutional Context of Family Therapists

Many theories exist to help bridge the gap between the application of nursing and family theory to the family and broader social action on behalf of communities of families. Most family theorists view the family as a system that interfaces with outside suprasystems or institutions only when a problem is to be addressed, such as in the school or a courtroom. The following three approaches go beyond the family as a system to address the interaction between the family and the larger social system:

- Ecological framework
- Network therapy
- Transactional model

Ecological Framework

The **ecological framework** is a blend of systems and developmental theory with an individual's understanding of his or her environment. This approach indicts the specialization and fragmentation seen in the social and health service structure based on Western concepts of time and space. This approach focuses on providing a more complex and flexible structure. Helping families transcend rigid boundaries established by health care providers and agencies is essential, as is changing the social and health service structure. For example, Kogan and others (2004) investigated parent–health care

provider discussions of family and community health risks during well-child examinations. Additionally, they studied the gaps in issues discussed by the practitioner and the information the parent desired. Based on the results of the National Survey of Early Childhood Health, health topics for discussion were identified: family financial difficulties, the presence of a support partner, parent's emotional support, alcohol and/or drug use in the home, cigarette smoking in the home, the parent's physical health, and community violence. Cigarette smoking was discussed nearly 80% of the time, and alcohol and drug use was discussed 45% of the time; however, community violence was discussed less than 10% of the time and financial needs 12%. The results indicate the need for better communication and education between health care providers and clients.

Network Therapy

Network therapy involves changing the network of families, be it extended family or friends, who tend to maintain a dysfunctional status quo in the nuclear family. This is done by replacing the network with others from the wider system that would be able to provide more support and enhance the functioning of the family. The concept of social network is related to social support. "Social network refers to a web like structure comprising one's relationships and social support focuses on the nature of the interactions taking place within social relationships" (Friedman et al., 2003, p. 462). A family's social network includes friends, community groups, church, and agencies. Social network also can be explained as the structure of relationships and social support as the function of relationships. Examples of network therapy are drawn from community mental health. In an early study evaluating the social networks of 24 people with schizophrenia 1 year after social network therapy, 12 of the 24 people showed significant improvement in their social network (Gillies et al., 1993). In comparison with the unimproved group, the improved group had an increase in the number of reciprocal relationships, an increase in the number of confidants, and improvement in scales measuring psychotic symptoms, anxiety, and depression.

In a 2005 study, Voorhees, Murray, Welk, and others studied the relationship between peer social network and physical exercise in adolescent girls. The study found that younger adolescent girls were more active than older girls and that physical activity was significantly increased in both groups when it was supported by peer networks. The study supports the idea of building support systems for at-risk populations, as proposed by social network theory.

Transactional Model

In the **transactional model**, the term *transaction* refers to a system that focuses on process as opposed to a linear approach. This may lead to blaming or labeling. The family as an institution, along with other institutions (e.g., religious, educational, recreational, or governmental), is culturally anchored (i.e., each holds a distinct set of beliefs and values about the nature of the world and human existence). An awareness of culture (e.g., beliefs and values) as it is expressed in

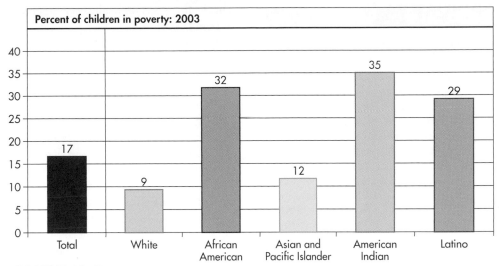

FIGURE 18-8   Percentage of children in poverty by race/ethnic groups: 2003. (From Annie E. Casey Foundation: *10 key indicators of child well-being, by race and ethnicity,* KIDS COUNT 2004 Data Book Online, The Author, http://www.aecf.org/kidscount/databook/indicators.htm.)

each system is important (i.e., as it is expressed in mainstream U.S. values vs. the value patterns of the family).

The following are examples of research using the transactional model. Many studies support the importance of parent influences on the self-esteem and resiliency of children. A study of parent influences on the self-esteem of children from economically disadvantaged families used data from both parents and their children and reported the influence of the parents on the child's self-concept and self-esteem, parental support, children's competencies, child-rearing practices, and family conflict (Killeen, 1993). In a 1999 study, Killeen used a transactional model of adolescent self-esteem to study adolescent boys and girls between the ages of 11 and 15, whose mothers experienced depression. The adolescents reported perceptions of their own behaviors and the behaviors of other adolescents. The adolescents' behaviors were also observed and described by teachers. As hypothesized, there was a positive correlation between mothers with depression and adolescent behaviors exhibiting lower self-esteem. Katsurada and Bugental (2000) used a transactional model to explore the relationship of aggressive children and their mothers. In this study, negative parenting behaviors were found to contribute to low self-esteem and aggressive behaviors in children. A Parent Perception Inventory was used, which asked the children questions such as "How often does your mother…?" and asked mothers questions such as "How often do you…?" The results of the study indicated the need for helping mothers acquire parenting styles that improve parent-child communication.

Models of Social Class and Health Services

Social class places major limitations on access to medical care. In 1997, 15% of children had no health coverage of any kind. This accounts for 10.7 million children in the United States. In 2003, the uninsured rate for children reached 19.2%. The percentage and number of children (people under 18 years old) uninsured remained the same between 2002 and 2003—at 11.4%, or 8.4 million children. Children living in poverty were more likely to be uninsured in 2003 at 19.2% compared with 11.4%. Older children were more likely not to have a source of health care than were younger children, 12.7% as compared with 10.6% (U.S. Census Bureau, 2003).

Approximately 60% of Americans were covered by employment-based health insurance plans in 2003. This was a decline from 69.9% in 2002. During this time, there was also an increase in the number of people covered by Medicare and Medicaid. Medicaid coverage increased to 12.4% and Medicare to 13.7% (U.S. Census Bureau, 2003).

Most children in poverty are white and non-Hispanic; however, the percentages of black or Hispanic children living in poverty are higher than that of white families. Figure 18-8 illustrates the percentages of American children living in poverty, compared by ethnic and racial groups.

Among these groups, there are also differences in access to health care. For example, in 2003, Hispanic people were more than twice as likely as white people to be without health care coverage (32% vs. 11%, respectively) (U.S. Census Bureau, 2003). The majorities (93%) of these children are citizens by birth but are living in homes where at least one of the adults is a noncitizen.

A classic theoretical perspective used to explain the reasons for disparities among populations was suggested three decades ago by medical sociologists as a **culture of poverty** view of life that discouraged self-reliance (Lewis, 1966). Reasons for lack of use of health services included a crisis orientation, a living-for-the-moment attitude, a low value of health, and a lack of psychological "readiness." Another explanation is the structural view, which considers constraints that limit use of medical care, such as material constraints (i.e., money to buy services), and characteristics of health care settings for the poor in contrast to private office practices for the economically stable (e.g., available hours, waiting time, transportation, block appointments, specialty clinics, and disease-oriented rather than preventive care).

Brownstein (2000) stated that the 1980s and 1990s were a time when the "rich got rich and the poor got poorer." The result has been a shift in the distribution of money and resources. Since the 1990s, there has been a decrease in the number of social programs designed to target the poor, especially the working poor. The nature of poverty continues to change, with increased numbers of the working poor in the lower class (Seccombe, 2001). Families need more support and resources than ever before but have greater financial and systems barriers, which prevent them from using the current health care system. Evidence supports the findings that unequal use of health care is likely the result of the system of care rather than of individual characteristics of people seeking care Seccomber, 2001).

Models of Care for Communities of Families

Models exist to guide the community health nurse in providing care to communities of families in special need of services that improve access, equality between consumer and provider, and sensitivity to human need. There is generally an increase in the number and type of models that emerge, as traditional public and private models of health care decline due to funding and shrinking resources. Many of the programs develop as the result of community efforts or partnerships with existing health care providers. The following are examples of models.

The Kentucky Partnership for Farm Family Health and Safety

The Kentucky Partnership is a community coalition, originally funded by WK Kellogg Funds, involving farm families, universities, and various community-based organizations.

The coalition was originally established to improve the health of farm families in rural Kentucky. Farming is identified as one of the most dangerous occupations in the United States, and few resources have been developed to support the unique needs of farm families. The Partnership identified farm women as the primary "health officers" for farm families. The farm women were provided with opportunities to develop leadership skills, conflict resolution, and team-building skills. Nurse educators and nursing students provided health education and assisted the farm women in developing a self-sustaining structure to support their efforts to improve family health. CPR and first aid classes, the development of unique emergency medical subsystems, and other activities helped improve the health of the farm families. The local members reported an increase in personal knowledge, self-esteem, and personal satisfaction through the Partnership efforts. The Kentucky Partnership for Farm Family Health and Safety continues to affect the health of farm families in south central Kentucky. The efforts are supported through the help of the South Central Kentucky Area Health Education Center at Western Kentucky University. The coalition has been replicated in three states (Texas, Louisiana, and Florida) and continues to connect universities and farm families in research efforts. Outcome assessment research was conducted to evaluate the impact of the coalition efforts on farm family health (Palermo and Ehlers, 2001).

The Health Access Nuturing Development Services (HANDS) Program

The HANDS program is a voluntary home visitation program for new and expectant parents. Implemented through interdisciplinary teams consisting of social workers, nurses, and parent resource persons, the program serves first-time pregnant mothers and their families. HANDS was originally funded through tobacco settlement monies allocated through the state legislature to the Kentucky Cabinet for Health and Family Services. The program services are provided through district health departments and currently are available throughout the Commonwealth of Kentucky. Counseling, education, and support services are provided until the child reaches school age (4-5 years of age). Referrals to the program can be made through any primary care provider such as OB-GYNs, family physicians, and/or family nurse practitioners. The HANDS team completes an assessment to identify at-risk, first-time mothers, for example, teen mothers, older first-time mothers, pregnant women lacking social support or networks, mothers with substance abuse in the home, or mothers in abusive relationships. Such women qualify as candidates for HANDS services. Regardless of the risk level, all first-time mothers may receive the services. The goal is to support families in developing successful parenting. The program is based on evidence-based interventions that result in healthy families and children. Specific outcomes of this program have not been identified; however, the growth of the program supports the need for home visitation programs such as HANDS (Kentucky Cabinet for Health and Family Services, 2005).

These alternative health programs are strategies to change the structural barriers that prevent low-income families' access to care. Professional role functions changed as nurses, rather

The school nurse, Jana, works with multiple city schools including this inner city school. The school has a low-income, ethnically diverse population.

Jana assesses the community as she drives to the Garcia's home, noting the availability of resources such as the local groceria.

Local churches are a community resource, offering socialization and spiritual support for immigrant families in the United States such as the Garcia family,

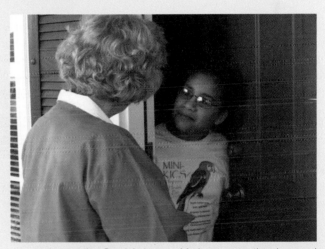

Jana arrives at the Garcia's house. Maria answers the door and invites Jana into the Garcia home.

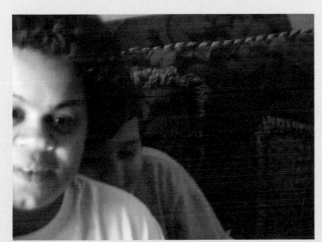

Miguel hides behind Mrs. Garcia shyly during the completion of the family assessment. Jana tries to include all family members present in the completion of the family assessment in order to develop a comprehensive family assessment.

Jana completes the family assessment of the Garcia family with the help of Maria as interpreter for Mrs. Garcia. Mrs. Garcia listens intently as Jana asks questions about the family's health needs.

Jana reviews the plan of care and confirms the family's commitment to the plan of care developed with Jana.

than physicians, provided health care. Active self-care was promoted, and health and medical knowledge was shared. Assistance by family and social networks was encouraged. Both of these programs address aspects of the health needs of populations at risk, but they do not "address the social determinants of disease." Neither program addresses the health-damaging conditions that poor people face, such as poor housing, malnutrition, and environmental hazards at the workplace and in the community. Although these programs represent steps in the right direction, changes in access to medical and health services are not enough. Social changes also are necessary.

APPLYING THE NURSING PROCESS

Home Visit

The Case Study presents the application of the nursing process to a family on a home visit. The example notes the use of the home visit to identify health needs of the family within the community and programs planned to meet those needs, which ultimately will benefit a population of families in the future.

The home visit is a crucial experience for the nursing student and family (Friedman et al., 2003). Important factors that may influence the home visit include the family's background experience with the health care system, the agency in which the nursing student is working, the family's experience with previous nursing students who have visited the family, and the student's background. For example, nursing student characteristics may vary; the student brings differing levels of knowledge of medical and nursing practice, self, and the community.

The nursing student brings previous learning about families, family-related theory, the growth and development of members of different ages within a family, disease processes, and access to the health care system. Curricula

within schools of nursing vary; therefore some students will also bring preparation in all specialties—medical-surgical nursing, childbearing, parent-child nursing, and psychiatric and mental health nursing—to the experience. Others may be taking basic clinical courses, such as pediatrics and psychiatric–mental health nursing, concurrently with community health. Thus the need for review of appropriate theory, health education, and standard assessment tools for individuals and families will vary.

The nursing student's knowledge of self, previous life experiences, and values also are important in planning for home visits. Nursing students must recognize their strengths and weaknesses in preparation for entering a new community and working with families. Additional preparation by all nursing students is necessary before the first home visit, depending on the content of the referral. The student should gather referral information, review assessment forms, and gather intervention tools (e.g., screening materials, supplies) before going to the home. Flexibility is important in working with families because the nursing student will not know the family's priority needs until the home visit.

SUMMARY

This chapter highlighted the community health nurse's work with families and identified the major family-related health care needs that the health care system has not adequately addressed. The nature of the family is changing and challenging traditional definitions and configurations. Approaches to meeting the health needs of families must go beyond that of the traditional health care system, which addresses the individual as the unit of care. Strategies were given in this chapter for expanding notions of care from the individual to the family and from the family to the community. To guide intervention with families, nurses have traditionally relied on common theoretical frameworks from the disciplines of psychology or social psychology. These frameworks often target individuals;

Text continued on p. 383

CASE STUDY | Application of the Nursing Process

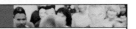

Jana Parks is a community health nurse employed by the District Health Department. She is a school health nurse, providing services for six schools in a moderately sized community. After receiving a referral from school officials related to a student's absenteeism, Jana plans to assess the student and family. (see the photo novella on pp. 379-380 for photo that defict this case study.)

ASSESSMENT

Jana knows that the school is located in the inner city, with approximately 360 students in the first through sixth grades; nearly 75% have a median family income at or below the federal poverty level. The school population is significantly more ethnically diverse than the overall community; the surrounding neighborhood frequently houses newly immigrated families. English is the second language for approximately 25% of the students, and 5% are not fluent in spoken or written English. Each year, more than 20% of the student body moves into or out of the school district.

She reviews the school records for the student, Maria Garcia, and learns that this is the first year of enrollment for the sixth grader and her second-grade brother, Miguel. Maria's family moved to the area 6 months ago from the Dominican Republic. School records note that the girl is adequately fluent in spoken English but that the parents do not speak English. The student's father works part-time at a local furniture manufacturer. There has been a noticeable decline in grades over the previous quarter, there have been no disciplinary actions, and teacher comments are positive regarding the student's classroom performance. The health record indicates that she is up-to-date with required immunizations; no chronic illnesses are noted on the school physical exam record. Jana notes that Maria's brother does not have the same school absence pattern.

Jana contacts the family and identifies her role as school health nurse. She explains the need for a meeting with the student and family to discuss concerns about Maria's school attendance. A time is scheduled when both parents and the student are available. She confirms the home address and directions.

As she drives through the neighborhood, Jana notes both single-family and multifamily dwellings; the streets are lined with parked vehicles, trash bins, and household items. As she approaches the student's home, she observes that an older model sedan is parked in the drive. The house is in need of paint and some windows have been replaced with cardboard; however, the yard is free of clutter and there are containers of blooming plants on the small porch.

Jana knocks on the door and, after a moment, states, "It's Jana Parks, the school nurse." Maria Garcia opens the door, and Jana enters a small, dimly lit room. As the student makes introductions, Mr. Garcia stands and greets Jana with a nod and handshake while Mrs. Garcia remains recumbent on the sofa but raises her hand in greeting. Mrs.

Garcia's appearance surprises Jana, as she appears much older than Mr. Garcia. Her skin color is pale, eyes are sunken, and she appears frail, with a distended abdomen and generalized muscle wasting.

Jana is aware that the exchange of social conversation is important in establishing a relationship with Hispanic clients. She mentions the beautiful picture in the room and learns that a family member painted it as a wedding gift for the Garcias. Jana learns that the family has no other relatives in the community and moved to the city through the work of a refugee assistance organization. She asks where they would like her to sit and, after a few minutes, begins to transition to a focused question interview. In this interview, Jana plans to collect information related to individual, family, and/or community functioning.

Throughout the conversation, Jana has noted that both Maria and Mr. Garcia appear tense; Mrs. Garcia is quiet and rarely speaks or smiles. Maria has translated throughout the conversation, although Jana senses that the parents may have limited understanding of spoken English. To lessen anxiety, Jana begins the interview by saying, "I am here because the school and I are concerned about Maria's absences. I want to learn why Maria misses school and to see if there are ways that the school can help."

Through the interview process, Jana learns that Maria likes school and has made friends there. She observes that Miguel stays close to Maria and frequently hides his face into her shoulder when Jana speaks to him. She also notes that Mr. and Mrs. Garcia rarely look at each other, and Mr. Garcia chooses a seat on the opposite side of the room. The family rents the home, and the father has been able supplement his part-time income by working as a day laborer for a lawn service. The family was beginning to establish connections at a local church and with neighbors when Mrs. Garcia was diagnosed with an abdominal tumor that has required numerous surgeries over the past 3 months. She is still receiving home care visits for a surgical wound that has not healed. Although Medicaid has covered most physician and hospital expenses, the family has experienced out-of-pocket expenses for noncovered medications. These problems have contributed to family financial stress. Mr. Garcia has to drive his wife to medical appointments; as a result, he is in danger of losing his job. Maria also attends these appointments to serve as the interpreter, resulting in her frequent school absences.

In addition, Jana learns that Maria has assumed responsibility for the household cooking, cleaning, and laundry since her mother's illness. Mr. Garcia shops at a small neighborhood groceria. Jana determines that with food stamps the family has adequate resources to purchase food, although Maria admits that she is still learning to cook. The family eats the evening meal together, frequently rice and beans. Maria and Miguel are eligible for subsidized breakfast and lunch at school. Maria believes that it is her responsibility to help Miguel complete his homework, get to bed on time, and attend school regularly. Mr. Garcia disciplines both children.

Continued

CASE STUDY   Application of the Nursing Process (cont'd)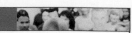

Jana asks questions regarding family health practices and learns that they see a provider at the health department only when ill or for school requirements and do not seek dental care. She observes a number of medication bottles on a table near the sofa.

DIAGNOSIS

Individual

- Caregiver role strain related to time-consuming activities, insufficient finances, and insufficient recreation (Mr. Garcia and Maria)
- Risk for injury related to improperly stored medications (Miguel)
- Knowledge deficit related to language and cultural differences (Mr. and Mrs. Garcia)
- Alterations in health maintenance related to lack of routine dental hygiene (Mr. and Mrs. Garcia, Maria and Miguel)

Family

- Risk for interrupted family processes related to change in Mrs. Garcia's ability to function, financial burden of treatments for ill family member, and disruption of family routines
- Impaired parenting related to mother's illness
- Risk of family crisis secondary to mother's prolonged illness

Community

Inadequate systematic programs for linking Hispanic families to community resources

PLANNING

A plan of care is developed to meet the needs of the individuals, family, and community. Planning involves mutual goal setting between the nurse and family; mutual setting of objectives to meet goals; prioritizing, or setting short- and long-term goals with the family; **contracting,** or establishing the division of labor between nurse and family that will meet the objectives; and evaluation of the process and outcome.

Individual

Long-Term Goals

- Mr. Garcia will recognize appropriate roles and responsibilities for Maria. He will identify and use resources to allow her to resume suitable educational, social, and family duties.
- Mr. Garcia will identify and use community resources to assist with transportation needs and medication costs.
- Mr. and Mrs. Garcia need long-term dental care and education. Jana noted a long-term need to discuss dental care.
- Mr. and Mrs. Garcia will improve their English comprehension and speaking skills.

Short-Term Goals

- Relieve Maria of interpreting at medical appointments by identifying alternate interpretive resources.
- Store medications in a secure location.

Family

Long-Term Goal

- The family will be able to find and use appropriate services for physical and social support.

Short-Term Goal

- The family will learn to appropriately express their feelings related to the mother's illness, social isolation, role strain, and/or fear.

Community

Long-Term Goal

- The community will establish programs to support immigrant family needs for transportation, interpretation, and enculturation to the American medical system.

Short-Term Goal

- Mr. Garcia will identify existing programs available to support Hispanic immigrants.

INTERVENTION

- Jana recognizes that many interventions must be carried out at the individual, family, and community levels.

Individual

- Education regarding safe medication storage
- Referral to the Refugee Assistance Society or local churches for interpretive assistance

Family

Direct nursing interventions directed at family functioning include the following levels:

- Cognitive: new information is provided to the family usually educational that promotes problem solving by the family. An example is referring the Garcias to the community free clinic for medical and dental care.
- Affective: families are encouraged to express their feelings that may be blocking their efforts at problem solving. An example of this would be Jana's planned validation of Mr. Garcia's concerns regarding finances and the threat of losing employment.
- Behavioral: tasks are negotiated to be carried out either during the family interview or as homework between visits. An example is Mr. Garcia's planned call to the Refugee Assistance Society.

Community

Jana recognizes that her referral of Mr. Garcia to the Refugee Assistance Society to obtain support through existing

Continued

CASE STUDY   Application of the Nursing Process (cont'd)

programs is also an intervention at the community level. She engages in ongoing parafamily work to identify how the community can be mobilized to provide physical, mental and social support to immigrant families. Does anyone at the community free clinic speak Spanish? Are interpreters available at health care facilities? Where do most immigrant families receive health care and social support? Are classes on English as a second language free-of-charge for Hispanic families? Are job skill training or courses available for Mr. Garcia? Questions such as these bring up many areas of assessment that Jana will need to make with the Garcia family and the community in the future.

EVALUATION

Individual/Family

Jana assists the Garcias to obtain a small lockable box in which to store medication. Mr. Garcia establishes contact with a local church that provides a volunteer interpreter and driver for medical visits and twice-weekly delivery of meals. Mr. Garcia takes Maria and Miguel to the free clinic where dental sealants are applied to molars. The social worker at the community's free clinic meets with Mr. Garcia to offer him assistance in obtaining low-cost medications. Through this conversation, Jana identifies his reluctance to ask for financial assistance. He states that he should provide for his family and that Maria should not have to assume the role of mother for Miguel. However, he does not see any other options at this time. She identifies that Mr. Garcia may be in need of ongoing support and suggests that he talk with a counselor about his concerns. Mr. Garcia refuses to see a counselor, but agrees that he will talk to the pastor of his church. Maria and Miguel meet with the school counselor as needed to discuss feelings related to the mother's illness and resulting family strain.

Community

Jana identified that many community resources are available to immigrant families; however, information is limited and not readily accessible. She contacts the director of the Refugee Assistance Society, and together they initiate a community coalition to address this issue.

LEVELS OF PREVENTION

Society's expectations of the family are in transition. Application of the levels of prevention to families by the community nurse must take into account the changing family configuration; the financial, emotional, and physical burdens often compounded in the single-parent family; and the lack of resources such as non-existing health insurance or inadequate health insurance.

Developed by Mary Kovar, RN, MSN, and Barbara Minix, RN, MSN.

---

frameworks are needed that go beyond the individual to the family and community and address social and policy changes needed to alter the social, economic, and environmental conditions under which families must function. This chapter provided tools for assessing the family and the family within the community, and gave examples of the extension of family health intervention to larger aggregates, which involves social action to overcome constraints to accessing health services. Non-nursing and community health nursing models of care provided for communities of families were presented and critiqued. The nursing process was applied at the individual, family, and community levels on a home visit. Examples of interventions by the community health nurse at individual, family, and community levels were presented.

Families remain the core of society, with diversity as the constant for families in the United States. Family nursing must be understood and practiced by community health nurses. An understanding of family theory provides a mechanism for assessing and intervening with families to improve their level of wellness and increase the health of the community as a whole.

LEARNING ACTIVITIES

1. Define the term *family* with a group of three colleagues. Compare definitions and list similarities and differences. Develop a list of criteria for being a member of a family.

2. Complete a personal genogram. What are the high-risk factors in the family history? Current risk factors? Categorize current risk factors into physical, interpersonal, and environmental. Identify needed health education and determine who needs the education. Identify sources of appropriate screening in the community for the identified risk factors.

3. Complete a personal ecomap. Is the family an "open" or "closed" family system? What resources do families currently use for mental, physical, emotional, social, and community health? What referrals are needed?

4. Identify family types or situations (e.g., families of different cultures, gay or lesbian families, or never-married mother families) that elicit "discomfort" in working situations. Identify ways to overcome barriers in working with these types of families.

REFERENCES

Allen DR, Fine MA, Demo HD: An overview of family diversity: controversies, questions, and values. In Demo DH, Allen KR, Fine MA, editors: *Handbook of family diversity,* New York, 2000, Oxford Press.

Allen JK, Blumenthal RS: Risk factors in the off-spring of women with premature coronary heart disease. *Am Heart J* 135:3:428-34, 1998.

Allmond BW, Buckman W, Gofman HF: *The family is the patient,* St. Louis, 1979, Mosby.

American Association of Retired Persons (AARP): Help for grandparents raising grandchildren, The Author, http://www.aarp.org/families/grandparents/raising_grand child/.

Anderson MP, O'Grady RS, Anderson IL: Public health nursing in primary care: impact on home visits, *Public Health Nurs* 2:145, 1985.

Annie E. Casey Foundation: *10 key indicators of child well-being, by race and ethnicity,* KIDS COUNT 2004 Data Book Online, http://www.aecf.org/kidscount/databook/indicators.htm.

Auger, JR: *Behavioral systems and nursing,* Englewood Cliffs, NJ, 1976 Prentice-Hall.

Beard M: Home nursing, *Public Health Nurs Q* 7:44-51, 1999.

Black C, Ford-Gilboe M: Adolescent mothers: resilience, family health work and health-promoting practices, *J Adv Nurs* 48(4):351-160, 2004.

Brownstein R: Government should work harder to help those left behind by booming economy, *Los Angeles Times,* Oct 11, 1999:A5.

Capps R, Fix M, Passell JS: *The dispersal of immigrants in the 1990s,* Washington, DC, 2002, The Urban Institute.

Capps R et al: *The health and well being of young children of immigrants,* Washington, DC, 2004, The Urban Institute.

Carter E, McGoldrick M: The family life cycle and family therapy: an overview. In Carter E, McGoldrick M, editors: *The family life cycle: a framework for family therapy,* New York, 1980, Gardner Press.

Carter E, McGoldrick M, editors: *The changing family life cycle: a framework for family therapy,* ed 2, New York, 1988, Gardner Press.

Cody WK: Nursing frameworks to guide practice and research with families, *Nurs Sci Q* 13(4):277-284, 2000.

Cohen PN: *Racial-ethnic and gender differences in returns to cohabitation and marriage: evidence from the current population survey,* Washington, DC, 1999, US Census Bureau.

Conger RD et al: Angry and aggressive behavior across three generations, *J Abnormal Child Psychol* 31:143-161, 2003.

Cook E: *The life of Florence Nightingale,* vol 2, London, 1913, MacMillan.

Curran D: *Traits of a healthy family,* Minneapolis, Minn, 1983, Harper and Row.

Diekelmann N: *Primary health care of the well adult,* New York, 1977, McGraw-Hill.

Dreher MC: The conflict of conservatism in public health nursing education, *Nurs Outlook* 30:504, 1982.

Dunn HL: *High-level wellness,* Arlington, Va, 1961, RW Beatty.

Duvall EM: *Marriage and family relationships,* ed 5, Philadelphia, 1977, JB Lippincott.

Duvall EM, Miller BC: *Marriage and family development,* ed 6, New York, 1985, Harper and Row.

Erikson E: *Childhood and society,* ed 2, New York, 1963, WW Norton.

Families USA: *Children in jeapardy,* Special Report, Washington, DC, 2002, The Author, http://www.familiesusa.org.

Freeman R: *Public health nursing practice,* ed 3, Philadelphia 1963, WB Saunders.

Friedman MM: *Family nursing: theory and assessment,* ed 3, East Norwalk, Conn, 1998, Appleton-Lange.

Friedman MM, Bowden VB, Jones EG: *Family nursing: research, theory and practice,* ed 3, Upper Saddle River, NJ, 2003, Prentice Hall.

Gillies LA et al: Differential outcomes in social network therapy, *Psychosoc Rehabil J* 16:141, 1993.

Glaser B, Strauss AL: *Chronic illness and the quality of life,* St. Louis, 1975, Mosby.

Hanson S, Mischke KB: Family health assessment and intervention. In Bomar PJ, editor: *Nurses and family health promotion: concepts, assessment, and interventions,* ed 2, Philadelphia, 1996, WB Saunders.

Hanson SH: Family and family nursing in the 21st century. In Hanson SH, editor: *Family health care nursing: theory, practice and research,* ed 2, Philadelphia, 2001, FA Davis.

Hartman A: Diagrammatic assessment of family relationships, *Soc Casework* 59:465, 1978.

Hartman A: *Finding families: an ecological approach to family assessment in adoption,* Beverly Hills, 1979, Sage.

Hopia H, Paavilainen E, Astedt-Kurki P: Promoting the health for families of children with chronic conditions, *J Adv Nurs* 48(6):575-583, 2004.

Jordheim AD: Alternative life-styles and the family. In Reinhardt AM, Quinn MD, editors: *Family-centered community nursing: a sociological framework,* St. Louis, 1982, Mosby.

Kentucky Cabinet for Health and Family Services: HANDS program, Frankfort, Ky, 2005, The Author, http://chfs.ky.gov/dph/ach/hands/htm.

Killeen MR: Parent influences on children's self-esteem in economically disadvantaged families, *Issues Ment Health Nurs* 14:323, 1993.

Killeen MR: A transactional model of adolescent self-esteem, *J Fam Psychol* 12(1):132-149, 1999.

Klever P: The multigenerational transmission of nuclear family processes and symptoms, *Am J Fam Ther* 32:337-351, 2004.

Kogan MD et al: Routine assessment of family and community health risks: parent views

and what they receive *Pediatrics* 113(6):1934-1943, 2004.

Leahey M et al: The impact of a family systems nursing approach: nurses' perceptions, *J Cont Educ Nurs* 25(5):219-225, 1995.

Lewis O: The culture of poverty, *Sci Am* 215:19, 1966.

Manley M, Graber A: Coronary prevention program in a community hospital, *Heart Lung* 6:1045, 1977.

Maslow A: *Motivation and personality,* ed 2, New York, 1970, Harper and Row.

Miller FM: *Coping with chronic illness: overcoming powerlessness,* Philadelphia, 2000, FA Davis.

Minuchin P: Looking toward horizon: present and future in study of family systems. In McHale JP, Grolnick WS, editors: *Psychological study of families,* Mahwah, NJ, 2002, Lawrence Erlbaum.

Montalvo B: Useful coincidences and family strengths, *Contemp Fam Ther* 26(2):117-119, 2004.

Murray CI: *Nursing concepts for health promotion,* ed 4, Thousand Oaks, Calif, 2004, Sage.

National League for Nursing: *A curriculum guide for schools of nursing,* New York, 1937, The Author.

Neis MA, McEwen M: *Community health nursing: Promiting the health of populations,* ed 3, Philadelphia, 2001, WB Saunder

Otto H: A framework for assessing family strengths. In Reinhard A, Quinn M, editors: *Family-centered community health nursing,* St. Louis, 1973, Mosby.

Palermo T, Ehlers J: *Coalitions: building partnerships to promote agricultural health and safety,* Washington DC, 2001, National Institutes for Occupational Health and Safety, http://www.cdc.gov/nasd/doc/d001701-d001774.html.

Palermo T, Ehlers J: Coalitions: Partnership to promote agricultural health and safety, *J Agr Safety Health,* 8(2):161-174, 2002.

Patterson CJ: Lesbian and gay parent-hood in Bornstein M, editors: *Handbook of Parenting* ed 2, Mahwah NJ, 2002, Erlbaum.

Patterson JM: Healthy American families in a postmodern society: an ecological perspective. In Green WH et al, editor: *Health and welfare for families in the 21st century,* Boston, 1999, Jones and Bartlett.

Pratt L: *Family structure and effective health behavior,* Boston, 1976, Houghton Mifflin.

Puskar KR, Lamb JM, Bartolovic M: Examining the common stressors and coping methods of rural adolescents, *Nurs Pract* 18:50, 1993.

Rodriquez N, Hagan J, Capps R: *The effects of recent welfare and immigration reforms on immigrants,* Washington DC, 2004, The Urban Institute.

Ross MM, Helmer H: A comparative analysis of Neuman's model using the individual and family as the units of care, *Public Health Nurs* 5:30, 1988.

Saksvig B, Jobe JB: The role of peer social network factors and physical activity in adolescent girls, *Am J Health Behav* 29(2): 183-190, 2005.

Saluter AF: *Marital status and living arrangements: March 1993,* Current Population Reports P20-478, Washington, DC, 1994, US Census Bureau.

Sameroff AJ: Developmental systems and family functioning. In Parke RD, Kellam SG, editors: *Exploring family relations with other social contexts,* Hillsdale, NJ, 1994, Lawrence Erlbaum.

Seccombe K: Families in poverty in the 1990s: Trends, causes, consequences, and lessons learned. In Milardo RM, editor: *Understanding families into the new millennium,* Minneapolis, Minn, 2001, National Council on Family Relations.

Stern PN: Affiliating in stepfather families: teachable strategies leading to stepfather-child friendship, *West J Nurs Res* 4:75, 1982a.

Stern PN: Conflicting family culture: an impediment to integration in stepfather families, *J Psychosoc Nurs Ment Health Serv* 20:27, 1982b.

Swanson JM, Nies MA: *Community health nursing: promoting the health of aggregates,* ed 3, Philadelphia, 2001, WB Saunders.

Teachman JD, Tedrow LM, Crowder KD: The changing demographics of America's families. In Milardo RM, editor: *Understanding families in the new millennium: a decade in review,* Minneapolis, Minn, 2001, National Council on Family Relations.

US Census Bureau: *Current Population Survey,* Washington, DC, March 2003, The Author, http://www.uscensus.gov.

US Census Bureau: *How we're changing: demographic state of the nation 2005,* Washington DC, April 2005, The Author, http://www.census.gov.

US Census Bureau: *Population profile of the nation: dynamic version 2005,* Washington DC, April 2005, The Author, http://www.census.gov/population/www/pop-profile/profiledynamic.html.

US Department of Health and Human Services: *Healthy People 2010,* Washington, DC, 2000, US Government Printing Office, http://www.healthypeople.gov/.

US Department of Health and Human Services: New family history tool promotes prevention, *Nation's Health* 34(10):33, 2005.

Voorhees CC, Piercy RC, Fred P: Children of separation: an annotated bibliography for professionals. *J Marital Fam Ther* 22(1): 149; 1996.

von Bertalanffy L: *General systems theory: foundations, development, applications,* New York, 1968, George Braziller.

von Bertalanffy L: The history and status of general systems theory. In Klir G, editor: *Trends in general systems theory,* New York, 1972, Wiley.

von Bertalanffy L: General systems theory and psychiatry. In Arieti S, editor: *American handbook of psychiatry,* New York, 1974, Basic Books.

Wald L: The family as a unit of care: a historical review, *Public Health Nurs* 3: 427-428, 515-519, 1904.

Women's Educational Media: *It's elementary: why address gay issues with children,* The Author, http://www.womedia.org/ic_why address.htm.

World Health Organization: *The family health nurse: context, conceptual framework and curriculum for the European region for the 21st century* ERU/00/5019309/1300074, Denmark, 2000, The Author.

World Health Organization: *Health 21: The health for all policy framework for the WHO Europoean region.* Copenhagen, WHO/EURO, No 6, p 139.

Wright LM, Leahey M: *Nurses and families: a guide to family assessment and intervention,* Philadelphia, 1984, FA Davis.

Wright LM, Leahey M: *Nurses and families: a guide to family assessment and intervention,* ed 2, Philadelphia, 1994, FA Davis.

Wright LM, Leahey M: Maximizing time, minimizing suffering: the 15-minute (or less) family interview, *J Fam Nurs* 5(1):259, 1999.

Wright LM, Leahey M: *Nurses and family: a guide to family assessment and intervention,* ed 3, Philadelphia, 2000, FA Davis.

Yarnell J et al: Family history, longevity, and risk of coronary heart disease, *Inter J Epidemiol* 32:71-77, 2003.

UNIT 5

Vulnerable Populations

Populations Affected by Disabilities

Linda L. Treloar ▪ Barbara M. Artinian

MEDIA RESOURCES

Additional Material for Study, Review, and Further Exploration

evolve Website at http://evolve.elsevier.com/Nies

❖ Quiz ❖ Case Studies ❖ Content Updates ❖ Glossary ❖ WebLinks

OBJECTIVES

Upon completion of this chapter, the reader will be able to do the following:

1. Differentiate between medical model and social construct definitions for disability.
2. Describe historical attitudes and perspectives surrounding disability that have contributed to devaluation and disempowerment of people with disabilities.
3. Compare and contrast short- and long-term, health-related, disabling conditions.
4. Discuss key federal legislation applicable to people with disabilities.
5. Identify selected health care and social issues that influence the ability of people with disabilities to live and thrive in the community.
6. Apply a nursing model that integrates a holistic focus promoting the health and well-being of people with disabilities and their families.

KEY TERMS

activities of daily living (ADLs)
Americans With Disabilities
   Act (ADA)
disability

handicap
functional activities
impairment

Individuals with Disabilities
   Education Act (IDEA)
instrumental activities of daily

living (IADLs)
Intersystem Model
reasonable accommodations

CHAPTER OUTLINE

SELF-ASSESSMENT: RESPONSES TO DISABILITY

DEFINITIONS AND MODELS FOR DISABILITY
   National Agenda for Prevention of Disabilities Model
   Quality of Life Issues in Disability

CHARACTERISTICS OF DISABILITY
   Measurement of Disability
   Prevalence of Disability
   Health status of the Elderly
   Health Status and Causes of Disability

COSTS ASSOCIATED WITH DISABILITY
   Economic Well-Being and Employment
   Long-Term Care and Personal Assistance Support
   Health Insurance and Public Health Programs

***HEALTHY PEOPLE 2010* AND THE HEALTH NEEDS OF PEOPLE WITH DISABILITIES**

A HISTORICAL CONTEXT FOR DISABILITY
   Early Attitudes Toward People With Disabilities
   Attitudes Toward People With Disabilities
    in the Eighteenth and Nineteenth Centuries

   Disability in the Twentieth Century
   Contemporary Conceptualizations of People
    With Disabilities

DISABILITY AND PUBLIC POLICY
   Legislation Affecting People With Disabilities

RECONCEPTUALIZING HEALTH CARE FOR PEOPLE WITH DISABILITIES

THE PERSONAL EXPERIENCE OF DISABILITY
   Family and Caregiver Responses to a Disabled Member

THE INTERSYSTEM MODEL

STRATEGIES FOR THE COMMUNITY HEALTH NURSE IN CARING FOR PEOPLE WITH DISABILITIES

ETHICAL ISSUES FOR PEOPLE AFFECTED BY DISABILITIES
   Nursing Education and Practice When the Nurse
    Is Disabled

After developing an incomplete spinal cord injury following an automobile accident, a 29-year-old man named Jim progressed from visible physical disability and paralysis to continued disability without the use of a wheelchair. Jim explained his progression, which follows:

> You know it's really weird. In some ways it's hard to enter into that wheelchair life, to go into that life and then come back out of it again. I entered into a whole other realm [life with paralysis] that I'd only observed. I stepped into the unknown and pulled back out of it again. Yet, one foot is still in that world (Treloar, 1999c, p. 189).

According to Jim, disability may create a "whole other realm," or an "unknown" world. Like Jim, most people lack awareness of the divergence of perceptual worlds that disability creates and the historical, sociopolitical context and culture that surround disability. Nurses may think they understand disability, but this may not be true. Attitudes toward disability influence people's responses to and care for others; therefore nurses should consider the following self-assessment.

SELF-ASSESSMENT: RESPONSES TO DISABILITY

What comes to mind when you think of *someone with a disability?* Focus on those sights, sounds, and smells. What are your thoughts and feelings? List characteristics using adjectives or short phrases to describe people with disabilities. What values, customs, and traditions are promoted or blocked by members of the group?

Picture yourself as a *person with a disability.* What do you notice? What concerns you? How do others respond to you? Who or what kinds of supports can you rely on for help? What do you wish others understood about disability?

Now imagine living in a *family affected by disability.* How does disability affect you and your family? What activities does your family engage in that are associated with disability? What family or personal activities are more difficult to perform with a disability? How do people respond to your disability or your family member's disability? What do you wish others understood about living in a family affected by disability? What kinds of social and personal supports do you have? What kinds of supports do you wish were available to families like yours?

Think about your health as a *person with a disability.* What are your health care concerns and needs? What has been your experience with the health care system and its providers? What do you want nurses and others to understand about living with disability? How might health care professionals devalue and disempower you? How can nurses and other health care providers care for you in a way that conveys respect and concern for you as a person?

What is the experience of *living with disability within your community?* What social or environmental barriers related to disability exist? How can nurses intervene to reduce or eliminate these barriers? What major roles can nurses perform in working within an interdisciplinary team model that forms alliances with the client and family affected by disability?

What implications exist for health care policy and research related to disability?

Health care professionals are taught to assess and provide interventions that promote health and they usually believe they know what people with disabilities need. However, the actions of health care professionals may convey different messages to people with disabilities and their families. Regardless of their professional experience or familiarity with disability, clients may ask how they can understand disability if they are not themselves disabled.

Disability affects people irrespective of class, culture, race, or economic level. Depending on the term's definition, disability affects about 20% of Americans. Disability increases with age, often influencing a person's ability to maintain self-care, essential to living in their preferred living environment. This chapter provides content that community health nurses can use in a variety of settings to provide knowledgeable, appropriate care for people with disabilities and their families.

DEFINITIONS AND MODELS FOR DISABILITY

In 1980, the World Health Organization (WHO) developed a tool for classifying the consequences of disease, called the International Classification of Impairments, Disabilities, and Handicaps (ICIDH) (WHO, 1980). Although the tool was modified and renamed in 2001 as The International Classification of Functioning, Disability, and Health (ICF), the following definitions remain in use (WHO, 2001). A **disability** involves any restriction or inability (resulting from an impairment) in performing an activity in a normal manner or within the normal range. An anatomical, mental, or psychological loss or abnormality is an **impairment.** A **handicap** is a disadvantage resulting from an impairment or disability that prevents fulfillment of an expected role. In comparing these concepts, an impairment affects a human organ on a micro level; disability affects a person on an individual level; and a handicap involves society on a macro level of analysis (Batavia, 1993). Table 19-1 compares and contrasts these definitions related to disability.

A similar framework for disability is described by the Nagi model, which uses functional limitations to determine disability (Pope and Tarlov, 1991). Whether a disability becomes a handicap depends on how the person functions in the community. Impairments do not necessarily result in disabilities and disabilities do not necessarily produce handicaps. Although the WHO and Nagi frameworks recognize that a person's ability to perform a socially expected activity reflects characteristics of the individual and the larger social and physical environment, they are commonly criticized for their medical emphasis and definitional inconsistencies.

National Agenda for Prevention of Disabilities Model

The Committee on a National Agenda for the Prevention of Disabilities (NAPD) conceptualized a model for disability (Figure 19-1) that extends the ICIDH (ICF) and Nagi

TABLE 19-1   Terminology for Impairment, Disability, and Handicap

CHARACTERISTIC	IMPAIRMENT	DISABILITY	HANDICAP
Definition	Physical deviation from normal structure, function, physical organization, or development	Restricted ability to perform an activity in normal or expected manner; what activity the person cannot perform	Disadvantage imposed by impairment or disability related to environment
Measurability	Objective and measurable	May be objective and measurable	Not objective or measurable; is an experience related to the responses of others
Illustrations	Spina bifida, spinal cord injury, amputation, and detached retina	Cannot walk unassisted; uses crutches and/or a manual or power wheelchair; blindness	Reflects physical and psychological characteristics of the person, culture, and specific circumstances
Level of analysis	Micro level (e.g., body organ)	Individual level (e.g., person)	Macro level (e.g., societal)

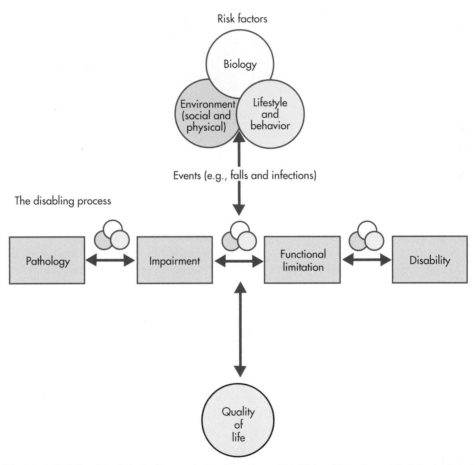

FIGURE 19-1   Model of disability. (Reprinted with permission from Pope AM, Tarlov AR, editors: Disability in America: toward a national agenda for prevention, Washington, DC, 1991, Institute of Medicine, National Academy Press. Copyright 1991 by the National Academy of Sciences. Courtesy National Academy Press, Washington, DC.)

frameworks. In the NAPD model, disability occurs when a person's physical or mental limitations, in interaction with physical and social barriers in the environment, prevent the person from taking equal part in the normal life of the community (Pope and Tarlov, 1991). Furthermore, disability develops through a complex, interactive process involving biological, behavioral, and environmental (i.e., social and physical) risk factors and quality of life (QOL). In this social model for disability, *bodily impairments and functional limitations are not necessarily accompanied by disability.* Disability

may be preventable and preventive measures can promote an improved QOL and reduce costs related to dependence, lost productivity or unemployment, and medical care.

Risk Factors

Three categories of risk factors for disability are identified in this model. These include *biological* (e.g., Rh type), *environmental* (e.g., access to care or exposure to lead paint), and *lifestyle and behavioral* characteristics (e.g., overeating or smoking) that influence health-related conditions.

The Disabling Process

The model provides an alternative framework for viewing four related and distinct stages in the disabling process. *Pathology* at the cellular and tissue level may produce an *impairment* in structure or function at the organ level. An individual with an *impairment* may experience a *functional limitation,* which restricts his or her ability to perform an action within the normal range. The functional limitation may result in a *disability* when certain socially defined activities and roles cannot be performed.

Although the model appears to indicate unidirectional progression from pathology, to impairment, to functional limitation, to disability, stepwise or linear progression may not occur. Disability prevention efforts can address any of the risk factors or stages in the disabling process. Health promotion efforts include primary prevention of disability, secondary reversal of disability and restoration of function, and tertiary prevention of complications.

Quality of Life Issues in Disability

Quality of life perspectives cannot be separated from considerations related to the disabling process. Enabling or disabling influences created by environmental and social barriers often affect QOL for people with disabilities. Barriers to access may be geographical (e.g., location of services), financial (e.g., cost of care), organizational (e.g., appointment difficulties, prolonged waiting room time, transportation or referral difficulties), and cultural (e.g., language barriers or differences in health belief models) (Lawthers, et al., 2003). Denied, delayed, or inappropriate access to needed health services negatively affects quality of life, and contributes to other detrimental effects for the health, well being, and independence of persons with disabilities (Neri & Kroll, 2003). The text insets provide illustrations of common barriers and their impact on living with disability. Community nurses who are sensitive to challenges inherent to living with disability, can partner with clients and families to remedy barriers that negatively affect quality of life for this population. Most important, quality of life is promoted when nurses "consider all aspects of an individual's life rather than focusing narrowly on health issues" (Northway and Jenkins, 2003, p. 62).

CLINICAL EXAMPLE

Cathy sought an eye examination at an optical center in a local department store where she did much of her shopping. Although the receptionist advised her that no one could see her for several months, she noted that the woman in line behind her received an appointment for the following day. Cathy left the store feeling puzzled and angry. She called several optical offices and advised them that unless their equipment could accommodate her motorized wheelchair, someone would need to lift her into the examining chair and hold her upright throughout the eye examination. The limitations of the optical equipment required someone to assist Cathy during the examination. After she contacted several potential providers, Cathy finally obtained an appointment.

One optometrist chose to see Cathy when the others failed. Physically disabled himself, the optometrist had a mobility impairment as evidenced by a limp. Although his functional limitations and the

RESEARCH HIGHLIGHTS

Disability, Spiritual Beliefs, and the Church

Perhaps you've wondered: Why is it that some people affected by disabilities become embittered, while others choose to live with joy? In the presence of a well-established literature on coping with disabilities, little is known about how people use spiritual beliefs to establish meaning for and respond to life with disability. While holism is a major tenent of nursing practice, many nurses may find it easier to address concerns of the body and the mind, as compared with those of the spirit.

The author interviewed 30 persons, comprised of parents with disabled children and adults with disabilities, leading to recommendations for caregivers and leaders in the Christian church. Although the qualitative research design limits generalizability of the findings, this study and the literature support recognition of spiritual beliefs as a stabilizing force for people affected by disabilities. Trial or difficulty contributed to spiritual challenges and the breaking of self, leading to reliance on God, and strengthened faith in God. The participants in the study viewed their lives with purpose; they chose to live with joy and thankfulness, despite difficulties associated with disability.

Consistent with an emphasis on holism, nurses should ensure that spiritual needs and resources are considered in caring for persons affected by disability. This includes collaboration with pastoral caregivers. Assisting this population to achieve spiritual well-being promotes health that transcends physical, cognitive, or emotional limitations.

Treloar, LL: Disability, spiritual beliefs and the church: the experiences of adults with disabilities and family members. *J of Adv Nurs* 40(5): 594-603, 2002.

extent of his disability were much less severe than Cathy's, he also experienced societal bias and discrimination related to disability. Unfortunately, when people saw Cathy's wheelchair or heard about her potential need for accommodation, their attitudes may have transformed her disability into a handicap. ■

CHARACTERISTICS OF DISABILITY

Whether someone has a disability depends on the criteria used. The Americans With Disabilities Act (ADA) of 1990 and the Rehabilitation Act of 1973 defined a disability by the limitations in carrying out a major life activity. Physical disabilities, sensory disabilities (e.g., being deaf or blind), intellectual disabilities (i.e., contemporary terminology for mental retardation), serious emotional disturbances, learning disabilities, significant chemical and environmental sensitivities, and health problems such as AIDS and asthma are examples of disabilities that may substantially limit at least one *major life activity.* Major life activities include the ability to breathe, walk, see, hear, speak, work, care for oneself, perform manual tasks, and learn.

DISABILITY: A SOCIALLY CONSTRUCTED ISSUE

Much of the complexity in defining disability stems from its socially constructed nature. If disability were a fixed medical or social fact, it could be relatively easily determined. However, because disability is more usefully conceptualized as the inability to perform important life functions, it becomes a product of interaction between health status and the demands of one's physical and social environment. Thus using a wheelchair is disabling in a workplace with steps and narrow doorways, but much less so in one with ramps and wide passageways. Similarly, cultural beliefs and attitudes shape the extent to which an impairment is disabling, and the extent to which people with physical or mental impairments are able to function in jobs and more broadly in public life (Scotch, 1994, p. 172). ∎

Measurement of Disability

The U.S. Census Bureau defines disability as a long-lasting physical, mental, or emotional condition that creates a limitation or inability to function according to certain criteria. It collects disability data through four household surveys. One of these, the Survey of Income and Program Participation (SIPP) that includes an extensive set of disability questions which include limitations in **functional activities** (e.g., seeing, hearing, speaking, walking, using stairs, and lifting and carrying items), **activities of daily living (ADLs)** (e.g., getting around inside the home, getting in and out of a bed or chair, bathing, dressing, eating, or toileting), and **instrumental activities of daily living (IADLs)** (e.g., going outside the home, shopping, tracking money or bills, light housecleaning, and preparing meals). It gathers data on whether people use an adaptive mobility device (e.g. wheelchair, cane, crutches, or walker) for 6 or more months; have a mental or emotional disability; have an impairment that produces on-the-job limitations or the inability to perform housework, or that involves the disability status of children (U.S. Census Bureau, SIPP, 2004b). Small sample size limits application of SIPP data estimates to regional areas, select states, and metropolitan areas. More importantly, poor test-retest reliability in follow-up surveys and divergent reporting by respondents limits the use of SIPP data by researchers (Disability Statistics Center, 2005).

A second instrument, the American Community Survey (ACS), gathers estimates of demographic, housing, social, and economic characteristics for both long and short terms for the civilian household population, *excluding* those in group settings, such as institutions and college dormitories. This survey asks respondents whether they have a disability limitation in six areas that affect a certain function or activity, such as sensory perception, physical activities, mental and emotional state, self-care, ability to leave home, and employment options (U.S. Census Bureau, ACS, 2004a). Eventually, the ACS will be implemented annually in all states, providing changes in estimates over time for small geographic areas and population groups.

A third instrument used by the U.S. Census Bureau, the Current Population Survey (CPS), while not designed to measure disability, asks questions to determine if people are less able or unable to work because of a health condition or disability. The final source of disability data collected by the U.S. Census Bureau comes from the Decennial Census of Population and Housing. Limited data on disability is collected through two major questions, which aim to identify people with a sensory or other impairment that limits one or more

basic physical activities, and determine whether these people have long-lasting functional limitations as a result.

Disability Measurement Challenges

Variation in definitions and measurement parameters for disability make uniform measures of disability difficult. In 2003, ACS changed the layout of the questions, therefore data obtained from the 2003 and later ACS surveys are not comparable to findings in earlier versions of the ACS or to previous decennial census items. To illustrate, U.S. Census 2000 data revealed that 48.9 million people (19.2%) who were 5 years old or older and living in housing units had a disability. This compares with an estimated 39.7 million (15.6%) of the population surveyed by the Census 2000 Supplementary Survey (C2SS), a sample that used the ACS design (Stern, 2004a; 2004b). Prevalence rates were similar for sensory, physical, mental, self-care, and go-outside-home disability, but varied dramatically for employment disability (9.4% for C2SS and 12.9% for Census 2000). Stern and Brault (2005) suggest that relatively minor differences in survey methodology contributed to statistical differences in measurement. Similarly, comparisons between Census 1990 and Census 2000 data are not recommended because of major differences in disability questions used in each survey.

In addition to the U.S. Census Bureau, many organizations collect disability data (see the U.S. Census Bureau disability home page [http://www.census.gov/hhes/www/disability/disability.html] for an extensive list). For example, the National Health Interview Survey on Disability (NHIS-D) conducted by the National Center for Health Statistics (NCHS) in 1994 and 1995 measured disability according to limitations in activity associated with chronic health conditions and particular age groups. Levels of severity also varied. In comparison, the SIPP focuses on an inability to perform physical activities, whereas the NHIS-D measured the need for assistance in activities. This discussion illustrates ongoing challenges with measurement of disability data.

Prevalence of Disability

According to Census 2000 estimates (U.S. Census Bureau, 2003), about 50 million people (19.3%) of the civilian non-institutionalized population aged 5 years and older, nearly 1 in every 5 persons, have a long-lasting condition or disability. As indicated in Table 19-2, the majority report physical limitations (8.2%), with fewer people reporting sensory limitations that impair sight or hearing (3.6%), or a mental condition causing difficulties in learning, remembering, or concentrating (4.8%). Of the 212 million people aged 16 years and older, 8.6% reported a condition that made it difficult to go outside their home, whereas 11.9% of the 178.7 million people aged 16 to 64 years had a condition that affected their ability to work at a job or business.

These estimates are comparable to 1994-1995 SIPP data estimates that 20.6% of the noninstitutionalized general population, nearly 54 million people, had a disabling condition that interferes with life activities (U.S. Census Bureau, 1997b).

TABLE 19-2 Six Types of Disability, Census 2000

DISABILITY LIMITATION	NUMBERS
Sensory, involving sight or hearing	3.6 % (9.3 million), ages 5 and older
Physical (e.g. walking, climbing stairs, reaching, lifting, or carrying)	8.2% (21.2 million), ages 5 and older
Mental (e.g., learning, remembering, or concentratingdue to physical, mental or emotional condition)	4.8% (12.4 million), ages 5 and older
Self-care (e.g., dressing, bathing, getting around home due to physical, mental, emotional condition)	2.6% (6.8 million), ages 5 and older
Go-outside-home disability	8.6% (18.2 million) of 212 million, ages 16 and older
Employment disability	11.9% (21.3 million) of 178.7 million, ages 16-64 years

From U.S. Census Bureau: *Disability status: 2000—Census 2000 brief*, Issued March 2003, The Author, http://www.census.gov/hhes/www/disability/disabstat2k.html.

TABLE 19-3 Characteristics of the Civilian Noninstitutionalized Population by Age, Disability Status, and Type of Disability: 2000

CHARACTERISTIC	TOTAL NUMBER	TOTAL PERCENT	MALE NUMBER	MALE PERCENT	FEMALE NUMBER	FEMALE PERCENT
Population 5 and older	**257,167,527**	**100.0**	**124,636,825**	**100.0**	**132,530,702**	**100.0**
With any disability	49,746,248	19.3	24,439,531	19.6	25,306,717	19.1
Population 5 to 15	**45,133,667**	**100.0**	**23,125,324**	**100.0**	**22,008,343**	**100.0**
With any disability	2,614,919	5.0	1,666,230	7.2	948,689	4.3
Sensory	442,894	1.0	242,706	1.0	200,188	0.9
Physical	455,461	1.0	251,852	1.1	203,609	0.9
Mental	2,078,502	4.6	1,387,393	6.0	691,109	3.1
Self-care	419,018	0.9	244,824	1.1	174,194	0.8
Population 16 to 64	**178,687,234**	**100.0**	**87,570,583**	**100.0**	**91,116,651**	**100.0**
With any disability	33,153,211	18.6	17,139,019	19.6	16,014,192	17.6
Sensory	4,123,902	2.3	2,388,121	2.7	1,735,781	1.9
Physical	11,150,365	6.2	5,279,731	6.0	5,870,634	6.4
Mental	6,764,439	3.8	3,434,631	3.9	3,329,808	3.7
Self-care	3,149,875	1.8	1,463,184	1.7	1,686,691	1.9
Difficulty going outside the home	11,414,508	6.4	5,569,362	6.4	5,845,146	6.4
Employment disability	21,287,570	11.9	11,373,786	13.0	9,913,784	10.9
Population 65 and older	**33,346,626**	**100.0**	**13,940,918**	**100.0**	**19,405,708**	**100.0**
With any disability	13,070,118	41.9	5,634,282	40.4	8,343,836	43.0
Sensory	4,738,479	14.2	2,177,216	15.6	2,561,263	13.2
Physical	9,545,680	28.6	3,590,139	25.8	5,955,541	30.7
Mental	3,592,912	10.8	1,380,060	9.9	2,212,852	11.4
Self-care	3,183,840	9.5	1,044,910	7.5	2,138,930	11.0
Difficulty going outside the home	6,795,517	20.4	2,339,128	16.8	4,456,389	23.0

From U.S. Census Bureau: Census 2000 Summary File 3, The Author.

Approximately half of these people, 26 million, had a severe disability and fit the following criteria:

- Were age 15 years or older
- Were unable to perform one or more functional activities, or
- Depended on the help of others to perform one or more ADLs or IADLs, or
- Used an assistive device on a long-term basis

In addition, people with Alzheimer's disease or a developmental disability, those aged 16 to 67 years who are unable to do housework or work at a job or business, or those who receive federal disability benefits meet the criteria for a severe disability.

Disability Prevalence by Age, Gender, Race/Ethnicity, Region

The proportion of the U.S. population with disabilities continues to *rise with age for both sexes,* as indicated in Table 19-3. Overall disability rates increased from 5.8% of children ages 5

to 15 years, to 18.6% of the population aged 16 to 64 years, to 41.9% of people aged 65 years and older. Difficulty going outside the home affected 6.4% of working age adults as compared with 20.4% of older adults. Similarly, rates for physical disability rose from 6.2% in working age adults to 28.6% in older adults. Likewise, rates for sensory disabilities, self-care limitations, and difficulties in learning, remembering, or concentrating were highest in adults aged 65 years and older. Although overall disability rates remained lowest for children of ages 5 to 15 years, mental limitations (4.6%) far exceeded rates for sensory (1%) or physical (1%) disabilities.

In general, males in most age-groups have higher disability rates than females of the same age. For example, in 2000 there were approximately 1.7 million (7.2%) males aged 5 to 15 years with a disabling condition, as compared to 949,000 (4.3%) girls this age. However, by age 65 years, demographic shifts associated with an aging population (a greater per-

TABLE 19-4 Percentage of Civilian Noninstitutionalized Population With a Disability by Age, Selected Race, and Hispanic/Latino Origin, Census 2000

RACE AND HISPANIC/LATINO ORIGIN	TOTAL POPULATION AGES 5 AND OLDER*	PERCENTAGE WITH A DISABILITY			
		5 AND OLDER	5 TO 15	16 TO 64	65 AND OLDER
Total	257	19.3	5.8	18.6	41.9
White alone	195	18.5	5.6	16.8	40.6
Black or African American alone	30.3	24.3	7	26.4	52.8
American Indian and Alaska Native alone	2.2	24.3	7.7	27	57.6
Asian alone	9.5	16.6	2.9	16.9	40.8
Native Hawaiian and Other Pacific Islander alone	0.338	19	5.1	21	48.5
Some other race alone	13.6	19.9	5.2	23.5	50.4
Two or more races	6.2	21.7	7.1	25.1	51.8
Hispanic or Latino (of any race)	31	20.9	5.4	24	48.5
White alone, not Hispanic or Latino	180	18.3	5.7	16.2	40.4

*Rounded number in millions.
From U.S. Census Bureau: *Disability status: 2000—Census 2000 brief*, modified from Table 2, issued March 2003, The Author, http://www.census.gov/hhes/www/disability/disabstat2k.html.

TABLE 19-5 Percentage Distribution of Noninstitutionalized Civilians Ages 5 and Older and People With Disabilities by Geographical Region, Census 2000

	NORTHEAST	MIDWEST	SOUTH	WEST
% of total*	19.2	22.9	35.5	22.4
% of people with disabilities**	19.0	21.0	38.3	21.6

From U.S. Census Bureau: *Disability Status: 2000—Census 2000 Brief*, modified from Figure 4, issued March 2003, The Author, http://www.census.gov/hhes/www/disability/disabstat2k.html.
Population U.S. Census, 2000.
NOTE: Since numbers are rounded, totals may not equal 100%.

centage of women outlive men) coincide with higher disability rates in women (43%) than men (40.4%).

Whites reported a low rate of disability (18.5%), compared with the overall rate of 19.3% for all persons aged 5 years and older, as indicated in Table 19-4. Asian Americans had the lowest overall disability rate (16.6%), whereas blacks or African Americans, and American Indians and Alaskan Natives reported the highest overall disability rates at 24.3% each, as well as the highest rates across each age category. Hispanics or Latinos of any race (20.9%) had a higher disability rate overall as compared with whites who were neither Hispanic nor Latino (18.3%).

As illustrated in Table 19-5, the largest percentage of people with disabling conditions lived in the South, with significantly lower rates (about one in five disabled persons) in other areas of the country. Although 35.5% of the civilian, noninstitutionalized population aged 5 years and older lived in the South in 2000, 38.3% of this population reported disabling conditions. This disparate rate for disability, coupled with the South's total population, produced the largest regional number of people with disabilities in 2000, with 19.1 million. The Northeast had the fewest people with disabilities, 9.5 million (U.S. Census Bureau, 2003). Increasing disability rates were correlated with coal mining areas in Southern states (i.e., Kentucky, West Virginia, and Virginia) or older industrial cities with high concentrations of blacks, Hispanics, and other racial/ethnic groups with high disability

rates. Areas with a small proportion of residents aged 65 years and older or high concentrations of families with children had the lowest disability rates.

Disability rarely limits itself to one aspect of personal functioning. In fact, respondents who noted one disability measure from Census 2000 were likely to report one or more additional measures. For example, a person with a physical disability may experience a self-care disability, or have difficulty leaving home, which could contribute to an employment disability. In fact, of the 43.6% of people reporting an employment disability, 56.4% reported an additional disability. Nearly all (97%) of respondents with a self-care limitation reported one or more other measures of disability (U.S. Census Bureau, 2003).

Health Status of the Elderly

Although there is continuing debate about whether the elderly population is more or less healthy over time, longitudinal data collected over the past 20 years through the National Long-Term Care Survey (NLTCS) indicate "clear, overwhelming evidence that the average health of the elderly population is improving. Between 1982 and 1999, the share of the elderly with severe disabilities, measured roughly as the ability to function independently with ease, declined from 26.2% to 19.7%. The cumulative reduction in disability is 25%, or 1.7% per year" (Cutler, 2001, p. 6546). Disability in elders is declining more rapidly over time, and

TABLE 19-6   Top 21 Main Conditions as Cause for Disability, by Self-Report in Civilian, Noninstitutionalized Persons Ages 18 and Older, U.S. Survey of Income and Program Participation, 1999

MAIN CONDITION	ALL PERSONS NO.*	%	MEN NO.*	%	WOMEN NO.*	%
Arthritis/rheumatism	7,207	17.5	1,955	11.0	5,235	22.4
Back, spine problem	6,780	16.5	2,903	16.3	3,877	16.6
Heart trouble/hardening of arteries	3,209	7.8	1,666	9.4	1,543	6.6
Lung, respiratory problem	1,931	4.7	883	5.0	1,048	4.5
Deafness, hearing problem	1,794	4.4	1,183	6.7	611	2.6
Limb/extremity stiffness	1,747	4.2	842	4.7	905	3.9
Mental, emotional problem	1,541	3.7	733	4.1	808	3.5
Diabetes	1,399	3.4	610	3.4	789	3.4
Stroke	1,160	2.8	592	3.3	567	2.4
Broken bone/fracture	885	2.1	373	2.1	512	2.2
Mental retardation	827	2.0	507	2.9	320	1.4
Cancer	792	1.9	303	1.7	489	2.1
High blood pressure	692	1.7	255	1.4	437	1.9
Head or spinal cord injury	408	1.0	257	1.4	150	0.6
Learning disability	408	1.0	257	1.4	150	0.6
Alzheimer's disease/senility/dementia	354	0.9	110	0.6	244	1.0
Kidney problems	348	0.8	172	1.0	177	0.8
Paralysis	310	0.8	175	1.0	135	0.6
Missing limbs	299	0.7	211	1.2	–	–
Stomach/digestive problems	279	0.7	112	0.6	167	0.7

*In thousands. All percentages were reported to be at 95% confidence interval or higher.
From Centers for Disease Control and Prevention: Prevalence of disabilities and associated health conditions among adults: United States, 1999, *MMWR Morb Mortal Wkly Rep* 50(07):120-125, 2001.

between 1989 and 1999 it fell at a higher rate for blacks than nonblacks (Manton & Gu, 2001). These findings are accompanied by a large relative and absolute drop in institutional use (nursing home) and an increase in number of years of schooling for both blacks and nonblacks. After 1990, while per capita use of Medicare increased for blacks, whites received more care from specialists and high-tech services, leading to overall better health.

A number of factors influence the trend toward "large disability reductions," as shown in the NLTCS in the U.S. elderly population (Cutler, 2001; Manton & Gu, 2001). These include improved medical treatments for arthritis (e.g., joint replacements), heart disease (e.g., surgical procedures), hypertension (e.g., improved medications), cataracts (e.g., outpatient surgery), and other common causes of activity limitations. Lifestyle modifications, which include a decline in cigarette smoking and reduction in dietary fat intake, contribute to decreased morbidity and mortality associated with hypertension, cardiovascular, respiratory, and cerebrovascular disease. Increased availability and use of assistive devices decrease ADL and IADL limitations, and assisted living facilities and other in-home care options make it easier for elderly disabled persons to safely remain in the community, avoiding a nursing home.

A variety of socioeconomic and cultural variables influence differences in disability prevalence rates related to aging, gender, race/ethnicity, and geographical area. In caring for people affected by disabilities, the community health nurse must closely monitor overall health status and promote well-being. The next section continues the discussion on health status and common causes of disability.

Health Status and Causes of Disability

Arthritis or rheumatism, back or spine problems, and heart trouble or hardening of the arteries were the leading reported causes of activity limitation or functional disability (vision, hearing, or speech disabilities were excluded) for civilian noninstitutionalized persons aged 18 years or older, according to a 1999 SIPP data report (Centers for Disease Control and Prevention, 2001) summarized in Table 19-6. Women had higher rates of arthritis and "other" associated health conditions, whereas men had higher rates for heart trouble or hardening of the arteries, and deafness or hearing problems. These findings should be considered with caution, however, becausse the data may not reflect current population statistics. Methodological issues, restriction of the population (to civilian, noninstitutionalized population, aged 18 years or older), and reporting of only one major disability (many persons have multiple disabilities) are limiting factors. However, it is clear that *disability rates increase with higher rates of chronic disease*. Activity limitations increase with age, consistent with self-reported high rates for arthritis, back or spine problems, and cardiovascular disease. Similarly, chronic respiratory conditions, hearing and vision disabilities, stroke, and fractures (both pathological, caused by osteoporosis, and accidental, from falls) increase with aging. Cognitive impairments, such as dementia, are clearly recognized for their disabling potential. Americans in all age-groups and cultures who are sedentary and overweight or obese are more likely to develop type 2 diabetes. This discussion illustrates the connection between *increasing rates for chronic health problems and aging and associated functional disability*. This finding heralds the importance of nurses' involvement in health promotion and disease prevention, particularly as life expectancy increases.

National Health Interview Survey (NHIS) data indicate that although 7 in 10 persons in the civilian, noninstitutionalized population reported themselves to be in excellent or very good health in 2002, 12% of the population, or approximately 34 million people, reported a limitation in their usual activities due to one or more chronic health conditions (Schiller & Bernadel, 2004). In addition, nearly 4 million persons (2% of the population) required assistance with ADLs (e.g., eating, dressing, and bathing), and 7.5 million (4% of the population) required help with IADLs (e.g., shopping and household chores). Prevalence of limitation in usual activities increased with age, consistent with other surveys. Indeed, 10% of adults aged 75 years and over required assistance with ADLs, and 20% needed help with IADLs.

For both adults and children, the number of persons with activity limitations and poorer health status increased with lower education levels and low family incomes. *America's Children 2003* (ChildStats.gov, 2003), a report based on NHIS 2001 data, found that approximately 8% of children aged 5 to 17 years had activity limitations due to chronic conditions. Six percent (4.3 million) were identified as having activity limitations due to their participation in special education or early intervention services. Boys were nearly twice as likely to receive services as girls. A number of factors probably explain these differences, including maturational, behavioral, social, and diagnostic reasons. Children who received Medicaid services were more likely to receive special education or early intervention services when compared with children who had private or no health insurance.

Causes of activity limitation vary considerably based on age. According to the NHIS (LaPlante and Carlson, 1996), the five leading causes of activity limitation for children and adolescents under 18 years of age include the following: asthma (19.8% of all limiting conditions), learning disability and mental retardation (19.2%), mental illness (8.8%; roughly two thirds is related to hyperkinetic syndrome of childhood), speech impairments (6.7%), and hearing impairments (3.8%).

Although estimates for mental retardation range from 0.67% to 3.0% depending on age and the definition used, the most commonly accepted estimates indicate that 1% of the noninstitutionalized U.S. population (2.5 million people) have mental retardation. In addition, approximately 695,000 people with mental retardation lived in residential settings, nursing homes, and other institutions in 1995 (Kraus, Stoddard, and Gilmartin, 1996).

Estimates for the number of people disabled by mental and emotional disorders vary widely for many reasons. These include a lack of standard criteria for the disorders and their associated limitations, and the stigma associated with mental illness and substance abuse that leads to underreporting. Mental and emotional disorders are sometimes described as "hidden" disabilities because they cannot be detected by observation alone. However, whether a mental disorder is disabling depends on how disability is defined.

According to Jans and Stoddard (1999), the NHIS-D estimated that in 1994 and 1995, 23.5 million people in the United States had mental disorders. The findings suggested that approximately 70% of people with mental disorders have a functional disability, a work limitation disability, a perceived disability, and/or receive one or more governmental support services (e.g., Social Security Disability Income [SSDI], Supplemental Security Income [SSI], a disability pension, or special education services).

Regardless of the causes of disability, the nurse must see beyond the disabling impairment, carefully assessing people's perceptions of the disability experience. Sociocultural biases and traditions may influence the personal and family meaning of disability. Ultimately, the personal belief system of the individual and the family, and the traditions of the community influence the individual's lived experience with disability and his or her participation in health care.

COSTS ASSOCIATED WITH DISABILITY

Disability is associated with costly medical, social, public health, and moral issues. Specific impairments and their accompanying limitations often are of minor importance to people with disabilities when compared with societal issues of exclusion, blocked access, discriminatory practices, educational segregation, poverty, and unemployment. Although people with disabilities have seen noteworthy improvements in the past 15 years, they continue to lag behind nondisabled Americans in many of the basic aspects of life. These include gaps in employment, income, education, access to transportation, health care, frequency of socializing, entertainment, attendance at religious services, and political participation (National Council on Disability, 1999; National Organization on Disability and Louis Harris and Associates, 2000). According to a 1997 IOM publication, *Enabling America,* disability consumes an estimated 4% of the gross domestic product, approximating an annual aggregate cost of $300 billion, which includes medical care expenditures and lost productivity costs (Brandt and Pope, 1997). Today, those numbers may be higher, based on limitations associated with increasing rates for type 2 diabetes, obesity, and aging.

Economic Well-Being and Employment

Many people with disabilities live at or near the poverty level (Jans and Stoddard, 1999). Nearly one third (29%) of the adults with disabilities in a Harris Survey (National Organization on Disability and Louis Harris and Associates, 2000) reported living in households having a total income of $15,000 or less, compared with only 10% of those who are nondisabled. According to Census 2000 data, 8.7 million people with disabilities, or 17.6% of disabled persons aged 5 years and older are impoverished, as compared with 10.6% of the nondisabled population (U.S. Census Bureau, 2003). In both the disabled and nondisabled populations, children aged 5 to 15 years have the highest poverty rates: 25% for children with disabilities compared with 15.7% for children without disabilities. There are approximately twice as many people aged 16 to 64 years who are both impoverished and

TABLE 19-7   Employed Men and Women Ages 16-64 as a Percentage of the Civilian Noninstitutionalized Population by Disability Status: 2000

	MEN	WOMEN
With a disability	60.1	51.4
Without a disability	79.9	67.3

From U.S. Census Bureau: *Disability status: 2000—Census 2000 brief*, modified from Figure 7, issued March 2003, The Author, http://www.census.gov/hhes/www/disability/disabstat2k.html.

disabled (18.8%), compared with those who are poor but not disabled (9.6%). Similar contrasts occur in older adults, although the overall rates remain lower (13.2% for poverty/disability and 7.4% for poverty/no disability).

Working age persons are less likely to be employed if they are disabled (U.S. Census Bureau, 2003) as seen in Table 19-7. Over the past 20 years, the employment rate for people with disabilities has hovered around 30%, much lower than the national average for nondisabled persons (Employment and Disability Institute, Cornell University, 2003-2005). A national survey performed by Louis Harris and Associates (National Organization on Disability and Louis Harris and Associates, 2000) found that working-age adults with disabilities made only limited employment gains compared with 10 years previous. The Harris Survey reported that only 32% of disabled people aged 18 to 64 years worked full- or part-time, compared with 81% of the nondisabled population. Among working-age Americans with disabilities, two thirds of those unemployed said they would prefer to work. In comparing gender differences, women face double jeopardy, because they are less likely to participate in the workforce and they receive lower earnings (Jans and Stoddard, 1999). These findings can be compared to CPS data for 2002, which estimated an employment rate of 20.8% for people aged 21 to 64 years who reported a work-limiting health problem or disability. Unemployment issues are complex, involving more than civil rights protection, which promotes equal opportunities for all people, regardless of their disability status. Increasing opportunities for employment by those who want to work requires removal of disabling barriers (whether environmental or attitudinal) and addition of social support to do so (continuation of necessary benefits for health care, caregiver assistance, etc.). Governmental efforts include President George W. Bush's New Freedom Initiative, directing federal agencies to create a central information gateway, http://www.DisabilityInfo.gov, a website with links of interest to people with disabilities, employers, service providers, and other community members.

Long-Term Care and Personal Assistance Support

Of the 9.3 million people aged 15 years and older who require assistance in performing ADLs or IADLs, family members provide about 80% of the personal assistance support (U.S. Census Bureau, 1997a). Nearly half of these primary helpers live with the person who has a disability (U.S. Census Bureau, 1997a, 1997b). Not surprisingly, the need for assistance increases with age. However, despite the high rate of disability among people aged 80 years and older (71.5% had a disability and 53.5% had a severe disability), only 34.1% receive personal assistance.

U.S. public policy is limited by the absence of an affordable system for long-term services and supports for individuals and families affected by disabilities. An institutional bias exists in the Medicaid statute; therefore nursing home care is mandatory in every state and home, whereas community-based care is optional. Institutional services receive approximately 80% of the funding for long-term services and supports (National Council on Disability, 1999). Although the vast majority of people with disabilities and their families prefer that services are delivered in the "most integrated" home- and community-based settings, the current system offers few real choices for people with disabilities who need long-term support.

Health Insurance and Public Health Programs

People with disabilities are more likely to participate in public health programs (e.g., Medicare and Medicaid) compared with nondisabled people. In addition, they are less likely to have private health insurance (Schiller & Bernadel, 2004). Growth in Medicaid program enrollment by disabled and aged populations continues to increase at 2.5% per year or more (Holahan and Bruen, 2003). A rise in health care and prescription drug costs, a decrease in employer-subsidized private health insurance, an increase in the use of home and community based waiver services, and an increase in disability secondary to life-extending medical technology are other factors that may explain continued increases in Medicaid program enrollment by disabled and aged people. These findings are not surprising, considering socioeconomic factors, employment rates, and prevalence data related to disability.

Total Medicaid spending increased by about 25%, which is over $50 billion, between federal fiscal years 2000 and 2002, with nearly 60% of the spending growth in aged and disabled populations (Holahan and Bruen, 2003). Overall increases in Medicaid expenditures are related to loss of income associated with the U.S. economic downturn (after the terrorism attacks on September 11, 2001), and to rising health care costs, especially hospital and prescription drugs. Nearly half of all Medicaid drug costs were incurred by disabled and aged people who also received Medicare benefits. Although Medicaid enrollment rates for children and non-disabled adults far exceeded enrollment rates for aged and disabled people, the latter populations are more expensive per enrollee, and their costs are increasing proportionally at a much greater rate than costs in the general population. According to Holahan and Bruen (2003), aged and disabled enrollees account for more than 70% of total Medicaid spending, 85% of Medicaid spending on prescription drugs, more than 50% of Medicaid spending on combined inpatient and outpatient services, and nearly all Medicaid long-term

HEALTHY PEOPLE **2010** | Selected Objectives for People With Disabilities and Secondary Conditions

Objective	Baseline (i.e., 1998)	% Target
6-2: Reduce the proportion of children and adolescents with disabilities who are reported to be sad, unhappy, or depressed.	31%	17%
6-5: Increase the proportion of adults with disabilities reporting sufficient emotional support.	70%	79%
6-6: Increase the proportion of adults with disabilities reporting satisfaction with life.	87%	96%
6-7: Reduce the number of people with disabilities in congregate care facilities, consistent with permanency planning principles.	NA	NA
6-8: Eliminate disparities in employment rates between working-aged adults with and without disabilities.	52%	82%
6-9: Increase the proportion of children and youth with disabilities who spend at least 80% of their time in regular education programs.	45%	60%
6-10: Increase the proportion of health and wellness and treatment programs and facilities that provide full access for people with disabilities.	NA	NA
6-11: Reduce the proportion of people with disabilities who report not having assistive devices and technology needed.	NA	NA
6-12: Reduce the proportion of people with disabilities reporting environmental barriers to participation in home, school, work, or community activities.	NA	NA

US Department of Health and Human Services: *Healthy people 2010*, Updated November 10, 2000, Office of Disease Prevention and Health Promotion, USDHHS, www.health.gov/healthypeople.

care expenditures. Growth in public health programs, such as Medicaid, pressures state budgets strained by declining revenues. States' efforts to curtail Medicaid spending, together with a decline in employer-sponsored health insurance has contributed to record increases in uninsured lower income adults. The 2002 CPS results (based on 2001 data) show the number of uninsured adults increased by 1.5 million (Holahan and Bruen, 2003). This trend is expected to continue.

By 2030, elderly persons are estimated to increase from 13% to 20% of the population. By 2050, the frail elderly, those aged 85 years and over, will increase from 2% to 5% of the population, leading to profound impacts on future health care and long-term care costs. Recent research indicates a declining age-adjusted rate for chronic disability among older U.S. adults, which has the potential to moderate future health care costs. However, greater longevity may mean more years of disability with associated long-term care and medical costs. Spillman (2004) urges researchers to explore the underlying causes of the observed declines in chronic disability and to examine the changing use of services and costs. If reported reductions in less severe disabilities, particularly in IADLs, primarily reflect improvements in the environment (consistent with increased use of assistive equipment), rather than overall health, costs are unlikely to decrease. Earlier diagnosis and improved treatment may contribute to fewer disabilities for certain conditions; however, this may increase, rather than decrease health care costs, at least short term. Further study is required to understand "what is driving the trends in specific aspects of disability before we can understand the implications for health care and long-term care costs" (Spillman, 2004, p. 185).

HEALTHY PEOPLE 2010 AND THE HEALTH NEEDS OF PEOPLE WITH DISABILITIES

People with disabilities experience increased health concerns and are more likely to develop secondary conditions (e.g., medical, physical, social, emotional, spiritual, or societal). Disability increases the population's need for fully accessible health care that promotes health and well-being, prevents secondary conditions, and provides support for long-term health conditions. One of the 26 major goals of *Healthy People 2010* is to promote the health of people with disabilities, prevent secondary conditions, and eliminate disparities between people with and without disabilities and the U.S. population (US Department of Health and Human Services [USDHHS], 2000). Selected *Healthy People 2010* objectives for people with disabilities and secondary conditions are shown in the table above.

A disabled person's ability to perform a socially expected activity reflects the characteristics of the individual and the larger social and physical environment; therefore considerations for each of these elements must be incorporated into community health programs that serve people affected by disability. For example, nurses may consider how to promote access to food and medication labeling for people with visual disabilities. Nurses must also be sensitive to environmental and social barriers that could prohibit any person's participation in health promotion activities. For example, current estimates indicate that women with functional limitations are less likely to participate in preventative screening for breast and cervical cancer (Jans and Stoddard, 1999). Hopefully, efforts to reduce barriers in the community specified in *Healthy People 2010* will result in more accessible provider offices and diagnostic equipment (Neri and Kroll, 2003). Community health nurses might ask the following:

Can a woman who uses a wheelchair obtain mammography for breast cancer screening, or is the lack of adaptive equipment a barrier to her participation?

What is the availability and cost of accessible transportation to the screening site?

The United States leads the world in the "community imperative," the deinstitutionalization of persons with disabilities, moving this population from institutions into private homes, small group and independent living centers. However, in the United States and world-wide, unrecognized health care problems frequently go untreated in people with intellectual or other cognitive disabilities who cannot easily communicate their symptoms, exhibit behavioral problems that discourage health care providers from adequate caring, or resist attempts to care for them because of their discomfort or unfamiliarity with the health care setting or equipment. Other problems include difficulties in obtaining a client history and in determining the nature and cause of a health care problem, along with inexperience and inadequate training by health care providers in specific health care problems that accompany intellectual disabilities (Jansen et al., 2004). Health care providers at whatever level, whether nurse's aide, nurse, therapist, or physician, would benefit from increased education that addresses issues on caring for people with disabilities. For example, general practitioners in an Australian study (Phillips, Morrison, and Davis, 2004) reported inadequate prior education in the same areas that they reported substandard care of clients with intellectual disabilities. These areas were behavioral or psychiatric conditions, syndrome-specific medical problems, human relations and sexuality issues, and collaboration with government services (social programs). In addition, medical care for complex medical problems and primary health care of clients with intellectual disabilities reportedly fell below acceptable standards for health care practice. Improving the care of people with intellectual disabilities in today's fast-paced health care climate is a serious concern that deserves further study.

Although this chapter focuses on health promotion for people with disabilities, primary prevention of disability for nondisabled people must not be minimized. Prevention of osteoporosis in nondisabled women, or in women who are mobility impaired from a physical disability, may prevent secondary health problems, such as hip and spine fractures that produce significant morbidity and mortality in older women. The health care concerns of nondisabled people may differ from those of people with disabilities: they may be accentuated or minimized. Epidemiological studies are needed to augment information on health promotion strategies specific to people with disabilities, as well as to those who are able-bodied.

Health care for people with disabilities must incorporate remedies that address issues surrounding access to health care and the removal of environmental and social barriers that prevent full participation in society. Nurses who

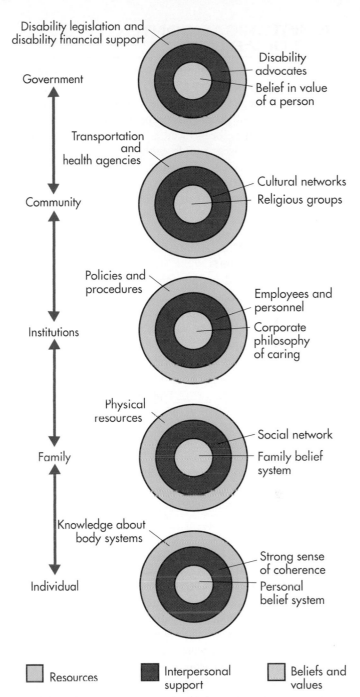

FIGURE 19-2   Systems of support for people with disabilities.

practice holistic nursing will recognize that caring for people affected by disabilities requires a perspective that transcends the individual. The community health nurse will use a range of support systems that promote the health of the person with a disability and the health of his or her family. Figure 19-2 illustrates these support systems. The importance of governmental public policies, including disability legislation and financial support, cannot be overemphasized. It is only when the nurse considers a broad approach to disability that he or she can realize the objectives of *Healthy People 2010.*

A HISTORICAL CONTEXT FOR DISABILITY

Current models and definitions for disability cannot be understood apart from their historical-sociopolitical context. As cultures changed, and with them images of beauty and value, "exceptional" people have experienced a wide range of treatment. They have been loved as mascots and fascinating freaks. In other cases, people with disabilities have been isolated, ridiculed, and discriminated against, or worse, marked for extermination (Bogdan, 1986). The following section explores some of the images and attitudes that surround people with disabilities.

Early Attitudes Toward People With Disabilities

Societal bias toward people with disabilities has ancient roots. Since the beginning of recorded history, people with disabilities were set apart from others and viewed as different or unusual. Carvings on the walls of Egyptian tombs contain pictures of dwarfs and blind or disabled musicians and singers. Early Greek and Roman cultures emphasized bodily and intellectual perfection. Babies who were sick, weak, or born with obvious disabilities were typically killed or left to die (Barnes, 1996). In Biblical times, many people with disabilities were outcasts. Commonly viewed as unclean and/or sinful, people with disabilities were frequently isolated and separated from others. However, the Jewish culture prohibited infanticide based on sanctity of life beliefs. In European history, people with disabilities sometimes served as royal court pets, entertainers, circus performers, and sideshow exhibitions.

Attitudes Toward People With Disabilities in the Eighteenth and Nineteenth Centuries

In the absence of a scientific model for understanding and treating disability, people saw disability as an irreparable condition caused by supernatural agency (Longmore, 1987). People with disabilities were viewed as sick and helpless. They were expected to participate in whatever treatment was deemed necessary to cure or produce a reasonable level of social or vocational performance. This treatment typically followed the emerging "medical model" (Gartner and Joe, 1987). Although contemporary perspectives for disability in Western civilizations do not support these ancient views, they continue to persist, varying across cultures and within populations.

During the nineteenth century, the Industrial Revolution stimulated a societal need for increased education. Those who could not reach the minimum educational level (i.e., equivalent to a contemporary third-grade education) were labeled as "feebleminded" (Pfeiffer, 1993). Although this included people with mental disabilities, soon the label transferred to those with sensory and communication disorders (e.g., vision, hearing, and speech) and mobility impairments.

Schools for people who were deaf and blind were established in the early 1800s. In 1849, Dr. Samuel Gridley Howe established the Massachusetts School for Idiotic Children and Youth in Boston. Although these early efforts demonstrated that people with disabilities could be educated and integrated into society, institutionalization and segregation of people with disabilities was the norm (Pfeiffer, 1993; Shapiro, 1993).

Disability in the Twentieth Century

World War I stimulated application of economic concepts surrounding disability (Hahn, 1985). The first federal vocational rehabilitation legislation for veterans with disabilities in 1918 and for civilians in 1920 focused on limitations in the amount or type of work that people with disabilities could perform (Longmore, 1987). Special interest groups for this population developed at about the same time. For example, the Association for Retarded Citizens (ARC) used its collective power to advocate for the needs of people with intellectual disabilities (Turnbull, 1990).

In the early 1900s, social Darwinism and the eugenics movement promoted involuntary sterilization of those with intellectual disabilities (Pfeiffer, 1993; Shapiro, 1993). Hitler's attempts to exterminate "inferior" people in World War II, including those who were disabled or weak, are well known. These activities confirmed the medical model view of disability as undesirable and abnormal person-centered pathology (Hahn, 1985).

By the 1950s and 1960s, many groups worked on behalf of people with disabilities and focused on the delivery of needed services. In the 1960s and 1970s, parents' groups and professionals worked together to improve institutional care and establish community-based independent living centers (Longmore, 1987; Shapiro, 1993). However, professionals and parents, rather than people with disabilities, commonly assumed leadership roles within these groups. The public retained the predominant assumption that people with disabilities were *dis*-abled. In classic sociological writings on stigma and social identity, Goffman (1963) associated stigma with blemish and moral inferiority. In the social deviance model of disability, the stigmatized person was "not quite human," which necessitated avoidance by others.

Contemporary Conceptualizations of People With Disabilities

Common stereotypical images of people with disabilities are found in contemporary literature and the media. These portrayals range from pitiful and pathetic, to sinister or evil. They may be portrayed as laughable, curious, burdensome, or heroic (e.g., "super crip") (Friedberg, Mullins, and Sukiennik, 1985). People with disabilities are seldom presented with a full range of personalities and abilities. Even when the media portrays people with disabilities as fully functioning, integral members of society, society may perceive this as unusual or unexpected, rather than normal and expected.

A survey was performed to determine the changes in media portrayals of people with disabilities (Martin and Catlett, 1999). The study examined the content from 191 articles for themes associated with disability issues. Table 19-8 describes the findings from the study and suggests that media images

TABLE 19-8 Changing Media Portrayals of People With Disabilities

LOGICAL	FALLACY	FREQUENCY (%)	RELIABILITY (%)
Pathos or pity	69 articles	36.1	92.7
Normalization	44 articles	23	77
Super human	26 articles	13.6	100
Challenging the system	22 articles	11.5	91
Devaluation	16 articles	8.3	81.6
Non sequitur (i.e., cause and effect does not necessary follow)	11 articles	5.6	100

Data from Martin SS, Catlett SM: *Same window, new view: print media and persons with disabilities*, Unpublished paper presented at 1999 TASH Conference, Chicago, Ill, 1999.

appear to be changing positively following the passage of the ADA of 1990. A continuing emphasis on inclusion, normalization, and deinstitutionalization of people with disabilities appears to have contributed to this change. Although pathos or pity remains the predominant societal response, the lives and stories of people with disabilities are increasingly viewed as "normal."

Common responses toward people with disabilities range from ambivalence and avoidance to pity and paternalism. Some reported responses follow:

Being deaf is an accident of nature. Being indifferent is very often a deliberate choice of mankind. Of these two wounds in our society, one is at least curable (Nanette Fabray cited in Friedberg, Mullins, and Sukiennik, 1985).

Society does not value our bodies, which makes it difficult for us to value ourselves. We constantly hear that we are faulty, malformed, broken and sick. Many people with disabilities respond in kind, hating their bodies and their disabilities, wishing they were different (Creamer, 1995, p. 60).

In a society focused on activities, on doing and on fixing, people with chronic illnesses and disabilities are an enigma. We cannot be fixed. We find that generally people want to do something when what we need is someone just to be near, to accompany us. Some are willing to help for a while, but usually people expect us to get better and get discouraged when we do not (Caron, 1996, p. 24).

Stigmatizing influences continue to shape perceptions of disability. Johnson and Johnson (1995) coined the word "disaphobia" to describe the "prejudice, ignorance, fear and anxiety that persons feel in their interaction with the disabled, based on societal stigmatization" (p. 31). Murphy (1990), an anthropologist, reports the following in *The Body Silent*:

One cannot . . . . shelve a disability or hide it from the world. A serious disability inundates all other claims to social standing, relegating to secondary status all the attainments of life, all other social roles, even sexuality. It is not a role; it is an identity, a dominant characteristic to which all social roles must be adjusted. And just as the paralytic cannot clear his mind of his impairment, society will not let him forget it (Murphy, 1990, p. 106).

Murphy's description sharpens an understanding of the marginalized status often attributed to people with disabilities. People using wheelchairs are commonly noticed by others, but are seldom acknowledged. Parents often teach their children not to look at a person who is obviously disabled,

TABLE 19-9 Language Usage Surrounding Disability

LESS DESIRABLE LANGUAGE	MORE DESIRABLE LANGUAGE
Confined to a wheelchair; wheelchair-bound	Uses a wheelchair
Afflicted with or suffers from cerebral palsy	Has cerebral palsy
The blind, the deaf, and the disabled	People who are blind, deaf, or disabled
Mentally handicapped or mentally retarded	People with intellectual disabilities
Handicapped students and normal classmates	Students who are disabled and nondisabled or students with and without disabilities
The spinal-cord injury in room 232	John, in room 232, has a spinal cord injury

which reinforces "deviance disavowal" of disability. A community health nurse describes societal stigma experienced by the families of children with disabilities, which follows:

It's a huge amount. The teasing in schools. Kids are brutal to normal kids. We try to run some groups on teasing and how to cope with that . . . . Families talk about going to the grocery store and being sick of answering questions or having people stare at the child. I don't know that any of the families really always know how to deal with that (Treloar, Unpublished interviews, 1999e).

Contemporary language and actions may convey a lack of respect for people with disabilities (Blaska, 1993). For example, people continue to use the term *handicap* improperly to refer to people with disabilities whether or not these people are handicapped by their environments (Batavia, 1993). Table 19-9 provides further information on uses of language related to disability. To help the reader understand this aggregate, Box 9-1 lists common misconceptions surrounding disability. Finally, Table 19-10 notes reminders that promote effective interactions between people with and without disabilities.

DISABILITY AND PUBLIC POLICY

Since the 1980s, parallels have been drawn between people with disabilities and other groups who have been subjected to discrimination and oppression. Disability has been reconceptualized as a socially constructed and stigmatized role. Gartner and Joe (1987) wrote the following:

Persons with disabilities are not treated seriously because they have limited power and are seen as neither whole nor equal. And they are seen that way because they have limited power. Work then needs to be carried out on both sides of the equation: in changing the images and in changing the opportunity structure. At present, the disabling images constrain opportunities and the resulting limited achievements confirm the images. It can be different (p. 208).

Redefinition of disability, the disability rights movement, and growing recognition of disability's impact on the U.S. economy and population have contributed to the development of Disability Studies as an emerging discipline. Practitioners and scholars from a broad interdisciplinary base share concerns about disability policy and issues that affect people with disabilities. Box 19-2 contains foundational values and ideologies that underlie public policy related to people with disabilities.

Disability policy attempts to minimize disadvantages related to impairments and disabilities and to maximize opportunities for people with disabilities to live productively in their communities (Batavia, 1993). According to DeJong (1994), disability policy includes civil rights protections (e.g., Title 504 of the Rehabilitation Act and the ADA), skill enhancement programs (e.g., special education and vocational rehabilitation), and income and in-kind assistance programs (e.g., Social Security Disability Insurance, Medicare, and Medicaid).

People with disabilities use disproportionately more health care services than those who are nondisabled; therefore public health perspectives related to epidemiology and disability prevention have assumed increasing importance (DeJong, 1994). People's health and well-being reflects the resources available to them; therefore community health nurses must be knowledgeable about public health and social support programs that affect a disabled person's ability to live in the community.

Legislation Affecting People With Disabilities

Consistent with historical and social changes and the recognition of barriers and discrimination, key federal legislation supports the rights of people with disabilities. The following section presents a few of the most significant acts.

BOX 19-1 Misconceptions Surrounding Disabilityy

Disability = cannot have fun
Disability = want to be pitied
Disability = cannot live in the community
Disability = menace to society
Clear voice = clear mind
You can always tell if someone has a disability by looking at the person
All parents want to care for a child with a disability
Wheelchair = hard of hearing
Wheelchair = blind
Wheelchair = mentally retarded
Learning disabled = mentally retarded
Mentally retarded = cannot learn
People with disabilities do not know when someone makes fun of them
Most disabilities and disabling diseases are contagious

BOX 19-2 Public Policy Values Related to Disability

Equal protection: All deserve equal protection under the law.
Egalitarianism: Regardless of differences in abilities, all people should receive equal treatment through equal opportunities.
Normalization: People with disabilities should be treated like nondisabled people, minimizing differences wherever possible.

TABLE 19-10 Do's and Dont's for Interactions With People With Disabilities

DON'T	DO
Assume anything or offer expert advice or assistance based on what you think the person needs or can do	Ask if the person needs help and how to assist; listen and follow his or her instructions; allow him or her to do what he or she can
Ignore or exclude the person	Treat him or her like any other person or friend; approach and include him or her
Be afraid of joking with or offending the person	
Be afraid to ask questions	Recognize that educating others helps remove attitudinal barriers; children who ask are less likely to be afraid of people with disabilities
Focus on differences	See the person as able; accept differences and be patient; seek out similarities and shared interests
Lean on or move the person's wheelchair	Respect a wheelchair as part of the person's personal space; sit on kneel at eye level when communicating with the person
Assume that a person who is blind knows who is speaking or who is present	Inform the person of who is present; say good-bye when leaving
Grab the arm of a person who is blind	Let the person take your arm so he or she does not lose balance
Become impatient and complete the speech or the action of the person	Acknowledge that the person has something important to say or do; take time to listen and understand
Repeat loudly what you want to say	Face the person; speak distinctly and slightly more slowly (this is particularly important for the person who lip reads)
Pet a working dog; there are service dogs for people with physical, hearing, or visual disabilities	Ask for permission to pet the dog; better yet, do not interrupt the dog's work
Assume that the person can participate	Consider possible environmental obstacles (e.g., sensory, architectural, colognes or fragrances for people with chemical sensitivities)
Assume that "bad" parenting explains children's behavior	Recognize that autism and other invisible disabilities influence behavior
Assume that disability and failure to be healed reflects unresolved sin and lack of faith in God	Recognize that humans as holistic beings benefit from interventions that address spiritual meaning for disability

The Individuals With Disabilities Education Act (IDEA)

The Education for All Handicapped Children Act (EHA) of 1975 (20 USC 1401 or PL 94-142), later renamed the **Individuals With Disabilities Education Act (IDEA),** established legislation designed to ensure a *free appropriate public education* (FAPE) in the *least restrictive setting* to children with disabilities *based on their needs.* The IDEA reauthorizations of 1997 and 2004 continue that process, serving as both a grants statute and a civil rights statute, providing federal funding through state administered programs from preschool through secondary education for children with disabilities. Addressing special education needs requires appropriate evaluation and transition services. Parents, students, and professionals participate in decision making, developing an Individualized Education Program (IEP) that includes measurable special educational goals and related services for the child.

In addition to IDEA legislation, exclusionary or discriminatory practices by schools have spurred a multitude of judicial remedies designed to protect the rights of children with disabilities (U.S. Department of Justice, 2000). For example, the Supreme Court, in *Cedar Rapids Community School District v. Garret F.,* ruled that the school must provide extensive health care (although not medical/physician) services during the school day for Garret, a cognitively intact child paralyzed from the neck down as a result of a motorcycle accident (Jones & Apling, 2004). Faced with tight budgets and limited funds, school districts complain that they cannot afford to fund the kinds of care required by severely disabled children, such as that represented by the case of Garret F.

In IDEA 2004, state and school officials received more power to shape the terms for providing services to children with disabilities, leading to concerns that the rights of parents and the nation's 6.5 million disabled students would be eroded. However, most agree that the legislation restores a balance of power between schools and disabled children and their families. For example, schools may find it easier to remove disruptive students whose misbehavior is unrelated to their disability, while potentially reducing costs, bureaucratic rules, and legal challenges by dissatisfied parents (Schemo, 2004).

The Americans With Disabilities Act

The most comprehensive civil rights legislation for people with disabilities, the **Americans with Disabilities Act (ADA)** (PL 101-336), became law in July 1990, although most provisions took effect in the first half of 1992. This landmark civil rights legislation provides a clear and comprehensive mandate against discrimination toward people with disabilities in everyday activities (U.S. Department of Justice, 2000). The ADA uses the authority of the federal government to guarantee equal opportunities for people with disabilities related to employment, transportation, public accommodations, public services, and telecommunications. In addition, it provides protections to people with disabilities similar to those provided to any person on the basis of race, color, sex, national origin, age, and religion. The U.S. Equal Employment Opportunity Commission (EEOC) is the federal agency charged with enforcement for the employment provisions found in Title 1 of the ADA.

The ADA refers to a *qualified* individual with a disability as a person with a physical or mental impairment that substantially *limits* one or more *major life activities,* a person with a record of such an impairment, or a person who is regarded as having such an impairment. The ADA also prohibits discrimination against people who have a known association or relationship with an individual with a disability (U.S. Department of Justice and Commission, and U.S. Equal Employment Opportunity Commission, 1996).

A *qualified* individual with a disability must meet legitimate skill, experience, education, or other requirements of an employment position. The person must be able to perform the *essential functions* of the job, such as those contained within a job description, with or without *reasonable accommodation.* Provided that the person is *qualified* under these conditions, except for limitations caused by a disability, the employer must consider whether the person could perform these functions with reasonable accommodation (U.S. Department of Justice and Commission, and U.S. Equal Employment Opportunity Commission, 1996).

Reasonable accommodations are necessary to allow a qualified person to participate in an educational program (Treloar, 1999a) or an employment setting at a level equal to a nondisabled person. These include modifications of equipment or instructional materials; job restructuring or placement in an available, alternate job; altered work schedules; providing readers, interpreters, or note takers; and other activities that promote architectural accessibility of the physical environment. The organization must provide reasonable accommodations unless it can demonstrate that the accommodation will cause significant difficulty or expense, producing an *undue hardship* (U.S. Department of Justice and Commission, and U.S. Equal Employment Opportunity Commission, 1996). A number of factors influence whether an accommodation may be burdensome. Possible remedies may involve other funding sources (e.g., through the state vocational rehabilitation office) and other financial incentives that could include tax credits and deductions for small businesses.

The ADA is landmark legislation that confirms U.S. leadership in protecting the rights of people with disabilities. Additional refinements and interpretations of this and other legislation will continue to shape disability policy. Some disability advocacy groups, along with the 15-member presidential-appointed National Council on Disability, criticize the Supreme Court for various decisions that have dramatically affected the interpretation of the ADA (National Council on Disability, 2002). Some of these Supreme Court decisions have helped and others hindered implementation of the ADA. It is clear that continuing emphasis on the issue that must continue to realize the law's promise.

Rather than attempt to become an expert on disability law, the community health nurse should develop a resource network that includes disability resource center specialists, public interest law firms, and legal advocacy groups. High-priority interventions include helping people with disabilities learn about their rights and empowering them to act on their own behalf.

The United States needs other public policies to ensure that all Americans, disabled or not, have equal opportunities to become productive citizens. Historically, national public policy has defined disability as the inability to work. Typically, people with disabilities could only qualify for such benefits as health care, income assistance programs, and personal care attendant services if they chose not to work. Unfortunately, neither the ADA nor other legislation, such as the Workforce Investment Act of 1998, have increased employment rates for persons with disabilities (National Council on Disability, 2005). The next act discussed directly addresses employment and benefit issues for persons with disabilities.

Ticket to Work and Work Incentives Improvement Act

In 1998 President Clinton created the Presidential Task Force on Employment of Adults with Disabilities (Presidential Task Force on Employment of Adults With Disabilities, 1998), whose purpose was to create a national policy that would increase the employment rate of adults with disabilities to the rate of nondisabled Americans. In December 1999, the U.S. Congress passed the bipartisan Jeffords-Kennedy-Roth-Moynihan Ticket to Work and Work Incentives Improvement Act (TWWIIA) and signed it into law.

Among other provisions, this legislation removes guidelines that typically result in the termination of Medicaid and Medicare benefits for people with disabilities when they return to work. The TWWIIA modernizes the employment services system for people with disabilities, reducing disincentives to work by increasing access to vocational services, and providing new methods for retaining health insurance after leaving benefit rolls and returning to work. Through the TWWIIA, public health care programs such as Medicare and Medicaid become "tools rather than barriers," as people with disabilities seek opportunities for employment and increased self-sufficiency (Young, personal communication, 1999). Although successful implementation of the TWWIIA at federal and state levels offers people with disabilities increased options in reentering the workforce, the complexity of the law suggests that "explaining it and empowering people to use it remains daunting" (National Council on Disabilities, 2003). At this time, the TWWIIA and other measures have yet to improve employment rates for people with disabilities.

CLINICAL EXAMPLE: THE DILEMMA OF CHOOSING EMPLOYMENT VS. HEALTH CARE AND COMMUNITY SUPPORT ASSISTANCE

John uses a power wheelchair because he has what he calls "spastic quadriplegia" from cerebral palsy. John is college educated and chooses not to work. John weighed his options and acknowledged that if he worked, he would lose the state-supported social service benefits that provide his health care services and attendant caregiver services. Unfortunately, until public policy provides adequate health and social support programs, John's disability will remain a handicapping condition (Treloar, 1999c). ∎

RECONCEPTUALIZING HEALTH CARE FOR PEOPLE WITH DISABILITIES

Disability rights advocates and scholars commonly criticize the medical model of disability for its assumptions about people with disabilities (Hahn, 1991; Kirby, 2004). They argue that this perspective has done the following:

Played a role in the segregation of people with disabilities, and in the labeling of those people—often as aberrant, deviant, or contaminated, and certainly as abnormal . . . . has discouraged full citizenship for people with disabilities (Monaghan, 1998, p. A15).

In the medical model, the health professional prescribes interventions to ameliorate functional limitations of the ill person. Social, psychological, economic, or political factors receive limited attention. This perspective focuses on problems and solutions at the level of the individual rather than the environment or society. Although client autonomy receives increasing attention, professionals who operate from the medical model tend to disempower the person with a disability (Northway, 1997). Table 19-11 summarizes these contrasting perspectives.

The social construct paradigm for disability differs from that traditionally used by the health sciences, rehabilitation, medical sociology, special education, and related fields. Disability may not be pathological or require disease management. Functional limitations do not necessary result in a handicapping condition. This model implies the following:

Disability stems from the failure of a structured social environment to adjust to the needs and aspirations of disabled citizens rather than from the inability of a disabled individual to adapt to the demands of society. . . . The devaluation of disabled persons has not resulted from a lack of economic productivity or from their alleged biological inferiority. . . . this inequality has resulted from the reluctance of society to recognize their dignity and worth as human beings or to grant them civil rights as members of a political community (Hahn, 1985, p. 93).

Rather than emphasize personal deficits like the medical model, contemporary *sociopolitical perspectives for disability* focus on the modification of attitudinal, architectural, sensory, and economic barriers in the environment. This approach attempts to remediate inadequate support services to overcome barriers and empowers the individual, decreasing possible overdependence on professionals and others. Solutions include self- and system-advocacy, removal of barriers, and control by the person with a disability based on desired outcomes.

Nursing education and practice must move beyond the traditional rehabilitation model to incorporate the social construction of disability. According to Woodill (1994), nurses who are disability-conscious can speak out against oppression when they encounter it, use their nursing skills to provide needed support and services for organizations of persons with disabilities, and tell others about issues and concerns of people with disabilities. However, as able-bodied persons, nurses must first "learn to see the world from the perspective of a person with a disability" (Woodill, 1994, p. 47).

Richardson (1997) urges nurses to establish working alliances with families affected by disabilities and develop

TABLE 19-11 Disability Paradigm Influences Policy and Actions

DEFINING CHARACTERISTIC	MEDICAL MODEL	SOCIAL CONSTRUCT
Framework or paradigm	Disability as pathology; emphasizes functional limitations; physical limitations are primary source of problems	Disability as expected (i.e., normal); emphasizes minority-group model (i.e., discrimination and oppression) related to social attitudes and other barriers
Focus of concern	Person	Environment
Problem	Personal deficits (e.g., an impairment, lack of a vocational skill, poor adjustment, or lack of motivation)	Environmental barriers (e.g., attitudinal, architectural, sensory, economic, and inadequate social supports)
Person with a disability	Patient in need of professional help	Person is expert, knowledgeable about self, may or may not seek professional assistance
Role of the health professional	Expert and expects advice to be followed	Collaborating partner; mutually negotiated role reflects needs and desires of person and resources of professional
Perspective of discipline	Medicine, nursing, rehabilitation, medical sociology and psychology, special education, and allied health	Disability studies and disability policy
Model for decision making	Hierarchical (i.e., professional on top)	Collaboration for empowerment of person
Plan of care	Professional centered	Person centered
Desired outcomes	Reflect professional's goals	Reflect person's goals

TABLE 19-12 Conceptualization of Chronic Health Conditions

	SHORT-TERM CONDITIONS	LONG-TERM CONDITIONS		
DIMENSION		MODEL CASE	RELATED CASE	CONTRARY CASE
	Acute illness	**Chronic illness**	**Disabling condition**	**Life-threatening Illness**
Cellular	Inflammation	Inflammation; degeneration	Destruction or atrophy	Proliferation
Time	Short	Long	Long	Short or long
Purpose of Rx	Rx to remove problem (i.e., cure)	Rx to alleviate symptoms	Rx to improve functioning	Rx to kill cancer cells (i.e., cure)
Examples of immediate effect of treatment	Severe pain of surgery; immobility	Weight gain of prednisone therapy; dietary restrictions	Discomfort of splinting; pain of retraining muscles	Loss of hair, nausea, and weight loss
Anticipated outcome	Cure expected	Cure not expected	Cure not expected	Cure hoped for or death feared
Trajectory	Short	Exacerbations and remissions; slow progressive decline; shortened life span	Steady	Remission or cure or death
Effect on ADLs	Severe during Rx or none after	Regimen required	Modifications required	Severe during Rx or none during remission or cure
Mental outlook	Temporary problem	Depression or challenge	Stigma or challenge	Fear or hope
Metaphorical interpretation	A temporary setback	Chain binding; a prisoner of uncertainty because body is unreliable	Obstacle to overcome	Sword hanging over head; a sentence

goals and interventions that address disabling environmental and social barriers. Turnbull and Turnbull III (1996) stated that nurses must work with families affected by disabilities to promote "collaboration for empowerment," which combines an increased control over an individual's life with the dynamic process of connecting families' resources within an empowering context to make decisions collectively. This requires the nurse to view people with disabilities and their families as collaborators and enable them to move beyond a position limited to decision making or receiving professionals' expert judgments. Such collaboration promotes self-determination and allows choices that promote personal values and preferences.

THE PERSONAL EXPERIENCE OF DISABILITY

Persons with disabilities are commonly thought to constitute the largest minority group in the United States (Olkin, 1996). In fact, most people whose lives do not end abruptly will experience disability. Regardless of the disease or condition that precipitates a disability, many experiences are common to lived experience with disability. However, the personal experience (i.e., the personal meaning of disability) differs significantly, based on the time frame and the event or disease process. Table 19-12 compares differences between short-term disability and long-term conditions characterized by disability.

It is clear that those who develop a temporary disability, such as from a sprained or broken ankle, have a very different experience than those who are permanently disabled. Although they may experience the frustrations of mobility associated with the use of a wheelchair or crutches, they do not enter the world of people with disabilities, because they know they will soon reenter society as able-bodied. They often do not develop the skills of living with a disability, such as walking on crutches expertly, obtaining a disabled parking placard, and learning to perform daily activities with a disability. They view it as a temporary problem and a temporary setback.

In contrast, those who develop a permanent disability from an accident or disease process, such as a stroke, must learn to incorporate the modifications required for living into their daily living and identity. Silvers, Wasserman, and Mahowald (1998) describe their situation in the following way: "Their difference from other people is inescapable and can be concealed—if at all—only at formidable cost to their energy and self esteem" (p. 2).

Two people who have not attempted to conceal their disabilities and are nationally recognized for their creative response to disability are Joni Eareckson Tada and Christopher Reeve (now deceased). Although cure is unlikely, their impairments do not prohibit their ability to perform useful work. Their disabilities become a challenge and an obstacle to overcome. Their disabilities are visible and definitive; therefore they did not make decisions about disclosing disability or using assistive devices.

People who become disabled from the progressive decline of a chronic illness often put off accepting the assistive devices that would make life easier for them. They believe that accepting the device would mean accepting the label of disabled. In one study of people with chronic obstructive pulmonary disease (COPD) (Artinian, 1995), many clients reported continuing to work without using oxygen, long after adequate oxygenation was necessary, to avoid the associated stigma. Others reported reluctance to use a cane or wheelchair because they did not want to appear disabled. Others reported reluctance to use a disabled parking placard because they appeared physically fit and did not want people to accuse them of abusing the placard.

In many progressive diseases, a benchmark event forces the person to accept the label of disabled (e.g., failure to wean from the ventilator, a driving accident caused by failing eyesight or mental capacity, a leg amputation from diabetic complications, or a fall when a degenerative disease such as multiple sclerosis impairs mobility). For these people, their bodies have become unreliable. They can no longer plan daily activities and expect to accomplish them independently. Although some young adults experience this type of disability, many of the elderly have chronic illnesses that end in disability.

Family and Caregiver Responses to a Disabled Member

Disability remains poorly understood by the public. Those who are uninitiated into the culture of parents of children with disabilities may wonder *how and why* a parent cares for a child with serious disabilities. We quickly recognize that such caring entails great personal expense, which many of us fear and may be loathe to assume, although we run from such thoughts. We cannot grasp the profound influence the experience will have on us. All members of the family are affected. Parents will redefine their image and expectations for the child, and also themselves as individuals, parents, marital partners, and members of a culture and society (Treloar, 2004). Sibling responses to a disabled brother or sister may be influenced by such factors as age of sibling, reservoir of coping strategies, strength of peer relationships, perception of parent's burden in caring for the disabled child, desire of sibling to protect parents from their concerns about the disabled child, and the impact of the disabled child on family plans and social activities. Grandparents and other extended family, like parents, may grieve the loss of the anticipated child, although this has not been as well studied. Perhaps most important, the occurrence of disability in a family member or close friend *stimulates transformational changes in our implicit and explicit views of the world, producing different attitudes and behaviors, and reassessment of our beliefs about the meaning of disability*. The comments of a mother with two children, the youngest one with serious disabilities, illustrate these points (Dwight, 2001):

> My first son, Timmy. . . . had taught my husband, Phil, and me many things. . . . But I don't think I came face to face with the true meaning of motherhood until Aidan entered our lives (p. 18). As I poured over the books and talked with these other parents, I found the factual side of Down syndrome fairly easy to piece together. . . . Of course, there was nothing in those reference books that could fully explain the other side of the story—the ups and downs of raising a child with Down syndrome in our society. That's what we've been learning from Aidan himself (pp. 34-35).
>
> In many ways, our lives have been transformed. We have found loving support from people who used to be strangers. We look at the world differently. . . . We have an appreciation for a slower pace. . . . And we have a newfound understanding of the preciousness of all people (p. 37).

Current research literature clearly establishes various benefits, along with challenges in families who care for disabled children. Previous studies emphasized pathology, personal deficits and impaired family functioning. Newer family research suggests that the lives of families with disabled children resemble those of other families, exhibiting variability comparable to the general population with respect to outcomes, including parenting stress, family function, and marital satisfaction (Ferguson, Gartner, and Lipsky, 2000). Parental narratives and related research describe lived experience marked by joy amid chronic sorrow (Kearney and Griffin, 2001). Families quickly learn that neither governmental social support nor private health plans offer adequate community-based or in-home assistance for disabled family members. However, parents with satisfying emotional and instrumental support by families, friends, and professionals tend to experience fewer potentially negative effects of unplanned or distressing events (Treloar, 2002).

How can nurses help parents and families adjust to disability in a child? Parents benefit from information about

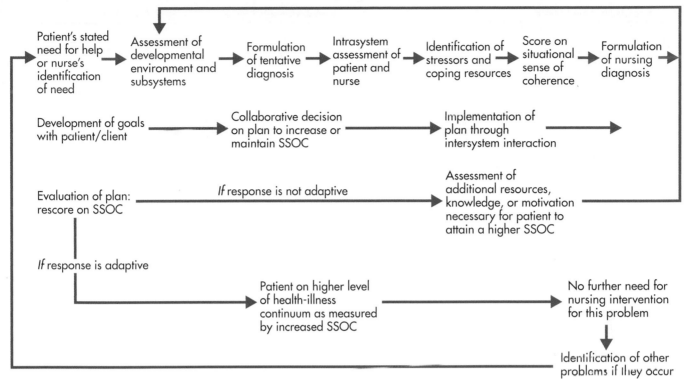

FIGURE 19-3 A summary of the clinical decision-making process used to implement the Intersystem Model. (Reprinted with permission from Artinian BM: The development of the intersystem model, *J Adv Nurs* 16:164-205, 1991. Copyright Blackwell Publications, Inc.).

the child's condition and educational and social services, together with emotional support from professionals, informal and formal social networks, and support groups (Rahi et al., 2004). Empowering and enabling the parent for decision-making on behalf of the child, and establishing a partnership between the parent and health care team, are other important strategies. The next section discusses a model for assessing the needs of the client and family and the nurse.

THE INTERSYSTEM MODEL

The community health nurse working with clients from any of these groups must look beyond the actual limitations to the meaning these limitations hold for the client. The **Intersystem Model** (Artinian, 1997) provides a framework that assists the nurse in understanding the client's knowledge about the disability, the values the person has regarding life with the disability, and the skills the person has for managing the disability. Taylor (1997) used this model to design a program for clients with spinal cord injuries, based on health-related principles in contrast to pathogenic principles. Each person in the rehabilitation team was a teacher, and the client was an active participant in the process. The program focused on partnership as it helped people live with disability.

The Intersystem Model focuses on the interaction between the nurse and the person who is faced with a stressor that cannot be resolved without nursing assistance. The goal of the interaction is to establish a joint plan of care that is congruent with the values and beliefs of the client to increase his or her Situational Sense of Coherence (SSOC) in relation to the

defined problem. SSOC is measured on the basis of comprehensibility (i.e., knowledge about the problem), motivation (i.e., the willingness to work on the problem), and resources to manage the problem. Each aspect can be scored on a scale of 1 to 3 (1 being low and 3 being high).

The interaction begins with a clear definition of the problem that concerns the client or nurse. The client can be an individual, a family, an institution, or a community. Each has a biological subsystem, a psychosocial subsystem, and a spiritual subsystem. Problems can arise from any of these subsystems, and a problem in one subsystem can affect other subsystems. The nurse assesses the client's subsystems, including beliefs, values, past experiences, coping mechanisms, support systems, religious preferences, physical conditions, and current needs. A strength of the model is that the nurse assesses both the client's and the nurse's knowledge about the problem, the values they hold in relation to the problem, and the resources they bring to the situation.

Both client and nurse are active participants in the process. Collaboration is required to develop a plan of care that both the client and nurse find acceptable. Sometimes the nurse must be flexible in his or her expectations. In the final analysis, *the client will only accomplish what he or she agrees to accomplish*. This model produces a shift from an authoritarian relationship to a collaborative and supportive relationship between the client and nurse. Figure 19-3 presents a summary of the decision-making process in this model. Nurses who use the Intersystem Model in working with clients or their families describe their interactions in the following way:

Knowledgeable Patient   Knowledgeable Nurse

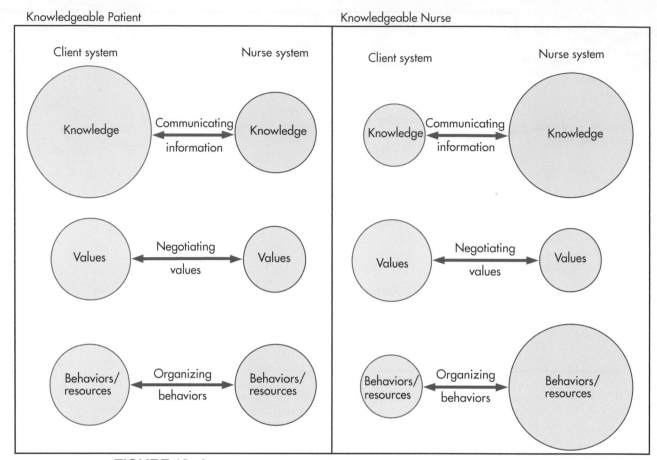

FIGURE 19-4 Knowledgeable client and knowledgeable nurse in the Intersystem Model.

The first thing is sensitivity. As one nurse observed, "Sensitivity is being able to listen, being able to hear families, being able to respond to where they're at. Not your own agenda, and that's real hard for nurses. You have such an agenda, what you think you need to do for health care and you really lose track of where the family is and put all kinds of things onto family that are experts in their child's own care. They may not do it the way we want, but they're experts in their own child's care" (Treloar, unpublished interviews, 1999e).

Another nurse who works with the frail elderly in a rural community said the following: "I give them many options, but they need to decide what will work best for them because they know what their situation is and what they have already tried" (Artinian, unpublished interviews, 1999).

A nurse who works with newborns and children up to 3 years old helps families who are just learning about their children's disabilities navigate "the system." She states that although many parents become very capable, they do not know what to do about the disability in the beginning (Treloar, unpublished interviews, 1999e).

These examples illustrate how clients and their families interact with the community health nurse from very different perspectives. In one case a client has been living with disability for a long time and has become sensitive to the needs of his or her body. This client wants the nurse to listen to these concerns and may benefit from a referral to health-related resources. However, this client *does not need to be told how to manage*

the disability. Figure 19-4 describes this client as the "knowledgeable client." The nurse must ask the client what works best for him or her and what goals the client is pursuing. In contrast, the newly diagnosed client can use the nurse's information about the disability and the available community and governmental resources for the client and family. Figure 19-4 describes this as the "knowledgeable nurse."

If the nurse attempts to tell the knowledgeable client what to do, the client may become angry with the health care system and seek help from other sources. *If the nurse is unable to help a newly diagnosed client learn how to manage the disability and accept himself or herself as disabled, the nurse may lose the opportunity to help the person come to terms with the disabled state.* For example, the staff at a clinic for congenital amputees believed it was important to contact the family before friends and relatives could present a negative image of the child. The case study at the end of this chapter applies the nursing process using The Intersystem Model.

STRATEGIES FOR THE COMMUNITY HEALTH NURSE IN CARING FOR PEOPLE WITH DISABILITIES

Nurses who partner with people with disabilities and their families provide nursing care using a number of strategies in a variety of community-based sites. The individual, his or her family, and the community may be the primary client.

People affected by disabilities have health care needs and resources common to people without disabilities; others are unique to disability. In comparing disabled and nondisabled people, the person with a disability is *both the same as a nondisabled person and different* (Treloar, 1999b). Lawthers et al. (2003) state that "good quality service delivery means that choice of services should be appropriate to the individual, the results effective, and the services delivered in a safe and timely manner" (p. 290). They identified five major quality of care issues for the disabled population: underutilization of age-appropriate preventive health care, undertreatment of comorbid health care conditions, inadequate health care provider knowledge of appropriate and effective treatments, barriers to effective communication between client and family and providers, and risk factors for accidental injury.

The nurse's role should reflect the needs and resources of the client and his or her family. Data from interviews conducted with nurses who provide care to this population and people with physical disabilities illustrate the following guiding principles (Treloar, unpublished interviews, 1999e):

- *Do not assume anything.* The nurse should collect data from the perspective of the person and family with a disability. A nurse case manager for families with disabled children explains:

  Look at each person, client, family, each situation as a totally new and different one. Not assuming anything. Not lumping people into categories. I know we learn cultural things, we learn stereotypes. You have to put that out of your mind. There are cultural things that you would want to respect. But, do not assume anything . . . . And then, listen to what is not said. I watch people . . . . You go into a home and you can learn a tremendous amount by not even asking any questions at times.

- *Adopt the client's perspective.* If the nurse operates from his or her agenda or personal cultural norms rather than from those of the client, less productive and satisfactory outcomes will result. More importantly, the nurse will fail to establish a relationship that respects the client as expert in his or her own health status. Recognize that people's situations may not exist as expected or as they appear. Further, what appears to be a barrier or a limitation may not reflect the true situation or the client's perspective. Another nurse comments

  There can be very good families that are taking excellent care of their children in poverty situations. That does not mean that is a bad place for that child. I think we become very quick to pull children out of what visually is not good from our perspective. It may be the most loving thing that child is going to ever have.

- *Listen and learn from the client.* Gather data from the perspective of the client and family. If the client has severe mental disabilities and cannot offer reliable information, ask the family or caregiver. Nurses must establish relationships that are responsive to the person's methods and the family's methods for dealing with disability. One adult who uses a wheelchair said the following about the difficulties she experienced with health care providers:

Health care providers who have training of some sort, at whatever level, already have set ideas of how things are supposed to be done. I prefer someone that has no idea what they are supposed to do . . . . They do it exactly how they are being told, to the best of their ability, and they do it like a human being instead of like a robot that's going by a list of instructions.

An experienced nurse explained that she does not consider herself the expert, states:

That parent or caretaker is the one that is there for that child all the time. They know that child far better. I may know something medical that they do not know. How can we share that information? That is where you get down to sharing those kinds of things. Teach me. I am always there to learn.

- *Care for the client and the family, not the disability.* The style and intent of client and provider communication influences the acceptability of the interaction. A "conversational" style that establishes an equal partnership with the client is preferable to an "open up the textbook" approach that tells the client "here is what you need to do." The nurse should ask what the client needs help with, what the client is capable of doing, what the client would like to do, and how he or she can help. This approach is dramatically different from saying, "Okay, I can see that you cannot do this, this, and this. This is what I am going to do."

A community health nurse illustrates these ideas in working with families of children with disabilities:

Are they able to develop a health care plan of their own for their child? This, again, may not be ours [plan]. Are they able to follow through on the important pieces of health care for their child, or at least identify that they don't have the resources to do that? . . . . At times we make families feel that if they don't follow our plan, then they're bad parents. So then they don't talk to us about the fact that they can't follow our plan or it's not their plan.

- *Be well informed about community resources.* Learning about resources by reading a community manual is less helpful than meeting with the staff and agencies in person. People often respond differently to requests by someone they know and respect; therefore it may be beneficial for the community health nurse to contact agency personnel about a client and family need. A nurse explains the following:

[When the nurse understands the community resources, she can direct families to] the better systems . . . . Help them identify who the crucial people in those systems are to perhaps help them through them. [She can assist families to] positively interface with systems and get support so that they don't become so embittered.

Lawthers et al. (2003) describe care coordination as the "lubricant" that facilitates links for all areas of quality for a person with a disability, and provides the most significant opportunity for improvement in care delivery by multidisciplinary health care providers.

- *Become a powerful advocate.* The community health nurse's advocacy for the person affected by a disability extends beyond a resource and referral coordinator role, or speaking on the other's behalf. People with disabilities *want to speak for themselves.* They *want to be in control of their lives and their health care.* One person with a disability stated:

They [health care providers who act in an advocacy role] provide the information, but they leave the choice up to the person. And then even if the person chooses against what has been suggested, they still provide the same support.

According to this person with a disability, advocacy implies that the community health nurse's support continues even when the client or family's health care decisions conflict with the health care provider's recommendations.

The community health nurse's perspective on disability will influence the nursing role and the level of care he or she provides to people with disabilities and their families. A variety of systems, ranging from government, community, institutions, family, and the individual (see Figure 19-2), influence the experience of living with a disability. Whether the nurse chooses to work in a setting that specializes in health care services for people affected by disabilities, disability is a common experience that all practicing nurses will encounter.

ETHICAL ISSUES FOR PEOPLE AFFECTED BY DISABILITIES

People with disabilities and their families are concerned about the same contemporary ethical and legal issues that concern nondisabled people. However, some of the associated issues carry particular interest for people with disabilities and their families, including questions and problems surrounding definitions of personhood, respect for human beings, and the rights of people with disabilities.

Associated issues include choosing between abortion and continuing the pregnancy when prenatal screening suggests the presence of impairments and health problems, and determining the appropriate medical care for infants, children, and adults with disabilities. People's spiritual perspectives play an important role in decision-making with a change in health status or life-threatening illness. People who establish hope and meaning in their lives may choose to positively reframe the difficulties associated with functional limitations that others may find intolerable (Treloar, 1999c). Holistic caregiving requires the nurse to assess and promote spiritual health, along with physical and psychological well-being as illustrated in Box 19-3.

Differences in QOL and justice perspectives intersect with concerns about the control of health care costs. For example, people with disabilities and their families may be concerned with how many and what kind of health care services they should be entitled to receive and whether or not these expenditures should be capped, and if so, under what criteria. Many people with life-long disabilities establish a "disability identity" in their adaptation to their limitations and desire (costly) life-sustaining treatment. In contrast, people who are either newly disabled or nondisabled may see any future life as a disabled person as so burdensome that they may refuse extraordinary medical treatments and/or actively seek to end their lives (Hahn and Belt, 2004).

New genetic technologies offer hope for the prevention and cure of disease. However, people with disabilities caution that these scientific advances could be used to eliminate people with disabilities, similar to Hitler's attempts to exterminate

---

BOX 19-3 Spiritual Issues and Disability

Assessment: Theresa is a 29-year-old, single, separated mother of two children, an 8-year-old daughter and a 5-year-old son. Her husband left her shortly after the premature birth of Joseph. He has cerebral palsy with serious intellectual and physical disabilities. In the months and early years following Joseph's birth, Theresa experienced an intense and prolonged questioning of God. Theresa remarks:

In the beginning, I used to ask Him, "Why me?" I was upset. I had little hope, little faith, but I stuck to it. I knew it was going to get better, I just didn't know when . . . . It's been tough for me as a single parent. What I've been through has made me stronger. Now I thank God for my boy. But when he was born, I thought God was punishing me. I couldn't believe it! I really had a rough time. I didn't understand how God could give me a problem like this, when I had so many problems to begin with (Treloar, 1999c, p. 111).

Nursing Diagnosis: Spiritual distress related to establishing meaning for disability as manifested by repeated questioning and blaming of God

Commentary: Disability in oneself or others is an unexpected event, often with what feel like tragic consequences. While disability at any age may not be easy to adapt to, declining capabilities more commonly occur with aging and chronic illness. However, we do not expect disability to strike in the prime of our lives, or with the birth of a new child.

Regardless of our religious perspectives, we are all spiritual beings who seek to establish meaning for the events that occur in our lives. Even people with established spiritual beliefs may question their relationship to a higher power. Community health nurses who are comfortable with their own spirituality should assess for spiritual needs and provide appropriate spiritual care for people affected by disabilities. In talking directly with the person or family about these needs, the nurse does not push his or her version of spiritual beliefs. The nurse creates a climate that invites people to incorporate religious rituals, connect with clergy, or address spiritual needs according to their preferences. However, when people's spiritual needs go unrecognized and unmet, spiritual distress may linger, causing disruption in other parts of their lives.

---

undesirable peoples in World War II. Disability advocacy groups, including Not Dead Yet, have taken a strong stance against physician-assisted suicide, fearing it will lead to the early or forced death of people with disabilities (Burgdorf, 1998). Parents who seek cochlear implants for their deaf children often encounter opposition by deaf advocacy groups. These groups argue that people should accept deafness because deafness benefits the client through deaf culture and additional skills, such as sign language. Similarly, the use of Ritalin and other stimulant medications for children or adults with attention deficit hyperactivity disorder carry pro and con arguments that include ethical considerations.

An emphasis on self-determination, the deinstitutionalization movement, and the accompanying expansion of community-based independent living centers and other residential settings for people with disabilities create other perplexing issues. Disabled people needing assistance with ADLs and IADLs commonly find that social welfare programs have limited funding for community-based living, finding it less expensive to place these disabled persons in long-term care settings. Imagine living in a nursing home when you are 25 years old, intellectually intact, yet physically disabled! In fact, according to Hahn and Belt (2004), the disability rights

ETHICAL Insights

When Is Life Worth Continuing?

The world watched while Terri Schiavo's situation unfolded amid numerous legal and legislative challenges surrounding whether her feeding tube should be discontinued, and conflict developed between her parents and her husband and guardian, Michael. Disability rights groups and right-to-life advocates kept vigil for weeks outside the nursing home where Terri resided. Terri, a 41-year-old brain-damaged woman, died on March 31, 2005, 7 years after experiencing an anoxic event that led to her condition. Although previous court decisions have clearly established a person's right to discontinuation of treatment, including the provision of food and fluids, there was no documentation or advanced directive indicating Terri's wishes. Terri's parents offered to assume guardianship of their daughter, believing her to be both responsive to her environment and desiring life in her current condition. Michael fought to have her feeding tube removed, stating that in previous discussions, Terri said that in a similar situation, she would not want to continue living. Medical discussions focused on the extent of her "vegetative state" and capacity to respond to her environment. Seven years later, amid numerous court challenges and Michael's obtaining a reported million-dollar plus malpractice settlement designated for his wife's care, the court ordered that Terri's feeding tube and all hydration be stopped as requested by her husband. She died several days later.

What do you think? When does life become meaningless and not worth continuing? What are the relevant issues when families are in conflict about what medical treatment the person with a severe disability would want in the absence of written advanced directives? What values and ethical principles should be considered? Williams (2005), a physician, suggests that a key question to be considered is: "How should we have looked at Terri? Was she a person (or nonperson) in a persistent vegetative state, perhaps with diminished rights, or was she a severely handicapped person with rights that were not considered fairly?" When medical care is futile (i.e. useless or burdensome), it *should* be stopped; however, what guides our practice when treatment, such as artificial nutrition through a feeding tube, is withdrawn because a life is seen to have no value or care of that person is excessively burdensome?

Consider the words of a writer with a severely disabled daughter, Claire, and a mother, both in a "vegetative state" with feeding tubes: Columnist and law professor Marianne M. Jennings (2005) writes:

Doctors are almost always wrong. While I have the highest respect for the physicians who have treated our daughter and my mother and will be forever grateful for their selfless efforts and care, I know, and perhaps they do, too, that these patients are unique.

Doctors are inevitably taken aback at some point by Claire and patients like her who fight for their lives. If I had dug my daughter's grave each time a doctor told me she wouldn't live, I'd be in China by now . . . . When Claire turned 10, the good docs called her an outlier and threw in the towel on death predictions. Claire turned 18 two months ago. Doctors read CAT scans, MRIs and EEGs and conclude that, clinically, there ain't nothin' there.

But doctors are not with these patients 24/7. Our Claire has a perfectly flat EEG . . . . Terri Schiavo was higher functioning than our Claire. Yet each morning, when we touch the bottom of her shirt to prepare for her shower, she closes her eyes in anticipation of that shirt coming over her face. She clinches her teeth if you put a washcloth to her face because washcloths mean a good mouth cleaning . . . . She turns her head when you say her name. Claire's smiles come mostly in response to her mother's and father's voices.

They feel, they flinch, they startle, they turn, they moan, they react, they have some memory, and no one truly knows how much gets through, what is serendipitous and what is a real responses. When in doubt, doubt the doctors.

Spirituality engulfs the vegetative . . . . The life that exists . . . . has had the judicial imprimatur of "So not worth it" placed upon it and the plug (tube) pulled. Yet the life that resides in these bodies so ravaged by immobility scares the livin' daylights out of me. If you already believe in a god, these souls will confirm your faith. If you don't believe, well, I have seen atheists and agnostics humbled, silenced and in tears as they stumbled upon a spiritual experience that caught them unawares. These are the very elect of beings.

Those who allow these lives to be taken, especially in reliance upon clinical reports, engage in the sentencing of innocents . . . . We are not here for them. They are here for us . . . . My family and I have learned more from these two [daughter and mother] non-speaking souls than in any of our many studies for degrees . . . . I fear for the clinical callousness of this [Schiavo's] tube removal . . . . The removal of this feeding tube, with the resulting death, gives me pause about the precedent for our Claire and my mom. I fear for us . . . . Her [Schiavo's] death dulls our collective conscience and eases us into the taking of life in the name of inconvenience (Jennings, 2005, pp. V1-2).

Many hoped that the Patient Self-Determination Act of 1990 would motivate more people to prepare advance directives for decision-making in life-threatening illness; however, many people do not consider these issues, leaving families, as surrogates, to decide what the individual would want. Hopefully Terri's case, which polarized the nation on what *should* be done in her case, may stimulate people to think through, discuss with loved ones, and complete advance directives that are communicated to a health care provider.

---

movement was started by the students who refused to live in nursing homes.

Like any ethical problem, issues related to disability do not have easy solutions. However, societal attitudes and bias toward people with disabilities may negatively influence policies and decisions related to the interests and fair treatment of people with disabilities. Disability rights proponents worry that the devaluation of people with disabilities may promote their unnecessary and untimely deaths. Ethical decision making cannot be separated from discussions that include the meaning associated with life and life's accompanying challenges. The case of Terri Schiavo described in the Ethical Insights box illustrates some of these issues.

Nursing Education and Practice When the Nurse Is Disabled

What are the *essential functions* for professional nursing practice? What specific behaviors and work functions characterize the practice? Under the ADA, nursing education programs and employers must provide *reasonable accommodations* for *qualified* students and nurses, unless this would present an *undue burden or hardship* on the institution or employer as established by law. A *qualified* student or nurse must be able to meet the requirements of the clinical experience or job with reasonable accommodations, removal of barriers, and provision of appropriate aids (e.g., amplified stethoscope for someone with a hearing impairment) and

Creative wheelchair transport. People with disabilities and their families become experts at adapting to their environment. The author's husband, Bob, built these folding ramps for use with daughter Joy's wheelchair. Unfortunately, many families lack easy access to a vehicle equipped with a wheelchair lift, or accessible public transportation. This affects their ability to obtain health care, accomplish instrumental activities of daily living, and to compete with others on an equal level.

Father Bob adjusting Joy's wheelchair. Obtaining durable medical equipment that fits properly and meets a disabled person's specific needs often challenges therapist and client alike. Commonly, families with disabled members learn to modify and repair wheelchairs and other adaptive equipment. This illustrates another aspect in which family and client become experts in the care of the person with a disability.

I want a ride, too! Joy rents a home which she shares with her caregiver family. The Hispanic couple's children began riding on Joy's lap in a carrier harness when they were babies. As young children, they delight in climbing onto Joy's wheelchair and helping her shop for groceries at the corner fruit and vegetable market. Joy comments: "When children see me they ask questions out of curiosity, while adults practice avoidance." Joy comments further: "Being in a wheelchair is one part of me—it doesn't define who I am. After a while, people don't see my wheelchair."

Preparing teacher lesson plans. Joy teaches underprivileged students in an inner city grade school. As a college student, she faced bias by education faculty who questioned the appropriateness of her dream to be a teacher. Admittedly, they lacked experience in working with a teacher or student with a disability. A few advocated for her, and she persevered and fulfilled her career goal. Despite the ADA, discrimination and misunderstanding continue to influence the lives of people with disabilities, stimulating some to fight, while others give up.

Photos taken by the chapter's lead author, Dr. Linda Treloar, of her family.

Science fair preparations.

Teacher Joy and her class. Joy's students like the fact that they are at her eye level (although some tower over her). Students quickly learn to actively help their teacher and one another. Joy uses a variety of resources to teach concepts that may be challenging due to her physical limitations. This includes the use of volunteers like Joy's dad (Bob) who assist students with science experiments.

Unloading after a day of teaching. Joy uses "Dial-A-Ride" (commonly described as "Dial-A-Wait") to travel to and from her job and to run errands. Local bus service is another option, but can be problematic due to bus route scheduling, broken-down lifts, and sometimes surly bus drivers.

Weiners go with everything, even bingo! Joy lives in a multicultural world where Spanish is the dominant language spoken by people in her home and at school. Joy contributes to and benefits from being part of two families—that of her parents (the author) and her Hispanic caregiver family. Nurses with a community focus recognize and support human networks that encourage and move one another toward well-being.

services (e.g., scribe or translator). Institutions are not expected to lower their standards for an *unqualified* student or nurse.

Rather than focusing on "technical" aspects of nursing practice (e.g., bed-making) that tend to discriminate against nurses with physical or sensory disabilities, the argument has been made that nursing should emphasize its "humanistic" capacities (Carroll, 2004). The art and science of nursing practice reflects a specialized knowledge base applied through interpersonal caring. Skilled nurses continuously gather and critically analyze data about their clients and families; they

know the client and they *know about* the client. These characteristics of nursing practice are not limited to nondisabled persons. The type of setting influences whether a nurse who is disabled is *qualified to* perform the *essential functions of the job*. For example, a nurse who has serious physical disabilities, although functionally impaired, may not be *handicapped* or *unqualified* as a nurse performing telephone triage. However, the same nurse may be *unqualified* to practice nursing in a medical-surgical setting or emergency department, where physical lifting and similar movements are *essential functions* of the job.

CASE STUDY   Application of the Nursing Process

NOTE: Names and demographic information have been changed to protect the privacy of the client.

INTERSYSTEM MODEL: CLIENT CARE PLAN

During his regular urology clinic visit at a large medical center it was discovered by ultrasound that Juan, a client with spina bifida, had small bladder stones. Juan refused to have surgery to have the stones removed. When he made his regular visit to the spina bifida clinic in a health department several months later, he explained the reasons for his refusal to the nurse coordinator. The first reason was that he had not been informed that stones were a probable complication of the bladder augmentation surgery that had produced a stoma on his abdomen for catheterization. He also wanted to wait until all the stones had formed and have them all removed at the same time. The nurse coordinator was concerned that without surgery, Juan would continue to have urinary tract infections.

Focus of Situational Interaction (Either Client Concern or Nurse Concern)

Juan refused to have minor ultrasound surgery to have the bladder stones removed while they were still small because the doctor had told him they might develop again. The State Children's Services (SCS) nurse coordinator believed it should be done at this time.

ASSESSMENT

Developmental Environment
Biological Subsystem

Juan, age 18 years, is paraplegic because of spina bifida with hydrocephaly. He has neurogenic bladder and bowels and dislocated hips. He is wheelchair-dependent. He was referred to SCS by the county hospital when he was 5 years old because of a urinary tract infection (UTI). He has been attending the spina bifida clinic since then. Juan has had surgery to release the tendons in his legs and also surgery on his bladder. Juan developed bladder stones 2 years after his bladder augmentation surgery.

Psychosocial Subsystem

Juan has an older brother who is living at home. Juan speaks Spanish and English, but his parents speak Spanish only. His brother plays basketball with him on a daily basis. Juan is trying to accomplish his young adult task of separating himself from his parents so that he can be independent in life. He is presently studying computer science at a technical training school.

Spiritual Subsystem

The family is Catholic and has a strong religious heritage.

Situational Environment
Intrasystem Analysis of the Client

Detector Function: Knowledge (What does the client know about the problem?)

Juan does not know what the surgery will be like, how much pain he will experience after the surgery, or what the outcome will be. He does not understand that if he waits he risks frequent UTIs and will need major abdominal surgery in the future.

Selector Function: Attitudes and Values (What are the client's attitudes and values about the problem?)

Juan is fearful of any surgery because he previously had surgery for contracture releases for his legs. The surgery was more painful than he had been led to believe. Also, before the stoma surgery he was not told that bladder stones might develop. Therefore he is distrustful of doctors. He also expresses concerns over taking pain medications because he fears becoming addicted. In his previous surgery he had thought he could cope with the pain without pain medication but found that he could not. Therefore he does not want to go through another painful experience again. In addition, because he needs to make his own decisions, he does not want to be pressured into the surgery by his parents.

Effector Function: Behaviors (What skills or resources does the client have to deal with the problem?)

Juan is very familiar with the catheterization procedure and does it consistently every 4 hours. He also drinks more water to prevent development of bladder stones. These behaviors promote health following the surgical procedure.

Intrasystem Analysis of the Nurse

Detector Function: Knowledge (What do I know about the problem?)

The nurse is aware of the potential problems that can occur if the surgery is not done and that the relative risk is small at this time.

Selector Function: Attitudes and Values (What are my attitudes and values about the problem?)

The nurse believes that Juan's insistence on making his own decision is very positive. She has observed that persons with spina bifida make the least successful transition to adulthood of the clients in her clinics and supports his desire to manage his own life. In fact, she fosters this type of behavior for all clients in her clinics as soon as they are 14 years of age, to prepare them for their adult role. At that age, she starts communicating directly with the clients rather than the parents so that they can learn to be responsible for their own care. She engages them in problem solving long before they are 21 years old to prepare them for the transition to adult services and responsibilities.

Effector Function: Behaviors (What skills or resources do I have to deal with the problem?)

Because of her history of communicating directly with Juan, he is able to trust the nurse's judgments and respects her opinions. She also knows the resources in the community that can help Juan.

ANALYSIS

Identification of stressors
  Previous negative experiences with surgery
  Unresolved separation issues with parents
Coping resources
  Supportive family
  Good relationship with SCS nurse
  Financial resources from SCS

SCORING ON SITUATIONAL SENSE OF COHERENCE

(High = 3, Medium = 2, Low = 1)

Comprehensibility: In relation to what the client needs to know about the situation, how much is known?

SCORE: 1

The patient does not know what to expect about the surgery or the relative risk of having the surgery or not.

Meaningfulness: In relation to motivation, how much effort is the client willing to put into resolving this problem?

SCORE: 1

The patient believes that a wait-and-see approach is better and wants to postpone the surgery until all the potential stones are formed, so that he can have just one surgery.

Manageability: In relation to resources, what is available to manage this problem?

SCORE: 3

Medical and financial resources are available for the surgery.

DIAGNOSES

Individual

- Knowledge deficit about the surgical procedure
- At risk for repeated urinary tract infections
- Anxiety due to autonomy issues

Family

- Change in parenting tasks to allow client to take responsibility for his care and make decisions

Community

- Need for support programs that allow young adults autonomy in treatment decisions
- Scarcity of resources and programs to allow clients to be independent, such as modification of car so that he can drive using his hands

PLANNING

Since the nurse and client are not in agreement about what should be done, **Nursing goals** are made:

Individual

Long-Term Goal

- After making the decision, the client will demonstrate or verbalize trust in the nurse coordinator.

Short-Term Goals

- The patient will be offered the opportunity to learn more about the surgery so that he can make an informed decision.
- The nurse will continue to honor the decision of the client.

Family

Long-Term Goal

- The nurse will collaborate with the family and his physician, who has followed the client for many years, to encourage client autonomy and cooperation with future medical care.

Short-Term Goal

- Parents and physician will not pressure Juan to undergo surgery until Juan makes his own decision.

Community

Long-Term Goal

- The community will provide additional programs to prepare disabled university students for entering the work community.

Short-Term Goal

- The community will work with Juan to initiate use of rehabilitation resources that are in place.

INTERVENTION: INTERSYSTEM INTERACTION (CLIENT AND NURSE INTERACTION)

Communication of Information: The SCS nurse referred Juan to the Clinical Nurse Specialist (CNS) at the urology clinic near the hospital where the surgery would be performed. This CNS is a male Hispanic who is very skilled in communication and has expertise in this surgery. He provided relevant information about the surgery. The SCS nurse purposefully involved the CNS because of Juan's age. Juan will be transitioned to adult services after he is 21 years old, and this nurse could be a resource person after Juan is discharged from SCS.

Negotiation of Values: When Juan understood the relative risk of having the surgery versus waiting, he agreed to have the surgery done. During the time this information was being given to Juan, the SCS nurse told the clinic urologist and his parents, "Just give him time, I know he will make the right decision."

Organization of Behaviors: (A mutual plan of care). Juan agreed to have the surgery and it was done without difficulty.

Continued

CASE STUDY   Application of the Nursing Process (cont'd)

EVALUATION: (RESCORING ON SITUATIONAL SENSE OF COHERENCE)

Comprehensibility: In relation to what the client needs to know about the situation, how much did he learn?

SCORE: 3

Juan now understands the procedure and knows about future problems that could occur.

Meaningfulness: In relation to motivation, how willing was the client to accept the challenge of the problem and work to overcome it?

SCORE: 3

Juan is willing to follow the treatment regimen and also wants other clients to know about the whole treatment program, so that they will not experience the same problems he did.

Manageability: In relation to resources, how adequate were they in helping Juan and his family manage the problem?

SCORE: 3

This problem was managed with adequate resources.

LEVELS OF PREVENTION

The following are examples of the three levels of prevention as applied to the individual, family, and community.

Primary

- In relation to the bladder stones, encourage client to drink fluids to prevent occurrence of more stones and to follow a consistent schedule of irrigation of bladder and catheterization to adequately drain the bladder.
- Use available resources for independent living.

Secondary

- Initiate self-care behaviors for follow-up after discharge from hospital to monitor progress.

Tertiary

- Arrange independent transportation for Juan to limit the effects of his disability.
- Continue to work with the family about Juan's need to have autonomy over his life decisions.
- Offer community support to enable Juan and other clients with mobility problems to attend college for career possibilities.

COMMENTS

Because the SCS nurse was willing to help Juan make his own decision in this matter, Juan was willing to work with her on other problems associated with his disability in making his transition to adulthood responsibilities.

Although concerns about client safety and competing rights (individual versus societal) must be considered, people with disabilities are excluded too often from nursing educational programs and practice based on what the person *cannot do,* rather than how or where **access** could be created to practice nursing. Nurses must consider how personal attitudes toward people with disabilities influence not only their client care, but their responses to nursing students and colleagues with disabilities. Sowers and Smith (2004) surveyed 88 nursing faculty members in eight programs on their perceptions, knowledge, and concerns regarding nursing students with disabilities. They write:

> *Perhaps the most positive and hopeful finding of this study was that respondents recognized that they needed to learn more about disability issues and how to teach and accommodate students with disabilities. . . . There is still a desperate need for faculty training, not only about the law, but also about the ability of people with disabilities to successfully complete nursing school and to be practicing nurses, as well as about the strategies that are effective in making this a reality for them (p. 218).*

Moore (2004) challenges nurses to consider their answer to the ultimate question: "What is the core and essence of nursing, held by all nurses, in all settings, in all roles, and in all parts of the world?" (p. 201). She contends that through answering this question, nursing education programs will

capture the essential components and technical standards that comprise the essence of nursing.

SUMMARY

To address these issues, community health nurses must recognize that there are a variety of personal and societal perspectives on disability with accompanying moral or ethical issues. They should practice holistic nursing care that incorporates mind, body, and spiritual care considerations into health care practice (Treloar, 1999d). To this end, nurses can do the following:

- Become familiar with a variety of ethical frameworks for decision making, and learn a strategy to analyze ethical problems related to health care for people with disabilities.
- Help the client and family access needed information from the health care team to make informed decisions that reflect their interests.
- Help educate the public on health care issues within the nurse's scope of practice and knowledge and skill level.
- Participate in the development of institutional policies and procedures for ethical and legal issues related to disability.
- Take a position on an ethical issue with political implications.
- Work to influence governmental policies and laws related to disability.

LEARNING ACTIVITIES

1. Interview a person with a disability or a family with a disabled family member about their experiences with health care providers and the health care system.

2. Shadow a nurse in a community-based health clinic that serves children with disabilities. Observe the roles and the interactions of the multidisciplinary team members. Follow a family through clinic. If possible, meet the family at their home before clinic and observe their preparations before coming to clinic. Accompany them from clinic check-in to departure. After returning to their home, ask them for their thoughts on the clinic experience.

3. Interview a community resident who has a serious disability. How does he or she view himself or herself? What challenges or concerns does the resident mention? Interview a caregiver about the caregiving experience.

4. Ask an experienced nurse about his or her encounters with people with disabilities. Listen to his or her language and perceptions of disability. Compare these to the perspectives reflected in the social construct model for disability.

5. Visit with the residents and staff in a community-based living environment for people with disabilities. Assist with caregiving for the residents.

6. Visit one or two community-based agencies that provide services to people with disabilities. How do families gain access to services and what services are offered? How do available services and resources address the needs of people affected by disabilities (a person with a disability and his or her family)?

7. Spend time in the home of a family who has a child with intellectual disabilities. Note the family relationships. Interview the parents and siblings about their experiences with a child with special needs. Spend time with the child.

REFERENCES

Artinian B: The process of regaining control: outcome of a pulmonary rehabilitation program for patients with advanced COPD, Paper presented at the California Society of Pulmonary Rehabilitation, San Francisco, Calif, 1995.

Artinian BM: Overview of the Intersystem Model. In Artinian BM and Conger M, editors: *The intersystem model: integrating theory and practice,* Thousand Oaks, Calif, 1997, Sage.

Batavia AI: Relating disability policy to broader public policy: understanding the concept of "handicap," *Policy Stud J* 21(4): 735-739, 1993.

Barnes C: Theories of disability and the origins of the oppression of disabled people in Western society. In Barton L, editor: *Disability and society: emerging issues and insights,* New York, 1996, Longman.

Blaska J: The power of language: speak and write using "person first." In Nagler M, editor: *Perspectives on disability: text and readings on disability,* Palo Alto, Calif, 1993, Health Markets Research.

Bogdan R: Exhibiting mentally retarded people for amusement and profit: 1850-1940, *Am J Ment Defic* 91(2):120-126, 1986.

Brandt EN Jr, Pope AM, editors: *Enabling America: assessing the role of rehabilitation science and engineering,* Washington, DC, 1997, Committee on Assessing Rehabilitation Science and Engineering, Institute of Medicine, National Academy Press.

Burgdorf RL Jr: Assisted suicide: a disability perspective position paper, March 24, 1997, Updated September 14, 1998, National Council on Disability, http://www.ncd.gov/publications/suicide.html.

Caron C: Making meaning out of the experiences of our lives, *Womens Educ des Femmes* 12(2):22-25, 1996.

Carroll, SM: Inclusion of people with physical disabilities in nursing education, *J Nurs Educ* 43(5):207-212, May 2004.

Centers for Disease Control: *Prevalence of disabilities and associated health conditions among adult: United States, 1999.* MMWR Weekly, February 23, 2001/50(07); US Department of Health and Human Services, http://www.cdc.gov/mmwr/preview/mmwrhtml/mm5007a3.htm.

ChildStats.gov: *America's Children 2003,* 2003, The Author, http://www.childstats.gov/ac2003/indicators.asp?IID=121&id=4.

Creamer D: Finding God in our bodies: theology from the perspective of people with disabilities, part II, *J Religion Disabil Rehabil* 2(2):67-87, 1995.

Cutler DM: The reduction in disability among the elderly, *Proc Natl Acad Sci USA* 98 (12): 6546-6547, 2001.

DeJong G: Toward a research and training capacity in disability policy, *Policy Stud J* 22(1):152-160, 1994.

Disability Statistics Center: *Survey of income and program participation,* University of California, San Francisco, http://dsc.ucsf.edu/main.php?name=sipp.

Dwight V: Aidan's gift. In Klein SD, Schive K, editors: *You will dream new dreams: inspiring personal stories by parents of children with disabilities,* New York, 2001, Kensington, pp. 31-37.

Employment and Disability Institute: *Unemployment rate IS NOT equal to 70%,* 2003-2005, Cornell University, http://www.ilr.cornell.edu/ped/disabilitystatistics/issues.cfm#unemployment.

Ferguson PM, Gartner A, Lipsky DK: The experience of disability in families: a synthesis of research and parent narratives. In Parens E, Asch A, editors: *Prenatal testing and disability rights,* Washington, DC, 2000, Georgetown University Press, pp. 72-94.

Friedberg JB, Mullins JB, Sukiennik AW: *Accept me as I am: best books of juvenile nonfiction on impairments and disabilities,* New York, 1985, RR Bowker.

Gartner A, Joe T, editors: *Images of the disabled, disabling images,* New York, 1987, Praeger.

Goffman E: *Stigma: notes on the management of spoiled identity,* Englewood Cliffs, NJ, 1963, Prentice-Hall.

Hahn H: Toward a politics of disability: definitions, disciplines, and policies, *Soc Sci J* 22(4): 87-105, 1985.

Hahn H: Theories and values: ethics and contrasting perspectives on disability. In Marinelli RP, Orto AED, editors: *The psychological and social impact of disability,* ed 3, New York, 1991, Springer.

Hahn H, Belt, TL: Disability identity and attitudes toward cure in a sample of disabled activists, *J Health Soc Behav* 45:453-464, Dec 2004.

Holahan J, Bruen, B: *Medicaid spending: what factors contributed to the growth between 2000 and 2002?* September 2003, Kaiser Commission on Medicaid and the Uninsured, http://www.kaisernetwork.org/health_cast/uploaded_files/4139.pdf#search='Bruen, %20holahan,%20Medicaid%spending%20and%20disability.

Jans L, Stoddard S: Chartbook on women and disability in the United States, 1999, Updated July 21, 1999, Department of Education, National Institute on Disability and Rehabilitation Research, http://www.infouse.com/disabilitydata.

Jansen DEMC et al: People with intellectual disability and their health problems: a review of comparative studies, *J Intellect Disabil Res* 48(Pt 2):93-102, 2004.

Jennings, MM: Souls that give us a glimpse of the divine, *The Arizona Republic* April 3, 2005, pp. V1-2.

Johnson AF, Johnson LS: Shame and spirituality: taboo topics in the disability community, *J Religion Disabil Rehabil* 2(3):29-38, 1995.

Jones NL, Apling RN: The Individuals with Disabilities Education Act (IDEA): comparison and analysis of selected provisions in H.R. 1350 as passed by the House and by the

Senate, 108th Congress, May 25, 2004. http://digitalcommons.ilr.cornell.edu/key_workplace/35.

Kearney PM, Griffin T: Between joy and sorrow: being a parent of a child with developmental disability, *J Adv Nurs* 34:582-592, 2001.

Kirby JC: Disability and justice: a pluralistic account, *Soc Theory Pract* 30(2),:229-246, April 2004.

Kraus LE, Stoddard S, Gilmartin D: *Chartbook on disability in the United States, 1996, An InfoUse Report*, Updated November 12, 1998, US National Institute on Disability and Rehabilitation Research, http://www.infouse.com/disabilitydata/chartbook.choices.html.

LaPlante MP, Carlson D: *Disability in the United States: prevalence and causes*, 1996, Disability Statistics Rehabilitation Research and Training Center, Institute for Health and Aging, School of Nursing, University of California, http://dsc.ucsf.edu/UCSF/pub.taf?_function=search&recid=65&grow=1.

Lawthers et al: Rethinking quality in the context of persons with disability, *Int J Qual Health Care* 15(4): 287-299, Aug 2003.

Longmore PK: Uncovering the hidden history of people with disabilities, *Rev Am Hist* 15(3):355-364, 1987.

Manton KG, Gu X: Changes in the prevalence of chronic disability in the United States black and nonblack population above age 65 from 1982 to 1999, *Proc Natl Acad Sci USA* 98(11): 6354-6359, 2001.

Martin SS, Catlett SM: Same window, new view: print media and persons with disabilities, Unpublished paper presented at 1999 TASH Conference, Chicago, Ill, 1999.

Monaghan P: Pioneering field of disability studies challenges established approaches and attitudes, *Chron High Educ* XLIV(20):A15-16, 1998.

Moore, CA: Disability as difference and the nursing profession, *J Nurs Educ* 43(5):197-201, May 2004.

Murphy RF: *The body silent,* New York, 1990, Henry Holt.

National Council on Disability: *National disability policy: a progress report: November 1, 1997 to October 31, 1998*, February 16, 1999, The Author, http://www.ncd.gov/publications/policy97-98.html.

National Council on Disability: *National Council on Disability Recommendations Workforce Investment Act Reauthorization*, March 17, 2005, The Author, http://www.ncd.gov/newsroom/publications/2005/workforce_investment.htm.

National Council on Disability: *National Council on Disability says employment for people with disabilities remains far tooLow*, August 1, 2003, http://www.ncd.gov/newsroom/news/2003/r03-427.htm.

National Council on Disability: *Supreme Court decisions interpreting the Americans with Disabilities Act,* updated September 17, 2002, The Author, http://vlcd.gov/newsroom/publications/2002/supremecourt_ada.htm.

National Organization on Disability, Louis Harris and Associates: *N.O.D./Harris 2000 survey of Americans with disabilities, 2000,* The Author, http://www.nod.org/attitudes.html.

Neri MT, Kroll T: Understanding the consequences of access barriers to health care: experiences of adults with disabilities, *Disabil Rehabil* 25(2): 85-96, 2003.

Northway R: Disability and oppression: some implications for nurses and nursing, *J Adv Nurs* 26(4):736-743, 1997.

Northway R, Jenkins R: Quality of life as a concept for developing learning disability nursing practice? *J Clin Nurs* 12:57-66, 2003.

Olkin R: *What psychotherapists should know about disability,* New York, 1999, Guilford Press.

Pfeiffer D: Overview of the disability movement: history, legislative record, and political implications, *Policy Stud J* 21(4):724-734, 1993.

Phillips A, Morrison J, Davis RW: General practitioners' educational needs in intellectual disability health, *J Intellect Disabil Res,* 48(Pt 2):142-149, Feb 2004.

Pope AM, Tarlov AR, editors: *Disability in America: toward a national agenda for prevention,* Washington, DC, 1991, IOM, National Academy Press.

Presidential Task Force on Employment of Adults with Disabilities: *Recharting the course: first report of the presidential task force on employment of adults with disabilities,* November 15, 1998, The Author, http://www.dol.gov/dol/_sec/public/programs/ptfead/rechart.html.

Rahi JS et al: Meeting the needs of parents around the time of diagnosis of disability among their children: evaluation of a novel program for information, support, and liaison by key workers, *Pediatrics* 114(4):e477-e482, Oct 2004.

Richardson M: Addressing barriers: disabled rights and the implications for nursing of the social construct of disability, *J Adv Nurs* 25(6):1269-1275, 1997.

Schemo, DJ: Parts of special-ed bill would shift more power to states and school districts, *The New York Times,* November 22, 2004, http://www.aapd-dc.org/News/IDEA/analysisIDEA.html.

Schiller, J.S. and Bernadel, L. *Summary health statistics for the U.S. population: National health interview survey, 2002,* National Center for Health Statistics, Vital and Health Statistics, 10(220). 2004, http://www.cdc.gov/nchs/data/series/sr_10/sr10_220.pdf.

Scotch RK: Understanding disability policy: varieties of analysis, *Policy Stud J* 22(1):170-175, 1994.

Shapiro JP: *No pity: people with disabilities forging a new civil rights movement,* New York, 1993, Times Books.

Silvers A, Wasserman D, Mahowald MB: *Disability, difference, discrimination: perspectives on justice in bioethics and public policy,* Lanham, Mass, 1998, Rowman & Littlefield.

Sowers J, Smith MR: Nursing faculty members' perceptions, knowledge, and concerns about students with disabilities, *J Nurs Educ* 43(5): 213-218, May 2004.

Spillman BC: Changes in elderly disability rates and the implications for health care utilization and cost, *Milbank Q* 82(1):157-194, 2004.

Stern, S.M., U.S. Census Bureau: 2003 ASA presentation: *Counting people with disabilities: a comparison of estimates in Census 2000 and the Census 2000 Supplementary Survey*, released August 2004a, U.S. Census Bureau, http://www.census.gov/hhes/www/disability/whatsnew.html and http://www.census.gov/acs/www/Downloads/ACS/asastern.pdf.

Stern, S.M., U.S. Census Bureau, Poverty and Health Statistics Branch: *Counting people with disabilities: how survey methodology influences estimates in Census 2000 and the Census 2000 Supplementary Survey,* released August 2004b, U.S. Census Bureau, http://www.census.gov/hhes/www/disability/whatsnew.html and http://www.census.gov/acs/www/Downloads/ACS/finalstern.pdf.

Stern, S.M., & Brault, M., U.S. Census Bureau, Housing and Household Economic Statistics Division, *Disability data from the American community survey: A brief examination of the effects of a question redesign in 2003,* released February 2005, U.S. Census Bureau, http://www.census.gov/hhes/www/disability/whatsnew.html and http://www.census.gov/hhes/www/disability/ACS_disability.pdf.

Taylor D: The implications of sense of coherence for the early treatment of people who have had a traumatic spinal cord injury, Unpublished doctoral dissertation, University of Wollongong, Wollongong, Australia, 1997.

Treloar LL: Lessons on disability and the rights of students, *Community College Rev* 27(1): 30-40, 1999a.

Treloar LL: People with disabilities: the same, but different: implications for health care practice, *J Transcult Nurs* 10(4):358-364, 1999b.

Treloar LL: Perceptions of spiritual beliefs, response to disability, and the church, Unpublished doctoral dissertation, The Union Institute, Cincinnati, Ohio, 1999c.

Treloar LL: Spiritual care: assessment and intervention, *J Christ Nurs* 16(2):15-18, 1999d.

Treloar LL: Disability, spiritual beliefs and the church: the experiences of adults with disabilities and family members, *J Adv Nurs* 40(5): 594-603, 2002.

Treloar LL: Response to Chapter 9 and 10: On the significance of caring, co-published in *The Journal of Religion, Disability, and Health,* 8(3/4): 181-190, 2004, and Swinton, J editor, *Critical reflections on Stanley Hauerwas' theology of disability: disabling society, enabling theology,* Binghamton, NY, 2005, Haworth Pastoral Press.

Turnbull AP, Turnbull HR III: *Families, professionals, and exceptionality,* Upper Saddle River, NJ, 1996, Merrill.

Turnbull HR III: *Free appropriate public education: the law and children with disabilities,* Denver, Colo, 1990, Love.

US Census Bureau: *Census brief 97-5: disabilities affect one-fifth of all Americans,*

December, 1997a, The Author, http://www.census.gov:80/prod/3/97pubs/cenbr975.pdf.

US Census Bureau: *Current population reports: Americans with disabilities: 1994-1995*, August 1997b, The Author, http://www.census.gov/prod/3/97pubs/p70-61.pdf.

US Census Bureau: *Disability Status: 2000—Census 2000 Brief*, Issued March 2003, http://www.census.gov/hhes/www/disability/disabstat2k.html.

US Census Bureau: *American community survey, subject definitions, disability*, August, 2004a, the Author, http://www.census.gov/acs/www/UseData/Def/Disabili.htm.

US Census Bureau: *The survey of income and program participation (SIPP)*, December 10, 2004b, The Author, http://www.census.gov/hhes/www/disability/sipp.html.

US Department of Health and Human Services: *Healthy people 2010*, Updated November 10, 2000, Office of Disease Prevention and Health Promotion, USDHHS, http://www.health.gov/healthypeople.

US Department of Justice: *A guide to disability rights laws*, Pub No 466-728/20269, Pueblo, Colo, 2000, Consumer Information Center.

US Department of Justice and US Equal Employment Opportunity Commission: *The Americans With Disabilities Act: questions and answers*, Pub No 412-943/50507, Pueblo, Colo, 1996, Consumer Information Center.

Williams, H: *Afterthoughts on Terri Schaivo*, May 5, 2005, Center for Bioethics and Culture Electronic Newsletter, http://www.thecbc.org/enewsletter/index.html.

Woodill G: The role of an able-bodied person in a disability movement, *Disabil Stud Q* 14(2):48, 1994.

World Health Organization: *The international classification of impairments, disabilities, and handicaps*, 1980, WHO Division of Mental Health and Prevention of Substance Abuse, and WHO Collaborating Centres, http://www.alternatives.com/wow/who-old.htm.

World Health Organization, Report by the Secretariat: *The international classification of functioning, disability, and health*, 2001, The Author, http://216.239.57.104/u/who?q=cache:5lMPNgZh-4wJ:www.who.int/gb/ebwha/pdf_files/WHA54/ea5418.pdf+definition+for+disability&hl=en&ie=UTF-8.

Homeless Populations

Nellie S. Droes ▪ Diane C. Hatton

MEDIA RESOURCES

Additional Material for Study, Review, and Further Exploration

evolve Website at http://evolve.elsevier.com/Nies

❖ Quiz ❖ Case Studies ❖ Content Updates ❖ Glossary ❖ WebLinks

---

OBJECTIVES

Upon completion of this chapter, the reader will be able to do the following:

1. Discuss two meanings of the term *homeless*.
2. Describe the scope of homelessness in the United States.
3. Analyze factors that contribute to homelessness.
4. Identify major health problems among various homeless aggregates.
5. Discuss access to health care for the homeless.
6. Analyze the health problems of the homeless using upstream thinking and a social justice perspective.
7. Apply knowledge about the homeless when planning community health services for this aggregate.

KEY TERMS

acceptability
accessibility
accommodation

affordability
availability
disconnectedness

dual diagnosis
homeless

market justice
social justice

CHAPTER OUTLINE

DEFINITIONS, PREVALENCE, AND DEMOGRAPHIC CHARACTERISTICS OF HOMELESSNESS
    Definitions of Homelessness
    Prevalence of Homelessness
    Demographic Characteristics

FACTORS THAT CONTRIBUTE TO HOMELESSNESS
    Shortage of Affordable Housing
    Income Insufficiency
    Inadequacy and Scarcity of Supportive Services

HEALTH STATUS OF THE HOMELESS
    Homeless Men
    Homeless Women

    Homeless Children
    Homeless Adolescents and Youth
    Homeless Families
    Homeless People With Mental Health and Substance
      Abuse Problems

ACCESS TO HEALTH CARE FOR THE HOMELESS

CONCEPTUAL APPROACHES TO HEALTH OF THE HOMELESS

RESEARCH AND THE HOMELESS

The presence of homeless people continues a trend that began in the early 1980s. The number of homeless individuals has increased, and the demographic profile of this population has changed. Joining the "traditional" homeless, predominantly composed of single males, are the "new homeless," which include families (Wright, Rubin, and Devine, 1998).

The purpose of this chapter is to describe the scope of this problem. The chapter presents definitions, prevalence, and demographic characteristics of homelessness; analyzes factors that contribute to homelessness; and describes the health status of various aggregates of the homeless population. The chapter also addresses issues of health care access, explores conceptual approaches to understanding health among the homeless, and proposes community health nursing strategies for the primary, secondary, and tertiary prevention of homelessness and its associated problems.

DEFINITIONS, PREVALENCE, AND DEMOGRAPHIC CHARACTERISTICS OF HOMELESSNESS

Definitions of Homelessness

Many meanings exist for the term **homeless.** Some view the term *home* as a synonym for the place where an individual's family resides. People without family ties, such as those living in single-room-occupancy hotels without family contacts, are, from this perspective, "homeless" (Jencks, 1994). However, government agencies' definitions of *homeless* focus on living quarters, or more specifically sleeping places, and not family ties. Official governmental reports continue to use the definition put forth by the federal McKinney-Vento Homeless Assistance Act, which was originally authorized in 1987 and defines *homeless* in two different sections.

One section defines homeless as the following (U.S. Department of Housing and Urban Development, 2001):

1. *an individual who lacks a fixed, regular, and adequate nighttime residence; and*
2. *an individual who has a primary nighttime residency that is the following:*
   A. *a supervised publicly or privately operated shelter designed to provide temporary living accommodations (e.g., welfare hotels, congregate shelters, and transitional housing for the mentally ill);*
   B. *an institution that provides a temporary residence for individuals intended to be institutionalized; or*
   C. *a public or private place not designed for or ordinarily used as a regular sleeping accommodation for human beings.*

The education subtitle of the McKinney-Vento Homeless Education Assistance Improvements Act of 2001 (U.S. Department of Education, 2004) contains definitions that relate to children and youth.

2. *The term homeless children and youths*
   A. *means individuals who lack a fixed, regular, and adequate nighttime residence (within the meaning of section 103(a)(1)); and*
   B. *includes*
      i. *children and youths who are sharing the housing of other persons due to loss of housing, economic hardship, or a similar reason; are living in motels, hotels, trailer parks, or camping grounds due to the lack of alternative adequate accommodations; are living in emergency or transitional shelters; are abandoned in hospitals; or are awaiting foster care placement;*
      ii. *children and youths who have a primary nighttime residence that is a public or private place not designed for or ordinarily used as a regular sleeping accommodation for human beings (within the meaning of section 103(a)(2)(C));*
      iii. *children and youths who are living in cars, parks, public spaces, abandoned buildings, substandard housing, bus or train stations, or similar settings; and*
      iv. *migratory children (as such term is defined in section 1309 of the Elementary and Secondary Education Act of 1965) who qualify as homeless for the purposes of this subtitle because the children are living in circumstances described in clauses (i) through (iii).*

However, many Americans use another definition of *homelessness.* This colloquial usage reflects the more traditional view of the homeless as the shabbily dressed people they notice in public places during the day (O'Flaherty, 1996). Homeless advocates argue that it is also important to consider those who are poor and tenuously housed. This includes those who are without their own shelter but have "doubled up" with a family member or friend. An estimate of this population is difficult at best. Definitions of *homelessness* vary and consequently give rise to many interpretations and confusion regarding research findings and policy implications (Shinn and Baumohl, 1999).

Prevalence of Homelessness

The homeless are intrinsically difficult to count. There are no recent national studies indicating the number of homeless people in the United States. The most frequently used sources of national data are the federally funded Urban Institute studies conducted in 1987 and 1996 (Burt et al., 2001). The U.S. Census Bureau (Smith and Smith, 2001) collected national data on the homeless population in Census 1990 and Census 2000. However, the Bureau has indicated that the information generated by these efforts should not be used as counts. A brief description of the Census Bureau's efforts, including the limitations, in enumerating the homeless population is presented next. This is followed by a brief account of the Urban Institute studies, including an estimate of homeless prevalence.

The earliest effort by the U.S. Census Bureau (Smith and Smith, 2001) to collect data related to the homeless population occurred during Census 1990. On "Shelter and Street Night (S-Night)" in March 1990, the U.S. Census Bureau enumerators counted people in shelters, which served adults, youth, and abused women, and visible in pre-identified street locations. Although the Bureau had indicated the results of this 1990 effort were limited and not to be used as a count, "census stakeholders and data users" (p. 1) expressed concern as to the meaning and use of the data.

Attempting to clearly indicate that Census 2000 would not produce a count of the homeless population, the Bureau used the term "people without conventional housing." On March 27, 2000, enumerators gathered information from individuals located in emergency and transitional shelters, including hotels and motels used to provide shelter for people without conventional housing. The next day, March 28, enumerators counted people at soup kitchens and mobile food vans. On March 29, 2005, the Bureau enumerated people at targeted, nonsheltered outdoor locations. The Bureau's report of the Census 2000 efforts is limited to the data obtained on the first night, March 27, with one very important exception.

The "report does not include data for the population counted in shelters for abused women or shelters against domestic violence" (Smith and Smith, 2001, p. 4). Consequently, this report is severely limited and is not an appropriate source of valid information regarding the homeless population.

Given the limitations of U.S. Census data, the Urban Institute studies of 1985 and 1996 (Burt et al., 2001), although more than 10 years old, remain as important sources of national data on the homeless population. Both of these federally funded studies were point prevalence studies. In other words, they obtained data during a limited point in time, in contrast to collecting data over an extended period. It is important to note that it was not the purpose of either study to directly count the number of people who were homeless. However, based on data collected during the two studies, the researchers estimated the number of homeless people for the two different years. Based on the 1987 study, they estimated between 500,000 and 600,000 people were homeless at any given time. Using data from the 1996 study, they estimated the number of homeless for a one-week period to be between 444,000 and 842,000. Based on the 444,000, they projected that 2.3 million people experienced a spell of homeless and used homeless assistance programs over the course of a year. Care needs to be used in interpreting this last number. It does not mean that there were 2.3 million people homeless at one time in 1996 (Burt et al., 2001; Urban Institute, 2000).

There are several other sources, although not national in extent and lacking prevalence data that present information on the extent of homelessness. These reports are based on the use of homeless assistance services by homeless people.

The U.S. State Conference of Mayors releases annual reports of its survey of providers of food and shelter assistance in 27 major cities in the United States. During 2004, requests for emergency shelter increased by an average of 6%. Requests from homeless families increased by 7%, and estimates indicate that 23% of the requests by homeless people overall and 32% of requests by families went unmet. About 46% of the cities indicated that the amount of time people remain homeless increased during the year, with people remaining homeless an average of 8 months (U.S. Conference of Mayors, 2004).

The National Student Campaign Against Hunger and Homelessness (2005) surveyed emergency food and shelter providers in urban, rural, and suburban areas in 32 states and 426 cities and towns during 2004. The survey found that 65% of agencies surveyed reported an increase in request for shelter and that 77% indicated they turned away requests for shelter due to a lack of resources.

For the reader attempting to grasp the various nuances involved in counting the homeless, Wright et al. (1998) offer the following helpful metaphor:

> Given the episodic nature of much homelessness, trying to count the homeless is a little like trying to count the number of flies in a house whose windows and doors are wide open. At any one moment, there is a definite number of flies in the house and that number is theoretically countable. Practically speaking, however, the rapid movement of flies in and out means that no count can be definitive or even very useful. Likewise, while there is some finite and theoretically countable number of literally homeless people in the United States at any one time, they are but a fraction of a much larger number of persons who are at risk of homelessness and who are destined to be homeless at some other time. In this sense, the number of flies or of homeless people is a less pertinent question than the transition probabilities that govern movement in and out of the condition being counted. (p. 63)

Although the homeless population is difficult to define and count, the federal government, in an attempt to improve the quality and availability of information, has mandated a Homeless Information Management System (HMIS). To receive federal funding, the U.S. Department of Housing and Urban Development (HUD) (2005) has required local communities to install HMISs. The intent is to obtain national data including counts and basic demographic information. In April 2006 HUD announced that the First Annual Homeless Assessment Report (AHAR) was being finalized (US Department of Housing and Urban Development 2006).

In summary, data that are available indicate that the number of homeless people is not decreasing. Kozol (1988) argued more than 15 years ago:

> We would be wise . . . to avoid the numbers game. Any search for the "right number" carries the assumption that we may at last arrive at an acceptable number. There is no acceptable number. Whether the number is 1 million or 4 million . . . there are too many homeless people in America. (p. 10)

Demographic Characteristics

Most national and local studies reveal that demographic characteristics of homeless people are highly variable. Moreover, the information that is available varies by data source, including the locale, collection methods, analysis, and presentation. Although there is considerable variation, there are trends in some basic demographic characteristics that can be identified based on several national and local studies (Burt, 1999). An overview of these trends is presented next.

Families with children are estimated to comprise between 35% to 40% of the homeless population. A large majority of theses families are headed by single women with children 8 years or younger. African Americans are overrepresented compared to the general population. Men make up the largest group of single homeless people. Unaccompanied youth are most likely underrepresented due to their reluctance to use shelter services (Burt, 1999).

Presented next are "snapshots" of homeless people by family status and racial/ethnic categories. These views are from reports of several different national and local studies and reflect the configuration and presentation employed by the authors or sponsors.

The Urban Institute's researchers categorized homeless people in the 1996 study by family status: clients with children, single clients, and other clients (Burt et al., 2001). Single men were 60.7% of the whole sample; single women were 14.9%. Women with children were 12.2%; men with children were 2.3%. Among other clients, those with someone other than own minor children; men were 5.3% and women 4.6%.

BOX 20-1 Twenty-Seven Major Cities Included in U.S. Conference of Mayors Survey (2004)

Boston	Kansas City	Portland
Burlington	Louisville Metro	Providence
Cedar Rapids	Los Angeles	St. Paul
Charleston	Miami	Salt Lake City
Charlotte	Nashville	San Antonio
Chicago	New Orleans	San Francisco
Cleveland	Norfolk	Santa Monica
Denver	Philadelphia	Seattle
Detroit	Phoenix	Trenton

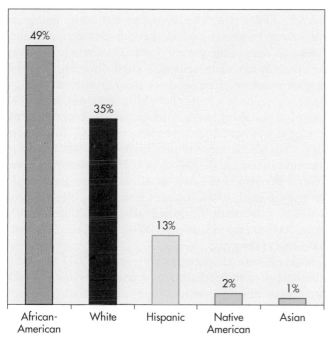

FIGURE 20-1 Proportion of persons seeking shelter by ethnicity/race. (From US Conference of Mayors—SODEXHO USA: *Hunger and Homelessness Survey 2004: a status report on hunger and homelessness in America's cities*, Dec 2004, The Author, http://www.usmayors.org/uscm/hungersurvey/2004/onlinereport/HungerAndHomelessnessReport2004.pdf.)

Racial/ethnic characteristics of the homeless population surveyed have been reported by the U.S. Conference of Mayors in their annual reports for more than 15 years. Across the 27 cities surveyed in the 2004 report (Box 20-1), the racial/ethnic characteristics of the homeless population were: 49% African American, 35% white, 13% Hispanics, 2% Native-American and 1% Asian (U.S. Conference of Mayors, 2004) (Figure 20-1).

This section has presented the federal definition of homelessness; a discussion of the challenges in obtaining a count of homeless populations; and a brief outline of selected demographic characteristics. A discussion of factors contributing to homelessness follows.

FACTORS THAT CONTRIBUTE TO HOMELESSNESS

In the larger society, there are three broad factors that contribute to homelessness: (1) shortage of affordable housing, (2) incomes insufficient to meet basic needs, and (3) inadequate and scarce support services. Over the past 25 years, the interaction among these factors has been largely responsible for the increase in homelessness.

Shortage of Affordable Housing

Housing is considered affordable if it costs a renter or owner no more than 30% of his or her income. The U.S. Department of Housing and Urban Development (HUD) operates, in cooperation with state and local governments and nonprofit housing organizations, programs that provide financial housing assistance to low-income families. This assistance may be provided as (1) direct payment to apartment owners, who in turn lower rents for low-income tenants; (2) access to an apartment located in a public housing facility; (3) or housing choice vouchers, which may be used by low-income persons to "pay" all or part of the rent. Option (3) continues to be more commonly known as "Section 8 housing." Although these programs are intended to alleviate housing problems for low-income renters, the demand for these assisted housing programs has far exceeded the supply. Factors contributing to the shortages include market forces that inhibit the private housing sector's production of affordable rental housing, decreases in the federal government's spending on assisted housing for low-income families, and the increasing inequality of incomes among groups within the larger population (Children's Defense Fund 2004, 2005a; Hockett et al., 2005; National Law Center on Homelessness and Poverty, 2004; Pitcoff et al., 2004; U.S. Dept of Housing and Urban Development, 2005).

Income Insufficiency

Homeless clients have reported that insufficient incomes and lack of employment prevented them from leaving homelessness (Burt et al.,1999 2001). The U. S. Census Bureau's report (DeNavas-Walt, Proctor, and Mills, 2004) reveals that, in 2003, the real median household income remained at $43.318, its 2002 level, following 2 consecutive years of decline. However, between 2001 and 2003, both the number of people in poverty and the poverty rate increased each year. Overall, the percentage of people living below the poverty line increased from 12.1% in 2002 to 12.5% in 2003, and during this same period, the number increased from 34.6 million to 35.9 million. The poverty rate among children younger than 18 years increased from 16.7 to 17.6 between 2002 and 2003. Moreover, among the poor, those in extreme poverty—classified as those having income below half of the poverty line—increased to 43%. This is the highest level since 1975 (Center on Budget and Policy Priorities, 2004; DeNavas-Walt et al., 2004).

As a consequence of the shortage of affordable housing and insufficient income, an increasing number of low-income people end up paying much more than they can afford for rent. In many areas of the country, wages needed to afford housing are three to five times higher than the minimum wage of $5.15 per hour. This wage has remained the same since 1997. Paying too much of their income for rent leaves low-income people without adequate resources for other necessities, such as food, clothing, and health care, and increases the risk of homelessness.

Inadequacy and Scarcity of Supportive Services

Accompanying the previously described factors, shortage of affordable housing and insufficient income, is the scarcity of supportive services for low-income people who need them. Some low-income people need services to maintain their housing status, whereas others need services in order to work and earn money. Those that need services to maintain their housing status include those with serious chronic mental health and/or substance abuse problems. In addition to needing income assistance, this group requires comprehensive and accessible health care, both physical and behavioral.

There are other homeless people who, without the serious physical and mental disabilities of the former group, are able to function in the workforce. These people need assistance in the forms of child care, transportation, and vocational training.

What the two groups have in common is the need for affordable health care, that is, health care in its broadest sense as outlined by the World Health Organization (WHO) (WHO, 1948). Unfortunately, the number of people in the general population without health insurance increased in 2003 by a rate of 15.6%, and a third of those whose incomes are below federal poverty levels are without health insurance. Rates of homeless shelter clients and clients receiving other homeless services who do not have health insurance are reported to range from 55% to 70%. Consequently, lack of health insurance is a significant factor in preventing people from leaving homelessness and may, indeed, be a major risk factor for homelessness. A serious illness or disability can lead to a downward spiral into homelessness as a result of job loss, use of savings to pay for care, and inability to pay rent (Burt et al., 1999, 2001; DeNavas-Walt et al., 2004; National Health Care for the Homeless Council, 2005).

The three broad factors contributing to homelessness—shortage of affordable housing, insufficient income, and scarcity of supportive services—are conditions in society. Singularly and more importantly, the interaction among these factors has serious consequences for low-income people. These conditions potentiate the vulnerability factors found among certain individuals and families and increase the probability of homelessness.

HEALTH STATUS OF THE HOMELESS

As discussed in Chapter 1, the WHO has defined health from a broad perspective. This classic definition, which purports that health is "a state of complete physical, mental, and social well-being and not merely the absence of disease or infirmity" (WHO, 1948, p. 2), is particularly useful when considering the health status of the homeless. For these individuals, a continual interaction exists among these three dimensions (physical, mental, and social) that has enormous consequences for health. The boundaries of these dimensions overlap; therefore, it is difficult, if not impossible, to address health among the homeless without a concomitant analysis of physical, mental, and social dimensions. Therefore this section addresses the health status of various homeless aggregates from this broad WHO interpretation. Specifically, the subgroups discussed include men, women, children, and adolescents. Special groups considered are homeless families and homeless people in the community with mental health and substance abuse problems.

Homeless Men

Homeless men experience acute physical health problems, respiratory infections, trauma, and skin disorders at higher rates than men in the general population. Chronic disorders including hypertension, musculoskeletal disorders, gastrointestinal problems, peripheral vascular disease, respiratory problems (asthma, chronic bronchitis, emphysema), neurological disorders including seizures, and poor dentition are also more prevalent among homeless populations. In addition, HIV and AIDS, tuberculosis, hepatitis C, and sexually transmitted diseases (STDs) occur at higher rates than in the general population (Culhane et al., 2001; Douglass et al., 1999; Goss et al., 2003; Institute of Medicine, 1988; Robertson et al., 2004; Sachs-Ericsson et al., 1999; Solliday-McRoy et al., 2004; Stein and Nyamathi, 2004; Stratigos and Katsambas, 2003; Tulsky et al., 2004).

Burt (1999) and colleagues (Burt et al., 2001) relate that homeless people reported physical acute and chronic health problems similar to those identified by health care providers. They also note that clients' self-reports may underestimate problems because there is a lack of knowledge of medical conditions or reluctance to admit to some conditions.

Many of these acute and chronic conditions are exacerbated by alcoholism, which occurs more frequently among homeless than nonhomeless men; alcoholism may be the single most prevalent health problem among the homeless. Likewise, serious mental illnesses occur more frequently among the homeless than in the general population. In addition, minor emotional problems (e.g., personality disorders) are also more frequent among homeless than nonhomeless men. Drug abuse, like alcohol abuse, occurs more frequently among the homeless, and considerable overlap of alcohol and drug abuse exists. Men are more likely than women to report alcohol abuse (Glasser, 1994; Institute of Medicine, 1988; Reardon et al., 2003; Wright, 1990b; Wright et al., 1998).

Studies comparing homeless and housed poor people indicate that homeless adults are more likely to be male and have veteran status than the housed poor. Homeless adults are more likely to be unemployed, or if employed, the job is temporary or at a low wage and without benefits. Consequently, their income is insufficient to maintain housing costs. Although a lack of monetary resources is a variable related directly to becoming and remaining homeless, additional deficits in social resources contribute to the condition. Many of the homeless have relied on social support from families and friends to provide housing. Homelessness results when both monetary resources and social support are exhausted (Wilder Research Center, 2004a, 2004b; Wright et al., 1998).

Data from the National Health Care for the Homeless Program, an initiative funded by the RWJ Foundation and the Pew Charitable Trust Fund in the late 1980s, are the basis of much of the earliest information on the health status of men. Although dated, these data nevertheless stand as major sources of information on the health status of the homeless population (Wright, 1990a). The more recent reports substantiate this earlier report.

Homeless Women

Homeless women have diverse backgrounds and a variety of health needs. The National Survey of Homeless Assistance Providers and Clients (NSHAPC) has identified the following three subgroups among homeless women and their percentages: 38% have a minor child, 47% are by themselves, and 15% are with another person/not a minor child ("other clients"). In the survey, women from all three groups reported health and nutrition needs that far exceeded those of women in the general population. Women with minor children and single women were more likely to use shelters and less likely to sleep on the streets; women designated as "other clients" were the least likely to receive services. The latter were the most reclusive of the three subgroups—they typically slept on the streets and generally avoided shelters and soup kitchens (Burt et al., 2001). Although the health problems of many homeless women cluster around problems of substance use/abuse, mental illness, history of violence, and/or childhood risks, women who do not have custody of their children tend to present more health-related vulnerability than do women with their minor children (Metraux and Culhane, 1999; Page and Nooe, 2002).

Homeless women have higher rates of pregnancy, including unintended pregnancy, than their housed counterparts, and researchers have demonstrated that the severity of homelessness increases the likelihood of preterm births and low-birth-weight infants. Although increased access to prenatal care may improve the health of homeless women, preventing homelessness in the first place is even more critical for birth outcomes, as women bring to pregnancy stressors that have a cumulative effect over the life course for reproductive health (Stein, Lu, and Gelberg, 2000).

In the 1990s, research clearly documented the extraordinary histories of violence, from childhood through adulthood, among women experiencing homelessness (Anderson, 1996; Bassuk et al., 1997; Bassuk, Melnick, and Browne, 1998). Bassuk et al. (1996) reported that an estimated 92% of homeless women have experienced physical or sexual assault sometime in their lives. Other researchers have reported a study in which 13% of the homeless women participants were raped during the previous year—half of these were raped at least twice that year. These sexually assaulted women fared far worse on every physical and mental health measure used in the study and were more likely to use/abuse alcohol and other drugs (Wenzel, Leake, and Gelberg, 2000).

As may be expected, women living in unsheltered locations on the street have increased risk for victimization than women living in shelters. Unsheltered women also have greater odds of having multiple sexual partners and are less likely to utilize health services. Other factors that increase risk of physical and sexual victimization include history of mental illness, substance use/abuse, and engaging in survival strategies including selling sex and drugs (Nyamathi et al, 2000a; Wenzel, Koegel, and Gelberg, 2000).

Research indicates that homeless women report less satisfaction with their health care than their housed counterparts; in addition, they prefer care from shelter and outreach clinics designed specifically to meet their needs rather than care from county/government clinics (Swanson, Andersen, and Gelberg, 2003). Because of their sexual and reproductive health needs, homeless women face complex health-related burdens. Up to two thirds report gynecological problems, including STDs and pelvic inflammatory disease, related to forced sex and subsistence sex. In addition, women often lack information regarding STDs and health care and find negative attitudes of providers toward them unacceptable (Gelberg et al., 2004; Hatton, 1997).

Social support also influences homeless women's physical and mental well-being and their ability to access health services. They often report a **disconnectedness** beginning in childhood that continues in adult life (Anderson, 1996). As adults, they score lower than their nonhomeless counterparts on measures of social support as well as intimacy and reciprocity (Anderson and Rayens, 2004). They have fewer persons in their social networks and these persons often experience similar emotional distress and have high-risk behaviors (Bassuk et al., 1996; Nyamathi, Flaskerud, and Leake, 1997). Women who have substance nonusers in their social support networks report better psychosocial status and increased health services utilization than those who have only substance users (Nyamathi et al, 2000b). Other research has suggested that individuals within social networks, including shelter staff, health professionals, and even other homeless women, are critical for facilitating access to health care by acting as "brokers" to appropriate services (Hatton, 2001).

Over a decade ago, Dr. Ellen Bassuk, president of the National Center on Family Homelessness, summarized the health-related problems from which homeless women suffer. They do not differ from the problems that impede many women in the United States, she argued, although their problems are likely to be more intense, frequent, and apt to occur in concert. Often, homeless women have limited education, limited earning power, and fragmented support networks. Trapped by a lack of economic and social opportunities, homeless women profoundly experience society's inequities (Bassuk, 1993).

Homeless Children

As indicated earlier in this chapter, the number of homeless families continues to increase in many areas of the United States with a concomitant increase in the number of homeless children. Comparison of homeless children's physical and mental health and educational attainment with children in the general population follows.

Children born to mothers who are homeless are more likely to be preterm or of low birth weight than children in the general population (Stein et al., 2000). More homeless children than those in the general population experience immunization delays, upper respiratory tract and ear infections, asthma, skin disorders, diarrhea, anemia, and hunger (Berti, Zylbert, and Rolnitzky, 2001; Nabors et al., 2004; National Policy and Advocacy Council on Homelessness, 2005; Partington, Nitzke, and Csete, 2000; Weinreb et al., 2002; Wilder Research Center, 2004a, 2004b; Wright et al., 1998).

In addition to having physical health problems, homeless children also experience mental health problems and developmental delays at greater rates than other children. Many have experienced events that adversely affect their mental health, for example, domestic violence, repeated moves, and family separations. More homeless than nonhomeless children experience depression, anxiety, and withdrawal (Berti et al., 2001; Buckner et al., 1999; Children's Defense Fund, 2005a,b; Huang and Menke, 2001; Nabors et al., 2004; National Policy and Advocacy Council on Homelessness, 2005; Weinreib et al., 2002; Wilder Research Center, 2004a, 2004b).

The previously outlined physical, mental, and developmental problems interact and adversely affect homeless children's educational achievement on standardized tests covering reading, language usage, and/or mathematics. Missing days of school, due to family mobility, homeless children are more likely than other children to repeat grades. Homeless children may lack resources for clothing and school supplies and access to facilities for personal hygiene maintenance. As a consequence, they may be at risk of nonacceptance or teasing by other students, thereby compounding the effects of their physical and mental problems (Julianelle and Fascarinis, 2003; National Policy and Advocacy Council on Homelessness, 2005; O'Neil-Pirozzi, 2003; Rafferty, Shin, and Weitzman, 2004; Roschelle and Kaufman, 2004; Wilder Research Center, 2004a, 2004b).

Homeless Adolescents and Youth

This next section describes the health problems of adolescents in general, the health problems of homeless adolescents, and the health problems of several homeless adolescent subpopulations. Several researchers note that the literature on homeless adolescents is limited and lacks rigorous research. A large majority of the studies were conducted in metropolitan areas and on the West Coast. The age-group varied; some studies included young adults up to 24 years of age (Haber and Toro, 2004; Robertson and Toro, 1999).

As reported in the National Youth Risk Behavior Survey, 2003, adolescents from all sectors of society engage in health-risk behaviors that result in serious health problems (Centers for Disease Control and Prevention, 2004). These problems include unintended pregnancy, STDs (including HIV/AIDS), alcohol and drug abuse, depression, and suicide. These problems are, for the most part, related to risk-taking behaviors. However, homeless adolescents experience these problems at higher rates than the general adolescent population (American Academy of Pediatrics, 2004; Rew, 2005; Wilder Research Center, 2005).

Homeless adolescents experience STDs, physical and sexual abuse, skin disorders, anemia, drug and alcohol abuse, and unintentional injuries at higher rates than adolescents in the general population. Depression, suicidal ideation, and disorders of behavior, personality, or thought also occur at higher rates among homeless adolescents. Family disruption, school failures, prostitution or "survival sex," and involvement with the legal system indicate that homeless adolescents' social health is severely compromised (Baer, Ginzler, and Peterson, 2003; Barkin et al., 2003; Baron, 2003; Cameron, Racine, Offord and Cairney, 2004; Cauce, Tyler, and Whitbeck, 2004; Feldmann and Middleman, 2003; Greene et al., 2002; Rew, Taylor-Seehafer, and Fitzgerald, 2001; Roy et al., 2004; Ryan et al., 2000; Taylor-Seehafer, 2004; Tyler and Cauce, 2002; Whitbeck et al., 2004; Wilder Research Center, 2005).

Homeless adolescents who are pregnant, engage in prostitution, or identify themselves as gay, lesbian, bisexual, or transgender experience more health problems than other homeless adolescents. Pregnant homeless adolescents have more severe mental health problems and use alcohol and drugs more than nonpregnant homeless adolescents. Not surprisingly, they have higher rates of negative pregnancy outcomes than nonhomeless adolescents (Haley et al., 2004).

Runaway or homeless adolescents, both female and male, make up a large percentage of all youth involved in prostitution. Many become involved because they need money to meet subsistence needs, which is the source of the term "survival sex." These adolescents are more likely to have serious mental health problems and to be actively suicidal. Alcohol and drug use occurs at higher rates among this group than among homeless adolescents not engaged in prostitution. Youth involved in prostitution are more likely to report histories of physical and sexual abuse (Cauce et al., 2004; Greene et al., 2002; Rew et al., 2001; Ryan et al., 2000).

Rates of attempted suicide are higher among gay homeless adolescents. A large majority of males involved in survival sex identify themselves as gay or bisexual. Many of these youth are on the streets because of effects of homophobia and prejudice. Facing problems similar to other homeless adolescents, gay-identified youth face an additional set of problems as a result of others rejecting them because of their sexual orientation (Cochran et al., 2002).

The previously cited studies are quantitatively descriptive of samples of various sizes and locations of homeless youth. These types of studies are an important part of the literature on homeless youth; however, they lack the poignancy and detail found in qualitative case-study types of research. Finley and Finley (1999) present homeless youth "in their own voices" in a research story titled "Sp'ange," the street term for "spare change." Their account includes themes of "formation by homeless youth of family-like structures, the use of cocaine and heroin, early use of alcohol and primacy of alcohol as the drug of choice, and attitudes toward government economic structures and work" (p. 313), thereby bringing the life of

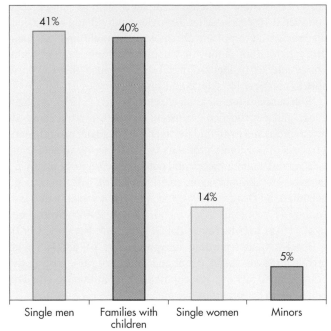

Breakdown of Persons Seeking Shelter: US Conference of Mayors, 2004

41% — Single men
40% — Families with children
14% — Single women
5% — Minors

FIGURE 20-2   Breakdown of persons seeking shelter. (From US Conference of Mayors—SODEXHO USA: *Hunger and Homelessness Survey 2004: a status report on hunger and homelessness in America's cities,* Dec 2004, The Author, http://www.usmayors.org/uscm/hunger survey/2004/onlinereport/HungerAndHomelessnessReport2004.pdf.)

throwaway youth into sharp focus. Bourgois, Prince, and Moss's (2004) account provides details of what life on the street is like for young women. Using field research techniques, this study yields a glimpse into the "everyday violence" experienced by young "street women."

Adolescents in the general population are at risk, homeless adolescents are at even higher risk, and the special subgroups of adolescents—including those who are gay identified, those who are pregnant, and those who are practicing survival sex—are particularly vulnerable. Health for many of these youth is severely jeopardized.

Homeless Families

In the 1980s, much discussion ensued about the "old homeless" and the "new homeless"—a situation whereby young families with children joined the "homeless population" composed of predominantly single men with substance use disorders living on the streets (Rossi, 1990). Many thought improved economic conditions would eventually eradicate this problem. Yet, family homelessness persists. During 2004, the U.S. Conference of Mayors reported that families with children made up 40% of the homeless population (Figure 20-2). In that year, family requests for shelter increased in 78% of the survey cities. The average increase for family emergency shelter beds was 16%, and, in a majority of survey cities, families continued to break up to meet shelter requirements. Fifty-two percent of the cities continued to

report shelters where families can stay only at night and leave during the day. With the average wait for public housing at 20 months, access to public housing remained beyond the reach of many poor families. In 59% of the survey cities, at least one assisted housing program stopped accepting applications altogether because of lengthy waiting periods (U.S. Conference of Mayors, 2004).

Many families experience more than a brief crisis spell of homelessness. Indeed, the NSHAPC has reported that only 36% of families fit into a brief crisis group. Thirty-five percent have, instead, episodic homelessness and 28%, chronic homelessness. The NSHAPC also reports that among many poor families, more than one spell of homelessness during the course of a year has become commonplace (Burt et al., 2001). Because so many shelters, especially transitional shelters, now serve this repeatedly homeless aggregate, some have asked: "A shelter is not a home . . . or is it?" (da Costa Nunez, 2004).

The Worcester Family Research Project has extensively documented the situations of homeless families headed by single mothers. These families experience substandard living conditions, social isolation, and myriad physical and health problems. Over 40% of the mothers in this project reported a major depressive disorder and over 33% experienced post-traumatic stress disorder. Nearly 33% had attempted suicide at least once, and nearly 50% reported substance abuse problems. Rates of asthma, anemia, and ulcers were also disproportionately high (Bassuk et al., 1996). These mothers' physical, mental, and social health problems have enormous consequences for family stability and, ultimately, for the health of their children.

The NSHAPC findings show that single women head 84% of homeless families with minor children. These researchers note that the men in the other 16% of families have notably low educational attainment, limited work skills/history, and frequent histories of incarceration. Thus Burt and colleagues (2001) argue that, in spite of the serious situations faced by single-parent families headed by women, the two-parent homeless families may actually be "worse off than the female headed families" (p. 94).

U.S. policies on assistance to the poor often view children as the most "blameless" and "deserving" of support; thus, many of the services funded for the homeless target families with minor children. Yet, conditions remain dire with homeless families reporting, for example, much higher levels of hunger and food insecurity than housed families (Burt et al., 2001). Moreover, the Personal Responsibility and Work Opportunity Reconciliation Act of 1996, or "welfare reform," has further exacerbated the impoverished living situations of many families and has eliminated the safety net that prevented at least some families from falling into homelessness (Bassuk, 1996; National Coalition for the Homeless, 2001; Stevens, 2000). Without policy changes, advocates project that families will continue to experience chronic homelessness. According to the Coalition for the Homeless, "Children now make up nearly half (44%) of the total shelter population in New York City, and for an entire generation, a shelter may be their only home" (as cited in da Costa Nunez, 2004, p. 1).

Homeless People With Mental Health and Substance Abuse Problems

This section describes problems that homeless people experience with mental health and substance abuse and examines inherent risks for health status. Several authors (e.g., Folsom and Jeste, 2002; Wright et al., 1998), in substantial reviews of multiple studies on homelessness and the mentally ill, note that the rate of psychiatric disorder is higher among the homeless compared with the domiciled population. Estimates of mental illness among homeless people have varied from 10% to 90%. In a 1996 national survey of clients of homeless service providers, 45% of respondents self-reported experiences with mental health problems in the previous year (Burt et al.,1999; 2001; North et al., 2004).

Variations in rates of mental illness are attributed to different measurement methods (Bellavia and Toro, 1999; Martens, 2001). For example, using hospitalization rates ignores those homeless who have not entered the hospital; samples consisting of service provider clients exclude those who do not use such services. Consequently, these estimates may be at the low end. Conversely, many of the measurements employed fail to consider the context of homelessness. Unhappiness, discouragement, worry, and fatigue are components of frequently used measurements of mental health. These feelings are common among the homeless. As Wright et al. (1998) note, if homeless people were happy about their circumstances, their "grasp on reality" (p. 107) would be in doubt. Lay people frequently label behaviors that are necessary for survival (e.g., rummaging in garbage cans and urinating in public) as crazy or abnormal. However, when the homeless lack money for food or lack access to public restrooms, such behaviors may demonstrate survivability.

Wright et al. (1998) allege that the estimated rate of alcohol abuse exceeds 40% among the nation's homeless and is near 50% among homeless men. An extensive study of the homeless in New Orleans estimated that 75% of the city's homeless abuse alcohol and more than half abuse other drugs (i.e., mostly crack). Substance abuse was a critical factor in determining homelessness because those with more resources consumed more drugs and those with fewer resources consumed fewer drugs. The nature of the disorder prevented these homeless people from using the resources that they had for improved social or housing alternatives (Nwakeze et al., 2003; Wright et al., 1998). In the previously mentioned 1996 national survey (Burt, 1999; Burt et al., 2001), 46% of the adult respondents reported problems with alcohol and 38% reported problems with other substances within the previous year.

Moreover, for a sizable proportion of the homeless, severe mental illness exists concomitantly with the problems of alcohol or other drug use, which is a phenomenon known as *comorbidity* or **dual diagnosis** (California Department of Mental Health, 2003; U.S. Department of Health and Human Services, 2003). In a review of epidemiological studies, Fischer (1991) concluded that 10% to 20% of homeless single adults suffer from this combination of a psychiatric disorder and substance use, or comorbidity. Among homeless adults in Los Angeles, Koegel and colleagues (1999) found that 77% of

people with a severe or chronic mental disorder were also chronic substance abusers. They also note that this rate was nearly a twofold increase compared with a study they conducted 10 years earlier. Homeless individuals with a dual diagnosis may represent the most vulnerable and the most difficult to treat among the homeless; they are especially vulnerable to residential instability because they are less able to compete for scarce housing resources.

Substance abuse carries considerable health risks. Alcohol abuse and dependence are associated with a wide range of health problems involving the liver, nervous system, and heart. The loss of economic productivity, vulnerability to accidents, and victimization are common outcomes. Drug use involving intravenous administration carries risks of infections (e.g., hepatitis), STDs (e.g., HIV), and significant social, legal, and economic problems (Galea and Vlahov, 2002; Goldfinger et al., 1998; McMurray-Avila, Gelberg, and Breakey, 1999).

Recent data regarding the prevalence of persons with mental illnesses and alcohol and other drug use among the homeless are lacking. Recent literature continues to cite data collected in the previous decade.

ACCESS TO HEALTH CARE FOR THE HOMELESS

Proposing to clarify "access" as it relates to health care services, Penchansky and Thomas (1981) noted that access is a general concept that represents the "degree of 'fit' between the clients and the system" (p. 128). Furthermore, the general term *access* summarizes the following five specific areas of "fit between the patient and the health care system" (p. 128):

1. **Availability** refers to the relationship between the amount (i.e., number of providers and facilities) and type of health care services to the amount and type of client needs.
2. **Accessibility** connotes the relationship between the location of the services and the client's location.
3. **Accommodation** indicates the relationship between how services are organized (e.g., hours of operation and appointment systems) and the client's ability to accommodate to these factors. The client's perception of the appropriateness of these factors is a component of accommodation.
4. **Affordability** refers to the price of provider services or payment requirements and the client's ability to pay.
5. **Acceptability** represents the relationship between the client's attitudes about providers and providers' attitudes about acceptable client characteristics.

These five factors are used as a framework for exploring problems in accessing health care by people who are poor but housed, homeless people in general, and special aggregates of the homeless.

Poor but housed people experience considerable problems related to each of the five access dimensions; however, the primary problem is affordability. Many poor people lack any form of health insurance, including Medicaid. For those who do meet Medicaid eligibility requirements, the low reimbursement rate discourages or prohibits health care providers from participating. As a consequence of the inability to afford the services of a market-driven system, those who are excluded from the private fee-for-service arrangement must rely on public hospital systems' outpatient clinics, emergency rooms, and inpatient services. Heavy demands on these less-than-adequate facilities frequently result in less-than-desirable or appropriate accommodations. Long waits for services in overcrowded, uncomfortable settings may discourage people from seeking care at an earlier and more easily treated stage.

Notwithstanding such difficulties, these facilities are frequently situated some distance from the client's shelter or work. Although the inner-city resident may access such facilities through a public transportation system, those individuals who reside in rural areas lack such services and must find other resources (e.g., relatives, neighbors, and friends) or do without health care. Providers in many public systems are under considerable stress working in less than optimal conditions with heavy workloads and find it difficult to provide care to poor clients who frequently have complex problems and different cultural and language expectations. Consequently, these clients may find such services unacceptable and may fail to seek care until illnesses are intolerable (Aday, 2001; Institute of Medicine 1988; Wright, 1990b).

Like people who are poor but housed, homeless people experience considerable difficulty accessing the health care system. However, the homeless face more severe problems than the housed poor. Eligibility for many services frequently requires forms of documentation that homeless people find difficult to provide because they are homeless. Lacking secure storage space makes it difficult to protect personal papers from loss, theft, or weather. Frequently, homeless people must walk to service sites because use of public transportation is too costly. Consequently, accessibility is even more problematic for the homeless than for those who are housed and have a more intact system of transportation (e.g., transportation vouchers, relatives, neighbors, and friends). Without a permanent mailing address or message center, accommodating a health care system that relies on mailed notification of appointments or results of health care procedures is unlikely. Furthermore, the hours of service may force the homeless to choose between obtaining health care and obtaining food and shelter (Aday, 2001; Institute of Medicine, 1988; Wright, 1990b).

Special aggregates within the homeless population experience additional problems in obtaining health care services. The following section describes the problems of homeless people who are chronically mentally ill and homeless pregnant women.

Although physical health services available to the poor are inadequate, mental health services are even less available. Several researchers have investigated access to mental health and substance abuse services by community-based homeless adults. As a group, homeless people with chronic mental illness or substance abuse continue to experience difficulty in obtaining access to needed services. These researchers stress that attention to systems-level features is necessary to provide access for this especially vulnerable group of homeless people (Bird et al., 2002; Fortney et al., 2003; Koegel et al., 1999; Wenzel et al., 2001). The historic

conditions of deinstitutionalization, whereby community-based mental health services failed to materialize, and the current policy, whereby Medicaid and managed care plans reimburse less for mental health services than for physical health services, cause the need for mental health services for homeless mentally ill clients to far exceed the supply.

The homeless mentally ill also require physical health services. Obtaining such care from these two disconnected and complex systems requires considerable skill in negotiation. The nature of the illness frequently compromises this skill. Notwithstanding the lack of services, the chronically mentally ill, from the intrinsic nature of their health problems, frequently experience significant problems related to dimensions of accommodation and acceptability. Frequently distrustful of established institutions, the chronically mentally ill find the traditional services provided by mental health agencies inappropriate. Many providers find their bizarre manner of dress, lack of personal hygiene, and inappropriate physical appearance difficult to accept (Aday, 2001; Institute of Medicine, 1988; USDHHS, 1992).

Given the conditions of homelessness and the necessity of obtaining food and shelter, pregnant homeless women frequently find seeking early prenatal care a lesser priority. Compounding the lower priority are the problems of obtaining prenatal and obstetric care. Some obstetric providers refuse to see or limit the number of women on Medicaid they will see because low reimbursement rates, complex billing requirements, and increased risk associated with malpractice suits exist. Consequently, the availability of prenatal and obstetric services is severely compromised. Long waits for initial appointments and long waits at each visit impose considerable stress on homeless women obtaining prenatal care. Many providers find the unhealthy lifestyles, lack of compliance with provider advice, and failure to keep appointments unacceptable (Aday, 2001; Anderson and Hatton, 2000; Curry, 1989; Institute of Medicine, 1988). Multiple complex factors reduce access to health care for this vulnerable, underserved aggregate.

CONCEPTUAL APPROACHES TO HEALTH OF THE HOMELESS

The following discussion provides a conceptual and theoretical framework for exploring health care of the homeless and outlines the market justice and social justice approaches to the distribution of benefits and burdens. It provides an explanation of social justice as the absence of structural violence and discusses upstream versus downstream approaches to homeless health care.

Models of justice provide a blueprint for considering the health problems of the homeless. Beauchamp (1979) distinguished between the two types of justice (i.e., market justice and social justice) that influence public health policy in the United States. **Market justice** has been the dominant model and purports that people are entitled to valued ends (i.e., status, income, and happiness) according to their own individual efforts. Moreover, this model stresses individual responsibility, minimal collective action, and freedom from collective obligations other than respect for another person's fundamental rights. In contrast, under a **social justice** model, all people are equally entitled to key ends (i.e., access to health care and minimum standards of income). Consequently, all members of society must accept collective burdens to provide a fair distribution of these ends. Moreover, social justice is a foundational aspect of public health (Krieger and Birn, 1998).

Additional explication of social justice is found in Galtung's analysis of violence. Distinguishing between physical and structural violence, Galtung (1969) defined violence as "present when human beings are being influenced so that their actual somatic and mental realizations are below their potential realization" (p. 168). The difference is between the actual and the possible. He further distinguished between physical and structural violence according to whether a person who acts is present. Galtung noted that when an actor is present who commits the violence, this is personal or direct violence. In contrast, structural violence is indirect because it lacks an actor. More specifically, the violence is built into the social structure and is displayed as unequal power and unequal life chances. Stated differently, resources are unevenly distributed (e.g., access to medical services from ability to pay or from location). Presence of structural violence is also known as social injustice. Conversely, its absence is social justice.

Butterfield in Chapter 3 discusses McKinlay's (1979) use of the metaphor depicting illness as a river; health workers focus exclusively on pulling people out of the river rather than going upstream to find out why people are in the river. Hence, the predominant mode of approaching societal problems is a downstream mode of intervention.

As McKinlay and Marceau (2000) note, a social philosophy that is focused on an individualistic approach is the dominant approach to public health problems in the United States. In this approach, individual people are the center of concern. Collectivism is a contrasting approach that focuses on "categories (age, sex, social class, race/ethnicity) or places and social positions in society" (p. 26), which is the more dominant theme in Europe.

McKinlay and Marceau (2000) argue that the market justice model, accompanied by an individualistic social model, results in a downstream approach to problems and contributes to structural violence. This model holds individuals responsible for their own conditions and negates the responsibility of all individuals and groups to share in the burdens of prevention. In contrast, the social justice model, which seeks to reduce the structural conditions contributing to the problem through collective action, supports upstream thinking.

Building on McKinlay's "river" metaphor, McKinlay and Marceau (2000) suggest conceptualizing homelessness as the river and the people in the river as the homeless. They purport that government and private efforts to address homeless health care problems largely focus on "pulling the bodies out of the river of homelessness." Such downstream interventions aimed at treating or alleviating health care problems such as physical disease and mental illnesses are worthy and needed. However, these interventions are far less adequate in alleviating homeless people's social health problems. To improve the social health of the homeless, it is necessary to go upstream and focus on the primary contributors to homelessness itself (i.e., lack of affordable housing, inadequate income, and insufficient services).

Some purport that affordable housing and income support are sufficient to relieve homelessness (Timmer, Eitzen, and Talley, 1994). Timmer and colleagues argued that the homeless are not different from other people in physical and mental health status. The research reviewed here does not support these conclusions; it indicates that the homeless have more health problems than the poor who are housed. Although we agree that the primary mode of preventing homeless health problems is to prevent homelessness, they also believe that secondary and tertiary types of interventions are necessary.

RESEARCH AND THE HOMELESS

Many factors complicate research with persons experiencing homelessness. As noted earlier in the chapter, much of the data available on homeless persons are collected at one point in time. Information about individuals and families over time, therefore, is somewhat limited, and the transient nature of the population makes longitudinal studies particularly difficult. The presence of substance use disorders, other mental illnesses, and additional physical health problems compound this difficulty. To improve studies with difficult-to-reach and hidden populations, researchers have identified special research strategies, including locator forms that identify personal contact information, incentives for participation, rapport with participants, and peer data collectors (Hatton and Kaiser, 2004; McKenzie and Tulsky, 1999).

Locating study participants and recruiting them into research projects can be daunting. Because many community agencies that serve the homeless struggle for adequate funding, staff turnover is commonplace. Yet, developing ongoing relationships with agency staff that, in turn, can introduce researchers to potential participants can increase research effectiveness. Staff members can also assist the informed consent process by encouraging participants to ask questions about the investigation and about their risks and benefits as potential participants (Anderson and Hatton, 2000; Hatton and Kaiser, 2004).

In spite of these obstacles, a considerable body of research with the homeless has developed over the past two decades and represents a variety of disciplines, including nursing. Nurse scientists, who bring both their clinical and research perspectives to investigations, have considerable expertise to conduct research with this aggregate. For example, Dr. Adeline Nyamathi and her colleagues at the Center for Vulnerable Populations Research, UCLA, have examined drug and alcohol use, social support, HIV prevention education, perception of health status, victimization, and acculturation among the homeless (Nyamathi et al, 2000a; Nyamathi et al, 2000b; Nyamathi, Flaskerud, et al., 2001; Nyamathi et al, 2001c; Nyamathi et al, 2004). In addition, researchers from nursing and medicine have advocated innovative research approaches and developed theoretical perspectives to guide future work (Flaskerud and Nyamathi,

CASE STUDY APPLICATION OF THE NURSING PROCESS

Katie Brown, a public health nurse (PHN), has just received a new referral from a transitional shelter for mothers and children located near the County Health Center where she is a member of the nursing staff. The shelter staff requests an assessment of a new client, Annie Jones, who is "having difficulty adapting to communal living." The referral indicates that Annie is a 33-year-old Caucasian mother of four children, although she currently has custody of only one child, a newborn girl. Her three other children reside in foster care.

ASSESSMENT

When Katie visits the shelter, she finds Annie sobbing in her room. Annie tells her she has a history of severe depression and has been hospitalized "many times." Annie reports that after the birth of her daughter, her physician recommended she not take her medications because she intended to breast-feed the infant. Annie also informs the PHN that she has a long history of alcohol and methamphetamine use and that she left the father of the baby because he repeatedly assaulted her.

The shelter's case manager impatiently says that Annie's behavior disrupts the other shelter residents. She adds that the shelter cannot manage clients with psychiatric problems. Annie has a newborn, however, so they decided to give her special consideration. Tensions among Annie, the staff, and other clients clearly have begun to escalate, and Katie's past clinical experience reminds her that the community has few agencies that provide shelter and services to mothers with mental illness.

DIAGNOSIS

Individual
- *Client:* At risk for ineffective health maintenance
- *Infant:* At risk for delayed development

Family
- Impaired home maintenance
- At risk for impaired parenting

Community
- Inadequate mental health services for women with children
- Inadequate affordable housing

PLANNING

Individual
Long-Term Goal
- Client will, in the next 6 months, engage in actions designed to maintain health of infant and self.

Short-Term Goal
- Client will, in the next week, follow-through with scheduled appointments for identified health and social services.

Family
Long-Term Goal
- Client will adhere to plan she, shelter staff, and PHN formulated to assist in her adapting to shelter living and parenting.

Short-Term Goal
- Client will, in the next week, meet with shelter staff, and PHN to develop a 6-month plan designed to assist her in adapting to shelter living and parenting.

Community
Long-Term Goal
- Increased capacity of mental health agencies to provide services for women with co-morbidities and their children,

Short-Term Goal
- Enhanced ability of shelter staff to assist women who have co-morbidities and are accompanied by children.

INTERVENTIONS

Individual and Family
Katie consults with colleagues in the community who have experience working with persons who have co-occurring disorders (substance use disorder and other mental illness) and identifies resources for treatment. She discusses the importance of managing mental health problems with Annie and the case manager. Based on Annie's desires for care for herself and baby, Katie contacts the Family Nurse Practitioner (FNP) at the County Health Center and arranges for an appointment the next day for health maintenance care both Annie and her baby.

For psychiatric evaluation and treatment, Katie refers Annie to a community mental health agency that provides services to low-income and homeless persons. This agency has services especially designed for individuals with co-occurring disorders. Annie's case manager facilitates her care by assisting her to reestablish her Medicaid eligibility and begins to explore her eligibility for disability benefits under SSI (Supplemental Security Income).

Katie develops specific guidelines with Annie's case manager to monitor her progress in the shelter.

Community
Katie continues to work with the shelter staff to develop strategies for caring for Annie and her newborn. One

Continued

strategy that Katie and staff used to provide care was to identify clear expectations for Annie in the shelter, including household tasks, management of her illness, and care of her newborn. As Annie gradually adapts to shelter living, Katie and staff assist her in keeping appointments for health and social services.

As a member of the local Interagency Council on Homelessness, Katie volunteered to serve on an ad hoc committee formed to identify housing needs of women with mental illness and substance use problems with special emphasis on women who had young children.

EVALUATION

Individual and Family

Over the 6-month period, the case manager, Annie, and Katie met on a biweekly basis to review the overall situation and address any concerns that emerged.

Annie attended parenting classes with other shelter residents and weekly Narcotics Anonymous meetings. She also enrolled in the shelter's program that addresses intimate partner violence. Annie left her infant for short periods in the shelter's day care facility and attended a day treatment program at the community mental health agency. She resumed a prescribed anti-depressant and initiated formula-feeding her baby. Gradually she adapted to shelter living. Having successfully met her goals, Annie was at the end of 6 months beginning to plan for moving to a more independent living facility.

Community

At the shelter's manager's request, Katie, in collaboration with colleagues at the Community Health Center, developed an in-service educational program for shelter staff. The program was designed to enhance the staff's

skills in assisting women residents with mental illness and substance use problems who had young children. Staff indicated, in their self-reported evaluations, that the program provided helpful information. Katie also noted that the shelter was now providing services to several more women with problems similar to Annie's.

The Interagency Council on Homelessness ad hoc committee completed the needs survey related to housing needs of women with mental illness and substance use problems. The committee has recommended to the Council that advocating for an increase in the supply of available housing for this at-risk population deserves a high priority as it has the potential of preventing homelessness at all levels—primary, secondary, and tertiary.

LEVELS OF PREVENTION

Primary
- Immunizations for Annie and her infant.
- Promotion of policies designed to increase supply of affordable and accessible housing, health, and social services.

Secondary
- Provision of services that enhance Annie's ability to maintain a residency for herself and her infant at the transitional shelter.
- Periodic health screening services for Annie and her infant.
- Advocating for policies and programs to assist homeless persons.

Tertiary
- Treatment for Annie's mental illness and substance use disorder in order to prevent further deterioration.
- Shelter program that addresses intimate partner violence.

2002; Flaskerud and Winslow, 1998; Gelberg, Andersen, and Leake, 2000).

Notably, the research that describes the characteristics of individuals and families who experience homelessness, as well as interventions designed to prevent disease transmission and access to health care, informs community health program planning for this vulnerable population. Farmer (1999, 2003), however, reminds us that research must not have an undue focus on the psychological or cultural peculiarities of vulnerable persons. An individualistic focus, he argues, limits the research to the effects of larger societal problems rather than on their causes. Similarly, Burt and her colleagues (2001) emphasize the importance of understanding the role that U.S. policies play in the problem of homelessness. In particular, they point to government-supported programs such as Supplemental Security Income (SSI), food stamps, general assistance, and welfare that help prevent many from slipping into homelessness, especially chronic homelessness. They

advocate innovative housing programs that target persons known to be at risk for homelessness. Thus, future research that explores not only individual characteristics and risk factors for homelessness but also considers the impact of community structural factors will provide the broad knowledge base essential for effective community health nursing practice and advocacy with this vulnerable aggregate.

SUMMARY

Homelessness evolves from the interaction of complex factors at the societal level and among vulnerable individuals. Consequently, these individuals and families find themselves living in the streets, abandoned buildings, other public places, and shelters. Homeless people are heterogeneous, difficult to count, and suffer from a variety of complex health problems. Their access to health care is problematic at best, and interventions to deal with this enormous problem represent largely downstream endeavors. Future research with members of this aggregate, which explores the complexity of their lives from a variety of methodological perspectives, will generate the knowledge necessary for more upstream community health nursing interventions.

LEARNING ACTIVITIES

1. Compare the information contained in the most recent U. S. Conference of Mayors Annual Report on Hunger and Homelessness with the information contained in the previous 3 years. What has changed?
2. Analyze at least three or four factors that contribute to homelessness in the United States.

3. Discuss common health problems found among homeless men, women, children, and adolescents.
4. Identify two special subgroups of the homeless and describe their health problems.
5. Describe the five specific areas of access identified by Penchansky and Thomas (1981). What is the significance of these areas for community health nursing practice with homeless individuals and families?
6. Use a market justice model and a social justice model to analyze how the United States has approached the health problems of the homeless.

REFERENCES

Aday LA: *At risk in America: the health and health care needs of vulnerable populations in the United States,* San Francisco, 2001, Jossey-Bass.

American Academy of Pediatrics, Committee on School Health: School-based mental health services: policy statement, *Pediatrics* 113(6): 1839-1845, 2004.

Anderson D. Homeless women's perceptions about their families of origin, *West J Nurs Res* 18(1):29-42, 1996.

Anderson DG, Hatton DC: Accessing vulnerable populations for research, *West J Nurs Res* 22(2):244-251, 2000.

Anderson DG, Rayens MK: Factors influencing homelessness in women, *Public Health Nurs* 21(1):12-23, 2004.

Baer J, Ginzler J, Peterson P: *DSM*-IV alcohol and substance abuse and dependence in homeless youth, *J Stud Alcohol* 64(1): 5-14, 2003.

Barkin S et al: Health care utilization among homeless adolescents and young adults, *J Adolesc Health* 32(4):253-256, 2003.

Baron S: Street youth violence and victimization, *Trauma Violence Abuse* 4(1):22-44, 2003.

Bassuk EL: Social and economic hardships of homeless and other poor women, *Am J Orthopsychiatry* 63(3):340-347, 1993.

Bassuk EL: Welfare reform and the real lives of poor women, *Am J Orthopsychiatry* 66(4): 490-582, 1996.

Bassuk EL, Melnick S, Browne A: Responding to the needs of low-income and homeless women who are survivors of family violence, *J Am Med Womens Assoc* 53(2):57-64, 1998.

Bassuk EL et al: The characteristics and needs of sheltered homeless and low-income housed mothers, *JAMA* 276(8):640-646, 1996.

Bassuk EL et al: Homelessness in female-headed families: childhood and adult risk and protective factors, *Am J Public Health* 87(2):241-248, 1997.

Beauchamp DE: Public health as social justice. In Jaco EG, editor: *Patients, physicians, and illness,* ed 3, New York, 1979, Free Press.

Bellavia CW, Toro PA: Mental disorder among homeless and poor people: a comparison of assessment methods, *Community Ment Health J* 35(1):57-67, 1999.

Berti LC, Zylbert S, Rolnitzky L: Comparison of health status of children using a school-based health center for comprehensive care, *J Pediatr Health Care* 15:244-250, 2001.

Bird C et al: Predictors of contact with public service sectors among homeless adults with and without alcohol and other drug disorders, *J Stud Alcohol* 63(6):716-725, 2002.

Bourgois P, Prince B, Moss A: The everyday violence of hepatitis C among young women who inject drugs in San Francisco, *Hum Organ* 63(3):253-264, 2004.

Buckner J et al: Homelessness and its relation to the mental health and behavior of low-income school-age children, *Dev Psychol* 35(1). 246-257, 1999.

Burt M: *Five questions for...,* Washington, DC, 2005, Urban Institute, http://www.urban.org/toolkit/fivequestions/fivequestions.

Burt M et al: *Helping America's homeless: emergency shelter or affordable housing?* Washington, DC, 2001, Urban Institute.

Burt, M et al: *Homelessness: programs and the people they serve: a summary report of the findings of the National Survey of Homeless Assistance Providers and Clients.* Washington DC, 1999, Urban Institute, http://www.urban.org/publications/310291.html.

California Department of Mental Health: *Effectiveness of integrated services for homeless adults with serious mental illness: report to the Legislature,* 2003, The Author, http://www.dmh.cahwnet.gov/AOAPP/Int_Services/docs/Leg_Report_2003.pdf.

Cameron K, Racine Y, Offord D, Cairney J: Youth at risk of homelessness in an affluent Toronto suburb. *Can J Public Health* 95(5): 352-356, 2004.

Cauce A, Tyler K, Whitbeck L: Maltreatment and victimization in homeless adolescents: out of the frying pan and into the fire, *Prev Res* 11(1):12-14, 2004.

Center on Budget and Policy Priorities: *Census data show poverty increased, income stagnated, and the number of uninsured rose to a record level in 2003,* News release, Aug 27,

2004, The Author, http://www.cbpp.org/8-26-04pov.html.

Centers for Disease Control and Prevention: Surveillance summaries, *MMWR Morb Mortality Wkly Rep* 53(SS-2), May 21, 2004.

Children's Defense Fund: *Basic facts on assisted housing,* Jan 2004, The Author, http://www.childrensdefense.org/familyincome/housing/basicfacts.aspx.

Children's Defense Fund: *Bush administration policies exacerbate growing housing crisis for families with children,* 2005a, The Author, http://www.childrensdefense.org/familyincome/housing/housing_crisis.pdf#xml=http://childrensdefense.org.master.com/texis/master/search/mysite.txt?q=families+with+children&order=r&id=2031780174a40e4b&cmd=xml.

Children's Defense Fund. *Increasing the minimum wage: an issue of children's well-being,* 2005b, The Author, http://www.childrensdefense.org/familyincome/jobs/minimumwagereport2005.pdf.

Cochran BN et al: Challenges faced by homeless sexual minorities: comparison of gay, lesbian, bisexual, and transgender homeless adolescents with their heterosexual counterparts, *Am J Public Health* 92(5):772-777, 2002.

Culhane D et al: The co-occurrence of AIDS and homelessness: results from the integration of administrative databases for AIDS surveillance and public shelter utilisation in Philadelphia, *J Epidemiol Community Health* 55(7): 515-520, 2001.

Curry MA: Nonfinancial barriers to prenatal care, *Womens Health* 15:85, 1989.

da Costa Nunez R: *A shelter is not a home...or is it? Lessons from family homelessness in New York City,* New York, 2004, White Tiger Press.

dela Cruz FA, Brehm C, Harris J: Transformation in family nurse practitioner students' attitudes toward homeless individuals after participation in a homeless outreach clinic, *J Am Acad Nurse Pract* 16(12): 547-554, 2004.

DeNavas WC, Proctor BD, Mills RJ: *Income poverty and health insurance coverage in the United States: 2003,* Current Population Reports P60-226, 2004, http://www.census.gov/prod/2004pubs/p60-226.pdf.

Douglass RL et al: Health care needs and services utilization among sheltered and unsheltered Michigan homeless, *J Health Care Poor Underserved* 10:5-18, 1999.

Farmer P: *Infections and inequalities: the modern plagues,* Berkeley, 1999, University of California Press.

Farmer P: *Pathologies of power: health, human rights, and the new war on the poor,* Berkeley, 2003, University of California Press.

Feldmann J, Middleman A: Homeless adolescents: common clinical concerns, *Semin Pediatr Infect Dis* 14(1):6-11, 2003.

Finley S, Finley SJ: Sp'ange: a research story, *Qual Inq* 5:313-337, 1999.

Fischer PJ: *Alcohol, drug abuse, and mental health problems among homeless persons: a review of the literature, 1980-1990,* Rockville, Md, 1991, National Institute on Alcohol Abuse and Alcoholism.

Flaskerud JH, Nyamathi AM: New paradigm for health disparities needed, *Nurs Res* 51(3):139, 2002.

Flaskerud JH, Winslow BJ: Conceptualizing vulnerable populations health-related research, *Nurs Res* 47(2):69-78, 1998.

Folsom D, Jeste V: Schizophrenia in homeless persons: a systematic review of the literature, *Acta Psychiatr Scand* 105:404-413, 2002.

Fortney J et al: Measuring continuity of care for clients of public mental health systems, *Health Serv Res* 38(4):1157-1175, 2003.

Galea S, Vlahov D: Social determinants and the health of drug users: socioeconomic status, homelessness, and incarceration, *Public Health Rep* 117(suppl 1):S135-S145, 2002.

Galtung J: Violence, peace, and peace research, *J Peace Res* 16:167-191, 1969.

Gelberg L, Andersen RM, Leake BD: The behavioral model for vulnerable populations: application to medical care use and outcomes for homeless people, *Health Serv Res* 34(6):1273-1302, 2000.

Gelberg L et al: Access to women's health care: a qualitative study of barriers perceived by homeless women, *Women Health* 40(2):87-100, 2004.

Glasser I: *Homelessness in global perspective,* New York, 1994, GK Hall.

Goldfinger S et al: *HIV, homelessness and serious mental illness: implications for policy and practice,* Delmar, NY, 1998, National Resource Center on Homelessness and Mental Illness, Policy Research Associates, http://www.nrchmi.samhsa.gov/pdfs/publications/HIV.pdf.

Goss C et al: Cost and incidence of social comorbidities in low-risk patients with community-acquired pneumonia admitted to a public hospital, *Chest* 124(6):2148-2155, 2003.

Greene JM et al: *Sexual abuse among homeless adolescents: Prevalence, correlates, and sequelae,* Report of the Administration of Children, Youth, and Families, 2002, US Department of Health and Human Services, http://www.acf.hhs.gov/programs/opre/fys/sex_abuse/reports/sexabuse_hmless/sex_abuse_hmless.pdf.

Haber MG, Toro PA: Homelessness among families, children, and adolescents: an ecological developmental perspective, *Clin Child Fam Psychol Rev* 7(3):123-164, 2004.

Haley N et al: Characteristics of adolescent street youth with a history of pregnancy, *J Pediatr Adolesc Gynecol* 17:313-320, 2004.

Hatton D: Managing health problems among homeless women with children in a transitional shelter, *Image J Nurs Sch* 29(1):33-37, 1997.

Hatton DC: Homeless women's access to health services: a study of social networks and managed care in the USA, *Women Health* 33(3/4):149-162, 2001.

Hatton DC, Kaiser L: Methodological and ethical issues emerging from pilot testing an intervention with women in a transitional shelter, *West J Nurs Res* 26(1):129-136, 2004.

Hockett D et al: *The crisis in America's housing: confronting myths and promoting a balanced housing policy,* Washington, DC, Jan 2005, Center for Community Change, http://www.nlihc.org/research/housingmyths.pdf.

Huang C, Menke E: School-aged homeless sheltered children's stressors and coping behaviors, *J Pediatr Nurs* 16(2):102-109, 2001.

Institute of Medicine: *Homelessness, health, and human needs,* Washington DC, 1988, National Academy Press.

Jencks C: *The homeless,* Cambridge, Mass, 1994, Harvard University Press.

Julianelle PF, Foscarinis M: Responding to the school mobility of children and youth experiencing homelessness: the McKinney-Vento Act and beyond, *J Negro Educ* 72(1):39-54, 2003.

Koegel P et al: Utilization of mental health and substance abuse services among homeless adults in Los Angeles, *Med Care* 37(3):306-317, 1999.

Kozol J: *Rachel and her children: homeless families in America,* New York, 1988, Fawcett Columbine.

Krieger N, Birn AE: A vision of social justice as the foundation of public health: commemorating 150 years of the spirit of 1848, *Am J Public Health* 88(11):1603-1606, 1998.

Martens W: A review of physical and mental health in homeless persons, *Public Health Rev* 29(1):13-33, 2001.

McKenzie M, Tulsky JP: Tracking and follow-up of marginalized populations: a review, *J Health Care Poor Underserved* 10(4):409-429, 1999.

McKinlay JB: A case for refocusing upstream: the political economy of illness. In Jaco EG, editor: *Patients, physicians, and illness,* ed 3, New York, 1979, Free Press.

McKinlay JB, Marceau LD: To boldly go . . . public health matters, *Am J Public Health* 90(1):25-33, 2000.

McMurray-Avila M, Gelberg L, Breakey WR: Balancing act: clinical practices that respond to the needs of homeless people. In Fosburg LB, Dennis DI, editors: *Practical lessons: the 1998 National Symposium on Homelessness Research,* Washington, DC, Aug 1999, US Department of Housing and Urban Development and US Department of Health and

Human Services, http://www.aspe.hhs.gov/progsys/homeless/symposium/8-Clinical.html.

Metraux S, Culhane DP: Family dynamics, housing, and recurring homelessness among women in New York city homeless shelters, *J Fam Issues* 20:371-396, 1999.

Nabors LA et al: Assessment, prevention, and intervention activities in a school-based program for children experiencing homelessness, *Behav Modif* 28(4):565-578, 2004.

National Coalition for the Homeless: *Homeless families with children,* NCH Fact Sheet #7, 2001, The Author, http://www.nationalhomeless.org/families.html.

National Health Care for the Homeless Council: The left hand giveth. The right hand taketh away, *Health Care for the Homeless Mobilizer* 10(2), Feb 12, 2005, http://www.nhchc.org/2005mobilizerpdf/Mobilizer021205FY06Budget.pdf.

National Law Center on Homelessness and Poverty: *Key data concerning homeless persons in America,* July 2004, The Author, http://www.nlchp.org/FA_HAPIA/HomelessPersonsinAmerica.pdf.

National Policy and Advocacy Council on Homelessness: *Facts about homelessness,* 2005, The Author, http://npach.org/.

National Student Campaign Against Hunger and Homelessness: *Communities in crisis: survey of hunger and homelessness in America 2004,* Feb 2005. Retrieved April 16, 2005, The Author, http://www.studentsagainsthunger.org/hunger.asp?id2=15761.

North C et al: Are rates of psychiatric disorders in the homeless population changing? *Am J Public Health* 94(1):103-108, 2004.

Nwakeze P et al: Homelessness, substance misuse, and access to public entitlements in a soup kitchen population, *Subst Use Misuse* 38(3-6):645-668, 2003.

Nyamathi A, Flaskerud J, Leake B: HIV-risk behaviors and mental health characteristics among homeless or drug-recovering women and their closest sources of social support, *Nurs Res* 46(3):133-137, 1997.

Nyamathi A et al: Two-year follow-up of AIDS education programs for impoverished women, *West J Nurs Res* 21(3):405-425, 1999.

Nyamathi A, Leake B, Gelberg L: Sheltered versus nonsheltered homeless women: differences in health, behavior, victimization, and utilization of care, *J Gen Intern Med* 15:565-572, 2000.

Nyamathi A, Leake B, Keenan C, Gelberg L: Type of social support among homeless women: its impact on psychosocial resources, health and health behaviors, and use of health services, *Nurs Res* 49(6):318-326, 2000.

Nyamathi A, Flaskerud JH et al: Evaluating the impact of peer, nurse case-managed, and standard HIV risk-reduction programs on psychosocial and health-promoting behavioral outcomes among homeless women, *Res Nurs Health* 24(5):410-422, 2001.

Nyamathi A, Leake B et al: Reliability of homeless women's reports: concordance between hair assay and self report of cocaine use, *Nurs Res* 50(3):165-171, 2001.

Nyamathi A, Wenzel SL et al: Comparison of psychosocial and behavioral profiles of victimized and nonvictimized homeless women and their intimate partners, *Res Nurs Health* 24(4):324-335, 2001.

Nyamathi A et al: Perception of health status by homeless US veterans, *Fam Community Health* 27(1):65-74, 2004.

Page T, Nooe RM: Life experiences and vulnerabilities of homeless women: a comparison of women unaccompanied versus accompanied by minor children, and correlates with children's emotional distress, *J Soc Distress Homeless* 11(3):215-231, 2002.

O'Flaherty B: *Making room: the economics of homelessness*, Cambridge, Mass, 1996, Harvard University Press.

O'Neil-Pirozzi TM: Language functioning of residents in family homeless shelters, *Am J Speech Lang Pathol* 12:229-242, 2003.

Partington S, Nitzke S, Csete J: The prevalence of anemia in a WIC population: a comparison by homeless experience, *J Am Diet Assoc* 100(4):469-471, 2000 [erratum appears in *J Am Diet Assoc* 100(6):629, 2000].

Penchansky R, Thomas JW: The concept of access: definition and relationship to consumer satisfaction, *Med Care* 19:127, 1981.

Pitcoff W et al: *Out of reach 2004*, Washington, DC, 2004, National Low Income Housing Coalition, http://www.nlihc.org/oor2004/index.htm.

Portnoy FL, Dumas L: Nursing for the public good, *Nurs Clin North Am* 29(3):371-375, 1994.

Rafferty Y, Shinn M, Weitzman B: Academic achievement among formerly homeless adolescents and their continuously housed peers, *J School Psychol* 42(3):179-200, 2004.

Reardon M et al: Alcohol use and other psychiatric disorders in the formerly homeless and never homeless: prevalence, age of onset, comorbidity, temporal sequencing, and service utilization, *Subst Use Misuse* 38(3-6):601-644, 2003.

Rew L: *Adolescent health: a multidisciplinary approach to theory, research and intervention*, Thousand Oaks, Calif, 2005, Sage.

Rew L, Taylor-Seehafer M, Fitzgerald M: Sexual abuse, alcohol and other drug use, and suicidal behaviors in homeless adolescents, *Issues Compr Pediatr Nurs* 24:225-240, 2001.

Robertson MJ, Toro PA: Homeless youth: research, intervention, and policy. In Fosburg LB, Dennis DI, editors: *Practical lessons: the 1998 National Symposium on Homelessness Research*, Washington, DC, Aug 1999, US Department of Housing and Urban Development and US Department of Health and Human Services, http://www.aspe.hhs.gov/progsys/homeless/symposium/3-Youth.html.

Robertson M et al: HIV seroprevalence among homeless and marginally housed adults in San Francisco, *Am J Public Health* 94(7):1207-1217, 2004.

Roschelle A, Kaufman P: Fitting in and fighting back: stigma management strategies among homeless kids, *Symbolic Interaction* 27(1):23-46, 2004.

Rosenheck R: *Homelessness in America* (editorial), *Am J Public Health* 84(12):1885-1886, 1994.

Rossi PH: The old homeless and the new homelessness in historical perspective, *Am Psychol* 45:954-959, 1990.

Roy E et al: Mortality in a cohort of street youth in Montreal, *JAMA* 292(5):569-574, 2004.

Ryan KD et al: Psychological consequences of child maltreatment in homeless adolescents: untangling the unique effects of maltreatment and family environment, *Child Abuse Negl* 24(3):333-352, 2000.

Sachs-Ericsson N et al: Health problems and service utilization in the homeless, *J Health Care Poor Underserved* 10:443-452, 1999.

Shinn M, Baumohl J: Rethinking the prevention of homelessness. In Fosburg LB, Dennis DI, editors: *Practical lessons: the 1998 National Symposium on Homelessness Research*, Washington, DC, Aug 1999, US Department of Housing and Urban Development and US Department of Health and Human Services, http://www.aspe.hhs.gov/progsys/homeless/symposium/13-Preven.html.

Shoenberger JM, Houpt JC, Swadron SP: Occult trauma in high-risk populations, *Emerg Med Clin North Am* 21(4):1145-1163, 2003.

Smith AD, Smith DI: *Emergency and transitional shelter population 2000*, Special Reports CENSR/01-2, 2001, US Census Bureau, http://www.census.gov/prod/2001pubs/censr01-2.pdf.

Solliday-McRoy C et al: Neuropsychological functioning of homeless men, *J Nerv Ment Dis* 192(7):471-478, 2004.

Stein J, Lu M, Gelberg L: Severity of homelessness and adverse birth outcomes, *Health Psychol* 19(6):524-534, 2000.

Stein J, Nyamathi A: Correlates of Hepatitis C virus infection in homeless men: a latent variable approach, *Drug Alcohol Depend* 75(1):89-95, 2004.

Stevens P: A nursing critique of US welfare system reform, *Adv Nurs Sci* 23(2):1-11, 2000.

Stratigos A, Katsambas A: Medical and cutaneous disorders associated with homelessness, *Skinmed* 2(3):168-172, 2003.

Swanson KA, Andersen R, Gelberg L: Patient satisfaction for homeless women, *J Womens Health* 12(7):675-686, 2003.

Taylor-Seehafer M: Positive youth development: reducing the health risks of homeless youth, *MCN Am J Matern Child Nurs* 29(1):36-40, 2004.

Timmer DA, Eitzen S, Talley KD: *Paths to homelessness: extreme poverty and the urban housing crisis*, Boulder, Colo, 1994, Westview Press.

Tulsky J et al: Can the poor adhere? Incentives for adherence to TB prevention in homeless adults, *Int J Tuberc Lung Dis* 8(1):83-91, 2004.

Tyler KA, Cauce AM: Perpetrators of early physical and sexual abuse among homeless and runaway adolescents, *Child Abuse Negl* 26:1261-1274, 2002.

US Conference of Mayors—SODEXHO USA: *Hunger and Homelessness Survey 2004: a status report on hunger and homelessness in America's cities*, 2004, The Author, http://www.usmayors.org/uscm/hungersurvey/2004/onlinereport/HungerAndHomelessnessReport2004.pdf.

US Department of Education: *McKinney-Vento Homeless Education Assistance Improvements Act of 2001*, 2004, The Author, http://www.ed.gov/policy/elsec/leg/esea02/pg116.html.

US Department of Health and Human Services: *Ending chronic homelessness: strategies for action*, Report from the Secretary's Work Group on Ending Chronic Homelessness, March 2003, The Author, http://aspe.hhs.gov/hsp/homelessness/strategies03/.

US Department of Health and Human Services, National Institute of Mental Health: *Outcasts on main street: report of the Federal Task Force on Homelessness and Severe Mental Illness*. ADM 92-1904. Washington, DC, Interagency Council on Homeless, 1992.

US Department of Housing and Urban Development. Homeless Management Information Systems (HMIS) Technical Assistance News. *HMIS.INFO* (14), April 2006, The Author, http://www.hmis.info/news_docs/April%202006%20Newsletter%2014.pdf.

US Department of Housing and Urban Development: *General definition of homeless individual* (Sec. 103 of PL 100-77, July 22, 1987, 101 Stat. 482, known as the McKinney-Vento Homeless Assistance Act), 2001, The Author, http://www.hud.gov/offices/cpd/homeless/rulesandregs/laws/title1/sec11302.cfm.

US Department of Housing and Urban Development: *National HMIS Standards/HMIS Research*, 2005, The Author, http://www.hud.gov/offices/cpd/homeless/hmis/standards/index.cfm.

Urban Institute: *A new look at homelessness*, Feb 2000, The Author, http://www.urban.org/urlprint.cfm?ID=7476.

Weinreb L et al: Hunger: its impact on children's health and mental health, *Pediatrics* 110(e41), 2002, http://www.pediatrics.org/cgi/content/full/110/4/e41.

Wenzel S et al: Access to inpatient or residential substance abuse treatment among homeless adults with alcohol or other drug use disorders, *Med Care* 39(11):1158-1169, 2001.

Wenzel SL, Koegel P, Gelberg L: Antecedents of physical and sexual victimization among homeless women: a comparison to homeless men, *Am J of Community Psychol* 28(3):367-390, 2000.

Wenzel SL, Leake B, Gelberg L: Health of homeless women with recent experience of rape, *J Gen Intern Med* 15:265-268, 2000.

Whitbeck LB et al: Mental disorder and comorbidity among runaway and homeless adolescents, *J Adolesc Health* 335:132-140, 2004.

Wilde MH et al: Development of a student nurses' clinic for homeless men, *Public Health Nurs* 21(4):354-360, 2004.

Wilder Research Center: *Homeless adults and children in Minnesota: statewide survey of people without permanent shelter,* Saint Paul, Minn, Sept 2004a, The Author, http://www.wilder.org/download.0.html?report=484.

Wilder Research Center: *Homeless in Minnesota: a closer look at families and children,* Saint Paul, Minn, June 2004b, The Author, http://www.wilder.org/download.0.html?report=558.

Wilder Research Center: *Homeless youth in Minnesota: 2003 Statewide survey of people without permanent shelter,* Saint Paul, Minn, Feb 2005, The Author, http://www.wilder.org/download.0.html?report=410.

World Health Organization: *WHO definition of Health,* Preamble to the Constitution of the World Health Organization as adopted by the International Health Conference, New York, 19-22 June, 1946; signed on 22 July 1946 by the representatives of 61 States (Official Records of the World Health Organization, no. 2, p. 100) and entered into force on 7 April 1948, http://www.who.int/about/definition/en/.

Wright JD: The health of homeless people: evidence from the National Health Care for the Homeless Program. In Brickner P et al, editors: *Under the safety net: the health and social welfare of the homeless in the United States,* New York, 1990a, WW Norton.

Wright JD: Poor people, poor health: the health status of the homeless, *J Soc Issues* 46:49-64, 1990b.

Wright JD, Rubin BA, Devine JA: *Beside the golden door: policy, politics and the homeless,* New York, 1998, Aldine de Gruyter.

Rural and Migrant Health

Kathleen Chafey ▪ Wade G. Hill ▪ Glenna R. Burg

MEDIA RESOURCES

Additional Material for Study, Review, and Further Exploration

evolve Website at http://evolve.elsevier.com/Nies

❖ Quiz ❖ Case Studies ❖ Content Updates ❖ Glossary ❖ WebLinks

OBJECTIVES

Upon completion of this chapter, the reader will be able to do the following:

1. Describe features of the health care system and population characteristics common to rural aggregates.
2. Explain why rural populations and geographical areas must be defined specifically.
3. Discuss the impact of structural barriers vs. personal barriers on the health of rural aggregates.
4. Identify factors that place farmers and migrant workers at risk for illness and accidents.
5. Discuss the importance of the informal care network to rural health and social services.
6. Describe the characteristics of rural community health nursing practice.
7. Apply an upstream perspective to health promotion, illness prevention, and premature death and disability.

KEY TERMS

acute pesticide poisoning
Community-Oriented
  Primary Care (COPC)
disparities
frontier
informal care systems
metropolitan
micropolitan
migrant workers
noncore
rural
seasonal workers

CHAPTER OUTLINE

RURAL HEALTH RESEARCH
Capacity of Rural Public Health to Manage
Improvements in Health
Information Technology in Rural Communities

Performance Standards in Rural Public Health
Leadership and Workforce Capacity for Rural Public Health
Interaction and Integration of Community Health
Systems, Managed Care, and Public Health

RURAL UNITED STATES

There are many different versions of rural America, in that each rural area is somewhat unique but shares certain features with other rural regions. Geographic, demographic, environmental, economic, and social factors all influence health, access to health care and quality of health care; and when aggregated, these characteristics may be contrasted with those of urban populations. In this section, we present a "snapshot" of rural population and health characteristics that contribute to challenging health **disparities** for many of the people living in the most rural areas of America.

Although the urban growth rate has been steadily climbing since 1890, with numbers of urban dwellers surpassing those in rural areas around 1920, the number of rural residents is the highest in the country's history. The number and size of rural counties are highest in the Midwest and West, and rural Americans comprise about 25% of the nation's population (Ricketts, Johnson-Webb, and Randolph, 1999). Current census estimates are that 17% of the nation's children under age 18 years live in rural areas (United States Department of Agriculture [USDA], 2005), as do 15% to 20% of the nation's elderly (Rogers, 2002), and over 50% of the nation's poor (USDA, 2005)

The economic base of rural America is changing rapidly. Whereas rural residents have long been thought to be family farmers and ranchers, today, demographers and economists consider trends in farm and farm-related employment much more broadly. They characterize agriculture as a "food and fiber system" that encompasses all aspects of agriculture, from core materials sectors (farm, food processing, textiles, and other manufacturing) to wholesale and retail trade and the food service sector (Edmondson, 2004). Considered as such, the system accounted for 30% of the U.S. Gross National Product in 2001, and 21% of jobs in nonmetropolitan areas (USDA, 2002). However, the 1990 census classified only 8% of the rural population (less than 2% of the total U.S. population) as farm or ranch operators, compared with 62% in 1920 (Ricketts et al., 1999). In addition, 80% of farm and ranch operators work full-time in off-farm jobs (Whitener and McGranahan, 2003). Despite the shrinking number of family farms and full-time farmers, agriculture continues to be an important part of the rural and U.S. economy. Today however, rural economies are increasingly dependent on other sources of business to attract people and jobs, especially recreation, tourism, retirement living, and light manufacturing (Whitener and McGranahan, 2003). Farm owners often sell long-held family farms because land values and taxes may be higher than agricultural profitability; the younger generation may not want to invest in a business known for small profits and long hours; and, particularly when the land is located in less rural areas, prices for farm and ranch land may make selling an attractive option.

The rural population is undergoing rapid change. Not only is the economic base shifting, but the age composition is as well. Many rural areas are growing, especially in the West and South, and many rural counties, especially in the Great Plains states are losing population because of a decline in agricultural and manufacturing jobs. Younger people are leaving rural areas for jobs in urban centers, so that those who remain behind are increasingly older and isolated, and have diminished access to health care (Whitener and McGranahan, 2003). Recent demographic changes in rural areas have also included an influx of retirees and escapees from urban areas, who are able to live in rural areas and conduct business through modern telecommunication and airline travel (Purdy, 1999). Recent demographic data (2001) indicate that the number of rural persons aged 60 years and older comprise 20% of the population of nonmetropolitan areas, in contrast to 15% of the population of urban areas (Rogers, 2002). Of the nation's rural elderly, the largest clusters live in the South (45%) and the Midwest (31%) (Rogers, 2002). The trends of "aging-in-place, out-migration of young adults, and immigration of older persons from metro areas" (Rogers, 2002, p. 2) present challenges to already stressed communities that must provide adequate health care, housing, transportation, and other human services.

Poverty, a key health determinant, continues to be greater in rural America than in urban areas. Whereas the metropolitan population had a poverty rate of 11% in 2002, the rural population had a poverty rate of 14%. This overall gap may not seem large, but when the *degree* of rurality or the poverty rate for particular subpopulations (e.g., minorities, children under 18 years of age, or the elderly) are examined, the gap increases greatly. For example, the poverty rate for non-Hispanic blacks in nonmetropolitan areas in 2002 was 33%, compared to a rate of 23% for the same group in metropolitan areas. The poverty rate for people in the rural South was 18%, versus 13% for Southerners living in and around metropolitan areas (USDA, 2004).

The rural population is also becoming more ethnically diverse. Generations ago, many families began farming when they came to the United States as European immigrants. In the 1990s, new immigrants began buying and operating their own small family farms, and others found employment in rural agriculture and manufacturing. Between 1992 and 1997, the number of immigrant Hispanics who owned small farms doubled. Like those before them, these immigrants want something for themselves. For example, the 2000 census shows that Hispanics accounted for a quarter of the growth of the nonmetropolitan population of the United States. This growth occurred in such areas as Texas, Arizona and California, which traditionally had large Hispanic populations. But today, nearly one half of rural Hispanics live outside the Southwest, and "high-growth Hispanic counties" are mostly in the South and Midwest (Kandel and Cromartie, 2003). Hispanics are now the most rapidly growing demographic group in rural and small-town America.

Policies and programs developed to close the health disparities gap must take a population health view of the special circumstances of rural life. Although 75% of U.S. counties are classified as rural, they contain only 20% of the U.S. population. Members of rural populations also are more likely to be older, be less educated, live in poverty, lack health insurance, and experience a lack of available health care providers and access to health care. Only 10% of U.S. physicians practice in rural counties (Gamm, Castillo, and Pittman, 2003), and the ratio of medical specialists to rural population size is 40 per 100,000 people (compared with 134 per 100,000 in urban settings) (Berkowitz, 2004).

Rural residents more often assess their health as fair or poor, and have more disability days associated with acute conditions than their urban counterparts. Rural people also tend to have more problems related to negative health behaviors (e.g., obesity and alcohol, tobacco, and drug use) that contribute to excess deaths and chronic disease and disability rates. The literature suggests, for example, that the highest death rates for children and young adults were in the most rural counties. Residents of rural areas are nearly twice as likely to die from unintentional injuries, including motor vehicle accidents, when compared with their urban counterparts (National Rural Health Association [NRHA], n.d.).

Noting a prominent and persistent pattern of risky health behaviors in rural dwellers, Hartley (2004) has suggested that "rural culture" may itself be a key determinant of health in rural communities. However, the same "rural culture" that may tolerate risky behavior may also be harnessed to create positive change in rural communities. Berkowitz (2004) has written about disparities in the structure and ability of rural health departments to carry out core public health functions in rural communities. She concludes the following: "Models that stress collaboration among rural public health departments and community partners hold promise for meeting the challenges of rural public health leaders" (Berkowitz, 2004, p. 1681). Rural dwellers do tend to enjoy a strong sense of community and demonstrate the capacity to work together to improve their own infrastructure and health care programs (e.g., diabetes education, smoking cessation, community alcohol control, and community exercise programs). Without access to the services that many urban residents take for granted, a spirit of community is essential to address local problems of isolation, lack of health care access, economic depression, and unhealthy behaviors that worsen the health of community members (Eberhardt et al., 2001; Institute of Medicine [IOM], 2005).

RESEARCH HIGHLIGHTS

Defining Rural Areas: Old and New Classifications

Defining rural areas: Old and new classifications

Old system (before Census 2000)

Metropolitan (metro) areas:
- Cities of 50,000 or more residents, or
- Urbanized areas of 50,000 or more residents and total area population of 100,000 or more

Nonmetropolitan (nonmetro) areas:
- All counties not classified as metro

New core-based system (starting with Census 2000)

Metropolitan (metro) areas:
- Central counties with 50,000 or more residents, regardless of total area population. Includes outlying counties with 25% or more of the employed population commuting daily

Micropolitan (micro) areas:
- Central counties with one or more urban clusters of 10,000-50,000 persons. Includes outlying counties with 25% or more of the employed population commuting daily.

Noncore areas:
- All counties not meeting the new "metro" or "micro" classification are classified as "outside core based statistical areas."

From Slifkin RT, Randolph R, Ricketts TC: The changing metropolitan designation process and rural America, *J Rural Health* 20(1):1-6, 2004.

Defining Rural Populations

Multiple definitions of rural populations have been formulated to describe the characteristics of low population density areas. Previous definitions have simply included either those towns with a population of less than 2500 or towns located in open country as **rural**. This definition has often been further differentiated into subcategories of farm and rural nonfarm. A second classification of interest used the term *rural* for populations with less than 45 persons per square mile, and the term **frontier** for geographical areas with less than 6 people per square mile (Elison, 1986). Many counties of the Great Plains, Intermountain West, and Alaska are designated frontier. The foregoing definitions are still commonly found in journal articles and on websites about rural America. The terms *rural* and *urban* are commonly used synonymously with *non-metropolitan* and *metropolitan*.

Census maps and statistical reports in use since the 1990s used the term Metropolitan Statistical Areas (MSAs) to differentiate nonmetropolitan and metropolitan areas. In June 2003, however, the Office of Management and Budget (OMB) released a new classification scheme, developed in 2000, to better reflect trends in population distribution across the nation (OMB, 2000). The MSA designation has been replaced by county-level Core Based Statistical Areas (CBSAs), which make up a new classification scheme to simplify the multilevel designations in use since 1990. The new CBSA system includes two categories of counties: **metropolitan** areas and **micropolitan** areas. Counties that are neither metropolitan nor micropolitan are called "outside CBSAs" also known as **noncore** areas. Within CBSAs, metropolitan areas are those counties that contain at least one urbanized area of 50,000 or more people. A micropolitan area contains a cluster of 10,000 to 50,000 persons. Rural researchers and policy makers are concerned that the new classification scheme may lead to "lumping metropolitan and micropolitan together because of their common designation as CBSAs" (Slifkin, Randolph, and Ricketts, 2004, p. 1). Others are concerned that tracking long-term trends will be difficult with changes in classification, and there is concern that this classification scheme tracks the urban growth of the nation . . . but pays little attention to the places that are outside CBSAs altogether" (Slifkin et al., 2004, p. 1) Because the MSA classification is used extensively for congressional policymaking and funding decisions, the change could have serious ramifications for health care financing within rural market areas.

Describing Rural Health and Populations

Rural populations differ in complex geographical, social, and economic areas. Although older, poorer, and less educated people are usually overrepresented in rural areas, this may not apply to all rural areas or to everyone in a particular rural area. Remembering there are many "rural Americas in rural America" is paramount to a successful community health nursing practice (Miller, Farmer, and Clarke, 1994).

The health profiles discussed below are shared by rural areas in general and may be contrasted with overall patterns of health, health habits, and health care in urban settings. However, the reader should note that it is difficult to interpret differences between urban and rural health. First, statistically significant differences between urban and rural health indicators may seem small when data are aggregated to "rural areas" in general. The differences tend to become larger when data are available for particular rural areas (e.g., certain counties), particular rural subgroups (e.g., minorities), or specific characteristics (e.g., percentage of uninsured children). Second, heterogeneity of race, age, economic status, regional distribution, and cultural groupings makes health data for rural populations useful only as estimates of individual health. For example, a 2005 AARP public policy publication listed the percent of persons in the United States at or below the poverty level for 2004 as 11% (average of all ages) (Flowers et al., 2005). This publication also provided state-by-state data. For example, Montana, a rural Western state, had a poverty level for persons under age 65 of 15.4%. In Oregon, a state with both urban and rural areas, 12.9% of the population under age 65 was at or below the poverty level. The highest poverty level in the nation was in Mississippi (56.6% rural), which was considered rural and had a poverty rate of 18.4%, among the highest in the nation for a geographic area (Flowers et al., 2005). Farmer, Clark, and Miller (1993) showed that infant mortality, a major health status indicator, varies greatly by geographical area, even within rural areas. Mortality for white infants in rural areas adjacent to a population center with less than 2500 people varied from a high of 9.85 per 1000 in the South, to 6.46 per 1000 in the West. Although the infant mortality rates have changed since 1993, this fine-grained approach to infant mortality data

provides insight into the heterogeneity of rural populations, and shows why national or even regional data such as infant mortality may or may not reflect the status quo for a particular county or local population.

One might also consider the health disparities that exist among rural racial and ethnic minorities. Although limited because the phenomenon is understudied, research findings support the conclusion that rural racial and ethnic minorities—Native Americans, Alaska Natives, Hispanics/Latinos, and African Americans—concentrated in the South and West are more disadvantaged not only relative to rural majority members but also relative to urban racial and ethnic minorities. The disparities include all of the key indicators listed above as examples: employment, income, education, health insurance, mortality, morbidity, and access to care. (Probst et al., 2004).

Because population numbers are small, national rural data, limited as it is, can only suggest the health needs of a particular area, racial or ethnic mix, or age distribution, for example. Program planners will still need to determine whether certain health or health care delivery problems apply to their specific service area. Useful data sources include state, county, and census tract level data on health and demographics available from state and federal government agencies, such as those cited in the reference section of this chapter. In planning for health-related programs, nurses can also gather community-level data from health care providers, local records, focus groups, and older residents who know the area's history.

RURAL *HEALTHY PEOPLE 2010*

Minority Health and *Healthy People 2010*

Healthy People 2010, like its predecessor, *Healthy People 2000*, represents the health promotion and disease prevention agenda for the nation (U.S. Department of Health and Human Services [USDHHS], 2000). Additionally, *Healthy People 2010* is the United States' contribution to the World Health Organization's (WHO) "Health for All" program. The framework for *Healthy People 2010*, developed through public consensus, builds upon the national health program established since the 1980s. It includes the broad goals of increasing quality of life and years of life, eliminating disparities in health among different population groups and increasing access to preventive health services (Figure 21-1).

Healthy People 2010 is based on the premise that the health of the individual is almost "inseparable from the health of the larger community and that the health of every community in every State and territory determines the overall health status of the Nation" (USDHHS, 2000, p. 2). The new 10-year plan takes a bold step forward by presenting only one set of standards for the health of all racial, ethnic, income, gender, and age-groups. The new goal is to eliminate health disparities, achieve access to preventive health services, and add years of life for all groups. The challenges are great, but public health professionals and planners in every state have,

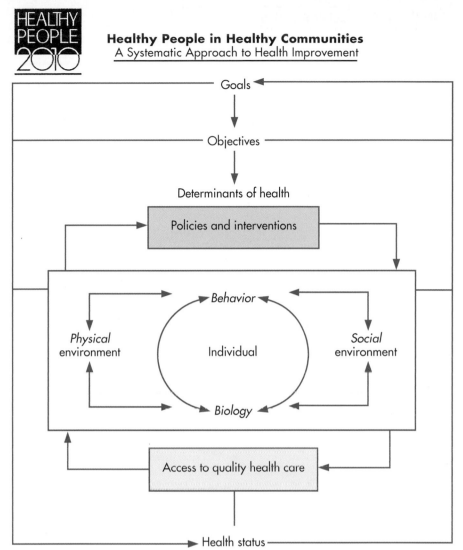

Healthy People in Healthy Communities
A Systematic Approach to Health Improvement

FIGURE 21-1   Diagram of the *Healthy People 2010* approach to health improvement. (From US Public Health Service: *Healthy People 2010: healthy people in healthy communities,* Washington, DC, 1997, US Government Printing Office.

or soon will have, a plan patterned on *Healthy People 2010* goals to direct their efforts. Figure 21-1 presents a diagram of the *Healthy People 2010* approach to health improvement. Recently, a three-volume companion document to *Healthy People 2010*, entitled *Rural Public Health 2010*, has been published. These reports are designed to "better inform readers on current rural health conditions, provide insights into possible points of attack, and offer examples of models that might be employed in practice to improve health conditions" (Gamm et al., 2003 p. vi) (see *Healthy People 2010* table). This valuable resource is also available online at: http://www.srph.tamushsc.edu/centers/rhp2010/.

Rural Health Disparities: Context and Composition

In current rural research and policy discussions, there is an increased focus on population health, public health, environmental health, and the differences between urban and rural

health behaviors (Hartley, 2004). The idea behind population health is captured in the preface to this text and is based on empirical evidence that medical care contributes little to health improvement when compared with sociocultural, economic, environmental, and genetic factors. Examples of such factors include health behaviors, population density, income and employment, education, and ethnicity.

To better understand the health of populations and health disparities, there is also a growing emphasis on the distinction between context, which is defined by the characteristics of places of residence, and composition, which is the collective health effects that result from a concentration of persons with certain characteristics (Probst et al., 2004). Most public health problems include elements of both context and composition, though they may be predominately one or the other (Phillips, 2004; Probst et al., 2004).

Health issues in rural areas are contextual when they derive from characteristics of place. Characteristics of place include

HEALTHY PEOPLE 2010 | Rural Health Priorities

Rural Priorities (Identified by 25% or More)	Percent of Respondents (N = 44)
Access to health care (includes one of the following):	73%
Access to emergency medical services	32%
Access to health workforce	29%
Access to health services (general)	29%
Access to health insurance	26%
Access to primary care	24%
Mental health	49%
Oral health	41%
Educational and community-based programs	29%
Diabetes	26%
Injury and violence prevention	26%
Nutrition and overweight	21%
Public health infrastructure	21%
Tobacco	21%
Maternal, infant, and child health	18%
Occupational safety and health	18%
Cancer	15%
Environmental health	15%
Heart disease and stroke	15%

Data from Gamm LD, Hutchison L, Dabney RJ, Dorsey AM, Editors: *Rural Healthy People 2010: A Companion Document to Healthy People 2010, Volumes 1-3.* College Station, Texas: The Texas A&M University System Health Science Center, School of Rural Public Health, 2003, Southwest Rural Health Research Center.

not only natural features of geography and environment, but also the political, social, and economic institutions that build and support communities within a given geographic areas. For example, limited economic opportunities, low wages, or agricultural accidents might be considered to have contextual effects on the health of populations. Problems in rural areas are compositional when they derive from individual characteristics of groups of people residing in rural settings. Examples of compositional sources of health disparities include such characteristics as age, education, income, ethnicity, and health behaviors.

Consideration of both context and composition enable us to take a more fine-grained approach to study, plan programs, and deliver health care services to rural populations. There is a complex relationship between place, or context, and health characteristics of people in those places. The high rate of death and disability from automobile crashes in a given area could be thought of as both contextual (long distances to travel over rural roads in bad weather) and compositional (involving high rates of speed, the use of alcohol or drugs, or failing to use seat belts or car seats for children).

Although the overall health of rural Americans is worse when compared with that of urban Americans, the relationship between rurality and health is not necessarily linear, that is, there are many differences between rural areas in both the

nature and extent of health problems. Furthermore, some rural populations share more in common with people in urban core areas than with other rural areas. Effective planning depends on understanding and documenting needs that take into account context, composition, and their interaction (Eberhardt and Pamuk, 2004). The next section presents data for problems of both contextual and compositional sources of health disparities in rural America.

Context: Health Disparities Related to Place

Regardless of their diverse demographic and geographical attributes, rural groups share certain health patterns, difficulties, and delays in obtaining health care (see Ethical Insights box). Many of the contextual issues that contribute to rural health disparities are described in the introduction to the chapter ("Rural United States"). Many rural regions that are already sparsely populated are losing residents, which often triggers a downward spiral. People leave and services are lost; the local drugstore closes; the tax base will not support an ambulance service; most seriously ill persons must be transported long distances to get health care; jobs become scarce and younger people leave the area. Retirees may be attracted to the lower costs, but they need public health and other services provided by counties without the tax base to support

ETHICAL Insights

Racial and Ethnic Disparities in Health Care

Because public health is a societal approach to protecting and promoting health that usually acts through social rather than individuals means (Kass, 2001), many of the most pressing ethical dilemmas are considered in public domains. Perhaps no more important ethical challenge facing our public today revolves around the just distribution of health care resources.

For example, among 34.6 million rural minority adults in 2000, 32% of black, 35% of "other" race persons, and 45% of Hispanics were uninsured, compared with only 18% of whites (Glover et al., 2004). These data may help explain why minorities are more likely to be denied authorization for care (Lowe, 2001), use less prenatal care (Barfield, Wise, and Rust, 1996), and have fewer visits to physicians (Tai-Seale, Freund, and LoSasso, 2001).

Differences in care resulting from patient or care process-level variables (e.g., patient attitudes, preferences, or expectations; provider bias, stereotyping, or uncertainty) are problems of professional ethics. *Disparities in care* resulting from system level variables, such as financing, accessibility and geographic location, are problems of justice (Institute of Medicine, 2003). Subsequently, solutions for justice issues in *disparities in care* require public discourse aimed at solving system level problems.

From an ethical perspective, the theory of justice as fairness was formulated to specify terms of social cooperation that are "fair" and ensures that people of equal basic liberties have equal opportunity (Daniels, Kennedy, and Kawachi, 1999). The Civil Rights Act of 1964 specifically bars discrimination in health care for all entities that receive federal funds, and both the American Nurses Association and American Medical Association codes of ethics eschew the principle of justice. However, despite overall agreement that justice is an important practice concept, difficulty arises in implementing changes in the health system to address *disparities in care*.

Solutions to disparities in care have been suggested by the Institute of Medicine (2003) and include the following policy, health system, and patient education and empowerment interventions:

➤ Policy interventions
1. Medical care financing should discourage fragmentation of health care into separate tiers of providers who adhere to different standards of care and serve separate racial and ethnic minority segments of society. Government programs that require enrollment in managed care should be prepared to pay plans at rates comparable to privately insured patients.
2. Strengthen the stability of patient-provider relationships in publicly funded health plans and create policy to create consistency, limit patient loads for providers, and provide reasonable time allowances for initial and follow-up visits.
3. Increase the proportion of underrepresented U.S. racial and ethnic minorities among health professionals.
4. Apply the same managed care protections to publicly funded HMO enrollees that apply to private HMO enrollees.
5. Provide greater resources to the U.S. Department of Health and Human Services Office for Civil Rights to enforce civil rights laws.

➤ Health systems interventions
1. Promote the consistency and equity of care through evidence-based guidelines. These guidelines should be published to allow public and professional scrutiny.
2. Construct payment systems to enhance available services to minority patients, and limit provider incentives that may promote disparities.
3. Enhance patient-provider communication and trust by providing financial incentives for practices that reduce barriers.
4. Support the use of interpretation services where community need exists.
5. Institute programs that use community health workers among medically underserved and racial and ethnic minority populations.
6. Support greater use of multidisciplinary treatment and preventive care teams to improve and streamline care for racial and ethnic minority patients.

➤ Patient education and empowerment interventions
1. Implement patient education programs to increase patients' knowledge of how to access care and participate in treatment decisions.

Barfield WD et al: Racial disparities in outcomes of military and civilian births in California, *Arch Pediatr Adolesc Med* 150(10):1062-1067, 1996; Glover, S et al: Disparities in access to care among rural working-age adults, *J Rural Health* 20(3):193-205, 2004; Institute of Medicine: *Unequal treatment: confronting racial and ethnic disparities in healthcare*, Washington, DC, 1988, National Academy Press; Kass, NE: An ethics framework for public health, *Public Health Matters* 91(11):1776-1782, 2001; Lowe RA et al: Effect of ethnicity on denial of authorization for emergency department care by managed care gatekeepers, *Acad Emerg Med* 8(3):259-266, 2001; Tai-Seale M, Freund D, LoSasso A: Racial disparities in service use among Medicaid beneficiaries after mandatory enrollment in managed care: a difference-in-differences approach, *Inquiry* 38(1):49-59, 2001.

them. Racial and ethnic minorities are migrating to rural areas to find employment opportunities. Structural, financial, and personal barriers to accessing health care services exist in all environments, but rural residents are unique in how they experience structural barriers.

Access to Care

In a survey of 90 national and state rural health experts, Gamm and Hutchison (2004) reported that access to health care was the number one priority identified by the majority (73%) of rural health care leaders. Access was the leading priority regardless of rural region (Northeast, Midwest, South, West) and regardless of type of organization represented in the survey (state organization, public health units, centers and clinics or rural hospitals).

Primary Care

Many rural counties have no primary care providers, and there are fewer physicians (other than family practitioners and general practitioners) in rural areas of every region of the country. Only 10% of physicians, 22% of nurse practitioners, and 23% of physician assistants practice in rural areas (Gamm, Castillo; and Pittman, 2003). Availability of providers and health care facilities in rural areas is an important determinant of the quality of the health care delivery system and the likelihood of positive health outcomes for rural residents (Eberhardt et al., 2001). A good example of the lack of specialists is the lack of mental health services available for rural dwellers of any age. "The availability of mental health services in frontier areas . . . . is vastly inferior to other areas . . . ." (Ricketts et al., 1999,

p. 174). Although need for services is approximately the same in rural and urban areas, "rural areas suffer shortages in mental health infrastructure and supply of mental health professionals" (Gamm, Stone, and Pittman, 2003, p. 166). Primary care doctors, nurses, and physician assistants, rather than mental health specialists, provide most of the mental health care in rural regions.

General Health Services

Population decline in rural areas in the Great Plains and lower South for example has resulted from an out-migration of younger people, leaving a greater concentration of older people in a dwindling population. A recent Institute of Medicine study reported rural medical access problems in these areas, with some hospital and pharmacy closures, greater distances to travel for physician services, and limited if any choice of providers (IOM, 2005). Lack of local access to primary care and health care facilities forces rural residents to either go without or travel long distances—often over rural roads in dangerous weather conditions—to access needed care. Access to health care may become a particularly challenging and expensive proposition for the elderly who do not drive and are dependent on limited public transportation. Geography, health care costs, and lack of available services also are contextual problems that keep many rural adults and children from obtaining needed primary, secondary, and tertiary preventive services.

Health Insurance

With economic decline and rising costs of health care, health insurance, or more importantly the lack of health insurance, for Americans has become a major issue for the health of the nation. An estimated 45 million people were without health insurance in 2003 (Nevas-Walt, Proctor, and Mills, 2003). Although the number of uninsured persons had begun to decline, estimates for 2004 indicate the trend is continuing in the direction of more uninsured persons (17.7% were estimated to have been uninsured for at least part of 2004) (Cohen, Martinez, and Hao, 2005, and U.S. Census Bureau, 2004a).

As with poverty and unemployment data, insurance coverage varied with race and ethnicity coverage in 2004, as did age and residence (rural or urban). For example, an estimated 33% of Hispanics were uninsured for all or part of 2004; young adults were more likely to lack health insurance than older persons; 14% to 15% of poor or near-poor children lacked coverage. Lack of insurance coverage was greatest in the South (16.6%) and West regions (18.2%) in 2001 (Cohen et al., 2005), and in general, rural residents were more likely than urban residents to lack insurance (20% versus 17%) (IOM, 2005). Two thirds of the persons living in the most rural counties are low-income families, and 30% are children (USDA, 2004).

Health insurance coverage influences health patterns and often poses financial barriers to adequate health care for rural dwellers. Research points to a "strong nexus between health insurance status, chronic illnesses and poverty." (Bolin and Gamm, 2003, p. 19). Rural people are often employed in industries characterized by seasonal work, economic uncertainty and decline, high unemployment risk, and occupational accidents and death (e.g., agriculture, mining, forestry, and fisheries). Rural industries are often small and offer low wages, thereby contributing to the increasing number of uninsured rural families. For example, self-employed farm families need to purchase private health insurance; however, in periods of hardship they often cannot afford the increasingly high premium costs. Farm families also tend to be two-parent households, so they are less likely to qualify for Medicaid, even with incomes below the federal poverty level. Because of the high percentage of elderly in rural areas, Medicare recipients are more apt to live in rural than in urban areas, yet Medicare spends less on rural than urban beneficiaries. The reasons for this difference could be that rural beneficiaries use fewer health care services than enrollees in urban areas, and providers have lower reimbursement rates in rural settings. Medicare payments per enrollee in 1998 ranged from a low of $3,600 to $3,800 in sparsely populated states such as Montana, North Dakota, South Dakota, to a high of $6,800 to $7,100 per enrollee in Louisiana and the District of Columbia (Eberhardt et al., 2001). Finally, 46% of the Medicare population in rural counties lack any form of prescription drug coverage, but only 31% of Medicare recipients in urban counties are similarly deficient (Mueller and Schur, 2004).

Health insurance has been identified as one of the 10 leading health indicators because it is generally a reliable predictor of overall health status (Cohen and Bloom, 2005). Public health professionals and health planners are most concerned with the impact of increasing numbers of uninsured children. In 1998 the overall percentage of children who were uninsured was 13.2% (Cohen and Bloom, 2005). Of the uninsured, 21% were rural children (Dunbar and Mueller, 1998). In the absence of health insurance, poverty becomes an even more powerful predictor of poor health for all age-groups and particularly for children.

In 1997, the Children's Health Insurance Program (CHIP) was enacted to improve health insurance coverage of children under 19 years of age in poor and near poor families (see the "Legislation and Programs Affecting Public Health in Rural Areas" section in this chapter). In the years following passage of this program, 1998-2003, the overall percentage of children who were uninsured fell from 13.2% to 10.2% (Cohen and Bloom, 2005). The decrease must be viewed with caution because it is represents a national average. Health insurance coverage of children as well as adults varies from state to state and is influenced by employment patterns, the percentage of children in the population, state Medicaid policies, poverty levels, and racial and ethnic composition. For example, an estimated 19.2% of children in Montana were living in poverty in 2002, according to census estimates (U.S. Census Bureau, 2004b).

Composition: Health Disparities Related to Persons

To review, health problems in rural areas are compositional when they result from a concentration of persons with certain characteristics (Probst et al., 2004). Examples of compo-

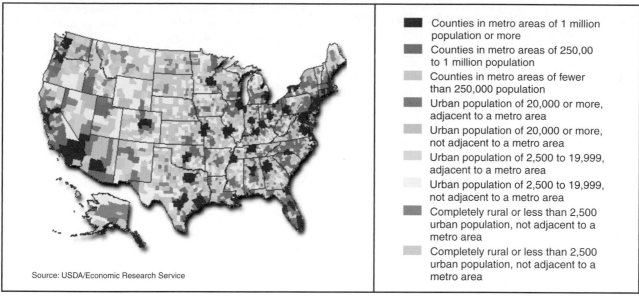

Legend:
- Counties in metro areas of 1 million population or more
- Counties in metro areas of 250,00 to 1 million population
- Counties in metro areas of fewer than 250,000 population
- Urban population of 20,000 or more, adjacent to a metro area
- Urban population of 20,000 or more, not adjacent to a metro area
- Urban population of 2,500 to 19,999, adjacent to a metro area
- Urban population of 2,500 to 19,999, not adjacent to a metro area
- Completely rural or less than 2,500 urban population, not adjacent to a metro area
- Completely rural or less than 2,500 urban population, not adjacent to a metro area

Source: USDA/Economic Research Service

FIGURE 21-2   Rural-urban continuum of poverty, 2003. (From USDA, Economic Research Service: *Profiles of America: data*, 2003, The Author, http://www.maps.ers.usda.gov/Profiles/index.aspx#graphic_area.)

sitional sources of health disparities include such characteristics as income, health behaviors, education, occupation, gender, and ethnicity. In the RHP2010 survey cited previously, 73% of respondents listed access to health care as the top rural health priority (Bolin and Gamm, 2003). An additional 13 priorities listed by respondents as leading health problems are largely compositional but may also have a contextual dimension. For example, such problems as obesity, chronic pulmonary disease, and higher levels of infant mortality have a strong compositional component because their variation is related to the health behaviors, and educational, socioeconomic, racial, and ethnic characteristics of the rural groups. The variation may also be contextual, because the groups have fewer educational opportunities, have low-wage jobs, lack insurance, or have genetic propensities for certain health problems.

Income and Poverty

Education, income, and type of employment help determine socioeconomic status, and in the aggregate, rural dwellers have lower educational levels, higher unemployment rates, longer unemployment periods, higher poverty rates, and lower income levels than urban aggregates. The poverty rate is one of the most important indicators of the health and well-being of all Americans, regardless of where they live (see Ethical Insights box). The U.S. Department of Agriculture's Economic Research Service (ERS) tracks economic trends and demographic characteristics of rural dwellers to help develop policies and services for rural people. In the most recent report, the ERS contrasted the economic growth and downward trend in poverty rates during the 1990s with those of the current decade. In the last 10 years, rural poverty declined on average from a decade high of 17% (1993) to a low of 11% (2000). Since 2000, the rate of rural poverty has been climbing. In 2003, 14% of the general rural population lived in poverty (compared with 12% of urban dwellers (USDHHS,

2005). Poverty rates for rural people have always been higher than those of urban dwellers (Figure 21-2). As noted earlier in this section, however, data averaged across all rural counties in the United States do not give planners and providers much information about their own counties, or even regions. On the following pages are examples of data that are available to make a more fine-grained analysis of local and regional conditions and characteristics.

Rural Poverty: Regional Differences

Consistent with the idea that there are many rural Americas in rural America, rural poverty varies by rural region (Box 21-1). For example, rural counties make up 340 of 386 (88%) counties with persistent poverty rates in the United States (persistent poverty is defined as counties in which 20% of the population has been in poverty over the last 30 years). Of the 340 rural counties with persistent poverty, 280 (82%) are in the South, and 60 (18%) in the West and Midwest (USDA, 2004). Poverty is also highest in the most rural areas. In completely rural counties (i.e., not adjacent to any metropolitan counties) the poverty rate is 16.8%.

Rural Poverty: Racial and Ethnic Minorities

When poverty rates among rural dweller are analyzed by race, ethnicity, age, and family structure, the statistics on poverty are even more dramatic than residence or region. Racial and ethnic minorities (mainly non-white Hispanics, blacks, and Native Americans) constituted 17% of the rural population, according to the 2000 Census (USDA, 2004). This segment of the rural population has grown 30% in the last decade, largely due to the dramatic increase in non-white Hispanics (up 70.4% from 1990 to 2000) (IOM, 2005). In 2002, according to the Economic Research Service (ERS), poverty rates among rural and racial minorities were two to three times higher than poverty rates for rural whites (11 percent) (Jolliffe, 2004).

BOX 2-1 The 2006 Health and Human Services Poverty Guidelines

In concept, the poverty guidelines are determined by estimating the minimum income level needed by a family or individual to just meet the basic needs of food, shelter, clothing, and other essential goods and services. Official poverty guidelines adjusted for family size and composition are set by the Department of Health and Human Services (DHHS) for use by all federal agencies to determine financial eligibility for certain federal programs (e.g., Medicaid). Some programs (e.g., State Childrens' Health Insurance Program) also use multiples of the guidelines to determine eligibility of participants. For example, participants may be eligible for programs if they are classified as being at or near poverty, where poverty is defined as 100%, and near poverty as 125% or 150% of the poverty level. Poverty guidelines are adjusted periodically by DHHS to reflect price changes, and are published in the *Federal Register*. The 2006 guidelines reflect just the size of the "family unit" rather than the family composition. The poverty level for a family unit of one, for example, was $9,800; it was $20,000 for a family unit of four, and $33,600 for a family of eight. Each household's cash income (including pretax income and cash welfare assistance, but excluding in-kind welfare assistance, such as food stamps and Medicare) is compared to the poverty line for the household.

From US Department of Health and Human Services: *The 2006 HHS poverty guidelines: one version of the [U.S.] federal poverty measure*, 2006, The Author, http://aspe.hhs.gov/poverty/06poverty.shtml.

Rural Poverty: Family Composition

Families with two or more adults are less likely to be poor, whether in rural or urban areas, because they are more likely to have multiple sources of income. Families with more than one adult have lower out-of-pocket child care costs and are less likely to have to limit their working hours. Over 75% of rural families are headed by a married couple, and these constitute only 7% of families living in poverty. On the other hand, people living in female-headed families (15%) have the highest poverty rates (37%), which is 10 percentage points greater than in female-headed families in metro areas. The Economic Research Service attributes the high rate of poverty for female-headed families to "lower labor force participation rates, shorter average work weeks, and lower earnings" (USDA, 2004).

Rural Poverty: Children

Children are particularly vulnerable to outcomes of poverty, and are among the poorest citizens in rural America, constituting 36% of the overall population of rural poor in 2003. The heaviest concentrations of child poverty are in the South and West. Understanding how poverty is distributed in rural populations is important for planning and delivering programs that ameliorate the impact of poverty, such as food stamps, school lunch programs, school health nursing interventions, and health insurance coverage (USDA, 2005). When race and ethnicity are taken into account, the poverty profile of children worsens dramatically. Racial and ethnic minorities fare far worse than the general rural population of children from birth to18 years of age. When family composition is taken into account, we find that almost half of non-

Hispanic black children, 34% of Native American children, and 18% of rural children who live in a female-headed household are poor (USDA, 2005).

Health Risk, Injury, and Death

"Improving health behaviors to reduce the risk of disease and disability poses distinct challenges for....the most rural counties with more dispersed and older populations" (Eberhardt et al., 2001, p. 3). Notable health behaviors vary along the rural-urban continuum and within rural populations by geographical area. For example, researchers have noted that adults in non-metropolitan areas use seat belts less often and are less likely to use preventive screening (although the latter trend is confounded by access problems). Rural residents in the Southern states are more likely to be obese, smoke more heavily if they do smoke, use smokeless tobacco, and engage in sedentary lifestyles. In the rural West, smoking, seat belt use, and obesity are lower, and alcohol and smokeless tobacco use are higher (Eberhardt et al., 2001). For example, 19% of adolescents living in the most rural counties are smokers, compared with 11% in large metropolitan counties. Among adults living in the most rural counties, 27% of women and 31% of men smoke, compared with 20% of women and 25% of men in large metro areas. Tobacco use is increasing for men and women in the South.

Other risk factors include alcohol use (higher in rural areas and highest among persons living in the most rural areas, and more commonly among men than women), obesity (higher in rural areas, most particularly rural areas of the South), and physical inactivity during leisure time, which varies by level of urbanization and also by region for both men and women (highest level of inactivity in the South and in central counties of large metro areas of the Northeast) (Eberhardt et al., 2001).

Infant mortality rates dramatize the importance of both contextual and compositional data. For non-Hispanic whites, the rates of infant deaths per 1,000 live births continued a downward trend. For black Americans the rate of infant deaths is 2.5 times that of whites and Hispanics. In both the South and West, rural counties experienced the highest rates (24% and 30% higher than fringe areas of large metro areas) (Hoyert, et al., 2005).

Unintentional injuries are the leading cause of death in the United States for both sexes, all races and ethnicities, and for all age-groups from ages 1 to 44 years. In the latest available reports, unintentional injuries continue to be higher in rural areas of the United States. The mortality rate for unintentional injuries reported in the *Urban and Rural Health Chartbook* was 54.1 per 100,000 rural residents, which is twice the rate for large metropolitan counties (Eberhardt et al., 2001) Unintentional injuries are highest among males and in rural counties with the lowest population densities (Peek-Asa, Zwirling, and Stallones, 2004).

According to the CDC's National Center for Health Statistics (NCHS), unintentional injuries ranked 5th in the leading causes of death in both 2002 and 2003. This category of death includes "transport accidents," including motor vehicle accidents, and "non-transport accidents," including falls, firearm accidents, drowning, fire-related deaths, accidental poisoning, and other accidental deaths (Hoyer, Kung, and Smith, 2005). Males aged 15 to 24 years are the most likely victims of unintentional injuries.

In four of the least populated states, the percentage of deaths from unintentional injuries was much higher than the national average, with 7.7% in Idaho, 8.0% in Montana, 9.1% in Wyoming, and 14.3% in Alaska. Overall, deaths from unintentional injuries were approximately 80% to 85% higher for females and males in the most rural counties than for suburban areas of metropolitan counties in 1996 to 1998, and highest of all in the West (Eberhardt et al., 2001). Driving at high speeds, driving long distances, driving in winter conditions, not using seat belts, and consuming alcohol have been cited as contributing to greater levels of injury deaths and disability by rural residents in the West. Lack of ready access to counseling, emergency medical services, and rehabilitation are also thought to be contributing factors to these high levels.

Suicide is also a major public health problem in rural areas. In rural areas adjacent to a small city, suicide rates were 31% higher than suburban rates and 43% higher in rural areas that were not adjacent to small cities (Eberhardt et al., 2001). Nationally, suicide was the 11th leading cause of death overall, 8th for males, and 17th for females. Little regional variation was found, except in the most rural parts of the West (especially in the least populated states of Wyoming, Alaska, Montana, and Idaho), where rates were 80% higher than those in metropolitan areas (Eberhardt et al., 2001). There was also variation by race and ethnicity. Decreased access to mental health services for treatment of depression may contribute to these higher rates (Eberhardt et al., 2001). As reported by the Centers for Disease Control and Prevention (2002, p. 1), *Injury Fact Book 2001-2002,* "It is also believed that men are less likely to ask for help, especially emotional help . . . . Because men seldom reach out for help with depression they are more socially isolated and vulnerable to suicide. Males attempting suicide are also more likely to use more lethal means, such as guns, which increase their likelihood of completing the act" (Centers for Disease Control and Prevention, 2002, p. 2).

Vulnerable Age-Groups

Demographic and personal characteristics, such as age, education, gender, race, ethnicity, language, and culture, round out the examples of factors that affect health and may block access to existing services (Braden and Beauregard, 1994). Age is an important consideration in planning health care services for rural communities. As noted in previous sections, many retirees are moving into rural areas, and many younger people are moving out. Because the incomes of many elderly may be lower, the tax base of counties and municipalities may be inadequate to cover the disproportionate share of the health care services used by the elderly (age 65 years and over) (Eberhardt et al., 2001).

According to demographer Carolyn Rogers, the elderly (the majority of whom are women) make up 20% of the rural population, compared with 15% of the urban population. The elderly are concentrated in the South, with large groups also found in the Midwest. The "oldest old" (generally referring to those aged 85 and above) are a growing component of the population of elderly (5.9% in 1991 and 7.6% in 2001). The population of elderly is expected to double by 2050 (Rogers, 2002). Elderly women tend to live at or near the poverty level and achieve poverty status twice as often as men. Along with educational attainment, this is a critical indicator of well-being for the elderly and the young. The elderly poor tend to be isolated and lack access to support services, health care, prescription drugs, adequate nutrition, and transportation.

The number of children in rural areas increased by 3% in the decade from 1990 to 2000 (USDA, 2005). In addition to population growth, racial and ethnic diversity increased in the 1990s. Today, the proportion of Hispanic children is the fastest growing component of the rural population regardless of region. The population of black children has remained steady, and the majority of rural black children are still concentrated in the South. Native American children constitute only 3% of the total nonmetropolitan population, although in areas of the country (mainly West and Central) with high concentrations of Native Americans, this percentage is, of course, much higher. Evidence suggests that fetal, infant, and maternal mortality are slightly higher in nonmetropolitan than metropolitan areas, and that care in the later prenatal stages is problematic. Nonmetropolitan children, like adults, are more likely to live in poverty, and proportionately fewer rural children were covered by health insurance in 2001, despite the enactment of CHIP in 1997 (Kandel and Cromartie, 2003; USDA, 2005).

Rural children are involved in farm and highway accidents and deaths. Data from a 1992 report by the National Vital Statistics System revealed that "fatal injuries were 44% higher among rural children aged 1 to 19 years compared with their urban counterparts" (Ricketts et al., 1999, p. 155).

Youth substance abuse (including alcohol, tobacco, and illicit drug use) is perhaps the greatest problem of rural youth in America today. Lisnerski et al. (1991) reported on the use of smokeless tobacco by elementary school children in a rural Southeastern state. Roughly one third of male first graders had experimented with smokeless tobacco; by the seventh grade, 70% of these rural males had experimented with or were regular users of smokeless tobacco. Use was attributed to "perceived flavor" but was also predicted by "self-concept" and presentation to peers' and "family influence." Furthermore, Long and Boik (1993) reported that nearly 60% of sixth and seventh graders in their rural sample reported using alcohol. Although these studies took place some years ago, we know from more current data that tobacco use (either smoking or smokeless tobacco) and alcohol use are still significant problems for rural youth. For this reason, substance abuse has been identified as one of the 10 "leading health indicators" by the U.S. Department of Health and Human Services (USDHHS, 2000). In the recent RHP2010 survey, substance abuse was of particular concern to rural public health leaders in Western and Northeastern regions. In rural regions that already have heavy alcohol use, these areas now have the second highest rate of illicit drug use (5.8%), which is slightly less than the rate of 7.65% seen in large metropolitan counties. However, the pattern of drug use among youth shows a

High school completion rates, 2000 (adults 25 and older)

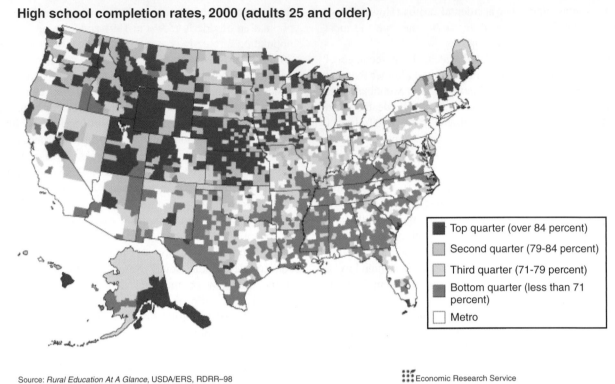

Source: *Rural Education At A Glance*, USDA/ERS, RDRR–98   ⣿ Economic Research Service

FIGURE 21-3 High school completion rates for adults. (From USDA, Economic Research Service: *High school completion rates, 2000 (adults 25 and older),* The Author, http://www.ers.usda.gov/Publications/RDRR98/ChartsMaps.htm.

different and more alarming pattern. Survey data published in 2001 revealed that the prevalence of illicit drug use was 14.4% among rural youth, and 10.4% in both small and large metropolitan areas (Hutchison and Blakely, (2003).

Education and Employment

Research on the socioeconomic determinants of health has revealed a strong positive correlation between health and length of schooling (Fuchs, 1998). As Swanson (1999, p. 2) discussed, "Demographic characteristics of a minority group both affect and result from their economic and social status. Age structure and education combine as an indication of the level of employment a group might be able to enjoy." For the aged and for ethnic and racial minorities, a pattern of lower educational attainment and unfavorable economic circumstances emerges with increasing rurality (Figure 21-3). Although the education picture is changing, many elderly women in their 70s and 80s grew up before public education was mandatory. Families could not afford to send them to school, or they were simply expected to learn to read and write, seek employment, and marry. Education, with its links to economic and health variables, is still a serious problem for rural America (Figure 21-4). Low education and employment levels characterize all rural minority groups except Asians. "Children of all racial and ethnic groups who live in precarious economic conditions have additional challenges to doing well in school and remaining in school through high school graduation" (Swanson, 1999, p. 4). In 2000, 77% of rural dwellers held high school diplomas or Graduate Equivalency Diplomas (GEDs) (compared with

Nonmetro poverty rates by educational attainment, 2000

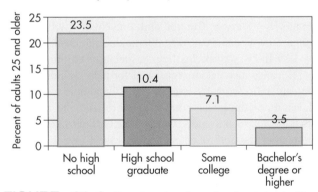

FIGURE 21-4 Poverty rates by educational level. (From USDA, Economic Research Service: *Non-metro poverty rates by educational attainment,* 2000, The Author, http://www.ers.usda.gov/Emphases/Rural/Gallary/index.htm#pov.)

70% in 1990) (USDA, 2003). The major difference between these two groups was in the percentage of rural students who held college degrees. The college completion rate of rural students was almost half that of urban students. There are also large gaps in educational completion by region, race, and ethnicity (see Figures 21-3 and 21-4), with the West and Midwest students exceeding the high school completion rates of students in the rural South (USDA, 2005). Rural and central city students, especially minorities other than Asians, lag behind suburban children on most indicators of adequate progress in schools (IOM, 2005). Low educational attainment is a challenge in rural America. Skill requirements for rural employment continue to rise, lack of education is correlated with persistent poverty, and poverty is a predictor of poor health.

Furthermore, counties that have a low-wage economy have difficulty providing the infrastructure needed to provide education, public health and health care services for low-wage families. They also have difficulty attracting new employers who might contribute to the economic development of a rural area, but need a more highly educated workforce.

Occupational Health Risks

In the United States, approximately 65,000 workers die each year of work-related illnesses and injuries (Herbert and Landrigan, 2000). Fatal occupational injuries declined 23.1% from 1992 to 2002. The rate (number of fatal injuries per 100,000 workers) decreased from 5.2 in 1992 to 4.0 in 2002 (National Institute for Occupational Safety and Health [NIOSH], 2004).

Occupational injuries, fatalities, and illnesses play a significant role in rural health, since rates of disabling injuries and injury-related mortality are dramatically higher in the rural population, particularly in the West and South (NCHS, 2004). Industries with the highest death rate were mining, agriculture, forestry, and fishing, followed by construction, transportation, and public utilities (Eberhardt et al., 2001). The majority of job-related deaths due to workplace injuries in 2003 were in the following categories: transportation-related motor vehicle accidents, machinery-related events, homicides, falls, electrocution, and chemical and thermal injuries. Two industries accounted for more than 40% of fatal occupational injuries in 2002: construction (22.6%) and transportation and public utilities (18.3%). Three Western states, Alaska, Wyoming and Montana, had the highest fatality rates (over 10 per 100,000 persons) for 2002 (Eberhardt et al., 2001).

Occupational death and disability can also be attributed to nonfatal injuries, and occupational diseases, such as cancer, asbestosis, silicosis, and anthracosis associated with both organic and inorganic exposures (NCHS, 2004; NIOSH, 2004). Work-related injuries, deaths, and illness data must be interpreted with caution. Although surveillance of occupational injuries, illnesses, and fatalities has improved through the collaboration of the states and NIOSH, data still come from many sources, and underreporting continues to be problematic.

Gender, Race, and Ethnicity

Both rural men and women are less likely than metropolitan residents to report their health as good or excellent. Rural areas, particularly in the rural South, have higher incidents of heart disease and cancer. Higher prevalence of chronic disease is consistent with the composition of rural populations, which tend to be older, poorer, and less educated (Gosschalk and Carozza, 2003). Rural men and women also smoke or use smokeless tobacco more. In the aggregate they exercise fewer preventive behaviors, have less contact with physicians, and often have less access to care than people with similar problems in urban areas (Gamm et al., 2003, Vol. 1). Rural men

and youths are also more likely to die or become disabled from unintentional injuries due to risky behavior or work-related causes, and are more likely to commit suicide than women or urban men and youths.

Although rural populations overall are at lower risk for most cancers, certain rural subpopulations are at greater risk. For example, Appalachia has a much higher rate than the national figure. Residents in low-income areas and the uninsured, particularly African Americans, tend to have more late-stage cancer diagnoses; and rural residents in general may have less access to quality health care, including both medical care and screening and prevention programs (Gamm et al., 2003, Vol. 1). A particularly serious problem for minorities and the elderly is the lack of cancer screening, including breast and cervical cancer for women, and prostate cancer for men. Preventive care is especially important for African-American men, for whom prostate cancer is higher than for any other racial or ethnic group.

From 1987 to 2000 the age-adjusted percentage of women over 40 years of age who had a mammogram improved from 29% to 70.3% according to the CDC's National Center for Health Statistics (CDC/NCHS, 2004). The percentage was lower for all racial and ethnic minorities, with 67.8% for African-American women and 47.3% for American Indian and Alaska Native women. Use of mammography was the lowest among the poor, most particularly in the 40- to 49-year old age bracket (47.4%), and among the least educated (CDC/NCHS, 2004). Health objectives for the year 2010 called for at least 80% of American women aged 40 years and older to have received a mammogram and clinical breast exam in the previous 2 years (USDHHS, 2000). Similarly, women who are poor, elderly, and less educated are less likely to receive Pap tests. In racial and ethnic groups, the percentages of women who get Pap tests are lower for Hispanics, American Indians, and Alaska Natives. The lowest percentage is found in Asian women.

Rural-dwelling men suffer the long-term effects of having poor health habits, lacking consistent primary health care, and participating in hazardous occupations, as mentioned previously. In rural areas, particularly the Mountain West, men (especially older white men and younger American-Indian men) have the highest suicide rates of any group (Pickle et al., 1996). Rural men in the South suffer higher rates of ischemic heart disease and cancer. Adult males on the whole were twice as likely as females to lack a usual source of health care in 2000 to 2001. In the West the percentage of adults without a usual source of care was 19.4% in 2001 to 2002, and has changed little over the past 10 years (NCHS, 2004). In fact, among rural working-age adults, 45% of Hispanics, 32% of blacks, and 18% of whites were uninsured, and similar percentages had not visited a health care provider in the previous year (Glover et al., 2004).

Interacting with poverty and lack of access to care, rural minorities are among the nation's least healthy citizens. African-American and Native-American children and children of migrant workers are among the poorest of rural residents. By almost any measure or index (e.g., AIDS incidence, birth-weight, blood pressure, cholesterol level, cancer incidence, and substance abuse), rural poor African Americans, Hispanics, American Indians, and Alaska Natives are less healthy than whites. They also suffer food insecurity and hunger more frequently and have less access to quality health care (Probst et al., 2004).

Perhaps no other group better illustrates the many problems that characterize rural health care than Native Americans. The following are excerpts from a special report entitled "A Health Crisis," which was compiled by faculty and students from the University of Montana School of Journalism (1993):

- *In Montana, Indians die prematurely at a rate almost twice that of the general population.*
- *Death rates among Indians as a result of heart disease, cancer, accidents, cirrhosis, suicide, and diabetes are higher for Indians than for other citizens of this state.*
- *This terrible toll afflicts Native-Americans from the moment of their birth. The state's infant mortality rate for Indian babies is 43 percent higher for Montana Indian infants than for babies born of other ancestry.*
- *Montana Indians live in poverty at a rate three times that of their fellow residents.*
- *Half of those Indians who are poor are children and adolescents, and they are more than three times more likely to come from homes where a mother is the only parent present. Yet Indians get free health care, so why are they so sick?*

Because, as the American Indian Health Care Association found, Indians face significant barriers to getting that health care. Only enrolled tribal members living on a reservation can get full health care benefits supplied by the federal government. And that health care is rationed. Many Indians live long distances from Indian Health Service facilities. That becomes a factor when studies show that more than twice as many Montana Indians than white people have no access to a vehicle. And almost half the Indians in the state are without a telephone. A third of tribal and Indian Health Service facilities in Montana have no emergency and ambulance services, a critical need on Montana's large and rural reservations (School of Journalism, 1993, p. 1).

The percent of Hispanics and Latinos in the U.S. population was about equal to African Americans (12.5% vs. 12.3% during the year 2000) and will soon become the largest minority group in the United States. They are already the predominant minority in the West. Hispanics have a diverse culture, history, and socioeconomic and health status. The largest Hispanic subgroups are of Mexican, Cuban, and Puerto Rican descent, although Mexican is the largest by far (58% of the Hispanic population living in the United States). In nonmetropolitan areas, the population of Hispanics has doubled, and almost half of all Hispanics that live in rural areas are living outside the traditional areas of settlement in the Southwestern states. As emphasized previously, this growing segment of the population continues to be overrepresented among the rural poor. In 1999, the U.S. Census Bureau reported that just over 25% of Hispanics live below the federal poverty level, compared with 8.2% of the white, non-Hispanic population. Of those under age 18, the percentage living below the poverty level was 34% for Hispanics, compared to 10.6% of white non-Hispanics. The elderly were also two and one half times more likely to live below the poverty line

than white non-Hispanics. Hispanics are most likely to report barriers in obtaining needed health care and are least likely to have a usual source of care; for those blacks and Hispanics reporting a usual source of care, the source is most likely to be hospital-based (Kass, Weinick, and Monheit, 1999).

SPECIFIC RURAL AGGREGATES

Agricultural Workers

By 2005, 20 states had posted their *Healthy People 2010* plans to the project's website. The plans are built upon national objectives, but they have been tailored to each state's particular needs and population configurations. To eliminate disparities among different population groups, the health care system will need to undertake programs to dramatically improve the health of minority groups on no fewer than 93 health indicators that show a 25% or greater disparity in various health statistics. These statistics are based on race and ethnicity, socioeconomic status, gender, age, and geographical location. Rural states struggling with structural and economic deficits will face daunting challenges in meeting the 2010 targets.

Health Disparities

An example of health disparities among agricultural workers rural is the group of farm workers that support fruit and vegetable production. In general, migrant and deasonal farmworkers (MSFW) may have the poorest health of any aggregate in the United States, and the least access to affordable health care. Eighty-five percent of the MSFW are Hispanic, Latino, or African-American. The rest are largely white seasonal workers who follow the harvests to drive combines or haul crops from the fields to storage, market, or seaports. These populations, estimated between three and five million people each year, are vulnerable to a host of health problems and diseases that center on occupational and environmental hazards and other health correlates as described in the section about agricultural workers.

Accidents and Injuries

Working in highly variable environmental conditions (e.g., temperature extremes, a wide variety of work tasks, and unpredictable circumstances) is associated with an increased frequency of accidents and fatalities. Farm-related activities are extremely heterogeneous and vary significantly with the season, types of crops produced, and types of machinery used. Farmers are located in geographically isolated areas and often work alone. This constellation of factors places farmers and their families at increased risk for accidental injury and delayed access to emergency or trauma care.

The 2001 to 2002 rate of fatal injury for those employed in the agricultural sector was 21.3 per 100,000 workers, compared with a rate of 4.2 per 100,000 for all types of U.S. workers. According to NIOSH, agricultural machinery is the most common cause of fatalities and nonfatal injuries of U.S. agricultural workers, including on-farm fatalities among youth under 20 (NIOSH, 2004). Tractor-related accidents, especially rollovers, are the most frequent causes of farm accidents and account for more than one fourth of farm fatalities. The actual causes of death and serious injury are associated with rollovers of equipment that lack of rollover protective structures (ROPS) and seat belts (Struttmann et al., 2001). It is easy to see why accident prevention programs for farm children and families have focused heavily on tractor safety awareness.

Acute and Chronic Illnesses

Several types of farming activities are associated with higher than expected occurrences of acute and chronic respiratory conditions. People with long-term exposure to grain dusts, such as grain elevator and dairy workers, have diminished respiratory function and increased frequency of respiratory symptoms, such as cough or phlegm production (Cotton et al., 1989). Occupational asthma and more exotic fungal or toxic gas-related conditions also occur in higher frequency in agricultural than nonagricultural populations (Warren, 1989). Community health nurses, who are familiar with local farming practices in rural areas, often make links between farm work and respiratory symptoms. In such situations, the role of the nurse is to refer patients to appropriate health care providers and provide support and education for affected people and their families.

Exposure to pesticides, herbicides, and other chemicals is also a major concern for farmers and their families. From an occupational perspective, farming is unusual because the home and the work site are the same. Exposure risks to children and spouses may be heightened when farmers wear contaminated clothing and boots into the home. Homes are often located in close proximity to fields and animal containment facilities, which are treated with a variety of chemicals.

Nurses in rural emergency rooms or other ambulatory care settings may be the first providers to encounter farmers and others with **acute pesticide poisoning**. During discussions with farmers, ranchers, or other high-risk groups (e.g., nursery workers and tree planters), community health nurses may note a pattern of headaches and nausea that occur during planting or spraying seasons. In such an instance, the nurse can serve as an important resource by obtaining a careful history of signs and symptoms, the temporal nature of symptom occurrence, and the types of pesticides and personal protection used (e.g., respirators and protective clothing). When evidence suggests pesticide-related illness, appropriate referral and follow-up are imperative to ensure the safety of the affected person and the family.

Signs and symptoms of acute pesticide poisoning are fairly clear and most health providers in rural communities should recognize them. Although there are exceptions, it frequently follows exposure to insecticides classified as organophosphates or carbamates. These products, which are sold under a wide variety of trade names (e.g., Parathion, Vapona, Sevin, and Dursban), kill insects by inhibiting the enzyme acetylcholinesterase; this leads to an accumulation of acetylcholine in the neuromuscular junction (Environmental Protection Agency [EPA], 1989). Common symptoms include headache, dizziness, diaphoresis, nausea, and vomiting. If left untreated,

those affected may experience a progression of symptoms including dyspnea, bronchospasm, and muscle twitching. Deaths are relatively uncommon, but they do occur.

Overall, farmers have a lower rate of cardiovascular disease because of the secondary protection of demanding farm work. In addition, the prevalence of smoking in farmers is generally lower than in the general population (Blair and Zahm, 1995). National and international data addressing cancer risks in farmers provide evidence that farmers have lower rates of some cancers and elevated rates of other cancers. Generally, rates of lung, bladder, and esophageal cancers are lower in farmers. Higher than expected rates of non-Hodgkin's lymphoma, prostate cancer, leukemia, brain tumors, multiple myeloma, and cancer of the lip have been observed by cancer epidemiologists in the United States and Canada (Blair and Zahm, 1995; Gabos, Fincham, and Berkel, 1995; Morrison et al., 1995).

Migrant and Seasonal Farmworkers

Although the discussion of agricultural issues has focused primarily on farmers and farm families, it is important to understand the role of **migrant** (i.e., migrate to find work) and **seasonal** (i.e., reside permanently in one place and work locally when farm labor is needed) farmworkers in U.S. agricultural production and the health risks to this population. Older references to farmworkers often referred to three "migrant streams," in which workers entered the country through Mexico and migrated north. The present reality is that migrant workers enter the country through a variety of access points and follow any route necessary to obtain work. Seasonal workers permanently reside in agricultural areas and take various farm jobs during harvesting times. For example, a seasonal worker may be employed in restaurant work during the winter and may spend the summer months picking apples or working in a local apple shed or cannery.

MSFW comprise a vulnerable population in regard to health risks because they have low income and migratory status. In many rural areas, community health nurses form the central link between farmworkers and health services. Through standing or mobile clinic sites, nurses have established a leadership role in the provision of episodic and preventive services for workers and their families. Lacking access to many types of preventive services, farmworkers often visit a migrant clinic with any number of health problems including severe dental problems, unresolved communicable diseases, and untreated injuries. In addition to the direct provision of care, nurses in many communities have served as important advocates on behalf of farmworkers and have worked to ensure health care access to those traveling through their areas.

Cultural, linguistic, economic, and mobility barriers all contribute to the nature and magnitude of health problems observed in farmworkers. Cultural and linguistic barriers are the most overt because many of the communities where farmworkers work consider them outsiders. In many settings, migrant workers live isolated from the agricultural communities they serve. Although some workers travel in extended family groups and have the support that comes

TABLE 21-1 Available State Data for Numbers of MSFWs

STATE	ADJUSTED MSFW FARMWORKER ESTIMATES	MSFW FARMWORKERS AND NONFARMWORKERS	MSFW CHILDREN (<20 YEARS OF AGE)
Arkansas	16,613	27,613	8,682
California	732,109	1,302,797	416,289
Florida	197,182	286,725	91,953
Louisiana	8,392	12,349	3,569
Maryland	7,934	9,522	1,648
North Carolina	100,960	156,893	45,608
Mississippi	11,762	18,191	5,263
Oklahoma	8,201	14,202	4,217
Texas	197,393	362,724	129,591
Washington	186,976	289,235	91,394

Data from Bureau of Primary Healthcare: *Migrant and seasonal farmworker enumeration profiles study,* 2000, The Author, http://bphc.hrsa.gov/migrant/Enumeration/EnumerationStudy. htm.

with being together, other workers leave their families at home. Often these are male workers who work and live together. A common misconception among U.S. health care providers is that these farmworkers are from Mexico and Spanish is their primary language. Farmworkers originate from many communities in Mexico, the Caribbean, Central and South America, and they may speak the language of their home country, English, or several languages.

Enumeration of Migrant and Seasonal Farmworkers

To increase access to primary and preventative care for MSFW populations, information is needed on the numbers and distribution of farmworkers at the national, state, and local levels. Because MSFWs move frequently for work, census estimates generally provide a poor assessment of needs for health care services for this population. Additionally, the legislation that created the Migrant Health Program (MHP) (Section 330g of the Public Health Service Act), under the direction of the Bureau of Primary Health Care (BPHC) (2000) and the Health Resources and Services Administration (HRSA), requires that priorities be established based on where the greatest need exists. Hence the MHP has supported the ongoing and comprehensive assessment of the numbers of MSFWs and published the most recent estimates in the Migrant and Seasonal Farmworker Enumeration Profile Study (MSFWEPS) (Bureau of Health Professions, 2000).

Enumeration data from the MSFWEPS is available for Arkansas, California, Florida, Louisiana, Maryland, North Carolina, Mississippi, Oklahoma, Texas, and Washington. Table 21-1 summarizes the latest available data for numbers of MSFWs (as well as nonfarmworkers living in MSFW households) in each state whose work is associated with agriculture, nurseries, greenhouses, food processing, or reforestation. Although populations sizes of MSFWs range from relatively small numbers in such states as Maryland and Oklahoma, to very large numbers in California and Washington, it is important to recognize that primary and preventative care services must be appropriately planned for those not engaged in farm and seasonal work, including other household members and children. For example, the state of Califor-

nia has an estimated population of 732,109 MSFWs, but an additional 570,688 nonfarmworkers must be considered in planning and evaluating services.

Health Needs and Opportunities for Preventive Care

Similarities in exposure and work practices make some of the farmworkers' health needs similar to those of farmers and their families. Generally, these health needs reflect the increased rates of accidents and injuries, dermatological conditions, and pulmonary problems observed in both populations. However, there are additional challenges in both the identification and treatment of farmworkers with health problems. One of the biggest problems that nurses face in designing health programs is understanding the full magnitude of their problems. Many farmworkers who become ill eventually return to their countries of origin to obtain treatment and to be with family. This phenomenon makes it difficult to get complete, reliable numbers about disease rates. A variety of public health indicators are likely to undercount farmworkers as a group, ranging from tumor registries to Workers' Compensation injuries (Schenker, 1995). In addition, farmworkers may be less likely to seek treatment for health problems that do not require emergency treatment or surgery.

Studies of farmworkers' health status have provided data indicating that farmworkers are less likely to receive preventive care from any health source (Schenker, 1995). Preventive needs include dental care, vision screening and treatment, and gynecological and breast exams. In addition, children of farmworkers are likely to receive incomplete sets of immunizations by the age of 5 years (Schenker, 1995). Many farmworkers, because they move from community to community, are often unaware of clinical and social services they could receive at reduced or no cost to low-income families.

Because agriculture is one of the most dangerous industries in which to work in the United States, MSFWs bear a disproportionate burden of environmentally related illnesses and occupational injuries. Contact with herbicides, insecticides, and fertilizers may put farmworkers at increased risk for acute and chronic health problems such as eye injuries, cancer, respiratory illnesses, and dermatitis associated with exposure to these chemical agents. There is some evidence that, like farmers, farmworkers have elevated rates of multiple myeloma and cancers of the prostate, stomach, and testes. A few smaller studies indicate that rates of oral, lung, and liver cancer may also be elevated in farmworkers (Zahm and Blair, 1993), though cancer incidence is not well documented among farmworker populations (Larson, 2001). Occupational injuries also significantly affect the health of MSFW populations and the effects are not limited to adults. Because child labor laws do not always prevent children for working in fields either alone or with adults, many children can be affected by the same types of musculoskeletal and traumatic injuries that adults face. In a study of almost 300 MSFWs, about 12% had experienced an injury in the past 3 years, and many of these considered medical attention necessary but unavailable (Villarejo and Baron, 1999).

Hearing Farmworkers' Voices

Several studies and pilot projects have used focus groups, community meetings, or other qualitative research methods to listen to farmworkers' concerns and give these concerns a voice through publication and advocacy. Several years ago, the Farmworker Justice Fund brought female farmworkers together in a national effort to give them a forum for their concerns and their impressions of health needs. The women identified priority concerns in the areas of child and family issues, health care services, workplace issues, and empowerment. The group's recommendations in the area of health care included the following directives: keep clinics open during evening hours, provide transportation to clinics, increase access through mobile health units, provide social and health services in one building, increase home visits by students, encourage careers in farmworker health, enhance nutrition education to families, teach first aid, enforce farm labor health laws, and give farmworkers a copy of the record after each clinic visit (Wilk, 1995). It is interesting to note that a group of baccalaureate nursing students in Georgia documented similar concerns. During an immersion course, the students listened to and documented the concerns of farmworker families. The need to restructure health services was a predominant theme voiced by the workers, who noted the importance of health care worker field visits and evening home visits (Bechtel and Davidhizar, 1999).

Involving MSFWs as active participants in the planning and provision of care may become more challenging since the terrorist attacks of September 11, 2001. Following this unprecedented event, policy makers began discussing broad changes to current immigration laws to protect the United States by securing the borders. In short, discussions have focused on limiting access of foreign workers to jobs in the United States and providing those already here with limited provisions for continuing in their current role. Concerns raised by public health advocates center around the idea that an increasingly punitive system of immigration will discourage seasonal workers and farmworkers from accessing health care or encourage them lie to health care providers about critical issues (Mautino, 2004).

APPLICATION OF RELEVANT THEORIES AND "THINKING UPSTREAM" CONCEPTS TO RURAL HEALTH

Upstream and prevention-oriented approaches have several implications for nurses in rural practice. Three strategies for upstream interventions follow: attack community-based problems at their roots, emphasize the "doing" aspects of health, and maximize the use of informal networks.

Attack Community-Based Problems at Their Roots

Upstream approaches to community health problems direct the nurse toward an understanding of the precursors of poor health within populations of interest. Individual nurses can be effective forces in uncovering and enhancing community awareness of health-endangering situations. Environmental health issues in rural communities, such as pesticide exposure or health hazards from point-source factory emissions, are more effectively assessed and remedied on a community level than on a case-by-case basis. Nurses' involvement in helping people understand health problems in a larger context can be the genesis of change. Nurses and other community members can take social action on behalf of those affected. For example, by heightening awareness of sulfur dioxin levels from a local refinery and the relationship of those emission levels to respiratory problems in vulnerable populations, nurses can help citizens gain an understanding of the collective rather than individual burden of the refinery on their community's health.

Emphasize the "Doing" Aspects of Health

There are consistent differences between the way rural and non-rural residents perceive health. The primary one may be the relative importance of "work" and "being able to work" in self-reported definitions of health (Weinert and Long, 1987). Rural attitudes generally emphasize the "doing" aspects of health by functioning and performing the daily activities fundamentally important in their daily lives. The high value placed on "being able to do" can provide astute nurses with intervention opportunities for both families and communities. Examples of nursing intervention strategies that capitalize on this include accident prevention programs for children, exercise and nutrition programs for seniors, and local industry participation in risk reduction programs for workers. Active involvement of the target population in all phases of program planning and implementation is key to the success of these programs.

Maximize the Use of Informal Networks

Recognizing and using informal networks in the community is essential to the "doing" concept of prevention programs. The name used, such as empowerment models or community action models, is less important than soliciting the involvement of informal networks and local leaders in planning health interventions. As most people who have been involved in community empowerment programs will attest, the involvement of these important entities is not easy or straightforward. Turf issues and collateral agendas can sometimes seem to obstruct rather than facilitate change. However, failure to elicit community involvement in population-based health interventions will result in unfavorable consequences; frequently, superimposed change tends to fit poorly with the community it is intended to serve. Rural change strategies will be short-lived unless members understand them and invest in their own well-being.

RURAL HEALTH CARE DELIVERY SYSTEM

In the past, rural illness care was modeled after urban areas. Urban models emphasize specialist providers and in-hospital acute care with many high-tech, expensive procedures. Many rural hospitals can no longer compete with the larger facilities. This brief overview discusses past and present characteristics of the system and how many community members, providers, and health policy analysts believe it should be changed.

In the 1980s rural health was focused almost exclusively on hospitals, with the emphasis on making them financially viable. Health administrators and health policy analysts, who recommended that the community hospital become the community's health center, examined the rural small hospital crisis. To many public health professionals, this appeared to be a contradiction of terms. Public health providers assert that hospitals deliver treatment for illness and ignore health promotion and disease prevention. Providers and institutions delivering acute care and those promoting public health have long mistrusted one another. Public health, with its commitment to disease prevention, health promotion, and universal access to community-oriented primary health care, had little in common with cure-oriented hospitals.

In the late 1980s and 1990s many hospitals developed wellness programs and some additional increased services. For example, at the request of the county government, a small frontier hospital surmounted the barrier between the hospital and public health by taking over the following basic public health services: home visits, school nursing, and immunization clinics. Hospital-employed nurses make school visits for health education and screening and home visits for prenatal follow-up. The shift toward public health orientation served to broaden the hospital's commitment to the community (Clancy, 1992).

The new century brings substantial changes within rural hospitals and in their communities. Numerous hospitals have elected to provide a full continuum of care ranging from preventive services to long-term care. Many are joining networks and merging or affiliating with other rural hospitals, physicians, advance practice nurses, and other providers to benefit from managed care systems. Increasingly, rural health care is being delivered across integrated networks that benefit from greater availability of resources. The addition of new partners, lower transaction costs, and improved legitimacy increase a network's chance of survival (Moscovice, Wellever, and Christianson, 1997).

Health Care Provider Shortages

The Bureau of Health Professions (BHPr) (2003) states that the size and characteristics of the future health workforce are determined by the interaction of various forces acting on the health environment, including economic factors, technology, regulatory and legislative actions, epidemiological factors, the health care education system, and demographics. Current shortages of health care professionals in rural areas are likely to become worse with increased demand caused by population aging and increasing racial and ethnic diversity. In actual numbers, the shortage has been growing since 1990. Although approximately 25% of the U.S. population lives in nonmetropolitan counties, only 18% of registered nurses (RNs) practice there. In addition, the supply of physicians has not equaled service need in rural areas, and only 8.7% of the 675,047 active physicians in the United States provided services in rural areas in 1998 (Pasko, Seidman, and Birkhead, 2000). For nonphysician primary care professionals, such as nurse practitioners (NP), physician assistants (PAs), and certified nurse midwives (CNMs), trends are similar to physicians except for physician assistants. Gamm, Castillo, and Pittman (2003) report that there are about 25 NPs per 100,000 people in urban areas and only 20 NPs per 100,000 people in rural areas, with a slightly greater disparity for CNMs and about the same numbers for PAs.

Clearly the growing nursing shortage will affect all of America. This is both a supply and a demand shortage. Declining school enrollments, retirement of current nurses, and the increased need for care of an aging population make the situation especially critical (Sigma Theta Tau International, 2006). A survey by the American Organization of Nurse Executives (AONE) found that in small hospitals, usually located in rural areas, it takes significantly longer to fill vacancies than in larger urban facilities (Beyers, 1999). Rural nurses earn less than their urban counterparts, which compounds recruitment difficulties. Nurses with baccalaureate and masters degrees, other than masters prepared NPs, are compensated less for this additional education (Pan, Straub, and Szigeti, 1998).

A solution proposed for the shortage of health care providers is for rural communities to "grow their own." A rural community, a group of small communities, or a county could support local students attending college and recruit students currently attending professional schools. The students make a commitment to work in the community in return for monetary support for their educations (Jones and Brand, 1995). Tuition reimbursement and access to distance learning programs can assist practicing nurses. Continuing education and baccalaureate and masters degrees are available through e-mail, Internet-based courses, interactive video classes, and by-mail videos. Some programs are provided exclusively via the Internet. Nebraska rural communities are enthusiastic about the University of Nebraska College of Nursing Internet courses. The program is helping them grow their own nurses. Research shows that nurses educated in rural communities are more apt to stay and work there than those who move away to attend school (Pullen, 1998).

Communitywide Health Care Systems

To cope with provider shortages and fewer acute care facilities, community members, rural health care planners, and health care professionals are recommending the development of a communitywide health care system with the hospital as one component. The central focus of this system is community-based care in the form of **Community-Oriented Primary Care (COPC)** services (Van Hook, 1992; Welton, Kantner, and Katz, 1997). COPC is a model in which for-profit health care providers can function in concert with public agencies. Similar to the old axiom that all politics are local, it is also appropriate to consider health care as a local affair. Rohrer (1999) provides guidelines for building the local health care system within the context of community.

- *The delivery system needs to enhance the health of the community.*
- *The system should be frugal, because communities do not appreciate wasted resources.*
- *The critical health care delivery organization is not a physical institution, such as a hospital, nursing home . . . but is a local system of primary care (e.g., a community network).*
- *The mission of the local health care system must be optimization of the community's health. The emphasis is on primary care, health promotion and prevention, and coordination with public health agencies.*
- *Some key concepts for health systems based on "community" are community governance, population-based planning, information systems, accountability, and community-oriented primary care.*

(Rohrer, 1999, p. 22)

Primary care is first-line care a provider (e.g., physician, nurse, NP, PA, mental health counselor, or other health care professional) gives in an office or clinic setting. A recommended model for rural communities combines the primary care model with that of COPC services. COPC is often called primary health care. A primary health care model assumes that providers address the health and illness concerns of not just the clients they see in the clinic or office, but of the community as a whole, using an epidemiological orientation. Providers integrate aspects of public health, health promotion, and disease prevention into their primary care practices. This model moves the provider's orientation from individual clients in the office or clinic practice to population health. For example, this community-oriented, or upstream, approach to prevention will help providers establish a community education program on farm safety and provide the immediate cleaning and suturing of a client's hand lacerated by a piece of farm machinery.

The formation of a community health care system that includes primary care and a community-oriented primary health care focus may bring accessible and affordable illness care to "the country." This system bases health promotion and disease prevention on the needs of the community. Bringing a holistic and integrated approach to both health and illness care,

it appears to resemble a nursing model rather than a medical model (Van Hook, 1992). This approach is cooperative rather than market driven and competition based. The community-oriented model complements the public health philosophy of optimal allocation of limited resources and the social justice ethic of equitable access to health and illness care.

Rural communities struggle to define what illness care services they need, want, and can afford. Although outsiders are not always trusted, some communities have successfully enlisted trained facilitators to help develop and execute an effective, practical plan for maintaining or eliminating local services. These facilitators help communities determine how many and what kinds of services to implement. This process is a type of community organization model that includes community participation, needs assessment, and leadership training (Amundson, 1993).

Rural and frontier community health nurses, with their knowledge of advocacy, community assessment, aggregates, and community involvement strategies, can be an excellent local resource for the planning process (Shreffler, 1996). Currently, most planning is related to illness care. Involvement by community health nurses and other local and state health department personnel is integral to a community-wide health care system. Community-based care is central to the development of such a system (American Nurses Association, 1996). Optimal models for reformed rural health care systems are those in which the community is the central organizing and sponsoring group for the system. The essential feature of these models is a community-primary care orientation under local leadership (NRHA, 1998).

Managed Care in the Rural Environment

Managed care has recently changed health care delivery in the United States. In rural areas, health care delivery networks with managed care elements are being developed. An NRHA issue paper has identified potential benefits and risks of managed care to rural areas. Possible benefits include lowering primary care costs, improving the quality of care, and stabilizing the local rural health care system. Risks are also apparent, including probable high start-up and administrative costs, and the volatile effect of large, urban-based for-profit managed care companies (NRHA, 1995).

Outside of Medicaid, managed care has yet to become a major presence in much of rural America, because small disperse populations, few visits per individual, and large numbers of elderly on Medicare with low-level reimbursements do not make the aggregate financially attractive to an managed care organization (MCO) In fact, despite the existence of at least one health maintenance organization (HMO) in more than 82% of rural counties in 1995, very few rural people were enrolled (Mueller, Coburn, and Cordes, 1999). Providers in rural markets face severe financial constraints as HMOs increasingly cope with smaller numbers of enrollees and continue to decrease provider reimbursement. The NRHA recommends that "communities or networks develop community health plans, combining delivery and financing systems at the local level. Assuming responsibility for the financing of care for prepaid enrollees is accomplished either by rural communities obtaining their own HMO licenses or by establishing strategic partnerships with HMOs or insurance companies that allow local assumption of financial risk" (NRHA, 1998, p. 4). In frontier communities, a partnership to reach a critical mass of enrollees would be the most appropriate strategy for meeting the challenge of managed care. Communities that make the most progress toward partnerships or integration are those whose local leaders and providers have strong incentives to work together and are motivated to bring about change to the health care system (Fasciano et al., 1999). Authorities in rural health and managed care report that it is too soon to know whether managed care will become a significant way of delivering health care in rural areas, like it has become in urban America (Voelker, 1998).

COMMUNITY-BASED CARE

In the mid-1990s, the phrase *community-based care* became a popular term for the myriad of services provided outside the walls of an institution. Health care services are no longer provided exclusively in the hospital setting. Community-base care includes services that are provided where individuals live, work, or go to school. Examples of community-based services are home health and hospice care, occupational health programs, community mental health programs, ambulatory care services, school health programs, faith-based care, and elder services, such as adult day care. The concept also includes community participation in decisions about health care services, a focus on all three levels of prevention, and an understanding that the hospital is no longer the exclusive health care provider.

Home Care and Hospice

Home health and hospice programs vary in structure. In a national study on Medicare hospice use, only one third of rural counties have a hospice based within the county, but nearly two thirds of urban counties do (Vernig et al., 2004). Urban hospices are more likely to be free-standing, whereas rural hospices tend to be hospital-based. Larger communities may support a hospital-based home care agency with hospice service, a free-standing, full-service agency, or both. In sparsely populated rural locations, home health and hospice services may be contracted from a larger regional agency, with a local nurse hired to provide services. Public health agencies may also provide home health and hospice care. A successful Utah model for hospice service development combines external resources based in a city with those of a small community. The large urban-based facility provides administrative support for local nurses hired to work in the hospice program (Memmott, 1991).

A study by Buehler and Lee (1992) reported that family caregivers for cancer patients in the most rural areas believed they had limited formal resources. Vernig et al. (2004) found the more remote the rural environment, the less likely hospice services were used. Nurse case management and development of local resources, using the county extension services as a bridge for outreach services, can improve home care for these patients and provide support for their families. A partnership between the public health nurse and county extension service could provide support and information groups and caregiving classes for the important informal provider network. Chapter 31 discusses home health and hospice in greater detail.

Faith Communities and Parish Nursing

Rural residents are perceived as having strong traditional values. At the heart of these values is a strong sense of community, family life, and religious faith (W. K. Kellogg Foundation, 2001). Faith communities in rural America have a long and positive legacy. Because they reflect the local customs, rural residents trust them (Griffin, 1999). For these reasons, they can be valuable partners in improving overall community health.

Since the conceptualization of parish nursing in the early 1980s, RNs have developed and expanded the role. Parish nurses integrate nursing expertise and faith-based knowledge to provide holistic care to members of congregations. Over 7000 nurses have completed formal training programs in parish nursing. The exact number of parish nurses working as paid and unpaid staff in both urban and rural faith communities is not known, because many nurses have not been formally prepared for the role (International Parish Nurse Resource Center, n.d.). Both professional nursing and parish nursing are based on health and healing (ANA, 1998).

In a comparison of experiences of rural and urban parish nurses, Chase-Ziolek and Striepe (1999) found rural nurses more likely to be involved in case management and coordination of services than their urban counterparts. In urban settings, contact with parishioners was primarily at the church, whereas contacts in rural settings were most often in the home, on the phone, or in other community based settings. Collaboration between faith communities and other organizations can help extend limited rural community health resources. Such partnerships have been promoted by federal and state governments to enhance the public health efforts (Zahner and Corrado, 2004). Chapter 30 provides an in-depth discussion of parish nursing.

Informal Care Systems

Limited availability and accessibility of formal health care resources in rural areas combined with self-reliance and self-help traits of rural residents have resulted in the development of strong rural community informal care and social support networks. Rural residents are more apt to entrust care to established informal networks than to new formal care systems (Weinert and Long, 1987, 1990). One study reported that rural residents sustain a higher level of social health than urban residents. They attributed this social health to their higher level of family and community involvement (Eggebeen and Lichter, 1993), which may contribute to the formation and use of informal systems.

Informal care systems or networks include people who have assumed the role of caregiver based on their individual qualities, life situations, or social roles (Figure 21-5). People who participate in these networks may provide direct help, advice, or information. Rural residents identify spouses, adult

FIGURE 21-5 Traditional models of care. *"Grandfather Spirit gave us knowledge to use the things in the environment for food and for medicine. Our tribal ceremonies are prayers for spiritual direction and good health...."* (Photograph courtesy Caring for Our Own Program, Montana State University-Bozeman College of Nursing; Linda Best, photographer. Quote courtesy Dr. Henrietta Mann, Southern Cheyenne Elder.)

children, other family members, friends, and neighbors as informal providers of care (Buckwalter et al., 2002).

Informal caregivers often find themselves in stressful circumstances. Rural residents who are in need of assistance are usually elderly, have chronic illness, have few resources, and must travel long distances for health care. Caregivers are often elderly individuals with physical and mental health concerns of their own. Sanford and Townsend-Rocchiccioli (2004) found that informal caregivers in the rural south have significantly lower perceived health status than the general population. The implications of this finding are numerous. Caregivers also need care. Caregivers should be taught health promotion and prevention techniques to increase or maintain their level of health. The Maine Primary Partners in Caregiving is an example of collaboration by various community-based agencies to identify needs of caregivers in rural Maine. The Area Agency on Aging, the Center on Aging at the University of Maine, and several primary care provider practices have joined together to identify caregivers early in their caregiving experience and to offer support in a variety of ways, including education, support groups, and case management (Kaye et al., 2002).

It is especially significant that community-based providers identify and combine informal services with formal systems (Weinert and Long, 1987, 1990). Both institution- and community-based professional health care providers must recognize the strengths and positive contributions of informal care providers, as well as provide support for these valuable community resources.

Rural Public Health Departments

There are over 2800 local health departments in the United States. Many of these serve populations of less than 50,000 people (Rosenblatt, Casey, and Richardson, 2002). The purpose of *Healthy People 2010* objective 23-11 is to increase the proportion of state and local public health departments that meet national performance standards for public health services (USDHHS, 2000). The standards are based upon the core public functions of assessment, policy development, and assurance. Data from 2004 indicate that only 11% of 2315 local public health agencies used the national standards, with only 3% fully or substantially meeting the model national standards (USDHHS, 2004).

In 2002, approximately 3.3% of all money spent on health care in the United States was spent on public health services. Public health expenditures have steadily decreased since 1960. This trend is unlikely to improve given limited public resources, the aging of the population with the subsequent need for acute illness care, and changing Medicaid from public to private providers (NCHS, 2004).

In a study of 99 local health departments in three rural states, Rosenblatt et al., (2002) found that public health nurses were the core provider of public health services. Many smaller local health departments do not have the economic base to employ other professional public health providers, such as physicians, epidemiologists, sanitarians, and nutritionists at the local level. Frequently these services are provided at the state level or collaboratively between groups of local health departments. A local physician may serve as a part-time, unpaid health officer. The lack of additional onsite public health providers poses two problems. First, the ability to collaborate with others about potential or actual public health problems is decreased or nonexistent. Second, the ranges of services provided are less comprehensive. Often, these small facilities can only offer federally funded programs with few locally funded services. Environmental health, maternal and child health, and communicable disease control are the three highest priority programs of rural local health departments (Berkowitz, 2004).

Since rural health departments are not always able to provide all the needed public health services, their role is to fulfill the core public health function of assurance. To develop the most comprehensive services possible for the population, rural community health nurses need to develop partnerships with other health provider agencies. Others agencies that provide public health services in rural communities include rural health clinics (RHCs), migrant health centers (MHCs), public schools, parish nurses, family planning centers, Head Start programs, and public hospitals.

Rural Mental Health Care

The economic crisis that affected much of the rural population in the 1980s contributed to mental health problems (American

Psychological Association, 1995). Natural disasters, such as drought and flood, and economic downturns in the late 1990s have contributed to continuing chronic stress. Those affected are most apt to work in the traditional ranching, farming, mining, forestry, and fishing industries. They have not enjoyed the good economic times generated by the information and technology age (NRHA, 1999). Although mental health disorders widely affect rural and urban residents across the life span, factors such as poverty, race, age, and rural dwelling lower the prospect of accessing mental health services (Gamm, Stone, and Pittman, 2003). Clearly, large sections of at-risk rural populations are without mental health care (NRHA, 1999).

There are three key factors that have been identified as contributing to mental illness in rural areas (Gamm, Stone, and Pittman, 2003). First, there is a lack of specialized mental health providers in rural areas. The most recent figures show that 75% of rural counties with populations between 2500 and 20,000 do not have a psychiatrist, and 95% do not have a child psychiatrist. Next, because of the lack of qualified mental health care providers, rural residents often receive services from primary care providers. McCabe and Macnee (2002) found that many rural primary care providers are ill-equipped to provide mental health services. Both specialized mental health care and primary health care providers are confronted with barriers related to rural practice. These include a more diverse practice, fewer opportunities for ongoing education, and fewer professionals to consult than their colleagues in urban practice.

Lastly, rural residents often do not seek mental health services because of perceived stigma. They do not always recognize a need for mental health services (Gamm, Stone, and Pittman, 2003).

Sowing Seeds of Hope is a collaborative model for practice that addresses the mental health care needs of rural farm families in seven Midwestern states. Services are provided to individuals and families who lack the needed financial resources to access care (i.e., inadequate or no insurance coverage). At the state level, coalitions of individuals, agencies, and organizations have been developed to carry on the work of project. Because of the shortage of qualified professionals, the use of informal care networks has been instrumental at the local level. See an overview of the project in Gamm, Stone, and Pittman (2003, pp. 175-178).

Emergency Services

Access to emergency medical services (EMS) has been identified as one of the most significant health care issues for rural residents (Rawlinson and Crews, 2003). Emergency medical services include pre-hospital care, hospital or health center-based emergency care, and trauma systems.

Rural residents depend on EMS because of their high risk for unintentional injury. Low population density has been shown to be a strong predictor of increased injury-related morbidity and mortality rates in rural areas (Peek-Asa, Zwerling, and Staliones, 2004). In medically underserved areas, EMS systems play an increasingly important role in decreasing the morbidity and mortality of individuals needing emergency care. Getting patients from the place of injury to the trauma center within the "golden hour" is frequently not possible in rural areas because distance, terrain, climatic conditions, and communication methods produce barriers. Some rural facilities are more than 2 hours away by air from the nearest trauma center or tertiary care hospital (Furlow, 1999).

Challenges faced by rural EMS systems include a shortage of volunteers, a lower level of training than among urban providers, training curricula that often do not reflect rural hazards (e.g., farm equipment trauma), lack of guidance from physicians, and lack of physician training and orientation to the EMS system (Rawlinson and Crews, 2003). Low population density, large, isolated, or inaccessible areas, severe weather, poor roads, and lower density of telephones or other communication methods also contribute to difficult public access for emergency care. These problems make the challenges of developing EMS in rural and frontier areas substantial (NRHA, 1997).

An example of a model for practice is the TENKIDS EMS Computer Network. The purpose of this project is to provide continuing education, training, and improved communications to remote and volunteer EMS providers throughout the state of Montana, with the overall goal of improving patient care. The success of this project was dependent upon the collaborative efforts of many organizations. Personal computers were placed with each of the 123 EMS agencies throughout the state. Asynchronous training is provided to 4000 EMS providers, many of whom are volunteers, using CD-ROM and web-based technologies. Data, used for epidemiological purposes, can be collected and transmitted using this system (Rawlinson and Crews, 2003).

LEGISLATION AND PROGRAMS AFFECTING PUBLIC HEALTH IN RURAL AREAS

Programs That Augment Health Care Facilities and Services

Several programs are particularly important for meeting the public health needs of rural people. One is the Community Health Centers (CHC) program, administered by the United States Public Health Service (USPHS). The CHC Program benefits underserved areas and populations by providing primary health care and, in some cases, supplemental secondary and tertiary health care, such as hospital care, long-term home health care, and rehabilitation. Rural health clinics (RHCs) are designed to improve access to primary care. As an incentive to rural communities to apply for RHCs, Medicare and Medicaid are reimbursed at a higher rate than usual.

The Migrant Health Clinic (MHC) program and the Migrant Health Program (MHP) also come under the Division of Community and Migrant Health and HRSA. The MHC program provides comprehensive nursing and medical care and support services to migrant and seasonal farmworkers and their families. The centers provide culturally sensitive care to a racially and culturally diverse farm labor force from many countries in Latin America and the Caribbean. Bilingual,

BOX 21-2   Critical Access Hospitals (CAH) for Rural Communities

During a 5-year period (1987 to 1991), 193 rural hospitals closed nationally. Fortunately, the trend toward rural hospital closure did not continue through the 1990s. They numbered 28 from 1994 through 1997 (Ricketts and Heaphy, 1999). In the more populated rural areas, another hospital was often available within 20 miles. However, for populations in frontier counties, there were very real problems with finding basic primary care. In the United States, 11% of rural hospitals are in frontier areas. These hospitals serve a wide geographical area (46% of the total U.S. land area) where 1% of the U.S. population resides.

Closure of the local hospital can result in the loss of physicians and other providers, and the reduction or curtailment of primary care services and emergency medical services. To adapt to the realities of health care management and to improve access to care in frontier areas, new rural hospital models are being developed.

Medicare's Rural Hospital Flexibility (RHF) grant provides funding to states to establish limited-service hospitals that can obtain designation as Critical Access Hospitals (CAH) in rural communities. Grants are awarded for planning, implementing, and establishing networks of care and improving emergency medical services. The Office of Rural Health Policy and the Health Resources and Services Administration administer this program. There is also assistance for small communities to adjust to changes in clinical practice patterns and in-hospital use, shifts from hospital- to community-based care, and changes in emergency care delivery patterns. These federal grants help address the top priority need of rural communities, that is, access to health care.

From U.S. Department of Health and Human Services, Centers for Medicare and Medicaid Services: http://www.cms.hhs.gov/CertificationComplianc/04; and U.S. Department of Health and Human Services, Health Resources and Services Administration, Rural Health Policy. http://www.ruralhealth.hrca.gov/funding/flex. htm.

bicultural health personnel including lay outreach workers use culturally appropriate protocols for providing primary care, preventive health care, transportation, dental care, pharmaceuticals, and environmental health. The MHCs must provide the same services as the CHC and may also offer supplemental services, such as environmental health services, infectious disease and parasite control, and accident prevention programs.

Medicare's Rural Hospital Flexibility (RHF) grant program replaces earlier demonstration programs during the 1990s (Box 21-2). According to information provided by the Office of Rural Health Policy (ORHP), the RHF program "allows small hospitals the flexibility to reconfigure operations and be licensed as Critical Access Hospitals (CAHs)" (Office of Rural Health Policy, n.d.). The program also provides cost-based reimbursement for inpatient Medicare and outpatient service. Grants are also awarded for planning, implementing, and establishing networks of care, and improving emergency medical services. The ORHP and HRSA administer this program (Office of Rural Health Policy, n.d.).

Primary care cooperative agreements facilitate the development of primary care services and attract primary care providers to rural HPSAs. Special legislation for HPSAs has also created programs to provide acute care facilities and services. The Rural Transition Grants Program, administered

by HCFA, helps small rural communities with nonprofit hospitals adjust to changes in clinical practice patterns and in-hospital use, shifts from hospital- to community-based care, and changes in emergency care delivery patterns.

RURAL COMMUNITY HEALTH NURSING

Perhaps a more accurate title than rural community health nursing would be "community health nursing along the rural continuum." Nonmetropolitan areas are at one end of the continuum, whereas metropolitan areas are at the other end.

Practice in a rural area may require working as the only nurse at a health department in a remote Western Great Plains frontier county with a population of 6000, at a full-service health department in a town of 50,000 people, or at a large health department in a rural area next to an urban population. A practice in a rural area adjacent to a large metropolitan area often appears to have more in common with the urban end of the continuum in terms of agency size, distances, and resources. For the purposes of this discussion, the practice setting is at the more "rural" end of the continuum.

The following definition illustrates the broad-based, generalist focus of the modern rural community health nurse. It includes the important geographical and cultural environment where community health practice is implemented and helps define appropriate nursing interventions.

> Rural nursing is the practice of professional nursing within the physical and sociocultural context of sparsely populated communities. It involves the continual interaction of the rural environment, the nurse, and his or her practice. Rural nursing is the diagnosis and treatment of a diversified population of people of all ages and a variety of human responses to actual (or potential) occupational hazards or actual or potential health problems existent in maternity, pediatric, medical/surgical and emergency nursing in a given rural area (Bigbee, 1993, p. 132).

Characteristics of Rural Nursing

Dolphin (1984) reported that the several positive aspects of rural nursing were "ability to give holistic care, to know everyone well, and to develop close relationships with the community and with coworkers." Autonomy, professional status, and being valued by the agency and community have been reported components of positive job satisfaction (Davis and Drocs, 1993; Dunkin et al., 1992).

Of those components identified as negative, agencies and professional organizations are most actively addressing professional isolation. The use of distance education technologies is one way to address the isolation many rural nurses experience. University degree programs and continuing education courses are readily available online or by full-motion interactive television. Using these technologies, rural nurses are able to update their skills and network with other nurses without having to leave their home communities.

Scharff (1998) discussed the distinctive nature of the rural nurse's practice. She found that the rural nurse is a generalist, and generalist is not synonymous with boring. Interviews with rural nurses show that they feel an "intensity of purpose" that makes rural nursing distinctive. Nurses living and practicing in the same place have a strong sense of integration and continuity between practice and community.

> The newcomer practices nursing in a rural setting, unlike the old-timer, who practices rural nursing. Somewhere between these extremes lies the transitional period of events and conditions through which each nurse passes at her or his own pace. It is within this time zone that nurses experience rural reality and move toward becoming professionals who understand that having gone rural, they are not less than they were, but rather, they are more than they expected to be. Some may be conscious of the transition, and others may not, but in the end, a few will say, "I am a rural nurse." (Scharff, 1998, p. 38).

Rural community health nursing is rewarding and challenging. Services can include maternal and child health, elder health, school health, mental health, and occupational health. The nurse practicing with the autonomy common in rural practice brings knowledge and competence in other clinical specialties. The work requires a discriminating, solid practitioner who can perform general nursing at a skill level beyond that of the outdated "mile wide and inch deep" general nursing. The rural nurse must be an "expert generalist."

RURAL HEALTH RESEARCH

Contemporary developments in the healthcare delivery system and advances in science suggest the need for an active agenda in rural health research. Berkowitz, Ivory, and Morris (2002) comment that rural health policy and research agendas must at the very least address the following issues:

1. The capacity of rural public health to manage improvements in health.
2. Information technology capacity in rural communities.
3. Developing and monitoring performance standards in rural public health.
4. Developing leadership and public health workforce capacity within rural public health.
5. Interaction and integration of community health systems, managed care, and public health in rural America.

Capacity of Rural Public Health to Manage Improvements in Health

Healthy People 2010 (USDHHS, 2000) outlines health related objectives for Americans and forms the rationale for efforts to intervene with trends in disease to improve health. The status of health indicators, such as rates of morbidity, mortality from common diseases or injury, and perhaps more importantly, access to healthcare services, allow for priorities to be determined for which improvements in health are needed. Importantly, *Healthy People 2010* objectives have been analyzed for rural-urban disparities that may exist along geographic, demographic, and cultural dimensions to provide a more specific picture of potential research priorities concerning improvements in health for rural areas alone (Gamm et al., 2003, Vol. 1). The *Healthy People table* presents data from a survey of 44 national and state rural health experts that identifies percents of respondents indicating priority status for various health issues.

Research questions directed towards improving health may be suggested along any of the *Health People 2010* objectives, but may have the greatest potential to address salient rural trends if they relate to issues of access to care, mental health, oral health, educational and community based programs, diabetes, or injury and violence prevention. Additionally, investigators may want to consider how these established rural priorities may be consistent or different within specific populations of concern. Because availability of surveillance data are often limited as researchers concern themselves with increasingly smaller populations (e.g., from state to county), efforts to gather additional primary data may be needed to set research priorities for improvements to health.

Information Technology in Rural Communities

As the distribution of technology expands across rural populations more research is needed to examine the impacts of readily accessible information to both rural citizens and the healthcare delivery system. Rural patients are able to access specialty services such and radiological or dermatological exams through telemedicine, and rural people are increasingly taking advantage of the World Wide Web to access information to make health decisions. Recent federal efforts directed toward disaster and terrorism preparedness have strengthened rural technological infrastructure so that communication pathways remain open during times of need. Just as patients access health care services from isolation, rural citizens are accessing health education through distance programs for both continuing education as well as entry-level and advanced degree programs in various health sciences. The need to address new research questions has grown alongside rapid expansion of information technology (IT), and questions abound relating to the application and evaluation of technology for both improving systems of care and care outcomes (see Research Highlights box). Berkowitz, Ivory, and Morris (2002) suggest that the following questions be answered with respect to information technology (IT) for public health in rural areas:

> What is the role of telehealth in public health?
> * What impact is distance learning having on the skills of rural public health professionals?
> * What are the costs and infrastructure implications of ensuring access to IT in rural areas?
> * How can IT be used to fill the gaps in epidemiology and surveillance capacity in rural health departments?

Performance Standards in Rural Public Health

The National Public Health Performance Standards Program (NPHPSP) is a collaborative effort, organized through the CDC, whose mission is to improve the quality of public health practice and the performance of local public health systems by providing and evaluating standards of performance.

The NPHPSP utilizes the Ten Essential Public Health Services to establish three assessment instruments that can be used by local and state public health systems for evaluation

CASE STUDY | Application of the Nursing Process

All three levels of prevention (i.e., primary, secondary, and tertiary) are reflected in rural practice. These are applied to individuals, families, and aggregates. The generalist nature of the rural community health practice gives the nurse an excellent opportunity to assess health needs and help improve health status at all levels of prevention. The following case study includes short-term individual and family approaches. It also focuses on upstream interventions developed to handle the identified problems. Upstream interventions focus on population and prevention. They deal with political, economic, and environmental factors that are precursors to health problems.

At 4:30 PM on a hot fall day, community health nurse Mary Fieldson, RN, drove up a narrow gravel township road 40 miles from her office in the county courthouse. She had just completed her sixth home health visit. By the time Mary returned home, she traveled more than 150 miles, but she enjoyed the drive. She worked in a rural county of 6000 where she grew up. She made a skilled visit to Joe Lingh, the father of a high school friend. On her way home, she traversed the valley where she once lived. She recently returned "home" after a 15-year absence to live, work, and raise her 12-year-old daughter.

When she approached the Connelly farm, Mary saw Eliza Connelly standing by the road waving her down. Mary stopped to say hello. Eliza said, "I called Ruth Lingh and she said you had just left. How is Joe's leg?" Mary was aware that this was a friendly inquiry about a neighbor of 40 years, but she was mindful of the need for confidentiality. Mary told Eliza that Joe was glad to be home from the hospital. Eliza asked if Mary had heard about her husband's accident Monday evening. "He cut his hand up in the silage chopper and is in the hospital in Spring City," she told Mary tearfully. "I just knew something was going to happen someday. I worry so much about them working with all that machinery and the men work in the fields alone so much. I feel about ready to fall apart. Thank God Jim [their son] was working with him when it happened!"

Mary had a cup of coffee with Eliza, who regained her composure. Eliza continued to talk about long-standing fears for the safety of her family in doing the farm work. She asked Mary to stop by and check on her husband, Austin, when he returned home the following week. Mary told Eliza to request a referral from the primary care physician so insurance would pay for the visits. At 5:30 PM Mary began the drive back to her office in Wolsey, the county seat.

Monday afternoon Mary received a telephone call from Dr. Lobban, the local primary care physician. He requested weekly skilled nursing visits for Austin for the next 3 weeks to assess the wound for infection and to teach Eliza how to change the dressings and recognize signs and symptoms of infection. Austin was discharged from the Spring City hospital the following day, 6 days after the injury. Dr. Lobban sent Mary the emergency room records and the hand specialist's discharge summary.

ASSESSMENT

The medical records provided the following information. The first finger was severed at the metacarpophalangeal joint (i.e., the third joint) and reattached. The second, third, and fourth fingers were severed distal to the proximal interphalangeal joints (i.e., between the first and second joints). The severed portions of the second, third, and fourth fingers could not be reattached because they were too badly mangled. At discharge, infection was not evident. The injuries were healing well.

The Connelly family provided additional information about the circumstances of the accident. At approximately 6:30 PM, Austin and his son, Jim, were chopping oats for silage. Seeing rain clouds on the horizon, Jim and Austin hurried to finish before rain fell on the unchopped grain. The silage chopper was not working well. Austin shut it off and hurriedly reached into the inspection hole. The still-turning blades caught his right hand, severing the fingers. Jim wrapped his father's hand tightly in his shirt, retrieved the fingers, and drove his father to their house two miles away. Jim went back to the field to finish chopping the oats. Eliza drove her husband 23 miles to the primary care hospital emergency room. The family physician cleaned and dressed Austin's hand, gave him medication for pain, and packed the severed fingers for transport to the hand specialist in Spring City. A family friend and his son drove Mr. and Mrs. Connelly 150 miles to the Spring City hospital where Austin was admitted and underwent surgery. Eliza went home with their friend and his son after the surgery. She spoke to Austin by telephone daily and drove to Spring City on Tuesday to bring him home.

On her first home visit Mary assessed the following:
- Individual client, Austin, for signs and symptoms of infection, pain control, and functional positioning
- Eliza's comfort level and knowledge of dressing changes and signs and symptoms of infection (i.e., she is the primary caregiver)
- Stress and grief processing of all family members
- Ability of family members to provide physical and emotional support during crisis resolution
- Risk-taking behaviors, especially those related to work, of all family members
- Assessment of neighborhood groups and neighbors who can provide support and help the family with the fall harvest work

DIAGNOSIS

Individual
- At risk for infection, pain, and loss of hand function (Austin)
- At risk for grief related to loss of fingers, some use of hand, and decreased ability to do farm work (Austin)
- Anxiety related to ongoing fear of injury of family members (Eliza)

Continued

- Stress related to new responsibilities for farm management (Jim)

Family
- At risk for family crisis related to instability caused by the injury

Community
- Inadequate programs for farm injury prevention
- Nonexistent EMS or first-response service

PLANNING

A plan of care is developed at the individual, family, and community levels. Mutual goal setting and contracting are essential if the outcomes are to be optimal.

Individual
Long-Term Goal
- Client will experience successful rehabilitation.

Short-Term Goals
- Client will remain free of infection.
- Individual family members will be able to express grief.

Family
Long-Term Goals
- Family will demonstrate coping skills appropriate to the crisis.
- Family will identify risky behavior related to farm work.

Short-Term Goals
- Identify support to help with farm work.
- Identify ways to keep in contact with each other when family members are working alone in the fields.

Community
Long-Term Goal
- Program will be established for farm injury prevention education for populations at risk.

Short-Term Goals
- Begin the health planning process to put into place a farm injury primary prevention program.
- Explore the potential for a volunteer EMS response team.

INTERVENTION

Mutual goal setting between Mary Fieldson and the Connelly family made it possible for them to carry out interventions collaboratively.

Individual
Mary taught Eliza how to change dressings and monitor Austin's hand for infection and function. Austin was involved in his care during healing and was able to monitor and manage the pain. He was most concerned about rehabilitation. He especially wanted to know when he could return to work and how disabled he would be. The local physician monitored Austin's progress. With Austin and Eliza present, the local physician consulted with the hand specialist by two-way interactive video conferencing. This enabled them to confer, thereby eliminating a 150-mile trip to Spring City. The home care PT visited the farm once to set up a program of hand exercises. Austin, who plays the piano, wanted to know if piano playing would be a good exercise. "Playing 'Moonlight Serenade' would sure stretch that right hand," he told the therapist. The therapist told him that he should play three times a day as part of the rehabilitation care plan.

Family
Mary worked with the family to find ways to finish the fall work. They decided to hire part-time help, and two workers helped full-time until the crop was harvested. While in the hospital, Austin was able to assist his son by supporting his ability to make the necessary decisions about farm management. After discharge, he also was able to participate in the process. The family identified the need for more awareness about the dangers of farm work. They immediately purchased a cellular phone to take to the field. Eliza felt this would relieve her anxiety about being out of touch with Austin and Jim and not knowing why they were later than expected for meals. There was much discussion about the cost of the telephone and service. Eliza convinced the men that her peace of mind was worth the cost.

The stress and grief reactions were minimal. Most of the stress centered on getting the fall farm work done and seeing that Austin recovered enough to work "the way he is used to doing." Support from neighbors and the rehabilitation program helped them deal with stress and grief.

Community
When an accident happens in a small rural community, it brings home the dangerous nature of farm work. People begin recalling their own "close calls" and remembering friends and family members who have been injured. This period of high awareness is an excellent time to bring people together to discuss accident prevention. During the annual fall 4-H Achievement Days, Mary Fieldson set up an information booth in the exhibit hall and asked for volunteers to plan and implement a farm safety program in the county.

Austin's accident was handled appropriately by the family without EMS intervention. However, others had recently required trained personnel at the site to stabilize the injured person and minimize damage during transport to the primary care hospital. For Mary, her home care visits to farm families reinforced the need for EMS in these remote areas. She met with the county health department, local physicians, and county commissioners to investigate the feasibility of establishing an EMS.

CASE STUDY | Application of the Nursing Process (cont'd)

EVALUATION

Individual

Individual members of the Connelly family used the home care nurse, PT, and local physician appropriately as evidenced by Austin's successful healing and rehabilitation. Austin returned to work with minimum disability. During a drop-in visit by Mary 3 months after the accident, Austin treated her to a rousing piano rendition of "Stars and Stripes Forever."

Family

With Mary's guidance, the family wrote down a list of hazards and strategies to improve safety on the farm. Interestingly, one of the items was to wear seat belts in the car and truck. The family installed seat belts in a 40-year-old farm truck still in regular use. They purchased the cellular phone and used it to keep Eliza in touch with Austin and Jim while they were in the field. This has proven so successful that several neighbors have also bought cellular phones.

The family continued to demonstrate good coping skills as Austin progressed in his rehabilitation. Communication between father and son was excellent after the initial concern that Austin would feel like his position as farm manager was being usurped. He became involved with daily decision making as soon as he returned home from the hospital. The family effectively solved the problem of getting the fall work done by requesting the help of friends and neighbors. They borrowed money from the bank to hire a part-time farm hand until Austin could work again.

Community

Mary's information booth at the 4-H Achievement Days attracted the attention of several women from the County Extension Club. As a result of their interest, the club made farm safety education their service project for the following year. Lack of community support halted development of a volunteer emergency medical first-response team.

LEVELS OF PREVENTION

The following are examples of the three levels of prevention as applied to the individual, family, and community.

Primary

- Assessment and teaching about farm accident prevention to family
- Initiation of a program of farm safety information at the community level
- Use of a cellular telephone to decrease anxiety about family members' locations and well-being

Secondary

- Infection prevention and pain management of injured hand
- Screening at family and community level for farm hazards (i.e., a component of the overall primary prevention education program)

Tertiary

- Rehabilitation of Austin to limit disability
- Assessment and counseling to help family and injured individual cope with stress and grief reactions
- Attempted development of an EMS system to facilitate stabilization and safe transport

---

and improvement. Standards describe an optimal level of performance by public health systems, which include all public, private, and voluntary entities that contribute to activities directed toward public health in an assessment area. The assessment can be used to improve collaborations among key public health partners, educate participants about public health, strengthen the network of public health partners, identify strengths and weaknesses, and provide benchmarks for public health practice improvements (CDC, 2004a). Research questions that need to be addressed in rural areas may focus on the extent to which state and local performance assessments outlined by NPHPSP have been carried out, as well as the ability of rural public health systems to respond to needed changes to comprehensively address essential services. Additionally, rural areas may benefit from research examining resource constraints and the need to expand partnerships to address essential services that may be challenging to provide within isolated populations.

Leadership and Workforce Capacity for Rural Public Health

In 2003, the IOM published results of a project intended to improve our understanding of what is needed to prepare the public health workforce for the twenty-first century (Gebbie, Rosenstock, and Hernandez, 2003). Workforce capacity challenges cited by the IOM report include globalization, which increases travel and allows for distribution of emerging and reemerging diseases (e.g., HIV and AIDS, tuberculosis, hepatitis B, malaria, cholera, diphtheria, and Ebola); advances in scientific and medical technologies that challenge the public health workforce in areas of ethics, data security, and communication; and demographic transformations that require new skills and services as our population ages and becomes more diverse.

The Public Health Workforce Development initiative (CDC, 2004b), created jointly by the CDC and the Agency for Toxic Substances and Disease Registry (ATSDR) to address future challenges to public health workforce development, outlines six strategies to prepare a competent workforce that will be able to perform the essential public health services in light of new challenges. This initiative suggests that an initial strategy is to monitor workforce composition and conduct research to validate methodology for public health worker enumeration. Other areas of needed research for workforce development include understanding discipline-specific competencies, developing and testing educational curricula, expanding and testing technology-supported learning systems, and testing the basic assumption that improvements in both quantity and quality of the public health workforce will translate to better performance of core public health functions.

Interaction and Integration of Community Health Systems, Managed Care, and Public Health

The evolution of managed care into rural environments has limited the safety-net role of some local health departments to provide primary care by preventing fee-for-service reimbursement and contracting care to networks of providers or organizations. This is especially true for Medicaid managed care, which serves that same population of people that are traditionally served with primary care services through local public health departments. As Hurley, Crawford, and Praeger (2002) note, Medicaid's importance for rural areas is likely to grow as broader health care developments, such as declining inpatient use of rural hospitals and reductions in Medicare reimbursement, provoke more interest in using the Medicaid system to support threatened rural infrastructure.

Consequently, the administration of the Medicaid program will increasingly seek the cost savings promised by managed care, and the role of rural public health departments may increasingly narrow into areas that are currently without any type of reimbursement. Because of this, Berkowitz, Ivory, and Morris (2002) argue that finding ways to integrate public health in the rural primary care at the community level will become increasingly important. There will be many questions to be answered by additional research. What are the factors associated with successful integration of public health and managed care in rural environments? What capacity do rural health departments have for contracting arraignments with managed care organizations? What are the effects of local public health and managed care contracts on direct provision of services?

SUMMARY

This chapter provides an overview of rural and migrant health. People who live in rural areas make up 61 million, or approximately 25%, of the U.S. population. The reader must not assume that all rural people are similar; diversity exists in age, ethnicity, income, education, and geography.

Not all rural residents are disadvantaged. The data show that in some ways they are penalized as a whole, no matter how diverse the rural population. Health care access and income levels are areas where disadvantages generally exist. Provider shortages, an ineffective health care system, hospital-based

and community-based care, and little health promotion and disease prevention services represent a marginal health care network. One half of the poor in the United States live in rural areas. The combination of poor health care access and low income level results in higher morbidity and mortality rates in rural populations. The high-risk nature of such occupations as farmworkers, miners, and loggers also contributes to disability and death rates. This chapter describes the structural, financial, and personal barriers contributing to poor health care access.

Nurses who work with rural people must assess each aggregate's characteristics. A ranching community in Wyoming will have different needs than a migrant community in Arizona. Demographic information, aggregate morbidity and mortality data, emerging rural nursing theory, knowledge of barriers, and rural health care research are all necessary to plan appropriate upstream community health nursing interventions. Integrating these concepts gives nurses the tools to improve the health of rural people.

LEARNING ACTIVITIES

1. University libraries commonly subscribe to newspapers published within the state. Visit the library and select three to four small town or rural county newspapers. Read them for information about health care activities and concerns related to the health of the individuals, families, and community.
   * Report findings to the class about rural health concerns and activities.
   * Identify one priority problem that could be researched in the community and has relevance to rural community health nursing practice.
2. Select a rural community health nurse (i.e., public health or home care), and conduct an interview in person or by telephone if distance prohibits a face-to-face meeting.
   * Identify what the nurse sees as the pros and cons of rural nursing.
   * If negative aspects of rural nursing are identified, discuss how the nurse deals with them.
   * Ask the nurse to discuss the three highest priority efforts related to his or her rural practice.
3. Choose one of the major causes of morbidity and mortality in migrant populations.
   * On the basis of risk factor and natural history, specify interventions for primary, secondary, and tertiary prevention of this problem.
   * Identify which of these interventions are examples of upstream thinking.
4. Locate a telephone book or community resource directory from a rural community.
   * List and evaluate the resources that are available for prevention, assessment, intervention, and follow-up care for the major cause of mortality and morbidity identified in Learning Activity 3.
   * Would it be necessary to go outside the rural town or county for any of the needed resources? Which ones? Where might they be located?

REFERENCES

American Nurses Association: *Rural/frontier nursing: the challenge to grow,* Washington, DC, 1996, The Author.

American Nurses Association: *Scope and standards of parish nursing practice,* Washington, DC, 1998, The Author.

American Psychological Association, Office of Rural Health: *Caring for the rural community,* Washington, DC, 1995 The Author.

Amundson B: Myth and reality in the rural health service crisis: facing up to community responsibilities, *J Rural Health* 9:176-187, 1993.

Association of State and Territorial Directors of Nursing: *Quad Council PHN Competencies,* 2003, The Association, http://www.astdn.org.

Baer LD, Smith LM: Nonphysician professionals and rural America. In Ricketts TC, editor: *Rural health in the United States,* New York, 1999, Oxford University Press.

Bechtel GA, Davidhizar R: Community health strategies: an innovative education strategy in a migrant farm community, *Nurse Educ* 24(1):23-24, 1999.

Berkowitz, B. Rural public health service delivery: Promising new directions. *Am J Public Health,* 94(10): 1678-1681, 2004.

Berkowitz B, Ivory J, Morris T: Rural public health: policy and research opportunities. *J Rural Health,* 18(suppl):186-196, 2002.

Beyers M: The new nursing shortage, *JONAS Healthc Law Ethics Regul* 1(3):22-24, Sept 1999.

Bigbee J: The uniqueness of rural nursing, *Nurs Clin North Am* 28:131-144, 1993.

Blair A, Zahm SH: Epidemiologic studies of cancer among agricultural populations. In McDuffie H et al, editors: *Agricultural health and safety: workplace, environment, sustainability,* Boca Raton, Fla, 1995, CRC Press.

Bolin J, Gamm LG. Access to quality health services in rural areas: insurance. In *Rural Healthy People 2010: A Companion Document to Healthy People 2010. Volume 1.* College Station, Tex: The Texas A&M University System Health Science Center, School of Rural Public Health, 2003, Southwest Rural Health Research Center.

Braden J, Beauregard K: *Health status and access to care of rural and urban populations,* AHCPR Pub No 94-0031, National Medical Expenditure Survey Research Findings 18, Rockville, Md, February, 1994, PHS.

Buckwalter KC et al: Telehealth for elders and their caregivers in rural communities, *Fam Community Health* 25(3):31-40, 2002.

Buehler J, Lee H: Exploration of home care resources for rural families with cancer, *Cancer Nurs* 15:299-308, 1992.

Bureau of Health Professions: *Changing demographics: implications for physicians, nurses, and other health workers,* 2003, The Author, ftp://ftp.hrsa.gov/bhpr/nationalcenter/changedemo.pdf.

Bureau of Primary Healthcare: *Migrant and seasonal farmworker enumeration profiles study,* 2000, The Author, http://bphc.hrsa.gov/migrant/Enumeration/EnumerationStudy.htm.

Centers for Disease Control and Prevention: *National Public Health Performance Standards Program,* 2004a, The Author, http://www.cdc.gov/od/ocphp/nphpsp/.

Centers for Disease Control and Prevention: *The Public Health Workforce Development Initiative,* 2004b, http://www.phppo.cdc.gov/owpp/workforcedev.asp#Workforce%20Development%20Library.

Centers for Disease Control and Prevention, National Center for Health Statistics: *HHS issues report on community health in rural, urban areas: HHS News,* 2001, the Center http://www.cdc.gov/nchs/pressroom/01news/hus01.html.

Centers for Disease Control and Prevention, National Center for Injury Prevention and Control: *CDC fact book: different People, different injuries, 2002,* pp. 1-7. The Author, http://www.cdc.gov/ncipc/fact-book.

Chase-Ziolek M, Striep J: A comparison of urban versus rural experiences of nurses volunteering to promote health in churches, *Public Health Nurs* 16(4):270-279, 1999.

Clancy F: Rural rx, *Harrowsmith Country Life* 2:31-37, 1992.

Cohen RA, Bloom B: *Trends in health insurance and access to medical care for children under age 19 years: United States, 1998-2003.* Advance data from vital and health statistics; no 355, Hyattsville, Md, 2005, National Center for Health Statistics.

Cohen RA, Martinez ME.and Hao, CK K: *Health insurance coverage: estimates from the National Health Interview Survey, January-September, 2004,* Centers for Disease Control and Prevention, Division of Health Interview Statistics, National Center for Health Statistics, http://www.cdc.gov/nchs/nhis.htm.

Cotton DJ et al: *Grain* dust and alveolar macrophages: an experimental study of the effects of grain dust on the mouse lung. In Dosman JA and Cockcroft DW, editors: *Principles of health and safety in agriculture,* Boca Raton, Fla, 1989, CRC Press.

Daniels N, Kennedy BP, Kawachi I: Why justice is good for our health: the social determinants of health inequalities. *Daedalus* 128:215-251.

Davis D, Droes N: Community health nursing in rural and frontier counties, *Nurs Clin North Am* 28:159-169, 1993.

Division of Shortage Designation, Bureau of Primary Health Care: *Selected statistics on health professional shortage areas: as of December 31, 1998,* Bethesda, Md, 1998, Health Resources and Services Administration, USDHHS.

Dolphin N: Rural health. In Logan B, Dawkins C, editors: *Family centered nursing in the community,* Menlo Park, Calif, 1984, Addison-Wesley.

Dunbar J, Mueller C: *Anticipating the 1997 state children's health insurance program: what's current in five rural states?* Bethesda, Md, January 1998, The Project HOPE Walsh Center for Rural Health Analysis.

Dunkin J et al: Job satisfaction and retention of rural community health nurses in North Dakota, *J Rural Health* 8:268-275, 1992.

Eberhardt MS et al: *Urban and Rural Health Chartbook, 2001,* Department of Health and Human Services, Centers for Disease Control and Prevention, National Center for Health Statistics. Hyattsville, Md, National Center for Health Statistics, http://www.cdc.gov/nchs/pressroom/01news/hus01.htm.

Eberhardt MS, Pamuk ER: The importance of place of residence: examining health in rural and nonrural areas, *Am J Public Health* 94(10):1682-1686, 2004.

Edmondson W: *Economics of the food and fiber system, 2004,* amber waves, US Department of Agriculture, Economic Research Service, http://www.ers.usda.gov/AmberWaves/February04/DataFeature/.

Eggebeen D, Lichter D: Health and well-being among rural Americans: variations across the life course, *J Rural Health* 9:86-98, 1993.

Elison G: Frontier areas: problems for delivery of health care services, *Rural Health Care* 8:1-3, 1986.

Environmental Protection Agency: *Recognition and management of pesticide poisonings, ed 4,* EPA Pub No 540/9-88-001, Washington, DC, 1989, US Government Printing Office.

Farmer F, Clark L, Miller M: Consequences of differential residence designations for rural health policy: the case of infant mortality, *J Rural Health* 9:17-26, 1993.

Fasciano MK et al: Preparing rural communities for managed care: lessons learned, *J Rural Health* 15(1):78-86, 1999.

Flowers L, Gross L, Kuo P, Sinclair S: *State profiles: reforming the health care system, ed 13,* Washinton, DC, 2005, American Association of Retired Persons Public Policy Institute. http://www.aarp.org/research/health/care-financing/reform_profiles.html.

Fuchs VR: *Who shall live? Health, economics and social choice,* River Edge, NJ, 1998, World Scientific Publishing.

Furlow L: Crisis in the country: addressing the challenges of rural trauma care, *Texas J Rural Health* 17(1):4-6, 1999.

Gabos S, Fincham S, Berkel J: The interaction between farming occupation and exposure to smoking in squamous carcinomas of the lip. In McDuffie H et al, editors: *Agricultural health and safety: workplace, environment, sustainability,* Boca Raton, Fla, 1995, CRC Press.

Gamm LD, Castillo G, and Pittman S: Access to Quality Health Services in Rural Areas-primary care: A Literature Review. In Gamm LD, Hutchison L, Dabney RJ, Dorsey AM, editors: *Rural Healthy People 2010: a companion document to Health People 2010,* Volume 2. College Station, Tex, 2003, The Texas A&M University System Health Science Center, School of Rural Public Health, 2003, Southwest Rural Health Research Center.

Gamm LD, Hutchison L: Rural Healthy People 2010: evolving interactive practice, *Am J Public Health* 94(10):1711-1712, 2004.

Gamm LG, Stone S, Pittman S: *Mental health and mental disorders: a rural challenge, Rural Healthy People 2010: a companion document to Healthy People 2010,* Volume 1. College Station, Tex: The Texas A&M University System Health Science Center, School of Rural Public Health, 2003, Southwest Rural Health Research Center.

Gamm LD, Hutchison L, Dabney RJ, Dorsey AM, editors: *Rural Healthy People 2010: a companion document to Healthy People 2010,* Volumes 1-3, College Station, Texas, 2003, The Texas A&M University System Health Science Center, School of Rural Public Health, 2003, Southwest Rural Health Research Center.

Gebbie K, Rosenstock L, Hernandez LM: *Who will keep the public healthy? Educating public health professionals for the 21ˢᵗ century,* Washington, DC, 2003, The National Academies Press.

Glover S et al: Disparities in access to care among rural working-age adults, *J Rural Health* 20(3):193-205, 2004.

Gosschalk A, Carozza S: Cancer in rural areas. In Gamm, LD, Hutchison L, Dabney RJ, Dorsey AM, editors: *Rural Healthy People 2010: a companion document to Healthy People 2010,* Volumes 1-3. College Station, Tex, 2003, The Texas A&M University System Health Science Center, School of Rural Public Health, Southwest Rural Health Research Center.

Griffin J: Parish nursing in rural communities. In Solari-Twadell PA, McDermott MA, editors: *Parish nursing: promoting whole person health within faith communities,* Thousand Oaks, Calif, 1999, Sage Publications.

Hartley D: Rural health disparities, population health, and rural culture. *Am J Public Health* 94(10):1675-1678, 2004.

Herbert R, Landrigan PJ: Work-related death: A continuing epidemic. *Am J Public Health* 90(4):541-545, 2000.

Hoyer, DL, Kung, HC, Smith, BL: Deaths: Preliminary data for 2003, *Natl Vital Stat Rep* 53(15). Hyattsville, Md, 2005 National Center for Health Statistics.

Hurley RE, Crawford H, Praeger S: Medicaid and rural health care. *J Rural Health* 18(suppl): 164-175, 2002.

Hutchison L, Blakely C: Substance abuse: trends in rural areas. In Institute of Medicine: *Community oriented primary care,* Washington, DC, 1983, National Academy Press.

Institute of Medicine: *Quality through collaboration: the future of public health,* Washington, DC, 2005, National Academy Press.

International Parish Nurse Resource Center: *Information for clergy,* http://ipnrc.parishnurses.org/forcl.phtml. Retrieved April 21, 2005.

Jones HP, Brand MK: Providing rehabilitative services in rural communities: report of a conference, *J Rural Health* 11(2):122-127, 1995.

Kaiser Family Foundation: *State health facts,* 2004, The Author, http://www.statehealthfacts.org/.

Kandel W, Cromartie J: *Hispanics find a home in rural America,* 2003, Amber Waves, US Department of Agriculture, Economic Research Service, http://www.ers.usda.gov/AmberWaves/.

Kass BL, Weinick RM, Monheit AC: *Racial and ethnic differences in health*: 1996, MEPS Chartbook No 2, Pub No 99-0001, Rockville, Md, 1999, Agency for Health Care Policy and Research.

Kaye LW et al: Early intervention screening for family caregivers of older relatives in primary care practices: establishing a community health service alliance in rural America, *Fam Community Health* 26(4):319-328, 2002.

Larson A: *Migrant health issues: nvironmental/occupational safety and health,* 2001, http://www.ncfh.org/docs/02%20-%20environ-ment.pdf.

Lisnerski DD et al: Demographic and predictive correlates of smokeless tobacco use in elementary school children, *Am J Health Promot* 5:426-431, 1991.

Long K, Boik R: Predicting alcohol use in rural children: a longitudinal study, *Nurs Res* 42: 79-86, 1993.

Mautino K: Law watch: the new amnesty, *J Immigr Health* 6(3):101-102, 2004.

McCabe S, Macnee C: Weaving a new safely net of mental health care in rural America: a model of integrated practice, *Issues Ment Health Nurs* 23(3):263-278, 2002.

Memmott R: Developing hospice programs in frontier communities. In Bushy A, editor: *Rural nursing,* Volume 2, Newbury Park, Calif, 1991, Sage Publications.

Miller M, Farmer F, Clarke L: Rural populations and their health. In Beaulieu J, Berry D, editors: *Rural health services: a management perspective,* Ann Arbor, Mich, 1994, AUPHA Press, Health Administration Press.

Morrison HI et al: Mortality among Canadian fruit and vegetable farmers. In McDuffie H et al, editors: *Agricultural health and safety: workplace, environment, sustainability,* Boca Raton, Fla, 1995, CRC Press.

Moscovice I, Wellever A, Christianson J: Understanding integrated rural health networks, *Milbank Quarterly* 75(4): 563-588, 1997.

Mueller K, Coburn A, Cordes S: The changing landscape of health care financing and delivery: How are rural communities and providers responding? *Milbank Q* 77(4):485-510, 1999.

Mueller C, Schur C: Insurance coverage of prescription drugs and the rural elderly, *J Rural Health,* 20(1):17-25, 2004.

National Center for Health Statistics: *Health, United States, with chartbook on trends in the health of Americans,* 2004, Centers for Disease Control and Prevention, http://www.cdc.gov/nchs/hus.htm.

National Institute for Occupational Safety and Health, *Worker health chartbook,* 2004. NIOSH Pub No. 2004-146., Cincinnati OH, 2004, The Author.

National Rural Health Association: *Managed care as a service delivery model in rural areas,* Issue paper, Kansas City, Mo, 1995, The Author.

National Rural Health Association: *Rural and frontier emergency medical services toward the year 2000,* Issue paper, Kansas City, Mo, 1997, The Author.

National Rural Health Association: *A vision for health reform models for America's rural communities,* Issue paper, Kansas City, Mo, 1998, The Author.

National Rural Health Association: *Mental health in rural America,* Issue paper, Kansas City, Mo, May 1999.

National Rural Health Association: *What's different about rural health care?* The Author, http://www.nrharural.org/about/sub/different.html.

Nevas-Walt C, Proctor BD, Mills RJ: *Income, poverty, and health insurance coverage in the United States: 2003,* US Census Bureau, Current Population Reports P60-226, Washington, DC, US Government Printing Office.

Office of Management and Budget: Standards for defining metropolitan and micropolitan statistical areas, *Fed Reg* 65(249):82228, 2000.

Office of Rural Health Policy, Health Resources and Services Administration: *Rural Hospital Flexibility Grant Progam,* Rockville Md, 1999, USDHHS. http://ruralhealth.hrsa.gov/funding/flex.htm. Retrieved April 29, 2005.

Pan S, Straub L, Szigeti E: Factors influencing nurses to practice in rural areas, *Texas J Public Health* 16(2):5-14, 1998.

Pasko T, Seidman B, and Birkhead S: *Physician characteristics and distribution in the U.S.* Chicago, Ill, 2000-2001, American Medical Association.

Peek-Asa C, Zwerling C, Stallones L: Acute traumatic injuries in rural populations, *Am J Public Health* 94(10):1689-1693, 2004.

Phillips CD: Health in rural America: Remembering the importance of place. *Am J Public Health,* 94(10):1661-1663, 2004.

Pickle LW, et al: *Atlas of United States mortality,* Hyattsville, Md, 1996, Centers for Disease Control and Prevention, NCHS.

Probst JC et al: Person and place: the compounding effects of race/ethnicity and rurality on health, *Am J Public Health* 94(10): 1695-1703, 2004.

Pullen C: Modern technology brings nursing education into rural students' homes, *Rural Clinician Q* 8(3):3-5, 1998.

Purdy J: The new culture of rural America, *The American Prospect,* December 20, 1999, pp 26-31.

Rawlinson C, Crews P: Access to quality health services in rural areas: emergency medical services. In Gamm LD, Hutchison L, Dabney RJ, Dorsey AM, editors: *Rural Healthy People 2010: a companion document to Health People 2010,* Volume 1. College Station, Texas, 2003, The Texas A&M University System Health Science Center, School of Rural Public Health, Southwest Rural Health Research Center.

Reschovsky JD, Cunningham PJ: *CHIPing away at the problem of uninsured children,* Issue Brief No 14, Washington, DC, 1998, Center for Studying Health System Change.

Ricketts TC, Heaphy P: Hospitals in rural America. In Ricketts TC, editor: *Rural health in the United States*, New York, 1999, Oxford University Press.

Ricketts TC, Johnson-Webb KD, Randolph RK: Populations and places in rural America. In Ricketts TC, editor: *Rural health in the United States*, New York, 1999, Oxford University Press.

Rogers, CC, The older population in 21st century rural America, *Rural America* 17(3), 2002, http://www.ers.usda.gov/publications/ruralamerica/ra173/ra173b.pdf.

Rohrer JE: *Planning for community oriented health systems,* ed 2, Washington, DC, 1999, American Public Health Association.

Rosenblatt RA, Casey S, Richardson M: Rural-urban differences in the public health workforce: local health departments in 3 Western states, *Am J Public Health* 92(7):1102-1105, 2002.

Sanford JT, Townsend-Rocchiccioli J: The perceived health of rural caregivers, *Geriatr Nurs* 75(3):145-148, 2004.

Scharff KE: The distinctive nature and scope of rural nursing practice: philosophical bases. In Lee HJ, editor: *Conceptual basis for rural nursing*, New York, 1998, Springer.

Schenker MA: General health status and epidemiologic considerations in studying migrant and seasonal farmworkers. In McDuffie H et al, editors: *Agricultural health and safety: workplace, environment, sustainability*, Boca Raton, Fla, 1995, CRC Press.

School of Journalism, University of Montana: *A health crisis,* Missoula, Mont, 1993, The Missoulian.

Shreffler MJ: An ecological view of the rural environment: levels of influence on access to health care, *Adv Nurs Sci* 18(4):48-59, 1996.

Sigma Theta Tau International: *Facts on the nursing shortage,* 2006, The Author, http://www.nursingsociety.org/media/facts_nursing shortage.html.

Slifkin RT, Randolph R, Ricketts TC: The changing metropolitan designation process and rural America, *J Rural Health* 20(1):1-6, 2004.

Struttmann TW et al: Equipment dealers' perceptions of a community-based rollover protective structures promotion campaign, *J Rural Health* 17(2):131-139, 2001.

Swanson LL: Minorities represent growing share of tomorrow's work force, *Rural Cond Trends* 9(2):1-5, 1999.

Turner T, Gunn I: Issues in rural health nursing. In Bushy A, editor: *Rural nursing,* volume 2, Newbury Park, Calif, 1991, Sage Publications.

US Census Bureau: *Historical health insurance tables,* 2004a, The Author, http://www.census.gov/hhs/www/hlthins/historic/hihistt1.html.

US Census Bureau: *Small area income and poverty estimates: annual estimates for states, counties and school districts,* 2004b, http://www.census.gov/hhes/www/saipe/saipe.html.

US Department of Agriculture, Economic Research Service: *The economics of food, farming, natural resources, and rural America, United States farm and farm-related employment,* 2002, The Author, http://www.ers.usda.gov/Data/FarmandRelatedEmployment/.

US Department of Agriculture, Economic Research Service: *Rural education at a glance,* 2004, Rural Development Research Report, No 98, http://www.ers.usda.gov/publications/rdrr98.

US Department of Agriculture, Economic Research Service: *Rural poverty at a glance,* 2004, Rural Development Research Report, No 100, http://www.ers.usda.gov/Publications/rdrr100/.

US Department of Agriculture, Economic Research Service: *Rural children at a glance,* Economic Information Bulletin, No 1, March 2005, http://www.ers.usda.gov/Emphases/Rural.

US Department of Health and Human Services, Public Health Service: *Healthy People 2010: Volume I, Understanding and Improving health,* 2000, US Department of Health and Human Services, Leading Health Indicators, 2002, The Author, http://www.healthypeople.gov/LHI/.

US Department of Health and Human Services, Public Health Service: *Progress review public health infrastructure,* 2004, http://www.healthypeople.gov/LHI/.

US Department of Health and Human Services, *The 2006 HHS poverty guidelines: one version of the [U.S.] Federal Poverty Measure,* 2006, The Author, http://www.aspe.hhs.gov/poverty/06poverty.shtml.

US Department of Health and Human Services, Centers for Medicare and Medicaid Services, 2004, the Author, http://www.cms.hhs.gov/CertificationCompliance/04.

US Department of Health and Human Services, Health Resources and Services Administration: *Rural health policy: Rural Hospital Flexibility Grant Program,* The Author, http://www.rural-health.hrsa.gov/funding/flex.html.

Van Hook R: Foreword. In Straub L, Walzer N, editors: *Rural health care: innovation in a changing environment,* Westport, Conn, 1992, Praeger Press.

Villarejo D, Barron SL: The occupational health status of hired farmworkers, *State Art Rev Occup Med* 14:613-635, 1999.

Voelker R: Does managed care fit for rural America? *Adv RWJ Newslett,* Issue 4, 1998.

Warren CP: Overview of respiratory health risks in agriculture. In Dosman JA, Cockcroft DW, editors: *Principals of health and safety in agriculture,* Boca Raton, Fla, 1989, CRC Press.

Weinert C, Long KA: Understanding the health care needs of rural families, *Fam Relat* 36:450-455, 1987.

Weinert C, Long KA: Rural families and health care: refining the knowledge base, *J Marriage Fam Rev* 15:57-75, 1990.

Welton WE, Kantner TA, Katz SM: Developing tomorrow's integrated community health systems: a leadership challenge for public health and primary care, *Milbank Q* 75(2): 261-288, 1997.

Whitener LA, McGranahan DA: *Rural America: opportunities and challenges,* 2003, Amber Waves, US Department of Agriculture, Economic Research Service. http://www.ers.usda.gov/AmberWaves/.

Wilk VA: Reducing health risks; farmworker women working together. In McDuffie H et al, editors: *Agricultural health and safety: workplace, environment, sustainability,* Boca Raton, FL, 1995, CRC Press.

W.K. Kellogg Foundation: *Perceptions of rural America,* 2001, The Foundation, http://www.wkkf.org.

Zahm SH, Blair A: Cancer among migrant and seasonal farmworkers: an epidemiologic review and research agenda, *Am J Ind Med* 24(6):753-766, 1993.

Zahner SJ, Corrado SM: Local health department partnerships with faith-based organizations, *J Public Health Manag Pract* 10(3): 258-265.

22

Populations Affected by Mental Illness

Melanie McEwen ▪ Jane Mahoney

MEDIA RESOURCES

Additional Material for Study, Review, and Further Exploration

evolve Website at http://evolve.elsevier.com/Nies

❖ Quiz ❖ Case Studies ❖ Content Updates ❖ Glossary ❖ WebLinks

OBJECTIVES

Upon completion of this chapter, the reader will be able to do the following:

1. Explain the concept of mental health and discuss the importance of mental health promotion.
2. Discuss the influence of deinstitutionalization on mental health aggregates.
3. Describe some of the most common types of mental illnesses encountered in community settings.
4. Discuss the problem of suicide and recognize risk factors.
5. Describe different types of treatment for mental disorders, including use of psychotherapeutic medications, psychotherapy, and behavior therapy.
6. Describe the role of mental health nurses in the community.

KEY TERMS

agoraphobia
anorexia nervosa
anxiety disorder
attention deficit disorder
attention deficit hyperactivity disorder
bipolar disorder
bulimia nervosa
Community Mental Health

Centers Act
deinstitutionalization
depression
dysthymia
generalized anxiety disorder (GAD)
major depression
marginalization

Mental Health Equitable Treatment Act
mental health
mental illness
obsessive-compulsive disorder
panic disorder
phobia

posttraumatic stress disorder
Program of Assertive Community Treatment (PACT)
psychotherapeutic medications
schizophrenia

CHAPTER OUTLINE

OVERVIEW AND HISTORY OF COMMUNITY MENTAL HEALTH
Age of Confinement
Mental Health Reform
Medicalization of Mental Illness
Community Mental Health and Deinstitutionalization
Decade of the Brain

HEALTHY PEOPLE 2010 AND MENTAL HEALTH

FACTORS INFLUENCING MENTAL HEALTH
Biological Factors
Social Factors
Political Factors

MENTAL DISORDERS ENCOUNTERED IN COMMUNITY SETTINGS
Overview of Selected Mental Disorders

IDENTIFICATION AND MANAGEMENT OF MENTAL DISORDERS
Identification of Mental Disorders
Management of Mental Disorders

COMMUNITY-BASED MENTAL HEALTH CARE

ROLE OF THE COMMUNITY MENTAL HEALTH NURSE

"Mental health is a state of successful performance of mental function, resulting in productive activities, fulfilling relationships with other people, and the ability to adapt to change and to cope with adversity" (U.S. Department of Health and Human Services [USDHHS], 2000, p. 18-3). Mental health refers not only to the absence of mental disorders but also to the ability of an individual to negotiate daily challenges and social interactions of life without experiencing cognitive, emotional, or behavioral dysfunction. Mental health and mental disorders can be affected by numerous factors, such as biological and genetic vulnerabilities, acute or chronic physical dysfunction, environmental conditions, and stressors. Consider the following statistics (USDHHS/ Substance Abuse and Mental Health Services Administration [SAMHSA], 2005):

- Mental disorders affect approximately 20% of the U.S. population.
- Each year, almost 10% of the adult population will experience "serious psychological distress."
- About 20% of children and adolescents (9 to 17 years of age) have a diagnosable mental disorder (e.g., depression, autism, and attention deficit hyperactivity disorder [ADHD]) during a given year.
- Schizophrenia affects about 1% of the adult population at any one time.
- Major depression is a leading cause of disability (measured by the number of years lived with a disabling condition among persons age 5 and older).
- Depression and associated affective/mood disorders affect about 5% of the population of the United States at any one time; approximately 14.7% of the population has experienced at least one episode of major depression.
- Suicide, a potential outcome of mental illness and mental disorders, was the 11th leading cause of death in the United States in 2001, and the third leading cause of death among 15- to 24-year-olds.
- Only about 25% of persons with a mental disorder obtain help for their illness in the health care system.
- Persons hospitalized with major depression account for more bed days than any impairment except cardiovascular disorders.
- Individuals with job-related stress and depression miss an average of 16 work days annually.

Community health nurses face the challenge of providing mental health services to an increasing number of clients with fewer resources. Historically, people with mental illness have been treated in acute care settings, but now the vast majority reside in the community where most have only limited access to mental health services. Across the nation, acute care settings have downsized, private insurance reimburses fewer mental health services, and waiting lists in publicly funded mental health centers grow longer. This state of affairs is a result of the following factors: decreased state and federal funding, managed care, discriminate private insurance coverage, and the influence of deinstitutionalization (Torrey, 1997). The purpose of this chapter is to illuminate critical issues that affect the mental health of communities and explore the potential influence that nurses have on these issues. It also provides basic information on mental illnesses encountered in community settings and explores the environmental, biological, social, and political factors that influence mental health. Finally, some of the most commonly encountered options for management of mental illness are discussed.

OVERVIEW AND HISTORY OF COMMUNITY MENTAL HEALTH

Words used to describe people with mental illness have been a source of social and political debate. Historically, words and labels assigned to people with mental illness have been a source of discrimination and stigma (Corrigan and Penn, 1999). For example, the words *crazy, insane,* and *deranged* conjure images of violence, fear, and intellectual inadequacy. Others, such as *nuts, crackers,* or *flake,* appear to trivialize or even minimize the impact of mental illness.

The stigma and discrimination many people diagnosed with mental illness experience are unfounded and based on faulty assumptions and misinformation. People diagnosed with mental illness are neighbors, colleagues, and family members. Most people diagnosed with mental illness are productive members of the community and have meaningful lives.

Throughout this chapter, the concepts of mental health and mental illness are used frequently. Mental health is more than absence of mental illness. There are varying degrees of mental health; not one characteristic is indicative of good mental health nor can lack of one characteristic indicate a mental illness. In general, **mental health** is determined by how a person feels about himself or herself, how a person feels about others, and how a person meets the demands of everyday life (National Mental Health Association, 1996). Further, mental health incorporates the ability to adapt to distress by mobilizing internal and external resources to minimize tension. Mentally healthy individuals are independent, have positive self-image, are self-actualized and autonomous, and are able to form meaningful interpersonal relationships (Antai-Otong, 2003; Stuart & Laraia, 2005). **Mental illness**, in contrast, refers to maladaptive responses to distress and an inability to mobilize resources. The mentally ill person is often dependent, has low self-esteem, and has difficulty forming interpersonal relationships (Antai-Otong, 2003).

Since recorded history, communities have been both formally and informally caring for members with mental illness. The evolution of community mental health is discussed in the following five phases: Age of Confinement, mental health reform, medicalization of mental illness, deinstitutionalization, and Decade of the Brain. Identification and treatment of people with mental illness in communities during each phase has generally been based on the ability to characterize individual behavior or personality as different from the social norm.

Age of Confinement

The "Age of Confinement" refers to the very early years of establishment of the colonies and the republic. During this time period, individuals who behaved in ways inconsistent with social norms were labeled "mad," separated from their communities, and placed in the custodial care of the state. Poverty, homelessness, alcoholism, seizure disorders, and mental illness were all illnesses or life conditions that created rationale for placement in asylums.

Conditions in the early asylums were frequently deplorable. Individuals residing in these asylums were often restrained, whipped, ill fed, unwashed, and treated with bloodletting, purgatives, and other "curative" therapies. In addition, madness was attributed to idleness; therefore treatment included forced labor. The early asylums became places of harborage and indentured servitude for individuals labeled with mental illness. Those confined were commonly required to bear the labor of public works. Often, the same places that confined the mentally ill served as places of incarceration for those who committed crimes against the state (Foucault, 1965; Hunter, 1963).

Mental Health Reform

By the end of the eighteenth century, inhumane conditions and treatment in houses of confinement gained the attention of philanthropists and humanists. In the late eighteenth and early nineteenth century France, Phillipe Pinel worked to dramatically change conditions in mental asylums. He replaced many of the horrifying practices of the time (e.g., bleeding, purging, blistering) and employed a psychologically oriented approach, encouraging gentleness and understanding when caring for mentally ill patients. In 1796, a Quaker merchant family, headed by William and Samuel Tuke, opened the York Retreat in England. Their desire was to demonstrate that humane treatment could abate mental illness. Pinel and Tuke sought to liberate individuals with mental illness from confinement and create a milieu of human kindness and moral treatment. Humanistic person-centered principles replaced indentured servitude and confinement (Grob, 1991).

In the mid nineteenth century, Dorthea Dix took up the cause of reform in the United States. Aided by changed attitudes toward suffering and social welfare, she helped effect reform in American hospitals and prisons. She established Saint Elizabeth's Hospital, in 1885 in Washington, DC, and eventually 32 state mental hospitals (Grob, 1983).

Medicalization of Mental Illness

After treatment reform in the mid to late eighteenth century, societies convened to govern conduct at asylums. The American Society of Superintendents of Mental Institutions of the Insane became the American-Medico-Psychological Association in the late eighteenth century. Its membership included neurologists, psychologists, and asylum-trained psychiatrists and nurses. The association of psychiatry with neurology proved to be a seminal event in the historical development of psychiatry and community mental health. Neurologists had publicly chastised psychiatry as an inexact science without empirically based standards for which other branches of medicine were held accountable. In response, psychiatrists attempted to formulate associations between insanity and biological or organic causes.

Benjamin Rush, an American physician, proposed the first physiological etiology of insanity in 1835. Rush believed the cause of insanity was positioned primarily in the vessels of the brain. Rush theoretically linked mental illness to other physical ailments involving arterial abnormalities. In 1845, Wilheim Griesinger published *Pathology and Therapy of Mental Diseases,* which established psychiatry as a medical specialty specifically concerned with diseases of the brain. In the late eighteenth century, insanity also was linked to the ingestion of intoxicating substances, trauma to the brain, and neuritis. Scientific and political respectability for psychiatry depended on a biomedical perspective (Grob, 1983).

Numerous somatic treatments for mental illness followed biomedical theories. Those treatments included lobotomy, electroconvulsive therapy, insulin shock therapy, and hydrotherapy (Deutsch, 1949). As discussed by Grob (1983), Egas Moniz, a Portuguese neurologist and neurosurgeon, introduced prefrontal lobotomy in 1935 for the treatment of mental illness. Moniz assumed that the synapse was the organic foundation of thought; therefore normal psychic thought was dependent upon proper functioning of the synapse, and mental disorders were a result of synaptic derangement. Moniz believed it was necessary to alter these synaptic paths to modify corresponding ideas and force thought into different channels. Insulin shock therapy, hydrotherapy, and electroconvulsive therapy were thought to have the same organic outcome. Moniz won the Nobel Prize in 1949 for the therapeutic use of prefrontal lobotomy (Grob, 1994). It was not until the early 1950s that the antipsychotic medication Thorazine (chlorpromazine) was discovered; this medication alleviated, in a more humane fashion, some of the most troubling symptoms experienced by individuals with psychotic disorders (Deutsch, 1949; Grob, 1991).

Community Mental Health and Deinstitutionalization

Treatment reform was based largely on the premise that mentally ill people were not bad or morally flawed, but sick and in need of treatment. The Great Depression of the 1930s continued to force the issue of treatment reform based primarily on financial concerns. States could no longer afford the vast expense of the custodial and institutional care for people diagnosed with mental illness. Caregivers, families, and communities became viable alternatives to costly institutional care.

In recognition of the need to improve research to identify effective treatment for mental illness, in July 1946, President Truman signed the National Mental Health Act, which established the National Institute of Mental Health (NIMH). A few years later, the Mental Health Study Act of 1955 (PL 84-182) called for "an objective, thorough, nationwide analysis and reevaluation of the human and economic problems of mental health." These efforts continued to point to the need to assess and evaluate mental health resources throughout the United States and to develop a national program to help meet the needs of the mentally ill.

The **Community Mental Health Centers Act** of 1964 (PL 88-164) provided significant federal support for mental health services. Among other things, this Act supported measures to implement facilities to care for those who were mentally retarded and to construct community mental health centers. The Act also mandated **deinstitutionalization,** or a halt to the long-held policy of keeping the severely mentally ill hospitalized. The process of deinstitutionalization was intended to reduce long-term care of seriously mentally ill persons, by transferring their treatment to a community setting. As a result, between 1955 and 1980, the number of patients confined to state and county mental hospitals declined from 559,000 to 138,000 (Sharfstein, Stoline, and Koran, 2002).

This mass exodus of individuals from institutions across the nation, often after many years of hospitalization, resulted in a situation in which individuals with serious mental illness were returned to families and communities who were ill prepared to care for them. In addition, alternative community mental health resources had not yet been established (Grob, 1994). With ill-prepared families and minimal community services, many individuals with mental illness found themselves homeless, in shelters, or in prisons or jails.

In the mid 1970s, the federal government acknowledged the relative inadequacies of the Community Mental Health Centers Act and made recommendations to link community mental health services with informal community support services. The idea was to improve inpatient, outpatient, emergency and day treatment, and consultation and education services for persons with mental disorders.

Decade of the Brain

The Community Mental Health Centers Act and subsequent legislation improved environmental conditions in institutions. Medical treatment for mental illness, on the other hand, remained relatively unchanged since the accidental discovery of Thorazine in the early 1950s. In 1952, a physician in a military hospital prescribed Thorazine for nausea to a patient who was also hearing voices. After the administration of Thorazine, the voices dissipated. Thorazine was reclassified as an antipsychotic medication and used extensively for decades to treat individuals diagnosed with mental illnesses such as schizophrenia (Grob, 1994).

The development of neuroimaging in the 1980s provided new data on the anatomical and neurochemical nature of the brain (Buchsbaum and Haier, 1982). These data rendered the foundation for developing pharmacological agents to treat mental illness that had a mechanism of action different from Thorazine. In the late 1980s, the National Advisory Mental Health Council—a policy advisory group that counsels the Secretary of Health and Human Services, the Director of the National Institutes of Health, and the Director of NIMH—recommended that the Decade of the Brain be initiated for the 10 years preceding the year 2000 (USDHHS, 1999). During that decade, the annual research budget of the NIMH increased, and much of the funding was allocated to research aimed at uncovering the biomedical etiology of schizophrenia and continuing to develop new pharmaceuticals. By the end of the twentieth century, several new psychiatric medications had been developed that have vastly improved the quality of life for those diagnosed with mental illness (Kandel, 1998).

Thus, over the past 50 years, psychiatry and mental health services have changed dramatically. Until the mid nineteenth century, treatment of the mentally ill was largely carried out first in mental asylums and then in long-term psychiatric hospitals. The development of psychotropic drugs, beginning in the 1950s, led to dramatic breakthroughs in the treatment of mental illness and enabled thousands of clients to be treated on an outpatient basis.

In 1955, 75% of patient care for mental illnesses took place in state hospitals. Today, 75% of client care for mental disorders occurs in community-based settings (Sharfstein et al., 2002). Ambulatory, or outpatient, care for mental disorders can be provided in many settings and by a variety of professionals, paraprofessionals, and volunteers. Persons with mental problems may seek assistance from physicians and other professional clinicians (e.g., psychologists, counselors) in private practice, hospital outpatient departments, mental health centers or clinics, alcohol and drug units or outpatient clinics, emergency departments, family or social service agencies, crisis centers, volunteer services such as self-help programs (e.g., Alcoholics Anonymous [AA], Narcotics Anonymous [NA]), and clergy or religious counselors.

HEALTHY PEOPLE 2010 AND MENTAL HEALTH

The evolution of mental health care in the United States is ongoing. Most recently, the U.S. Surgeon General has proposed a series of objectives addressing mental health and illness in *Healthy People 2010* (USDHHS, 2000). The *Healthy People 2010* table lists several objectives from *Healthy People 2010* that cover issues related to mental health. (see *Healthy People 2010* box on p. 472)

FACTORS INFLUENCING MENTAL HEALTH

Although treatment of mental disorders has dramatically improved, the exact cause of most mental illnesses is not well understood. Research has identified a number of factors—biological, sociological, and political—that contribute to mental health and mental illness. Some of these will be presented in this section.

Biological Factors

The explosion of research since 1990 indicates that the biological foundation of mental illness involves complex and evolving factors. Although several key studies have led to fundamental changes in the way mental illness is comprehended, science has yet to fully explain its biological basis. Contemporary views on the biological etiology of mental illness can be grouped into the following three areas: genetic factors, neurotransmitters, and structural brain abnormalities.

Genetic Factors

The success of the Human Genome Project in mapping the structure of deoxyribonucleic acid (DNA) markers has made it possible to examine human genes to investigate sites

HEALTHY PEOPLE 2010 Objectives Related to Mental Health		
Objective	Baseline (1998)	Target
18-1: Reduce the suicide rate	11.3 suicides per 100,000	5 suicides per 100,000
18-3: Reduce the proportion of homeless adults who have serious mental illness	25%	19%
18-5: Reduce the relapse rates for persons with eating disorders including anorexia nervosa and bulimia nervosa	NA	NA
18-9a: Increase the proportion of adults aged 18 to 54 years with serious mental disorders who receive treatment	47%	55%
18-14: Increase the number of states, territories and the District of Columbia with an operational mental health plan that addresses mental health crisis interventions, ongoing screening and treatment services for elderly persons	24 states	50 states and the District of Columbia

From US Department of Health and Human Services: *Healthy People 2010*, ed 2, Washington, DC, 2000, Government Printing Office.

NA, Data not available.

potentially linked to mental illness. For example, studies have indicated that some mental disorders (e.g., schizophrenia, bipolar disorder, ADHD, depression) have a genetic basis. Other studies show variation associated with mental illness in genes at specific neurotransmitter receptor sites in the brain, but the actual mechanism associated with variations and its contribution to mental illness is unknown. A key question remaining in the search for a genetic basis for mental illness is how genes that convey greater susceptibility for mental illness actually produce specific symptoms. A synthesis of the genetic research on mental disorders suggests that multiple genes convey a small amount of genetic susceptibility (Weinberger, 1997).

Neurotransmitters

Before the advent of neuroimaging, the role of amino acids and neurotransmitters in mental disorders was poorly understood. In recent years, defects or dysregulation in one or more neurotransmitter systems have been implicated in mental illness. For example, it is thought that symptoms of schizophrenia are related to disturbances of the neurotransmitters dopamine, serotonin, norepinephrine, acetylcholine, cholecystokinin, glutamate, and gamma-aminobutyric acid (Fortinash, 2004; Laraia, 2005; Pearson, 2006). Similarly, dysregulation of either norepinephrine or serotonergic neurotransmitter systems appears to contribute to the development of depression (Lewin, 2003).

Structural Brain Abnormalities

In the Decade of the Brain, identifying abnormalities in brain development as a factor in mental disorders became an increasingly popular topic for research. Evidence indicates that structural brain abnormalities seem to occur more often in those with mental illness. An increase in ventricular spaces and cortical volume deficits in the cerebral cortex are associated with mental illness. Research concerning the association with general structural abnormalities in schizophrenia suggests a decrease in brain volume in the left temporal and right frontal regions of the brain (Lim, 1996; Marsh, 1994).

Although a number of theories of the etiology of mental disorder have been developed from research during the Decade of the Brain, many have not been replicated. Information from studies to date is insufficient to establish a definitive biological cause for mental illness. Scholars have concluded that mental disorders are multifactorial, complex physiological phenomena. To provide holistic care, health providers must consider the interaction of many elements, including the genetic, anatomical, physiological, and biochemical factors, as well as life events, developmental factors, and the environment on mental health and mental illness (Mohr and Mohr, 2001).

Social Factors

Throughout history, the symptoms of mental illness have been perceived as permanent, dangerous, frightening, and shameful. People diagnosed with a mental illness have been described as lazy, idle, weak, immoral, irrational, and feigning illness. Based on these characterizations and assumptions, many people diagnosed with a mental illness have experienced widespread social rejection (Hanson, 1998; Holiday, 1996). People with a mental illness experience stigma and discrimination. **Marginalization** the process of social and political peripheralization of individuals or groups based on real or perceived differences from the majority. Marginalization makes access to the goods and services of a community more difficult (Hall, Stevens, and Meleis, 1994).

Although mental illness is assumed to have a biological basis, it is also a complex and abstract cultural construct. The myths associated with mental illness have historical, political, economic, and social roots. Individuals diagnosed with mental illnesses are shunned, less likely to be hired, and less likely to be accepted as neighbors (McCrae, 1996). Also, because of deinstitutionalization, many people with severe mental illness left state institutions to live in communities that were ill prepared to provide treatment. Consequently, many of individuals are homeless, incarcerated, or living in residential boarding homes. With the ongoing decrease in community services, this trend continues, leaving people with mental illness vulnerable to victimization.

Political Factors

Political factors can dramatically influence how mental disorders are managed. One significant factor in the politics of mental illness is parity in health care coverage. Parity refers to equal access to health care for physical and mental illnesses. For example, mental and physical illness affecting the same physiological symptoms is often treated with disparity. Although both illnesses affect the same neurotransmitter (i.e., dopamine), a person diagnosed with Parkinson's disease might have full insurance coverage and a person diagnosed with schizophrenia might have no coverage (NIMH, 1998).

In 1999, legislation was introduced to Congress to end disparity in health care coverage. The **Mental Health Equitable Treatment Act** of 1999 (SB 796) was written to require equal health care benefits for individuals diagnosed with severe mental disorders. Explicit in that legislation was a prohibition of limits on lifetime and annual mental health benefits, inpatient hospital stays, outpatient visits, and inequitable co-payments. That bill eventually died in Congress, but it was resurrected in 2003 as the Paul Wellstone Mental Health Equitable Treatment Act. For the next 3 years, a majority of House members approved the legislation, but it was rejected in the Senate. The most recent version (HR 1402) was reintroduced in Congress in March 2005, and is pending (American Hospital Association, 2005). Proponents argue that this legislation will increase insurance premiums by less than 1% and that these costs would be recouped by lower absenteeism and higher productivity of workers who are properly treated. Further, they observe that 34 states have already enacted parity laws similar to the Paul Wellborn Act but that federal legislation is necessary to ensure parity for all Americans (National Association for the Mentally Ill [NAMI], 2003).

MENTAL DISORDERS ENCOUNTERED IN COMMUNITY SETTINGS

The influence of untreated mental illness on communities and their social structure has been vastly understated. The NIMH estimates that the prevalence of diagnosable mental disorders in the U.S. population is about 22% at any given time (USDHHS/SAMHA, 1999). Mental illness accounts for more than 10% of the disease burden worldwide, ranking it second, following all forms of cardiac disease (USDHHS/SAMHSA, 2005). In the United States, the estimated cost of mental illness exceeds $150 billion yearly: $69 billion for costs of diagnosing and treating mental disorders; $75 billion in lost productivity and disability insurance payments; and $6 billion due to criminal justice costs and property loss (USDHHS, 2000).

Given these data, and recognizing that most mental illnesses are identified and managed in noninstitutional settings, it is essential that community health nurses be very familiar with the most commonly occurring mental disorders. They should understand the prevalence and risk factors for these disorders, as well as how to identify and manage them. Further, a recent government-sponsored report underscored

TABLE 22-1 1-Year Prevalence Rates for Mental Disorders*

DISORDER	PERCENT
Anxiety disorders	**16.4**
Simple phobia	8.3
Social phobia	2.0
Agoraphobia	4.9
Generalized anxiety disorder	3.4
Panic disorder	1.6
Obsessive-compulsive disorder	2.4
Posttraumatic stress disorder	3.6
Mood disorders	**7.1**
Major depressive episode	6.5
Unipolar major depressive	5.3
Dysthymia	1.6
Bipolar I	1.1
Bipolar II	0.6
Schizophrenia	1.3
Nonaffective psychosis	0.2
Somatization	0.2
Anti-social personality disorder	2.1
Anorexia nervosa	0.1
Severe cognitive impairment	1.2
Any disorder	**21.5**

From US Department of Health and Human Services: *Mental health: a report of the surgeon general*, Rockville, Md, 1999, The Author, http://www.surgeongeneral.gov/library/mentalhealth/chapter2/sec2_1.html.

*Individuals may report more than one mental disorder at a given time and more than one per year.

the need for screening, referring, and follow-up for those with actual or potential mental disorders to ensure that the mental health needs of the community are being met (Unutzer et al., 2006).

Overview of Selected Mental Disorders

In the *Diagnostic and Statistical Manual of Mental Disorders* (fourth edition, text revision) (American Psychiatric Association, 2000), the APA has classified mental illnesses and outlined diagnostic criteria for more than 300 mental disorders. Table 22-1 presents data on U.S. prevalence rates of the most commonly identified mental disorders encountered in community settings. This section provides a summary of some of these disorders, including risk factors, diagnostic criteria, and basic treatment recommendations.

Schizophrenia

Schizophrenia is the most serious and profound of all mental illnesses; globally, it affects about 1% of the population (NIMH, 2005b). The effect of this condition on the community is enormous in terms of social and economic burden. To the individual and families affected by schizophrenia, the impact is incalculable. Schizophrenia is the most common psychotic disorder. It presents with (1) positive symptoms that include hallucinations, delusions, disorganized thinking and speech, and bizarre behavior and (2) negative symptoms such as flat affect, poor attention, lack of motivation, apathy, lack of pleasure, and lack of energy. Onset typically occurs during late adolescence and early adulthood in males and somewhat later in females. There is an increased risk for alcohol use, depression, suicide, and diabetes among persons with schizophrenia. These factors compound the problems associated with living with a psychotic disorder.

Diagnostic criteria for schizophrenia are two or more of the following (each present for a significant portion of a 1-month period): delusions, hallucinations, disorganized speech (e.g., frequent derailment or incoherence), grossly disorganized or catatonic behavior, affective flattening, alogia, and avolition (APA, 2000). There are several subtypes of schizophrenia: paranoid type, disorganized type, catatonic type, undifferentiated type, and residual type. The subtype diagnosis is based on careful evaluation and may change over time. For additional information, the American Psychiatric Association has published a quick reference to the assessment and treatment of schizophrenia that is available online at http://www. psychiatryonline.com.

Michael Nye, a photographer, has spent hundreds of hours photographing and taping illness narratives of individuals living with schizophrenia and other serious mental illness. Viewing his photographs and listening to the accounts of those living with these conditions are valuable experiences for nurses who care for this population (http://michaelnye.org/fineline/index.html).

Depression

Depression is the most frequently diagnosed mental illness in the United States and is one of the leading causes of disability. In 2004, more than 17 million adults experienced at least one major depressive episode (USDHHS/SAMHSA, 2005). In addition, depression is often a complication of serious physical disorders such as heart attack, stroke, diabetes, and cancer.

It is estimated about 25% of all women and 12% of all men will suffer at least one episode or occurrence of depression during their lifetime, and approximately 3% to 5% of teenagers experience clinical depression each year. Most people (almost two thirds) with a depressive illness do not seek treatment, although most, even those with the most severe disorders, can be helped (NIMH, 2000).

The most prevalent types of depression are the following:
- *Major depression:* Manifested by a combination of symptoms that interfere with the ability to work, sleep, eat, and enjoy once-pleasurable activities
- *Dysthymia:* Long-term (minimum of 2 years), chronic symptoms that do not disable but keep the individual from functioning or from feeling good; some people with dysthymia also experience major depressive episodes
- *Bipolar disorder (manic-depressive illness):* Produces cycles of depression and mania (APA, 2000)

Risk Factors and Symptoms

Nurses working in community-based settings should be aware of risk factors for developing depression and of symptoms that might indicate a depressive episode. They can then work to reduce risk factors and teach others to be

RESEARCH HIGHLIGHTS

Improving Care for Depressed and Suicidal Individuals

Raingruber (2002) performed a phenomenological study examining 50 clients to identify the issues that influence the care of depressed and suicidal individuals. For this project, she interviewed involved clients, licensed mental health professionals, primary care physicians, police officers, high school teachers, counselors, and parents. She determined that the stigma of being diagnosed with a mental illness had a major influence on whether depressed or suicidal individuals were willing to seek care and to continue in treatment. Further, she found that open communication, community awareness, education and prevention, and community-centered services were ways to minimize stigma and enhance care.

To help reduce stigma, Raingruber suggested widespread use of public service/education ads (e.g., television, radio, billboards) designed to emphasize the treatable nature of depression and "normalize" it. She further advocated that hospitals and others sponsor programs related to the prevention of depression and suicidal ideation to decrease associated stigma. Finally, she encouraged modifying health care providers' attitudes toward depression and advocated the use of community-centered and in-home services in the management of this condition.

From Raingruber B: Client and provider perspectives regarding the stigma of and nonstigmatizing interventions for depression, *Arch Psychiatr Nurs* 16(5):201-207, 2002.

aware of these symptoms. Health education should also include information on when and how to obtain treatment. Symptoms of depression and mania are included in Box 22-1. The following are risk factors for depression (USDHHS/Office of Disease Prevention and Health Promotion [ODPHP], 1998):
- Prior episode(s) of depression
- Family history of depressive disorder
- Prior suicide attempt(s)
- Female gender
- Postpartum period
- Medical comorbidity
- Lack of social support
- Stressful life events
- Personal history of sexual abuse
- Current substance abuse

The highest rates of depressive disorders are found among those 25 to 44 years of age, with rates apparently increasing among those born after 1945. This trend may be the result of psychosocial factors (e.g., single parenting, changing roles, stress). Married people and those in ongoing intimate relationships have a lower rate of clinical depression than do those living alone. Overall, however, unhappily married people have the highest rates, whereas happily married men have the lowest. Finally, studies indicate that almost one third of clinically depressed individuals have some form of substance abuse or dependence.

Depression in Children and Adolescents

According to the National Mental Health Association (2006), between 2% and 4% of prepubertal children and as many as 12% of adolescents may have depression. A family history of

BOX 22-1   Symptoms of Depression and Mania

Depression

- ➤ Persistent sad or empty mood
- ➤ Feelings of hopelessness, pessimism
- ➤ Feelings of guilt, worthlessness, helplessness
- ➤ Loss of interest or pleasure in ordinary activities, including sex
- ➤ Decreased energy, fatigue, being slowed down
- ➤ Difficulty concentrating, remembering, making decisions
- ➤ Insomnia, early-morning waking, or oversleeping
- ➤ Appetite loss, weight loss, or overeating and weight gain
- ➤ Thoughts of death or suicide; suicide attempts
- ➤ Restlessness, irritability
- ➤ Persistent physical symptoms that do not respond to treatment (e.g., headaches, digestive disorders, chronic pain)

Mania

- ➤ Abnormal or excessive elation
- ➤ Unusual irritability
- ➤ Decreased need for sleep
- ➤ Grandiose notions
- ➤ Increased talking
- ➤ Racing thoughts
- ➤ Increased sexual desire
- ➤ Markedly increased energy
- ➤ Poor judgment
- ➤ Inappropriate social behavior

From National Institute of Mental Health: *Depression*, NIH Pub No 00-3561, Rockville, Md, 2000, The Author.

depression is a major risk factor for childhood depression. Other associated factors that may increase the risk of depression in children and adolescents include a history of verbal, physical, or sexual abuse; frequent separation from, or loss of, a loved one; poverty; mental retardation; ADHD; hyperactivity; and chronic illness. Complications of depression in children and adolescents include poor school performance, poor peer relations, alcohol and drug abuse, promiscuity, teenage pregnancy, other psychiatric illnesses, and suicide (USDHHS/ODPHP, 1998). It should be noted that suicide is the third leading cause of death among persons 15 to 25 years and that the rate of suicide among young males is five times that among young females. Health care providers should recognize the symptoms of depression and refer for treatment as appropriate. Box 22-2 summarizes characteristics of depression that may be seen in all age-groups.

Treatment

Treatment for depression includes pharmacological therapy, psychotherapy, behavior therapy, electroconvulsive therapy, or a combination of these (APA, 2005; NIMH, 2004a). In general, the most effective, first line treatment is a combination of antidepressant medication and psychotherapy. A quick reference is also available, provided by the American Psychiatric Association, at http://www.psychiatryonline.com. Treatment for all mental disorders is addressed in greater detail later in this chapter.

Bipolar Disorder

Bipolar disorder refers to a group of mood disorders that present with changes in mood from depression to mania. The depressed phase is manifested by symptoms seen in major depressive disorder. The manic phase is characterized by a persistent abnormally elevated or irritable mood, impaired judgment, flight of ideas, pressured speech, grandiosity, distractibility, excessive involvement in goal-directed activities, few hours sleeping, and impulsivity. These symptoms may co-occur with psychotic features such as hallucinations and delusions. Persons with bipolar disorder are at increased risk for alcohol and substance abuse as well as increased risk for suicide. The presence of bipolar disorder results in poor occupational and social functioning.

Management of bipolar disorder must be ongoing and involve close monitoring. Goals of treatment of manic or "mixed" episodes are to control symptoms to allow the individual to return to usual levels of functioning and to manage agitation, aggression, and impulsivity. Treatment generally involves use of medication—frequently lithium, often in combination with other medications (e.g., antipsychotics such as olanzapine and/or valproate), depending on the severity of the symptoms. For management of depression, goals are to achieve remission of the symptoms of major depression and return the individual to usual levels of functioning and to avoid a precipitating manic or hypomanic episode. For some individuals, treatment of depressive episodes will necessitate addition of an antidepressant to the pharmacological regimen (APA, 2005). When working with persons with bipolar disorder, nurses need to monitor symptoms and response to psychopharmacological treatment—this is discussed in more detail later in the chapter. For additional information, see http://www.psychiatryonline.com/content.aspx?aID=110111.

Anxiety Disorder

Anxiety disorder refers to a group of mental illnesses characterized by feelings of severe anxiety, resulting symptoms, and efforts (sometime extreme) to avoid those symptoms. Anxiety disorders affect up to 16% of the general population at any time. Anxiety disorders may be attributed to genetic makeup and life experiences of the individual. Some of the more commonly encountered anxiety disorders are generalized anxiety disorder, panic disorder (sometimes accompanied by agoraphobia), phobias, obsessive-compulsive disorder, and posttraumatic stress disorder (USDHHS/Public Health Service [PHS], 1999). These are discussed briefly here.

Generalized Anxiety Disorder

Generalized anxiety disorder (GAD) is characterized by chronic, unrealistic, and exaggerated worry and tension about one or more life circumstances lasting 6 months or longer without anything seeming to provoke it (USDHHS, 1999). Approximately half of cases of GAD begin in childhood or adolescence, and it is more common in women than in men.

Symptoms of GAD include trembling, twitching, muscle tension, headaches, irritability, sweating or hot flashes, dyspnea, nausea, and feeling a lump in the throat. It typically

BOX 22-2 Characteristics of Depression Across the Life Span

Infants and Preschoolers
- ➤ Insidious onset
- ➤ Apathy, fatigue, withdrawal
- ➤ Poor appetite, weight loss
- ➤ Agitation, sleeplessness
- ➤ Rarely, spontaneous disclosure of feeling sad

Prepubertal Children
- ➤ Possible disclosure of sadness, suicidal thoughts
- ➤ Irritability, self-criticism, weepiness
- ➤ Decreased initiative and responsiveness to stimulation, apathy
- ➤ Fatigue, sleep disturbance
- ➤ Enuresis, encopresis
- ➤ Weight loss, anorexia
- ➤ Somatic complaints
- ➤ Poor school performance
- ➤ Social withdrawal, increased aggressiveness

Adolescence
- ➤ Feelings of sadness (less frequent than in other age-groups)
- ➤ Unhappy restlessness, boredom, irritability
- ➤ Intense, labile affects
- ➤ Low self-esteem, hopelessness, worthlessness
- ➤ Associated anxiety
- ➤ Feelings of loneliness and being unloved
- ➤ Pessimism about the future
- ➤ Loss of interest in friends and activities, apathy
- ➤ Low frustration tolerance
- ➤ Poor school performance
- ➤ Argumentativeness
- ➤ Increased conflict with peers
- ➤ Acting-out behavior (e.g., running away, stealing, physical violence)
- ➤ Sexual activity
- ➤ Substance abuse
- ➤ Complaints of headaches, abdominal pain
- ➤ Hypersomnia

Early and Middle Adulthood
- ➤ Depressed mood
- ➤ Anhedonia
- ➤ Feelings of worthlessness, hopelessness, guilt
- ➤ Reduced energy, fatigue
- ➤ Sleep disturbance, especially early morning awakening and multiple nighttime awakenings
- ➤ Decreased sexual interest and activity
- ➤ Psychomotor retardation
- ➤ Anxiety
- ➤ Decreased appetite and weight loss or increased appetite and weight gain

Later Adulthood
- ➤ Unlikely to complain of depressed mood or present with tearful affect
- ➤ Feelings of helplessness
- ➤ Pessimism about the future
- ➤ Ruminating about problems
- ➤ Critical and envious of others
- ➤ Loss of self-esteem
- ➤ Guilt feelings
- ➤ Longer and more severe depressions than in middle adulthood
- ➤ Perceived cognitive deficits
- ➤ Somatic complaints
- ➤ Constipation
- ➤ Social withdrawal
- ➤ Loss of motivation
- ➤ Change of appetite

Core Symptoms Across Age-Groups
- ➤ Suicidal ideation
- ➤ Diminished concentration
- ➤ Sleep disturbance

From Tommasini NR: The client with a mood disorder (depression). In Antai-Otong D, editor: *Psychiatric nursing: biological and behavioral concepts,* Philadelphia, 1995, WB Saunders, pp. 157-190.

fluctuates with periods of increasing symptoms that are usually associated with life stressors or impending difficulties.

Panic Disorder

Some 2% to 4% of the population will suffer from panic disorder during their lifetime; women experience it at approximately double the rate of men (USDHHS, 1999). Panic disorder can occur at any age, but it most often begins in young adulthood (average age, 17-30 years). **Panic disorder** typically develops in three stages, with clients potentially stopping at any stage or progressing through all three. Individuals often have their first attack or cluster of attacks after a variety of life stresses.

Panic attacks consist of a period of intense fear that develops abruptly and unexpectedly (Box 22-3). The initial attack may occur suddenly and unexpectedly while the client is performing everyday tasks. Typically, he or she experiences tachycardia; dyspnea; dizziness; chest pain; nausea; numbness or tingling of the hands and feet; trembling or shaking; sweating; choking; or a feeling that he or she is going to die, go crazy, or do something uncontrolled. This can be extremely frightening. A diagnosis of panic disorder is made when attacks occur with some degree of frequency or regularity.

During the second stage, the anxiety attacks become increasingly frequent and severe, and the individual develops anticipatory anxiety (fear of having a panic attack). During this phase, events and circumstances associated with the attack may be selectively avoided, leading to phobic behaviors (e.g., if a woman has an attack while driving, she may become anxious the next time she needs to drive, and she may begin to avoid driving and then refuse to drive altogether). In this phase, the client's life may become progressively constricted.

As the avoidance behavior intensifies, the third stage may develop, in which the client begins to withdraw further to avoid being in places or situations from which escape may be difficult or embarrassing or help may be unavailable in the

BOX 22-3 Criteria for Diagnosis of Panic Attack

Period of intense fear in which at least four of the following symptoms develop abruptly and reach a peak within 10 minutes:
- ➤ Palpitations, pounding heart, or accelerated heart rate
- ➤ Sweating
- ➤ Trembling or shaking
- ➤ Sensations of shortness of breath or smothering
- ➤ Feeling of choking
- ➤ Chest pain or discomfort
- ➤ Nausea or abdominal distress
- ➤ Feeling dizzy, unsteady, lightheaded, or faint
- ➤ Derealization (feelings of unreality) or depersonalization (being detached from oneself)
- ➤ Fear of losing control or going crazy
- ➤ Fear of dying
- ➤ Paresthesias (numbness or tingling sensations)
- ➤ Chills or hot flushes

From American Psychiatric Association: *Diagnostic and statistical manual of mental disorders*, ed 4, text revision, Washington, DC, 2000, The Author.

event of a panic attack (e.g., church, elevators, movie theaters). The fear of being in these situations or places can lead to **agoraphobia** (literally, fear of the marketplace or open places). Individuals with agoraphobia frequently progress to the point where they cannot leave their homes without experiencing anxiety. Agoraphobia is the most common phobia leading to the use of health services, particularly when accompanied by panic attacks. About one third of all people who experience panic attacks eventually develop agoraphobia.

Panic disorder is often accompanied by other conditions. If not treated, approximately 50% to 65% of clients with panic disorder will develop a major depression at some time in their lives (USDHHS, 1999). Alcoholism is also common among individuals with panic disorders. Cognitive-behavioral therapy and medication can help 70% to 90% of people with panic disorder.

Phobias

A **phobia** is an irrational fear of something (an object or situation), and as many as 8% of Americans are affected by phobias at any given time. Adults with phobias realize their fears are irrational, but facing the feared object or situation might bring on severe anxiety or a panic attack. Phobias may begin in childhood, but they usually first appear in adolescence or adulthood.

Social phobia, or social anxiety disorder, is a persistent and intense fear of, and compelling desire to avoid, something that would expose the individual to a situation that might be humiliating and embarrassing (APA, 2000). Its tendency is familial and may be accompanied by depression or alcoholism. Social phobia often begins in childhood or early adolescence. Individuals suffering from social phobia think that whereas others are very competent in public, they are not. Small mistakes are exaggerated. The most common social phobia is a fear of public speaking. Other examples include being unable to urinate in a public bathroom and not being able to answer questions in social situations. Most

people with social phobias can be treated with cognitive-behavior therapy and medication.

Simple phobias (excluding panic attack or social phobia) involve a persistent fear of, and compelling desire to avoid, certain objects or situations. Common objects of phobias are spiders, snakes, dogs, cats, and situations such as flying, heights, and closed-in spaces. The person often recognizes that the fear is excessive or unreasonable but nonetheless avoids the situation or endures it with intense anxiety. Systematic desensitization and normal exposure are the most effective treatments for simple phobias. Medication produces minimal benefit.

Obsessive-Compulsive Disorder

Obsessive-compulsive disorder (OCD) is characterized by anxious thoughts and rituals that the individual has difficulty controlling. The person with OCD is overcome with the urge to engage in some ritual to avoid a persistent frightening thought, idea, image, or event. Obsessions are recurrent thoughts, emotions, or impulses that cannot be dismissed. Compulsions are the rituals or behaviors that are repeatedly performed to prevent, neutralize, or dispel the dreaded obsession. When the individual tries to resist the compulsion, anxiety increases. Common compulsions include hand washing, counting, checking, or touching.

Obsessive-compulsive disease is diagnosed only when the compulsive activities consume at least an hour a day and interfere with daily life (APA, 2000). Most individuals recognize that what they are doing is senseless but are unable to control the compulsion. About 2% of Americans are afflicted with OCD, which often appears in the teenage years or early adulthood. Depression or other anxiety disorders often accompany OCD. Clomipramine (Anafranil) and fluoxetine (Prozac) have been effective in treating OCD. Behavioral therapy also has been found to be helpful.

Posttraumatic Stress Disorder

Posttraumatic stress disorder (PTSD) is a debilitating condition that follows a terrifying event. It affects about 3.6% of U.S. adults (NIMH, 2002a). Individuals with PTSD have recurring, persistent, frightening thoughts and memories of their ordeal. Traumatic incidents that trigger PTSD may have threatened that individual's life or the life of someone else. Incidents include "shell shock" or "battle fatigue" common to war veterans, violent attack (e.g., kidnapping, rape, mugging), serious accidents, natural disasters (e.g., earthquake, tornado), or witnessing mass destruction or injury, such as an airplane crash. Sometimes the individual is unable to recall an important aspect of the traumatic event. Interestingly, about 30% of Vietnam veterans have experienced PTSD at some point after the war (NIMH, 2002a).

People with PTSD repeatedly relive the trauma in the form of nightmares or disturbing recollections, flashbacks, or hallucinations during the day. As a result, they often have sleep disturbances, depression, and feelings of detachment or emotional numbness, or are easily startled. They may avoid places or situations that bring back memories (e.g., a woman raped in an elevator may refuse to ride in elevators), and anniversaries of the event are often very difficult. Post-traumatic stress disorder occurs at all ages and may be accompanied by depression, substance abuse, and/or anxiety. It usually begins within 3 months of the trauma, and the course of the disorder varies. Some individuals recover within 6 months; the condition becomes chronic in others. Infrequently, the illness does not manifest until years after the traumatic event.

Posttraumatic stress disorder is treated with antidepressants and antianxiety medications and psychotherapy. Support from family and friends can be very beneficial. A quick reference for PTSD from the APA (2005) can be found at http://www.psychiatryonline.com.

Eating Disorders

Eating disorders are becoming increasingly prevalent in the United States. Indeed, the most common eating disorders, anorexia nervosa and bulimia nervosa, affect about 3 million U.S. residents. Currently, it is estimated that anorexia affects 0.5% to 3.7% of girls and women during their lifetime (NIMH, 2001). Additionally, as many as 4% to 15% of female high school and college women have some symptoms of bulimia (Cochrane, 2005).

Eating disorders almost exclusively affect females; males account for only 5% to 10% of bulimia and anorexia cases, although this may be underreported. Most clients diagnosed with eating disorders are white. This, however, may be because of socioeconomic factors rather than race because females in middle and upper socioeconomic groups are most frequently affected. Anorexia and bulimia are often triggered by developmental milestones (e.g., puberty, first sexual contact) or another crisis (e.g., death of a loved one, ridicule over weight, starting college).

Bulimia Nervosa

"The essential features of **bulimia nervosa** are binge eating and inappropriate compensatory methods to prevent weight gain" (APA, 2000, p. 589). A binge is defined as eating an abnormal amount of food at a discrete time (usually less than 2 hours). For example, a person suffering from bulimia might eat an entire pie, half a cake, or a half gallon of ice cream at one sitting. Snacking throughout the day is not considered bingeing. To lose or maintain weight, the person with bulimia practices purging, which usually involves self-induced vomiting, caused by gagging, using an emetic, or simply mentally willing the action. Laxatives, diuretics, fasting, and excessive exercise may also be employed to control weight.

Bulimia Nervosa typically begins in adolescence or during the early 20s, usually in conjunction with a diet. High school and college students, as well as members of certain professions that emphasize weight and/or appearance (e.g., dancers, flight attendants, cheerleaders, athletes, actors, models), are at high risk (Decker and Freeman, 1996).

A number of health problems may result from bulimia. Electrolyte imbalance can result in fatigue, seizures, muscle cramps, arrhythmias, and decreased bone density. Vomiting can damage the esophagus, stomach, teeth, and gums.

Anorexia Nervosa

The person suffering from **anorexia nervosa** becomes obsessed with a fear of fat and with losing weight. Anorexia nervosa often develops with a fairly gradual decrease in caloric intake. However, the decrease in caloric intake continues until the anorexic is consuming almost nothing. Anorexia usually begins in early adolescence (12 to 14 years is the most common age-group) and may be limited to a single episode of dramatic weight loss within a few months, followed by recovery, or the illness may last for many years.

As stated earlier, anorexia nervosa almost exclusively affects white adolescent girls. Other risk factors for eating disorders are perfectionism, low self-esteem, stress, poor coping skills, sexual/physical abuse, poor self-image, dependency on others' opinions and deference to others' wishes, and being emotionally reserved (Cochrane, 2005).

In response to the severely decreased caloric intake, the body tries to compensate by slowing down body processes. Menstruation ceases; blood pressure, pulse, and respiration rates slow; and thyroid activity diminishes. Electrolyte imbalance can become very severe. Other symptoms include mild anemia, joint swelling, and reduced muscle mass. Anorexia nervosa can be life threatening and has a mortality rate of 5% to 21% (Zimmerman, Berchin, and Quallo, 2003).

In addition to the health threats directly related to the eating disorders themselves, multiple studies indicate that many individuals with anorexia also have symptoms of other mental disorders (e.g. OCD, panic disorder, social phobia, or GAD). Likewise, significant numbers of those suffering from bulimia have symptoms of depression, substance abuse, and personality disorders (Decker, 2006).

Treatment for eating disorders includes nutrition counseling, psychotherapy, and behavior modification and may take a year or more. Hospitalization may be required for clients with serious complications. Self-help groups and support groups can be very beneficial for both the client and the family. Many bulimics appear to respond to antidepressants. Anorexia nervosa, however, does not appear as responsive to medication.

Nurses need to be aware of the "ProAna" websites, which promote the lifestyle associated with eating disorders. Such knowledge is important, as community health nurses assess the social influences that contribute to the condition. Also, nurses who frequently work with adolescent girls and young women in community settings such as schools and clinics should be aware of the risk factors, signs, and symptoms of anorexia and bulimia and be prepared to intervene.

Attention Deficit Hyperactivity Disorder

Two of the most common conditions encountered by nurses who work with children in community settings are **attention deficit hyperactivity disorder** (ADHD) and **attention deficit disorder** (ADD). In the United States, ADHD/ADD affects 3% to 5% of all children (about 2 million) (NIMH, 2003a). Behaviors that might indicate ADHD/ADD usually appear before age 7 years and are often accompanied by related problems, such as learning disability, anxiety, and depression. The three major characteristics of ADHD/ADD are inattention, hyperactivity, and impulsivity.

The cause of ADHD/ADD is not known, but it is important to note that it is not caused by minor head injuries, birth complications, food allergies, too much sugar, poor home life, poor schools, or too much television. Maternal substance use and abuse (e.g., alcohol, cigarettes, cocaine) may affect the brain of the developing baby and produce symptoms of ADHD/ADD later in life. This, however, accounts for only a small percentage of those affected (NIMH, 2003a).

Attention disorders run in families, as children diagnosed with ADHD/ADD usually have at least one close relative who also has ADHD/ADD, and at least one third of all fathers who had ADHD/ADD as children have children with symptoms. Additionally, in the majority of sets of identical twins in which one has the disorder, the other does also (NIMH, 2003a). Although parents may notice symptoms and signs, it is often teachers who recognize the behaviors consistent with attention deficit disorders and suggest referral for assessment and treatment.

Experts caution that diagnosis of attention disorders should be made following a comprehensive physical, psychological, social, and behavioral evaluation and not based solely on anecdotal reports from parents. The evaluation should rule out other possible reasons for the behavior (e.g., emotional problems, poor vision or hearing, physical problems) and should include input from teachers, parents, and others who know the child well. Intelligence and achievement testing may also be performed to rule out or identify a learning disability.

Symptoms of ADHD/ADD are typically managed through a combination of behavior therapy, emotional counseling, and practical support. Use of medication is becoming increasingly commonplace in the management of ADHD/ADD. It is very important, however, that children with attention disorders and their families understand that medication does not cure the disorder; it just temporarily controls symptoms.

Curiously, stimulants are the medications that have been shown to be successful in treating attention disorders in both children and adults. The most commonly used medications are methylphenidate (Ritalin) and amphetamines (Dexedrine, Dextrostat, or Adderall). About 90% of children with ADHD/ADD show improvement when taking one of these drugs. Effective doses vary among children, and drug regimens for treatment of ADHD/ADD vary among physicians. Some physicians recommend keeping children on medication only during school and having the child stop taking the medication on weekends and during the summer vacation. Others prescribe medication every day, assuming that this regimen is more beneficial in helping establish positive behavioral patterns and work habits.

Medications used to treat ADHD/ADD have some potential adverse effects. Appetite suppression is fairly common and may contribute to growth retardation. Periodic assessment of height and weight is therefore important. Sleeping difficulties are also possible. There is concern that long-term use of pemoline (Cylert) may affect the liver. Therefore liver function must be assessed periodically in clients taking this medication (NIMH, 2003a).

BOX 22-4 Suicide Facts

Suicides Deaths (United States, 2001)

➤ Suicide was the 11th leading cause of death in the United States; it was the 8th leading cause of deaths for males and 19th leading cause of death for females.

➤ The total number of suicide deaths was 30,622.

➤ About 1.3% of all deaths were from suicide (in contrast, 29% of deaths were from heart disease, 23% from cancer, and 7% from cerebrovascular disease—the three leading causes).

➤ There were twice as many deaths due to suicide than deaths due to HIV/AIDS (14,175).

➤ Suicide by firearms was the most common method for both men and women, accounting for 55% of all suicides.

➤ More men than women died by suicide; the gender ratio was more than 4:1.

➤ More than 73% of all suicides were committed by white men.

➤ Nearly 80% of all firearm suicides were committed by white men.

➤ The highest suicide rates were for persons older than 85 years (rate 54/100,000).

➤ Suicide was the third leading cause of death among young people 15 to 24 years of age (following unintentional injuries and homicide) in this age-group.

Attempted Suicides

➤ There were an estimated 8 to 25 attempted suicides to one completion; the ratio was higher in women and youth and lower in men and the elderly.

➤ More women than men reported a history of attempted suicide (gender ratio 2:1).

➤ The strongest risk factors for attempted suicide in adults were depression, alcohol abuse, cocaine use, and separation or divorce.

➤ The strongest risk factors for attempted suicide in youth were depression, alcohol or other drug use disorder, and aggressive or disruptive behaviors.

Modified from National Institute of Mental Health: *Suicide facts and statistics 2001, 2004b,* The Author, http://www.nimh.nih.gov/suicideprevention/suifact.cfm.

Suicide

Undoubtedly, the greatest cost of mental illness in the United States is measured in human lives. Almost all people who commit suicide have a diagnosable mental illness (i.e., depression is most common). In 2004, the third leading cause of death among those aged 15 to 24 was suicide. Further, the highest rate of suicide is found in males over 65 year of age; white males over the age of 85 are particularly vulnerable. In any given year, approximately 31,000 people will die as a result of suicide in the United States (Box 22-4).

In 1999, the USDHHS and the Office of the Surgeon General identified suicide as a primary public health problem of the new millennium. Consistent with the select aims of *Healthy People 2010,* the Surgeon General's Call to Action attempts to "put into place national strategies to prevent the loss of life and the suffering suicide causes" (USDHHS, 1999, p. 7) through increased public awareness, expansion of mental health services, and continuation of support of research aimed at understanding and preventing suicide in the United States.

Risk and protective factors are identified in relation to suicide prevention. Risk factors include previous suicide

BOX 22-5 Suicide Risk Factors

➤ One or more diagnosable mental or substance abuse disorder(s) (greatest risk: previous suicide attempts, major depression, drug abuse, bipolar disorder)
➤ Impulsivity
➤ Adverse life events
➤ Family history of mental or substance abuse disorder
➤ Family history of suicide
➤ Family violence, including emotional, physical, or sexual abuse
➤ Prior suicide attempt
➤ Firearm in the home
➤ Incarceration
➤ Exposure to the suicidal behavior of others (e.g., family members, peers, and/or the media in news or fiction stories)

National Institute for Mental Health: *Frequently asked questions about suicide,* Dec 1999, The Author, http://www.nimh.nih.gov/suicideprevention/suicidefaq.cfm; National Institute of Mental Health: *In harm's way: suicide in America,* NIH Pub No 03-4594, 2003b, The Author, from http://www.nimh.nih.gov/publicat/harmaway.cfm.

BOX 22-6 Suicide Prevention Strategies

➤ Because suicide is a highly complex behavior, preventative interventions also must be complex and intensive to have lasting effects.
➤ Recognition of mental and substance abuse disorders and appropriate treatment are the most promising ways to prevent suicide in older persons.
➤ Limiting young people's access to firearms and performing other forms of responsible firearm ownership, especially in conjunction with the prevention of mental and addictive disorders, may be beneficial for prevention of firearm suicides.
➤ School-based, information-only prevention programs focusing on suicide may actually increase distress in the young people who are most vulnerable.
➤ School and community prevention programs designed to address suicide as part of a broader focus on mental health (e.g., incorporating coping skills in response to stress, substance abuse, aggressive behaviors) are most likely to be successful.

National Institute for Mental Health: *Frequently asked questions about suicide,* Dec 1999, The Author, http://www.nimh.nih.gov/suicideprevention/suicidefaq.cfm; National Institute of Mental Health: *In harm's way: suicide in America,* NIH Pub No 03-4594, 2003b, The Author, from http://www.nimh.nih.gov/publicat/harmaway.cfm.

attempts, mental illness, substance abuse, and barriers to accessing mental health treatment. Protective factors may decrease the risk of suicide and include appropriate mental health care, easy access to treatment, community support, and continuing support from medical and mental health care providers. Box 22-5 lists risk factors all community health nurses should be recognize, and Box 22-6 provides prevention strategies that will help reduce the burden of suicide.

To assess the possibility of suicide behaviors, community health nurses should question those they determine at risk in terms of thoughts, plans, lethality, means, and intent. Potential questions to ask, suggested by the APA (2005), include

• Did you ever wish you could go to sleep and just not wake up?
• Have things ever reached the point that you have thought of harming yourself?
• How often have those thoughts occurred (include frequency, obsessional quality, controllability)?
• What do you envision happening if you actually killed yourself (e.g. escape, reunion with significant other, rebirth, reactions of others)?
• Have you made a specific plan to harm or kill yourself? If so, what does the plan include?

For additional information on assessment and treatment of suicidal behaviors, see http://www.psychiatryonline.com.

IDENTIFICATION AND MANAGEMENT OF MENTAL DISORDERS

Early identification, appropriate treatment, and rehabilitation can significantly reduce the duration and level of disability associated with mental disorders and decrease the possibility of relapse. Interventions to promote mental health and decrease mental disorders include focusing on decreasing stressors and/or increasing the capacity of the individual to cope with stress. Other interventions include the use of pharmacological agents and psychosocial interventions such as strengthening interpersonal, psychological, and physical resources through counseling, support groups, and psychoeducation.

The accessibility of mental health service is pivotal in promoting and maintaining the health of aggregates. In the age of financial health care reform, privatization of mental health services, and managed care, community mental services have been deemed the "second wave of deinstitutionalization" (Pickens, 1998). Decreased funding for services, managed care limitations on mental health coverage, and the inequality of coverage by the insurance industry have caused downsizing or forced closure in the traditional places of treatment, such as community mental health and community hospitals. In most cases, the decrease in acute care services has not been balanced by an increase in community mental health services (USDHHS, 1999). Consequently, the accessibility to community mental health services has become an issue of significant concern. In addition, the symptoms of mental illness often interfere with an individual's ability to access services. Alterations in thoughts and perceptions, anxiety, and decreased energy are common symptoms of mental illness, and all interfere with negotiating the complex systems that currently surround mental health service provision. This section describes actions that may be taken by community health nurse to identify mental illness. It also outlines potential treatment options.

Identification of Mental Disorders

Whether the nurse is working in a physician's office, a clinic, home health, a school, occupational health, or another setting, recognition of signs and symptoms that might indicate a mental disorder is an important component of practice. For example, a student might come to the school nurse's office concerned about a friend who induces vomiting in the bathroom after lunch each day; an occupational health nurse might observe signs consistent with alcohol abuse in an employee; or a client might visit a clinic for a routine visit but mention that for the past several weeks she has been unable to sleep, has lost several pounds, and is no longer interested in her normal activities. In each of these situations, the nurse should continue to assess for other signs and symptoms that might indicate a mental disorder and be prepared to intervene should concerns be supported.

Often, the assessment process includes direct questioning or observation. At other times, a standardized assessment tool or questionnaire might be employed. Figures 22-1 and 22-2 contain examples of instruments that are available to elicit information about symptoms of anxiety or depression. Whenever using these or other screening tools, the nurse should be prepared in advance to intervene based on assessment data. Often, this incorporates referral to other health professionals for further assessment, testing, counseling, and treatment and follow-up by all health professionals involved, including the community health nurse.

For example, the nurse who suspects that a student has an eating disorder can talk with his or her parents and teachers, the school counselor, principal, and others to determine the best course of action to follow up on assessment findings and associated concerns. If a client describes signs and symptoms consistent with depression, the nurse should chart the reported information and explain to the client's physician the comments that were voiced. When an employee is suspected of alcohol abuse, the occupational nurse should follow company policy on how, when, and under what circumstances the employee and his or her supervisor should be informed of the concerns. The employee should be given information on available treatment options and support groups.

Management of Mental Disorders

The goals of treatment for mental illness are to reduce symptoms, improve occupational and social functioning, develop and strengthen coping skills, and promote behaviors to improve the individual's life. Basic approaches to the treatment of mental disorders include pharmacotherapy, psychotherapy, and/or behavior therapy (USDHHS 1999).

Psychotherapeutic Medications

Psychotherapeutic medications do not cure mental illness; they act by controlling symptoms. As with medications for physical health problems, the appropriateness of psychopharmacological agents and their prescribed regimen depends on the diagnosis, side effects, and client response. Table 22-2, p. 482 lists some of the most commonly used psychotherapeutic medications. Indications and adverse effects and nursing implications for the different types of medications are briefly discussed.

Antipsychotic Medications

Antipsychotic medications are used to reduce symptoms of schizophrenia and other mental disorders. Antipsychotics are quite effective, but like all medications they may produce side effects. The most common are drowsiness, tachycardia, orthostatic hypotension, weight gain, photosensitivity, and menstrual irregularities. Often, side effects diminish after a few weeks. The side effects will depend on the classification of the drug, whether it is a "typical" or "atypical" antipsychotic.

More serious adverse effects of antipsychotic medications include "extrapyramidal symptoms" (movement disorders resulting from the effect of the drug on the extrapyramidal motor system): these are most commonly associated with the older typical antipsychotics (Laraia, 2005; Sherr, 2004). Acute dystonia (characterized by spasms or cramping of the muscles of the tongue, face, neck, or back), pseudoparkinsonism (including bradykinesia, masklike face, drooling, tremor, rigidity, shuffling gait), and akathisia (restlessness characterized by constant pacing and squirming) are extrapyramidal reactions sometimes seen early in treatment with typical antipsychotic drugs (Levi et al., 2003; Pearson, 2006; Sherr, 2004). These adverse effects tend to decrease with time or can be managed with other medications (e.g., antiparkinsonian agents).

The most serious extrapyramidal adverse effect of use of typical antipsychotic agents, however, is tardive dyskinesia. Tardive dyskinesia develops in about 4% of clients during long-term therapy and produces involuntary movement of the tongue and face. Eating difficulty and weight loss may result. Tardive dyskinesia is permanent, although some symptoms decline after the dosage is reduced or the drug is withdrawn (Pearson, 2006; Sherr, 2004).

Clozapine (Clozaril), risperidone (Risperdal), olanzapine (Zyprexa), quetiapine (Seroquel), and ziprasidone (Geodon) are termed *atypical* antipsychotics. These are relatively new medications that have been shown to be more effective than traditional antipsychotic medications for some people with schizophrenia. These medications also have less risk of extrapyramidal side effects, including tardive dyskinesia, than other antipsychotics. Further, newer atypical antipsychotic drugs have fewer side effects, and those that occur tend to be dose-related. Commonly reported side effects include sedation, weight gain, insomnia, orthostatic hypotension, agitation, constipation, and dry mouth (Levi et al., 2003).

Very serious complications or adverse effects from atypical antipsychotics are possible, however. For example, clozapine is known to cause agranulocytosis in 1% to 2% of clients. Because this condition is potentially fatal, persons on clozapine must have weekly white blood cell counts performed to assess for signs of agranulocytosis. Treatment is stopped if the white blood cell count is below 3000 or the granulocyte count is under 1500 (Levi et al., 2003). Additionally, olanzapine and clozapine have been identified as significantly increasing development or exacerbation of type 2 diabetes in some individuals (Cohen, 2004; Lambert et al., 2005). The choice of therapeutic agents, therefore, is generally based on side effect profile; however, the cost of new medications often influences which drugs are available to patients through managed care.

Antimanic Medications

Lithium is the "gold standard" medication for treatment of bipolar disorders. Response to treatment with lithium varies

During the Past Week	Rarely or None of the Time (Less than 1 Day)	Some or a Little of the Time (1-2 Days)	Occasionally or a Moderate Amount of the Time (3-4 Days)	Most or All of the Time (5-7 Days)
1. I was bothered by things that don't usually bother me.	0	1	2	3
2. I did not feel like eating; my appetite was poor.	0	1	2	3
3. I felt that I could not shake off the blues even with the help of my family or friends.	0	1	2	3
4. I felt that I was just as good as other people.	3	2	1	0
5. I had trouble keeping my mind on what I was doing.	0	1	2	3
6. I felt depressed.	0	1	2	3
7. I felt everything I did was an effort.	0	1	2	3
8. I felt hopeful about the future.	3	2	1	0
9. I thought my life had been a failure.	0	1	2	3
10. I felt fearful.	0	1	2	3
11. My sleep was restless.	0	1	2	3
12. I was happy.	3	2	1	0
13. I talked less than usual.	0	1	2	3
14. I felt lonely.	0	1	2	3
15. People were unfriendly.	0	1	2	3
16. I enjoyed life.	3	2	1	0
17. I had crying spells.	0	1	2	3
18. I felt sad.	0	1	2	3
19. I felt that people disliked me.	0	1	2	3
20. I could not get "going."	0	1	2	3

From Radloff, L. S. (1977). The CES-D scale: A self-report depression scale for research in the general population. *Applied Psychologic Measurement,* 1,385-401. Copyright © 1977, West Publishing Company/Applied Psychological Measurement, Inc. Reproduced by permission.
Interpretation: A total score of 22 or higher is indicative of depression when this scale is used in primary care.

FIGURE 22-1 Center for Epidemiologic Studies depression scale. Interpretation: A total score of 22 or higher is indicative of depression when the scale is used in primary care. (From Radloff LS: The CES-D scale: A self-report depression scale for research in the general population, *Applied Psychological Measurement* 1:385-401, 1977. Copyright 1977, West Publishing Company/Applied Psychological Measurement, Inc.)

somewhat between individual clients. In addition, the range between an effective dose and a toxic dose is small, so serum lithium levels must be monitored closely. It is recommended that levels be checked routinely at the beginning of treatment and every few months thereafter to determine the optimal maintenance dosage (NIMH, 2005a; Pearson, 2006).

Side effects are often worse during the initial stage of lithium therapy and include drowsiness, weakness, nausea, vomiting, fatigue, hand tremors, increased thirst, sexual disturbances, and weight gain. Long-term lithium use may affect thyroid and renal function; therefore, tests to assess both thyroid and kidney function should also be performed periodically (Levi et al., 2003). Lithium toxicity poses a life-threatening situation. Early signs of toxicity include nausea, vomiting, coarse hand tremors, ataxia, and drowsiness. This can be followed by fever, decreased urinary output, and de-

Rank	Life Event	Mean Value	Rank	Life Event	Mean Value
1	Death of spouse	100	23	Son or daughter leaving home	29
2	Divorce	73	24	Trouble with in-laws	29
3	Marital separation	65	25	Outstanding personal achievement	28
4	Jail term	63			
5	Death of close family member	63	26	Wife begins or stops work	26
6	Personal injury or illness	53	27	Begin or end school	26
7	Marriage	50	28	Change in living conditions	25
8	Fired at work	47	29	Change in personal habits	24
9	Marital reconciliation	45	30	Trouble with boss	23
10	Retirement	45	31	Change in work hours or conditions	20
11	Change in health of family member	44			
12	Pregnancy	40	32	Change in residence	20
13	Sex difficulties	39	33	Change in schools	20
14	Gain of new family member	39	34	Change in recreation	19
15	Business readjustment	39	35	Change in church activities	19
16	Change in financial state	38	36	Change in social activities	18
17	Death of close friend	37	37	Mortgage or loan less than $10,000	17
18	Change to different line of work	36			
19	Change in number of arguments with spouse	35	38	Change in sleeping habits	16
			39	Change in number of family get-togethers	15
20	Mortgage over $10,000	31			
21	Foreclosure on mortgage or loan	30	40	Change in eating habits	15
22	Change in responsibilities at work	29	41	Vacation	13
			42	Christmas	12
			43	Minor violations of the law	11

Life Crisis Categories and LCU Scores*

No life crisis	0-149
Mild life crisis	150-199
Moderate life crisis	200-299
Major life crisis	300 or more

Reprinted by permission of the publisher from Holmes, T. H., and Rahe, R. H. (1967). The Social Readjustment Rating Scale, *Journal of Psychosomatic Research, 11.* Copyright 1967 by Elsevier Science Inc. *The LCU score includes those life event items experienced during a 1-year period.

FIGURE 22-2 Social readjustment rating scale. (From Holmes TH, Rahe RH: The social readjustment rating scale, *J Psychosom Res* 11:213-217, 1967, Elsevier Science Inc.)

creased blood pressure. Clearly, these signs and symptoms require immediate medical attention.

Anticonvulsants

Increasingly, anticonvulsants such as valproic acid (Depakote), carbamazepine (Tegretol) and gabapentin (Neurontin) are used to treat mania. The most common side effects of anticonvulsants include drowsiness, dizziness, confusion, visual disturbances, memory impairment, weight gain, and nausea. Periodic blood tests are needed to monitor white blood cell counts and for anemia (NIMH, 2001).

Antidepressants

Antidepressants are used most often for serious depression, but they also can be helpful for mild depression and anxiety. The choice of medications is usually based on the individual client's symptoms. Most medications take 2 to 4 weeks before improvement is seen. If little or no change occurs in symptoms after 5 to 6 weeks, a different medication should be tried. Treatment is usually continued for a minimum of several months and may last up to a year or more. There

are three main categories of antidepressants: tricyclic antidepressants, monoamine oxidase inhibitors and selective serotonin reuptake inhibitors.

In the past, tricyclic antidepressants, such as imipramine (Tofranil), amitriptyline (Elavil) and nortriptyline (Pamelor) were commonly used for treatment of major depression, and they continue to be an effective treatment. However, the side effect profile of these agents, particularly the cardiovascular side effects, makes them less desirable than other, newer agents. Tricyclic antidepressants generally take 2 to 4 weeks to provide significant effect. Side effects vary somewhat between medications and the reaction of the individual to the medication. Potential side effects include drowsiness, blurred vision, dry mouth, constipation, weight gain, orthostatic hypotension, dysuria, fatigue, and weakness. Often, side effects diminish or disappear during the course of treatment. Tricyclics may interfere with other medications and substances, including thyroid hormone, antihypertensives, oral contraceptives, sleeping medications, antipsychotic medications, diuretics, antihistamines, aspirin, vitamin C, alcohol, and tobacco.

TABLE 22-2 Medications for Management of Mental Illnesses

GENERIC NAME	TRADE NAME
ANTIPSYCHOTIC MEDICATIONS	
Chlorpromazine	Thorazine
Chlorprothixene	Taractan
Clozapine	Clozaril
Fluphenazine	Permitil, Prolixin
Haloperidol	Haldol
Loxapine	Loxitane
Mesoridazine	Serentil
Molindone	Lidone, Moban
Olanzapine	Zyprexa
Perphenazine	Trilafon
Pimozide (for Tourette's syndrome)	Orap
Quetiapine	Seroquel
Risperidone	Risperdal
Thioridazine	Mellaril
Thiothixene	Navane
Trifluoperazine	Stelazine
Triflupromazine	Vesprin
Ziprasidone	Geodon
ANTIMANIC MEDICATIONS	
Carbamazepine	Tegretol
Divalproex sodium (valproic acid)	Depakote
Gabapentin	Neurontin
Lamotrigine	Lamictal
Lithium carbonate	Eskalith, Lithane, Lithobid
Lithium citrate	Cibalith-S
Topiramate	Topamax
ANTIDEPRESSANT MEDICATIONS	
Amitriptyline	Elavil
Amoxapine	Asendin
Bupropion	Wellbutrin
Citalopram (SSRI)	Celexa
Clomipramine	Anafranil
Desipramine	Norpramin, Pertofrane
Doxepin	Adapin, Sinequan
Escitalopram (SSRI)	Lexapro
Fluvoxamine (SSRI)	Luvox
Fluoxetine (SSRI)	Prozac
Imipramine	Tofranil
Isocarboxazid (MAOI)	Marplan
Maprotiline	Ludiomil
Mirtazapine	Remeron
Nefazodone	Serzone
Nortriptyline	Aventyl, Pamelor
Paroxetine (SSRI)	Paxil
Phenelzine (MAOI)	Nardil
Protriptyline	Vivactil
Sertraline (SSRI)	Zoloft
Tranylcypromine (MAOI)	Parnate
Trazodone	Desyrel
Trimipramine	Surmontil
Venlafaxine	Effexor
ANTIANXIETY MEDICATIONS (ALL OF THESE MEDICATIONS EXCEPT BUSPIRONE ARE BENZODIAZEPINES)	
Alprazolam	Xanax
Buspirone	BuSpar
Chlordiazepoxide	Librax, Libritabs, Librium
Clonazepam	Klonopin

TABLE 22-2 Medications for Management of Mental Illnesses (cont'd)

GENERIC NAME	TRADE NAME
ANTIANXIETY MEDICATIONS (ALL OF THESE MEDICATIONS EXCEPT BUSPIRONE ARE BENZODIAZEPINES)	
Clorazepate	Azene, Tranxene
Diazepam	Valium
Halazepam	Paxipam
Lorazepam	Ativan
Oxazepam	Serax
Prazepam	Centrax
STIMULANTS	
Amphetamine with dextroamphetamine	Adderall
Dextroamphetamine	Dexedrine, Dextrostat
Dexmethylphenidate	Focalin
Methylphenidate	Ritalin
Methylphenidate (long-acting)	Concerta
Methylphenidate (extended release)	Metadate ER
Pemoline	Cylert

From National Institute of Mental Health: *Medications,* NIH Pub No 02-3929, 2002b, The Author, http://www.nimh.nih.gov/publicat/medicate.cfm.
ER, Extended release; *MAOI,* monoamine oxidase inhibitor; *SSRI,* selective serotonin reuptake inhibitor.

An overdose of tricyclic antidepressant medications may produce tachycardia, dilated pupils, and flushed face. In extreme cases, overdose may cause agitation, which may progress to confusion, loss of consciousness, seizures, arrhythmias, cardiorespiratory collapse, and death (NIMH, 2002).

Monoamine oxidase inhibitors (MAOIs) are more often used for atypical depression in which symptoms like anxiety, panic attacks, and phobias are present and for depression that is unresponsive to other drugs (Pearson, 2006). The MAOIs may cause a serious reaction with certain foods (e.g., aged cheeses, foods containing monosodium glutamate), beverages (e.g., red wines), and medications (e.g., antihistamines, decongestants, local anesthetics, amphetamines, insulin, some narcotics, and antiparkinsonian medications). Reactions may produce hypertension, headache, nausea, vomiting, tachycardia, confusion, psychotic symptoms, seizures, stroke, and coma (NIMH, 2002). Persons taking MAOIs should be given a list of restricted foods, beverages, and medications and encouraged to strictly comply with the restrictions. Because of the side effect profile, these agents are rarely used to treat depression.

Selective serotonin reuptake inhibitors (SSRIs) (also selective reuptake inhibitors [SRIs] and selective norepinephrine reuptake inhibitors [SNRIs]) are the newest class of antidepressants available in the United States, and the most popular. The SSRIs have a more rapid onset of action than do other antidepressants. Improvement is usually seen in 2 to 4 weeks after initiation of therapy (Pearson, 2006). Gastrointestinal problems, headache, insomnia, anxiety, and agitation are the most common side effects of SSRIs. Ejaculatory delay in men and skin rashes, which may be severe, also have been noted. In addition, SSRIs may decrease appetite (Pearson, 2006; Levi et al., 2003).

Serious complications have resulted when SSRIs are used in conjunction with other medications. In particular, fluoxetine (Prozac) should not be combined with MAOIs and should only be used with caution with tricyclic antidepressants (Pearson, 2006). Also, the Food and Drug Administration (FDA) issued a "Black Box" warning for SSRIs suggesting that these drugs may increase suicidal thoughts and behaviors in children and adolescents (FDA, 2004). This has been a controversial subject in the mental health community as many mental health professionals recognize the value of treating suicidal patients and understand the risks involved in denying treatment. Additionally, a landmark study (Simon et al., 2006) appears to refute the claim that suicide increases with the use of SSRIs.

Antianxiety Medications

Benzodiazepines are among the medications used to treat most anxiety disorders. They have been shown to be safe and effective and have low addictive potential. The most commonly used benzodiazepines are alprazolam (Xanax), diazepam (Valium), clonazepam (Klonopin), and lorazepam (Ativan). Antianxiety medications usually act rapidly. Dosage varies greatly, depending on the symptoms and the individual's body chemistry. Common side effects include drowsiness, loss of coordination, fatigue, and mental slowing or confusion. Combination of benzodiazepines and alcohol can produce serious interactions and potentially life-threatening complications, and clients should be warned accordingly.

Stimulants

Stimulants are primarily used to treat symptoms of ADHD and narcolepsy. The most common side effects are decreased appetite and difficulty in falling asleep. Some children report gastrointestinal problems, headache, and depression. Growth retardation has been documented in some children and careful, ongoing assessment of growth patterns is recommended while children are taking stimulants.

Psychotherapy

Psychotherapy refers to a process of discovery that helps alleviate troubling emotional symptoms and assists individuals in returning to a healthy life (APA, 2005). It involves the use of a professional, therapeutic relationship that employs structured conversation to change a client's attitudes, feelings, beliefs, defenses, personality, and behaviors. The therapist's procedures vary across schools of psychotherapy and with the nature of the client's problem. Psychotherapy is often used in conjunction with medication to treat many mental disorders. Various types of psychotherapy include the following (NIMH, 1994):

- *Individual or interpersonal therapy* focuses on the client's current life and relationships within the family, social, and work environments.
- *Family therapy* involves discussions and problem-solving sessions with every member of a family—sometimes with the entire group, sometimes with individual members.

- *Couple therapy* is used to develop the relationship and minimize problems through understanding how individual conflicts are expressed in the couple's interactions.
- *Group therapy* involves a small group of people with similar problems who, with the guidance of a therapist, discuss individual issues and help each other with problems.
- *Play therapy* is a technique used for establishing communication and resolving problems with young children.
- *Cognitive therapy* works to identify and correct distorted thought patterns that can lead to troublesome feelings and behaviors; it is often combined with behavioral therapy.
- *Behavioral therapy* uses learning principles to change thought patterns and behaviors systematically; it is used to encourage the individual to learn specific skills to obtain rewards and satisfaction. Stress management, biofeedback, and relaxation training are examples of behavior therapy

Short-term psychotherapy is often used when situational stresses (e.g., death in the family, divorce, physical illness) produce problems. In these cases, therapy may last only a few weeks or months, with the goal of helping the individual resolve the problem as quickly as possible. Long-term therapy may last for several months to several years and emphasize underlying problems that started in childhood (APA, 2005; NIMH, 1994).

COMMUNITY-BASED MENTAL HEALTH CARE

Over the past several decades, there have been a number of initiatives directed toward improving and promoting community-based care of those with mental illness. One of those initiatives is the President's New Freedom Commission on Mental Health (NFCMH, 2003).

The New Freedom Initiative was first envisioned during George W. Bush's 2000 campaign for the presidency as a promise to tear down the barriers to equality that face millions of Americans with disabilities, including those with mental illness. Following Bush's inauguration, the New Freedom Commission on Mental Health was formed to study the mental health service delivery system. This represented the first comprehensive study of the nation's mental health delivery system in 25 years. The goal of the Commission was to advise the president on strategies aimed at improving the mental health system so that persons with serious and persistent mental illnesses can enjoy full access to community life. The Commission determined that in a transformed mental health system (NFCMH, 2003, p. 8):

1. Americans understand that mental health is essential to overall health.
2. Mental health care is consumer and family driven.
3. Disparities in mental health services are eliminated.
4. Early mental health screening, assessment, and referral to services are common practice.
5. Excellent mental health care is delivered and research is accelerated.
6. Technology is used to access mental health care and information.

TABLE 22-3 Goals and Recommendations of the New Freedom Commission on Mental Health

GOAL	RECOMMENDATIONS
1. Americans understand that mental health is essential to overall health.	Advance and implement a national campaign to reduce the stigma of seeking care and a national strategy for suicide prevention. Address mental health with the same urgency as physical health.
2. Mental health care is consumer and family driven.	Develop an individualized plan of care for every adult with a serious mental illness and child with a serious emotional disturbance. Involve consumers and families fully in orienting the mental health system toward recovery. Align relevant federal programs to improve access and accountability for mental health services. Create a Comprehensive State Mental Health Plan. Protect and enhance the rights of people with mental illnesses.
3. Disparities in mental health services are eliminated.	Improve access to quality care that is culturally competent. Improve access to quality care in rural and geographically remote areas.
4. Early mental health screening, assessment, and referral to services are common practice.	Promote the mental health of young children. Improve and expand school mental health programs. Screen for co-occurring mental and substance use disorders and link with integrated treatment strategies. Screen for mental disorders in primary health care across the life span, and connect to treatment and support.
5. Excellent mental health care is delivered and research is accelerated.	Accelerate research to promote recovery and resilience and ultimately to cure and prevent mental illnesses. Advance evidence-based practices using dissemination and demonstration projects and create a public-private partnership to guide their implementation. Improve and expand the workforce providing evidence-based mental health services and supports. Develop the knowledge base in four understudied areas: mental health disparities, long-term effects of medications, trauma, and acute care.
6. Technology is used to access mental health care and information.	Use health technology and telehealth to improve access and coordination of mental health care, especially for Americans in remote areas or in underserved populations. Develop and implement integrated electronic health record and personal health information systems.

From New Freedom Commission on Mental Health: *Achieving the promise: transforming mental health care in America, Final report,* USDHHS Pub No SMA 03-3832, Rockville, Md, 2003, The Author, http://www.mentalhealthcommission.gov/reports/reports.htm.

ETHICAL Insights

Disparities in Children's Mental Health Care

A recent research study reviewed the records of more than 45,000 children from 13 states to assess use of mental health services and the need for mental health care. Findings showed that, in general, only a minority of vulnerable children and adolescents receive mental health services. This problem was greatly exacerbated among black and Hispanic children and among low-income children. Hispanic children, for example, had the highest unmet need for mental health services: In excess of 77% did not receive needed treatment. Black children, likewise, had significant unmet mental healthy needs, as almost 70% did not get the services they need. Economic situation also played a significant role in children receiving mental health services: The highest level of need was among children in poor families, but they received the lowest level of service. Indeed, children from high-income families were more likely to receive mental health service than children from low-income families.

The researchers concluded that disparities are likely the consequence of state policies and health care market characteristics. There were large differences across states in service use and unmet need. It was suggested that state policies should encourage delivering services to children with the highest need. This would focus care on black and Hispanic children and children from low-income families.

From Strum R, Ringel, JS, Andreyeva T: Geographic disparities in children's mental health care, *Pediatrics* 112(4): 308-318, 2003.

The Commission acknowledged that mental illness comprises the only type of illness that defies a comprehensive delivery approach. This is due to the way the state and local governments organize, manage, and carry out distinct treatment systems, making comprehensive care impossible in the larger health care system. Thus the Commission called for a shift in the fragmented system to an integrated comprehensive approach to mental health care delivery. To that end, they developed a series of recommendations; examples are listed in Table 22-3.

One of the areas addressed by the Commission pertained to the need for school-based mental health (SBMH) programs. In an overview of key elements related to SBMH, Paternite (2005) identified the need for (1) partnerships between and among schools, families, and communities; (2) a pledge to support a full continuum of mental health services that include education, health promotion, assessment, and early intervention; and (3) services for all children and adolescents.

Subsequently, national mental health leaders were surveyed to assess the participants' perceptions of the impact of the New Freedom Commission recommendations (von Esenwein et al., 2005). Results of this survey suggested that the Commission findings and suggestions for improved care had a significant influence on the mental health care organizations represented.

In another initiative, the Center for Mental Health Services (CMHS) was formed in the early 1990s to improve

TABLE 22-4 Center for Mental Health Services: Examples of Programs and Initiatives

PROGRAM/INITIATIVE	PURPOSE AND ACTIVITIES
National Strategy for Suicide Prevention	Collaborative effort of SAMHSA, CDC, NIH, HRSA, and IHS to reduce the incidence of suicide in the United States; supports and monitors state-based suicide prevention programs and provides information and resources
Center on Women, Violence and Trauma	Sponsored by SAMHSA to highlight the role of violence and trauma in the lives of people with behavioral health disorders; provides information and helps fund related studies
Youth Violence Prevention Program	Offers the Safe Schools/Health Students Initiative to prevent school violence and foster the healthy development of children. This is a collaborative grant program that supports community collaborations that prevent youth violence, substance abuse, suicide, and other mental and behavioral problems.
Homelessness Programs	Support of programs to assist people with mental illness who are homeless in obtaining treatment and other services (e.g., primary health care, substance abuse treatment, legal assistance)
State Planning and Mental Health Block Grants	Awards grants to states to provide mental health services. These grants are designed to improve access to community-based health care delivery systems for people with serious mental illnesses who quickly exhaust available resources.
Caring for Every Child's Mental Health Campaign	National public information and education campaign to increase public awareness about the importance of protecting and nurturing the mental health of young people, to foster recognition that many children have mental health problems, and to encourage caregivers to seek early, appropriate treatment

CDC, Centers for Disease Control and Prevention; *HRSA*, Health Resources and Services Administration; *IHS*, Indian Health Service; *NIH*, National Institutes of Health; *SAMHSA*, Substance Abuse and Mental Health Services Administration.

prevention and mental health treatment services for all Americans. The CMHS helps states improve and increase the quality and range of treatment, rehabilitation, and support for people with mental health problems, their families, and communities (SAMHSA, 2005).

One of the programs promoted by the CMHS is the Community Support System. The Community Support System uses case management strategies to comprehensively provide care for those with serious mental illness. Components of the Community Support System include client identification and outreach, mental health treatment, crisis response service, health and dental care, housing, income support and entitlement, peer support, family and community support, rehabilitation services, and protection and advocacy. The case management approach serves to link the service system to the client and to coordinate their service received (Huggins and Anderson, 2006). Other initiatives and programs sponsored by the CMHS are shown in Table 22-4.

The **Program of Assertive Community Treatment (PACT)** is another example of a community-based initiative to help meet the needs of those with mental illness. PACT, which has been in existence since the late 1960s, has become the exemplar of community mental health treatment models. The PACT program moves the traditional 24-hour treatment model of acute care settings into the community and serves people with mental illness in a highly individualized fashion (NAMI, 2005). The PACT model provides around-the-clock supportive therapy, mobile crisis intervention, psychiatric medications, hospitalization, education, and skill teaching for consumers and their families. PACT brings service to the consumer and is considered the model of effective community mental health treatment of the future. A NAMI PACT initiative encourages all states to have assertive community treatment. Currently, seven states and the District of Columbia have statewide PACT programs, and many more have at least one pilot project (NAMI, 2005). Box 22-7 gives additional details about PACT programs.

BOX 22-7 Key Features of the Program of Assertive Community Treatment

- ➤ Psychopharmacological treatment
- ➤ Individual supportive therapy
- ➤ Mobile crisis intervention
- ➤ Hospitalization
- ➤ Substance abuse treatment
- ➤ Behaviorally oriented skill teaching
- ➤ Supported employment
- ➤ Support for resuming education
- ➤ Collaboration with families and assistance to clients with children
- ➤ Direct support to help clients obtain legal and advocacy services

ROLE OF THE COMMUNITY MENTAL HEALTH NURSE

During and shortly after deinstitutionalization, mental health services were accessed through the following distinct points of contact: inpatient facilities, community mental health centers, and community support programs. In recent years, community mental health services have become more complex. Services are currently provided in diverse settings that often are not in direct communication with one another.

To understand the mental health needs of an aggregate, nurses must consider several divergent factors that affect the mental health of aggregates, such as genetic inheritance, life experience, and temperament. In addition, mental health and mental illness are not static concepts. Mental health is subject to multiple influences. Consequently, mental illness and mental health must also be assessed in the context of social environments that include family, community, peer reference groups, and physical and cultural surroundings. Formal and informal sources of community mental health support are equally important. Consumers and their families have been a valuable and often overlooked community resource. Enhanced efforts

CASE STUDY   Application of the Nursing Process

Kay Morton is a registered nurse working in a public-sponsored primary care clinic for indigent and homeless people in a large southwestern city. The clinic is housed in a center that provides comprehensive care for the poor. The Center employs family practice physicians, two registered nurses, one licensed vocational nurse, a mental health nurse practitioner, two counselors, and three social workers. Residents from an area medical school provide additional medical support. In addition to meeting the health care needs of the community, the team provides assistance with job training and employment as well as assistance with housing and child care.

Jeannie Smith is one of the clients served by the Center. Jeannie is a 25-year-old single mother of three young children (ages 8, 6, and 2) who has been receiving public assistance for more than 8 years. During that time, her children have been in foster care on several occasions. She admits to a history of using marijuana, methamphetamine, and alcohol as well as having multiple sexual partners. Two years ago, Jeannie was diagnosed with bipolar disorder and is currently taking medication to manage her symptoms.

On a recent visit to the Center to work with her case manager, Jeannie was also seen at the clinic. Kay greeted Jeannie and led her to a private room for her follow-up care. During this period, she casually asked Jeannie about her children. They discussed how Jeannie was managing three children and her new job as a clerk at a local bank.

ASSESSMENT

Kay noted that Jeannie answered questions appropriately. In her notes, Kay wrote that the client stated that her work was tedious and she did not feel like she "fit in" with the other people at work. Jeannie reported that she had been generally compliant with her medication regimen, although she stated she sometimes forgets to take her morning medications because she is in a rush to get the children to school and day care and herself to work. She had not observed any side effects from the medications, and she denied using any illicit drugs or alcohol since her last visit. However, Jeannie told Kay that she was having strong urges to drink beer when she came home from work and that she was having trouble "fighting" these feelings. She also reported that Macy, her 8-year-old daughter, was having trouble in school. The teacher had noted that Macy often did not complete homework assignments, was having trouble paying attention in class, and had few friends.

DIAGNOSIS

Individual
- History of mental illness (bipolar disorder) and substance abuse
- Potential for noncompliance with treatment regimen
- Social isolation
- Chronic low self-esteem

Family
- Potential for family dysfunction
- Potential for social isolation

Community
- Knowledge deficit regarding community resources for diagnosis and management of mental disorders

PLANNING

Planning for Jeannie involved reviewing her case management protocol and determining if she was following recommendations. Agency protocols required random drug screening for all clients. For clients on certain medications (including those taken by Jeannie), blood testing was required. Then Kay talked briefly with Jeannie's case manager to determine the time scheduled for her counseling session. Kay also obtained information about the local Alcoholics Anonymous (AA) and the National Depressive and Manic Depressive Association (NDMDA) support group meeting schedules. Kay also consulted with the case manager to determine ways to improve her daughter, Macy's school performance.

Individual
Long-Term Goal
- Jeannie will progress with her employment and be able to support her family without public assistance.

Short-Term Goals
- Jeannie will remain compliant with her medication and case management regimen.
- Jeannie will remain drug-free.

Family
Long-Term Goals
- Jeannie and her children will maintain a stable household.
- The children will progress well in school.

Short-Term Goal
- Daughter Macy will be evaluated for a learning or attention disorder.

INTERVENTION

Individual
Kay collected a urine specimen from Jeannie to be sent for drug screening. To ensure that Jeannie's lithium levels were in therapeutic range, the physician asked Kay to obtain a sample of blood. Kay drew a small sample from Jeannie's right arm using careful sterile technique and paying attention to universal precautions. She reviewed the purpose of the test with Jeannie and explained that the results would be back in a couple of days. While she was working with Jeannie, Kay listened to her concerns about how she was going to pay for

CASE STUDY   Application of the Nursing Process (cont'd)

new clothes and shoes for the children for the upcoming school year.

Kay suggested that Jeannie plan to attend an upcoming AA meeting and reestablish herself with the group, as this had been a successful strategy in the past for managing Jeannie's urges to drink. Kay reeducated Jeannie about the purpose and effects of lithium and discussed the importance of maintaining a therapeutic level of the drug to prevent breakthrough bipolar symptoms. Kay also referred Jeannie to the NDMDA support group as a resource for illness management.

Family

Kay suggested that Jeannie make an appointment with the school counselor to discuss Macy's progress as well as an appointment for Macy to be seen in the clinic for a physical examination. After Kay finished charting, she reported the findings to Jeannie's counselor and was careful to mention what Jeannie had told her about financial concerns. Kay arranged for a follow-up appointment with Jeannie and Macy in 2 weeks, as she was aware that Jeannie was at risk for deteriorating symptomatically and also understood the importance of assessing Macy further in order to reduce Macy's distress and identify additional community resources for her.

EVALUATION

Jeannie verbalized understanding the importance of following the recommendations and left to keep her appointment with her counselor. Jeannie's counselor reported that she would assist her client in finding sources that would help pay for school clothes and supplies. Kay would watch for the results of the tests and report back to both Jeannie and her counselor. Jeannine also reported that she would talk with Macy's teacher and school counselor.

LEVELS OF PREVENTION

Primary

* Assisting Jeannie in finding and maintaining employment
* Providing information on services and providers to assist with clothing and school supplies for the children

Secondary

* Evaluation of daughter Macy to determine cause of school difficulties

Tertiary

* Monitoring of Jeannie's lithium levels
* Testing Jeannie's urine for illicit drugs
* Counseling to encourage Jeannie to attend AA meetings and NDMAD support group

---

are needed to provide peer support and intensive educational programs about mental illness in schools, worksites, and elsewhere.

Community mental health nursing roles can be conceptualized as multidimensional (e.g., educator and activist or practitioner and coordinator). As an educator and activist, the community mental health nurse is charged with improving public awareness of effective treatments and existing community resources. Community mental health nurses as educators and activists can dispel myths and provide accurate information about mental illness. In addition, the educator and activist responsibility includes influencing policy and legislation to empower and advocate for the rights of those with mental illness.

As practitioner and coordinator, the nurse works directly with individuals, groups, and families. Unlike the acute care setting, the community mental health environment is generally the consumer's home. Besides intervening to assist consumers in controlling or alleviating the symptoms of mental illness, the practitioner and coordinator also helps the consumer "navigate" within the segmented web of agencies and other service providers. Community mental health nurses do not merely take action to solve an immediate problem. They plan and intervene within parameters that ensure safety, continuity, and quality of care for consumers. Therefore the practitioner and coordinator role requires skills in anticipating and evaluating the actions of other providers and communicating

with consumers, families, rehabilitation services, and government or social agencies.

Within this aspect of community mental health nursing, individual-, family-, and community-level crises are anticipated, prevented, and, failing these, contained. For example, as practitioners and coordinators, nurses might organize people taking psychotropic medications to share experiences about interacting with a psychiatrist. Consumers might understand all of their options and maximize the benefits of medications. This is proactive in preventing crises resulting from sudden self-discontinuation of medication. In the practitioner and coordinator role, community mental health nurses work toward matching consumers and families with culturally appropriate and sensitive providers to achieve the "best fit."

SUMMARY

Like all other aspects of nursing, community mental health nursing is evolving. At the beginning of the twenty-first century, conditions are in place that should promote dramatic improvement in the identification and care for those with mental illness. Improved information and the advent of evidence-based practice should result in greater understanding of the factors that contribute to mental disorders and lead to more effective treatment. Ultimately, there should be increased attention given to prevention of mental illness and promotion of mental health.

As discussed in this chapter, the vast majority of individuals with diagnosable mental disorders are found in the community, and many, if not most, never seek professional help. The framework for community mental health nursing presented in this chapter should prove useful in improving the lives of individuals, families, and groups of people with mental illness. Further, it is hoped that all nurses will become advocates for the mentally ill and support social and political change to improve the mental health of all.

LEARNING ACTIVITIES

1. Reflect on personal experience interacting with individuals with mental illness. What thoughts or feelings did these experiences produce?
2. Locate the NAMI chapter in your community. What services do they offer? How might those services be helpful in the community mental health nursing role?
3. List five ways to act as an educator and activist for mental health issues in the community.

REFERENCES

American Hospital Association: House bill to end insurance discrimination gains majority support. "Fairness Coalition" urges policy-makers to vote on mental health parity, Press release, Nov 14, 2005, http://www.aha.org/aha/key_issues/psych/content/20051114parity.pdf#search='paul%20wellstone%20mental%20health%20equitable%20treatment%20act.

American Psychiatric Association: *Diagnostic and statistical manual of mental disorders,* ed 4, text revision, Washington, DC, 2000, The Author.

American Psychiatric Association: *Practice guideline for the treatment of patients with major depressive disorder,* ed 2, 2005, The Author, http://www.psychiatryonline.com.

American Psychiatric Association: *Assessing and treating suicidal behaviors: a quick reference guide,* The Author, http://www.psychiatryonline.com/content.aspx?aID=111622.

American Psychiatric Association: *Psychotherapy,* The Author, http://healthyminds.org/psychotherapy.cfm.

Antai-Otong D: Foundations of psychiatric nursing practice. In Antai-Otong D, editor: *Psychiatric nursing: biological and behavioral concepts,* Clifton Park, NY, 2003, Delmar Publishing, pp. 81-106.

Buchsbaum MS, Haier RJ: Functional and anatomical brain imaging, *Schizophr Bull* 14:383, 1982.

Cochrane C: Eating regulation response and eating disorders. In Stuart GW, Laraia MT, editors: *Principles and practice of psychiatric nursing,* ed 8, St. Louis, 2005, Mosby.

Cohen D: Atypical antipsychotics and new onset diabetes mellitus: An overview of the literature. *Pharmacopsychiatry,* 37(1):1-11, 2004.

Corrigan PW, Penn DL: Lessons from social psychology on discrediting psychiatric stigma, *Am Psychol* 54:765, 1999.

Decker SD: The client with an eating disorder. In Mohr WK, editor: *Psychiatric-mental health nursing,* ed 6, Philadelphia, 2006, Lippincott Williams & Wilkins, pp. 553-576.

Decker WA, Freeman M: The journey challenged by eating disorders. In Carson VB and Arnold EN, editors: *Mental health nursing: The nurse-patient journey.* Philadelphia: WB Saunders, 1996.

Deutsch A: *The mentally ill in America: a history of their care and treatment from colonial times,* New York, 1949, Columbia University Press.

Food and Drug Administration: *Labeling change request letter for antidepressant medications,* Rockville, Md, 2004, The Author, http://www.fda.gov/cder/drug/antidepressants/SSRIlabelChange.htm.

Foucault M: *Madness and civilization,* New York, 1965, Random House.

Fortinash KM: Schizophrenia. In Fortinash KM, Holoday-Worret PA, editors: *Psychiatric-mental health nursing,* ed 3, St. Louis, 2004, Mosby.

Grob GN: *Mental illness and American society, 1875-1940,* Princeton, NJ, 1983, Princeton University Press.

Grob GN: *From asylum to community: mental health policy in modern America,* Princeton, NJ, 1991, Princeton University Press.

Grob GN: *The mad among us: a history of the care of America's mentally ill,* New York, 1994, Free Press.

Hall JM, Stevens PE, Meleis AI: Marginalization: a guiding concept for valuing diversity in nursing knowledge development, *Adv Nurs Sci* 13(3):16, 1994.

Hanson KW: Public opinion and the parity debate: lessons from the survey literature, *Psychiatr Serv* 49:1059, 1998.

Holiday SG: *Schizophrenia: breaking down the barriers,* Manchester, England, 1996, Wiley.

Holmes TH, Rahe RH: The social readjustment rating scale, *J Psychosom Res* 11:213-217, 1967.

Huggins M, Anderson JA: Community mental health, support and rehabilitation. In Mohr WK, editor: *Psychiatric-Mental Health Nursing,* ed 6, Philadelphia, 2006, Lippincott Williams & Wilkins, pp. 319-337.

Hunter RA: *Three hundred years of psychiatry: 1535-1800,* London, 1963, Oxford University Press.

Kandel ER: A new intellectual framework for psychiatry, *Am J Psychiatry* 155:457, 1998.

Lambert BL, Chou CH, Chang KY, Tafesse E, Carson: Antipsychotic exposure and type 2 diabetes among patients with schizophrenia: a matched case-control study of California Medicaid claims. *Pharmacoepidemiol Drug Saf* 14(6):417–425, 2005.

Laraia MT: Biological context of psychiatric nursing care. In Stuart GW, Laraia MT, editors: *Principles and practice of psychiatric nursing,* ed 8, St. Louis, 2005, Mosby.

Levi V, Antai-Otong D, Pennebaker DF, Riley J: Psychopharmacologic therapy. In Antai-

Otong D, editor: *Psychiatric nursing: biological and behavioral concepts,* Clifton Park, NY, 2003, Delmar Publishing, pp. 767-816.

Lewin L: The client with a depressive disorder. In Antai-Otong D, editor: *Psychiatric nursing: biological and behavioral concepts,* Clifton Park, NY, 2003, Delmar Publishing, pp. 195-227.

Lim KO: Gray matter volume deficits in young onset schizophrenia, *Biol Psychiatry* 40:4, 1996.

Marsh L: Medial temporal lobe structures in schizophrenia: relationship of size to duration of illness, *Schizophr Res* 11:25, 1994.

McCrae CN: *Stereotypes and stereotyping,* New York, 1996, Guilford Press.

Mohr WK, Mohr BD: Brain, behavior, connections and implications: psychodynamics no more, *Arch Psychiatr Nurs* 15(4):171-181, 2001.

National Association for the Mentally Ill: *Paul Wellstone Mental Health Equitable Treatment Act of 2003 introduced,* Arlington, Va, April 28, 2003, The Author, http://www.nami.org/Content/ContentGroups/E-News/2003/February_2003/Paul_Wellstone_Mental_Health_Equitable_Treatment_Act_of_2003_Introduced.htm.

National Association for the Mentally Ill: *PACT: Program of assertive community treatment,* The Author, http://www.nami.org/Template.cfm?Section=ACT-TA_Center&template=/ContentManagement/ContentDisplay.cfm&ContentID=28608.

National Institute for Mental Health: *Helpful facts about depressive illness,* NIH Publication No. 94-3875. Rockville, MD: National Institute of Mental Health, 1994.

National Institute for Mental Health: *Parity: the equivalence of mental illness with general medical illness,* Washington, DC, 1998, US Government Printing Office.

National Institute for Mental Health: *Frequently asked questions about suicide,* Dec 1999, The Author, http://www.nimh.nih.gov/suicideprevention/suicidefaq.cfm.

National Institute of Mental Health: *Depression,* NIH Pub No 00-3561, Rockville, Md, 2000, The Author.

National Institute of Mental Health: *Eating disorders,* 2001, the Author, http://www.nimh.nih.gov/publicat/eatingdisorders.cfm.

National Institute of Mental Health: *Facts about post-traumatic stress disorder,* 2002a, The

Author, from http://www.nimh.nih.gov/publicat/ptsdfacts.cfm.

National Institute of Mental Health: *Medications,* NIH Pub No 02-3929, 2002b, The Author, http://www.nimh.nih.gov/publicat/medicate.cfm.

National Institute of Mental Health: *Attention deficit hyperactivity disorder,* NIH Pub No 3572, 2003a, The Author, http://www.nimh.nih.gov/publicat/adhd.cfm.

National Institute of Mental Health: *In harm's way: suicide in America,* NIH Pub No 03-4594, 2003b, The Author, from http://www.nimh.nih.gov/publicat/harmaway.cfm.

National Institute of Mental Health: *Depression: a treatable illness,* 2004a, The Author, http://menanddepression.nimh.nih.gov/infopage.asp?id=15.

National Institute of Mental Health: *Suicide facts and statistics 2001,* 2004b, The Author http://www.nimh.nih.gov/suicideprevention/suifact.cfm.

National Institute of Mental Health: *Going to extremes: bipolar disorder,* 2005a, The Author, http://www.nimh.nih.gov/publicat/manic.cfm.

National Institute of Mental Health: *Schizophrenia,* 2005b, The Author, http://www.nimh.nih.gov/healthinformation/schizophreniamenu.cfm.

National Mental Health Association: Children's mental health statistics, 2006, The Author, http://www.nmha.org/children/prevent/stats.cfm.

National Mental Health Association: *Mental health and you,* Alexandria, Va, 1996, The Author.

New Freedom Commission on Mental Health: *Achieving the promise: transforming mental health care in America, Final report,* USDHHS Pub No SMA 03-3832, Rockville, Md, 2003, http://www.mentalhealthcommission.gov/reports/reports.htm.

Paternite CE: School-based mental health programs and services: overview and introduction to the special issue, *J Abnorm Child Psychol* 33(6):657-663, 2005.

Pearson G: Psychopharmacology. In Mohr WK, editor: *Psychiatric-mental health nursing,* ed 6, Philadelphia, 2006, Lippincott, pp. 243-286.

Pickens J: Formal and informal care of people with psychiatric disorders: historical perspectives and current trends, *J Psychosoc Nurs Ment Health Serv* 36(1):37, 1998.

Radloff LS: The CES-D scale: a self-report depression scale for research in the general population, *Applied Psychological Measurement* 1:385-401, 1977.

Raingruber B: Client and provider perspectives regarding the stigma of and nonstigmatizing interventions for depression *Arch Psychiatr Nurs* 16(5):201-207, 2002.

Sharfstein SS, Stoline AM, Koran, LM: Mental health services. In Kovner AR, Jonas S, editors: *Jonas & Kovner's health care delivery in the United States,* ed 7, New York, 2002, Springer, pp 238-262.

Sherr J: Psychopharmacology and other biologic therapies. In Fortinash KM, Holoday-Worret PA, editors: *Psychiatric and mental health nursing,* ed 3, St. Louis, 2004, Elsevier.

Simon GE et al: Suicide risk during antidepressant treatment, *Am J Psychiatry* 163:41-47, 2006.

Strum R, Ringel, JS, Andreyeva T: Geographic disparities in children's mental health care, *Pediatrics* 112(4), 308-318, 2003.

Stuart GW, Laraia MT: *Principles and practice of psychiatric nursing,* ed 8, St. Louis, 2005, Elsevier/Mosby.

Substance Abuse and Mental Health Services Administration: *Results from the 2004 National Survey on Drug Use and Health: national findings,* Office of Applied Studies, NSDUH Series H-28, USDHHS Pub No SMA 05-4062, Rockville, Md, 2005.

Tommasini NR: The client with a mood disorder (depression). In Antai-Otong D, editor: *Psychiatric nursing: biological and beha-* *vioral concepts,* Philadelphia, 1995, WB Saunders, pp. 157-190.

Torrey EF: *Out of the shadows: confronting America's mental illness crisis,* New York, 1997, John Wiley and Sons.

Unutzer J et al: Transforming mental health care at the interface with general medicine: report for the Presidents Commission, *Psychiatr Serv* 57:37-47, 2006.

US Department of Health and Human Services: *Mental health: a report of the Surgeon General,* Washington, DC, 1999, Government Printing Office, http://www.surgeongeneral.gov/library/mentalhealth/chapter2/sec2_1.html.

US Department of Health and Human Services: *Healthy People 2010,* ed 2, Washington, DC, 2000, US Government Printing Office.

US Department of Health and Human Services/Office of Disease Prevention and Health Promotion: *Clinician's handbook of preventive services,* ed 2, Washington, DC, 1998, US Government Printing Office.

US Department of Health and Human Services/Substance Abuse and Mental Health Services Administration: *Results from the 2004 National Survey on Drug Use and Health: national findings,* Washington, DC, 2005, The Author.

von Esenwein SA et al: A survey of mental health leaders one year after the President's New Freedom Commission report, *Psychiatr Serv* 56(5):605-607, 2005.

Weinberger DR: The biological basis of schizophrenia: new directions, *J Clin Psychiatry* 58(10):22, 1997.

Zimmerman ML, Berchin H, Quallo HT: The client with an eating disorder. In Antai-Otong D, editor: *Psychiatric nursing: biological and behavioral concepts,* Clifton Park, NY, 2003, Delmar Publishing, pp. 583-610.

UNIT 6

Population Health Problems

Communicable Disease

Deanna E. Grimes

MEDIA RESOURCES

Additional Material for Study, Review, and Further Exploration

evolve Website at http://evolve.elsevier.com/Nies

❖ Quiz ❖ Case Studies ❖ Content Updates ❖ Glossary ❖ WebLinks ❖ Resource Tools

23A Recommended Childhood and Adolescent Immunization Schedule by Vaccine and Age – United States, 2005; **23B** Recommended Adult Immunization Schedule by Vaccine and Medical and Other Indications-United States, October 2005-September 2006

OBJECTIVES

Upon completion of this chapter, the reader will be able to do the following:

1. Review principles related to the occurrence and transmission of infection and infectious diseases.
2. Describe the three focus areas in *Healthy People 2010* objectives that apply to infectious diseases.
3. Describe the chain of transmission of infectious diseases.
4. Apply the chain of transmission to describing approaches to control infectious disease.
5. Review types of immunity, including herd immunity.

6. Review principles of immunization, and specify the immunization recommended for all age groups in the United States.
7. Describe the legal responsibility for control of communicable diseases in the United States
8. Describe the chain of transmission and control for priority infectious disease.
9. Identify nursing activities for control of infectious diseases at primary, secondary, and tertiary levels of prevention.

KEY TERMS

acquired immunity
active immunity
agent
antigenicity
carrier
case
cold chain
communicable disease
communicable period
control
direct transmission
elimination
endemic
environment

epidemic
eradication
fomite
herd immunity
host
immunity
immunization
incidence
incubation period
indirect transmission
infection
infectious disease
infectivity
isolation

latency
multicausation
natural immunity
notifiable infectious diseases
outbreak
pandemic
passive immunity
pathogenicity
portal of entry
portal of exit
primary vaccine failure
quarantine
reservoir
resistance

secondary vaccine failure
subclinical infection
susceptible
toxigenicity
universal precautions
vaccination
Vaccine Adverse Events Reporting System (VAERS)
vector
virulence

CHAPTER OUTLINE

Throughout history, epidemics have been responsible for the annihilation of entire groups of people. Despite amazing advances in public health and health care, control of communicable diseases continues to be a major concern of health care providers. The emergence of new pathogens, the reemergence of old pathogens, and the appearance of drug-resistant pathogens are creating formidable challenges worldwide.

Despite global eradication campaigns, malaria and other vector-borne diseases, and life-threatening gastrointestinal infections continue to cause significant morbidity and mortality in the developing world. Tuberculosis infects one third of the world's population and has become a leading killer of young adults worldwide, particularly those infected with the human immunodeficiency virus (HIV) (World Health Organization [WHO], 2004). Measles, when coupled with vitamin A deficiency, is a leading cause of blindness in many developing countries in the Eastern Hemisphere. To add to the world's growing infectious disease burden, HIV and acquired immunodeficiency syndrome (AIDS) continue to spread unchecked throughout the world, as evidenced by estimates of 39.4 million adults and children living with HIV/AIDS throughout the world at the end of 2004, and that 4.9 million new infections occur every year (UNAIDS, 2004).

Great strides have been made in the United States with respect to vaccine-preventable diseases, yet segments of the population remain unimmunized or under-immunized. Both measles and pertussis are preventable with a vaccine, and indigenous measles has virtually been eliminated in the United States, with only 56 cases reported in 2003. In contrast, there were 11,647 cases of pertussis reported in the same year, the highest number since 1964 (Centers for Disease Control and Prevention [CDC], 2005a). Hepatitis A, B, and C have been significantly reduced since the 1990s, by administering vaccines for hepatitis A and B and testing the blood supply for hepatitis C. Yet these diseases persist. Treatable sexually transmitted diseases (STDs), such as syphilis and gonorrhea, have declined somewhat during the past decade, but they are far from eradicated. At the same time incidence of another treatable STD, chlamydia, has increased almost 70% since 1995, and the number of cases reached 304.7 per 100,000 people in 2003 (CDC, 2005a). In the United States, there have been significant accomplishments in preventing food- and water-borne infections through environmental sanitation, but there appears to be increasing incidence of vector-borne infections, such as Lyme disease, Rocky Mountain spotted fever, St. Louis encephalitis, and West Nile encephalitis. Further, while the advent of effective antiretroviral treatment for AIDS in the mid 1990s briefly slowed the incidence of AIDS diagnosis, about 45,000 new AIDS cases have been reported every year since 1999 (CDC, 2005a).

Probably one of the most profound failures in infectious disease control in the United States and elsewhere is that the successes are not equally disseminated in the general population. Infectious diseases continue to be differentially distributed by income and ethnic groups, and the poor and minorities continue to experience the greater burden.

Although there has been marked improvement, infectious and communicable diseases persist. Recent scientific discoveries on the infectious etiology of stomach ulcers, coronary artery disease, and cervical cancer, for example, suggest that infectious agents may be responsible for more morbidity and mortality than previously recognized. New concerns include the rapid proliferation of drug resistant organisms (Box 23-1) and the recent threat that deadly pathogens will be weaponized by terrorists (Box 23-2). Other threats are emerging infectious diseases, those diseases where the incidence in humans has increased within the past two decades or threatens to increase in the near future (Table 23-1).

This chapter is written to provide nurses with the knowledge necessary to help control infectious diseases. The terms *communicable disease* and *infectious disease* are synonymous, and will be used interchangeably (Heymann, 2004).

BOX 23-1 Drug-Resistant Pathogens/Diseases

- *Acinetobacter* spp.: Nosocomial bacteremia, septicemia
- *Bordetella pertussis:* Pertussis
- *Campylobacter* (fluoroquinolone-resistant): Enteritis
- *Enterococcus* spp. (multidrug-resistant, including vancomycin-resistant [VRE])
- *Enterobacter* spp.
- HIV: AIDS
- *Klebsiella* spp.
- *Mycobacterium tuberculosis* (multidrug-resistant [MDR-TB]): Tuberculosis
- *Neisseria gonorrhoeae* (fluoroquinolone-resistant): Gonorrhea
- *Pediculous humanus capitus:* Head lice
- *Plasmodium falciparum* and *P. vivax:* Malaria
- *Pseudomonas aeruginosa*
- *Salmonella* spp.: Typhoid fever and salmonellosis
- *Staphylococcus aureus* (methicillin-resistant [MRSA], vancomycin-resistant [VRSA])
- *Staphylococcus epidermidis* (VRSE, MRSE)
- *Streptococcus pneumoniae* (multidrug-resistant): Pneumonia, meningitis, and otitis media
- *Treponema pallidum* (azithromycin-resistant): Syphilis
- Other gram-negative bacteria developing drug resistance: *Citrobacter freundii, Escherichia coli, Morganella morganii, Providencia* spp., and *Serratia* spp.

From Centers for Disease Control and Prevention: Diseases connected to antibiotic resistance, 2005b, The Author, http://www.cdc.gov/drugresistance/diseases.html; Heymann DL, editor: *Control of communicable diseases manual,* ed 18, Washington, DC, 2004, APHA; Murray PR et al: *Manual of clinical microbiology,* ed 6, Washington, DC, 1995, ASM Press.

BOX 23-2 Centers for Disease Control and Prevention List of Potential Bioterrorism Agents and Diseases

- Anthrax *(Bacillus anthracis)*
- Botulism (botulinum toxin)
- Brucellosis *(Brucella* spp.)
- Cholera *(Vibrio cholerae)*
- Plague *(Yersinia pestis)*
- Q fever *(Coxiella burnetii)*
- Salmonellosis *(Salmonella* spp.)
- Shigellosis *(Shigella* spp.)
- Smallpox (variola virus)
- Tularemia *(Francisella tularensis)*
- Viral hemorrhagic fevers (Ebola, Lassa, and Marburg viruses)

From: Centers for Disease Control and Prevention: Bioterrorism agents/diseases, 2004, http://www.bt.cdc.gov/agent/agentlist.asp.

ETHICAL Insights

Nurse's Responsibility Regarding Communicable Diseases

Rapid proliferation of drug resistant organisms, bioterrorism, and emerging infectious diseases are all concerns that have great implications for nursing practice. *Every* nurse should be knowledgeable about recognizing, preventing and controlling infectious diseases. Infectious disease control can no longer be limited to the jurisdiction of the public health department or the hospital infection control nurse; it is every nurse's responsibility.

COMMUNICABLE DISEASE AND *HEALTHY PEOPLE 2010*

Healthy People 2010 contains 467 objectives to improve health; these are organized into 28 focus areas. Three of the focus areas (Immunization and Infectious Diseases, Sexually Transmitted Diseases, and HIV) are specific to infectious diseases (U.S. Department of Health and Human Services [USDHHS], 2000a,b,c). These objectives have been used for evaluating national prevention and control efforts and can guide local prevention and control efforts. The *Healthy People 2010* table on p. 498 shows examples of objectives for immunizations and infectious diseases, objectives related to sexually transmitted diseases, and a few of the objectives covering HIV/AIDS. These lists suggest strategies for prevention and control of infectious diseases. Additional information, including baseline and target data for all objectives, can be found on the *Healthy People 2010* website listed with the table.

PRINCIPLES OF INFECTION AND INFECTIOUS DISEASE OCCURRENCE

Nuses in all settings must be aware of potential threats related to communicable diseases and prepared to intervene (see Ethical Insights). To help prepare nurses for this responsibility, biological and epidemiological principles inherent in infection and infectious disease occurrence have been reviewed and major terms defined in this section.

Multicausation

During the early years of medical and nursing history, science promulgated cause and effect theories of disease that relied on specifying one cause for each disease. Today, it is understood that disease etiology is complex and multicausal. Infectious diseases are the result of interaction among the human **host,** an infectious **agent,** and the **environment** which surrounds the human host and where transmission is occurring. This interaction is pictured in the epidemiological triad of agent, host, and environment, described in Chapter 4 (Epidemiology). The principle of **multicausation** emphasizes that an infectious agent alone is not sufficient to cause disease; the agent must be transmitted within a conducive environment to a susceptible host.

Spectrum of Infection

Not all contact with an infectious agent leads to infection and not all infection leads to an infectious disease. The processes, however, begin in the same way. An infectious agent may contaminate the skin or mucous membranes of a host, but not invade the host. Or it may invade, multiply, and produce a **subclinical infection** (inapparent or asymptomatic) without producing overt symptomatic disease. Or the host may respond with overt symptomatic infectious disease. **Infection,** then, is

TABLE 23-1 Examples of Emerging Infectious Diseases in the United States

INFECTIOUS DISEASE	PATHOGEN	SIGNIFICANCE
American trypanosomiasis (Chagas' disease)	*Trypanosoma cruzi* (protozoan)	Once considered a tropical infection, the parasite is now known to be transmitted in blood donated by travelers from areas where the disease is endemic; causes chronic, irreversible manifestation late in life
Coccidioidomycosis (valley fever, San Joaquin Valley Fever)	*Coccidioides immitis* (fungus)	Marked increase since 1991 in desert areas of California; affects all segments of population (4870 cases in 2003)
Cryptosporidiosis	*Cryptosporidium parvum* (protozoan)	Increased among persons with immune suppression; major outbreaks associated with public water supplies and public pools
Hantavirus pulmonary syndrome	*Hantavirus* spp.	Outbreaks first appeared in 1993; cases still being reported; 40%-50% mortality rate
Hemorrhagic colitis	*Escherichia coli* 0157:H7 (enterohemorrhagic *E.coli*)	First recognized outbreak in 1993 from a single source of undercooked hamburger resulted in at least 4 deaths; continues to occur, with 2671 cases reported in 2003
Creutzfeldt-Jakob disease (subacute spongiform encephalopathy)	Believed to be caused by a prion protein, the reservoir being infected cattle	Cases have been reported worldwide; transmission to humans is hypothesized to be ingestion of infected meat and transplantation of infected organs
Lyme disease	*Borrelia burgdorferi* (spirochete)	First recognized in 1982; becoming endemic with over 21,000 cases reported in 2003; transmitted by ticks and leads to chronic disability if untreated
Epidemic viral gastrointestinal disease	Norwalk-like viruses	A self-limiting disease; increasing reports of outbreaks affecting entire populations in close proximity (e.g., on cruise ships or in shelters)
Severe acute respiratory syndrome (SARS)	SARS virus (coronavirus)	First outbreak in Asia in 2003; high fatality rate; travelers returned to United States with the disease; no new outbreaks since June, 2003
St. Louis encephalitis (SLE)	SLE virus	Transmitted by mosquitoes; number of reported cases are low but steadily increasing; elderly are at greatest risk for severe disease and death
West Nile fever	West Nile virus	First recognized in 1999 in the United States; transmitted by mosquitoes

Grimes, DE, Grimes, KA, Zack, CM: Infectious diseases. In Thompson, JM et al, editors: *Mosby's clinical nursing*, ed 5, St Louis, 2002, Mosby. Additional references: Centers for Disease Control and Prevention, 2005c; Heymann DL: *Control of communicable diseases manual*, ed 18, Washington, DC, American Public Health Association

the entry and multiplication of an infectious agent in a host. **Infectious disease** and **communicable disease** refer to the pathophysiological responses of the host to the infectious agent, manifesting as an illness. Such a person, when diagnosed, would be considered a **case.** Once infectious agents replicate in a host, they can be transmitted from the host irrespective of the presence of disease symptoms. Some persons become **carriers** and continue to shed the infectious agent without any symptoms of the disease.

Stages of Infection

An infectious agent that has invaded a host and found conditions hospitable will replicate until it can be shed from the host. This period of replication before shedding is called the latent period or **latency.** The **communicable period** or communicability, follows latency and begins with shedding of the agent. **Incubation period** is the time from invasion to the time when disease symptoms first appear. Frequently the communicable period begins before symptoms are present. Understanding the distinctions between these terms is important in controlling transmission. These stages of infection are depicted in Figure 23-1.

Spectrum of Disease Occurrence

The principles covered to this point apply to individuals and their acquisition of infections and infectious diseases. Control of infectious diseases in a population requires identifying and monitoring the occurrence of new cases **(incidence)** in a population. Some infectious diseases are **endemic** and occur at a consistent, expected level in a geographic area. Such is the case with some STDs and with tuberculosis (TB). An **outbreak** is an unexpected occurrence of an infectious disease in a limited geographic area during a limited period of time. Outbreaks of pertussis and salmonellosis are not uncommon. A **pandemic** is a steady occurrence of a disease over a large geographic area or worldwide, such as malaria in Africa. An **epidemic** is an unexpected increase of an infectious disease in a geographic area over an extended period of time. Epidemics are defined relative to the infectious agent and the history of the disease in the area. One case of smallpox anywhere will constitute an epidemic, whereas 1000 new cases

HEALTHY PEOPLE 2010 | *Communicable Disease*

Focus Area 14—Immunizations and Infectious Diseases

➤ Reduce or eliminate indigenous cases of vaccine-preventable diseases

➤ Reduce new cases of chronic hepatitis B virus perinatal infections in infants and young children

➤ Reduce new cases of hepatitis B in adults and high risk groups (injection drug users, heterosexually active persons, homosexually active men, and occupationally exposed workers)

➤ Increase the proportion of persons with chronic hepatitis C infection identified by state and local health departments

➤ Reduces new cases of tuberculosis (TB)

➤ Increase the proportion of patients with TB who complete curative therapy within 12 months

➤ Reduce the number of courses of antibiotics for ear infections in young children

➤ Achieve and maintain effective vaccination coverage levels for universally recommended vaccines among young children

➤ Increase hepatitis B vaccine coverage among high-risk groups (long-term hemodialysis patients, homosexually active men, and occupationally exposed workers)

➤ Increase the proportion of noninstitutionalized and institutionalized adults who are vaccinated annually against influenza

➤ Reduce vaccine-associated adverse events

Focus Area 25—Sexually Transmitted Diseases

➤ Reduce the proportion of adolescents and young adults with *Chlamydia trachomatis* infections

➤ Reduce new cases of gonorrhea

➤ Eliminate sustained domestic transmission of primary and secondary syphilis

➤ Reduce the proportion of adults with genital herpes infection

➤ Reduce the proportion of persons with human papillomavirus (HPV) infection

➤ Reduce neonatal consequences from maternal STDs, including chlamydial pneumonia, and gonococcal and chlamydial ophthalmia neonatorum, laryngeal papillomatosis (from HPV infection), neonatal herpes, and preterm birth and low birthweight associated with bacterial vaginosis

➤ Increase the proportion of adolescents who abstain from sexual intercourse or use condoms if currently sexually active

➤ Increase the proportion of sexually active females aged 25 years and under who are screened annually for genital chlamydia infections

➤ Increase the proportion of pregnant females screened for STDs (including HIV and bacterial vaginosis) during prenatal health care visits, according to recognized standards

➤ Increase the proportion of all STD clinic patients being treated for bacterial STDs (chlamydia, gonorrhea, and syphilis) who are offered provider referral services for their sex partners

Focus Area 13—HIV/AIDS

➤ Reduce new cases of AIDS among adolescents and adults

➤ Reduce the number of cases of HIV infection among adolescents and adults

➤ Increase the proportion of sexually active persons who use condoms

➤ Increase the number of HIV-positive persons who know their serostatus

➤ Increase the proportion of substance abuse treatment facilities that offer HIV/AIDS education, counseling, and support

➤ Increase the number of state prison systems that provide comprehensive education about HIV/AIDS, STDs, and TB

➤ Increase the proportion of adults with TB who have been tested for HIV

➤ Increase the proportion of adults in publicly funded HIV counseling and testing sites who are screened for common bacterial STDs (chlamydia, gonorrhea, and syphilis) and are immunized against hepatitis B virus

➤ Reduce the number of deaths from HIV infection

➤ Extend the interval of time between an initial diagnosis of HIV infection and AIDS diagnosis, to increase lifespan of HIV-positive individuals

➤ Reduce new cases of perinatally acquired HIV infection

From US Department of Health and Human Services: *Healthy People 2010: immunization and infectious diseases*, 2000, The Author, http://www.healthypeople.gov/document/html/volume1/14immunization; From US Department of Health and Human Services: *Healthy People 2010: sexually transmitted diseases*, 2000, The Author, http://www.healthypeople.gov/document/html/volume2/25stds; From US Department of Health and Human Services: *Healthy People 2010: HIV*, 2000, The Author, http://www.healthypeople.gov/document/html/volume1/13hiv.

Stages of Infection

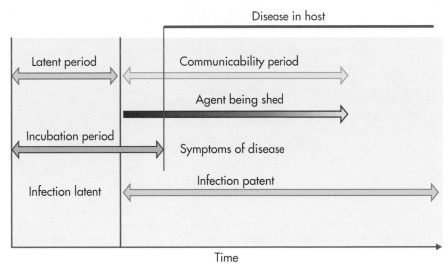

FIGURE 23-1 Stages of infection. (From Grimes, DE: *Infectious diseases,* St. Louis, 1991, Mosby.)

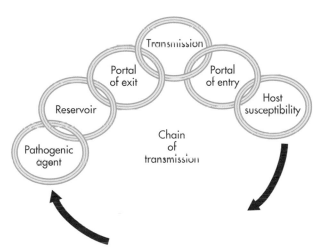

FIGURE 23-2 Chain of transmission. (From Grimes, DE: *Infectious diseases,* St. Louis, 1991, Mosby.)

of gonorrhea will not be considered an epidemic in an area where gonorrhea is common.

CHAIN OF TRANSMISSION

Transmission is frequently conceptualized as a chain with six links, all connected, as in Figure 23-2. Each of the links (infectious agent, reservoir, portal of exit, mode of transmission, portal of entry, and host susceptibility) represents a different component that contributes to transmission. The chain of transmission and its elements are summarized in Table 23-2.

Infectious Agents

Because the process of transmission is different for every infectious agent, one might envision a different configuration

of the chain and its links for each infectious agent and infectious disease that exists. Infectious agents act differently, depending on their intrinsic properties and interaction with their human host. For example, an agent's size, shape, chemical composition, growth requirements, and viability (ability to survive for extended periods of time) have an impact on transmission and the type of parasitic relationship it establishes with its host. These characteristics determine the classifications of different agents (e.g., prions, viruses, bacteria, fungi, and protozoa), and knowing the classification is helpful in understanding how specific agents are transmitted and produce disease. Also important is how the agent interacts with its host. What is its mode of action in the body? For example, *Mycobacterium tuberculosis* kills cells, but the spirochete that causes syphilis interferes with circulation. Or maybe it produces a toxin **(toxigenicity)** as does *Clostridium botulinum,* or stimulates an immune response in the host **(antigenicity),** as does rubella virus. Other considerations for understanding the action of agents include their power to invade and infect large numbers of people **(infectivity),** their ability to produce disease in those infected with the agent **(pathogenicity),** and their ability to produce serious disease in their hosts **(virulence).** Applying the above concepts, the chickenpox virus has high infectivity, high pathogenicity, and very low virulence. On the other hand, *M. tuberculosis* has low infectivity, low pathogenicity, but high virulence if untreated. Smallpox virus is high on all three concepts. Last, how adaptable is an agent to its human host, and does the agent change, or mutate, over time, as HIV does?

Reservoirs

The environment in which a pathogen lives and multiplies is the **reservoir.** Reservoirs can be humans, animals, arthropods, plants, soil, or any other organic substance. Some agents have more than one reservoir. Knowing the reservoirs for infectious

TABLE 23-2 Chain of Transmission

LINKS OF THE CHAIN	DEFINITION	FACTORS
Infectious agent	An organism (virus, rickettsia, bacteria, fungus, protozoan, helminth, or prion) capable of producing infection or infectious disease	Properties of the agent: morphology, chemical composition, growth requirements, and viability; interaction with the host: mode of action, infectivity, pathogenicity, virulence, toxigenicity, antigenicity, and ability to adapt to the host
Reservoirs	The environment in which a pathogen lives and multiples	Humans, animals, arthropods (bugs), plants, soil, or any other organic substance
Portal of exit	Means by which an infectious agent is transported from the host	Respiratory secretions, vaginal secretions, semen, saliva, lesion exudates, blood, and feces
Mode of transmission	Method whereby the infectious agent is transmitted from one host (or reservoir) to another host	*Direct:* Person to person *Indirect:* Implies a vehicle of transmission (biological or mechanical vector, common vehicles or fomites, airborne droplets)
Portal of entry	Means by which an infectious agent enters a new host	Respiratory passages, mucous membranes, skin, percutaneous space, mouth, and through the placenta
Host susceptibility	The presence or lack of sufficient resistance to an infectious agent to avoid contracting an infectious disease	Biological and personal characteristics (e.g., gender, age, genetics), general health status, personal behaviors, anatomical and physiological lines of defense, immunity

agents is important because, in some cases, transmission can be controlled by eliminating the reservoir.

Portals of Exit and Entry

Agents leave the human host through a **portal of exit** and invade through a **portal of entry.** Portals of exit include respiratory secretions, vaginal secretions, semen, saliva, lesion exudates, blood, and feces. Portals of entry are associated with the portal of exit, and include the respiratory passages, mucous membranes, skin and blood vessels oral cavity, and the placenta.

Modes of Transmission

Direct transmission is the immediate transfer of an infectious agent from an infected host or reservoir to an appropriate portal of entry in the human host through physical contact, such as a touch, bite, kiss, or sexual contact. Direct projections of mucous secretions by droplet spray to the conjunctiva, or mucous membranes of the eye, nose or mouth during coughing, sneezing, and laughing is also considered direct transmission. Direct person-to-person contact is responsible for the transmission of many communicable diseases (e.g., STDs).

Indirect transmission is the spread of infection through a vehicle of transmission outside the host. These may be contaminated fomites or vectors. **Fomites** can be any inanimate object, material, or substance that acts as a transport agent for a microbe (e.g., water, a telephone, or a contaminated tissue). The infectious agent may or may not reproduce on or in the fomite. Substances such as food, water, and blood products can provide indirect transmission through ingestion and intravenous transfusions. Botulism is an example of an indirectly transmitted food-borne enterotoxin disease.

Vectors can be animals or arthropods, and they can transmit through biological and mechanical routes. The mechanical route involves no multiplication or growth of the parasite or microbe within the animal or vector itself. Such is the case when a housefly carries gastrointestinal agents from raw sewage to uncovered food. Biological transmission occurs when the parasite grows or multiplies inside the animal, vector, or arthropod. Examples of diseases spread by this method of transmission include arthropod-borne diseases, such as malaria, hemorrhagic fevers, and viral encephalitis. Transmission from a vector to the human host is usually through a bite or sting. Such is the case with the mosquito vector that transmits St. Louis encephalitis.

Fecal-oral transmission can be direct and indirect. It can occur indirectly through the ingestion of water that has been fecally polluted or by consumption of contaminated food. Direct transmission occurs through engagement in oral sexual activity. Poliovirus and hepatitis A are spread through fecal-oral routes.

Airborne transmission occurs mainly through aerosols and droplet nuclei. The time frame in which an airborne particle can remain suspended greatly influences the virility and infectivity of the organism. The size of the particle can also determine how long it remains airborne and how successful it will be at penetrating the human lung. Aerosols are extremely small solid or liquid particles that may include fungal spores, viruses, and bacteria. Droplet nuclei, such as the spray from sneezing or coughing, may make direct contact with an open wound or with a mucous membrane, or they may be inhaled into the lung. TB is spread through inhalation of contaminated droplets.

Host Susceptibility

Not all humans are equally **susceptible** or at risk for contracting an infection or developing an infectious diseases. Biological and personal characteristics play an important role. Just as the young are at greater risk for diphtheria, older adults are at greater risk for bacterial pneumonia. General health status is important, as evidenced by the increased risk for gastrointestinal parasites in children living in poverty. Personal behaviors certainly influence susceptibility, as does the presence of healthy lines of defense. The immune system and immunization status play important roles in the increased number of infections in unimmunized and immunocompromised persons.

BREAKING THE CHAIN OF TRANSMISSION

Picture a situation in which one of the links in the chain of transmission is broken (see Figure 23-2). Breaking just one link of the chain at its most vulnerable point is, in fact, what is done to control transmission of an infectious agent. Of course, where the chain is broken depends on all of the factors that have just been discussed—characteristics of the agent, its reservoir, portals of exit and entry, how the agent is transmitted, and susceptibility of the host.

Controlling the Agent

Controlling the agent is an area where technology and medical science has been extremely effective. Inactivating an agent is the principle behind disinfection, sterilization, and radiation of fomites that may harbor pathogens. Antiinfective drugs, such as antibiotics, antivirals, antiretrovirals, and antimalarials, play important roles in controlling infectious diseases. Not only do they permit recovery of the infected person, but they also play a major role in preventing transmission of the pathogens to another. The first step in preventing transmission of tuberculosis and syphilis is to treat the infected person with antibiotics.

Eradicating the Nonhuman Reservoir

Common nonhuman reservoirs for pathogens in the environment include water, food, milk, animals, insects, and sewage. Treating or eliminating them is an effective method of preventing replication of pathogens, and thus preventing transmission.

Controlling the Human Reservoir

Treating infected persons, whether they are symptomatic or not, is effective in preventing transmission of pathogens directly to others. A **quarantine** is an enforced isolation or restriction of movement of those who have been exposed to an infectious agent during the incubation period; this is another method of controlling the reservoir. Quarantine was used effectively during the outbreak of severe acute respiratory syndrome (SARS) in 2003, when some hospitals required that their staff exposed to SARS patients remain at the hospital until proven to be symptom free at the end of the incubation period.

Controlling the Portals of Exit and Entry

The transmission chain may be broken at the portal of exit by properly disposing of secretions, excretions, and exudates from infected persons. Additionally, **isolation** of sick persons from others and requiring that persons with tuberculosis wear a mask in public can be effective.

The portal of entry of pathogens also can be controlled by using barrier precautions (masks, gloves, condoms), avoiding unnecessary invasive procedures, such as indwelling catheters, and protecting oneself from vectors, such as mosquitoes. In response to the risk of exposure to blood-borne pathogens (e.g., HIV, hepatitis B, and hepatitis C) in the late 1980s, the CDC developed a set of guidelines, called **universal precautions,** to prevent transmission of diseases found in blood and other body fluids. These guidelines were developed because infected people may be asymptomatic and have no knowledge of their conditions; therefore health care workers must assume that all patients are infectious and protect themselves.

Improving Host Resistance and Immunity

Many factors, such as age, general health status, nutrition, and health behaviors, contribute to a host's **resistance,** or ability to ward off infections. Immunity, however, is an incredible defense against infection. There are several kinds of **immunity,** each providing resistance in different ways to different pathogens. **Natural immunity** is an innate resistance to a specific antigen or toxin. **Acquired immunity** is derived from actual exposure to the specific infectious agent, toxin, or appropriate vaccine. There are two types of acquired immunity: active and passive. **Active immunity** is when the body produces its own antibodies against an antigen, either from infection with the pathogen or introduction of the pathogen in a vaccine. **Passive immunity** is the temporary resistance that has been donated to the host through transfusions of plasma proteins, immunoglobulins, or antitoxins, or transplacentally, from mother to neonate. Passive immunity lasts only as long as these substances remain in the bloodstream. Types of acquired immunity with examples are summarized in Table 23-3.

When administered according to established guidelines and protocols, vaccines provide acquired immunity in most cases. However, there are exceptions. **Primary vaccine failure** is the failure of a vaccine to stimulate any immune response. It can be caused by improper storage that may render the vaccines ineffective, improper administration route, or exposure of light-sensitive vaccines to light. Additionally, some immunized persons never seroconvert, either because of failure of their own immune system or for some other unknown reason. **Secondary vaccine failure** is the waning of immunity following an initial immune response. This often occurs in immunosuppressed patients and organ transplant patients in whom the immune memory is essentially destroyed.

Herd immunity is a state in which those not immune to an infectious agent will be protected if a certain proportion (generally considered to be 80%) of the population has been vaccinated or is otherwise immune (Figure 23-3). This effect applies only if those who are immune are distributed evenly in the population. This is especially true for the transmission of diseases, such as diphtheria, that are found only in the human host and that have no invertebrate host or other mode of transmission. Without the presence of a susceptible

TABLE 23-3 Types of Acquired Immunity

TYPE OF IMMUNITY	HOW ACQUIRED	LENGTH OF RESISTANCE
NATURAL		
Active	Natural contact and infection with the antigen	May be temporary or permanent
Passive	Natural contact with antibody transplacentally or through colostrum and breast milk	Temporary
ARTIFICIAL		
Active	Inoculation of antigen	May be temporary or permanent
Passive	Inoculation of antibody or antitoxin	Temporary

From Grimes DE, Infectious diseases, In Thompson JM et al, editors: *Mosby's clinical nursing*, St. Louis, 1991, Mosby.

Herd Immunity Example

Herd Immunity: 66% immunized (10/13 or 77%) protected

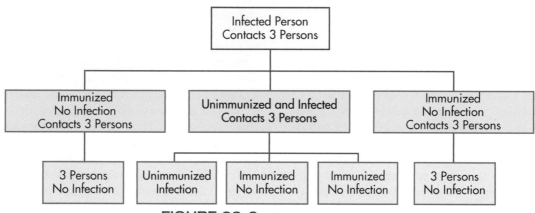

FIGURE 23-3   Example of herd immunity.

population to infect, the organism will be unable to live because the vast majority of the population is immune.

PUBLIC HEALTH CONTROL OF INFECTIOUS DISEASES

Most human diseases (e.g., cancer or diabetes) can be classified as personal health problems. Individuals with a personal health problem can be treated by the health care system one person at a time. By contrast, infectious diseases are categorized as public or community health problems. Because of their potential to spread and cause community-wide or worldwide emergencies, infectious diseases require organized, public efforts for their prevention and control.

Such organized public efforts are under the jurisdiction of official public health agencies at local, state, national, and international levels. Each government unit obtains its powers through a complex array of laws. It is important to remember is that, in areas of health within a state, state laws usually prevail over federal law. The reason for this hierarchy is that the U.S. Constitution did not address health, and the Tenth Amendment reserved power to the states over all issues not addressed in the Constitution (Schneider, 2006). Historically, states have

accepted this responsibility. For example, all states have laws addressing infectious disease control, such as what diseases must be reported and who has authority to implement quarantines. All states have a board of health and a department of health to implement state laws.

The CDC is the national public health entity responsible for infectious disease control across the states. The CDC has responsibility for monitoring infectious diseases and supporting local and state governments in control of outbreaks and epidemics, if such assistance is needed. Although there are many aspects of public health control of infectious diseases, only three are presented here—common control terminology, reporting diseases, and preventing diseases by vaccination

Terminology: Control, Elimination, and Eradication

Control of a communicable disease is the reduction of incidence or prevalence of a given disease to a locally acceptable level as a result of deliberate efforts (CDC, 1999a). The WHO's Expanded Programme on Immunizations (EPI) is a global attempt to control morbidity and mortality for many vaccine-preventable diseases, with each country adapting these guidelines as necessary. An example of control of pertussis would

BOX 23-3 Criteria for Disease Eradication

Criteria for disease eradication include the following:

➤ Human host only; no host in nature
➤ Easy diagnosis; obvious clinical manifestations
➤ Limited duration and intensity of infection
➤ Natural lifelong immunity after infection
➤ Highly seasonal transmission
➤ Availability of vaccine, curative treatment, or both
➤ Substantial global morbidity and mortality rates
➤ Cost-effectiveness of campaign and eradication
➤ Integration of eradication with additional public health variables
➤ Eradication imperative over control measures

From Centers for Disease Control and Prevention: Recommendations of the international task force for disease eradication, *Morb Mortal Wkly Rep* 42:1-38, 1993.

be to achieve 80% immunization coverage of children for pertussis.

Elimination of a communicable disease occurs when it is controlled within a specified geographical area such as a single country, an island, or a continent, and the prevalence and incidence of the disease is reduced to near zero. Elimination is the result of deliberate efforts, but continued intervention measures are required (CDC, 1999a). Such would be the case if no new cases of polio were reported in the United States during the year following an aggressive immunization campaign.

The International Task Force for Disease Eradication (ITFDE) defines **eradication** as reducing the worldwide incidence of a disease to zero as a function of deliberate efforts, without a need for further control measures (CDC, 1999a). Eradication is possible under certain conditions, which are listed in Box 23-3.

Smallpox was eradicated in 1977, and the virus now exists only in storage in laboratories. Many factors contributed to the successful eradication of smallpox, including the mode of transmission of the disease, the isolated geographical distribution of the infection, the ease of administration of the freeze-dried vaccine, the establishment of an effective surveillance system, the increase of national and international political will, and tremendous community participation.

Defining and Reporting Communicable Diseases

Standardized definitions of diseases are necessary for public health monitoring and surveillance across all levels of government. Diseases are defined and classified according to confirmed cases, probable cases, laboratory-confirmed cases, clinically compatible cases, epidemiologically linked cases, genetic typing, and clinical case definition. Once defined, disease occurrence can be compared across time, populations and geographic areas and appropriate control efforts can be implemented.

The CDC is responsible for monitoring communicable disease in the United States. Along with the Council of State and Territorial Epidemiologists, the CDC has designated **notifiable infectious diseases,** which health care providers who encounter these diseases must report to the local or regional health department. These notifiable diseases are listed in Box 23-4.

Because state health departments have the responsibility for monitoring and controlling communicable diseases within their respective states, they determine which diseases will be reported within their jurisdiction. Although not all nationally notifiable diseases are reportable in every state or territory, some states have notifiable disease lists that are longer than the CDC's list. So, all health professionals are advised to check the websites of their state health departments for specifics about reporting laws in their state. The processes for reporting also vary by state, and this information generally is available on the state health department's website. Generally, providers are encouraged to report cases of infectious diseases to their local or regional health departments, who will then report to the state and to the CDC.

The CDC publishes a weekly listing of notifiable diseases reported by region, state and nation in *Morbidity and Mortality Weekly Report* (MMWR). MMWR can be found in medical libraries, local health departments, infection control departments in hospitals and medical centers, and on the Internet at www.cdc.gov.

VACCINES AND INFECTIOUS DISEASE PREVENTION

This section contains comprehensive information on vaccines and vaccine-preventable diseases. Diseases for which there is a vaccine are listed in Box 23-5. Recommended vaccination schedules for selected groups are included.

Vaccines: Word of Caution

As with other areas of health care, information and recommendations on immunizations and vaccine usage change regularly. Therefore health care providers should seek the most current information on the CDC website. Recommendations, policies, and procedures concerning international immunization practices are determined by the WHO. In the United States, national governance is provided by the American Academy of Pediatrics (AAP) Committee on Infectious Diseases and the United States Public Health Service Advisory Committee on Immunization Practices (ACIP). Occasionally these agencies differ in their recommendations.

Precautions must be taken when giving any immunization. The most recent recommendations regarding which immunizations to give; who they should be given to; how they should be given; and how they are to be transported, stored, and administered can be obtained from the CDC. Additional information on vaccines can be obtained from the sources listed for this chapter in the WebLinks portion of the book's website.

The CDC produces Vaccine Information Statements (VISs) that explain the benefits and risks of a vaccine to vaccine recipients, their parents, or their legal representatives. Federal law requires that VISs be handed out whenever (before each dose) certain vaccinations are given. VISs can be downloaded from the Internet at http://www.cdc.gov/nip/publications/VIS.

BOX 23-4 Nationally Notifiable Infectious Diseases in the United States: 2005

- ➤ Acquired immunodeficiency syndrome (AIDS)
- ➤ Anthrax
- ➤ Arboviral neuroinvasive and nonneuroinvasive diseases: California serogroup virus disease, eastern equine encephalitis, Powassan virus disease, St. Louis encephalitis, West Nile virus disease, and western equine encephalitis
- ➤ Botulism (food-borne, infant, and other)
- ➤ Brucellosis
- ➤ Chancroid
- ➤ *Chlamydia trachomatis*
- ➤ Cholera
- ➤ Coccidioidomycosis
- ➤ Cryptosporidiosis
- ➤ Cyclosporiasis
- ➤ Diphtheria
- ➤ Ehrlichiosis (human granulocytic, monocytic, and unspecified agent)
- ➤ Enterohemorrhagic *Escherichia coli* (0157:H7, serogroup non-0157, and not serogrouped)
- ➤ Giardiasis
- ➤ Gonorrhea
- ➤ *Haemophilus influenzae* type B (HIB)
- ➤ Hansen's disease (leprosy)
- ➤ Hantavirus pulmonary syndrome
- ➤ Hemolytic uremic syndrome, postdiarrheal
- ➤ Hepatitis, acute (hepatitis A, hepatitis B, perinatal, hepatitis C)
- ➤ Hepatitis, chronic (hepatitis B and hepatitis C)
- ➤ HIV infection (adult and pediatric)
- ➤ Influenza-associated pediatric mortality
- ➤ Legionellosis
- ➤ Listeriosis
- ➤ Lyme disease
- ➤ Malaria
- ➤ Measles
- ➤ Meningococcal disease
- ➤ Mumps
- ➤ Pertussis
- ➤ Plague
- ➤ Poliomyelitis, paralytic
- ➤ Psittacosis
- ➤ Q Fever
- ➤ Rabies (animal and human)
- ➤ Rocky Mountain spotted fever
- ➤ Rubella
- ➤ Rubella, congenital syndrome
- ➤ Salmonellosis
- ➤ Severe acute respiratory syndrome (SARS)
- ➤ Shigellosis
- ➤ Smallpox
- ➤ Streptococcal disease, invasive, group A
- ➤ *Streptococcus pneumoniae*, drug resistant, invasive
- ➤ *Stroptococcus pneumoniae*, invasive, in children <5 years of age
- ➤ Syphilis (primary, secondary, latent, early latent, late latent, unknown duration, neurosyphilis, syphilis, late, and nonneurological)
- ➤ Syphilis, congenital (syphilitic stillbirth)
- ➤ Tetanus
- ➤ Toxic shock syndrome
- ➤ Trichinellosis (trichinosis)
- ➤ Tuberculosis
- ➤ Tularemia
- ➤ Typhoid fever
- ➤ Vancomycin-intermediate *Staphylococcus aureus* (VISA)
- ➤ Vancomycin-resistant *Staphylococcus aureus* (VRSA)
- ➤ Varicella (morbidity and death)
- ➤ Yellow fever

From Centers for Disease Control and Prevention: Nationally notifiable infectious diseases, 2005d, The Author, http://www.cdc.gov/epo/dphsi/phs/infdis1005.htm.

Types of Immunizations

Immunization is a broad term used to describe a process by which active or passive immunity to an infectious disease is induced or amplified. Immunizing agents can include vaccines, immune globulins, or antitoxins. **Vaccination** is a narrower term referring to the administration of a vaccine or toxoid to confer active immunity by stimulating the body to produce its own antibodies.

Vaccines can be prepared in several ways. They may be suspensions in a variety of solutions; protected with preservatives, stabilizers, or antibiotics; or mixed with adjuvants, which are used to increase immunogenicity. Vaccines can be live and attenuated, or they may be killed, or inactivated, with the virulence removed, leaving only the antigenic property necessary to stimulate the human immune system to produce antibodies. Types of inactivated vaccines include toxoids and polysaccharide vaccines. Inactivated conjugate vaccines, containing a chemically linked polysaccharide and protein and genetically engineered "recombinant" vaccines are also now being administered. Inactivated vaccines can be fractions or subunits or whole "killed" bacteria or viruses. Immune globulins and antitoxins are solutions that contain antibodies from human or animal blood and are introduced into a patient to provide passive protection without initiating the immune system to produce an immunogenic response. See Table 23-4 for information on types of available vaccines.

Vaccine Storage, Transport, and Handling

Vaccines should be safely stored, transported, and handled at all times to ensure the efficacy of the vaccine. A **cold chain** is a system used to ensure that vaccines are kept at a designated temperature from the time they are manufactured until they are used for vaccination. Failing to maintain the cold chain and exposing the vaccine to higher or lower temperatures than recommended may result in loss of potency and vaccine failure (CDC, 1996).

Several methods are available for ensuring that the appropriate temperature has been maintained throughout vaccine transport and storage. These include liquid crystal thermometers, dial thermometers, recording thermometers, digital thermometers, ice pack indicators, shipping indi-

BOX 23-5 Vaccine-Preventable Diseases

- Anthrax
- Diphtheria
- *Haemophilus influenzae* type b (Hib)
- Hepatitis A
- Hepatitis B
- Influenza
- Lyme disease
- Measles
- Meningococcus
- Monkeypox
- Mumps
- Pertussis
- Pneumococcus
- Poliomyelitis
- Rotavirus
- Rubella
- Smallpox
- Tetanus
- Tuberculosis
- Varicella (chickenpox)
- Yellow fever

From Centers for Disease Control and Prevention: Vaccine-preventable diseases and specific vaccines, 2005e, The Author, http://www.cdc.gov/node.do/id/0900f3ec8005df1f.

TABLE 23-4 Available Vaccines by Type

VACCINES	DESCRIPTION
Live Attenuated	
Viral	Measles, mumps, rubella, oral polio, vaccinia, yellow fever, and varicella
Bacterial	BCG
Recombinant	Oral typhoid
Inactivated	
Viral	Influenza, polio, rabies, and hepatitis A
Bacterial	Typhoid, cholera, and plague
Subunit (fractional)	Influenza, acellular pertussis, typhoid Vi, and Lyme disease
Toxoid	Diphtheria and tetanus
Recombinant	Hepatitis B
Conjugate polysaccharide	*Haemophilus influenzae* type b, and pneumococcal 7-valent
Pure polysaccharide	Pneumococcal 23-valent, meningococcal, and *Haemophilus influenzae* type b

From Centers for Disease Control: *Epidemiology and prevention of vaccine-preventable diseases (pink book)*, ed 6, Atlanta, 2000a, Public Health Foundation.

cators that change color if the temperature exceeds or falls below the recommended level, freeze-watch indicators, and cold chain monitors.

Vaccine Administration

The efficacy of the vaccine can be adversely affected if the vaccine is not administered appropriately. Therefore it is important to follow the same safety procedures one would use to administer any intramuscular (IM) or subcutaneous injection (i.e., use sterile technique, use the correct size needle, avoid injecting in a blood vessel, and dispose of the needle and syringe properly). Information on the correct dosage can be found on the package insert. If more than one vaccine is being administered simultaneously, different anatomical sites should be used.

Vaccine Spacing

Wherever possible, all children should be age-appropriately immunized and kept up to date according to current recommendations. Clinically stable premature infants should adhere to the same schedule as term infants, with the exception of hepatits B (Hep B). Low-birth-weight infants (less than 2000 g) born to hepatitis B surface antigen (HBsAg)-negative mothers should not be vaccinated with Hep B until they weigh 2 kg or are 2 months of age. Low-birth-weight infants born to HBsAg-positive mothers should receive hepatitis B immune globulin (HBIG) and Hep B at birth; however, the initial vaccine dose should not be counted in the required three-dose series (Pickering, 2000).

The number of injections for any one immunobiological substance should be administered according to ACIP recommendations. An interruption in the schedule does not require that the entire series begin again. However, if vaccines are administered at less than the recommended intervals, they should not be counted as part of the primary series of immunization. Completion of the primary vaccine series and receiving periodic booster doses as recommended are necessary to ensure protective levels of immunity. A specific alteration in immunogenicity has not been proven; therefore all vaccines can be administered simultaneously without contraindication, except for yellow fever and cholera vaccines, which must be separated by at least 3 weeks. Additionally, live injectable vaccines (e.g., measles-mumps-rubella [MMR] and varicella) must be separated by at least 4 weeks when not given simultaneously (Pickering, 2000).

Vaccine Hypersensitivity and Contraindications

Although adverse reactions are not common following immunization, they can occur in some individuals. These reactions can be from vaccine components such as eggs, egg proteins, antibiotics, preservatives, and adjuvants. Patient allergies should be considered before administration of specific vaccines. For additional precautions and contraindications, the vaccine package insert and the latest instructions from the CDC should be consulted.

Mild illness with or without low-grade fever is not a contraindication for vaccination. However, vaccination should be postponed in cases of moderate or severe febrile illness to avoid any confusion between a vaccine side effect and an unknown underlying cause.

Pregnancy is not a contraindication for immunization using inactivated vaccines, antitoxins, or immune globulins. However, pregnant women should avoid live vaccines, including MMR, varicella, and yellow fever, unless the risk of infection is very high (CDC, 2000a).

Immunocompromised patients should not receive live vaccines; however, MMR can be administered to asymptomatic HIV-infected people, and varicella can be given to people with humoral immunodeficiency and some HIV-asymptomatic people as determined by their physician (CDC, 2000a). Killed or inactivated vaccines can be given, but they may not produce an optimal antibody response.

Vaccine Documentation

Legal documentation of vaccinations is important for both the individual and the provider for future administration and follow-up of hypersensitivity reactions. Both individual and provider immunization records should be maintained. The health care provider is responsible for maintaining accurate records, including patient name, dates immunized, vaccine type, vaccine manufacturer, vaccine lot number, date of the Vaccine Information Statement (VIS), and the name, title, and address of the person administering the vaccine (CDC, 2000b).

Vaccine Safety and Reporting Adverse Events and Vaccine-Related Injuries

No drug is perfectly safe or effective and vaccines are no exception. They are biological rather than chemical and when introduced into the human biological system, they can and do produce a variety of responses, both positive and negative. Furthermore, vaccines are administered to healthy people; they are given to prevent illness and not treat it; and they are given to far greater numbers of people than other pharmaceuticals.

Public concern regarding the health risk associated with vaccines has increased in recent years as the risk of contracting the diseases has declined. For example, wild virus polio has been eliminated in the United States, yet each year 8 to 10 cases of vaccine-induced paralysis have been reported associated with use of the oral, live virus vaccine. The health risk of the oral vaccine exceeds that of the risk of the disease. This has led to a change in vaccine policy from the use of the live oral vaccine to the inactivated polio vaccine (IPV) (CDC, 1999b). Likewise, whole cell pertussis vaccine has been changed to an acellular pertussis vaccine because there are adverse side effects, most notably convulsions, associated with the whole cell vaccine.

To monitor actual and potential vaccine-related problems, health care providers must report specific postvaccination "adverse events" to the **Vaccine Adverse Event Reporting System (VAERS).** Information and reporting forms are available in both the U.S. Food and Drug Administration (FDA) *Drug Bulletin* and the *Physicians' Desk Reference*, and through a 24-hour recorded telephone message at 1-800-822-7967. The website for VAERS is http://www.vaers.org. The National Vaccine Injury Compensation Program reviews all VAERS reports and provides assistance for individuals and families who experience a vaccine-related injury, including disability and death. This program can be reached through a 24-hour recorded telephone message at 1-800-338-2392.

RESEARCH HIGHLIGHTS

Immunization Compliance: Beliefs and Actions Among RNs

McEwen and Farren (2005) conducted a survey of 1000 RNs in Texas to analyze the nurses' beliefs and actions related to hepatitis B and influenza immunization recommendations. They learned that only 8% of the responding RNs chose not to be vaccinated against hepatitis B. The primary reason the nurses chose not to be vaccinated were because they were not working in nursing, did not believe they were at risk of exposure, and were concerned about side effects or complications.

Similarly, 86% of the RNs reported that they had ever received a flu shot and 69% noted that they had been immunized during 2 of the previous 4 years. Rationales for receiving the immunization were belief in effectiveness, belief that they were at risk of exposures, and that the vaccine was free of charge. Reasons for declining influenza immunization included concerns about side effects, lack of concern about getting the illness, and doubts about the vaccine's effectiveness.

McEwen M, Farren E: Actions and beliefs related to hepatitis B and influenza immunization among registered nurses in Texas. *Public Health Nursing*, 22(3):230-239, 2005.

VACCINE NEEDS FOR SPECIAL GROUPS

Recommendation on immunizations and schedules for vaccination are routinely updated and published by the CDC on its website. Practitioners are encouraged to regularly check for updates.

Healthy Infants, Children, and Adolescents

The AAP, ACIP, and the American Academy of Family Physicians (AAFP) recommend that all children in the United States complete a schedule of 11 childhood vaccines by age 18 months. The schedule is complex and includes four doses of diphtheria, tetanus, and acellular pertussis vaccine (DTaP); three doses of IPV; one dose of MMR vaccine; three to four doses of *Haemophilus influenzae* type b (Hib) conjugate vaccine; three doses of Hep B vaccine; one dose of varicella vaccine; and four doses of a conjugated pneumococcal vaccine (CDC, 2005f). Hepatitis A vaccine is also recommended for children aged 2 to 18 years living in states, counties, or communities where hepatitis A rates are twice the national average. Recommendations are summarized in Table 23-5. Note that the pediatric immunization schedule has changed frequently in recent years. Therefore the reader should consult the CDC website (http://www.cdc.gov) for the most current recommendations.

AAP, ACIP, and AAFP all have recommended establishing a routine health care visit at 11 to 12 years of age to ensure that previously unvaccinated adolescents would receive Hep B, varicella vaccine (if no history of disease), a second dose of MMR vaccine, and a booster dose of tetanus and diphtheria vaccine (Td), if it has been more than 5 years since their prior dose. This visit would also provide an opportunity to administer any new vaccines that may be added to the vaccine schedule and provide an opportunity to offer other recommended preventive services.

Many colleges and universities across the United States are now requiring some minimal level of proof of immunizations before enrollment for new students. Two studies done by the

TABLE 23-5 Recommended Childhood and Adolescent Immunization Schedule,[1] by Vaccine and Age: United States—2005

VACCINE	BIRTH	1 MO	2 MOS	4 MOS	6 MOS	12 MOS	15 MOS	18 MOS	24 MOS	4–6 YRS	11–12 YRS	13–18 YRS
Hepatitis B[2]	Hep B #1	Only if mother HBsAg(−)	Hep B #2				Hep B #3				Hep B series	
Diphtheria, tetanus, pertussis[3]			DTaP	DTaP	DTaP			DTaP		DTaP	Td	Td
Haemophilus influenzae type b[4]			Hib	Hib	Hib[4]		Hib					
Inactivated poliovirus			IPV	IPV	IPV		IPV			IPV		
Measles, mumps, rubella[5]							MMR #1			MMR #2		MMR #2
Varicella[6]							Varicella				Varicella	
Pneumococcal[7]			PCV	PCV	PCV		PCV		PCV	PCV		
Influenza[8]					Influenza (yearly)		Influenza (yearly)			Influenza (yearly)		
Hepatitis A[9]										Hepatitis A series		

■ Range of recommended ages ■ Catch-up immunization ■ Preadolescent assessment

----Vaccines below red line are for selected populations----

From Centers for Disease Control and Prevention: Recommended childhood and adolescent immunization schedule—United States, 2005, *MMWR Morb Mortal Wkly Rep* 53:Q1-Q2, 2005.

The recommendations that appear on this table must be read along with the footnotes. **Resource Tool 23A** presents this table complete with all footnoted information. Please refer to **Resource Tool 23A** on the book's evolve website at http://evolve.elsevier.com/Nies.

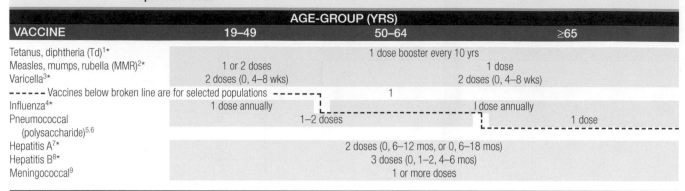

TABLE 23-6A Recommended Adult Immunization Schedule, by Vaccine and Age-Group: United States, October 2005—September 2006

VACCINE	AGE-GROUP (YRS)		
	19–49	50–64	≥65
Tetanus, diphtheria (Td)[1]*		1 dose booster every 10 yrs	
Measles, mumps, rubella (MMR)[2]*	1 or 2 doses		1 dose
Varicella[3]*	2 doses (0, 4–8 wks)		2 doses (0, 4–8 wks)
----- Vaccines below broken line are for selected populations -----		1	
Influenza[4]*	1 dose annually		I dose annually
Pneumococcal (polysaccharide)[5,6]		1–2 doses	1 dose
Hepatitis A[7]*		2 doses (0, 6–12 mos, or 0, 6–18 mos)	
Hepatitis B[8]*		3 doses (0, 1–2, 4–6 mos)	
Meningococcal[9]		1 or more doses	

☐ For all persons in this category who meet the age requirements and who lack evidence of immunity (e.g., lack documentation of vaccination or have no evidence of prior infection)

☐ Recommended if some other risk factor is present (e.g., on the basis of medical, occupational, lifestyle, or other indications)

From Centers for Disease Control and Prevention: Recommended Adult Immunization Schedule by Vaccine and Age Group: United States, October 2005–September 2006. The recommendations that appear on this table must be read along with the footnotes. **Resource Tool 23B** presents this table complete with all footnoted information. Please refer to **Resource Tool 23B** on the book's evolve website at http://evolve.elsevier.com/Nies.

CDC identified a slight increased risk for meningococcal disease among freshman dormitory residents. As a result the CDC recommends that vaccination against meningococcal disease be provided to freshman and other undergraduate students who request this vaccine, although routine vaccination is not recommended. Unfortunately, the current vaccine does not confer immunity against all meningococcal serogroups (CDC, 2000c).

Adults and the Elderly

Although immunization programs in the United States have greatly reduced morbidity and mortality rates among children, vaccine-preventable diseases continue to cause thousands of hospitalizations and deaths in the American adult and elderly populations. For example, adults aged 65 years and older account for 90% of the annual 20,000 to 40,000 deaths in the United States from influenza and pneumonia, many of which are preventable because effective influenza and pneumonia vaccines are available.

Missed immunization opportunities for this age group often occur during an office visit for acute or chronic health problems. Therefore the CDC recommends a routinely scheduled, preventive health care visit for the 50-year-old adult to assess immunization status, administer Td and influenza vaccines, and to assess risk factors and need for pneumococcal vaccine (CDC, 1995).

The pneumococcal and influenza vaccines can be administered during the same visit for those individuals needing both vaccines. With the emergence of serious new drug-resistant pneumococci, it is imperative that susceptible groups be immunized and protected from this group of bacteria. People needing the 23-valent pure polysaccharide pneumococcal vaccine are in the same risk groups as people needing influenza vaccine.

Recommended immunization schedules for adults and for health care workers are presented in Table 23-6 A and B and Table 23-7, respectively.

Immunosuppressed

Live virus or bacterial vaccines are not recommended for persons who are immunosuppressed for any reason (e.g., leukemia, lymphoma, HIV/AIDS, congenital immunodeficiency, radiation, therapy with an alkylating agent, or large doses of corticosteroids). The killed or inactivated vaccines can be given according to the same recommended administration schedule used for healthy people.

Pregnancy

The vaccines routinely indicated for susceptible pregnant women are detailed in Table 23-6. Although there are not any cases on record of congenital rubella syndrome or abnormalities in infants born to mothers who received these vaccines during pregnancy, MMR and varicella vaccines are both contraindicated when pregnancy is known. Other live virus vaccines (e.g., oral polio vaccine [OPV] and yellow fever) are not recommended during pregnancy, but they can be administered and are recommended for susceptible pregnant women who live in areas or may travel to areas where there is a high risk of exposure to these diseases. Inactivated vaccines, toxoids, and immune globulin preparations are not contraindicated during pregnancy. Hepatitis B, pneumococcal, meningococcal, and rabies vaccines are recommended for at-risk pregnant women (CDC, 1998b, 2005g).

Vaccines for International Travel

For individuals traveling outside of the United States into regions with specific endemic infectious diseases, vaccinations are sometimes recommended. The only vaccine required for travel to certain countries is yellow fever vaccine. These countries require a stamped and signed International Certificate of Vaccination, which can be obtained from any provider authorized to administer yellow fever vaccine (CDC, 1999-2000). Other vaccines (e.g., typhoid, Japanese encephalitis) may be recommended depending on the area, the season, and the likelihood of exposure. Travelers can obtain the most current

TABLE 23-6B Recommended Adult Immunization Schedule, by Vaccine and Medical and Other Indications: United States—October 2005–September 2006

Vaccine	Pregnancy	Congenital Immunodeficiency, Leukemia,[10] Lymphoma, Generalized Malignancy, Therapy With Alkylating Agents, Antimetabolites, Cerebrospinal Fluid Leaks, Radiation, or Large Amounts of Corticosteroids	Diabetes, Head Disease, Chronic Pulmonary Disease, or Chronic Liver Disease, Including Chronic Alcoholism	Asplenia[10] (Including Elective Splenectomy and Terminal Complement Component Deficiencies)	Kidney Failure End Stage Renal Disease, or Recipients of Hemodialysis or Clotting Factor Concentrates	Human Immunodeficiency Virus (HIV) Infection[2,10]	Health Care Workers
Tetanus diphtheria (Td)[1]*	1 dose booster every 10 yrs						
Measles, mumps, rubella (MMR)[2]*			1 or 2 doses				
Varicella[3]*			2 doses (0, 4–8 wks)				2 doses
Influenza[4]*	1 dose annually		1 dose annually			1 dose annually	1 dose annually
Pneumococcal (polysaccharide)[5,6]	1–2 doses		1–2 doses			1–2 doses	1–2 doses
Hepatitis A[7]*			2 doses (0, 6–12 mos, or 0, 6–18 mos)				
Hepatitis B[8]*	3 doses (0, 1–2, 4–6 mos)		3 doses (0, 1–2, 4–6 mos)			3 doses (0, 1–2, 4–6 mos)	
Meningococcal[8]	1 dose		1 dose			1 dose	

☐ For all persons in this category who meet the age requirements and who lack evidence of immunity (e.g., lack documentation of vaccination or have no evidence of prior infection)

☐ Recommended if some other risk factor is present (e.g., on the basis of medical, occupational, lifestyle, or other indications)

☐ Contraindicated

From Centers for Disease Control and Prevention: Recommended Adult Immunization Schedule by Vaccine and Medical and Other Indications: United States—October 2005–September 2006, http://www.cdc.gov/nip/recs/adult-schedule.htm.
* Covered by the Vaccine Injury Compensation Program.
The recommendations that appear on this table must be read along with the footnotes. **Resource Tool 23B** presents this table complete with all footnoted information. Please refer to **Resource Tool 23B** on the book's evolve website at http://evolve.elsevier.com/Nies.

TABLE 23-7 Immunizations Strongly Recommended for Health Care Personnel

VACCINE	DOSE SCHEDULE	INDICATIONS	MAJOR PRECAUTIONS AND CONTRAINDICATIONS	SPECIAL CONSIDERATIONS
Hepatitis B recombinant vaccine*	Three-dose schedule administered intramuscularly (IM) in the deltoid; 0, 1, 6-second dose administered 1 month after first dose; third dose administered 4 months after second. Booster doses are not necessary for persons who have developed adequate antibodies to hepatitis B surface antigen (anti-Hbs).	Health care personnel (HCP) at risk for exposure to blood and body fluids.	History of anaphylactic reaction to common baker's yeast. Pregnancy is not a contraindication.	No therapeutic or adverse effects on hepatitis B virus (HBV)-infected persons; cost-effectiveness of prevaccination screening for susceptibility to HBV depends on costs of vaccination and antibody testing and prevalence of immunity in the group of potential vaccinees; healthcare personnel who have ongoing contact with patients or blood should be tested 1–2 months after completing the vaccination series to determine serologic response. If vaccination does not induce adequate anti-Hbs (>10 mIU/mL), a second vaccine series should be administered.
Influenza vaccine (inactivated)	Annual single-dose vaccination IM with current vaccine.	HCP who have contact with patients at high risk or who work in chronic-care facilities; HCP aged ≥50 years or who have high-risk medical conditions.	History of anaphylactic hypersensitivity to eggs or to other components of the vaccine.	Recommended for women who will be in the second or third trimesters of pregnancy during the influenza season and women in any stage of pregnancy who have chronic medical conditions that are associated with an increased risk of influenza.§
Measles live-virus vaccine	One dose administered subcutaneously; second dose ≥4 weeks later.	HCP who were born during or after 1957 without documentation of (1) receipt of 2 doses of live vaccine on or after their first birthday, (2) physician-diagnosed measles, or (3) laboratory evidence of immunity. Vaccine should also be considered for all HCP who have no proof of immunity, including those born before 1957.	Pregnancy; immunocompromised† state (including human immunodeficiency virus [HIV]-infected persons with severe immunosuppression); history of anaphylactic reactions after gelatin ingestion or receipt of neomycin; or recent receipt of antibody-containing blood products.	Measles, mumps, rubella (MMR) is the recommended vaccine, if recipients are also likely to be susceptible to rubella or mumps; person vaccinated during 1963-1967 with (1) measles killed-virus vaccine alone, (2) killed-virus vaccine followed by live-virus vaccine, or (3) a vaccine of unknown type, should be revaccinated with two doses of live-virus measles vaccine.
Mumps live-virus vaccine	One dose subcutaneously; no booster.	HCP believed susceptible can be vaccinated; adults born before 1957 can be considered immune.	Pregnancy; immunocompromised† state; history of anaphylactic reaction after gelatin ingestion or receipt of neomycin.	MMR is the recommended vaccine.
Rubella live-virus vaccine	One dose subcutaneously; no booster.	HCP both male and female, who lack documentation of receipt of live vaccine on or after their first birthday, or lack of laboratory evidence of immunity can be vaccinated. Adults born before 1957 can be considered immune, except women of childbearing age.	Pregnancy; immunocompromised† state; history of anaphylactic reaction after receipt of neomycin.	Women pregnant when vaccinated or who become pregnant within 4 weeks of vaccination should be counseled regarding theoretic risks to the fetus; however, the risk of rubella vaccine–associated malformations among these women is negligible. MMR is the recommended vaccine.

TABLE 23-7   Immunizations Strongly Recommended for Health Care Personnel (cont'd)

VACCINE	DOSE SCHEDULE	INDICATIONS	MAJOR PRECAUTIONS AND CONTRAINDICATIONS	SPECIAL CONSIDERATIONS
Varicella-zoster live-virus vaccine	Two 0.5-mL doses subcutaneously 4–8 weeks apart if aged ≥1 3 years	HCP without reliable history of varicella or laboratory evidence of varicella immunity.	Pregnancy; immunocompromised state; history of anaphylactic reaction after receipt of neomycin or gelatin; recent receipt of antibody-containing blood products; salicylate use should be avoided for 6 weeks after vaccination.	Because 71%–93% of U.S.-born persons without a history of varicella are immune, serologic testing before vaccination might be cost-effective.

From Centers for Disease Control and Prevention: Immunizations strongly recommended for health care personnel (HCP). *Morb Mortal Wkly Rep* 52(RR-17):65, 2002, http://www.cdc.gov/mmwr/preview/mmwrhtml/rr5217a3.htm.
CDC: Immunization of health-care workers: recommendations of the Advisory Committee on Immunization Practices (ACIP) and the Hospital Infection Control Practices Advisory Committee (HICPAC). *MMWR* 1997;46(No. RR-18),
CDC: Prevention and control of influenza: recommendations of the Advisory Committee on Immunization Practices (ACIP). *MMWR* 2003;52:1-34.
CDC: Using live, attenuated influenza vaccine for prevention and control of influenza: supplemental recommendations of the Advisory Committee on Immunization Practices (ACIP). *MMWR* 2003;52(No. RR-13).
*A federal standard issued in December 1991 under the Occupational Safety and Health Administration requires that hepatitis B vaccine be made available at the employer's expense to all HCP occupationally exposed to blood or other potentially infectious materials. The Occupational Safety and Health Administration requires that employers make available hepatitis B vaccinations, evaluations, and follow-up procedures in accordance with current CDC recommendations.
†Persons immunocompromised because of immune deficiencies, HIV infection, leukemia, lymphoma, generalized malignancy, or persons receiving immunosuppressive therapy with corticosteroids, alkylating drugs, antimetabolites or persons receiving radiation.
§Vaccination of pregnant women after the first trimester might be preferred to avoid coincidental association with spontaneous abortions, which are most common during the first trimester. However, no adverse fetal effects have been associated with influenza vaccination.
¶A live attenuated influenza vaccine (LAIV) is FDA-approved for healthy persons aged 5-49 years. Because of the possibility of transmission of vaccine viruses from recipients of LAIV to other persons and in the absence of data on the risk of illness and among immunocompromised persons infected with LAIV viruses, the inactivated influenza vaccine is preferred for HCP who have close contact with immunocompromised persons.

recommendations from the Office of Overseas Travel at the CDC through their telephone hot line at 877-394-8747 or at their website at www.cdc.gov.

HEALTHY PEOPLE 2010 FOCUS ON IMMUNIZATION AND INFECTIOUS DISEASES

Healthy People 2010 objectives, discussed earlier in this chapter, detailed three focus areas for infectious diseases. Focus Area 14, seen previously in the *Healthy People 2010* table on 498, highlights vaccine-preventable and other priority infectious diseases, excluding STDs and HIV. This section provides tables summarizing the chain of transmission and control of the Focus Area 14 conditions. Table 23-8 covers childhood vaccine-preventable diseases, excluding hepatitis, which is summarized in Table 23-9. Table 23-10 summarizes tuberculosis.

HEALTHY PEOPLE 2010 FOCUS ON SEXUALLY TRANSMITTED DISEASES

Sexually transmitted diseases (STDs) include the more than 25 infectious organisms that are primarily transmitted through sexual activity (USDHHS, 2000d). STDs, even those for which treatment exists, continue to be a major public health problem. The rates of STDs in the United States are among the highest in the industrialized world, approaching those in some developing countries. An estimated 15 million cases of STDs occur each year in the United States, accounting for 87% of the top 10 infections reported to the CDC (USDHHS, 2000d).

Men and women of all ages, racial and ethnic backgrounds, and income levels contract STDs. However, the following populations are disproportionately affected: adolescents, young adults, women, minorities, and the poor (USDHHS, 2000d). Teenage girls in particular may be more susceptible to STDs because they have fewer protective antibodies to STDs and a cervix that is biologically immature. Women are at higher risk for contracting STDs than men because they have anatomical differences that enhance transmission of disease and make diagnosis difficult. In addition, they are also less likely to experience symptoms.

Complications from undiagnosed STDs occur more frequently and are more severe in women. For example, PID, largely resulting from an undetected STD, is diagnosed in more than one million women annually. Scarring from PID may lead to infertility, ectopic pregnancy, or chronic pelvic pain. An infected woman who transmits an STD to her fetus during pregnancy or childbirth may experience spontaneous abortion, premature delivery, stillbirth, neonatal death, and, in the infant, low birth weight, chronic respiratory problems, blindness, and mental retardation (USDHHS, 2000d). Finally, certain strains of HPV are strongly associated with cervical cancer; cervical cancer accounts for more than 4500 deaths annually.

Concern over the persistence and increases in STDs led those formulating the *Healthy People 2010* objectives to create a Focus Area 25 specific to STDs (see the *Healthy*

People 2010 table on p. 498). For easy reference, the chain of transmission and control of sexually transmitted diseases addressed in the *Healthy People 2010* objectives is presented in Table 23-11. The CDC regularly updates an excellent reference on STD treatment guidelines, which is available on the CDC website (CDC, 2002).

HEALTHY PEOPLE 2010 FOCUS ON HIV/AIDS

No other infection or infectious disease during recent history has inflicted as much destruction and pain to individuals, families, and communities, and created as many challenges for health care professionals as has HIV/AIDS. To this writer, HIV stands out as the one condition that touches nurses everywhere. HIV affects persons of every age, ethnicity, socioeconomic status, gender, and occupation. Eventually, HIV/AIDS has an impact on every organ and function of the human body. Every nurse, regardless of area of practice, will eventually care for someone with HIV infection. Currently, there is no cure or vaccine, and minimal hope of stemming the continuing spread throughout the world (Figure 23-4). It is not surprising, then, that *Healthy People 2010* objectives have an entire Focus Area 13 specific to HIV/AIDS (see the *Healthy People 2010* table on 498).

HIV, a retrovirus, is the organism that causes the syndrome known as AIDS. Following initial infection, the disease is typically asymptomatic for months to years. Usually the infected person does not know that he or she is infected, and continues to transmit the virus to others. The timeline for the usual course of HIV infection can be seen in Figure 23-5. HIV usually manifests gradually with conditions that result from inadequate immune system function, as the virus slowly attacks the body's immune system. Over time, the body loses its ability to fight illnesses, and opportunistic infections occur and become recurrent. A standardized case definition for AIDS was specified by CDC in 1993. This case definition is presented in Box 23-6, and the critical elements for both HIV and AIDS are summarized for easy reference in Table 23-12.

HIV infection is usually determined by the HIV antibody test, and the most commonly used form is the enzyme-linked immunosorbent assay (ELISA). There may be false-positive findings, so the Western blot is frequently used to verify the results. False-negative findings may also occur, especially before the body produces antibodies after exposure; therefore an exposed person should repeat the HIV antibody test at 1 month and 3 months after the original test. Additional tests are now available to detect the virus in the blood before antibodies are present (see Table 23-12).

Treatment for HIV and AIDS is complex and changes frequently. The FDA has approved many drugs for HIV infection and AIDS-related conditions. At present there are four classes of antiretroviral drugs, each corresponding to different mechanisms whereby HIV invades the cells of the immune system. It is beyond the scope of this chapter to review them all here. Current information on treatment is always available from the CDC. One source is the HIV/AIDS Treatment Information Service at http://www.aidsinfo.nih.gov.

Text continued on p. 519

TABLE 23-8 Chain of Transmission and Control: Childhood Vaccine-Preventable Diseases

	CHICKENPOX	DIPHTHERIA	PERTUSSIS	TETANUS	POLIO
Occurrence	Worldwide and universal in all populations, primarily in children	Rare where immunization rates are high; affects unimmunized children under 15 yr and adults whose immunity has waned	Worldwide and common in children; declined with immunization; some outbreaks in recent years in adults in the United States in those whose immunity has waned	Worldwide; occurs sporadically and affects all ages; more common in agricultural areas and among parenteral drug users; rare in areas with high immunization rates	Worldwide before immunization; it is now rare in countries with adequate immunization rates
Etiological agent	Human (alpha) herpesvirus 3 (varicella zoster virus)	*Corynebacterium diphtheriae*, of gravis, mitis, or intermedius biotypes	*Bordetella pertussis*	*Clostridium tetani* (an anaerobic pathogen)	Poliovirus, types 1, 2, and 3; all are paralytogenic
Reservoir	Humans	Humans	Humans	Intestines of humans and animals	Humans, particularly children with subclinical infections
Transmission	Direct and indirect contact with droplets from respiratory passage or vesicle fluid; extremely contagious	Direct or indirect contact with exudates from mucous membrane lesions of infected person or carrier; raw milk has served as a vehicle	Direct contact with droplets from respiratory passages	Tetanus spores enter body through a wound (usually puncture wound) contaminated with soil and feces; necrotic tissue favors the growth of the anaerobic bacillus	Direct and indirect contact with respiratory discharges and feces; fecal-oral route more common than respiratory transmission
Incubation period	14-16 days; range 2-3 wk; prolonged in immunocompromised persons	2-5 days; occasionally longer	9-10 days; range 6-20 days	10 days; range 3-21 days; rarely, several months	7-14 days; range 3-35 days
Communicability period	1-2 days before onset of rash to 5 days after lesions have crusted	Until bacilli have disappeared from discharges and lesions (usually 2 wk); effective antibiotic therapy interferes with shedding; a carrier may transmit for 6 mo	Highly communicable during early catarrhal and coughing stages; gradually decreasing until week 3; communicability is negligible after 5 days with effective antibiotic therapy	Not transmitted directly	Highly communicable during first days after onset of symptoms; virus is in throat secretions within 36 hr and in feces in 72 hr after infection; remains 1 wk in throat and 6 wk in feces
Susceptibility and resistance	General population not previously infected or vaccinated are at risk; can be severe and fatal in adults and immunocompromised persons	General unimmunized population are at risk; infants born of immune mothers have passive immunity for 6 mo; recovery from disease or asymptomatic infection usually confers lifetime immunity; immunization confers prolonged, but not lifetime, immunity	General unimmunized population are at risk; unimmunized children under 5 yr are most susceptible; no passive immunity from mother; disease confers prolonged, but not lifetime, immunity	General unimmunized population are at risk; active immunization from tetanus toxoid persists for 10 yr; tetanus immune globulin confers temporary immunity; infants born to immune mothers are protected at birth; active disease does not confer lifetime immunity	General unimmunized population is at risk; active immunization confers lifetime immunity; disease or subclinical infection confers type-specific lifetime immunity
Prevention and control	Single dose vaccination of children 12-18 mo, and for those up to 12 yr who have not had the disease	Immunization with diphtheria toxoid; (Tables 23-5 to 23-7); boosters every 10 yr	Immunization with whole cell vaccine; (Tables 23-5 to 23-7); prophylaxis with a 7-day course of erythromycin, should be given to all exposed persons, including health care workers, regardless of vaccination status	Active immunization with tetanus toxoid; (Tables 23-5 to 23-7); boosters every 10 yr, and as prophylaxis following penetrating injuries for those whose last booster was more than 10 yr ago	Active immunization with inactivated polio virus (IPV); (Tables 23-5 to 23-7)
Disease manifestations	Sudden mild fever and malaise, rash, or both; rash is progressive, changing from maculopapular to vesicular, and then forming a crust or scab; lesions tend to be more numerous on covered parts of the body; can be on all	Acute onset; usually affecting the upper respiratory tract; lesions are caused by the release of a cytotoxin and manifest as a patch or patches of inflammation surrounding a grayish membrane; complications may result in severe swelling of the neck,	Pertussis (whooping cough) begins with an upper respiratory cough and proceeds into a paroxysmal stage of coughing, often ending in vomiting; paroxysmal stage may last 1-2 mo or longer;	Tetanus (lockjaw) is an acute neurological illness caused by an anaerobic bacterium that produces an exotoxin in the portal of entry in the human host; tetanus causes gradually worsening neurological symptoms, including	Symptoms may range from inapparent illness to severe paralysis or death

Continued

TABLE 23-8 Chain of Transmission and Control: Childhood Vaccine-Preventable Diseases (cont'd)

	CHICKENPOX	DIPHTHERIA	PERTUSSIS	TETANUS	POLIO
	mucous membranes and are highly pruritic; complications are more common in persons over 15 yr old, infants less than 1 yr old, and immunocompromised persons; virus can persist in a dormant state in sensory nerve endings and can reactivate causing herpes zoster, or shingles	thrombocytopenia, neuritis, and myocarditis	complications include seizures, pneumonia, encephalopathy, and death	painful muscle contractions and spasms; frequently resulting in death	
Diagnosis	By symptoms	Bacteriological culture of nasal and throat secretions and from lesions	Bacteriological culture of nasal or throat secretions	History of injury plus clinical symptoms; bacterium is rarely found in wound cultures	Isolation of the virus from fecal or oropharyngeal specimens
Treatment	Antiviral drugs within 1 wk of exposure may modify severity; varicella-zoster immune globulin administered within 96 hr of exposure can modify or prevent the disease	Single dose of equine antitoxin followed by a full course of antibiotic therapy	Treatment with antibiotics reduces the period of infectivity and may lessen the severity of the disease if given before the paroxysmal stage	Tetanus antitoxin or tetanus immune globulin (TIG), preferably human; supportive care	Supportive care
Report to local health authority	Yes	Yes	Yes	Yes	Yes

Modified from Grimes DE, Grimes KA, Zack CM: Infectious diseases, In Thompson JM et al, editors: Mosby's clinical nursing, ed 5, St. Louis, 2002, Mosby. Data from Heymann DL, editor: Control of communicable diseases manual, ed 18, Washington, DC, 2004, APHA.

TABLE 23-8 Chain of Transmission and Control: Childhood Vaccine-Preventable Diseases (cont'd)

	MEASLES (RUBEOLA)	MUMPS	RUBELLA	HAEMOPHILUS INFLUENZAE TYPE B MENINGITIS	PNEUMOCOCCAL DISEASE	INFLUENZA
Occurrence	Worldwide; endemic and epidemic occurrences where immunization rates are low; still a major killer of children worldwide	Worldwide; incidence decreasing where immunization rates are high; one third of infected persons have subclinical infections	Worldwide and endemic where immunization rates are low; epidemics occur every 5-9 yr; primarily a disease of children	Worldwide; most common in children 2 mo to 5 yr of age; rare with widespread immunization	Worldwide; most common in children 2 mo to 3 yr of age, the elderly, and immunocompromised adults	Worldwide; in pandemics, epidemics, localized outbreaks, and sporadic cases
Etiological agent	Measles virus, a paramyxovirus	Mumps virus, a paramyxovirus	Rubella virus	*H. influenzae* serotype B (Hib)	*Streptococcus pneumoniae*	Three types of influenza virus (A, B, and C), each with many subtypes
Reservoir	Humans	Humans	Humans	Humans	Humans (often found in respiratory passages of healthy persons)	Humans; some mammals and birds suspected as sources of new subtypes
Transmission	Direct or indirect contact with nasal or throat secretions; highly communicable	Direct contact with saliva (airborne or droplets) from an infected person	Direct or indirect contact with nasopharyngeal secretions of infected persons; transplacental transmission leads to congenital rubella syndrome (CRS)	Direct or indirect contact with droplets of nasopharyngeal secretions	Direct or indirect contact with droplets of nasopharyngeal secretions	Airborne spread
Incubation period	10 days until fever; 14 days until rash; range 7-18 days	15-18 days; range 14-25 days	14-17 days; range 14-21 days	Unknown; probably 2-4 days	Unknown; probably 1-4 days	1-3 days
Communicability period	1 day before the prodromal period to 4 days after appearance of the rash	2 days before to 4 days after onset of parotitis; but the range can be 7 days before to 15 days after onset; can be transmitted by persons with subclinical infections	7 days before to 4 days after onset of rash; highly communicable; infants with CRS may shed virus for months after birth	Variable as long as organisms are in nasopharynx; noncommunicable within 24-48 hr after onset of effective antibiotic therapy	As long as organism is found in nasopharynx; may be prolonged in immunocompromised persons	3-5 days from clinical onset in adults; up to 7 days in children
Susceptibility and resistance	General population who have not had disease or immunization is at risk; lifetime immunity after illness; infants of mothers who have had the disease are protected for 6-9 mo; infants of immunized mothers have variable level of passive antibody; length of immunity following immunization is unknown	Lifetime immunity develops after subclinical and clinical illness	General unimmunized or previously uninfected population is at risk; lifetime immunity after illness; infants born to immune mothers are protected for 6-9 mo; longterm immunity following immunization	General unimmunized or previously uninfected population is at risk; immunity acquired transplacentally, from prior infection, and by immunization	General population is probably at risk; immunity is acquired transplacentally, from prior infection or from immunization	General population is at risk; infection and immunization produces immunity to only one subtype of the virus
Prevention and control	Active immunization with live, attenuated measles vaccine; (Tables 23-5 to 23-7)	Active immunization with live attenuated mumps virus vaccine; (Tables 23-5 to 23-7)	Active immunization with live, attenuated rubella virus vaccine in childhood (Tables 23-5 to 23-7); ensure immunity in adolescent girls	Active immunization with Hib conjugate vaccine (Tables 23-5 to 23-7)	Pneumococcal conjugate vaccine (PCV) for infants and children; pneumococcal polysaccharide vaccine (PPV) for high-risk groups; (Tables 23-5 to 23-7)	Active immunization yearly prior to influenza season

Continued

TABLE 23-8 Chain of Transmission and Control: Childhood Vaccine-Preventable Diseases (cont'd)

	MEASLES (RUBEOLA)	MUMPS	RUBELLA	HAEMOPHILUS INFLUENZAE TYPE B MENINGITIS	PNEUMOCOCCAL DISEASE	INFLUENZA
Disease manifestations	Acute-onset fever of 101° F or higher, cough, coryza, conjunctivitis, Koplik's spots on the buccal mucosa, and a red rash lasting longer than 3 days that begins on the face and becomes generalized; measles can progress into severe complications, including pneumonia, encephalitis, and death	Acute-onset fever and painful swelling of the salivary and parotid glands; may be asymptomatic; complications range from meningoencephalitis to permanent hearing impairment and orchitis in postpubescent males, but rarely sterility	Maculopapular rash and postauricular, occipital, and posterior cervical lymphadenopathy; children are usually relatively asymptomatic, but adults may experience fever, headache, and malaise; rare complications include encephalitis and thrombocytopenia; congenital defects in fetuses of pregnant women who are infected	Hib can affect multiple organ systems, resulting in meningitis, epiglottitis, otitis media, pneumonia, arthritis, and cellulitis, with symptoms associated with those conditions; complications are serious and include septic arthritis, life-threatening airway obstruction, fulminating infection, and death	Acute-onset symptoms of meningitis or pneumonia	Acute-onset dry cough, fever, headache, myalgia, sore throat, and other generalized symptoms; symptom severity depends on the subtype of the virus; complications include pneumonia, otitis media, meningitis, Reye's syndrome, and death.
Diagnosis	Tissue culture of nasopharyngeal secretions and serological testing	Isolation of virus from oral and throat spray, urine, and spinal fluid	Serological testing	Identifying organisms in blood or spinal fluid	Isolation of the organism from the blood or other sterile body site	Isolation of virus from nasal or pharyngeal secretions, serological testing, antigen detection, gene amplification, and rapid diagnostic test
Treatment	Supportive care	Supportive care	Supportive care	10-14 days antibiotics	Antibiotics	Antiviral drugs started within 48 hr of onset of symptoms
Report to local health authority	Yes	Yes	Yes	Yes	Epidemics only	Epidemics only

Modified from Grimes DE, Grimes KA, Zack CM: Infectious diseases, In Thompson JM et al, editors: *Mosby's clinical nursing*, ed 5, St. Louis, 2002, Mosby. Data from Heymann DL, editor: *Control of communicable diseases manual*, ed 18, Washington, DC, 2004, APHA.

TABLE 23-9 Chain of Transmission and Control: Hepatitis

	HEPATITIS A	HEPATITIS B	HEPATITIS C	HEPATITIS D	HEPATITIS E
Occurrence	Worldwide; sporadic and epidemic with cyclic recurrence; outbreaks in institutions where sanitation is poor	Worldwide; endemic; highest in young adults, homosexually active men, persons engaging in unprotected sex, injection drug users, health care and public safety workers	Worldwide; directly related to prevalence of injection drug use in the population, HCV in the donated blood supply, and lack of use of parenteral precautions in health care	Worldwide; occurs epidemically and endemically in population at risk for HBV infection; declining in areas where chronic carriers of HBsAG	Epidemic and sporadic cases, particularly in developing countries; highest in young adults; rare in children or the elderly
Etiological agent	HAV	HBV; made up of a core antigen, HBcAG, and a surface antigen, HBsAG; HBV has at least 8 different genotypes	HCV with 6 genotypes and 100 subtypes	HDV, consists of a coat of HBsAG and an internal antigen, the delta antigen	HEV
Reservoir	Humans and captive primates	Humans and possibly captive primates	Humans; virus has been transmitted experimentally to chimpanzees	Humans; virus can be transmitted experimentally to chimpanzees and to woodchucks	Humans and nonhuman primates, pigs, chickens, and cattle
Transmission	Person to person by fecal-oral route; contaminated food, water, shellfish, etc.	Direct and indirect contact with blood and serum-derived fluids; sexual contact; perinatal	Parenteral; sexual and mother-to-child transmission are less likely to occur	Similar to HBV; must co-infect with HBV	Person-to-person by fecal-oral route; contaminated food or water
Incubation period	28-30 days; range 15-50 days	60-90 days; range 45-180 days	6-9 wk; range 2 wk to 6 mo	2-8 wk	26-42 days; range 15-64 days
Communicability period	Latter half of incubation period to 1 wk after onset of jaundice	During incubation period and throughout clinical course of disease; carrier state may persist for years	Virus persists indefinitely	Throughout acute and chronic disease	Unknown; virus has been detected in stools 14 days after onset of symptoms and 4 wk after ingestion of contaminated food or water
Susceptibility and resistance	General population is at risk; usually affects children and young adults; probable lifetime immunity following infection	General population is at risk; disease is mild in children; lifetime immunity follows infection if antibody to HBV develops and HBV is negative	General population is at risk; degree of immunity following infection is not known	All person susceptible to HBV or who have an HBV infection and be coinfected with HDV	Unknown
Prevention and control	Eliminate common sources of infection by sanitation; improve hygienic practices and handwashing; cook shellfish; immunize high-risk groups or persons in high-risk situations; for post exposure: administer vaccine and IG within 2 wk; use universal precautions	Routinely immunize infants, children, and high-risk groups; at birth give HBIG and Hep B vaccine to infants born to HBsAg-positive mothers followed by additional vaccine doses at 1 and 6 months of age; immunize persons exposed to HBV; test all donated blood for HBV antigen; practice safe sex; use universal precautions	Apply HBV control measures except immunization: no vaccine exists at this time and IG does not prevent HCV infection	Apply HBV prevention and control measures; however, HBIG, IG and hepatitis B vaccine do not prevent HDV infection for those already infected with HBV	No vaccine; IG not effective; sanitation appears to be the only effective measure of prevention
Disease manifestations	Acute-onset fever, anorexia, malaise, dark urine, and jaundice, usually lasting 2 mo; it has a very low fatality rate and, although rare, it can last up to 6 mo	Insidious onset that ranges from asymptomatic illness to generalized nonspecific symptoms, such as anorexia, nausea, and vomiting followed by jaundice and occasionally resulting in fulminant fatal hepatitis	Like HBV, HCV has an insidious onset; symptoms vary from completely asymptomatic (80%) to the rare fulminating, fatal disease; mild symptoms are same as those for HBV; of those who are acutely ill, 75% to 85% develop chronic hepatitis	Abrupt onset with range of symptoms similar to HBV; always associated with HBV infection, either co-infection or as a superinfection in persons with chronic hepatitis B	Clinical course similar to hepatitis A; no chronic form

Continued

TABLE 23-9 Chain of Transmission and Control: Hepatitis (cont'd)

	HEPATITIS A	HEPATITIS B	HEPATITIS C	HEPATITIS D	HEPATITIS E
Diagnosis	Serum antibodies (anti-HAV) detectable 5-10 days postexposure	Presence in sera of HBsAG, anti-HBsAG (antibodies), HBc AG and anti-HBcAG, HBeAG and anti-HBeAG	Presence of serum antibodies to HCV (anti-HCV)	Presence of serum antibodies to HDV (anti-HDV)	Exclusion of other causes of hepatitis, particularly hepatitis A; presence of serum antibodies, anti-HEV; presence of HEV RNA in feces and serum
Treatment	Supportive care	Supportive care	Treatment with ribavirin and slow release interferons (pegylated interferons)	Supportive care	Supportive care
Case report to local health authority	Yes	Yes	Yes	Yes	Yes

Modified from Grimes DE, Grimes KA, Zack CM Infectious diseases, In Thompson JM, McFarland GK, Hirsch JE, Tucker SM, editors: *Mosby's clinical nursing*, ed 5, St. Louis, 2002, Mosby. Data from: Heymann DL, editor: *Control of communicable diseases manual*, ed 18, Washington, DC, 2004, APHA.

HAV, Hepatitis A virus; *HBV*, hepatitis B virus; *HCV*, hepatitis C virus; *HDV*, hepatitis delta virus; *HBIG*, hepatitis B immunoglobulin; *HBsAg*, hepatis B surface antigen; *HBcAG*, hepatitis B core antigen; *HBeAG*, hepatitis B early antigen.

TABLE 23-10   Chain of Transmission and Control: Tuberculosis

TUBERCULOSIS	
Occurrence	Worldwide; TB cases declined in United States since 1993; drug-resistant cases continue to be reported; most newly reported cases in the United States are reactivation of a latent infection and occur in older age-groups, children, and immunosuppressed persons; in areas of world with high incidence of new transmission, cases are in working-age adults and among disadvantaged populations
Etiological agent	*Mycobacterium tuberculosis;* less often *M. bovis* or *M. africanum*
Reservoir	Humans; diseased cattle for *M. bovis*
Transmission	Inhalation of airborne droplets from the sputum of persons with active disease; children rarely transmit because they do not cough forcefully; infrequently by ingestion or skin penetration

	INFECTION	ACTIVE DISEASE (CASE)
Incubation period	2-10 wk	Anytime during one's lifetime
Communicability period	Not communicable unless there are viable bacilli in the sputum	As long as bacilli are in sputum; inadequately treated persons may be communicable for years
Susceptibility and resistance	Anyone, such as healthcare workers, family members, or the institutionalized, working or living in close contact with a person with active disease can become infected	Vulnerable persons such as children, persons over 65 years old, those with chronic diseases or compromised immune systems, people who are malnourished, etc.
Prevention and control	Skin test in high risk groups, (e.g., health care workers), and treat those with new infections to prevent progression to active disease; routine skin testing, particularly of children, is no longer recommended in United States; Bacille Calmette-Guérin (BCG) vaccine is still used In some parts of the world	Promptly identify, diagnose and treat those with active disease; ensure compliance with treatment; initiate respiratory isolation until sputum is clear of bacilli; have patient wear a mask; examine close contacts of TB cases and treat, if infected
Disease manifestations	Initial infection goes unnoticed; 5%-10% of infected persons will eventually develop active disease, 50% of those within the first 2 yr	Onset of active disease can occur immediately following an initial infection or after a variable period of latency for untreated persons; disease onset is usually insidious with fever, night sweats, and weight loss; cough with pulmonary disease; extrapulmonary symptoms correspond with the location of disseminated bacilli and lesions
Diagnosis	TB skin test reaction within 2-10 wk of infection; the immune suppressed may have a negative skin test due to anergy; skin test results: 5 mm induration = + for immune suppressed and close contacts with active cases; 10 mm induration = + for infections < 2 yr and persons with high risk conditions; 15 mm induration = + for all low-risk persons	10%-20% have a negative skin test; demonstration of acid fast bacilli in stained smears of sputum or other body fluids; isolation of organism from cultured specimen; radiological evidence of TB in lungs or elsewhere
Treatment	Treat with isoniazid (INH) for 6-12 mo, or with other drug combinations for persons with HIV	Treat with combination of antimicrobial drugs, to which the strain of *Mycobacterium* is susceptible (INH, RIF, PZA, EMB) for 6-12 mo; monitor adherence carefully
Report to local health authority	No	Yes

Data from: Heymann DL, editor: *Control of communicable diseases manual,* ed 18, Washington, DC, 2004, APHA.

Exposure of health care personnel to HIV, although rare, remains a concern for the CDC and health care workers. The CDC continues to update recommendations for postexposure prophylaxis (PEP) for occupational exposures (CDC, 2005h). Although the principles of immediate treatment following exposure have not changed, the drugs and drug combinations have changed. These guidelines are among the many that can be downloaded from the website. Additional resources include the PEPline at 888-448-4911.

Before the onset of effective antiretroviral therapies in the late 1990s, reported cases of AIDS provided a good indicator of the progression of the epidemic. With effective treatment, persons with HIV infection have taken longer to progress to AIDS, and the incidence of AIDS has declined. This has given the false impression that the epidemic was coming under control.

Reporting cases of HIV infection has been incomplete and has varied by state. Whereas all states report AIDS cases by name, not all states report HIV infection cases by name. Recently, the CDC Director has made a plea for all state and territorial health departments to conduct HIV reporting using the same confidential, name-based approach currently used for AIDS surveillance nationwide (Gerberding, 2005).

TABLE 23-11　Chain of Transmission and Control: Sexually Transmitted Diseases

	GONORRHEA	CHLAMYDIA TRACHOMATIS	SYPHILIS	GENITAL HERPES	WARTS, HUMAN PAPILLOMAVIRUS (HPV) INFECTION
Occurrence	Worldwide; highest in males and females, 15-30 yr old	Worldwide; most prevalent STD	Worldwide and increasing; highest in males and females 20-30 yr old	Worldwide and increasing; highest in males and females 15-30 yr old	Worldwide
Etiological agent	Neisseria gonorrhoeae, the gonococcus	Chlamydia trachomatis	Treponema pallidum	Herpes simplex virus (HSV) type 2	Human papillomavirus (HPV); 70 types
Reservoir	Humans	Humans	Humans	Humans	Humans
Transmission	Contact with exudates from mucous membranes of infected persons; usually by direct sexual contact, although both pathogens can be transmitted during childbirth	Contact with exudates from mucous membranes of infected persons; usually by direct sexual contact, although both pathogens can be transmitted during childbirth	Direct sexual contact with infectious exudates from lesions; transplacentally; blood transfusion early in infection of donor	Direct contact with secretions from mucous membranes and lesions; transplacentally	Direct sexual contact; autoinoculation; during childbirth
Incubation period	2-7 days	7-10 days	3 wk; range 10 days to 3 mo	2-12 days	2-3 mo; range 1-20 mo
Communicability period	Months if untreated	Unknown	When moist lesions are present during the primary and secondary stages, generally 1 yr	During and up to 7 wk after primary lesions; transient shedding of virus in absence of lesions for years	Unknown, probably as long as lesions persist
Susceptibility and resistance	General population is at risk; antibodies are not protective against reinfection	General population is at risk; no acquired immunity	General population is at risk; however, only 30% of exposures lead to infection; some immunity develops over time	General population is at risk; immune response does not prevent recurrence	General population is at risk; immunosuppressed persons are more susceptible
Prevention and control	Safer sexual practices; detect and treat cases and contacts; test pregnant women for infection and treat			Safer sexual practices; cesarean delivery if lesions are present during late pregnancy	Safer sexual practices
Disease manifestations	Males: Urethritis with purulent discharge from anterior urethra; females: mucopurulent cervicitis, often asymptomatic; 20% progress to endometritis, salpingitis, and pelvic peritonitis; both genders may have pharyngeal or anorectal infections depending on their sexual practices; individuals are frequently co-infected with N. gonorrhoeae and C. trachomatis	Males: Urethritis with purulent discharge from anterior urethra; females: mucopurulent cervicitis, often asymptomatic; 20% progress to endometritis, salpingitis, and pelvic peritonitis; both genders may have pharyngeal or anorectal infections depending on their sexual practices; individuals are frequently co-infected with N. gonorrhoeae and C. trachomatis	Primary: moist lesion appearing within 3 wk at area of contact; secondary: symmetrical maculopapular rash in 4-6 wk; latency: indefinite time, no symptoms; tertiary: late lesions of bone, viscera, CNS, and cardiovascular system	Local, primary, vesicular lesions, period of latency and recurring, localized lesions; lesions start at area of contact but may spread to surrounding tissues or be disseminated in body, even to the CNS; other disease symptoms depend on extent of dissemination	Skin and mucous membrane lesions that are circumscribed, hyperkeratotic, and of varying sizes and shapes; certain types of HPV warts (16, 18, 31, 33, and 45) have been found to be associated with cervical cancer
Diagnosis	Gram stain of discharges, bacteriological cultures or tests that detect gonococcal nucleic acid	Failure to detect N. gonorrhoeae in discharges from symptomatic persons; mononuclear antibody tests on discharges	Serological testing of blood and CSF, if indicated	Detection of cell changes in tissue scrapings or biopsy; isolation of virus from lesions or other affected tissue; serological tests	Visualization of the lesion; excision and histological examination of the lesion
Treatment	Treat with antibiotics, preferably with single dose, IM antibiotics, such as ceftriaxone; treatment depends on extent of the infection; follow-up testing is recommended	Treat with antibiotics, such as single dose azithromycin or 7 days of doxycycline; advisable to treat for gonorrhea and chlamydia concurrently	Treat with antibiotics; treatment differs with stage of the disease	Treatment with antivirals; treatment varies depending on area of lesions and whether they are disseminated	Removal of the warts by freezing with liquid nitrogen or other chemical; removal reduces the risk of transmitting the virus
Report to local health authority	Yes	Yes	Yes, including congenital syphilis	No	No

Modified from Grimes DF, Grimes KA, Zack CM Infectious diseases. In Thompson JM et al. editors: Mosby's clinical nursing, ed 5, St. Louis, 2002, Mosby. Data from: Heymann DL, editor: Control of communicable diseases manual, ed 18,

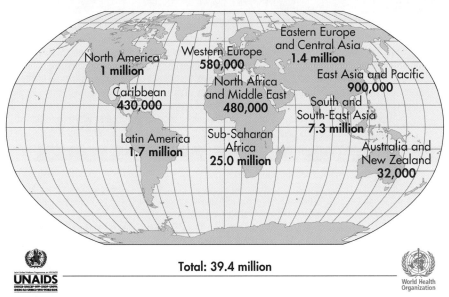

FIGURE 23-4 HIV/AIDS worldwide, 2004. (From UNAIDS: *2004 report on the global AIDS epidemic,* Geneva, 2004, The Author.)

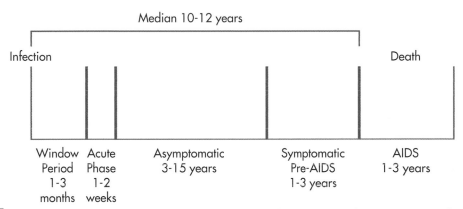

FIGURE 23-5 Usual course of HIV infection. (Modified from Grimes, DE, Grimes, RM: *AIDS and HIV infection*, St. Louis, 1994, Mosby.)

Eradication of AIDS is dependent on development of a vaccine and the infrastructure necessary to vaccinate populations at risk worldwide. Neither possibility is foreseen in the near future, although testing of vaccine in humans has been initiated.

PREVENTION OF COMMUNICABLE DISEASES

All practicing nurses have a role in primary, secondary, and tertiary prevention of communicable diseases. Examples of appropriate interventions are reviewed here and in Table 23-13.

Primary Prevention

Primary prevention of communicable diseases involves measures to prevent transmission of an infectious agent and to prevent pathology in the person exposed to an infection. All of the activities described in the section on breaking the chain of transmission are primary prevention activities. Immunization is primary prevention. Changing the behaviors that lead to exposure to a pathogen is primary prevention. See Tables 23-8 thru 23-12 for primary preventions specific to the conditions in those tables.

Secondary Prevention

Secondary prevention includes activities to detect infections early and effectively treat persons who are infected. Not only

TABLE 23-12 Chain of Transmission and Control: HIV/AIDS

HIV/AIDS	
Occurrence	Worldwide; in 2004 about 40 million persons estimated to be living with human immunodeficiency virus (HIV), 62% reside in sub-Saharan Africa, 18% in south and south east Asia, 5% in Latin America, and 2.5% in the United States
Etiological agent	HIV, a retrovirus with two serologically and geographically distinct types (HIV-1 and HIV-2); HIV-1 makes up 90%-95% of the world's cases; it may be more pathogenic, lead to more rapid disease progression, and have higher mother-to-infant transmission than HIV-2 does; multiple subtypes (sometimes called clades) have been identified for both HIV-1 and HIV-2
Reservoir	Humans; HIV may have evolved from a chimpanzee virus
Transmission	Direct person to person through unprotected sexual contact, mother to fetus or mother to infant (during birth or by breastfeeding); indirect by contact of abraded skin or mucous membranes with infected blood or body fluids; injection of contaminated blood or fluids, or through use of contaminated needles; transplant of organs from infected person

	HIV INFECTION	AIDS
Incubation period	1-3 mo before antibodies are detectable	<1 yr to 15 yr; may be longer with effective antiretroviral therapy
Communicability period	Presumed to be <10 days after infection and lasting throughout life; may be highest in early infection when viral load is highest, and again later when clinical status worsens	
Susceptibility and resistance	General population is at risk; increased risk for infection with untreated ulcerative STDs and in uncircumcised males; evidence that some persons are less susceptible because of chemokine-receptor polymorphisms; very small percentage of infected persons do not progress to AIDS for an unknown reason	
Prevention and control	Practice universal precautions and safer sex; treat pregnant women with antiretrovirals to prevent transmission to fetus; teach infected women to avoid breastfeeding; treat drug users and provide needle exchange programs for injection drug users; treat STDs to decrease chance of acquiring HIV through sores on mucous membranes; maintain a safe blood supply; encourage autologous blood transfusions, when possible	Adherence to effective antiretroviral therapy delays progression to AIDS; prophylactic treatment for opportunistic infections delays onset of conditions associated with AIDS diagnosis
Disease manifestations	Acute, self-limiting illness lasting for 1-2 wk with symptoms that mimic other conditions (fever, rash, pharyngitis, myalgia, lymphadenopathy, and malaise); although immune deficiency may progress, the person may be without further symptoms for years	Progressive immune-deficiency and increasing susceptibility to life-threatening infections and cancers
Diagnosis	*Early after infection:* The p24 and polymerase chain reaction blood tests identify the presence of viral nucleic acids; *within 1-3 months after infection:* Serologic tests (enzyme-linked immunosorbent assay, western blot) identify antibodies to HIV.	See Box 23-6 for case definition for AIDS
Treatment	Treatment with antiretroviral drugs to suppress the virus, not eradicate it; currently four classes of drugs are available: nucleoside reverse transcriptase inhibitors, nonnucleoside reverse transcriptase inhibitors, protease inhibitors, and fusion inhibitors; each attacks a different target in the reproduction process of the virus; current treatment strategies use at least 3 drugs from at least 2 classes; requires almost perfect adherence as development of drug-resistant HIV is common; treatment is very expensive and has many side effects; a person with AIDS will require additional treatment for infections and cancers that develop from impaired immune status	
Report to local health authority	Some states require reporting by name	Yes in all states

Data from Heymann DL, editor: *Control of communicable diseases manual,* ed 18, Washington, DC, APHA, 2004. UNAIDS: 2004 report on the global AIDS epidemic, Geneva, 2004, The Author.

does this prevent progression of the infectious disease, but it also prevents transmission of the pathogen to others. Reporting infectious diseases, investigating contacts, notifying partners, finding new cases, and isolating cases are examples of secondary prevention.

Tertiary Prevention

Tertiary prevention includes activities involved in caring for persons with an infectious disease to ensure that they are cured or that their quality of life is maintained. Maybe the most important part of the treatment process is to ensure that the person take their antimicrobials completely and effectively. In a time of increased resistance to pathogens, helping patients adhere to a drug regimen is critical. Additionally, caregivers should be taught to protect themselves and their environment

by using appropriate precautions when caring for an infected family member.

SUMMARY

This chapter has presented the challenges of infectious diseases that face community health nurses everywhere. It has reviewed principles that are the foundation for the occurrence, transmission, and control of infectious diseases, and applied those principles to infectious diseases that are emphasized in the *Healthy People 2010* objectives. Most importantly, because nurses will be impacted by infectious diseases wherever they practice, resources where any nurse can obtain up-to-date information on any infectious disease at any time have been included.

TABLE 23-13 Examples of Primary, Secondary, and Tertiary Prevention Activities for Control of Infectious Diseases at the Individual and Population Levels

INFECTIOUS DISEASE	INDIVIDUAL	POPULATION
PRIMARY PREVENTION		
Sexually transmitted disease	Teach safe sex practices	Place condom machines in accessible areas in places where young adults congregate
Diseases caused by blood-borne pathogens	Teach barrier precautions to all health care workers	Provide an adequate supply of gloves and sharps containers in patient care areas
	Teach injecting drug users about dangers of sharing needles	Initiate citywide needle exchange programs and methadone programs
Vaccine-preventable diseases	Ensure that all children who come to the clinic have age-appropriate immunizations	Work with community groups to cosponsor immunization clinics where immunization rates are low
Hepatitis A, gastrointestinal infections	Teach safe food handling practices in the home	Require, as part of the licensing of restaurants, that food handlers take a course in safe food handling
Hepatitis A and B	Provide immune globulin after exposure to hepatitis A or B	Mandate that health care workers are immunized for hepatitis A and B
SECONDARY PREVENTION		
STDs	Screen and treat for all STDs	STD partner notification program
Tuberculosis	Screen close contacts of persons with TB	Initiate a program of yearly testing of health care workers for TB
	Treat persons with a recent skin test conversion	Provide treatment to all recent converters free of charge at their workplace
HIV/AIDS	Provide testing and treatment for HIV in local clinics	Initiate reporting of HIV cases by name to the local health department to facilitate surveillance of HIV in population
Meningitis	Immunize and provide chemoprophylaxis for person exposed to meningitis	Provide immunization and chemoprophylaxis to all students in a school following an exposure
TERTIARY PREVENTION		
Tuberculosis	Provide therapy for person with active TB	Initiate a directly observed therapy (DOT) program in the community shelters and jails
	Teach patients to take all doses of prescribed antibiotics and monitor adherence	Initiate community education campaigns about the problem of drug resistance associated with incomplete antibiotic use

BOX 23-6 Case Definition for AIDS

According to the 1993 case definition, a diagnosis of AIDS is determined by repeatedly reactive HIV antibody tests, identification of HIV antigen in host tissue, or both, plus a combination of immunological status, as measured by CD4+ T-lymphocyte count (Categories 1-3), and clinical indicator conditions (Categories A, B, and C).

Any person who meets the following combination of criteria meets the case definition for AIDS:

1. Category 1, 2, or 3 CD4+ T-lymphocyte count, plus any Category C indicator condition
2. Category 3 CD4+ count plus any Category A, B, or C indicator condition

➤ Immunological marker categories:
   Category 1: >500 cells/μL
   Category 2: 200-499 cells/μl
   Category 3: <200 cells/μL

➤ Clinical indicator categories:
   Category A: Asymptomatic HIV infection; persistent generalized lymphadenopathy; acute primary infection
   Category B: Symptomatic conditions associated with HIV or complicated by HIV, but not necessarily limited to persons with immune suppression. These include:
      Bacillary angiomatosis
      Candidiasis, oropharyngeal; candidiasis, vulvovaginal
      Cervical dysplasia
      Fever or diarrhea lasting longer than 1 month
      Herpes zoster
      Idiopathic thrombocytopenic purpura
      Listeriosis
      Pelvic inflammatory disease

Category C: Conditions indicating severe immune suppression; these include:
   Candidiasis of bronchi, trachea, lungs, or esophagus
   Cervical cancer, invasive
   Coccidioidomycosis, disseminated or extrapulmonary
   Cryptococcosis, extrapulmonary
   Cryptosporidiosis, chronic intestinal
   Cytomegalovirus retinitis (with loss of vision)
   Encephalopathy, HIV-related
   Herpes simplex: chronic ulcers; or bronchitis, pneumonitis or esophagitis
   Histoplasmosis, disseminated or extrapulmonary
   Isosporiasis, chronic intestinal
   Kaposi's sarcoma
   Lymphoma, Burkitt's, immunoblastic, or primary of the brain
   Mycobacterium avium complex or any other species
   Mycobacterium tuberculosis, any site
   Pneumocystis carinii pneumonia
   Pneumonia, recurrent
   Progressive multifocal leukoencephalopathy
   Salmonella septicemia, recurrent
   Toxoplasmosis of brain
   Wasting syndrome

From Centers for Disease Control and Prevention: 1993 Revised classification system for HIV infection and expanded surveillance case definition for AIDS among adolescents and adults, *Morb Mortal Wkly Rep* 41:RR-17, 1992.

CASE STUDY   Assessment

Adrienne Zack is the Employee Health Nurse for a large city hospital. On a recent workday, she saw Beverly Yancy, a staff nurse in the newborn nursery of the hospital who presented to the employee health clinic with a productive cough, wheezing, low-grade fever, chills, and fatigue lasting over 1 month. Beverly stated that she had been treating her symptoms with over-the-counter (OTC) antihistamines, cough suppressants, and antipyretics. When weighed in the clinic, Beverly was surprised that she had lost 10 lb since she weighed last. She told Adrienne that she has no history of asthma or lung disease.

Beverly's employee health record revealed that she had had a positive tuberculin skin test (TBST) of 15 mm induration when she was screened 11 years earlier for employment at the hospital. A chest radiograph at that time showed no evidence of tuberculosis (TB) disease. Because Beverly was without TB symptoms at the time of employment and declined to take isoniazid (INH) for treatment of the latent tuberculosis infection (LTBT), she believed that the positive TBST was the result of having received Bacille Calmette-Guérin (BCG) vaccination at birth in the Philippines. Further, she has been negative for symptoms during her annual symptom screen by the Employee Health Clinic.

A chest x-ray showed suspicious areas indicating that Beverly most likely had active, infectious pulmonary TB. The diagnosis was confirmed when a sputum smear was positive for acid-fast bacilli (AFB). Based on the timing of her symptoms, Adrienne determined that Beverly probably has been communicable for 3 months.

DIAGNOSIS

Individual
- Active TB
- Potential for spread of TB to close contacts

Family
- Potential for undiagnosed TB

Community
- At risk for exposure to TB

PLANNING

Mycobacterium tuberculosis (MTB) is transmitted by airborne droplets of sputum from persons with active disease who cough or otherwise discharge respiratory droplets in the air. Health care workers are at risk for TB infection because of frequent exposure to patients with active TB disease. Beverly could not have been infected by the newborns in the nursery where she worked. Most likely she was exposed to TB before her screening 11 years previously. Her skin test of 15 mm induration suggested a latent TB infection rather than BCG vaccination at birth. Latent TB infection can become active

tuberculosis disease at any time. In this case, latency lasted more than 11 years.

Health care workers, like anyone with active TB, can transmit the infection to close contacts such as co-workers, high-risk patients, and personal contacts. Newborns and children under 2 years of age are at high risk for contracting TB infection and for progressing to TB disease. Such contacts must be found, screened and treated as soon as possible. The incubation period for a detectable infection is 2 to 10 weeks following exposure. Recent contacts that are skin-test negative now should be retested in 2 to 3 months.

GOALS

Individual
Short-Term Goals
- Beverly will begin her course of medications immediately.
- Beverly will take short-term disability and not return to work until cleared by the employee health clinic.

Long-Term Goals
- Beverly will complete her course of medications as directed.
- Beverly will provide sputum cultures and undergo chest x-ray examination at 3, 6, and 9 months and will be free of evidence of active TB.

Family
Short-Term Goals
- All of Beverly's family members will be tested for TB within 3 days.
- Any family member testing positive will be started on a course of medication as recommended by the health department and their health care provider.

Long-Term Goal
- All family members will be re-tested in 6 months.

Community (Hospital)
Short-Term Goals
- Beverly's co-workers will be tested for TB within 3 days.
- All of Beverly's patients from the past 3 months will be contacted to encourage them to be tested.
- Any contact or patient testing positive will be started on a course of medications as recommended by the local health department and their health care provider.

Long-Term Goal
- All contacts will be re-tested in 6 month.

INTERVENTION

Tuberculosis must be reported to local public health authorities who are responsible for control of TB in the

CASE STUDY   Assessment

community. Control relies on identifying and adequately treating all active TB cases and those with latent infections. The public health department will investigate Beverly's contacts inside and outside the hospital during the previous 3 months. This will be done to identify and treat persons, including the discharged newborns, to whom Beverly might have transmitted MTB. Adrianne and the other health clinic employees may be asked to assist with screening hospital workers exposed to Beverly and providing education about treatment.

Tuberculin skin tests are determined to be positive under the following conditions:

1. Induration of 5 mm in persons with HIV infection, those in close personal contact with someone with active TB or persons who have fibrotic chest radiographs
2. Induration of 10 mm in other high-risk persons, such as injecting drug users and persons with chronic disease or other causes of immune suppression and those from countries or communities where TB prevalence is high
3. Induration of 15 mm for anyone who does not meet the above criteria

All persons with a positive skin test should be tested for active disease. Those who have AFB in a stained smear of sputum, mycobacteria isolated from a cultured specimen or radiological evidence of TB must be treated for active disease with a combination of drugs according to protocols established by the Centers for Disease Control and Prevention (CDC).

Multidrug-resistant TB (MDRTB) is an ever-increasing problem. Of active TB, 1% to 2% is now resistant to all available drugs. Patients must be helped to meticulously adhere to the prescribed regimen. Studies have demonstrated that health care workers are as poor as the general public at adhering to long-term drug therapy.

Persons with a recent conversion to a positive TBST should undergo treatment for latency according to CDC protocols. Such treatment reduces lifetime risk of a latent infection converting to active disease. Persons taking isoniazid should be taught symptoms of side effects to the drug, including hepatotoxicity, peripheral neuropathy, and central nervous system (CNS) changes.

Teaching should include the following:
- The importance of isolating oneself from contact with others and wearing a mask in public until sputum is clear of bacilli—around 4 to 8 weeks with effective treatment.
- Proper discharge of sputum and materials contaminated with sputum.
- That drug therapy must be continued uninterrupted for designated time period even after sputum is negative for bacilli.
- That drug toxicity and side effects must be reported to physician immediately. These include, but are not limited to:

- *Isoniazid (INH):* Hepatotoxicity, peripheral neuropathy, CNS changes
- *Ethambutol:* Reduced visual acuity with inability to see the color green
- *Streptomycin:* Rash, fever, malaise, vertigo, deafness, gastrointestinal disturbance, CNS changes
- *Pyrazinamide:* Hypersensitivity, hepatotoxicity, gastrointestinal disturbances, renal failure
- *Rifampin:* Red-orange urine, hepatotoxicity, CNS symptoms
- *Ethionamide:* Gastrointestinal disturbance and symptoms of hepatotoxicity
- *Pyrazinamide:* Hepatotoxicity
- *Cycloserine:* CNS effects
- Sputum must be reexamined monthly until negative for bacilli, then every 3 months for duration of therapy

EVALUATION

Beverly others with active TB can return to work when they have had three negative AFB sputum smear results collected 8 to 24 hours apart, with at least one being an early morning specimen. Adrianne will refer to CDC's most recent guidelines for preventing transmission of tuberculosis in healthcare settings (CDC, 2005) and update the hospital's infection control plan in accordance with the guidelines.

LEVELS OF PREVENTION

Primary
- Educate health care workers and others about TB infection and disease.
- Educate staff on airborne precautions and the proper use of respiratory protection.
- Design and implement signage throughout the hospital to remind staff and patients about respiratory hygiene, cough etiquette, and hand hygiene.

Secondary
- Establish regular screening of health care workers for positive skin test conversions.
- Establish mechanisms for detection, referral, and treatment of staff with latent TB infections and with active TB.
- Implement procedures for rapid detection and treatment of patients with active TB.
- Coordinate efforts with the local health department.

Tertiary
- Monitor medication compliance and follow-up testing.

Centers for Disease Control and Prevention: Guidelines for preventing the transmission of *Mycobacterium tuberculosis* in health-care settings, *Morbid Mortal Wkly Rep* 54(RR17):1-141, 2005.

LEARNING ACTIVITIES

1. Subscribe to the e-mail listserv to receive *Morb Mortal Wkly Rep* (http://www.cdc.gov).
2. Attend an immunization clinic at your local health department to observe a nurse screening children for immunizations.
3. Obtain and evaluate health education materials regarding childhood immunizations from your local health department.
4. Log on to the website of an advocacy group against immunizations to understand the messages that they are communicating to the public.
5. Log on to your state health department website to learn about the process of reporting notifiable diseases in your state. Who is responsible for the reporting process? To whom do they report, what information is reported, and how often are diseases reported?
6. Log on to the CDC website to obtain the most recent guidelines for treating persons with HIV/AIDS, STDs, or tuberculosis.
7. Purchase a 1-year subscription to a public health nursing journal.

REFERENCES

Centers for Disease Control and Prevention: 1993 Revised classification system for HIV infection and expanded surveillance case definition for AIDS among adolescents and adults, *Morb Mortal Wkly Rep* 41(RR-17):1-23, 1992.

Centers for Disease Control and Prevention: Recommendations of the internal task force for disease eradication, *Morb Mortal Wkly Rep* 42(RR-16):1-38, 1993.

Centers for Disease Control and Prevention: *Epidemiology and prevention of vaccine-preventable diseases,* Atlanta, 1995, The Author.

Centers for Disease Control and Prevention: *Vaccine management: recommendations for handling and storage of selected biologicals,* Atlanta, 1996, CDC National Immunization Program.

Centers for Disease Control and Prevention: *Preventing emerging infectious diseases: a strategy for the 21st century,* Atlanta, 1998a, The Author.

Centers for Disease Control and Prevention: Guidelines for vaccinating pregnant women, *Morb Mortal Wkly Rep* 45(RR-4):1-18, 1998b.

Centers for Disease Control and Prevention: The principles of disease elimination and eradication, *Morb Mortal Wkly Rep* 48(SU01):23-27, 1999a.

Centers for Disease Control and Prevention: Recommendations of the advisory committee on immunization practices: revised recommendations for routine poliomyelitis vaccination, *Morb Mortal Wkly Rep* 48(27):590, 1999b.

Centers for Disease Control and Prevention: *Health information for international travel (yellow book),* Atlanta, 1999-2000, USDHHS.

Centers for Disease Control and Prevention: *Epidemiology and prevention of vaccine-preventable diseases (pink book),* ed 6, Atlanta, 2000a, Public Health Foundation.

Centers for Disease Control and Prevention: Vaccine information statements: state health departments, 2000b, The Author, http://www.cdc.gov/nip/publications/VIS.

Centers for Disease Control and Prevention: Meningococcal disease and college students, recommendations of the Advisory Committee on Immunization Practices (ACIP), *Morb Mortal Wkly Rep* 49(RR-07):11-20, 2000c.

Centers for Disease Control and Prevention: Sexually transmitted diseases treatment guidelines, 2002, *Morb Mortal Wkly Rep* 51(RR-6):1-84, 2002.

Centers for Disease Control and Prevention: Immunizations strongly recommended for health-care personnel (HCP), *Morb Mortal Wkly Rep* 52(RR17):65, 2003, http://www.cdc.gov/mmwr/preview/mmwrhtml/rr5217a3.htm.

Centers for Disease Control and Prevention: Bioterrorism agents/diseases, 2004, The Author, http://www.bt.cdc.gov/agent/agentlist.asp.

Centers for Disease Control and Prevention: Summary of notifiable diseases: United States, 2003, *Morb Mortal Wkly Rep* 52(54):1-86, 2005a.

Centers for Disease Control and Prevention: Diseases connected to antibiotic resistance, 2005b, The Author, http://www.cdc.gov/drugresistance/diseases.htm.

Centers for Disease Control and Prevention: Infectious disease information: emerging infectious diseases, 2005c, The Author, http://www.cdc.gov/ncidod/diseases/eid/disease_sites.htm.

Centers for Disease Control and Prevention: Nationally notifiable infectious diseases, 2005d, The Author, http://www.cdc.gov/epo/dphsi/phs/infdis1005.htm.

Centers for Disease Control and Prevention: Vaccine-preventable diseases and specific vaccines, 2005e, The Author, http://www.cdc.gov/node.do/id/0900f3ec8005df1f.

Centers for Disease Control and Prevention: Recommended childhood and adolescent immunization schedule: United States, 2005, *Morb Mortal Wkly Rep* 53(51): Q1-Q3, 2005f.

Centers for Disease Control and Prevention: Recommended adult immunization schedule: United States, October 2005-September 2006, *Morb Mortal Wkly Rep* 54(40):Q1-Q4, 2005g. http://www.cdc.gov/nip/recs/adult-schedule.htm.

Centers for Disease Control and Prevention: Updated US Public Health Service guidelines for the management of occupational exposures to HIV and recommendations for postexposure prophylaxis, *Morb Mortal Wkly Rep* 54, RR-9, 1-24, 2005h, http://www.cdc.gov/mmwr/preview/mmwrhtm./rr5409a1.htm.

Gerberding, JL: Dear colleague letter, July 5, 2005, http://www.cdc.gov/hiv/survellance.htm.

Grimes, DE: *Infectious diseases,* St. Louis, 1991, Mosby.

Grimes, DE, Grimes, RM: *AIDS and HIV infection,* St. Louis, 1994, Mosby.

Grimes, DE, Grimes, KA, Zack, CM: Infectious diseases. In Thompson JM et al, editors: *Mosby's clinical nursing,* ed 5, St Louis, 2002, Mosby.

Heymann DL, editor: *Control of communicable diseases manual,* ed 18, Washington, DC, 2004, American Public Health Association.

Murray PR et al: *Manual of clinical microbiology,* ed 6, Washington, DC, 1995, ASM Press.

Pickering LK, editor: *2000 red book: report of the committee on infectious disease,* ed 25, Elk Grove Village, Ill, 2000, American Academy of Pediatrics.

Schneider M-J: *Introduction to public health,* ed 2, Boston, 2006, Jones and Bartlett.

UNAIDS: *2004 report on the global AIDS epidemic,* Geneva, 2004, The Author.

US Department of Health and Human Services: *Healthy People 2010*: immunization and infectious diseases, 2000a, http://www.healthypeople.gov/document/html/volume1/14immunization.

US Department of Health and Human Services: *Healthy People 2010*: sexually transmitted diseases, 2000b, http://www.healthypeople.gov/document/html/volume2/25stds.

US Department of Health and Human Services: *Healthy People 2010*: HIV, 2000c, http://www.healthypeople.gov/document/html/volume1/13hiv.

US Department of Health and Human Services: *Healthy People 2010*: understanding and improving health, ed 2, Washington, DC: 2000d, US Government Printing Office.

World Health Organization: Tuberculosis: fact sheet No 104, 2004, The Author, http://www.who.int/gtb.

Substance Abuse

Joanne M. Hall ▪ Josephine Wade

MEDIA RESOURCES

Additional Material for Study, Review, and Further Exploration

evolve Website at http://evolve.elsevier.com/Nies

❖ Quiz ❖ Case Studies ❖ Content Updates ❖ Glossary ❖ WebLinks

OBJECTIVES

Upon completion of this chapter, the reader will be able to do the following:

1. Discuss the historical trends and current conceptions of the cause and treatment of substance abuse.
2. Describe the current social, political, and economic aspects of substance abuse.
3. Describe the ethical and legal implications of substance abuse.
4. Detail the typical symptoms and consequences of substance abuse.
5. Identify issues related to substance abuse in various populations encountered in community health nursing practice.
6. Apply the nursing process to substance abuse problems.

KEY TERMS

addiction
dual diagnosis
harm reduction

initiation
intervention
mutual help groups

professional enablers
social consequences

substance abuse
war on drugs

CHAPTER OUTLINE

HISTORICAL OVERVIEW OF ALCOHOL AND ILLICIT DRUG USE

PREVALENCE, INCIDENCE, AND TRENDS
Trends in Substance Use

ADOLESCENT SUBSTANCE ABUSE

CONCEPTUALIZATIONS OF SUBSTANCE ABUSE
Definitions
Etiology of Substance Abuse

SOCIOCULTURAL AND POLITICAL ASPECTS OF SUBSTANCE ABUSE

COURSE OF SUBSTANCE-RELATED PROBLEMS

LEGAL AND ETHICAL CONCERNS OF SUBSTANCE ABUSE

MODES OF INTERVENTION
Prevention
Treatment

Pharmacotherapies
Mutual Help Groups
Harm Reduction

SOCIAL NETWORK INVOLVEMENT
Family and Friends
Effects on the Family
Professional Enablers

VULNERABLE AGGREGATES
Preadolescents and Adolescents
Elderly
Women
Ethnocultural Considerations
Other Aggregates

NURSING PERSPECTIVE ON SUBSTANCE ABUSE
Nursing Interventions in the Community

Perhaps no other health-related condition has as many far-reaching consequences in contemporary Western society as substance abuse. These consequences include a wide range of social, psychological, physical, economic, and political problems. Health problems and disability associated with substance abuse total approximately $276 billion annually. Each year, it costs an estimated $1000 per person for health care, law enforcement, accidents, treatment, and lost productivity. More deaths, illnesses, and disabilities are attributed to substance abuse than any other preventable health condition in the United States (Substance Abuse and Mental Health Services Administration [SAMHSA], 2004c).

The **social consequences** of substance abuse include its role in crime (due to disinhibition), need for money to buy substances, and specific theft of drugs. Many offenders commit crimes while under the influence of drugs, alcohol, or both. Between 35% and 50% of inmates in correctional facilities reported that they had been under the influence of drugs when their crime was committed. Furthermore, almost 75% of inmates report prior drug use (Bureau of Justice Statistics [BJS], 2005).

All aggregates in society are potentially affected by substance abuse problems. Infants exposed in utero to alcohol, amphetamines, or opiates are at risk for with-drawal syndromes and later developmental problems. Indirect social effects of substance abuse include relationship conflicts, divorce, spousal and child abuse, and child neglect. Although well intended, many local and national efforts to fight substance abuse are often inadequate and ineffective (Drucker, 1999).

In the past, alcoholism and drug addiction were considered to be problems of the urban poor; society and most health professionals virtually ignored them. Substance abuse problems now pervade all levels of U.S. society, and awareness has increased. Community health nurses must be knowledgeable about substance abuse because it is a problem that frequently intertwines with other medical and social conditions.

This chapter focuses on helping community health nurses recognize substance abuse in their clients and in the larger community. The chapter reviews historical trends, the causes of substance abuse, the most common symptoms of these disorders, and treatment options. The authors suggest nursing interventions appropriate for assisting those with substance-related problems, in a community context.

HISTORICAL OVERVIEW OF ALCOHOL AND ILLICIT DRUG USE

During the twentieth century, fluctuations in the use of alcohol and illicit drugs were influenced by shifts in public tolerance and political and economic trends. In general, alcohol use gained more social acceptance than other drug use. Alcohol consumption in the United States was higher during World Wars I and II and decreased during Prohibition and the Great Depression. Alcohol use was highest during the 1980s when states lowered the drinking age to 18 years of age. Lawmakers became alarmed at the increased rate of drinking and the increased number of alcohol-related deaths among 18- to 25-year-olds after lowering the drinking age and thereby reversed the decision. During the late 1980s, alcohol use declined after the minimum drinking age was reinstated to 21 years of age. The decline in alcohol consumption through the 1990s and into the twenty-first century is attributed to less tolerant national attitudes toward drinking, increased societal and legal pressures and actions against drinking and driving, and increased health concerns among Americans. The identification of, and response to, driving under the influence is an example of a shift in thinking from addiction as the primary concern to other problems linked with, for example, alcohol use. These problems are thus termed *substance-related problems* and have become a significant community concern.

Public attitudes and governmental policies also have influenced the history of illicit drug use. Although nineteenth-century physicians prescribed morphine for a large variety of ailments, the discovery of the addictive properties of cocaine and opiates led to increased governmental regulation at the beginning of the twentieth century. The Harrison Narcotic Act of 1914, and subsequent laws, lessened the medical profession's control over the use of addictive drugs; the legislation specified that the physician could prescribe these drugs only in the course of general practice and not to maintain an addiction (Brecher, 1972). This limitation on the physician's power to prescribe and dispense addictive drugs, and restrictions on the importation of narcotics, limited the supply of these drugs until the 1950s and 1960s. At that time, an increase in illegal drug trafficking caused heroin use to proliferate, particularly in inner cities.

By the 1970s, drugs were increasingly available. During this period, a counterculture population, composed largely of young people, focused their efforts enhancing social justice, ending the Vietnam War, and lessening "repressive" sexual mores; many conceptualized drug use as a way to liberate the mind. Marijuana use took place in communal, social settings; alcohol use was less favored because it was associated with the "establishment" they were critiquing. Consequently, the use of hallucinogens, cannabis, and heroin spread beyond urban drug subcultures to the general population. Alarmed by the social and personal problems inherent in this change, the public grew less tolerant of drug use, and prevention and treatment programs were given more attention and resources. After peaking in 1979, illicit drug use decreased among most segments of the population throughout the 1980s, reaching a low in the early 1990s. Between 1995 and 2000, it increased slightly before dropping again in recent years (SAMHSA, 2005).

To combat concerns of the physical, social, and psychological impact of drug abuse and dependence, federal drug policy has emphasized law enforcement and interdiction—the **war on drugs**—to reduce the supply. Despite the large amounts of money spent toward reaching this goal, this strategy has been only somewhat effective (Drucker, 1999). Trends have shown renewed interest in prevention and

TABLE 24-1   Reported Percentage of Lifetime Substance Use by Age and Racial Group

SUBSTANCE	WHITE			HISPANIC			AFRICAN AMERICAN		
	2-17	18-25	≥26	12-17	18-25	≥26	12-17	18-25	≥26
Any illicit drug	23.4	65.0	48.6	21.2	57.5	35.5	18.9	54.2	44.8
Alcohol	45.7	89.0	90.3	41.3	77.8	78.8	34.3	76.6	75.1
Cigarettes	36.3	74.9	76.2	31.2	61.1	56.7	24.3	52.8	52.8
Marijuana	21.3	59.1	44.2	19.4	42.9	27.8	17.7	48.7	40.3
Inhalants	9.4	16.8	8.2	7.9	8.9	4.1	5.9	8.8	3.0
Hallucinogens	6.8	26.9	13.8	4.1	14.9	7.1	1.7	7.2	5.3

From Substance Abuse and Mental Health Services Administration: *Overview of findings from the 2002 National Survey on Drug Use and Health*, NHSDA Series H-21, USDHHS Pub No SMA 03–3774, Rockville, Md, 2003, The Author.

treatment efforts to decrease the amount of illicit drug use in society and to lessen its impact (SAMHSA, 2004c).

PREVALENCE, INCIDENCE, AND TRENDS

The increasing recognition of the widespread effects of substance abuse has initiated extensive collection of data by multiple agencies. This section describes selected statistics and current trends. The U.S. National Survey on Drug Use and Health (SAMHSA, 2005) is an annual survey conducted by the Substance Abuse and Mental Health Services Administration (SAMHSA), which estimates the prevalence of illicit drug and alcohol use in the United States. Findings from a recent report include the following (SAMHSA, 2003):

- About 8.2% of the general U.S. population over age 12 years were current drug users (compared to 7.1% in 2001).
- An estimated 50.1% of the U.S. general population age 12 years or older were current drinkers.
- Young adults ages 18 to 25 had the highest prevalence of binge drinking and heavy drinking.
- Of those ages 12 to 17 years, 8.2% used marijuana in the month before the survey.
- There were an estimated 2.6 million new marijuana users in 2002 (69% were under 18 and 53% female).
- Marijuana was the most commonly used illicit drug, especially among teens.
- More than one million people had recently used stimulants nonmedically.

Some alarming trends regarding substance use have been noted in recent years. One such trend is that dependence on, or abuse of, stimulants is most prevalent among young people ages 12 to 25. Stimulants most often abused are methamphetamine, prescription diet pills, cocaine, methylphenidate, and dextroamphetamine. Also, there has been a significant increase in lifetime nonmedical use of pain relievers, specifically hydrocodone, methadone, tramadol, and oxycodone (OxyContin). Reportedly, between 2002 and 2003 among persons age 12 and older, use of these pain relievers increased from 29.6 million to 31.2 million. Lastly, about 1% of the U.S. population use cocaine with smaller percentages using other drugs including heroin, hallucinogens, and inhalants (SAMHSA, 2003).

Notably, according to SAMHSA's (2003) Treatment Episode Data Set, the route of administration of heroin is changing. From 1992 to 2002, inhalation increased from 20% to 33% of primary treatment admissions, whereas injection decreased from 77% to 62%. Conversely, in those who are under 30, there was a 10% increase in heroin injection during the same period.

Demographic correlates show some regional, racial, and gender differences and changes over the past few years. For example, people living in the West have the greatest percentage of past month drug use at 9.3%, compared with 7.9% for those in the Midwest, 8.7% for those in the Northeast, and 7.4% for those in the South. Additionally, rates of current illicit drug use vary significantly among major racial/ethnic groups. Rates were highest among American Indians or Alaska Natives (12.1%), followed by African Americans (8.7%), whites (8.3%), and Hispanics (8.0%). Asians had the lowest rate at 3.8% (SAMSHA, 2003). Table 24-1 provides information about substance abuse among various racial and ethnic groups.

With relation to gender differences, 2.4% of males reported illicit drug dependence during the year before the survey, compared with 1.3% of females. Males were more likely to be dependent on or abusing alcohol or any illicit drug, except among youth ages 12 to 17 where the rates were the same for both males and females. There are distinctly different patterns for alcohol problems in women. Indeed, 70% of men and 61% of women age 12 and older consumed alcohol in the previous year. Although the majority of adult women drank alcohol occasionally, the group between 21 and 34 years of age reported the highest use (SAMSHA, 2003).

Trends in Substance Use

Research has revealed that problems associated with substance use may or may not relate to classically or clinically defined dependence or addiction. Many are turning to recovery before they have developed physiological dependence. Thus many in the field have begun to differentiate between *use* and *misuse* (*misuse* being interchangeable with *abuse*), and these terms now appear in the literature. This section describes significant trends in substances that are being abused and discusses substance abuse among special populations.

HEALTHY PEOPLE **2010** Selected Objectives for Substance Abuse		
Objective	**Baseline (1998)**	**Target**
13-3: Reduce the number of new AIDS cases among females and males who inject drugs	12,099 new cases in 1998	9,075
16-17a: Increase reported abstinence from alcohol in the past month by pregnant women	86%	94%
18-10: Increase the proportion of persons with co-occurring substance abuse and mental disorders who receive treatment for both disorders	NA	NA
26-1a: Reduce alcohol-related deaths in motor vehicle crashes	5.9 per 100,000	4 per 100,000
26-3: Reduce drug-induced deaths	6.3 per 100,000	1 per 100,000
26-6: Reduce the proportion of adolescents who report that they rode, during the previous 30 days, with a driver who had been drinking	33% (Grades 9 to 12)	30% (Grades 9 to 12)
26-9c: Increase the proportion of high school seniors never using alcoholic beverages	19%	29%
26-11b: Reduce the proportion of college students engaging in binge drinking of alcoholic beverages	39%	20%
26-20: Increase the number of admissions to substance abuse treatment for injection drug use	167,960	200,000
26-25: Extend legal requirements for maximum blood alcohol concentration levels of 0.08% for motor vehicle drivers aged 21 years and older	16 states	All states and the District of Columbia

From US Department of Health and Human Services: *Healthy People 2010*, ed 2, Washington, DC, 2000, The Author.

Healthy People 2010 and Substance Abuse

The U.S. Department of Health and Human Services (USDHHS) set goals and objectives related to substance abuse in *Healthy People 2010* (USDHHS, 2000). The objectives consist of norms and targets for the decade for health conditions for the U.S. population. The use of harmful substances is indirectly and directly related to all of the leading health indicators (i.e. tobacco use, alcohol and other drug abuse, physical activity, overweight and obesity, mental health, injury and violence, environmental quality, responsible sexual behavior, immunization, and access to health care). The *Healthy People 2010* table presents selected objectives and targets from *Healthy People 2010* related to substance abuse.

On review, there are mixed results related to progress toward the year 2010 objectives. Whereas overall drug use, particularly among adolescents, has declined, alcohol-related motor vehicle deaths have remained steady, at about 30% of all fatalities (USDHHS, 2000). A disturbing trend is the large increase in the use of methamphetamines, steroids, and inhalants by young people.

Methamphetamine

Since 1997, methamphetamine (MA) has evolved as the most widely produced controlled substance in the United States. It is appearing in mass quantities, in part because of the ease in which the fertilizer anhydrous ammonia can be converted into methamphetamine; this has resulted in attracting more individuals into this clandestine business. Illegal street forms of the drug, often called crank, crystal, or meth, are available as a powder that can be injected, inhaled, or taken orally. In addition, a smokable form, known as ice or glass, is widely available. Currently, the preferred route of administration is by injection. This is possibly due to the undesirable physical difficulties related to smoking MA (e.g., damage to the nasal tract, coughing up blood, or difficulty breathing) (Cretzmeyer et al., 2003).

There is new attention being paid to MA manufacture and use because of the alarming increase in rates of abuse. The incidence of MA use rose steadily between 1990 (164,000 new users) and 2000 (344,000 new users). The new users during this time were approximately evenly split between 12- to 17-year-olds and 18- to 25-year-olds. This shift in age distribution from previous decades was reflected in the average age of new users, which fell from 22.3 years in 1990 to 18.4 years in 2000 (SAMHSA, 2004c). Hospital admissions for abuse of stimulants, mainly MA, increased from 1% to 7% between 1992 and 2002 (SAMHSA, 2003).

The pleasurable effects of MA are due to the release of high levels of dopamine in the brain, leading to increased energy, a sense of euphoria, and increased productivity. Short-term effects are increased heart rate, insomnia, excessive talking, excitation, and aggressive behavior. Prolonged use results in tolerance and physiological dependence. There are multiple negative effects for users of MA, their families, and communities. It appears to damage the brain in ways that are different from, and more severe than, damage from using other drugs. Currently, there is rudimentary understanding of ways it affects brain, but, it is known that profound neurological changes occur even with first administration (Volm and de Araujo, 2004). Negative consequences range from anxiety, convulsions, and paranoia to brain damage (Block, Erwinn, and Ghoneim, 2002). Use of MA is associated with an increased incidence of violence such as domestic abuse, homicide, and suicide, whether as a victim or as a perpetrator (Logan, Fligner, and Haddix, 1998).

Methamphetamine is used predominantly by white young persons, with an overrepresentation of females. Thirty-six percent indicate that they were first introduced to the drug when they were under 16 years of age (SAMHSA, 2004a). Rates of admission for treatment of methamphetamine vary by region. The highest is Utah; however, most areas of the country are reporting an exponential rise of its manufacture and use.

The impact of MA abuse on communities, families, and social networks is considerable. Reported use is highest among 20- to 29-year-olds. This group often has young children, which puts these children at risk for abuse and neglect. The incidence of prenatal use is also rising, increasing the risk for children to be born with developmental problems, aggression, and attention disorders (Logan et al., 1998). Furthermore, exposure to combustible secondhand fumes puts children at risk of not only complications related to primary ingestion but also fatalities and injuries related to the highly combustible nature of the chemicals used in manufacture of the drug (Haight et al., 2005). Another pediatric issue is the growing number of teens recruited in manufacture and selling of MA (Block et al., 2002).

Steroids

Evidence suggests that steroid use among adolescents is on the rise. Between 1991 and 1998, the overall annual prevalence rate was fairly stable, but use jumped in 1999, from 1.2% to 1.7% in the 8th and 10th grades. Recent estimates found steroid use continuing to rise, as prevalence was 1.3%, 2.3%, and 3.3% for boys in Grades 8, 10, and 12, respectively, compared with 1.0%, 0.9%, and 1.7% for girls (National Institute on Drug Abuse [NIDA], 2005). Data are scarce on the extent of steroid use by adults, but it has been estimated that hundreds of thousands of people aged 18 and older use anabolic steroids at least once a year. Among both adolescents and adults, steroid use is higher among males than females (Gruber and Pope, 2000).

Use of steroids by popular sports figures may have influenced a generation of teenage athletes, girls as well as boys, to put themselves at risk. The health consequences of steroid use are well documented. Boys experience sexual changes, including decreased sperm count, impotence, shrinking of testicles, and difficulty urinating. In females, steroid use can manifest as masculinization, often producing increased facial hair and menstruation problems (Gruber and Pope, 2000). There are other more potentially fatal risks, including blood clots, liver damage, premature cardiovascular changes, and increased cholesterol (Sullivan et al., 1998). Evidence also points at behavioral changes leading to an increased potential for suicide and aggressive and risky behaviors among steroid users (Pope, Kouri, and Hudson, 2000). Most negative effects are reversible on discontinuation of the drug. Collaborative treatment programs that monitor both psychological and physical issues, including consideration of the drug use route as injection, are necessary to combat steroid abuse.

Inhalants

Inhalants are defined by mode of administration (inhalation of fumes) and encompass a range of substances as diverse as glues, aerosols, butane, paint thinner, and nail polish remover. These products are inexpensive, legal, and easy to obtain, making them attractive to younger adolescents who have less access to illicit drugs.

Use of inhalants has consistently been highest among eighth graders, but a recent survey showed that inhalant use has increased among older teens as well. Further, studies monitoring drug- and alcohol-related emergency department admissions show that the largest increase in admission between 1995 and 2002 were inhalants (186%) and amphetamines (166%) (NIDA, 2005).

ADOLESCENT SUBSTANCE ABUSE

Youth are a particularly susceptible aggregate for substance abuse. Individuals between 18 and 25 years of age have the highest prevalence of illicit drug use during their lifetime (65% of the population). One positive development is that teen use of cigarettes and smokeless tobacco has declined since the peak levels in the mid 1990s. Indeed, 30-day prevalence of smoking has declined by 56% in 8th grade, 47% in 10th, and 32% in 12th. It is noteworthy, however, that this significant decline in adolescent smoking and use of smokeless tobacco has decelerated sharply and seems to be on the verge of halting among 10th graders (NIDA, 2005). Cigarettes continue to be highly available to the young, and concerned groups continue to monitor advertising that targets new potential smokers, such as youth and women.

Virtually all major theories of the origins of adolescent substance abuse agree that the perceived acceptance of problematic drug-using behavior among family, peers, and society is an important influence on an individual's decision to use or not use alcohol, tobacco, and drugs. The perception that alcohol use is socially acceptable correlates with the fact that more than 80% of American youth consume alcohol before their twenty-first birthday, and the lack of social acceptance of other drugs correlates with comparatively lower rates of use. Similarly, widespread societal expectations that young people will engage in binge drinking may encourage this highly dangerous form of alcohol consumption (USDHHS, 2000). ∎

Trends in alcohol use by American teens are mixed. Throughout the early part of the century, there were drops in several indicators of alcohol use at all grade levels. In 2004, however, most drinking measures showed slight increases among 12th graders (NIDA, 2005)

Most of the movement in teen substance use has been in a downward direction, but generally the declines have been marginal (Johnston et al., 2005). Between 1995 and 2002, there was no consistent increase or decline in marijuana users. However, the percentage of adolescents reporting that it is easy to obtain marijuana declined slightly, from 55.0% to 53.6% (SAMHSA, 2003). In addition, initiation of both LSD and ecstasy declined. Use of PCP, or phencyclidine, has been at low levels for some time, and use fell further in 2004. The resurgence of inhalant use among the eighth graders was one of the more troublesome recent findings, as was the continued rise in use of the highly addictive narcotic drug oxycodone (OxyContin) among high school seniors and eighth graders (NIDA, 2005).

In order to effectively plan for the present and future needs of the community, the community health nurse needs the most current overall perspective. Information on the prevalence, incidence, and trends in the amount and types of substance abuse at the general, state, and local levels is readily available on the Internet. As harmful, illicit substances come in and out of vogue, particularly among young people, the community health nurse needs a good understanding of drug culture, terminology, and differing signs and symptoms.

CONCEPTUALIZATIONS OF SUBSTANCE ABUSE

Conceptualizations of substance abuse and dependence have changed over the years, often for political and social reasons rather than for scientific reasons. Some conceptualizations focus on the phenomenon of **addiction,** which is manifested by compulsive use patterns and the onset of withdrawal symptoms when substance use is abruptly stopped. Other views focus on the problems resulting from the substance use itself, regardless of whether an addictive pattern is present. Problematic consequences of substance use include intoxication, psychological dependence, relational conflicts, employment or economic difficulties, legal difficulties, and health problems. For example, addiction need not be present for individuals to experience legal consequences of illicit drug use, such as driving while intoxicated, or alcohol- or drug-related domestic violence.

Drawing fine distinctions among ideas of dependence, addiction, and abuse concerning substance use may seem irrelevant if there is evidence that the substance use has become problematic. However, broadly labeling all habitual or compulsive behavior patterns as addiction or dependence may obscure the fact that interventions could precede the development of addiction, for example, in cases where use has become misuse and a problem is evident. It is also becoming increasingly evident that specific interventions may be needed for each separate addictive problem (e.g., overeating and gambling). Moreover, in each specific group, there is wide individual diversity.

Definitions

The term **substance abuse** came into common usage in the 1970s. Earlier conceptualizations generally focused on either alcoholism or drug addiction as singular addictive disorders. Most substance abuse theories identify core commonalties that occur in regard to use of a variety of different substances or in relation to compulsive behavior syndromes (Leshner, 1997). There is also an emphasis on relapse prevention that may include moderate use goals and abstinence (Larimer and Marlatt, 1990).

There remains debate about how substance use and substance abuse should be defined and what substances should be included under each definition. Traditional conceptualizations of substance abuse focus solely on alcohol and illicit street drugs. Other conceptualizations include prescription medications such as tranquilizers or analgesics. In eating disorders, such as bulimia and compulsive overeating, food is viewed as the abused substance. Table 24-2 shows a classification scheme for commonly abused substances.

In addition to varying in their abuse potential, substances vary in their degree of potential harm to those who use them and to others in the immediate environment. Tobacco is an example of a substance that is unsafe to the smoker and to those who inhale secondhand smoke. Those who abuse alcohol may also harm others by driving under the influence, and lowering of inhibitions may foster violent activities in some (e.g., child or partner abuse).

Integrating the various opinions regarding the diagnosis of substance abuse, the American Psychiatric Association (APA) has classified substance use disorders as either "dependence" or "abuse" (APA, 2000). The APA focused on the following psychoactive substances that affect the nervous system: alcohol, amphetamines, caffeine, cannabis, cocaine, hallucinogens, inhalants, nicotine, opioids, phencyclidine, sedatives, and hypnotics or anxiolytics. Substance use disorders can also be categorized as being in partial or full remission. A diagnosis of substance abuse indicates a maladaptive pattern of substance use that is manifested by recurrent and significant adverse consequences related to repeated use of a substance. These adverse consequences include failure to fulfill major role obligations, repeated use in physically hazardous situations, multiple legal problems, and recurrent social and interpersonal problems. Boxes 24-1 and 24-2 list the criteria for diagnosis of substance dependence and substance abuse, respectively.

The criteria for the diagnosis of dependence include a cluster of cognitive, behavioral, and physiological symptoms that indicate continued use of the substance despite significant substance-related problems. A pattern of repeated, self-administered use results in tolerance, withdrawal, and compulsive drug-taking behaviors, which are frequently accompanied by a craving or strong desire for the substance. This craving then motivates the user to be preoccupied with supply, money to purchase drugs, and getting through time between periods of use, all of which take up mental energy, effort that is diverted from work or school and connectedness to significant others. This is how the use becomes problematic and how others around the user become confused and eventually often feel rejected, hurt, ignored, angry, or even responsible for the user's behavior.

Etiology of Substance Abuse

Substance abuse has an impact on virtually every aspect of individual and communal life, and many institutions and academic fields have addressed it. Several theories attempt to explain the cause and scope of these problems and offer solutions. Some theories address individual, physiological, spiritual, and psychological factors. Others deal with social influences involving family, ethnicity, race, access to drugs,

TABLE 24-2 Classification of Commonly Used and Abused Substances

SUBSTANCE	DESIRED EFFECT	POSSIBLE WITHDRAWAL SYMPTOMS
CNS DEPRESSANTS		
Alcohol	Euphoria, disinhibition, and sedation	Anxiety, irritability, seizures, delusions, hallucinations, and
Barbiturates	Retrograde amnesia	paranoia
Sedative-hypnotics (e.g., benzodiazapines [Rohypnol])	Sedation and amnesia	
Tranquilizers (e.g., GHB, the "date rape" drug)		
CNS STIMULANTS		
Amphetamines (e.g., methamphetamine)	Euphoria, hyperactivity, omnipotence, insomnia, and	Depression, apathy, lethargy, and sleepiness
Cocaine	anorexia	
Nicotine		
Caffeine		
NARCOTICS-OPIOIDS		
Codeine	Euphoria and sedation	Anxiety, irritability, agitation, runny nose, watery eyes,
Meperidine and acetaminophen (e.g., Demerol)		chills, sweating, nausea and vomiting, diarrhea,
Hydromorphone (e.g., Dilaudid)		tremors, and yawning
Fentanyl		
Heroin		
Methadone		
Morphine		
Opium		
Oxycodone (e.g., Percodan)		
HALLUCINOGENS		
Mescaline	Hallucinations, illusions, and heightened awareness	Depression
LSD	PCP: violent dissociative and anesthetic effect	
PCP (e.g., ketamine)		
STP and MDMA (e.g., ecstasy)		
Psilocybin (e.g., mushrooms)		
CANNABIS		
Marijuana	Relaxation, euphoria, and altered perceptions	Restlessness, insomnia, and anxiety
Hashish and THC		
INHALANTS		
Gasoline	Euphoria	Restlessness, anxiety, and irritability
Toluene acetate		
Cleaning fluids		
Airplane cement		
Amyl nitrate		

Modified from Faltz B, Rinaldi J: *AIDS and substance abuse: a training manual for health care professionals*, San Francisco, 1987, Regents of the University of California. Used with permission.
CNS, Central nervous system; *GHB*, gammahydroxybutyrate; *MDMA*, methylenedioxymethamphetamine; *PCP*, phencyclidine; *STP*, 2,5,dimethoxy,4,methyl amphetamine; *THC*, tetrahydrocannabinol.

environmental stressors, economics, political status, culture, and sex roles. Most theories suggest that a combination of factors is the underlying impetus for substance abuse.

Although physiological, medical model theorists have defined alcoholism as a loss of control over drinking or an individual malfunction, the cause of alcoholism was ambiguous in the past (Brown, 1969; Keller, 1972). Research has clearly identified genetic factors that increase a person's overall risk for alcohol abuse; there is strong evidence that alcoholism runs in families and that genetic factors play an important role (Kendler and Prescott, 1998; NIDA, 1997).

Individual and environmental factors also contribute to an increased risk for alcohol abuse. On the individual level, a person's inherited sensitivity to alcohol is a predictor for the development of alcohol abuse. Two broad personality dimensions are also associated with an increased risk for alcohol abuse. Impulsivity and ease of disinhibition add to risks for substance abuse. Proneness to anxiety and depression are also risks, and these comorbidities are not well understood. Alcohol expectancies (i.e., beliefs about anticipated consequences of drinking) are also a predictor of alcohol abuse. If one expects a certain effect, such as relief, one is more likely to feel it after

BOX 24-1 Diagnostic Criteria for Substance Dependence

A maladaptive pattern of substance use leading to clinically significant impairment or distress, as manifested by three (or more) of the following, occurring at any time in the same 12-month period:

1. Tolerance, as defined by either of the following:
   a. A need for markedly increased amounts of the substance to achieve intoxication or desired effect
   b. Markedly diminished effect with continued use of the same amount of the substance
2. Withdrawal, as manifested by either of the following:
   a. The characteristic withdrawal syndrome for the substance
   b. The same (or closely related) substance is taken to relieve or avoid withdrawal symptoms
3. The substance is often taken in larger amounts or over a longer period than intended.
4. There is a persistent desire or unsuccessful efforts to cut down or control substance use.
5. A great deal of time is spent in activities necessary to obtain the substance (e.g., visiting multiple doctors or driving long distances), use the substance (e.g., chain-smoking), or recover from its effects.
6. Important social, occupational, or recreational activities are given up or reduced.
7. The substance use is continued despite knowledge of having a persistent or recurrent physical or psychological problem that is likely to have been caused or exacerbated by the substance (e.g., current cocaine use despite recognition of cocaine-induced depression, or continued drinking despite recognition that an ulcer was made worse by alcohol consumption).
8. Specify if with or without physiological dependence (e.g., tolerance or withdrawal).

From American Psychiatric Association: *Diagnostic and statistical manual of mental disorders,* ed 4, text revision, Washington, DC, 2000, The Author.

BOX 24-2 Diagnostic Criteria for Substance Abuse

A maladaptive pattern of substance use leading to clinically significant impairment or distress as manifested by one (or more) of the following, occurring within a 12-month period:

1. Recurrent substance use resulting in a failure to fulfill major role obligations at work, school, or home (e.g., repeated absences or poor work performance related to substance use; substance-related absences, suspensions, or expulsions from school; neglect of children or household)
2. Recurrent substance use in situations in which it is physically hazardous (e.g., driving an automobile or operating a machine when impaired by substance use)
3. Recurrent substance-related legal problems (e.g., arrests for substance-related disorderly conduct)
4. Continued substance use despite persistent or recurrent social or interpersonal problems caused or exacerbated by the effects of the substance (e.g., arguments with spouse about consequences of intoxication, physical fights)
B. The symptoms have never met the criteria for substance dependence for this class of substance.

From American Psychiatric Association: *Diagnostic and statistical manual of mental disorders,* ed 4, text revision, Washington, DC, 2000, The Author.

use of a drug. The satisfied expectancies may set up neural pathways that are interpreted as pleasurable.

Medical models of alcoholism and other substance abuse conditions may not provide an understanding of commonalities among addictive behaviors (e.g., excessive drinking, gambling, eating, drug use, and sexual behavior). Cross-addiction, or multidrug use, is more prevalent now than in the past, and more studies point to the presence of both automatic and nonautomatic factors in physiological and psychological dependence. Specific biological medical models are giving way to multicausal models.

In the biopsychosocial model, risk factors interact with protective factors to develop a predisposition toward drug or alcohol use. This predisposition is then influenced by exposure to the substance, availability, and the experiential interpretation of the drug experience (e.g., pleasant or unpleasant). Continued availability of the substances and a social support system that enables or supports their use is also necessary. These factors combine to determine whether addiction develops and is maintained.

SOCIOCULTURAL AND POLITICAL ASPECTS OF SUBSTANCE ABUSE

Within community settings, substance-related problems are not always easy to identify. For example, the consequences of the sale and use of crack cocaine in an inner-city, African-American neighborhood may be apparent through media attention. The traffic of these drugs into the middle classes, on the other hand, is less easily recognized. The increasing tendencies of elderly persons to rely on alcohol and other, even illicit, drugs may be shocking to some nurses. It can be understood, however, contextually and may be the result of multiple factors, such as isolation, fears, uncontrolled chronic pain, anxiety, and sleep disturbances. Nurses must incorporate sociocultural and political dimensions into caring for clients in the community. Nurses must also possess knowledge that is useful in countering media stereotypes and can model a more holistic, multifaceted approach to prevention and management of substance abuse.

Although there are subcultural and regional variations, drinking norms of the dominant culture in the United States are relatively permissive. Traditional ethnic ceremonial and symbolic substance use patterns vary significantly. As acculturation occurs, however, cultural definitions of "appropriate" use of alcohol and drugs have been dulled, leaving a void regarding social expectations. Subcultural groups such as gay, lesbian, bisexual, and transgender persons have often had a social center that was a bar, and alcohol use was historically a way of demonstrating and celebrating differentiation from a more repressive majority. These cultural conditions create ambiguity in clearly determining when a substance abuse problem exists. Furthermore, each subculture may define abuse differently. It can be theorized that stigmatized minorities might be under more stress, and perhaps more likely to use substances, but this cannot be assumed in any individual case.

A particular drug experience can be understood as an interaction between the individual's subjective mood and the actual pharmacological effects of the drug, but this interaction does not take place in a vacuum. Rather, the expectations of a drug's effect are shaped by the user's culture and involve the adoption of roles taught by more experienced users and reinforced by other social groups, including health care providers in some cases (Montagne and Scott, 1993).

Substances are also given economic value and are bought and sold as commodities in a variety of social arenas, both legal and illegal. The ways in which drugs, including nicotine, medications and alcohol, are produced and distributed among the various segments of the population are determined largely by economic, cultural, and political conditions. For example, the economic realities of poor Colombians and Peruvians who rely on the growth and production of the coca leaf for financial survival can be understood as a confluence of larger, society-level and individual-level factors. The drug trade is very lucrative for some; it raises their societal status, gives them access to material things, and provides an enhanced sense of power in that society. Among urban poor minority youth in the United States, the fact that drug trafficking often precedes drug use suggests that involvement in the drug trade satisfies a need for status and economic power (Greenberg and Schneider, 1994).

These changes in power can have other consequences as various subgroups attain and maintain status. A group without cultural values, or with competing cultural values, suffers from chaos and disorganization. Competing value systems lead to cultural disintegration and a sense of powerlessness and hopelessness. The group becomes susceptible to forces that further threaten the group's ability to survive. When they are unable to organize or determine a collective direction because of conflicting values, the group and its members are separated and disempowered. The history of cocaine abuse and dependence among people of color is an example of how these conditions are interrelated. Indeed, cocaine use was epidemic in the 1980s and early 1990s, with crack cocaine most prevalent in poor communities, but its use has declined markedly in recent years (SAMHSA, 2004c).

COURSE OF SUBSTANCE-RELATED PROBLEMS

There is no predictable course of addictive illness and no "addictive personality type." When habitual use is well established, behaviors may be clinically visible and similar; this has led to assumption of a singular, addiction-prone personality. However, not everyone who initiates drug or alcohol use will progress to dependency or display associated behaviors. Because the path from **initiation** to dependency is multidimensional, the context of client and community experiences is key to understanding and responding to problems encountered. Nurses need to take a comprehensive health and substance use history and place this in a context of cultural, historical, family, and social factors. Neither addiction nor dependency is a unitary phenomenon with a single isolated cause; rather, it is the result of interactions among a host of variables.

The assessment process should include consideration of the triad: the person, the substance, and the context or environment. The person assessment includes demographic information, medical history, comorbidities, and known perceptions and meanings the individual displays. The drug assessment includes the qualities of the substance itself, physiopharmacological effects, pattern of use, availability, and toxicity. Context assessment should include family, social, employment, legal, cultural, and economic contingencies.

Hanson, Venturilli, and Fleckenstein (2002) categorize users of illicit substances as experimenters, compulsive users, or "floaters." Experimenters begin using substances largely because of peer pressure or curiosity; they are usually able to set limits. In contrast, compulsive users devote much of their time and energy to getting high and tend to immerse themselves in conversations and social interactions around drugs and alcohol. "Floaters" focus more on using other people's substances and generally have light to moderate use. This does not explain the meaning that substance use has for the individual, however, nor what kinds of experiences and perceptions are associated with use. The subjective experiences of using particular substances and other issues such as genetic predisposition, discrimination, past trauma, family strife, and economic status make each case of substance use or misuse as unique as one's fingerprint.

Genetic traits have been found to be associated with addiction to certain substances. For example, people of Chinese or Japanese extraction may become ill after ingestion of even small amounts of alcohol. A single nucleotide polymorphism (SNP) that encodes opiate receptors is more frequent among some heroin addicts, and an SNP that encodes dopamine receptors is more frequent in some alcoholics. Certainly there is a genetic and disease component to addiction, implying that prevention efforts can be more efficient when targeted at vulnerable individuals. As a result, prevention efforts should focus on children of addicts, who should be advised not to experiment (Goldstein, 2001).

The progression from initiation to continuation, transition to abuse, and, finally, addiction and dependency varies. Individuals often describe a progression that began with initiation through social interactions. For some, the substance and setting is reinforcing and primes the individual for a pattern of use. For others, the experience will be unpleasant enough to prevent further use. It cannot be assumed, however, that an unpleasant initiation will always be preventive. In the case of stimulants, such as methamphetamine, the drug produces such strong feelings of euphoria, alertness, control, and increased energy that future use is enticing, especially when the drug is easily accessible (Cretzmeyer et al., 2003).

The continuation stage of substance abuse is a subsequent period in which substance use persists but does not appear to be detrimental to the individual. In stimulant abuse, continued use often occurs in a binge pattern. Individuals are able to exercise some control over use, but use becomes more frequent. Neither the individual nor the social network views use during this stage as problematic.

A critical point is the transition stage from substance use to substance abuse. There may be evidence to both the users and their social networks that the use of the substance is having adverse effects. During this stage, users begin to use more often and in more varied settings. Rationalizations that deny the seriousness and consequences of the substance use are commonly constructed during this stage.

The research on correlates and antecedents of substance abuse points to a variety of personal and social motivations. For many young people, motivators are the attraction of a rebellious subculture, peer pressure, and nationwide fads. Considerable research exists on the self-medication aspects of individuals with comorbid mental illnesses. Once the addiction is established, unpleasant physical and emotional withdrawal symptoms are strong motivators to continue use. Abstinence in the stimulant abuser can result in symptoms such as depression, lethargy, and anhedonia (i.e., inability to feel pleasure). The depression experienced by the user when not using stimulants is contrasted with the recalled euphoria produced by the use of the drug. These factors, coupled with associated cues, help initiate the cycle of binge use, with increased craving and continued self-administration to relieve symptoms. Brain imaging techniques have demonstrated that abuse of drugs such as cocaine and amphetamine produce immediate and long-lasting physical changes that are likely to contribute to the maintenance of dependency (Obert, London, and Rawson, 2002).

The development of addiction or dependency is marked by changes in both behavior and cognition. There is an increasing focus on the substance and a narrowing of interests, social activities, and relationships. The process of becoming dependent or addicted requires the individual to deny or ignore evidence or information that may challenge their behavior or rationalization of their behavior. There is a preoccupation with the substance and its procurement during this stage, even in the face of negative consequences. Table 24-3 outlines the stages in the process of stimulant addiction.

LEGAL AND ETHICAL CONCERNS OF SUBSTANCE ABUSE

For the past 30 years, the United States has pursued a drug policy based on prohibition and the active application of criminal sanctions against the use and sale of illicit drugs. During this time, the number of criminal penalties for drug offenses has climbed to 1.5 million offenses. There has also been a tenfold increase in imprisonment for drug charges since 1979, despite an overall decline in drug prevalence (BJS, 2002).

This increase in drug-related imprisonment is a result of harsher enforcement policies and longer mandatory sentences for possession of smaller quantities of drugs. Although some individuals are in prison for violent crimes or major drug trafficking, many drug offenders are arrested for small-scale drug deals made to support their personal use (BJS, 2005).

Alcohol use and abuse are different issues because the possession and sale of alcoholic beverages is only illegal if the individual involved is a minor. Concerns arise when individuals are intoxicated during work, while driving, or in situations that may affect the welfare of others. Legal penalties have increased for driving under the influence of alcohol because groups such as Mothers Against Drunk Driving (MADD) influence legislation.

TABLE 24-3 Typical Course of Addictive Illness: Stages in Continuum From Initiation to Dependency

STAGE	CHARACTERISTICS
Initiation	First use of the substance
	Exposure frequently through family or friends
Continuation	Continued, more frequent use of substance
	Usually social use only, with no detrimental effects
Transition	Beginning of change in total consumption, frequency, and occasions of use
	More than just social use, with beginning of loss of control
Abuse	Adverse effects and consequences to substance use
	Rationalizations for continued use and denial of adverse effects present in user and significant others
	Unsuccessful attempts at control of use
Dependency and addiction	Physical or psychological dependence, or both, on the substance; marked by behavioral and cognitive changes
	Preoccupation with the substance and its procurement, despite negative consequences
	Narrowing of interests, social activities, and relationships to only those related to the substance use

ETHICAL Insights

Ethical Issues Related to Substance Abuse

Ethical issues regarding substance use and abuse relate to behaviors that present a risk to self, co-workers, or the public. A health care worker diverting medication from a patient, thereby depriving the patient of pain relief, is both unethical and illegal. Other ethical areas of concern include property theft or damage and the general welfare of others.

Drug testing, as part of preemployment assessment and random testing during employment, have become commonplace. Beginning in 1986, federal legislation, such as the Drug-Free Workplace Act and the Omnibus Transportation Employee Testing Act, has authorized drug and alcohol testing in specific job classifications. Although employees' attitudes toward workplace drug testing are mixed, it has been shown to have a positive effect, and currently about 90% of large U.S. companies have a drug screening policy in place (Levine and Rennie, 2004; Sweeney and Penner, 1997). There is evidence that the most effective deterrent to drug abuse in workers is a comprehensive program combining testing with an employee assistance program, supervisory training, employee education, and a clearly written substance use policy (Quazi, 1993). The legal conflict in testing is its opposition to rights of privacy; therefore testing is random rather than universal (Levine and Rennie, 2004).

One area that has also received the attention of the legal system is the use by pregnant women of substances known to increase risks to the fetus in terms of future long-term developmental and behavioral problems. Pregnant addicts have been imprisoned and forced into treatment, and their children have been removed from their custody after birth. Many treatment providers and patient advocates view this approach as punitive and counterproductive to assisting these women and their children. There is concern that such sanctions may prevent addicted women from seeking treatment, for fear of legal consequences (Chavkin et al., 1998; Paone and Alpern, 1998).

Heavy maternal use of alcohol during pregnancy can cause permanent birth defects, including fetal alcohol syndrome. Although alcohol-related defects are entirely preventable, the factors associated with maternal use of alcohol during pregnancy are complex and often resistant to change. The University of Washington has implemented a primary prevention and intervention program for those women identified as being at risk for producing children affected by prenatal alcohol exposure. Women identified as being at risk are referred to a multidisciplinary diagnostic clinic staffed by a physician, psychologist, language pathologist, occupational therapist, and social worker to facilitate diagnosis and comprehensive intervention for both the mother and affected children. This approach increases the potential for primary prevention of fetal alcohol syndrome by avoiding exposures and is a major protective factor in managing conditions among affected children (Astley, 2004; Cook, 2004). ■

MODES OF INTERVENTION

Correlating with the numerous theories about substance abuse is the wide variety of **intervention** strategies incorporating all levels of prevention. National, state, and local legislative measures have attempted to limit access to potentially addictive pharmaceuticals and illicit street drugs. The growing social demand for smoke-free environments in public buildings, restaurants, airplanes, and similar areas exemplifies how perceptions of tobacco and its risks have changed over the past 50 years. Alcohol taxes, zoning schemes for liquor outlets, a legal drinking age, and legal sanctions on driving while intoxicated are other examples of community efforts to prevent or contain substance abuse.

Media campaigns provide public service communications about the risks of substance abuse and the availability of treatment for these problems. However, these must include culturally relevant and realistic goals. Some have proven to be quite successful. For example, there was a long and substantial decline in the use of inhalants by adolescents after 1995, when the Partnership for a Drug-Free America conducted an anti-inhalant media campaign. This decline, however, has since reversed (Johnston et al., 2005).

One of the goals of *Healthy People 2010* (USDHHS, 2000) is to increase the proportion of middle, junior high, and senior high schools that provide school health education related to unintentional injury, violence, suicide, tobacco use and addiction, and alcohol and other drug use. Educational programs administered through schools and penal institutions have been developed, but evaluation and evidence of success or failure of the interventions have been sporadic.

The formation of national associations (e.g., the National Council on Alcoholism) and the establishment of federal research entities (e.g., the National Institute of Drug Abuse and the National Institute on Alcohol Abuse and Alcoholism) have facilitated centralized efforts in the areas of education, research, and treatment. At the state level, there have been legislative provisions to fund substance abuse treatment and rehabilitation. National organizations like Partnership for a Drug Free America and the National Alliance for the Mentally Ill, which have local chapters, are also important forces for community education, research, and support.

Recently, NIDA released a report aimed at addressing the community-level disaster of the September 11, 2001, attack and extended the report to include the 2005 hurricanes, Katrina and Rita, which displaced hundreds of thousands, and killed at least 1000. In the report, the experience of stress resulted in a sharp increase in the corticotrophin-releasing factor, setting in motion a host of biological changes related to posttraumatic stress and posttraumatic stress disorder. Stress may cause those with compulsive use patterns to relapse after a period of abstinence (NIDA, 2005) and may trigger those who have not previously misused substances to, at least temporarily, misuse them. These cases also delimit the efficacy of the "addictive personality" and the one-size-fits-all approach.

Prevention

The principles of prevention are paramount in community nursing practice. Primary prevention in the community includes working with other providers to perform a needs assessment. This will identify high risk situations and potential problems that threaten the integrity of the community and its inhabitants—in particular, what factors in the community are encouraging initiation of substance abuse, how effective are school- and community-based programs, and what political issues in the community may be influencing resource allocation.

On the federal level, primary prevention efforts have been overshadowed by the ongoing "war on drugs." A significant amount of fiscal resources has been allocated to law enforcement, interdiction, crop eradication, and harsh, punitive laws to prosecute drug users and manufacturers. Debate continues at both the state and federal levels regarding the cost-benefit ratio of drug legalization or decriminalization. Supporters argue that legalization and decriminalization would lead to a reduction in crime and would move the drug problem out of the realm of the moral failure of individuals toward more humane treatment approaches.

Opponents argue that decriminalization and legalization of drugs would do little to abate crime related to drug manufacture, sale, and use and that problems associated with use (e.g., domestic violence and drunk driving) would potentially increase (Goldberg, 2004). There is no question that substance abuse is a costly medical, social, and legal problem and that until society can effectively deal with the serious effects of two lethal but legal drugs (i.e., alcohol and nicotine), the argument for adding additional sanctions is difficult to accept and justify. Other preventive efforts at government and private levels include community-based programs, training

BOX 24-3 CAGE: An Alcoholism Screening Test

C "Have you ever felt that you should **C**ut down on your drinking?"

A "Have people **A**nnoyed you by criticizing your drinking?"

G "Have you ever felt bad or **G**uilty about your drinking?"

E "Have you ever had a drink, or an **E**ye-opener, first thing in the morning to steady your nerves or get rid of a hangover?"

➤ Two positive responses to these questions are considered a positive test and indicate that further assessment is warranted.

Modified from Ewing JA: Detecting alcoholism: the CAGE questionnaire, *JAMA* 252: 1905-1907, 1984.

of health professionals, faith-based initiatives, volunteer consumer groups, organized sports programs, and employer programs.

The secondary prevention role of the community health nurse includes screening and finding resources and solutions specific to his or her particular community. It is important for the community health nurse to be aware of the evidence base for certain programs and modify or discard those programs that have not proved successful over time.

Screening tools such as the CAGE test (Box 24-3) are brief and simple and allow health providers to talk about substance abuse by incorporating relevant questions into the interview and history (Cherpitel, 1997; Ewing, 1984). A positive response to any of the CAGE questions does not constitute a diagnosis of alcohol or drug dependence, but it should raise suspicion and mandate further investigation. Prevention efforts should be specific to aggregates, rather than directed at the general public.

Prevention efforts focusing on minority groups such as African Americans have produced results that are only marginally successful (Straussner, 2003). Possible reasons are that treatment programs fail to incorporate culturally sensitive and appropriate interventions and strategies. The demand for a culturally specific approach is evidence that previous approaches, and the assumptions that underlie them, are insufficient for understanding and explaining the etiology of substance abuse among members of minority groups. Successful prevention efforts are usually not focused solely on alcohol and drug abuse but are community controlled and work toward improving individuals' general competencies, communication skills, and self-esteem.

Treatment

Substance abuse problems are socially defined and frequently attributed to sufferers who do not recognize their substance use as a problem. Furthermore, the substance abuse treatment system has increasingly taken on social welfare and criminal justice tasks. In this sense, substance abuse differs from many other health-related problems. Most states have laws pertaining to involuntary treatment of substance abusers. Employers and families are often enlisted to assist or coerce the identified client into accepting treatment. This aspect of substance abuse as a health concern raises some crucial questions for health care providers in terms of the encroachment of therapeutic intervention on individual rights to privacy, informed consent, and self-determination.

On the individual level, those providing substance abuse treatment should take into consideration cultural and educational background, the resources of the person, the attitudes of significant others, the degree of invasiveness of the effects of the substance use, and the existence of alternatives. Interventions have been developed to assist some individuals in achieving moderation. Additionally, some research has shown that a small percentage of individuals who recognize a harmful pattern of substance use are able to stop using the substance or to achieve a controlled, nonpathological pattern of use. There are those who, because they experience an important life change, such as graduating from college or getting married, appear to change from excessive use to social alcohol use.

Nevertheless, many people exhibit serious problems related to their use of substances and are usually not able to stop or control their use without outside intervention. Research on identified problem drinkers' ability to return to social alcohol use is still inconclusive. Consequently, most scientists and health care providers advocate abstinence as a cornerstone of recovery.

Abstinence is difficult to maintain on a long-term basis. Therefore, an important area of continuing research is relapse prevention (i.e., a behavioral approach that aims to prepare the client for the relapse situation in the hope of preventing it or minimizing its impact on recovery). Relapse prevention models can be applied to alcohol, drug, and behavioral addictive problems (e.g., overeating and compulsive gambling) and can have either controlled use or abstinence as their goal. In relapse prevention, relapses are reframed as learning opportunities, and the client makes plans for coping with negative mood states, meeting the challenge of craving, and stopping a relapse quickly if it should occur.

Inpatient and outpatient are the two main types of treatment programs for substance abuse. Each of these programs may or may not include a detoxification component. Treatment programs also differ in the following ways: they may be voluntary versus compulsory and pharmacologically based versus drug free. In general, although treatment is intricately tied to the concept of recovery, disciplinary philosophy guides specific treatment approaches. There are a variety of treatment approaches and models, which are sometimes contradictory. The treatment models vary by such factors as the composition of staff and the philosophical approach (i.e., social vs. psychological vs. medical models) to substance abuse problems.

Inpatient treatment isolates individuals from the external world and provides an opportunity to focus only on substance abuse issues. Outpatient treatment is appropriate for those who do not require such structure and protection, those with strong supportive social networks and high levels of motivation, and those who need to continue working while in recovery.

The severity of the individual's alcohol or drug problems and pertinent cultural factors determine the necessity and type of treatment. Therefore the assessment process is of primary importance and begins with an accurate social and medical history. The history taking begins with more general questions about lifestyle, employment, relationships, and

RESEARCH HIGHLIGHTS

Stress Reduction and Treatment of Substance Abuse

A Mindfulness-Based Stress Reduction Intervention, employing various meditation practices (e.g., guided mediation, sitting mindfulness meditation, mindful Hatha yoga, walking meditation, and eating mediation), was used to help reduce psychological and physiological stress among residents of an in-patient, substance abuse treatment facility. During the 8-week program, the level of stress of the participants was determined by measuring their salivary cortisol levels and their scores on the Perceived Stress Scale (PSS).

Findings from the study showed that participates reported a decrease in stress over time (as measured by the PSS). Further, salivary cortisol levels were significantly lower following the intervention. The researchers concluded that the Mindfulness-Based Stress Reduction intervention may influence the physiological response to stress of individuals undergoing residential treatment for substance abuse. Federally funded research in this intervention is currently under way.

Marcus MT et al: Change in stress levels following a mindfulness-based stress reduction in a therapeutic community. *Addict Disord Their Treat* 2:63-68, 2003.

self-perception. This general line of questioning permits the development of a therapeutic relationship with the client.

A therapeutic relationship based on trust is essential to collecting information about sensitive issues such as drug and alcohol use. The assessment should then proceed to determining risky behavior patterns and stressors. The interviewer assesses dietary practices; prior health problems; allergies; hospitalizations, including psychiatric disorders; and family history of similar problems, including drug- and alcohol-related problems. This general line of questioning can be followed by more specific questions about harmful behaviors, such as smoking, drinking, and illicit drug use. This ordering of questions progresses from the more socially sanctioned behaviors to more "socially disapproved" behaviors and from the general to the more specific. Positive responses to questions about drug and alcohol use should be probed in a nonjudgmental, direct way and treated as "routine" in health care encounters.

A physical examination is another valuable tool in evaluating the client for potential or actual alcohol and drug problems. Although at-risk clients may not have physical signs of alcohol and drug problems and may even deny obvious consequences of such, certain physical findings warrant further investigation. Complaints such as vague, nonspecific abdominal pain, insomnia, depression, chronic fatigue, back pain, chronic anxiety, refractory hypertension, and night sweats require more intensive investigation. Spider angiomata on the thorax or face may be the result of long-term alcohol use. Poor dental health is common in injection drug and methamphetamine users. Although laboratory tests may not yield clues to drug or alcohol use, certain laboratory findings (e.g., abnormal liver function), in the absence of other etiological agents, may increase the index of suspicion.

Intervention strategies frequently begin with information about the effects of alcohol and drugs and a discussion of the solutions to substance abuse–related problems. This initial educational approach can defuse frequently encountered barriers to intervention such as shame, guilt, fear, and the client's erroneous perceptions regarding risks. Presenting information and solutions in a nonjudgmental and clear manner may help minimize defensiveness. Reframing interventions within the context of health maintenance or health promotion and education minimizes the sense of stigma.

Ambivalent clients may respond to education and decide to abstain from substances or seek treatment. Other clients, however, even when confronted with legal, financial, physical, and psychological consequences of substance abuse, may resist treatment offers. Therefore the clinician must continue to work with clients and involve important members of their social network to remove internal and environmental barriers and move clients toward readiness for change and treatment. Potential discrimination in group settings and logistical problems, such as lack of child care, may be barriers to treatment.

Much of the effort for substance abuse treatment has been invested in detoxification, residential, and outpatient treatment programs. Secondary problems related to drug and alcohol abuse are intoxication, overdose, and withdrawal. Overdose may be accidental or intentional and requires acute interventions to stabilize the client. As a client advocate, the community health nurse can be an important ally in ensuring that adequate follow-up is conducted for those admitted to emergency departments for overdose. Detoxification is best described as a short-term treatment intervention designed to manage acute withdrawal from the substance. It involves medical management to reduce the adverse side effects of the substance and help stabilize the client. This may be performed on an inpatient or outpatient basis, depending on the substance and severity of dependence.

Addressing acute withdrawal symptoms is of utmost importance in detoxification. The cocaine abuser may experience extreme depression with suicidal ideation. Withdrawal from central nervous system depressants, including alcohol, produces the most life-threatening medical consequences, including anxiety, tremors, delirium, convulsions, and possible death unless medically managed. Symptoms of withdrawal from narcotics, although less life threatening, are temporarily disabling and painful, including chills, sweating, cramps, and nausea. Such feelings may cause the individual who is withdrawing from treatment to begin the cycle of abuse again. Detoxification is one of the most crucial periods in the recovery process. Clinicians should be aware of the level of services offered in any detoxification program in order to make appropriate referrals.

Outpatient and inpatient treatment programs vary, but they usually include group and individual therapy and counseling, motivational interviewing, family counseling, education, and socialization into 12-step mutual self-help groups. Many programs are integrating psychotherapy, such as cognitive-behavioral therapy, with pharmacotherapy. These medications are discussed more fully in the next section. Other strategies include hypnosis, occupational therapy, confrontation, assertiveness training, blood alcohol–level discrimination training, and other behavior modification approaches. Relapses are common; therefore the most effective treatment programs incorporate some form of relapse prevention as a part of the healing process.

Therapy that involves the family has proven to be most effective in aiding recovery. Family and social contacts can be helped to initiate change in the abuser, to aid in recovery, and to assist in maintenance of treatment gains. A well-known family involvement motivational technique is the Johnson Institute Intervention, involving a confrontation of the abuser with guidance from therapists. A less coercive version of this is called A Relational Sequence for Engagement (ARISE), where significant others are educated and coached over a period of time. Another effective strategy is Community Reinforcement and Family Training (CRAFT). With this approach, a concerned significant other is trained in techniques such as positive reinforcement, identification of dangerous situations, and stress reduction (Fals-Stewart, O'Farrell, and Birchler, 2003). NIDA (1999) published a research-based guide to drug addiction treatment. Important points from this publication are listed in Box 24-4.

Treatment programs have been unprepared for the influx and unique problems associated with methamphetamine (MA). Prolonged use may lead to serious acute psychotic disorders, with intensive physical and psychological withdrawal characterized by protracted anhedonia and dysphoria, accompanied by severe craving (Kuyper et al., 2004). Currently, there are no medications to reverse overdoses and no reliable drugs to treat the paranoia and psychosis associated with MA. Complications of treatment include high dropout rates, severe behavioral and psychotic states, and severe craving (Rawson, Gonzales, and Brethen, 2002).

Various treatments for MA abuse and addiction are being tried with mixed results. The effect of MA on brain functioning suggests a need for longer treatment plans. The most promising is a long-term comprehensive case study approach, using home visits and assisting with transportation and emergency fund provision (Cretzmeyer et al., 2003). Cognitive-behavioral therapy and contingency management are other promising approaches for treatment of methamphetamine abuse and dependence (Rawson et al., 2002). Treatments currently being studied include aversion therapy, medication therapy, and matrix treatment plans.

Studies show that clients respond favorably to treatment, but because of the multiple dimensions, it is a very challenging problem. Women with MA problems who have young children require an increased level of care. Specific recommendations include a pretreatment and treatment safeplace center for social and emotional support (Cretzmeyer et al., 2003). Because many abusers lack a supportive environment, the potential for relapse is increased. Also, because of the MA addict's typical inability to recognize the problematic nature of their use, combined drug court and outpatient treatment strategies are being developed.

Having a substance abuse problem does not mean that problems are always attributable to the addiction. Many substance-abusing clients also have other psychiatric problems (e.g., schizophrenia, depression, bipolar affective disorder, dissociative disorder, posttraumatic stress disorder). Likewise, many of these clients have chronic medical problems. In cases with compounding problems, specialized attention involving a case management approach is warranted.

BOX 24-4 Guidelines for Drug Abuse Treatment

➤ A single treatment is not appropriate for all individuals. Treatment should be tailored to the specific needs of the individual because not all addicts and alcoholics are the same.

➤ Treatment must be readily available when people who are addicted are ready for treatment.

➤ Effective treatment attends to the multiple needs of the individual, not just his or her substance use. It must address associated medical, psychological, social, vocational, and legal problems. Treatment should stress the importance of interaction with family or significant others and attempt to engage important social network members in the process.

➤ An individual's treatment and services plan must be assessed continually and modified as necessary to ensure that the plan meets the individual's changing needs.

➤ Remaining in treatment for an adequate time is crucial for treatment effectiveness. For most patients, the threshold of significant improvement is reached in about 3 months.

➤ Individual or group counseling and other behavioral therapies are critical components of effective treatment for addiction.

➤ Medications are an important element of treatment for many patients, especially when combined with counseling and other behavioral therapies.

➤ Addicted or drug-abusing individuals with coexisting mental disorders should have both disorders treated in an integrated way.

➤ Medical detoxification is only the first stage of addiction treatment and does little to change long-term substance abuse.

➤ Treatment does not need to be voluntary to be effective.

➤ Possible drug use during treatment must be monitored continuously.

➤ Treatment programs should provide assessment for HIV and AIDS, hepatitis B and C, tuberculosis, and other infectious diseases and should provide counseling to help patients modify or change behaviors that place themselves or others at risk for infection.

➤ Recovery from drug addiction can be a long-term process and commonly requires multiple episodes of treatment. Relapses can occur, but participation in mutual help groups or self-help groups and ongoing support is helpful to maintain abstinence. Treatment is not recovery, but it is part of the recovery process and experience. Treatment programs must address the aftercare needs of the client to maintain the gains made in treatment.

From National Institute on Drug Abuse: *Principles of drug addiction treatment: a research-based guide,* NIH Pub No 99-4180, Washington, DC, 1999, Government Printing Office.

Research demonstrates that treatment for substance abuse can be more effective than no treatment, but evaluation of treatment alternatives requires establishment of appropriate criteria to measure effectiveness (Simpson, 2004). Examples of criteria that have been used are shown in Box 24-5. It is clear that treatment programs vary and that certain programs will be more culturally appropriate and therefore more effective than others for particular aggregates of individuals.

Pharmacotherapies

In the search for successful treatment of those susceptible to drug and alcohol problems, several pharmacotherapeutic adjuncts to formalized treatment have been developed. Medications include drugs used to assist in the initiation and maintenance of abstinence, drugs used as a substitute for illegal

BOX **24-5** Criteria for Measuring Effectiveness
of Substance Abuse Treatment Programs

➤ Number of days abstinent
➤ Number of days without negative consequences of substance use
➤ Employability or work attendance
➤ Self-image improvement
➤ Spouse's assessment of client's functionality
➤ Regular attendance at 12-step group meetings
➤ Compliance with follow-up appointments
➤ Absence of overt psychiatric symptoms such as depression or anxiety
➤ Self-reports of progress
➤ Evidence of personal satisfaction and growth

drug use, or drugs used to treat comorbidities. This section discusses pharmacotherapies that providers currently use. Good clinical judgment and patient motivation should guide the use of any pharmacotherapy, and therapy should be combined with psychosocial support.

Pharmacotherapy is used in detoxification, stabilization, and maintenance; as antagonists; and as treatment for coexisting disorders. Clinically, it is considered better to prevent withdrawal symptoms with medication than to wait for symptoms to appear. Methadone is the treatment of choice in withdrawal from heroin or other opiates. As a detoxification agent, methadone is dispensed over an 8-day period in a tapering dose. Dosage is dependent on the degree of opiate withdrawal symptoms present. A widely used example of the use of medication for long-term stabilization is methadone maintenance. The client is prescribed daily administration of a long acting opioid (methadone) as a substitute for the illicit use of opiates (typically heroin). A large body of research confirms its effectiveness in treatment retention and reduction of risks such as HIV (Carroll, 2003).

However, there are continuing varying philosophical opinions about abstinence versus sanctioned use in the debate over the use of methadone. Methadone maintenance is more controversial because the individual remains dependent on the drug. It is dispensed under medical supervision as part of a treatment program. Maintenance may minimize or abate illegal activity, eliminate the infection hazards of injection drug use, reduce the social disruption typically seen with opiate use, and facilitate increased levels of functioning. A myth about maintenance programs is that methadone produces a euphoric "high" and is therefore merely a legal substitute for heroin.

Naltrexone is a long-acting narcotic antagonist traditionally used as an adjunct in the treatment of opiate dependence. It blocks the effects of opiates via competitive binding, but it does not block the effects of other substances such as benzodiazepines, cocaine, and alcohol (Carroll, 2003). Recent studies indicate that naltrexone is also effective in reducing craving, rates of relapse to alcohol, and severity of alcohol-related problems (Carmen, 2004).

Buprenorphine is an opioid agonist-antagonist that has been used in the treatment of opiate-dependent clients and those with concurrent cocaine dependence. Buprenorphine does not produce severe withdrawal on abrupt cessation, which is an advantage over methadone. Its antagonist component helps reduce the possibility of lethal overdose. Clinical studies support the use of buprenorphine in reducing the frequency of heroin and cocaine self-administration.

Use of disulfiram (Antabuse) to promote cessation of alcohol abuse is rare today due to serious safety issues. A select group (i.e., those who are relapse prone, those who have supportive networks, and those who have histories of abstinence) may benefit from short-term use. Requests for disulfiram should not be granted in the absence of treatment and supportive relationships. Disulfiram, when combined with alcohol, produces the classic disulfiram ethanol reaction (DER) (i.e., flushing, tachycardia, nausea, headache, chest tightness, and chest pain). The DER is thought to be the result of a disturbance in alcohol metabolism. The response, which typically begins within minutes after alcohol consumption, is dose dependent and highly variable. Significant risks of the DER are cardiovascular symptoms of tachycardia, hypotension, dysrhythmia, and shock. Preexisting cardiac disease is an absolute contraindication. Emergency treatment of the DER is symptomatic.

Benzodiazepines are considered effective tools for alcohol withdrawal because they decrease the likelihood of seizures and delirium (Naegle and D'Avanzo, 2001). Acamprosate (calcium acetyl homotaurinate) has been used successfully in Europe over the past decade and recently allowed for use in the United States. The main efficacy is with reducing drinking frequency and abstinence maintenance. Acamprosate (Campral) reduces glutamatergic transmission and neuronal hyperexcitability during withdrawal from alcohol. This drug has a low incidence of side effects but should be used under the care of a physician and prescribed cautiously in patients with liver or kidney problems. No withdrawal syndrome or abuse has been shown as yet (Mann, Lehert, and Morgan, 2004).

Mutual Help Groups

Mutual help groups are associations that are voluntarily formed, are not professionally dominated, and operate through face-to-face supportive interaction focusing on a mutual goal. Many mutual help groups exist, and they are usually organized by recovering substance abusers or those recovering from compulsive behavior patterns. The first mutual help group was Alcoholics Anonymous (AA), founded in 1935. Initially, a small group of male alcoholics found a way to stay sober "one day at a time" through meeting regularly with others like themselves. The early AA members developed 12 steps to guide the recovery process (Kurtz, 1979). The process is summarized in Box 24-6.

As a nonprofessional ongoing source of assistance, AA is viewed as an invaluable resource to the community. However, not all of those with alcohol problems find AA comfortable, culturally relevant, and socially supportive. Because realities of social discrimination and regional variation in customs exist, AA should not be considered a universal form of assistance for

BOX 24-6 Basic Tenets of 12-Step Programs

➤ Admission of defeat and surrender to a higher power
➤ Inventory of past shortcomings and strengths
➤ Spiritual practices (e.g., prayer and meditation)
➤ Willingness to change
➤ Making amends
➤ Extension of this process into daily life

TABLE 24-4 Modes of Intervention for Substance Abuse

LEVEL	INTERVENTION
Individual and family levels	Education
	Treatment: detoxification, inpatient, outpatient, and residential
	Mutual help groups (e.g., AA, Narcotics Anonymous, Cocaine Anonymous, Al-Anon, and NarcAnon)
Community level	Law enforcement measures to limit access to and distribution of addictive substances (e.g., street drugs)
	Alcohol taxes and zoning schemes for liquor outlets
	Legal drinking age and legal sanctions on driving while intoxicated
	Education programs at schools and penal institutions
	Television and radio public service communications concerning the risks of substance abuse and the availability of treatment
State and federal levels	Formation of national associations such as the National Council on Alcoholism
	Establishment of federal research entities such as the National Institute of Drug Abuse and the National Institute on Alcohol Abuse and Alcoholism to centralize research, education, and treatment efforts
	Legislative provisions at the state level to fund substance abuse treatment and rehabilitation

alcohol problems. Predominantly in large cities, women and members of racial, ethnic, religious, or sexual preference minority groups with alcohol problems have formed their own AA groups and other mutual help organizations for support in recovery.

Other 12-step programs have developed through the adaptation of AA's approach to similar addictive problems. Narcotics Anonymous, Gamblers Anonymous, Debtors Anonymous, Cocaine Anonymous, Overeaters Anonymous, and Sex and Love Addicts Anonymous are examples. Because they became organized more recently than AA, these groups may not be as well known or as widely available, and they may not exhibit as much diversity among their membership as AA. Children, partners, and close associates of substance abusers have also founded self-help groups, such as Al-Anon, Codependents Anonymous, and Adult Children of Alcoholics. Although these groups initially had a predominance of female members, the trend is moving toward participation by equal numbers of men and women.

AA meetings are not standardized. Customs shaping the actual format and sequence of the meeting vary according to region, group size, ethnic and sex composition, and other cultural variations of the members. In general, 12-step meetings follow one of the following formats:

• Uninterrupted talks by one or more speakers about "what it was like, what happened, and what it is like now"
• Each person at the meeting has the opportunity to speak briefly during discussion
• A combination of the first two options
• Meetings may be either closed or open to the general public

At least two mutual help groups have developed in response to their founders' negative experiences in AA or their failure to succeed in AA. Women for Sobriety was organized in 1976 to replace or augment AA for women; it addresses women's needs to overcome depression, guilt, and low self-esteem. Secular Sobriety Groups were organized to meet the needs of individuals who are unable to accept the concept of, or to depend on, a "higher power" in their recovery from alcohol problems.

Other mutual help groups that do not follow the 12 steps are available for a variety of addictive problems. AA does not require dues or fees, but some groups, such as Weight Watchers, require monetary commitment. Other groups, such as Recovery Incorporated, have more professional involvement. Any of these groups could be a resource for selected people with substance abuse problems.

To be effective, interventions for substance abuse must take place at multiple levels and involve a number of indi-

viduals, activities, policies, and substances. Table 24-4 summarizes some of the many interventions for substance abuse at various levels.

Harm Reduction

New approaches reflecting a changing view of drug and alcohol addiction have been proposed for substance use problems that are not amenable to traditional approaches. Some of these have been grouped under the general term **harm reduction.** Harm reduction consists of individual and collective approaches to the treatment of substance use that are not primarily aimed at complete abstinence from all substances. Instead, incremental change is sought, which involves elimination of the more harmful effects of substance use through behavior and policy modifications. Harm reduction is a process rather than a static approach or an end in itself. It is used in various ways, depending on the context and the needs of individual clients (Erickson, 1999; MacCoun, 1998).

Harm reduction strategies remain controversial although some see them as a paradigm shift with the potential to significantly improve treatment results. They are often the only options that will preserve a therapeutic relationship when people continue to use or drink problematically. An early example of harm reduction is the substitution of methadone for heroin. Although they are still using an opiate, individuals taking methadone can be functional without getting high and without the need to engage in criminal activity for drugs.

Harm reduction psychotherapy aims to support the process of self-transformation through empathetic resonance, raising awareness of harm, setting goals, and understanding the multiple meanings of the substance (Tatarsky, 2003). Harm reduction has been used in response to alcohol, illicit drugs, and tobacco. In the case of alcohol, harm reduction might involve decreasing the number of drinks, decreasing the number of days in which drinking occurs, or avoiding drinking when driving.

On a community level, harm reduction may include attempts to legislate for decreased access to alcohol or raising the legal age for drinking. More controversial public health projects aimed at harm reduction are legalization of some illicit drugs and needle exchange programs. Needle exchange programs have had some success, and although they may not lead the intravenous drug user to abstinence, they do, in fact, serve to break the link in the deadly chain of AIDS exposure and transmission (Des Jarlais, 2004).

Viewed from a community health perspective, harm reduction involves planned social and policy changes. The goal of these changes is to decrease health risks consequent to alcohol and other drug use among specific aggregates (Kearney, 1999; Wodak, 1995). Although harm reduction strategies are not usually sanctioned by lay support systems (e.g., 12-step groups), they can have an important impact. Community health nurses using harm reduction strategies can help reduce drug- and alcohol-related social problems by advocating for programs that "bridge the gap" for those who cannot immediately reach the goal of abstinence.

People who drive while impaired by alcohol or other drugs are a public health hazard to themselves and others. During 2004, almost 16,700 deaths were due to alcohol- or drug-related motor vehicle accidents. Reduction in alcohol-involved motor vehicle–related fatalities requires a variety of interventions to change drinking and driving behaviors. These include altering drivers' perceptions of risk to themselves and to others riding with them, increasing efforts to screen for alcoholism among people convicted of driving while intoxicated, and changing public policy to deter adult drinking and driving (CDC, 2006). ∎

SOCIAL NETWORK INVOLVEMENT

Family and Friends

The social network of the substance abuser can either be highly influential in helping the individual alter behavior or aid and abet the substance abuser in self-destruction. There is evidence for both positive and negative effects of social support in either mitigating or supporting the behaviors of substance abusers (Latimer, 2003). Particularly among adolescents and young adults, evidence suggests that substance use and abuse often occur in the context of social interactions. Adolescents may use alcohol and other substances as a social lubricant during an often-troubled developmental period (Stinchfield and Winters, 2003). Family treatment is considered essential because of the potential for enabling behavior. In addition, the family has suffered the effects of substance abuse emotionally, socially, economically, physically, and spiritually. The family's wounds must be acknowledged and treated in order for the substance abuser to return to an environment supportive of recovery.

A user's social network may play a role in allowing the substance abuse to continue. Spouses may call work to report that their partner is "sick" or remain silent when evidence of abuse is discovered. Complex community and family interactions that serve to promote certain behaviors are commonly known as codependency and enabling. The boundaries between the nonaddicted family members and addict waver with the result that the excessive substance-abusing behavior is covered up or excused (Hanson et al., 2002). Social network members may compensate for the fact that the student is absent from school, the car payment is late, or an important appointment is canceled or forgotten. These distress signals are common but often go unrecognized because periods of use are often interspersed with periods of abstinence. This reinforces the individual's, and often the significant other's, perceived sense of control over the substance use. There are mutual help groups for addressing codependency that are founded on the principles of AA and provide opportunities to discuss the issues germane to the alcoholic or addicted family system or network. Families participating in treatment should also be encouraged to participate in these mutual help groups.

Codependency cannot be concretely defined the same way in each culture. Cultural groups vary in the degree to which individuals are expected to anticipate the needs of others and care for them. The danger in applying a rigid definition of codependency in all cases is that it might unfairly and inappropriately label it as a disease in some cultures that value interdependency over individualism.

Through development of a therapeutic relationship and comprehensive assessment, the community nurse should identify the important members of the social network for each client and the ways in which these individuals provide support for the client. The nurse must also recognize that the concept of family refers not only to nuclear families but also to alternative family systems. Whatever the constellation of family, significant others should be included in the treatment and intervention. Substance abuse, addiction, and recovery do not occur in a vacuum, and many relapses are precipitated by interpersonal conflicts.

Effects on the Family

Substance abuse has been called a family disease because it affects the entire family system and holds potential adverse psychological and physical consequences for the family members in addition to the abuser. Family theorists view families, whether the traditional nuclear form or an alternative, as social systems that try to stay in balance (Friedmann, Bowden, and Jones, 2003). Professionals may see families as either functional or dysfunctional depending on how well they fulfill the social tasks expected of them by society. Substance-abusing families are frequently observed to be dysfunctional in clinical terms. However, cultural and political factors should also be considered because families may have developed these patterns for historical reasons rather than as the effects of substance abuse.

A functional family system is open and flexible and allows its members to be themselves. In the nuclear family model, the parents model intimacy for the children, differences are negotiated, boundaries are defined and maintained, and communication is consistent and clear. In functional family systems, whether the traditional nuclear family or other nontraditional forms, there is trust, individuality, and accountability among family members. All family members are able to have their needs met in a reasonable way.

On the other hand, dysfunctional families are closed systems with fixed, rigid roles. In the case of substance abuse, a major purpose of the system is to deny the substance abuse of the affected family member and keep it a "shameful" family secret. Generally, ego boundaries between the family members are weakened or nonexistent, with enmeshment of the members and an intolerance of individual differences. Rules are rigid and communication is unbalanced; the dynamics are either always conflicting or always superficially pleasant. Children may become involved in a "role reversal" in which they act as caretakers of their parents.

When one or more family members are substance abusers, family functions revolve around the substance abuser and accommodate or compensate the abuser's behavior (Naegle and D'Avanzo, 2001). The individual needs of other family members are often unmet. Denial is central to a "dysfunctional" family system. The spouse of the substance abuser may gradually take over that person's role, functions, and control of the family. The children are cast into various roles (e.g., hero, junior parent, scapegoat, peacemaker, or caretaker) in their struggle for survival in this environment.

Adult children from dysfunctional families often carry these roles and coping mechanisms into adult life, with many becoming substance abusers or partners of substance abusers. The children of alcoholics are 4 to 9 times more likely to experience alcohol use disorders than are children of nonalcoholics (Anda, 2002). Frequently, they have difficulties with intimacy and parenting. Many have lifelong emotional problems such as depression and anxiety and physical illnesses often associated with these conditions (e.g., ulcers, colitis, migraine headaches, and eating disorders). However, some offspring exhibit thriving and resilient behavior. Using a strength-based approach, the community health nurse can work with resiliency factors (Mylant, 2002).

In addition to psychological burdens that substance abuse places on families, there are the financial burdens related to medical costs, loss of income from job difficulties or unemployment, and the financial losses attributable to divorce. Further, spousal violence and child abuse and neglect are strongly associated with substance abuse (Holtzworth-Munroe, 2004).

Professional Enablers

Health care professionals also can contribute to the initiation and continuation of substance abuse and dependency in various ways, becoming **professional enablers.** One obvious way is the physician's role in prescribing psychoactive medications. The medical model advocates the treatment of symptoms by medication. The relief of pain, anxiety, and insomnia are not exceptions. The addictive potential of narcotic analgesics and antianxiety agents is often ignored if quick symptom relief is the main goal. Long-term goals for the treatment of medical problems and nonmedication management of pain and anxiety are more thoughtful approaches. However, undermedication or refusal to use "addictive" medicines can lead susceptible clients to self-medicate with illegal drugs or alcohol.

Physicians and nurses are often the first to see the physical effects of substance abuse and are in an excellent position to intervene. By focusing on the health consequences of substance abuse, they can form trusting relationships, provide information, and refer patients to the appropriate treatment. Too often, this opportunity is missed because the health care professional is reluctant to bring up this taboo subject. This reluctance may be based on professionals' inability to examine their own drinking or drug-taking behaviors, or those of significant others, or concerns of negative responses by clients.

In the past, many psychiatrists and psychotherapists have focused on the reasons their client uses substances rather than on the dependency itself. The assumption was that insight would lead to a change in behavior. This approach has usually not proved to be effective, especially if the psychiatrist is concurrently prescribing other potentially addictive antianxiety medications or hypnotics. Complete abstinence from all mood-altering medication is a model for preventing the cross-addiction common in substance abusers (i.e., substituting one substance for another such as a benzodiazepine for alcohol). Exceptions to this approach are patients with serious medical conditions requiring pain medication and those who also have a second psychiatric disorder that requires medication (i.e., schizophrenia, depression, bipolar affective disorder). Recovering substance abusers often need support when they must take medication for these psychiatric conditions because others may criticize the use of any medication and place the client in a difficult situation.

Caregivers have become more aware of signs of client substance abuse. Some providers are willing to begin therapy with a nonabstinent client under the stipulation that if therapeutic gains are not made, the client will be referred for treatment or the caregiver will withdraw services. Clients who lack social support may succeed using this strategy, which allows the formation of a trusting relationship before taking the leap to abstinence. Clinical wisdom and research continue to point toward more tailored, individualized approaches to substance abuse.

VULNERABLE AGGREGATES

Substance abuse problems viewed from a community perspective clearly affect some populations more severely than others. Some groups are more susceptible to experiencing substance abuse problems, may tend to deteriorate more quickly in the process, or may have fewer sources of support for recovery. These groups are termed *vulnerable aggregates* and require special attention in terms of prevention, intervention, and rehabilitation strategies.

Current resources for prevention, treatment, and mutual support may not be flexible enough to meet the needs of various vulnerable aggregates who are at risk of experiencing substance abuse problems and are often excluded or alienated from services by policies, provider attitudes, economic constraints, and social isolation. This section describes the issues of substance abuse with several vulnerable aggregates, including adolescents, the elderly, women, and racial and ethnic minorities.

Preadolescents and Adolescents

Why do young people use drugs? It is clear that drug and alcohol use among adolescents is a pervasive problem with many devastating consequences. The trend data in some aspects are undoubtedly worse for adolescents than adults. The teenage years may be a turbulent time for some because of the necessary developmental tasks of discovering their own unique identity, learning how to form intimate relationships, and developing autonomy. Presently, this is accomplished in a confusing era when the cultural status of adolescents is undefined. Today's teenagers are an increasingly independent subculture with more money available than any time before, yet they have not attained full adult status.

The teenage years may be a time of experimentation, searching, confusion, rebellion, poor self-image, alienation, and insecurity. There is no such thing as the typical adolescent abuser, and there are multiple theories of causation. Researchers have concluded that adolescent drug use is a symptom and not the cause of maladjustment. Those with significant difficulty are usually using substances as coping mechanisms.

Studies have identified various predictors of adolescent substance abuse. For example, use of legal substances (e.g., tobacco, alcohol) almost always precedes use of illegal drugs. Poor school performance, a social setting where drug use is common, and drug use among peers are the strongest predictors of subsequent drug involvement, followed by strength of family bonds (Stinchfield and Winters, 2003). The younger the initiation the greater the probability of prolonged and accelerated use. Other contributing factors are the feeling of powerlessness and selling drugs as a viable economic solution to poverty (Hanson et al., 2002). Subculture theory describes the status and power that charismatic leaders have to influence members of peer groups. In drug-using peer groups, such leaders have influence over inexperienced drug users and acculturate them into the drug scene. Thus it is crucial that communities work to maintain strong family and social bonds.

Some vulnerable adolescents may become victims of a vicious cycle. Labels used to describe people can have a profound influence on their self-perception. Labeling theory posits that when a person is judged by conventional society to be immoral, their perception of themselves will begin to mirror the accuser's perceptions (Hanson et al., 2002). For example, the teenager who experiments with marijuana and

boasts about the amount may be perceived as a "stoner." In another example, teachers may find it difficult to have positive relationships with children with behavioral disorders. Research has shown that adolescents are at less risk for substance abuse if they have a positive relationship with their teachers (Stinchfield and Winters, 2003). Children with attention deficit disorder, traumatic brain injury, or psychiatric illness are known to be at increased risk because of impulsive behavior and difficulty gaining positive peer group acceptance (Ashman, 2004; Pelham, 2003). The community health nurse can play an important part in advocating for these vulnerable children and educating teachers on the vital importance of maintaining a validating, nonjudgmental attitude toward these students.

It is especially important that families are supported in the community. Substance abuse is less likely in families that give clear messages and have open communication and more likely in families where parents are alcoholic, condemning, overly demanding, or overly protective. Committed family involvement helps retain the adolescent in treatment. However, it must be remembered that many well-functioning families have children who succumb to substance abuse. These families also may experience significant community rejection and judgmental attitudes.

The preadolescent years are a particularly vulnerable time for initiation and subsequent problematic use. The number of teens between seventh and twelfth grades being offered drugs is increasing (NIDA, 2005). When drug use escalates in adolescents, it can have devastating long-lasting consequences. There is a strong relationship among adolescent behavior problems such as aggressiveness, delinquency, and criminal activity and heavy alcohol use between the ages of 12 and 17 years.

Ever use of marijuana has been acknowledged by 77% of teenagers (NIDA, 2005). One of the problems associated with this is that the strength of marijuana is much higher than it was in the mid twentieth century. A phenomenon termed *amotivational syndrome* is marked by apathy and school failure and is thought to be the result of heavy marijuana use. However, there is some dissension about to whether this precedes or is the result of use of marijuana. Of much concern is the rising incidence of combining marijuana with more lethal substances, such as crack cocaine and methamphetamine (SAMSHA, 2003). Indeed, marijuana use is a strong precursor to use of more dangerous substances, such as methamphetamine and heroin (Hanson, Venturelli and Fleckenstein, 2002). Escalating use of substances enhances the risk of school and social failure, criminal activities, violent behavior, sexual risk taking, sexual violence (such as date rape), depression, suicide, and unintended injuries. Further, 50% of motor vehicle injuries in teenagers are related to drug or alcohol use (SAMHSA, 2003).

Primary prevention for adolescents is typically focused on education aimed toward complete abstinence, which some say is unrealistic. Education plays an important role. A striking feature is the strong adverse relationship between perceived risk and drug use. For all drugs, with no change in drug availability, when students perceive a drug as harmful, fewer students actually use it (SAMSHA, 2005). Large-scale media efforts can bring about change but only with accompanying parental and community efforts. Early detection of predisposing factors, such as underlying psychiatric illness, is important. Other strategies are providing structured clubs and organizations and facilitating school success, career skills, family communication skills, and conflict resolution. Secondary prevention is targeted at inpatient and outpatient treatment and harm reduction.

However, almost as important as intervention and treatment is recognizing when treatment is unnecessary. Not all drug use requires therapy, nor is it even desirable. Not all young drug users are antisocial or mentally unstable, nor should they be labeled as such. For the most part, most will develop a responsible philosophy concerning substance use if given support and opportunity.

The increasingly sophisticated technology used to prepare for athletic competition has been a significant factor in the self-administration of performance-enhancing substances and associated risky injection practices. These substances include steroids and over-the-counter stimulant drugs and herbs, with steroids the most common. Non-medical use of steroids poses serious problems, because use is both illegal and dangerous. Behavioral and health problems that have been noted with steroid use include suicides, homicides, liver damage, and heart attacks.

Many substance abuse researchers believe that attempts to enhance athletic performance with steroids and other substances reduce the perceived negative consequences of substance abuse and increase the likelihood of using illicit drugs for other purposes. In addition, limited access to needles and other equipment results in a high rate of needle sharing among adolescent teammates who inject substances to enhance their performance (USDHHS, 2000). ■

Elderly

Elderly men and women are considered vulnerable to substance abuse problems because they have diminished physiological tolerance, increased use of medically prescribed drugs, and cultural and social isolation. Conservative estimates indicate that 6% to 11% of elderly patients admitted to hospitals exhibit symptoms of alcoholism, as do 20% of the elderly in psychiatric hospitals and 14% of elderly patients in emergency departments (Adams and Cox, 1997).

Misuse of prescription drugs may be the most common form of drug abuse among the elderly. According to NIDA (1999), elderly persons use prescription medications approximately 3 times as frequently as the general population. In addition, data from the Veterans Affairs Hospital System suggest that elderly patients may be prescribed inappropriately high doses of benzodiazepines. Alcohol and prescription drug use, especially benzodiazepines, are significant factors in geriatric trauma (Zautcke et al., 2002).

Substance abuse in the elderly is commonly missed by health care providers (Beullens, 2004). An important part of early intervention efforts is thorough assessment and appropriate diagnosis. This can be difficult with the elderly because they do not manifest problems with substance abuse in the same ways as younger people. Thoughtful and routine

use of assessment tools such as the MAST-G and the CAGE questionnaire can be valuable in determining the presence of substance abuse in the elderly (Beullens, 2004).

Women

Since the 1970s, much attention has been turned to substance abuse problems in women. Evidence is mounting that alcohol use and abuse affect women much differently than they affect men. Women absorb and metabolize alcohol differently than do men, partly due to body composition differences and the production of less gastric alcohol dehydrogenase by women (Cook, 2004). Specific aggregates of women may be more severely affected by substance abuse problems, including women from minority groups, low-income or no-income women, and working-class women. The increased risk stems from economic, social, and cultural factors.

Lesbians are another aggregate of women in whom substance abuse may be associated with marginalization and should be understood within the diversity of lesbians individually and culturally. This is especially heightened in periods when homosexuality is demonized through media, churches, and legislation linking homosexuality with pathology and when lesbians and gays are denied the right to marry (e.g., civil unions, partner benefits).

Women who were abused as children are more susceptible to substance abuse problems in adolescence and adulthood than are nonabused women. They also face many more distressing consequences in substance abuse treatment and recovery. Disclosure of abuse in group treatment contexts or 12-step meetings is risky. In some cases, women are told to compartmentalize the abuse issues and only speak of addiction. In other cases, women are told if they do not disclose in a group, they will fail in their recovery program (Hall, 1996b). However, many current-day treatment programs designed for women now routinely address interpersonal violence in individual and group settings, leaving disclosure up to the client.

Drug-dependent women report frequent physical and medical problems, many related to their reproductive systems (Wetherington and Roman, 1998). Women tend to experience symptoms of alcoholic hepatitis and cirrhosis sooner than men because they metabolize alcohol at a different rate. They also have higher blood alcohol levels relative to body weight and higher mortality rates from heavy drinking (Cook, 2004).

Excessive alcohol use, especially binge drinking, during pregnancy continues to have long-term developmental consequences on the newborn (Cook, 2004). Cocaine use during pregnancy is associated with increased risk of spontaneous abortion, premature delivery, and abruptio placentae. Infants who have been addicted to cocaine in utero are hyper-irritable, subject to seizures, and possibly at increased risk for SIDS (sudden infant death syndrome). Long-term learning disabilities, behavioral problems, mental retardation, and physical handicaps are other potential consequences associated with children of cocaine-using mothers (Messinger, 2004).

Getting the pregnant woman into treatment and managing her withdrawal are frequently problematic. The woman's fear of punitive legal actions complicates the process. Additionally, the addiction itself often interferes with obtaining adequate prenatal care. If addiction is linked with risky sexual behavior, or sexual assault, there is an increased risk of contracting HIV and hepatitis viruses that can infect the infant; testing should be recommended.

Ethnocultural Considerations

Community health nurses need to be culturally competent and aware of certain ethnocultural vulnerabilities and differing perspectives when considering treatments for individuals with substance abuse. Ethnocultural competency can be defined as "the ability of a clinician to function effectively in the context of ethnocultural differences" (Straussner, 2003, p. 7). Data on African Americans, Hispanics, and Native Americans suggest an increased risk for substance abuse. However, the usual ethnic/racial categories in research do not take into account the distinctions within each category. Consequently, there are limited data, especially about middle-class minorities. Creating another stereotype might undermine prevention and treatment strategies. However, it is true that, under the strain of poverty, underemployment, decreased job opportunities, macro-level and micro-level aggression, and ongoing racism, some members of these aggregates find the relief in using substances as use numbs the "social pain" caused by their environments. Racial and ethnic minorities are overrepresented among the economically disenfranchised. Limited financial resources may limit alternatives to public treatment settings, which are often understaffed, underfunded, filled to capacity, and have long waiting lists. The privatization of treatment has further decreased access.

Theories of stress, social causation, and oppressed status support the belief that discrimination and racism is a factor in the generation of mental illness and alcohol and drug problems in members of racial and ethnic minorities. Socioeconomic, political, and historical realities have encouraged some minorities to enter into the illegal drug trade as a means of economic survival. In working with ethnic and racial minorities, health care professionals must recognize the sociopolitical and socioeconomic factors that form the context of substance use, abuse, and dependency. These same factors will have an impact on help seeking, treatment, and outcome. Traditional substance abuse treatment modalities, designed primarily for white working males, sometimes overlook ethnic and racial minority experiences (Straussner, 2003). Recovery for minority groups might be contextually and experientially different from that of Caucasians, just as the environment that contributed to the initial abuse was different.

During periods of slavery, alcohol was used as a reward, and it was seen as a way to cope. The value themes for this aggregate are a oneness with nature and spirituality, the importance of extended family, a present orientation, and a spiral concept of time. Barriers to treating African Americans with substance abuse or addiction problems are listed in Box 24-7.

Myths about certain ethnicities must be critically examined. Native Americans, for example, fight the stereotype of the drunken, once-noble warrior. However, alcohol as the predominant drug of choice, does pose a threat to this population,

---

BOX 24-7 Barriers to Treating Substance Abuse and Addiction Problems in African Americans

- ➤ Weekend drinking as a reward
- ➤ Ongoing sociocultural violence
- ➤ Use of substances to escape the emotional pain caused by racism
- ➤ Poverty, underemployment, and unemployment
- ➤ Prevalence of both drugs and liquor stores within the community
- ➤ Cultural and community disintegration, which has altered traditional values and behaviors
- ➤ Allure and economic rewards of selling drugs
- ➤ Inadequate social support system for recovery
- ➤ Internalized racism harming the self-concept, along with anger and frustration
- ➤ More likely to be arrested than treated (3-6 times more than whites)
- ➤ Limited role models
- ➤ Unable to "change people and places" as advocated by 12-step programs

---

particularly among youth and young adults. Native-American adolescents use drugs and alcohol earlier and with more devastating consequences than other groups (NIDA, 2005). Evidence for a biological predisposition is conflicting, and many stop drinking when they reach adulthood and their sense of family and social responsibility increases. Interventions for this group must involve long-term outreach that gains respect from the community.

Mexican Americans come from a heritage of using hallucinogens, such as sacred mushrooms and peyote, in rituals. In addition, alcohol is woven into the fabric of family life. Sociocultural factors that the community nurse should understand when planning treatment for this group include the importance of religion, *familismo* (the significance of family), fatalism (things are inevitable, or meant to be), *machismo* (bravery, strength, being a good provider), and *personalismo* (one should be pleasant and engaging socially, with dignity and a sense of honor).

In contrast, among Chinese Americans there is an increased prevalence of narcotics and decreased use of alcohol (SAMSHA, 2003). This population has a very low use of treatment services. Individual counseling is preferred, as they have a strong desire for confidentiality. However, they are receptive of pharmacological treatment (Straussner, 2003).

Studies have identified that social support has a positive effect on treatment and outcome. Without this support, the individual completing treatment may return to the original social environment, undermining any gains made within the treatment setting. Environmental cues and conditioned reinforcement for continued drug and alcohol use may be extremely powerful. The individual may return to an environment of nonsupport, characterized by continued use by important members of the individual's social network. The individual needs a well-coordinated aftercare program that addresses these issues.

BOX 24-8   Intervention Approaches for Working With People From Diverse Cultures

➤ Recognize that interpersonal relationships affect motivation to change.
➤ Express genuine interest in cultural norms.
➤ Dispense with assumptions based on appearance.
➤ Be careful not to assume privilege by using client's first names prematurely.
➤ Show a willingness to understand the language of the client.
➤ Gradually request pertinent information.
➤ Be sensitive to words that might imply that the client is defective.
➤ Recognize the role of the elders and family.

Modified from Straussner SL: *Ethnocultural factors in substance abuse treatment,* New York, 2003, Guilford Press.

The treatment of ethnic and racial minority aggregates poses special challenges related to the individuals seeking treatment. Treatment providers must recognize that these vulnerable aggregates will encounter a host of barriers that will make treatment and long-term recovery extremely difficult. For example, providers should understand the effect of rituals, holidays, music, and customs and how they can hinder progress. Providers who work from the public health perspective of "thinking upstream," will examine larger macro-level issues that increase the susceptibility of people of color to alcohol and drug problems. Box 24-8 presents helpful information on working with people from diverse cultures.

Other Aggregates

Substance abuse is the most common psychopathological problem in the general population. Within this category is a smaller aggregate of people with one or more psychiatric diagnoses in addition to substance abuse; this is referred to as **dual diagnosis.** Nearly one third of adults with a mental disorder also experience a co-occurring substance abuse disorder (USDHHS, 2000). This may be less readily identified by health care providers, who may fail to recognize that both problems may coexist. Treatment of dual-diagnosis individuals is complicated when the individual must take prescribed psychotropic medications. It may be perceived as prescription drug abuse or as the substitution of one addiction for another. Special attention and flexibility are needed to meet the needs of the dual-diagnosis aggregate, and such strategies are still in the developmental phase.

Childhood maltreatment, including verbal, physical, emotional, and sexual abuse and neglect, frequently leads to the development of a wide array of difficulties in adulthood. Substance abuse is one of the most common aftereffects. Approximately one in four girls and one in six boys are sexually molested before age 18 (Hall, 1996b; Van der Kolk, McFarlane, and Weisaeth, 1996). Therefore substance abuse prevention and treatment should address these issues. However, caution should be taken to avoid forcing the disclosure of a traumatizing event in a group setting (Hall, 1996a).

In assessing the risks for substance abuse and the extent of its impact on the community, nurses must be aware that there frequently are several bases for the vulnerability occurring in one individual or group. The adolescent, the low-income Hispanic male, the lesbian African-American mother receiving public assistance, and the Native-American family living on reservation land are all facing multiple sources of vulnerability that contribute to an increased potential for substance abuse.

Special attention must be paid to the impact of sexually transmitted diseases (STDs) (e.g., HIV, herpes, genital warts, and syphilis) and their relationship to substance abuse. Substance abusers are at increased risk of STDs, including HIV, in the following ways:

- Substances may cloud judgment, which leads to high-risk sexual practices involving the exchange of body fluids (e.g., sex without the use of appropriate barriers such as condoms).
- Intravenous drug use may involve the sharing of hypodermic needles.
- Chronic substance use (e.g., alcohol, heroin, amphetamines, nicotine, and cocaine) impairs the immune system and facilitates infection by HIV or other pathogens that increase the chances of HIV infection.
- Substance abuse may hasten physical and mental deterioration from the condition of seropositivity to an AIDS diagnosis and, eventually, the terminal phase of the disease.
- Chronic substance abusers generally have few supportive relationships available to them in the process of coping with the hardships that accompany severe and chronic illnesses.
- People facing a stigmatizing, terminal, debilitating illness, in themselves or in a significant other, are more prone to experience substance abuse problems in an attempt to cope with distress.

Finally, substance abuse among health care professionals cannot be ignored. Physicians, nurses, dentists, and pharmacists are vulnerable to substance abuse; alcohol or narcotic use is most common (Trinoff and Storr, 1998). Health care professionals are assumed to be "immune" to dependency because they are knowledgeable about medications. However, their increased access to drugs, belief in pharmaceutical solutions, and work-related stress place them at increased risk for substance abuse. Typically, they gain access to drugs through their work settings by diverting medications for their own use or by abusing drugs obtained by prescription. State regulatory boards discover the abuse by these health care professionals following drug theft or when the effects of their substance abuse impair their professional functioning.

Community health nurses should be especially vigilant because colleagues are working in isolation and episodes of incompetence may not be easily observed. Most states have rehabilitation programs for health care professionals that consist of treatment and monitoring. They are allowed to retain their professional licenses during treatment. Despite their usually favorable recovery rate, it is difficult to get this population into treatment because they exhibit denial and shame related to their substance abuse. However, the threatened loss of their professional license to practice may be a good motivator to break through their denial of the problem and encourage them to seek treatment.

NURSING PERSPECTIVE ON SUBSTANCE ABUSE

Nurses have encountered substance abuse in clients whose health problems are clearly related to alcohol abuse, such as cirrhosis of the liver, heart disease, neurological syndromes, and nutritional deficits. Unfortunately, alcohol problems were often not addressed in these health encounters in the past because there is a stigma of alcoholism and a lack of effective treatments. The nursing literature did not clearly address substance abuse as a nursing problem until the late 1960s and did not address it as a significant problem until the 1970s. Before the 1970s, substance abuse was usually viewed as a moral problem or, if it involved illicit drugs, as a legal problem.

Since the 1970s, nursing has become more involved in the spectrum of compulsive behavior problems, including substance abuse. A specialized organization, the National Nurses' Society on Addiction has been established with the philosophy that alcohol abuse and other drug abuse; eating disorders; sexual and relational addiction; and compulsive gambling, working, and spending are closely related behavior patterns. Additionally, educational course work related to alcohol and drug abuse is now recommended for inclusion in general nursing school curricula (Naegle, 1994).

There is a tendency in society to deal with substance abusers in stigmatizing, devaluing, coercive, and punitive ways. Negative attitudes are ubiquitous in our culture. As part of the larger culture, nurses may reflect these attitudes and have difficulty providing care to these individuals. The moral view of substance abuse implies that individuals choose to become sick, injured, or addicted.

Strong negative feelings that conflict with nursing's humanistic stance may also stem from personal experiences. Being the emotionally or physically abused spouse or child of a substance abuser can have lasting effects on nurses' attitudes toward substance-abusing clients. If nurses use alcohol or drugs to relieve stress or self-medicate dysphoric states, they may overidentify with the patient and deny the severity of the client's substance abuse.

Frequently, substance abusers are difficult clients in health care settings. When intoxicated, they may be raucous, unco-operative, and antisocial. When not intoxicated, they may exhibit none of these negative behaviors, or they may be manipulative and demanding, using flattery or intimi-dation to hide drug-seeking behavior. Although nurses may initially be warm and understanding, once aware of manipulative attempts, they may have difficulty maintain-ing an accepting, non-judgmental attitude. Realizing that recovery from substance abuse often comes very slowly can help nurses feel less pressured to get patients into treatment and be more able simply to raise consciousness by presenting the facts about addictive illness and leaving the decision making to the client.

Nursing Interventions in the Community

The problem of substance abuse is so widespread that it affects every community and its inhabitants in varying degrees. Hence, the community health nurse is often involved with substance abusers or their significant others. Substance abuse nursing interventions with clients and their caregivers are necessary to ensure the success of other health interventions. Ignoring substance abuse problems frequently leads to lack of progress and clients' inability to perform needed health practices. This is especially frustrating for the community health nurse and other professionals who have collaborated on a comprehensive plan to allow an individual with a serious health problem to remain at home and avoid placement in an institution.

There are many ways in which community health nurses can assist individuals, families, and groups experiencing substance abuse problems. Community health nurses may be the first to identify or suspect an alcohol or drug problem in the clients and families with whom they are working. Nurses in all care contexts should routinely assess sub-stance use patterns when performing client histories. The client history is a critical assessment and screening tool that can identify those at risk. Using current knowledge and theories about substance abuse etiology and risk factors should help identify those individuals predisposed to alcohol and drug use.

The community health nurse can be alert to environmental cues in the home that indicate substance abuse, such as empty liquor and pill bottles. An indication of prescription medication abuse is the patient's involvement with several physicians from whom narcotic analgesics and tranquilizers are obtained. This type of assessment can help with case finding and treatment referral, although the individual may have denied the existence of a substance abuse problem initially.

Denial of substance abuse or dependence may range from completely blocked awareness of the problem to partial disavowal of the detrimental effects of the substance use and abuse. One of the primary tasks for intervention and treatment with the substance-dependent individual is to increase the individual's awareness of the problem. Family and significant others can assist with this process by being more honest and direct with the individual about the detrimental effects of the substance abuse. Before this occurs, the significant others must overcome their own denial of the problem and its associated shame and guilt. Referrals to community education programs on substance abuse and dependence and mutual help groups such as Al-Anon and NarcAnon are helpful interventions for families and significant others.

The community health nurse may also involve the social network in getting the client into treatment. Although indivi-duals who are forced to enter treatment may not be willing to admit the severity of the abuse, they can still benefit from exposure to the treatment program and eventually begin recovery. Experiencing serious health consequences related to dependency may constitute "hitting bottom" for the individual. This may break through denial or collusion on the part of the family.

CASE STUDY   Application of the Nursing Process

Evelyn Weaver, a 72-year-old widow, was referred to the Visiting Nurses Association for follow-up after hospitalization for a seizure and fall she experienced in her home. Her hospital discharge diagnoses were ethyl alcohol abuse, seizure disorder, hypertension, and bruises and contusions on her left arm and leg. Her discharge medications were phenytoin sodium (Dilantin), 900 mg orally at bedtime; one multivitamin orally every day; hydrochlorothiazide, 50 mg orally every day; and methyldopa (Aldomet), 250 mg orally every day.

Mrs. Weaver lives alone in a two-bedroom house in a middle-class suburb. Her husband died 10 years earlier. Until 4 years previous, her daughter lived nearby with her two children and visited frequently. However, after a divorce, her daughter and grandchildren moved several hundred miles away and visited only once or twice a year. Mrs. Weaver has a married son in the area. He pays her bills once or twice a month but otherwise has minimal contact. Mrs. Weaver's primary occupation was homemaker and mother. She stopped driving after her last automobile accident and is not involved in any local community organizations.

ASSESSMENT

Individual

The visiting nurse performed an in-home nursing assessment of the client and obtained information through the interview and physical assessment. Mrs. Weaver admitted to an alcohol abuse problem but minimized its severity. She reported that she stopped drinking for 2 days on her own and had a seizure. She denied any past alcohol treatment, such as counseling or attendance at AA meetings, and said she was not interested in treatment. She has been abstinent from alcohol since her discharge from the hospital and thought she would remain that way. She admitted to some loneliness and social isolation. She also reported sleep disturbances (i.e., difficulty falling asleep and staying asleep) and decreased nutritional intake with loss of appetite. She denied using other psychoactive medication, such as hypnotics, narcotic analgesics, and tranquilizers, or benzodiazepines. She agreed to a social work referral to investigate attendant care and food delivery service for seniors (e.g., Meals on Wheels [MOW]) to help her.

Family

Telephone contact between the nurse and the client's daughter revealed that the daughter was very concerned about her mother. She denied that alcohol abuse was her mother's problem but thought poor nutrition and health practices were the cause of the hospitalization. She was anxious for the social work referral to obtain attendant care to assist her mother in the home. It took several calls and messages before the nurse was able to speak with the client's son. He said his mother was an alcoholic and that he tried unsuccessfully in the past to get her to stop drinking. He was unwilling to do more than visit her twice a month to pay her bills.

Community

The client's middle-class suburb did not have alcohol treatment services geared toward the elderly. AA meetings and private substance abuse counselors were available, but none of them was willing to make home visits and assist an elderly, homebound client. The local senior center did not have programs or education involving substance abuse and refused to allow AA meetings in their building because they feared their clients would be offended. The client's physician was aware of her alcohol abuse problem but did not know how to assist her. Referral to an inpatient program for substance abuse would not help because Mrs. Weaver refused to attend.

DIAGNOSIS

Individual

- Altered cardiovascular status secondary to hypertension
- Altered neurological status secondary to alcohol withdrawal seizures
- Knowledge deficit about addictive disease and effects of alcohol abuse
- Sleep pattern disturbance
- Alteration in nutrition (i.e., less than body requirements)
- Social isolation
- Ineffective individual coping related to inability to adjust to role of widow and maintain involvement in community activities
- Knowledge deficit about the effects and side effects of all of her medicines

Family

- Knowledge deficit about addictive disease and effects of excessive alcohol intake
- Knowledge deficit of treatment approaches available for alcohol abuse and the recovery process
- Alteration in family process secondary to poor communication and denial of alcohol abuse in client

Community

- Knowledge deficit in senior center staff regarding the prevalence of alcohol abuse problems in the elderly population and adverse health effects of alcohol consumption in the elderly
- Knowledge deficits in community agencies that assist alcohol abusers (e.g., local AA and counselors) regarding the need to make home visits and provide services geared to the elderly

PLANNING

Planning for Mrs. Weaver's care involved collaboration among her family, her physician, the agency's social worker, and the community alcohol treatment resources. Health teaching and counseling were the main approaches used to directly assist the client and her family. Indirect approaches involved networking with community agencies and supervising other caregivers.

INDIVIDUAL

Long-Term Goals
* Mrs. Weaver will continue to abstain from using alcohol.
* Mrs. Weaver's health will improve as indicated by increased weight, decreased hypertension and reported improvement in sleep.
* Mrs. Weaver will become more involved in community/social activities.

Short-Term Goals
* Mrs. Weaver will follow her post-hospitalization treatment regimen.
* Mrs. Weaver correctly verbalize information related to all of her medications (e.g. rationale for taking the medication, when to take it, potential side effects).
* Mrs. Weaver will seek additional counseling/treatment (e.g., AA) to assist her in staying alcohol-free.

Family
Long-Term Goals
* Mrs. Weaver's son and daughter will become more active in her care.
* The family will seek counseling to resolve past issues.

Short-Term Goals
* Mrs. Weaver's daughter will acknowledge that her mother has a problem with alcohol abuse.
* Communication will improve between Mrs. Weaver and her children.

Community
Long-Term Goals
* Health providers will in area senior centers will become more knowledgeable about the problem of alcohol abuse among elders.
* Community agencies that assist alcohol abusers will recognize the need to enhance services to elders.

INTERVENTION

Individual
* Nursing visits two to three times weekly initially to monitor the client's medication issues or problems as related to maintaining abstinence or medication dosing, cardiovascular status, neurological status, and nutritional status
* Social work referral to establish attendant assistance in the home and food delivery service for seniors
* Health teaching regarding addictive illness, effects of excessive alcohol intake on the body, alcohol withdrawal seizures, no-added-sodium diet, and effect of medications
* Health teaching about the client's medications, their effects and side effects, and the necessity of following recommended dosing schedules

* Referral for alcohol treatment counseling and AA meetings when the individual is receptive

Family
* Continued contact with the client's daughter and son to involve them in her care
* Health teaching to the family on the course and treatment of addictive illness and the adverse effects of alcohol abuse on the client and the family as related to functioning, cohesion, and communication
* Role modeling by the visiting nurse of the use of clear, direct, and nonjudgmental communication about the client's alcohol abuse problems

Community
* List of local and national referral resources for clients with substance abuse problems made available to physicians, with a particular focus on resources providing services for older or elderly substance abusers
* Health teaching to community groups (e.g., senior center, AA fellowship, and substance abuse counselors) regarding the prevalence of alcohol abuse in the elderly population and treatment and counseling approaches useful with this aggregate
* Collaboration with community organizations that provide outreach for homebound elderly to assist in identification and referral
* Establishment of a referral network (i.e., telephone hotline) of concerned older or elderly individuals recovering from alcohol abuse

EVALUATION

Individual
Initially, interventions proceeded smoothly. Mrs. Weaver obtained attendant help for 2 hours per day, 3 times weekly and also received food from MOW. The visiting nurse filled her medication-organizing container, or Medi-Set, weekly. The attendant made sure that the client took her medications and ate her meals and assisted Mrs. Weaver with personal care. Mrs. Weaver remained abstinent from alcohol during this time but refused any treatment or counseling for her alcohol abuse problem. However, after 3 weeks, she was rehospitalized after falling at home again. She was diagnosed with phenytoin toxicity; this occurred because she had secretly been taking extra phenytoin at night to help her sleep.

After a few days, Mrs. Weaver was discharged from the hospital and the Visiting Nurses Association reopened the case. Private attendant care and MOW were also reinstated. This time, the physician discontinued the phenytoin and recommended that the client receive alcohol counseling. The client did follow-up with the counseling referrals given to her by the visiting nurse, but her social situation did not change. She remained very isolated and refused involvement with AA.

Continued

CASE STUDY   Application of the Nursing Process (cont'd)

Family

A third hospitalization occurred within a few weeks when Mrs. Weaver ingested an excessive amount of alcohol in combination with her hypertensive medications. She became physically ill and required treatment. After this hospitalization, her daughter decided to take action. She moved her mother into a retirement community that provided meals and social activities. The visiting nurse continued to follow the case in the new setting.

Her daughter encouraged her to become involved with the social activities at the community. The visiting nurse continued to remain active in the client's care by arranging for aftercare, focusing on providing goal-specific social support for abstinence and general support for addressing the client's concerns and issues, particularly as related to feelings of isolating loss and transitions. The nurse also worked with Mrs. Weaver's daughter and encouraged both to attempt to involve Mrs. Weaver's son.

Community

Staff from the retirement community contacted an area AA group and other agencies who work with substance abusers. A social worker agreed to explore ways make all involved more aware of this problem and to set up potential interventions.

LEVELS OF PREVENTION

Primary

- Involves health teaching to individuals and groups on risk factors, early symptoms of substance abuse, adverse health and social consequences, addictive disease process, and available treatment services
- Need to gear educational approaches to the more vulnerable aggregates (e.g., adolescents, minorities, mentally ill, women, and elderly)

Secondary

- Involves screening and early treatment approaches aimed at minimizing health and social consequences of substance abuse
- Involvement of physicians, nurses, and other health care professionals in various health care settings in this process
- Use of various screening and assessment tools and referrals to treatment services and mutual help organizations

Tertiary

- Involves more direct approaches (e.g., detoxification and inpatient or outpatient treatment) to halt the physiologically damaging effects of the substance abuse (e.g., liver disease, organic mental deficits, and gastritis)
- Frequent use of medications to treat the symptoms of substance abuse–related disorders or as part of aversion therapy (e.g., disulfiram)
- Services provided by medical practitioners, treatment services, and mutual help organizations generally advocate abstinence from the substance and improving the individual's health status

This case study illustrates the possible complexity and frustration involved in helping the substance abuser. Significant others and the medical community must be involved to help the community health nurse provide care. Often, the social situation, living situation, or social acquaintances must also change to maintain long-term recovery. However, with patience, persistence, and a caring, nonjudgmental attitude, the nurse can often be effective in helping clients with substance abuse problems attain recovery and improve their health status.

The trust that develops in a caring nursing relationship can support disclosure of substance abuse problems and decrease denial in the client or family members. A realistic and positive attitude toward the person with substance abuse can provide families with hope. Community health nurses must have knowledge of available community resources. One of the primary roles of the community health nurse in helping substance abusers is to facilitate contact with helping agencies such as local treatment programs or mutual help groups. Collaboration with the client's physician is helpful should medical detoxification be necessary. Community health nurses should assume a validating, nonjudgmental position toward the whole family and should avoid being confrontational, as it fans the fires of resistance. It is imperative that nurses ascribe a noble intention to their substance-abusing clients and families and avoid negativity or preaching.

Other traditional community health nursing roles and interventions also are appropriate to use with substance abusers. Examples follow:

- Health teaching regarding addictive illness and addictive effects of different substances
- Providing direct care for abuse-related and dependence-related medical problems
- Counseling clients and families about problems related to substance abuse
- Collaborating with other disciplines to ensure continuity of care
- Coordinating health care services for the client to prevent prescription drug abuse and avoid fragmentation of care
- Providing consultation to nonmedical professionals and lay personnel
- Facilitating care through appropriate referrals and follow-up

SUMMARY

This chapter provides an overview of the complex, multifaceted phenomenon of substance abuse and its manifestations in the community. The focus is on social, economic, political, and health-related aspects of substance abuse. In addition, the concept of substance abuse is related to the more general concept of addictive behaviors, not just those related to drug or alcohol abuse.

From the review of the various etiological theories, it is clear that there is not one causative factor in the development of substance abuse. Consequently, one treatment approach does not apply to all substance abusers. Recognition of multiple factors and issues specific to vulnerable aggregates, such as women, adolescents, the elderly, and people of color, must be considered when developing intervention plans and strategies and when evaluating outcomes. Resources for prevention and intervention at the individual, family, and community levels are outlined and should be familiar to nurses practicing in the community.

LEARNING ACTIVITIES

1. Attend a local AA, Narcotics Anonymous, or Cocaine Anonymous meeting and share impressions with classmates.
2. Attend a local Al-Anon, NarcAnon, or Adult Children of Alcoholics meeting and share impressions with classmates.
3. Visit a local treatment center that provides detoxification, inpatient, or outpatient treatment and determine the center's treatment philosophy and the types of services it provides to patients and their families.
4. Visit a treatment program for women and determine how the particular needs of this population are assessed and addressed.
5. Learn about the drug and alcohol education programs at a local community college or high school.
6. Contact mental health services or substance abuse treatment services at the county or city level and obtain a list of local treatment and education resources.

REFERENCES

Adams WL, Cox N: Epidemiology of problem drinking among elderly people. In Gurnack AM, editor: *Older adults misuse of alcohol, medicines and other drugs: Research and practice issues,* New York, 1997, Springer.

American Psychiatric Association: *Diagnostic and statistical manual of mental disorders,* ed 4, text revision, Washington, DC, 2000, The Author.

Anda R: Adverse childhood experiences, alcoholic parents, and later risk of alcoholism and depression, *Psychiatr Serv* 53(8):1001-1009, 2002.

Ashman TA: Screening for substance abuse in individuals with traumatic brain injury, *Brain Inj* 18(2):191-202, 2004.

Astley SJ: Fetal alcohol syndrome prevention in Washington State: evidence of success. *Paediatr Perinatal Epidemiol* 18:344-351, 2004.

Beullens J: Screening for alcohol abuse and dependence in older people using DSM criteria: a review, *Aging Ment Health* 8(1): 76-82, 2004.

Block RI, Erwin WJ, Ghoneim MM: Chronic drug use and cognitive impairments, *Pharmacol Biochem Behav* 73(3):491-504, 2002.

Brecher E: *Licit and illicit drugs,* Boston, 1972, Little, Brown.

Brown R: Vitamin deficiency and voluntary alcohol consumption, *Q J Stud Alcohol* 30: 592-597, 1969.

Bureau of Justice Statistics: *2002: at a glance,* Washington, DC, 2002, The Author, http://www.ojp.usdoj.gov/bjs/pub/pdf/bjsg02.pdf.

Bureau of Justice Statistics: *Drug use and crime,* The Author, http://www.ojp.usdoj.gov/bjs/dcf/duc.htm.

Carmen B: Efficacy and safety of naltrexone and acamprosate in the treatment of alcohol dependence: a systematic review, *Addiction* 99:811-828, 2004.

Carroll K: Integrating psychotherapy and pharmacotherapy in substance abuse treatment. In Rotgers F, Morgenstern J, Walters S, editors: *Treating substance abuse: theory and technique,* ed 2, New York, 2003, Guilford Press.

Centers for Disease Control and Prevention: Impaired driving fact sheet, 2006, The Author, http://www.cdc.gov/ncipc/factsheets/drving.htm.

Chavkin W et al: National survey of the states: policies and practices regarding drug-using pregnant women, *Am J Public Health* 88(1): 117, 1998.

Cherpitel CJ: Brief screening instruments for alcoholism, *Alcohol Health Res World* 21(4): 348-351, 1997.

Cook LJ: Educating women about the hidden dangers of alcohol, *J Psychosoc Nurs Ment Health Serv* 42(6):24-31, 54-59, 2004.

Cretzmeyer M et al: Treatment of methamphetamine abuse: research findings and clinical directions, *J Subst Abuse Treat* 24:267-277, 2003.

Des Jarlais DC: Assessing syringe exchange programs, *Addiction* 99(9):1081-1082, 2004.

Drucker E: Drug prohibition and public health: 25 years of evidence, *Public Health Rep* 114: 15-29, 1999.

Erickson PG: Introduction: the three phases of harm reduction: an examination of emerging concepts, methodologies and critiques, *Subst Use Misuse* 34(1):1-7, 1999.

Ewing JA: Detecting alcoholism: the CAGE questionnaire, *JAMA* 252:1905-1907, 1984.

Fals-Stewart W, O'Farrell T, Birchler G: Family therapy techniques. In Rotgers F, Morgenstern J, Walters S, editors: *Treating substance abuse: theory and technique,* ed 2, New York, 2003, Guilford Press.

Faltz B, Rinaldi J: *AIDS and substance abuse: a training manual for health care professionals,*

San Francisco, 1987, Regents of the University of California.

Friedmann MM, Bowden VR, Jones EG: *Family nursing: research, theory, and practice,* ed 5, New Jersey, 2003, Prentice Hall.

Goldberg R: *Taking sides: clashing views on controversial issues in drugs and society,* ed 6, Guilford, CT, 2004, McGraw-Hill.

Goldstein A: *Addiction: from biology to drug policy,* ed 2, New York, 2001, Oxford University Press.

Greenberg M, Schneider D: Violence in American cities: young black males is the answer, but what is the question? *Soc Sci Med* 39: 179-187, 1994.

Gruber AJ, Pope HG: Psychiatric and medical effects of anabolic-androgenic steroid use in women, *Psychother Psychosom* 69:19-26, 2000.

Haight W et al: "In these bleak days": parent methamphetamine abuse and child welfare in the rural Midwest, *Children Youth Serv Rev* 27(8):949-971, 2005.

Hall JM: Geography of childhood sexual abuse: women's narratives of their childhood environments, *Adv Nurs Sci* 18:29-47, 1996a.

Hall JM: The pervasive effects of childhood sexual abuse in lesbians' recovery from alcohol problems, *Subst Use Misuse* 31: 225-239, 1996b.

Hanson GR, Venturelli P, Fleckenstein A: *Drugs and society,* ed 9, Boston, 2002, Jones and Bartlett.

Holtzworth-Munroe A: Typologies of men who are maritally violent: scientific and clinical implications, *J Interpers Violence* 19(12): 1369-1389, 2004.

Johnston LD et al: *Monitoring the Future: National results on adolescent drug use: overview of key findings, 2004,* NIH Pub No 05-5726, Bethesda Md, 2005, National Institute on Drug Abuse.

Kearney MH: Drug treatment for women: traditional models and new directions, *J Obstet Gynecol Neonatal Nurs* 26(4):459-478, 1999.

Keller M: On the loss of control phenomenon in alcoholism, *Br J Addict* 67:153-166, 1972.

Kendler K, Prescott C: Cocaine use, abuse, and dependence in a population based sample of female twins, *Br J Psychiatry* 173:345-350, 1998.

Kurtz E: *Not god: a history of alcoholics anonymous,* Center City, Minn, 1979, Hazelden Educational Services.

Kuyper LM et al: Factors associated with sex trade involvement among male participants in a prospective study of injection drug users, *Sex Transm Infect* 80(6):531-535, 2004.

Larimer ME, Marlatt GA: Applications of relapse prevention with moderation goals, *J Psychoactive Drugs* 22:189-195, 1990.

Latimer W: Integrated family and cognitive-behavioral therapy for adolescent substance abusers: a stage I efficacy study, *Drug Alcohol Depend* 71(3):303-317, 2003.

Leshner A: Addiction is a brain disease and it matters, *Science* 278:45-47, 1997.

Levine MR, Rennie WP: Pre-employment urine drug testing of hospital employees: future questions and review of current literature, *Occup Environ Med* 61:318-324, 2004.

Logan BK, Fligner CL, Haddix T: Cause and manner of death in fatalities involving methamphetamine, *J Forensic Sci* 43:28-34, 1998.

MacCoun RJ: Toward a psychology of harm reduction, *Amer J Psychol* 53(11):1199-1208, 1998.

Mann K, Lehert P, Morgan M: The efficacy of acamprosate in the maintenance of abstinence in alcohol-dependent individuals: results of a meta-analysis, *Alcoholism* 28(1):51-63, 2004.

Messinger DS: The maternal lifestyle study: cognitive, motor, and behavioral outcomes of cocaine-exposed and opiate-exposed infants through three years of age, *Pediatrics* 113(6): 1677-1685, 2004.

Montagne M, Scott DM: Prevention of substance abuse problems: models, factors and processes, *Int J Addict* 28:1177-1208, 1993.

Mylant M: Adolescent children of alcoholics: vulnerable or resilient? *J Am Psychiatr Nurses Assoc* 8(2):57-64, 2002.

Naegle M: The need for alcohol abuse-related education in nursing curricula, *Alcohol Health Res World* 18:154-157, 1994.

Naegle M, D'Avanzo C: *Addictions and substance abuse: strategies for advance nursing practice,* Upper Saddle River, NJ, 2001, Prentice Hall.

National Institute on Alcohol Abuse and Alcoholism: *Ninth special report to the US Congress on alcohol and health,* Washington, DC, 1997, US Government Printing Office, http://www.niaaa.nih.gov.

National Institute on Drug Abuse: *The economic costs of alcohol and drug abuse in the United States, 1992,* NIH Pub No BKD265, Rockville, Md, 1997, US Department of Health and Human Services.

National Institute on Drug Abuse: *Principles of drug addiction treatment: a research-based guide,* NIH Pub No 99-4180, Washington, DC, 1999, Government Printing Office.

National Institute on Drug Abuse: *2000 Research report: steroid abuse and addiction,* NIH Pub No 00-3721, Washington, DC, April 2000, Government Printing Office.

National Institute on Drug Abuse: *Stress and substance abuse: a special report,* updated Sept 12, 2005, The Author, http://www.nida.nih.gov/stressanddrugabuse.html.

Obert JL, London ED, Rawson RA: Incorporating brain research findings into standard treatment: an example using the Matrix model, *J Subst Abuse Treat* 7(4):107-113, 2002.

Paone D, Alpern J: Pregnancy policing: policy of harm, *Int J Drug Policy* 9:101, 1998.

Pelham M: Childhood predictors of adolescent substance use in a longitudinal study of children with ADHD, *J Abnorm Psychol* 112(3):497-507, 2003.

Pope HG Jr, Kouri EM, Hudson MD: Effects of supraphysiologic doses of testosterone on mood and aggression in normal men, *Arch Gen Psychiatry* 57(2):133-140, 2000.

Quazi M: Effective drug-free workplace plan uses worker testing as a deterrent, *Occup Health Saf* 6:26-32, 1993.

Rawson R, Gonzales R, Brethen P: Treatment of methamphetamine use disorders: an update, *J Subst Abuse Treat* 23:145-150, 2002.

Simpson D: A conceptual framework for drug treatment process and outcomes, *J Subst Abuse Treat* 27(2):99-121, 2004.

Stinchfield R, Winters K: Predicting adolescent drug abuse treatment outcome with the Personal Experience Inventory (PEI), *J Child Adolesc Subst Abuse* 13(2):103-120, 2003.

Straussner SL: *Ethnocultural factors in substance abuse treatment,* New York, 2003, Guilford Press.

Sullivan ML, Martinez CM, Gennis P, Gallagher EJ The cardiac toxicity of anabolic steroids, *Prog Cardiovasc Dis* 41(1):1-15, 1998.

Substance Abuse and Mental Health Services Administration: *Overview of findings from the 2002 National Survey on Drug Use and Health,* NHSDA Series H-21, USDHHS Pub No SMA 03-3774, Rockville, Md, 2003, The Author.

Substance Abuse and Mental Health Services Administration: *Drug Abuse Warning Network, 2003: interim national estimates of drug-related emergency department visits,* DAWN Series D-26, USDHHS Pub No SMA 04-3972, Rockville, Md, 2004a, The Author.

Substance Abuse and Mental Health Services Administration: *Mortality data from the Drug Abuse Warning Network, 2002,* DAWN Series D-25, USDHHS Pub No SMA 04-3875, Rockville, Md, 2004b, The Author.

Substance Abuse and Mental Health Services Administration: *Results from the 2003 National Survey on Drug Use and Health: national findings,* NSDUH Series H-25, USDHHS Pub No SMA 04-3964, Rockville, Md, 2004c, The Author.

Substance Abuse and Mental Health Service Administration: *Overview of findings from the 2004 National Survey on Drug Use and Health,* NSDUH Series H-27, USDHHS Pub No SMA 05-4061, Rockville Md, 2005, The Author.

Sweeney M, Penner S: A study of employees' attitudes toward workplace drug testing: nursing implications, *J Addict Nurs* 9(4):156-163, 1997.

Tatarsky A: Harm reduction psychotherapy: Extending the reach of traditional substance abuse treatment, *J Subst Abuse Treat* 25(4):249-256, 2003.

Trinkoff A, Storr C: Substance abuse among nurses: differences between specialties, *Am J Public Health* 88(4):581-585, 1998.

US Department of Health and Human Services: *Healthy People 2010,* ed 2, Washington, DC, 2000, The Author.

Van der Kolk BA, McFarlane AC, Weisaeth L, editors: *Traumatic stress: the effects of overwhelming experience on mind, body and society,* New York, 1996, Guilford Press.

Volm BA, de Araujo IE: Methamphetamine activates reward circuitry in drug naïve human subjects, *Neuropsychopharmacology* 29(9): 1715-1722, 2004.

Wetherington C, Roman S: *Drug addiction research and the health of women,* NIH Pub No 98-4289, 1998, National Institute on Drug Abuse, www.health.org.

Wodak A: Harm reduction: Australia as a case study, *Bull N Y Acad Med* 72(2):339-347, 1995.

Zautcke JL et al: Geriatric trauma in the state of Illinois: substance use and injury patterns, *Am J Emerg Med* 20(1):14-17, 2002.

Violence

Linda Stevenson ▪ Alice Pappas

MEDIA RESOURCES

Additional Material for Study, Review, and Further Exploration

evolve Website at http://evolve.elsevier.com/Nies

❖ Quiz ❖ Case Studies ❖ Content Updates ❖ Glossary ❖ WebLinks ❖ Resource Tool
25A Planning for Safety

OBJECTIVES

Upon completion of this chapter, the reader will be able to do the following:

1. Describe the concept of community violence.
2. Identify long-term effects of violence on society.
3. Identify at-risk populations for violence and the role of public health in dealing with the epidemic of violence.
4. Describe the role of the nurse in primary, secondary, and tertiary prevention of violence.
5. Identify protection measures necessary for nurses and others working in situations where violence is prevalent.

KEY TERMS

cycle theory of violence	domestic violence	intentional injuries	physical neglect
date rape	elder abuse	intimate partner violence	sexual abuse
date rape drugs	emotional abuse	(IPV)	shaken baby syndrome
dating violence	emotional neglect	physical abuse	violence

CHAPTER OUTLINE

OVERVIEW OF VIOLENCE

HISTORY OF VIOLENCE

SCOPE AND PATTERNS OF ABUSE AND VIOLENCE
    Homicide
    Suicide
    Nonhomicide and Nonsuicide Abuse
    Influence of Firearms

VIOLENCE AND SELECTED AGGREGATES
    Youth-Related Violence
    Domestic Violence

    Child Abuse
    Elder Abuse

VIOLENCE FROM A PUBLIC HEALTH PERSPECTIVE
    Healthy People 2010 and Violence

PREVENTION OF VIOLENCE
    Primary Prevention
    Secondary Prevention
    Tertiary Prevention

SAFETY OF THE HEALTH PROFESSIONAL

Two adolescent males ambushed their high school classmates with guns, killing 13 and wounding many others before they killed themselves. A young woman who complained to the police about being stalked was killed when she opened a package delivered to her apartment. A deranged man opened fire on a Jewish preschool. A black male was dragged to death by five white supremacists. A mentally ill mother drowned her five children in the bathtub. Taking advantage of the anonymity of the Internet, a young male tracks down a former girlfriend and sends hundreds of violent and threatening emails. A drunken driver killed five family members as they returned home from church on Christmas Eve. Terrorists bombed a federal building to retaliate for perceived governmental injustices. Two college women visited a rape crisis center suspecting they were sexually assaulted by their dates, who tainted their drinks with a date rape drug. A 6-year-old boy shot and killed a 6-year-old girl because she yelled at him the day before.

The last four out of five U.S. Surgeon Generals have declared violence as a national public health epidemic. When viewed from a public health perspective, violence is clearly a learned behavior that can be changed and prevented.

The purpose of this chapter is to explore the influence of violence from a public health perspective as it relates to individuals, families, and communities. Included in this chapter are discussions of the effects of violence on society in terms of death, illness, and injury; homicides and suicides among emerging high-risk groups; death and injury from use of firearms; the direct influence of violence on individuals and society; public health interventions to reduce violence; the roles and responsibilities of the community health nurse in dealing with those experiencing violence; and measures to increase awareness of violence in the workplace.

OVERVIEW OF VIOLENCE

Violence is the intentional use of physical force against another person or against oneself, which results in or has a high likelihood of resulting in injury or death. Violence includes suicidal acts and interpersonal violence such as psychological, sexual, and/or physical abuse (Rosenberg, O'Connell, and Kenneth, 1992). In public health, injuries from violence are referred to as **intentional injuries**. Violence threatens the health and well-being of many people of all ages across the United States. On an average day in 2002, approximately 48 people died from homicide, and 87 people committed suicide. (Centers for Disease Control and Prevention, National Center for Injury Prevention and Control [CDC-NCIPC], 2004c).

The reasons for the high rate of violence in society are complex. "Alvin Toffler in his book *Powershift* identifies violence or the threat of violence as one of the three fundamental sources of all human power, the other two are money and knowledge. Of the three, violence is the lowest form of power because it can only be used to punish" (Koop and Lundberg, 1992, p. 3075).

The five most frequently cited underlying causes of or risk factors for violence are as follows:

1. Access to firearms
2. Polydrug and alcohol abuse
3. Poverty, unemployment, economic dependency
4. Specific personal characteristics of victims and perpetrators (e.g., between 15 and 34 years of age, 65 years of age or older, urban dweller, dependent upon caregivers, or socially isolated)
5. Having been a witness to violence (particularly as a child witnessing family violence)

Other causes mentioned less frequently include racism, lack of academic opportunity, gang membership, lack of realistic expectations regarding child development, absence of moral and behavioral guidance for young people, and exposure to media violence (Krug et al., 2004; Winett, 1998).

Research has demonstrated a link between violence in television shows that children watch and heightened aggressive behavior. Watching violent behavior on television makes it harder for children to distinguish between reality and fantasy. The public health community believes that repeated exposure to media violence leads to emotional desensitization to real-life violence (Cook et al., 2000). Media violence includes the exposure to and participation in violent video games that often distort the role of women and reward aggressive behavior.

Access to firearms is easy and even children are carrying guns to elementary schools to protect themselves. Nationwide, during 2005, 6.5% of children reported they had carried a weapon on school property (CDC, 2006). A high level of violence is associated with the sale of illegal drugs. Killings, either execution-style shootings or drive-by shootings, are often the result of a failed drug deal or drug turf battles.

Anger abounds in society among individuals, particularly adolescent males, who have not been taught how to control or deal with anger in a nonaggressive fashion (Chan et al., 2004). Adolescents and children are increasingly using violence as a means of resolving conflicts. Many studies link abuse during childhood with violent behavior in adult life. Children are often brutalized by a parent or other family member, or they may witness one parent beating the other. Research shows a strong correlation between childhood abuse and risk for exhibiting abusive behavior as an adult (CDC-NCIPC, 2004b). A study of adult male prisoners convicted of first-degree murder found that two thirds had experienced "continuous, remorseless brutality during childhood" (Mason, 1991).

HISTORY OF VIOLENCE

Violence is not limited to the present day or to the United States. Since the beginning of time, humans have dealt violently with other humans. In the Bible story, Cain killed his brother Abel out of jealousy and anger. Infanticide, or the killing of unwanted newborn children, has been practiced throughout history. For example, children were left to die from exposure or some other means when they were born a female, a twin, sickly, or deformed. Children, especially firstborn children, were often sacrificed for religious reasons. Infanticide was not condemned until early in the fifth century; however, this did not protect children in many societies. Children were the property of the father and he could do whatever he wanted with them (Campbell and Humphreys, 1993).

Throughout the ages, corporal punishment has been used as a means of controlling children. Biblical reference to corporal punishment has often been used as a justification for some types of child abuse. To some parents, "spare the rod and spoil the child" (Proverbs, 13:24) implies an imperative to abusively discipline an errant child. Physical child abuse has also been included in the education process. The idea of "beating some sense into him" was considered necessary to ensure that the lesson was learned. In 1874, the first legal protection against child abuse in the United States occurred when the Society for the Prevention of Cruelty to Animals (SPCA) intervened to protect an 8-year-old girl. As a result of the notoriety associated with this case, the New York Society for the Prevention of Cruelty to Children was organized later that year (Campbell and Humphreys, 1993).

Even nursery rhymes that adults read to small children seem to condone violence against them. Consider the following Mother Goose nursery rhyme:

There was an old woman who lived in a shoe.
She had so many children she didn't know what to do.
She gave them some broth without any bread,
And whipped them all soundly and sent them to bed.
         (Mother Goose Nursery Rhymes, 2000, pp. 195-196)

Wife beating was legal in the United States until 1824. Wives were seen as their husbands' chattel and could be beaten for such offenses as "nagging too much." In fact, the common phrase "rule of thumb" was derived from English law that allowed a man to beat his wife with a cane no wider than his thumb. Biblical interpretation of "wives be subject to your husband" (Ephesians, 5:22) still provides some males with a faulty rationalization for wife beating.

The silence that long surrounded domestic violence is derived from a historical perspective of women as their husbands' property. The problem of assault against women was not explored in America until the Civil Rights Movement of the 1960s. Marital rape was not considered an offense in the United States until 1980; marital rape is still not an offense in some states. In the last two decades, additional cultural issues have surfaced in the United States regarding domestic abuse. These include female circumcision and genital mutilation, abuse between gay partners, and the reality that men are also victims of domestic violence.

Elder abuse is also a problem that is not new. In pre-industrial Europe, legal documents were commonly drawn to allow the older parent to continue to sit at the family table and use the front door. The problem is of greater magnitude now because people are living longer, which results in increased cases of dependent and vulnerable adults. Elder abuse frequently goes undetected because there is a lack of awareness on the part of health care professionals and society. The exact prevalence of elder abuse is unknown because there is a lack of mandatory reporting in all states.

SCOPE AND PATTERNS OF ABUSE AND VIOLENCE

Homicide

One of America's greatest public health challenges is violence reduction. According to the CDC, the United States ranks first in the industrial world in violent death rates. Murder and suicide together claim the lives of approximately 50,000 individuals each year. The Federal Bureau of Investigation reported that in 2004 there were 586,558 arrests for violent crime (Federal Bureau of Investigation/U.S. Department of Justice [FBI/USDoJ], 2005). Furthermore, more than 70% of homicides are committed with a firearm. Many states and the District of Columbia report more deaths caused by firearms than motor vehicle accidents.

Homicide claimed the lives of 16,137 individuals in 2004. Certain populations are at greater risk for death by homicide. These include young people, women, and black and Hispanic males. Strikingly, although only 12% of U.S. residents are black, almost half of all murder victims are black, and in

RESEARCH HIGHLIGHTS

Physical Violence Among Poor Women

A prospective study of the multiple risk and protective factors for physical violence among impoverished women:

A sample of 810 women was taken from a group of women in Los Angeles shelters and in public housing; and was largely composed of minorities (84.9%). The researchers found that more than 30% of the women experienced physical or sexual abuse before the age of 18 years, and that 15% had experienced physical violence during the 6 months prior to the interview. Additional predictors of victimization include: previous experience of homelessness, experience of violence during childhood, history of two or more partners, alcohol or drug use by the woman and by the primary partner, and history of mental health problems (e.g., previous diagnosis of mental illness, reports of psychological distress).

Wenzel SL et al: Physical violence against impoverished women: a longitudinal analysis of risks and protective factors. *Women's Health Issues* 14(5):144-154, 2004.

almost 93% of cases, blacks killed other blacks (FBI/USDoJ, 2005).

Homicide and Youths

Homicide is the second leading cause of death among Americans aged 10 to 24 years and the leading cause of death among black males aged 15 to 34 years. In 2001 an average of 15 young people were murdered each day in the United States, a tragic loss of unfilled promise (CDC-NCIPC, 2004h). Children are not only victims of homicide, but increasingly younger children are committing murder. Incidents of school-related homicide have increased dramatically. Between 1994 and 1999, 172 students ages 5 to 18 years were killed on or near school grounds or at school-related activities (Anderson et al., 2001).

The United States has the dubious distinction of having the highest youth homicide rate among the 26 wealthiest nations (Palestra, 1999). In January 1999 the American Academy of Pediatrics labeled the incidence of violence in children an "epidemic," which was the first time a U.S. medical association identified violence as a health issue.

Women and Homicide

Homicide is the fourth leading cause of death from injury among females; the rate is substantially higher among black females than among white females. Domestic violence is the leading cause of homicide among women in all ethnic groups. Approximately 11% of murder victims are killed by an intimate, such as a spouse, ex-spouse, boyfriend, or girlfriend, and female murder victims are more likely to have been killed by an intimate than males (USDoJ, 2004). Women aged 20 to 29 years are at greatest risk of being killed by an intimate partner (Paulozzi, et al., 2001).

Suicide

Often ignored or overlooked, suicide is a leading cause of death for all Americans. More people die from suicide than from homicide in the United States; suicide took the lives of 31,655 people in 2002 (CDC-NCIPC, 2004g).

Suicide is becoming common in increasingly younger age-groups. For young people aged 10 to 24 years, suicide is the fourth leading cause of death, behind motor vehicle crashes, unintentional injury, and homicide (CDC, 2004). Suicide among the young is particularly problematic because young people do not completely fit the depression profile. Suicide is often an impulsive act that results from trouble at home, in school, or with the police; combined with weapons in the home, this creates a deadly combination.

Other high-risk populations include white males, who account for 72% of all suicides (83% of suicides among people aged 65 years or older); Native Americans and Alaskan Natives (particularly young males), whose rates are 1.5 times the national incidence; and unmarried jail inmates (CDC-NCIPC, 2000b).

Fifty-five percent of all suicides were committed with a firearm in 2001 (Anderson et al., 2003). Not surprisingly, research indicates that suicidal individuals are 5 times more likely to kill themselves if a gun is in the home (Kellerman et al., 1992). Women with a history of sexual assault are more likely to attempt or commit suicide than other women (Felitti et al., 1998). Women who attempt suicide are 3 times more likely to have been physically abused by intimate partners than women who made no attempt, and those who attempted were 3 times more likely to have posttraumatic stress disorder (El Bassel et al., 2001).

Nonhomicide and Nonsuicide Abuse

Each year, more than one million Americans visit emergency rooms for violent injury (CDC-NCIPC, 2004f). Assault, primarily in the context of marital or dating relationships, is a major source of injury among females. Studies of college (White and Koss, 1991) and high school (Gray and Foshee, 1997) students suggest that both males and females inflict and receive dating violence in equal proportion. However, the motivation for violence by women is more often for defensive purposes.

The 2000 National Violence Against Women Survey indicated that 1.5 million women are raped or physically assaulted by an intimate partner each year in the United States (Tjaden and Thoennes, 2000). The true incidence of women who are abused and seek emergency room help is unknown, but the incidence in studies ranges from 20% to 35% (Wilson, 1998). The exact incidence remains unknown, because a number of sources refute these statistics.

A new category of violence has arisen from the occasional news articles alluding to the hidden world of prison violence. These articles include allegations of physical abuse as well as horrifying reports of rape by both corrections officers and other inmates. The public and the judicial systems have expressed little sympathy for this population for a variety of reasons, including disbelief, denial, and the notion that "that the crime is a natural by-product of incarceration" (Michaels, 2005). There is no research available to reflect the long-term effects on these victims or society when they are released.

The impact of media violence continues to be debated. The first known quote related to entertainment violence is from St. Augustine, who commented in 380 BC that his society was addicted to gladiator games and "drunk with the fascination of bloodshed." In the early years of the twenty-first century, there is a growing consensus that something within media violence has changed (Media Awareness Network, 2005). There has been a significant increase in the amount of graphic sexual and sadistic displays of violence, particularly directed against women. This is evident in media games, music lyrics, television, and movies. The exposure of children to violence on television is dramatic; 87.9% of all violent acts appear before 9 AM, and 39% before 8 PM, which are prime viewing hours for children (Media Awareness Network, 2005).

Influence of Firearms

Approximately 192 million privately owned firearms exist in the United States, and 65 million are handguns. In 2002 almost 18,000 people were murdered in the United States; firearms were used in more than two thirds of those murders (CDC, 2005).

People may feel that they need a handgun in their home for protection; however, statistics do not support the logic of keeping a gun at home. Indeed, the risk of gun accidents and violence in the home far outweighs the protective factor. Guns kept in the home for self-protection are 43 times more likely to kill a family member or a friend than an attacker. Furthermore, the presence of a gun in the home triples the risk of homicide in the home and increases the risk of suicide fivefold (CDC, 1999a).

In 2002 almost 30,000 Americans were killed with firearms (combining numbers of homicides, suicides, and accidents), which made gun-related injuries the second leading cause of death from injury in the United States after motor-vehicle–related incidents (CDC, 2005). In comparison, 33,651 Americans were killed in the Korean War, and 58,148 Americans were killed in the Vietnam War. Palestra (1999) compared the number of deaths by handguns in the United States with other industrialized nations and found the following:

- New Zealand: 2 deaths
- Japan: 15 deaths
- Great Britain: 30 deaths
- Canada: 106 deaths
- Germany: 213 deaths
- United States: 9390 deaths

It is acknowledged that guns do not *cause* violence, but there is no question that they greatly raise the severity of the health consequences. Major trauma centers report that between 20% and 25% of nonfatal gunshot wounds cause permanent neurological impairment. The violence produced by guns is more severe and more likely to lead to death instead of injury alone.

The cost of violence from guns is staggering. Violence related to firearms costs the United States 1 billion dollars annually in direct costs. Indirect costs, including loss of productivity, mental health treatment, rehabilitation, legal and judicial costs, add more than 100 billion dollars to the cost of violence. To exacerbate the problem, approximately 85% of this is financed by taxpayers because many of the victims lack insurance (Cook and Ludwig, 2002).

TABLE 25-1   Risk Factors for Youth-Related Violence*

RISK FACTOR	COMMENT
Poverty	The risk factor most closely correlated with youth violence is low family income.
Repeated exposure to violence	Children in inner-city neighborhoods are often exposed to chronic and extreme violence, enough that inner-city children often exhibit the same symptoms of posttraumatic stress as children living in war-torn countries.
Drugs	Not only does a pharmacological connection exist between aggressive behavior and consumption of drugs and alcohol, but there is also a financial connection between the drug trade and violence.
Easy access to firearms	Approximately 50% of all households in the United States have a gun.
Unstable family life	Roughly 70% of juvenile offenders come from single-parent homes. Single-parent homes correlate with elevated rates of school dropout, which correlates with elevated violent crime rates.
Family violence	Juvenile delinquency has been found to correlate with a history of childhood abuse and neglect. Alcohol and/or drug use is closely associated with domestic violence.
Delinquent peer groups	Gangs are using more lethal weapons to engage in increasingly violent behavior.
Media violence	By the time a child reaches seventh grade, he or she has witnessed 8000 murders and more than 100,000 other acts of violence on television. Witnessing violence increases short- and long-term aggression, desensitization, and fear in children.

Modified from Ruttenberg H: The limited promise of public health methodologies to prevent youth violence, *Yale Law J* 103:1885, 1994.
*Multiple risk factors have a cumulative effect.

Discussion regarding firearms often evokes a heated response from opponents of gun control who see violence as the work of aberrant individuals. According to their view, the focus on guns as a major public health threat is misdirected in comparison with other health issues. Many opponents of gun control cite their constitutional "right to bear arms" and interpret efforts to control guns as an assault on their personal freedom. They believe that "law-abiding citizens" have a right to protect themselves despite the hazards of private gun ownership.

VIOLENCE AND SELECTED AGGREGATES

Youth-Related Violence

Violence is taking a toll on youth as an aggregate population. Violent crimes among youth are increasing, and such crimes as homicide, rape, robbery, and aggravated assault are much more prevalent among adolescents than adults. The rate of violence among adolescents is about twice that found among the general population. Assaults are significantly higher among adolescent males, higher for black than white teens, and higher for those with lower household incomes (USDHHS, 2000).

The average age of homicide offenders and victims has decreased in recent years. Most of the increased homicide rates among American youth are attributable to death caused by firearms. Teens are more likely to die from gunshot wounds than from all natural causes combined (Palestra, 1999). Table 25-1 lists risk factors for youth-related violence.

Violence among youth exists across the United States. It is not only a problem of minority communities and inner cities, although it is more concentrated there. It also puts a disproportionate burden on minority communities. Shooting or killing someone has become the symbol of a new rite of passage and the bestowing of manhood among some segments of society (Ozmar, 1994). Minority youth are particularly influenced, and violence among them is a large, complex problem. The toll of homicide and assault among young minority men, particularly blacks and Hispanics, is well known.

BOX 25-1   Violence in Schools

A national study on school violence was conducted in the late 1990s. Deaths were reported in 25 states and happened in both primary and secondary schools and communities of all sizes. Among the findings were the following:

➤ Less than 1% of all homicides among school-age children (i.e., 5 to 19 years of age) occur in or around school grounds or on the way to or from school.
➤ 65% of school-associated violent deaths were students, 11% were teachers or other staff members, and 23% were community members killed on school property.
➤ 83% of school homicide or suicide victims were males.
➤ 28% of fatal injuries happened inside the school building, 36% occurred outdoors on school property, and 35% occurred off campus.

From Centers for Disease Control and Prevention: Youth risk behavior surveillance: national alternative high school youth risk behavior survey, United States, 1998, *Morbid Mortal Wkly Rep* 48(SS07):1, 1999b.

Adolescents and children increasingly use violence to handle disputes. Many children are not taught nonviolent ways of resolving differences. Schools have become a common site for violence (Box 25-1). Factors influencing this include the availability of guns and drug trafficking on campuses, and the unfortunate reality of remote or absentee parents. A profile of a student who kills includes the following (Stewart, 1998):

• Male
• Unstable family environment
• Poor peer relationships, but a strong need for group belonging
• Deeply identified with violence

Retribution for perceived wrongs from peers has also been cited as a cause of school violence.

Fighting is a prominent cause of injuries among high school students and often precedes homicides. Studies have indicated that homicide or suicide by youths is almost always an impulsive act that is immediately regretted. Unfortunately, in the case of suicide, the impulsive act destroys one life; in homicide, it destroys two lives.

Many young people have become immune to violence and believe they are invincible. They experience tremendous peer pressure to experiment with guns; their impulsiveness and immaturity results in tragedy, which changes their lives forever.

Domestic Violence

Domestic violence is a pattern of coercive behaviors that are perpetrated by someone who is or was in an intimate relationship with the victim. These behaviors include battering resulting in physical injury, psychological abuse, and sexual assault. These acts contribute to progressive social isolation, deprivation, and intimidation of the victim. Abuse is typically repetitive and often escalates in frequency and severity.

Battering, spousal abuse, wife abuse, and *domestic violence* are terms used to describe violence within an intimate relationship. The CDC now uses the term **intimate partner violence (IPV),** which is defined as the intentional emotional or physical abuse by a spouse or ex-spouse, boyfriend or girlfriend, ex-boyfriend or ex-girlfriend, or date (CDC-NCIPC, 2000a). This term is more inclusive and may replace *domestic violence.* Partners do not need to be married; violence may begin in casual or dating relationships.

More than two million incidents of nonlethal IPV occur each year, and men direct violence against women approximately 85% of the time (CDC-NCIPC, 2004d; Tjaden and Thoennes, 2000). Violence may also be directed by women against women in lesbian relationships, men against men in homosexual relationships, and by women against men in a small percentage of cases.

IPV cuts across all ethnic, racial, socioeconomic, and educational lines. About 25% of women and 8% of men report being raped, physically assaulted, or both by a current or former spouse, cohabitating partner, or date at some point in their life (CDC-NCIPC, 2000a). The strongest predictor of IPV is alcohol use. Approximately 45% of males involved in IPV had been drinking, and 20% of the women had been drinking (CDC-NCIPC, 2004a). The following are risk factors for victims of IPV (CDC-NCIPC, 2000a):

- Female between 19 and 29 years of age
- Family with income below the poverty level
- Women who were abused as children
- Alcohol or drug use by the perpetrator (75% of the time alcohol or drugs were used at the time of the assault)
- Being stalked by a current or former husband or cohabiting partner

Domestic violence is the least reported crime in the United States and is the single greatest cause of injury to women. These physical injuries are frequently borne in silence and accepted as a transgenerational pattern of normative behavior. When children witness abuse between parents, they learn that violence is a means of control. Male perpetrators of IPV are abusive because "they can and it works" (K.L.D. Hakala, personal communication, November 20, 2000).

Sexual abuse occurs in almost half of the battered population. Often abusive partners believe it is their right to have sex whenever they want. Women may report that they were subjected to forced intercourse when they were ill or had

---

BOX 25-2 Considerations for Working With Victims of Violence

1. Working with victims of intimate partner violence (IPV):
   - ➤ Establish rapport and trust; this is essential
   - ➤ Deal with issues of confidentiality honestly
   - ➤ Provide the most current information regarding shelters and sources of support
   - ➤ Recognize and accept that clients may "choose" to stay in an abusive relationship
2. Working with victims of child abuse
   - ➤ As your primary obligation, protect the well being of the child
   - ➤ Report child abuse; it is a legal and ethical obligation in all states
   - ➤ Establish rapport and trust; this may take time
   - ➤ Remain objective when dealing with suspected family members
3. Working with victims of elder abuse
   - ➤ Establish rapport and trust; this may may take time
   - ➤ Report elder abuse; it is a legal and ethical obligation in all states
   - ➤ Remember that competent adults have the right to make decisions about their own care, even if it means staying in an abusive situation
   - ➤ Support efforts to create respite programs and support groups for caregivers
4. Advocating for the rights of vulnerable populations is the responsibility of all health care professionals
   - ➤ Support research on effective interventions for violence prevention and reduction
   - ➤ Lobby for decrease in media violence
   - ➤ Support community efforts to increase resources for victims of violence
   - ➤ Lobby for effective regulation of firearms and cyberstalking

---

recently given birth. They also report forced anal intercourse and other violent sexual acts.

IPV often increases in frequency and severity, reflecting an escalating cycle of abuse. In 2002 almost 4000 women were murdered in the United States, and almost 85% were killed by someone they knew. Of these, approximately half were murdered by a husband, ex-husband, or boyfriend, with 17% of the homicides occurring after the women left the relationship (CDC-NCIPC, 2004c). In recent years, well-publicized cases have been reported of battered women who have killed their partners. Although their legal appeal has been "self-defense," it is a controversial issue, which is often difficult to prove.

Box 25-2 presents considerations for working with victims of violence.

Dating Violence

Dating violence has become a national concern. **Dating violence** refers to the perpetration or threat of an act of violence (e.g., sexual assault, physical violence, or verbal or emotional abuse) by a member of an unmarried couple on the other member, within the context of dating or courtship. A national study of college students found that 27.5% of women suffered rape or attempted rape at least once since age 14 years. Between 80% and 95% of rapes that occur on college campuses are committed by someone the victim knows (Gray and Foshee, 1997).

Victims of dating violence are typically girls and women aged 12 to 18 years (women are 6 times more likely than men to experience violence at the hands of an intimate partner), have been associated with female peers who have been sexually victimized, have lower church attendance, have a greater number of dating partners, show acceptance of dating violence, and experienced a previous sexual assault. Perpetrators of dating violence are males with sexually aggressive peers; are heavy drug or alcohol users; show acceptance of dating violence; assume the traditional male roles of initiating the date by driving and paying expenses; show miscommunication about sex; had previous sexual intimacy with the victim; and have an interpersonal history of violence (CDC-NCIPC, 2000a).

A particularly alarming type of dating abuse involves the use of **date rape drugs,** such as gamma-hydroxybutyrate (GHB), Rohypnol, and ketamine to reduce inhibitions and promote anesthesia or amnesia in the victim. The preferred term for **date rape** is *drug-facilitated sexual assault* (National Women's Health Information Center, 2004). GHB is odorless, tasteless, and can easily be made at home. Instructions are available in libraries and on the Internet, which may explain the drug's rapid rise in popularity. Although illegal in the United States, it has become popular in many nightclubs where it is available in clear liquid form. GHB has been touted as an aphrodisiac and an anesthetic. It is actually a depressant that slows down the respiratory system and has been responsible for multiple deaths and numerous overdoses. When mixed with alcohol, it can be deadly.

Rohypnol (flunitrazepam), classified as a benzodiazepine, has been compared to Quaalude, the "love drug" of the 1960s and 1970s. Like GHB, Rohypnol is not legal in the United States, but many reports have been received of its use at fraternity parties, at other college gatherings, and in gay bars on both coasts. The ability to provide a quick, cheap high with long-lasting effects may explain its popularity. Combined with alcohol, serious side effects, including death, have been reported (Lyman, Hughes-McLain, and Thompson, 1998). Ketamine (ketamine hydrochloride) is an anesthetic used primarily in veterinary practice. It causes a lost sense of time and problems with memory. Alcohol may also contribute to sexual assault because it impairs the ability to think clearly, lowers inhibitions, and impair ability to evaluate an unsafe situation (U.S. Department of Justice, National Drug Intelligence Center [USDoJ-NDIC], 2004).

Abuse During Pregnancy

Pregnancy does not exclude women from the danger of abuse. Indeed, pregnancy may increase stresses within the family and provoke the first instances of battering. The actual incidence of battering during pregnancy is unknown, but it is estimated to be between 4% and 8% of all pregnant women (CDC, 2004d). The incidence of abuse is a public health concern because it may outrank diabetes and pregnancy-induced hypertension in common complications in selected populations. Societal awareness of IPV during pregnancy is a relatively recent phenomenon; the mention of abuse during pregnancy began to appear in the health literature in the 1980s.

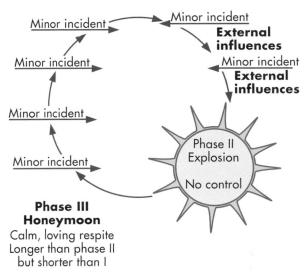

Phase I
Tension building
Limited control

Minor incident
Minor incident
External influences
Minor incident
Minor incident
External influences
Minor incident
Minor incident

Phase II
Explosion
No control

Phase III
Honeymoon
Calm, loving respite
Longer than phase II
but shorter than I

FIGURE 25-1 Walker's cycle of violence. (From Rawlins P, Williams S, Beck C: *Mental-health psychiatric nursing: a holistic life-cycle approach,* St. Louis, 1993, Mosby).

The image of a woman being battered during pregnancy shatters the idealized image of pregnancy as a time for nurturing and protection.

All pregnant women and adolescents should be routinely screened for abuse because pregnancy is a risk factor for battering. Common signs of IPV in pregnancy are: delay in seeking prenatal care, unexplained bruising or damage to breasts or abdomen, continued use of harmful substances (cigarettes, alcohol, drugs), recurring psychosomatic illnesses, and lack of participation in prenatal education (Lent, Morris, and Rechnen, 2000). Studies have shown that detection of abuse is more likely to occur when the health care provider routinely asks about abuse more than once during each prenatal visit. Abused pregnant women report blows to the abdomen, injuries to their breasts and genitalia, and sexual assault. Such violence can result in hemorrhage, intrauterine growth restriction, spontaneous abortion, stillbirths, preterm deliveries, and low-birthweight infants (Nichols and Zwelling, 1997).

Abusive Pattern

The **cycle theory of violence** was developed by Walker (1979) and explains a common abusive pattern of domestic violence. Depicted in Figure 25-1, this theory contains the following three phases: tension, explosion, and contrition (commonly known as the *honeymoon phase*).

During the *tension phase,* minor battering incidents may occur, such as slapping, kicking, and spitting. External influences that the batterer reacts to inappropriately (e.g., problems at the batterer's job, heavy traffic, or crying children) may trigger these minor incidents.

The second and most dangerous phase is the *explosive phase.* The explosive phase is inevitable as tension builds and is characterized by uncontrolled rage. The batterer may only stop when he or she becomes exhausted or is stopped by a third party (e.g., the police or other family member). Physical injuries occur during this phase; therefore the victim may seek health care. However, unless the injury is severe, the victim may not seek medical help because he or she feels shame or the need for secrecy.

Some women who have been through the violence cycle actually report provoking the batterer into the explosive phase. Such behavior, although startling to others, seems logical to the victim who has been through this before. By provoking the batterer into the inevitable explosive phase, the cycle can be completed and the tension relieved for a time.

The *honeymoon phase* is characterized by promises that the abuse will never happen again. The victim may be initially lulled into a sense of security as he or she receives apologies and the showering of gifts. This phase may also include pleas for forgiveness and a promise to seek counseling on the part of the batterer. The cycle of violence is characterized by the following (Sonkin and Durphy, 1997):

1. The more times the cycle is completed, the less time it takes to complete.
2. The longer the cycle goes uninterrupted, the worse the violence gets.
3. The longer the cycle goes uninterrupted, the shorter the third stage becomes.

Like many forms of violence, domestic violence is a learned behavior that is often modeled from transgenerational patterns. Children, especially males, who have witnessed their mothers being abused, are at high risk for imitating this behavior as adults with their own partners (CDC-NCIPC, 2004d). Although they may have tried to protect their mother from the abuse as children, they subconsciously learn that violence is a means of control. Lacking role models for developing healthy emotional relationships, these children often become adults who batter. Domestic violence is about control, not anger; therefore the objective of the abuse is to exert power and control over the victim. The victim may have also been exposed to domestic violence as a child. In these cases, the learned response may be one of helplessness that implies passivity and acceptance of abuse.

The Domestic Abuse Intervention Project in Duluth, Minnesota, has developed a wheel of violence that depicts the types of power and control that are used. These include emotional abuse and intimidation, minimization, denial and blaming, coercion and threats, isolation, economic abuse, and use of children. Male privilege is another excuse often given by men for abuse. They may cite biblical reference to rightful male authority over women or exploit cultural gender bias. Figure 25-2 depicts the power and control wheel.

Effects of Domestic Violence

Chronic stress characterizes the lives of people in relationships with violent partners. When subject to repeated abuse, the abuse victim experiences a variety of responses, including shock, denial, confusion, withdrawal, psychological numbing, and fear. He or she lives in anticipatory terror and often suffers chronic fatigue and tension, disturbed sleeping and eating patterns, and vague gastrointestinal and genitourinary complaints. Health care providers frequently overlook or misdiagnose this pattern of obscure symptoms. In many instances, providers may label the abuse victim as hypochondriacal or clinically depressed, which results in a sense of guilt, extreme passivity, and helplessness. Few victims spontaneously disclose that they are being abused; therefore the failure of health care professionals to assess for abuse in all emergency and routine health care visits significantly contributes to the missed diagnosis of abuse.

Fear, helplessness, and lack of knowledge regarding resources are primary reasons that many victims do not readily leave an abusive situation. The legal system is cumbersome and often inadequate. Victims who seek help through restraining orders or other judicial means find that such methods do not provide real safety or solutions. For example, after reporting abuse to the police, the partner may be jailed and given bail within 24 hours or less and return home, unannounced, to deliver another beating. After attempting to use the judicial system as a solution and experiencing its failure, the victim is unlikely to consider the legal system as a source of safety. He or she may also fear that legal intervention might be a threat to custody of his or her children.

Other factors that keep a victim in an abusive situation are culture, religion, and economics. Victims with few marketable skills who leave an abusive situation face serious economic problems and may fall into poverty. When children are involved in such economically dependent relationships, the victim may choose to remain in the setting as a means of economic survival for his or her children. Health care providers, including nurses, often ask the victim, "Why don't you just leave?" or "What did you do to deserve this?" These misdirected questions often reinforce the victim's sense of helplessness and guilt regarding his or her abusive situation. These questions reflect a lack of understanding regarding the dynamics of abuse and a lack of sensitivity toward the victim.

Victims who are most likely to leave a battering situation include the following (Campbell and Humphreys, 1993):

1. Those who have resources, such as money, friends, family, and support
2. Those who have power (e.g., a job, credit cards, and status outside the family)
3. Those without children
4. Those who were not abused as children
5. Those who did not see their mothers beaten
6. Those involved in battering situations that are frequent or severe
7. Those whose partner begins to beat children in the family

The most dangerous time for the victim is when he or she leaves or attempts to leave the relationship, because it is seen as an assault on the abuser's desire to control the victim. The victim is more likely to be killed at this time than at any other time in the relationship (Campbell and Humphreys, 1993).

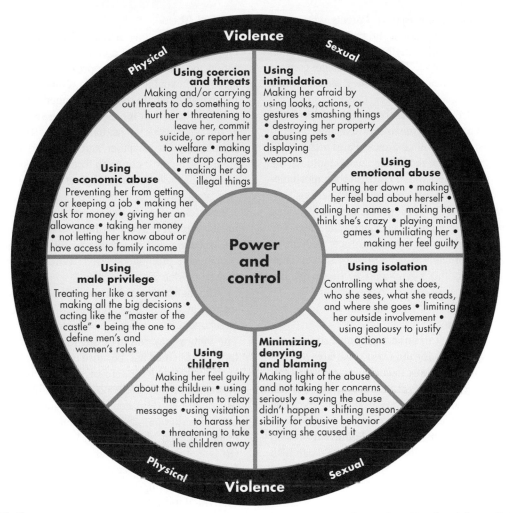

FIGURE 25-2 Power and control wheel developed by the Domestic Abuse Intervention Project (206 West Fourth Street, Duluth, MN 55806).

Child Abuse

Patterns of child abuse within families vary. In some family situations, all children are equal targets of abuse. In other families, one child might be selected as the designated recipient of abuse. The child may be singled out by a particular physical characteristic, such as hair color or resemblance to another family member who evokes negative emotions in the abusive parent. Child abuse, like domestic violence, is often a learned transgenerational behavior. Although statistical reporting of child abuse is mandatory throughout the country, reported numbers are likely an underestimation. Children are not likely to report the abuse because they fear reprisal, as with all other forms of abuse.

About 896,000 victims of child maltreatment lived in the United States in 2002. Girls are more likely to be victims than boys (CDC-NCIPC, 2004b). The five types of child abuse are as follows:

1. Physical abuse
2. Physical neglect
3. Emotional abuse
4. Emotional neglect
5. Sexual abuse

Physical Abuse

Physical abuse is an intentional injury inflicted on a child by another person and accounts for 20% of child abuse cases (Pillado, 2004). The most common type of physical abuse is beating, which can result in cuts, bruises, burns, and fractures. The type of physical injury varies only with the adult's imagination. Parents often select a method of meeting what they see as the child's disobedience. This may produce a "patterned" injury, which gives some clue to how the child was injured by leaving an imprint of the object on the child's skin. For example, a child who walks where he or she is not supposed to might have his or her feet dipped in scalding water; the burns would cover the stocking area of the foot. A child who touches a light cord or light plug might be beaten with it, producing a looped or linear pattern. A child who plays with matches or the stove might have his or her hand placed in the flame. A crying child or a child who talks back might have hot pepper or Tabasco sauce poured into his or her mouth or might be suffocated with a pillow.

Young children between 2 and 5 years of age are most frequently injured by physical abuse. This is most commonly explained by developmental behavior, such as the "terrible twos" and efforts toward physical autonomy and independence (e.g., toilet training and feeding issues). Parents who abuse often have unreasonable expectations of their children and misinterpret the child's behavior as threats to their parental self-esteem and need to control. Infants are in the greatest danger of severe injury or death because they are small and helpless.

An example of extreme infant abuse is **shaken baby syndrome.** Shaken baby syndrome is the leading cause of death from child abuse in the United States (Palusci, 2004). In this situation violent shaking of the infant causes trauma at the junction of the brain stem and spinal cord, and the morbidity and mortality rates for this injury are high. Serious and potentially permanent damage may occur, including retinal hemorrhages, spinal cord injuries, and brain injuries. The spouse or boyfriend of the mother typically inflicts this type of injury. Indeed, in approximately 65% to 90% of shaken baby cases the father or the mother's boyfriend is the perpetrator (Palusci, 2004).

Physical Neglect

Physical neglect is negligent treatment or maltreatment of a child by a person responsible for the child's welfare. It is the most common form of child abuse, which accounts for 60% of all cases (Pilado, 2004). Physical neglect includes the failure to provide basic needs, such as safety, food, clothing, and shelter by the responsible person. Failure to provide a nurturing environment for a child to thrive, learn, and develop and failure to provide for the health needs of a child can also be construed as neglect.

Emotional Abuse

Emotional abuse accounts for approximately 7% of all child abuse cases. It is the willful infliction of unjustifiable mental suffering on a child, which causes the child to be emotionally damaged (Pilado, 2004). The behavior evident in the child may demonstrate a substantial impairment in a normal range of performance and behavior, such as an overly compliant or passive child or the child who is very aggressive and apt to fly into a rage. Emotionally abused children frequently do not progress with the normal rate of physical, intellectual, and emotional development. Emotional abuse is almost always done in the home and is not witnessed by others. The symptoms displayed by the child can also occur in children who are not abused; therefore treatment of these children is difficult. Examples of emotional abuse include locking a child in a closet for a prolonged period of time, tying a child to a bedpost, or engaging in bizarre acts of torture. Subtle abuse might include name calling, such as "you're stupid," "you're a slut," "you're bad," or "you're evil." This type of name calling can irreparably harm a child's self-concept.

Emotional Neglect

Emotional neglect is the failure to nurture a child in developmentally appropriate ways. Some examples of emotional neglect are failure to cuddle and/or physically stimulate a newborn, failure to give positive feedback, failure to pay attention to the overall emotional needs of a child, or failure to show affection.

Sexual Abuse

Sexual abuse is any sexual activity between an adult and a child, including use of a child for sexual exploitation, prostitution, or pornography. Approximately 10% of child abuse cases are sexual abuse (Pilado, 2004). Sexual abuse can also involve an older child with a younger child, usually defined as a difference of 5 or more years of age between the two. Incest is the term used for sexual relations between close family members, such as father and daughter, mother and son, or siblings. The most common form of incestuous relationship is a stepfather with his stepdaughter or father with his daughter.

Sexual abuse often involves a person known to the child (i.e., a relative or friend). A growing concern is the sexual exploitation of children by Internet pedophiles who prey upon unsuspecting and naïve targets through chat rooms. It may occur over a prolonged period of time, and threats to the child may be used to ensure secrecy.

Although most of the research has focused on females as victims of sexual abuse, recent reports indicate that males are also targets. The incidence of male sexual abuse is unknown. The victim may refrain from reporting such abuse because they are ashamed and because cultural values expect males to be assertive and capable of self-defense. The aftermath of sexual abuse may predispose the victims to low self-esteem, psychiatric illness, depression, suicide ideation, drug and alcohol addiction, negative sexual esteem, sexual maladjustment, delayed developmental processes, and prostitution (Botash et al., 2005). The child may delay reporting the abuse for months to years because it may take that long for them to feel safe (Botash, 2004). Table 25-2 describes physical and behavioral indicators of child abuse and neglect.

Elder Abuse

Child abuse and IPV have been public health policy issues since the 1980s, but in many areas of the United States **elder abuse** lags far behind as a social and health care issue because society fails to recognize the inhumanity many older adults experience. This failure to recognize elder abuse is likely attributable to the elders as an "invisible" segment of the population. Three factors that relate to this invisibility of elders are their isolation, their reticence to admit to abuse, and society's negative views toward aging. Avoiding older persons and their circumstances often creates an atmosphere of nonexistence (Miller, 2004). As a result, the exact number of abused older adults is unknown because elder abuse is more underreported than child abuse. However, estimates indicate that 1% to 6% of the older adult population suffers some form of maltreatment (Miller, 2004). Reasons for this underreporting include shame on the part of the victim, social and physical isolation from resources, and the failure of health care providers to routinely assess for abuse and neglect during points of contact. A unique aspect of elder abuse is that the most vulnerable elders are in nursing homes. Periodic press reports of resident abuse in nursing homes most likely represents a very small percentage of the actual incidences. Chronic understaffing and high personnel turnover rates are likely contributing factors. The most likely victims of elder abuse are women over 70 years of age who are in poor physical or mental health, are dependent

TABLE 25-2   Physical and Behavioral Indicators of Child Abuse and Neglect

PHYSICAL INDICATORS	BEHAVIORAL INDICATORS
PHYSICAL ABUSE	
Unexplained bruises and welts in various stages of healing that may form patterns	Wary of adult contacts
Unexplained burns by cigars or cigarettes or immersion burns (e.g., socklike, glovelike, or on buttocks or genitalia)	Apprehensive when other children cry
	Constantly on alert
Burns in the shape of objects	Exhibiting extremes of behavior; aggressive or passive and withdrawn, or overly friendly to strangers
Rope burns	
Unexplained lacerations or abrasions	Frightened of parents
Unexplained fractures in various stages of healing; multiple or spiral fractures	Afraid to go home
Unexplained injuries to mouth, lips, gums, eyes, or external genitalia	Reporting injury by parents
PHYSICAL NEGLECT	
Hunger	Begging or stealing food
Poor hygiene	Alone at inappropriate times or for prolonged periods
Poor or inappropriate dress	Delinquent
Lack of supervision for prolonged periods of time	Stealing
Lack of medical or dental care	Arriving early to and departing late from school
Constant fatigue, listlessness, or falling asleep in class	Reporting having no caretaker
SEXUAL ABUSE	
Difficulty in walking or sitting	Exhibiting negative self-esteem
Torn, stained, or bloody underwear	Exhibiting inability to trust and function in intimate relationships
Genital pain or itching	Exhibiting cognitive and motor dysfunctions
Bruises or bleeding from the external genitalia, vaginal, or anal areas	Exhibiting deficits in personal and social skills
Sexually transmitted disease	Exhibiting bizarre, sophisticated, or unusual sexual behavior or knowledge
Drug and alcohol abuse	Delinquent or a runaway
Developmental delays	Exhibiting suicide ideation
	Reporting sexual assault
EMOTIONAL MALTREATMENT	
Failure to thrive	Exhibiting behavior extremes from passivity to aggression
Lags in physical development	Exhibiting habit and conduct disorders (e.g., antisocial behavior and destructiveness)
Speech disorders	
Developmental delays	Exhibiting neurotic traits
	Attempting suicide

upon others for physical or financial support, and who are often confused and depressed (Miller, 2004).

The five commonly described types of abuse and neglect of older adults are as follows:

1. Physical abuse (i.e., purposeful infliction of physical pain or injury or unnecessary physical restraint)
2. Psychological-emotional abuse (i.e., verbal assault, threats, provoking fear, or isolation)
3. Sexual abuse (i.e., unwanted sexual contact)
4. Physical neglect (i.e., withholding of personal care, food, or medications, intimidation, or humiliation)
5. Financial exploitation, theft, and misuse of money or property

Elder abuse tends to escalate in incidence and severity over time. When an older adult cannot provide self care because of the physical or mental infirmities of age, what happens to that person may depend on whether relatives can provide care, or whether the person has financial resources to purchase care in his or her own home, a retirement home, or a residential care facility. If none of these possibilities exist, the older adult may continue to live alone. This may be an unsatisfactory way of dealing with the problem because safety is an issue.

The caregivers are often adult children, nieces or nephews, or another relative of the older adult. This generation of individuals in their forties, fifties, and sixties are often called the *sandwich generation* because they are caring for their children at the same time they are providing care for their aging parents. As parents age, the role reversal is often painful and demanding on the part of the older adult and the caregiver.

Care of an aging parent may require more sacrifice and commitment than their children's care required. When providing care for children, their dependency on the caregiver usually lessens as the children grow older. However, an aging parent or relative becomes more dependent and may become cognitively or physically impaired, which may be a factor in the likelihood of abuse. Older adults may not know who they are, or they may suffer changes in personality that makes it difficult for their adult children to care for them. They may need to be lifted, which may be difficult for someone with limited strength. They may need assistance walking, using

TABLE 25-3   Indicators of Possible Elder Abuse

PHYSICAL INDICATORS	BEHAVIORAL INDICATORS
Any injury that has not been cared for properly	Fear
Any injury incompatible with the history	Withdrawal
Lack of care for injuries	Depression
Evidence of inadequate care	Helplessness
Evidence of inadequate or inappropriate administration of medicine	Resignation
Poor skin hygiene	Hesitation to talk openly
Hemorrhage beneath the scalp	Implausible stories related to injuries
Signs of confinement (e.g., tied to furniture, bathroom fixtures, or locked in room)	Confusion or disorientation
	Ambivalence; contradictory statements not caused by mental dysfunction
	Anger
	Denial
	Nonresponsiveness
	Agitation or anxiety

FAMILY OR CAREGIVER INDICATORS OF POSSIBLE ELDER ABUSE	FINANCIAL INDICATORS OF POSSIBLE ELDER ABUSE
Unwillingness to let the older adult speak for himself or herself, or see others without presence of the caregiver	Unusual activity in bank accounts
Aggressive behavior	Concern by relatives that too much money is being spent for the care of the older adult
Attitude of indifference or anger	Refusal to spend money on the care of the older adult
Blaming the older adult for things beyond his or her control, such as incontinence	Unexpected change in power of attorney
Problems with alcohol or drugs	Recent will change when the older adult is incapable of making a will
Conflicting accounts of incidents by the family and victim	Recent acquaintances expressing undying affection for a wealthy older adult
Unwillingness or reluctance to comply with service providers in planning care of the older adult	Recent change of title of house in favor of a "friend" when the older adult is incapable of understanding the nature of the transaction
Indications of inappropriate sexual relationship	Isolation of older adult from friends and family, causing the older adult to become alienated
Withholding affection	Promises of lifelong care in exchange for willing or deeding of all property or money to the caregiver
Lack of amenities such as grooming items and clothing when the estate can afford to buy it	Checks and documents signed when the older adult cannot write
	Missing personal belongings such as art, silverware, or jewelry
	Placement outside the home not commensurate with the financial ability of the older adult
	Signatures on checks that do not resemble the older adult's signature

Modified from Carlton L: *Elder abuse prevention protocol,* San Francisco, 1983, San Francisco Task Force.

the toilet, or eating, which takes time that the caregiver may not feel he or she has. There is also an intimacy to caring for a parent that the caregiver may not feel able to cope with. Another factor that can come to bear on aging parents is the care that they gave their children when they were young. If they were abusive to their children, adult children may use the older adult's dependency as an opportunity to finally respond in an abusive manner to them.

All of these factors cause stress, which is closely associated with abuse. This is especially true in families in which violence is a response to stress. Stress in the primary caregiver can be caused by the needs of the older adult exceeding the family's ability to meet them or personal stresses of the caregiver such as the interference with their job, illness, or other family problems.

In many ways a helpless older adult is in the same vulnerable position as an abused child, because he or she is dependent upon others to intervene. Until society becomes sensitized to this problem, elder abuse is likely to increase. The population of the United States is aging, and the number of frail older adults (i.e., over 85 years of age) is the fastest growing demographic segment with increasing dependency

needs. Recognition of possible indicators helps the professional become aware of possible abusive situations. None is conclusive in itself; however, they alert the professional to the need for careful and complete assessment. Table 25-3 lists the indicators of possible abuse of older adults.

VIOLENCE FROM A PUBLIC HEALTH PERSPECTIVE

Dealing with violence has traditionally been the U.S. criminal justice system's responsibility. However, violence has been called a *public health epidemic,* and efforts have been made to prevent and manage it using public health strategies. Violence has a tremendous influence on morbidity and mortality rates, quality of life indicators, and health care resources. Violence is a problem of such magnitude that it has reached beyond criminal justice methods of protecting the public. Public health has been challenged to go beyond its traditional work to embrace programs to decrease poverty, illiteracy, environmental degradation, and violence. Many of these problems are interrelated; therefore a coordinated approach should be used to address the issues.

HEALTHY PEOPLE **2010**	Selected Objectives Related to Violence		
Objective		**Baseline (1998)**	**Target**
15-32: Reduce homicides		6.2 per 100,000	3.2 per 100,000
15-33a: Reduce maltreatment of children under 18 years of age		13.9 per 1000	11.1 per 1000
15-33b: Reduce child maltreatment fatalities for children under 18 years of age		1.7 per 100,000	1.5 per 100,000
15-34: Reduce the rate of physical assault by current or former intimate partners for children 12 years of age and older		4.5 per 1000	3.6 per 1000
15-35: Reduce the annual rate of rape or attempted rape for children 12 years of age and older		0.9 per 1000	0.7 per 1000
15-36: Reduce sexual assault other than rape for children 12 years of age and older		0.6 per 1000	0.2 per 1000
15-37: Reduce physical assaults for children 12 years of age and older		31.1 per 1000	25.5 per 1000
15-38: Reduce physical fighting among adolescents grades 9 to 12		37%	33%
15-39: Reduce weapon carrying by adolescents on school property for grades 9 to 12		8.5%	6%

Healthy People 2010 and Violence

Violence was one of the areas addressed by *Healthy People 2010* and again in *Healthy People 2010*. Several objectives regarding violence and abuse prevention have been established for *Healthy People 2010*. The *Healthy People 2010* table lists a few of these (USDHHS, 2000). These objectives are intended to continue targeting causes of violence and abuse, improve national data collection and analysis, provide input for legislative funding, facilitate research efforts, and concentrate public health efforts on models that demonstrate effectiveness.

Many of the *Healthy People 2010* objectives are difficult to achieve because there are complex barriers. These barriers include lack of comparable data sources, standardized definitions, resources to adequately establish consistent tracking systems, and resources to fund promising prevention programs. The achievement of positive change in 13 of the original 19 objectives indicates that coordinated national efforts can bring about progress.

PREVENTION OF VIOLENCE

The nurse who cares for people experiencing violence must be a skilled clinician who is knowledgeable about both the problem and the community resources available to deal with the problem. The nurse may also work with individuals and families before abuse has occurred. He or she can educate families in the care and nurturing of family members, the growth and development of children, and the needs of older adults. Over the last 25 years a considerable body of knowledge has developed regarding the causes and trends in expressions of violence. Unfortunately, more peer-reviewed research that demonstrates effective interventions is needed (Arnetz and Arnetz, 2000). Table 25-4 provides the current components of a comprehensive program to reduce violence in the community.

Primary Prevention

One goal of primary prevention of violence is the promotion of optimal parenting and family wellness. Education plays a major part of primary prevention, from educating children in grade schools about a healthy family life and nonviolent methods of conflict resolution, to educating professionals to increase their awareness of violence and facilitate case detection and provision for early treatment. Community services are needed to provide care for families before serious injury occurs to any member. Nurses can be in the forefront in communities and act as an advocate for those in need of services. The nurse can work in the community to educate citizens about the problem of violence, potential causes of violence, and the community services that are necessary to serve those in need. Reduction of violence in the media and control of handguns and assault weapons are also essential.

Proposed changes range from banning private ownership of certain types of guns (especially assault rifles and small, cheap, poorly made handguns) to increasing manufacturers' and dealers' liability and holding gun owners responsible for the injury and loss of life caused by their weapons. Studies have shown a direct relationship between gun ownership and violent injuries. As discussed, availability of firearms is related to increased incidence of unintentional death, suicide, and homicide in states that have poor regulation of handguns (CDC-NCIPC, 2004c). More stringent measures to decrease gun violence include enforcement of sales restrictions to "high-risk" individuals, higher sales taxes for guns and ammunition, tighter federal dealer licensing standards, limits on the number of guns a person may purchase within a month, and promotion of new gun designs intended to reduce their lethality. Such design modifications include load indicators, magazine safety devices, push button locks, fingerprint or voice recognition chips, and a magnetic ring worn by the shooter that enables the gun to be fired (Palestra, 1999).

Primary prevention of abuse against women must begin at a societal level, helping to change attitudes toward violence and women. Children should be taught that no one has the right to beat another person or touch another person inappropriately. Each child has a right to be free from abuse. Children who witness their mothers being abused are at particular risk. Boys are at risk to grow to adulthood and abuse women with whom

TABLE 25-4 Components of a Comprehensive Program to Reduce Violence for Individuals, Families, and the Community

INDIVIDUALS	FAMILY	COMMUNITY
PRIMARY PREVENTION—GOAL: PROMOTION OF OPTIMAL PARENTING AND FAMILY WELLNESS		
Family life education in schools, churches, and communities Education of children on methods of conflict resolution Birth control services for sexually active teens Child care education for teens who babysit Preventive mental health services for adults and children Training for professionals in early detection of violence	Parenting classes in hospitals, schools, and other community agencies Provision of bonding opportunities for new parents Referral of new families to community health nurses for follow-up services after early discharge from the hospital Social services for families	Community education concerning family violence Reduction of media violence Development of community support services such as crisis lines, respite placement for children, respite care for families with dependent older adult members, shelters for battered women and their children, and development and vigorous enforcement of anti-stalking measures, including cyber-stalking Handgun control
SECONDARY PREVENTION—GOAL: DIAGNOSIS OF AND SERVICE FOR FAMILIES IN STRESS		
Nursing assessment for evidence of family violence in all health care settings A well thought-out safety plan for victims Knowledge of legal options to help ensure safety Shelter or foster home placement for victims	Social services for individuals or families Referral to self-help groups in the community Referral to community agencies that provide services for victims	All health professionals skilled in assessment of violence and equipped with protocols for dealing with the victims to help ensure their safety Hospital emergency rooms and trauma centers with 24-hour response, reporting, case intake, coordination with legal and medical authorities, coordination with voluntary agencies who have services, coordination with social services departments for provision of services Death review teams to review deaths from injury, especially for infants and children Public authority involvement by police, district attorneys, and courts Epidemiological tracking and evaluation of violence Handgun control
TERTIARY PREVENTION—GOAL: REEDUCATION AND REHABILITATION OF VIOLENT FAMILIES		
Empowerment strategies for battered women Professional counseling services for individuals	Parenting reeducation (i.e., formal training in childrearing) Professional counseling services for families Self-help groups	Foster homes, shelters, and care for older adults Public authority involvement Follow-up care for known cases of abuse Gun control

they have an intimate relationship. Girls are at risk for developing low self-esteem and ending up in an abusive relationship. Primary prevention must focus on stopping the transgenerational aspect of abuse.

Primary prevention of child abuse must include education about parenting. In a nation preoccupied by the need for education to meet the challenge of technological change, many people still do not value education for effective parenting. Parenting is the most difficult job that most individuals will undertake, yet there is a widespread myth that parenting "comes naturally." Reality and the disturbing statistics of abuse show that this is not true. Classes for parents should focus on more than preparation for labor and physical care of the infant. The realities of parenthood, including ways to soothe and manage a "fussy" baby, the effect of fatigue on a new mother, the need for support from a significant other or family member, and fears and questions of new parents must be addressed.

Changes in the health care delivery system cause nurses in the hospital to have far less time than they once did to help new mothers learn basic newborn care before discharge. Hospitals and public health agencies must provide follow-up to ensure that new parents can adequately care for their infant. This is

especially true of any person deemed to be high risk, including teenage mothers, mothers without supportive others, or women with a history of spousal abuse.

Educating professionals, caregivers, and the public on abuse is essential in primary prevention, and support for caregivers can help in the primary prevention of abuse of older adults. Education about the needs of older adults and the need for respite care for the caregiver should be available to those who face the care of aging parents. Just as a parent does not know everything about parenting simply by having a baby, an adult who may not have intimate contact with anyone of advanced age must be educated about the developmental processes and needs of the aging. Support groups for caregivers have been shown to be an effective outlet to vent frustration, and receive needed counseling. Caregiving is frequently a 24-hour responsibility. Institutional abuse occurs in a setting where workers provide care in shifts, but the stress for those who do not have that relief is much greater. Nurses need to help the caregivers care for themselves.

Prevention of abuse by the individual older adult would include the following (National Center on Elder Abuse, 2005):

1. WITHIN THE LAST YEAR, have you been hit, slapped, kicked, or otherwise physically hurt by someone?	YES	NO
If YES, by whom? _____		
Total number of times _____		
2. SINCE YOU'VE BEEN PREGNANT, have you been hit, slapped, kicked, or otherwise physically hurt by someone?	YES	NO
If YES, by whom? _____		
Total number of times _____		
MARK THE AREA OF INJURY ON THE BODY MAP. SCORE EACH INCIDENT ACCORDING TO THE FOLLOWING SCALE:		SCORE
1 = Threats of abuse including use of a weapon		_____
2 = Slapping, pushing; no injuries and/or lasting pain		_____
3 = Punching, kicking, bruises, cuts, and/or continuing pain		_____
4 = Beating up, severe contusions, burns, broken bones		_____
5 = Head injury, internal injury, permanent injury		_____
6 = Use of weapon; wound from weapon		_____
If any of the descriptions for the higher number apply, use the higher number.		
3. WITHIN THE LAST YEAR, has anyone forced you to have sexual activities?	YES	NO
If YES, by whom? _____		
Total number of times _____		

FIGURE 25-3 Abuse Assessment Screen. From McFarlane J, Parker B: Preventing abuse during pregnancy: an assessment and intervention protocol, *MCN Am J Matern Child Nurs* 19(6):321-324, 1994. (Developed by the Nursing Research Consortium on Violence and Abuse. Readers are encouraged to reproduce and use this assessment tool.)

- Seek help for self and family members for treatment of drug or alcohol abuse
- Maintain personal health
- Avoid social isolation
- Actively plan for your legal future with power of attorney, etc.
- Be aware of your legal rights

Although these are excellent suggestions for caregivers of the elderly, the current reality of prevention efforts leaves considerable room for improvement.

Secondary Prevention

The goal of secondary prevention related to violent behaviors is to provide assessment of and service to families in stress, which facilitates early diagnosis and treatment. Safety of family members is critical. Family violence is not just a nine-to-five event during weekdays; around-the-clock assistance is crucial. Women who do not have money must have access to legal options. Shelters should be available to offer sanctuary to a victim and to shield a woman and her children from danger.

Public health surveillance is important to obtain accurate numbers for intentional injuries of all individuals. Forming review teams can play an important part by analyzing the incidence of death from injury to determine whether the injury was intentional or unintentional. Removing guns from the hands of children and violent individuals is also an important facet in reducing deaths from violence. Some states have initiated gun "buy-back" programs to encourage community involvement in these efforts.

Secondary prevention begins with assessment of a battered victim. Consistent assessment of all women during health care visits will increase case finding and provide opportunities for earlier intervention. This is particularly crucial during pregnancy. Women should be interviewed in private when they are asked about battering. Questions should be asked in a matter-of-fact way and the health care provider should not show shock or dismay at their response. The Nursing Research Consortium on Violence and Abuse has developed a simple three-question abuse assessment screen (Figure 25-3).

These three questions should be asked of all women at each visit. If the woman responds "yes" to the questions about physical battering, she should be handed a pencil and allowed to mark the areas on a picture of a body, where she has been injured. If the nurse observes injuries, careful and detailed charting should be done. This screening tool may be reproduced and used for assessing women in a wide variety of settings. After disclosure of abuse, the nurse's response should include the following three statements:

1. "I am sorry this happened to you."
2. "This is not your fault."
3. "What is happening to you is illegal."

These three statements offer support and educate the victim about the dynamics of abuse (K. L. D. Hakala, personal communication, November 20, 2000).

By law the victim must be offered resources that may increase his or her safety once the existence of a violent situation is known. However, the victim may not be ready to leave the situation and it is wise to explore available options so that he or she can plan ahead. The victim should have knowledge of legal options and how to access them. The nurse should ask the victim about what resources he or she has, including friends and family, and if he or she could enlist their support if needed.

Some states that have mandatory reporting laws for spousal abuse have developed protocols for nurses who deal with the victims. Review of these protocols can help the nurse become familiar with the questions to ask the client and the suggestions that he or she should make to help the victim make a safety plan. A safety plan is essential in providing comprehensive care. The nurse should discuss the plan with the victim in privacy, and place it in the victim's hands if it is safe. Visit the book's website at http://elsevier.com/Nies, and see **Resource Tool 25A** for a sample of a safety plan that the nurse can use to help a victim explore his or her options.

Secondary prevention of child abuse begins with the discovery that the child has suffered from dysfunctional parenting or has been injured. The community health nurse in the home or school may be the one to discover the injured child and initiate the mandatory report to child protective or emergency services. The nurse can continue to support and educate the parent even though a report must be made. The primary focus should be obtaining a safe environment for the child.

In secondary prevention of abuse of older adults, the nurse's focus should be on the client and his or her needs. *Each time* an older adult is seen in the health care system, the nurse must make an opportunity to screen for the possibility of abuse. Elder abuse remains grossly unreported across the United States; therefore routine screening can begin to change attitudes and facilitate earlier intervention. A suggested screening protocol, such as the one shown in Figure 25-4, can provide an algorithm that the nurse can use in a variety of health care settings. Nurses can help raise professional and societal consciousness of elder abuse by participating in political activities to create or strengthen mandatory reporting laws and fund support groups for at-risk families.

The nurse must establish a trusting relationship when treating any person experiencing violence. A nurse working with the client over a long period of time can promote the most favorable climate for improved care. Time is required to gain an older adult client's confidence and to build a trusting relationship.

As individuals age, they confront ongoing losses. One of the most significant of these is the threat of losing their living arrangement. The feelings of grief and loss associated with this threat may influence an individual to tolerate abusive behavior from the caregiver in order to stay in their own home or apartment. The nurse must be aware of this need for independence because it may seem bewildering to others why an older adult would tolerate such behavior. It is important to keep in mind that as long as the client can make competent decisions, he or she has the legal autonomy to do so. As an outsider, it may take time to understand the family dynamics of a situation where issues such as dependency, anger, and helplessness intermingle to create abuse and exploitation.

The nurse should also work with all family members or caregivers who provide care for the older adult client and help promote healthier relationships. Stress is a contributing factor to abuse. Helping the caregiver deal with stress by finding respite care, a home health aide, or counseling may help. Most older adult victims live with the offender and are dependent on them; consequently, to help the victim, the nurse must also help the offender deal with the stresses that are causing or contributing to the abuse. The caregiver may also have problems, such as mental illness or drug or alcohol abuse. Until these problems are dealt with, the abuse will most likely continue.

The nurse should respect the patient's right to privacy and confidentiality. However, in states with mandatory reporting laws for the abuse of children, women, or older adults, the nurse must comply with the law. Nurses must be familiar with community resources for the client and family. The clinical issue of abuse is rarely managed by nursing alone, but rather in combination with other disciplines, which may include physicians, child and adult protective services, social workers, probation officers, chaplains, and police. The nurse should use an interdisciplinary approach whenever possible for optimal outcomes.

Precise charting is a crucial aspect of providing help to all victims of abuse and complying with medical-legal requirements. The nurse should record observations fully and completely and refrain from opinions and interpretations. This is especially important because court proceedings may use documentation that may have direct bearing on the victim's welfare.

When dealing with abuse, competing interests of the family, community, or institution often surface, such as the following:

- Financial dependency of caregivers upon the older adult
- Myths that an intact family is the ideal, children are better off in a two-parent home, and family problems should stay within the family
- Institutional short staffing that does not ensure the safe care of older adults

The nurse has the moral and legal obligation to prioritize the needs of the victim before all others. Depending upon the circumstances, this may require considerable courage and commitment.

Tertiary Prevention

The goal of tertiary prevention is to provide rehabilitative services to violent families. Involvement of a social service

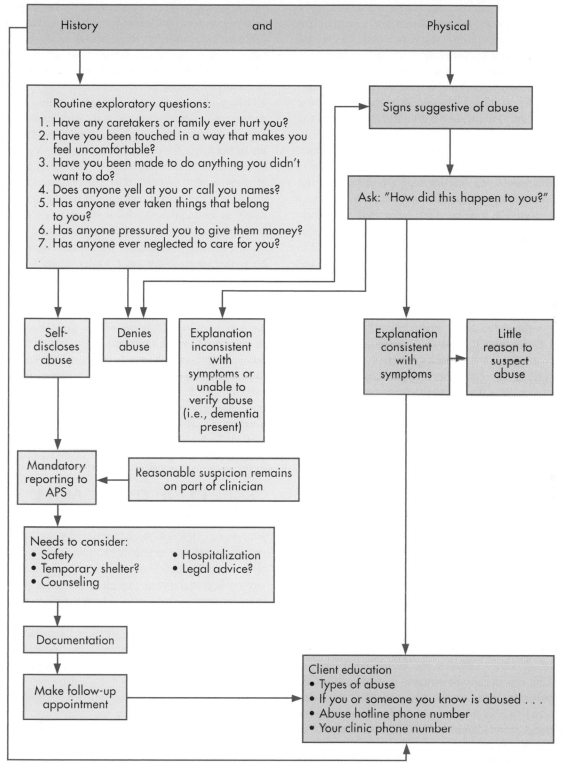

FIGURE 25-4 Clinical decision-making tree for detecting and treating elder abuse. (From Hakala KLD: Clinical decision making tree for detecting and treating elder abuse, unpublished manuscript, 1999.)

agency or local law enforcement members will be necessary if an injury has resulted in a report. Prosecution and punishment of the abuser or court-ordered removal of the victim from the family situation may occur. Professional counseling services and self-help or court-ordered groups can be helpful to the

family. Long-term follow-up and supervision may be necessary as in any rehabilitative situation.

Tertiary prevention is aimed at the rehabilitation of a victim who has been severely beaten. When dealing with an abused victim, the nurse should focus on the person first.

Accepting the victim and developing a trusting relationship is important for the patient and nurse to work together. The nurse should make community resources available to the patient. Telephone numbers for crisis lines and shelters need to be posted throughout the community in such areas as health clinic waiting rooms, public restrooms, bus stations, churches, and grocery stores. Nurses can carry cards in their pockets with referral numbers and give them to victims for future use.

Long-term care is necessary for an abuse victim. Maintaining contact with the individual and continuing support is essential for therapeutic nursing intervention. Support in the victim's ability to make decisions, even small ones, can help empower the abused victim. Many victims make the decision to remain in an abusive relationship; therefore health care providers may experience helplessness and possible anger toward the client. The nurse must understand the dynamics underlying the victim's decision to stay. The victim may take months or years to feel empowered to leave the situation. During this time, the nurse can provide crucial support and continue to offer resources. The nurse will be frustrated not knowing when or if these resources will be used; however, the nurse is most effective if he or she remains diligent in his or her support despite apparent lack of progress.

Tertiary care for a victim of child abuse usually entails a family involved in the court system. The courts or a local government agency such as protective services may refer the family to the community health nurse. The nurse may work with the parents while the child is in foster care after severe abuse; when a child is returned to his or her family, the nurse may provide ongoing care and supervision. The public health nurse must work with other health care providers and community agencies such as social workers, probation officers, and school nurses to provide coordinated care.

Tertiary prevention is important for children and adolescents who were sexually abused. Psychotherapy is usually necessary to resolve emotional problems that result from sexual abuse. These can be numerous and include anxiety, anger, eating disorders, and somatic complaints, such as headaches, abdominal distress, and concern with the genitourinary tract in younger children. Older children are at increased risk for substance abuse, sexual promiscuity, pregnancy, prostitution, depression, and suicide. They may become truants or run away from home. This behavior should be viewed as a way to escape the dysfunctional family situation and not as a means of normal adolescent rebellion.

Tertiary prevention may continue in the treatment of the adult woman who was sexually abused as a child. Sexuality issues often surface when these individuals require gynecological or mental health services. All of these patients require sensitivity during physical examinations and procedures. Some of the women may benefit from seeing a female practitioner to increase their comfort level. Depression and sleep disorders are common complaints. These women often experience anxiety and low self-esteem and may have chronic sexual problems dealing with fear of intimate relationships. Self-destructive behavior and substance abuse may also be evident.

The first step to receiving treatment is the recognition of the problem; nurses play an important role in recognition. After the nurse identifies the problem, he or she should refer the patient to a mental health professional for specific assistance. The nurse should remain available and in a supportive relationship with the patient.

Many obstacles may be present for the nurse in tertiary prevention of abusive situations in older adults. These include the reluctance to report the abuse, limited access to the client in his or her home, lack of consistent mandatory reporting laws, or lack of verifiable evidence. An additional factor is that the client is an adult and should be able to control his or her life as much as possible. An adult should be able to live freely and safely in the manner that he or she chooses. Care should not overly restrict the individual's freedoms.

Just as care is not forced on a battered woman, care cannot be forced on an older adult. Older adults who are deemed mentally incompetent have legal protection in many states similar to that provided for abused children. More research is necessary to develop appropriate care for older adult citizens because this is the fastest growing segment of the population. Current intervention for abused dependent older adults is primarily focused upon nursing home placement. Other alternatives need to be developed. Increased momentum for the protection of older adults is building as consumer groups such as the AARP and the Gray Panthers advocate for change. The aging of the baby boomers is also expected to accelerate political advocacy for protection of older adults.

SAFETY OF THE HEALTH PROFESSIONAL

Workplace violence tends to be higher in some service-oriented work environments including health care. Such violence is widely believed to be underreported, perhaps in part from beliefs that it is an expected part of the job, especially in specific settings (e.g., mental health and emergency departments). Nurses acting on their own have very little influence over the level of violence in their workplace, but through collective action they can influence policies designed to protect the health care workforce (McPhaul and Lipscomb, 2004).

In recent years, workplace violence has gained more attention because more dramatic incidents (e.g., shootings) and have occurred, and their frequency has increased. Nurses who work in public health roles are not immune to such risks because their work may bring them in contact with individuals prone to violent behavior. Identification of risk factors may offer some protection to the worker.

Simonowitz (1993) identified the following three risk factors for workplace violence that are applicable to the situation of the nurse dealing with violence in the family and community:

1. *Environment:* The nurse who works in the community must be aware of his or her environment, because a health care worker making home visits has little control over conditions of the community or the home. The nurse will some-

times find himself or herself in homes where violence is the rule.

2. *Work practices:* The greatest protection for the nurse is in careful work practices. Many involve common sense; others involve careful preparation. Preparing for the home visits, keeping the office aware of where he or she is at all times, and having emergency equipment such as a cellphone or a pager should be standard.

3. *Victim's and perpetrator's profiles:* Knowledge of previous violence by a member of a household may be the best indicator of the future potential for violence in that family. Interviewing a victim of violence, where the secrecy is broken, may put the nurse at risk if the perpetrator is on the premises or suddenly returns. In situations of suspected danger, the nurse should ask for a police escort. Box 25-3 offers safety tips for community health nurses.

SUMMARY

Violence is a major public health issue in the United States and affects individuals across the life cycle. Morbidity and mortality statistics indicate that violence is epidemic in many communities.

Violence at home, in the neighborhood, and at school affects countless numbers of individuals in the United States who live in fear for their lives. The easy access to and proliferation of handguns in the United States has been a major contributor to violence.

Violence can become transgenerational if the cycle of violence is not broken. This cycle causes indescribable pain to children, women, and older adults, who are the primary victims. The abuser is also a victim and the ultimate victim is society, which must care and pay for the results of violent acts.

Violence has been declared a public health epidemic; therefore national objectives for reducing violence have been identified. The efforts of public health have been mobilized to help stop this epidemic and bring healing to the nation. Health for all includes freedom from intentional injuries caused by violence. The core public health functions of needs assessment and surveillance, policy development, and assurance are useful methods of combating this epidemic. The literature in the area of violence mentions various interventions which focus on the three levels of prevention. The reality of the situation at present is that none of the suggested interventions are backed by rigorous research to validate outcomes. The need for meticulous research in violence intervention outcomes should be a priority for funding at the local, state, and national level. The disheartening reality of violence has already been validated. The public health nurse can be a crucial member of the team confronting violence. Commitment to caring about the problem is a first step. Careful assessment of all clients for evidence of injury is a second step. Teaching alternate methods of dealing with stress, improving parenting relationships, and considerately caring for older adults provide the essence of primary prevention. If an upstream approach of discovering the problem and then preventing it from occurring is used,

BOX 25-3 Safety Issues for the Community Health Nurse

Plan Ahead
- Know the area you are visiting.
- Schedule the visit ahead of time and get the correct address, directions, and information about who will be in the home.
- Tell the office where you will be and check in regularly.
- Carry a cell phone, possibly a pager, and a small amount of money
- Dress for function and mobility and wear a name tag. Avoid any provocative clothing.
- Ensure that the vehicle you drive is in good repair, has a full gas tank, and has emergency equipment. Always carry two sets of car keys.

Approaching the Home
- Notice the environment, animals, fences, activity, possible indicators of crime, and places you could go for assistance if necessary.
- Walk with confidence and maintain a professional attitude.
- Listen for signs of fighting before knocking. If you hear sounds of fighting, leave!
- Do not enter a home if you suspect an unsafe situation.

In the Home
- Be aware of who is in the home and what is going on. If angry people are in the home, use your professional and social skills. Do not expect the client to protect you.
- Note the exits and sit between the client and an exit of the home. Be prepared to leave quickly if the situation changes suddenly.
- If someone in the home is violent, leave and call 911.

Handling a Tight Situation
- Do not show fear; control your breathing.
- Speak calmly and in a soothing manner. Be assertive but not aggressive.
- Repeat the reason for your visit and find a reason to leave.

Leaving the Home
- Take all of your belongings and keep your car keys in your hand.
- Watch for cars following you when you leave. Do not stop. If you feel that you are in danger, go to the nearest police station or well-lighted business and ask for help.
- Trust your instincts. Never forget your own safety.

Modified from Oregon Public Health Association, Public Health Nursing Section, Seattle-King County Department of Public Health, Washington State Public Health Association: *Public health nursing domestic violence protocol (booklet)*, Seattle, Wash, and Salem, Ore, 1993, The Authors.

ultimately the transgenerational cycle will be broken, and society as a whole will be healthier.

LEARNING ACTIVITIES

1. Determine professional responsibilities in the state by securing a copy or reviewing the reporting laws for child abuse, women battering, spousal rape, and elder abuse.

2. Using the telephone directory or computer search engine, find three public or private agencies in the community that provide help for victims of violence. Make a list of the telephone numbers.

3. Call a child abuse hotline in the community and ask them what services they provide.

CASE STUDY Application of the Nursing Process

Caryn is a 23-year-old mother of two children, ages 3 years, and 2 months. She was separated from her husband of 4 years for a few months, but they recently reunited. He works as a computer programmer and is the sole supporter of the family. She is a patient at the local Planned Parenthood clinic today, scheduled for a postpartum exam and contraceptive counseling. During her physical exam, she is observed to have numerous bruises on her upper torso and external genitalia and a black eye. When asked about possible abuse, she avoids eye contact and refuses to answer the questions. Looking over her history, the clinic nurse notes that Caryn has completed high school, but has not worked outside the home for the past 3 years. This is Caryn's fourth visit to the clinic and the same nurse has seen her each time. The clinic is located in a small town where "everyone knows each other." Caryn refuses to leave her husband, stating, "I have place to go and I that he loves me," despite having a bad temper. Caryn is given a card with the phone number of the domestic violence hotline. She agrees to take the card but declines any further conversation about abuse. Caryn is fitted with a diaphragm and given spermicidal gel. She is able to effectively perform a return demonstration indicating appropriate insertion and removal, and she is scheduled to return in 6 months for a follow-up appointment.

Seen in the clinic 2 months later for amenorrhea and pregnancy testing, Caryn denies any further injuries, stating that things are going very well at home. A follow-up exam reveals that Caryn is 6 weeks pregnant. Caryn states that her husband refused to allow her to use contraception because it interferes with spontaneity. Although unplanned, she expresses acceptance of the pregnancy and says that things will work out for the best. The clinic nurse is frustrated with Caryn's situation and the patient's refusal to take control over her life. She struggles to maintain objectivity in her conversations with Caryn and offers information regarding safe shelters for abused women with children. Caryn denies a need for this service.

Caryn misses two consecutive prenatal visits and a follow-up phone call is made to arrange a home visit. The public health nurse notes facial bruising on Caryn, a very clean apartment, and 2 quiet children who appear well cared for. Caryn's husband questions the necessity for the visit stating, "You should have better things to do than snoop into people's homes." He refuses to leave the room when the public health nurse asks to speak with Caryn alone. Caryn explains her bruising by stating, "I am so clumsy. I walked into the door when I was getting up to go to the bathroom." She promises to keep her next clinic visit, which is rescheduled for the following week. Caryn's husband is present, so the nurse is unable to discuss the subject of abuse at this time.

When Caryn comes to the clinic, she reveals that her husband is reluctant for her go out alone, saying that she might be seeing other men when he is at work. She also says that she is starting to fear his unprovoked temper outbursts, which sometimes result in physical abuse. His drinking on the weekends frequently makes things worse. She makes a point of saying that he always apologizes for what he does and asks her to forgive him. She feels that she can handle the situation because of her deep faith in God. When asked about abuse, Caryn does acknowledge that she has held onto the abuse hotline card.

Caryn delivers her third child at 36 weeks' gestation, after "falling down the stairs" in her apartment. Both Mom and baby are physically well at her 6 weeks postpartum visit, though Caryn reports fatigue in keeping up with the three children and the apartment. She is breastfeeding, but reports that this baby is an additional challenge because he has colic. Her husband is disappointed that she does not always have dinner ready when he gets home, and she seems preoccupied with the children. Caryn asks for information about sterilization, stating that "three kids are probably all that I can handle. I am so tired all the time." She takes information regarding both tubal ligation and a vasectomy, stating that she wants to discuss them with her husband.

Caryn calls the clinic the following week sobbing and stating that her husband has beaten both her and the baby. He accused her of infidelity and poor mothering after she brought up the subject of sterilization. The baby's crying "gets on his nerves because he is under a lot of pressure at work and needs to relax when he gets home." Three months later, Caryn returns to the clinic to be placed on an oral contraceptive. She is no longer interested in sterilization, stating that her husband is adamantly opposed to the idea. She states that things are currently "pretty calm" in her life because they attended a marriage enrichment course at church and he is trying to be calmer at home. Caryn expresses some disillusionment with her life circumstances, but adds, "I do not have job skills aside from taking care of my children, so I need to make the best of it for now."

ASSESSMENT

The above information tracks the pattern of abuse for Caryn and her children over a period of a year. During that time, two community health nurses have worked with Caryn to provide contraceptive, prenatal and postpartum care, and abuse intervention. Signs of IPV were present from the first contact. But in a pattern that is not uncommon with IPV, Caryn later denied abuse and reported that things were better in her marriage. The same clinic nurse was able to see her on follow-up, and repeatedly encouraged her to seek help.

The IPV has now escalated to include reported child abuse. The following are the summary assessment points:

- Child abuse has been reported on 7-week-old male infant
- Family has a repeated history of IPV
- Caryn is a stay-at-home mom, with three children under the age of 5 years
- Caryn reports loss of friends due to husband's disapproval
- Caryn's deep faith in God is a source of strength
- The husband has a strong need for control
- Caryn believes she lacks employable skills

- Both sets of grandparents live 2 to 3 hours away and are unable to assist because of health issues
- The husband's abuse is aggravated by drinking

DIAGNOSES

Individual
- Risk for severe injury or death related to spousal abuse
- Risk for severe injury or death related to parental abuse

Family
- High risk for physical and emotional trauma from dysfunctional family dynamics

Community
- High risk for isolation from fear and shame

PLANNING

Individual
Long-Term Goals
- Caryn and her family will be free of IPV and child abuse.
- Caryn will enter individual counseling.

Short-Term Goals
- Infant will receive medical care and be placed in a safe environment.
- Caryn and her other children will be assessed for possible injury.
- Spouse will be referred for anger management classes.

Family
Long-Term Goals
- Family will demonstrate appropriate coping skills.
- Family will enter counseling.

Short-Term Goals
- Identify support to help Caryn with the children.
- Identify a setting where Caryn and the children can be safe.
- Identify resources for Caryn and the children.

Community
Long-Term Goals
- Programs on family violence will be presented in local churches.
- "Mother's-day-out" programs will be established in community churches.

Short-Term Goal
- Begin the planning process to establish community programs for IPV.

INTERVENTION

Mutual goal setting:

Individual and Family
Since Caryn's phone call indicates a possible life threatening situation, the immediate action is to call the police. The nurse also has an obligation to follow up with the police to ensure that child protective services has been notified. The baby was hospitalized for a fractured arm and skull. The other two children were removed from the home and placed in foster care. Caryn was treated in the emergency department and released with a referral to public nursing services for facial and head wound care. She declined to press charges or to go to a shelter. Caryn's husband immediately agreed to go to counseling with the church pastor, but initially refused to attend anger management classes. Both Caryn and her husband were devastated by the removal of the other children.

The baby was hospitalized for 2 weeks, and Caryn remained at the hospital during the hospitalization. Police filed charges because of the baby's injury. Her husband was found guilty and sentenced to 2 years probation and mandatory anger management classes. When the baby was discharged from the hospital, he was placed in foster care within the community. Supervised weekly visits for both Caryn and her husband were authorized. Caryn agreed to enter counseling and sought legal assistance to have a restraining order issued against her spouse. Over the next 2 weeks, the community health nurse visited Caryn three times weekly because of her need for dressing changes. The nurse's goals were centered upon Caryn's ongoing physical and emotional well-being.

During these visits, the nurse was able to engage Caryn in conversation regarding her future and that of her children. They discussed the role of a womens shelter and the impact of the foster care placement upon both Caryn and her children. Caryn indicted that this most recent episode of violence had both frightened her and caused her to question the wisdom of her decision to stay with her spouse in the past. The nurse arranged for Caryn to visit a womens shelter. After visiting the center, Caryn agreed to consider this option. She entered the shelter a week later, after a series of harassing phone calls from her spouse who was pressing her for reconciliation.

Community
The community health nurse arranged to speak at the the monthly breakfast meeting of the community pastors. She offered to present an informational program on intimate partner violence as a community service project to area churches. Within 3 weeks she received invitations from four of the nine chuches represented at the meeting. The first of the programs will take place in the next month. Two of the chuches have mother's day out available to church members. After an appeal from the community health nurse, one of the churches has expressed a willingness to open their program to non–church members.

EVALUATION

Individual, Family, and Community
The community health nurses jointly focused upon safety as a priority of care for both Caryn and her children. The

Continued

CASE STUDY   Application of the Nursing Process (cont'd)

call to the police started the chain of events that resulted in hospitalization for the baby and placement in foster care for the other two children. Caryn's injuries created an opportunity for the community health nurse to maintain contact and provide psychosocial support. Caryn's social isolation, which had been created by her husband, was lessened by the restraining order. During the nurse's visits, she was able to speak openly with Caryn and offer options that would enhance her coping skills. Caryn reported receiving parental support on the phone for her decisions. Her pastor has encouraged her to focus on her children and her own future.

When Caryn left for the womens shelter, the community health nurse offered her card and asked her to contact her when she was ready to return to the community. During her 6-week stay at the shelter, Caryn received intensive counseling and initial job skill training to prepare for beginning job placement. Paperwork was initiated to begin divorce proceedings, and to petition the court for the return of her children after she is settled in a job for 3 months.

Six months after Caryn's return to the community, she visited Planned Parenthood for an annual Pap test and exam. She tells the clinic nurse that her children have been returned to her. The two older children have received counseling through play therapy. The baby's recovery from the fractured skull and arm appear to have left no residual damage. Caryn is now working full-time as a receptionist at a law firm. The divorce proceedings are on hold as she and her husband are discussing a possible reconciliation. Caryn's husband continues to fulfill the requirements of his probation. Caryn offered that her husband's current remorse includes the fact that he wants to break the cycle that began with his father's abuse of him and his mother. He acknowledges that this will be an ongoing recovery process.

LEVELS OF PREVENTION

Primary
Goal: Promote safety and prevent violence.
- Encourage contact with friends in the neighborhood and at church
- Provide services of community health nurse
- Provide community education programs on anger management
- Provide community education programs about IPV

Secondary
Goal: Assess for signs of IPV and possible child abuse.
- Facilitate hospitalization for treatment of injuries
- Facilitate removal of children at risk for abuse
- Provide both physical and psychosocial support for injuries
- Provide referral for anger management
- Provide individual and family counseling
- Provide a 24-hour abuse hotline

Tertiary
Goal: Promote development of healthy family dynamics.
- Encourage continued use of community resources
- Provide information regarding local women's shelters
- Encourage community involvement with other young families
- Encourage establishment of mother's day out programs at area churches
- Provide community education programs on the cycle of violence

---

4. Call a battered women's shelter and determine the procedure for securing shelter placement for a battered victim and children.

5. Visit a respite center for older adults and observe the clients and the activities that are provided for them. What observed behaviors would contribute to stress in the caregiver?

6. Follow the newspapers for 1 month and clip articles that deal with violence. Determine how many individuals were killed or injured during that period in incidents of violence. How many of them were gun related and what type of weapon was used?

7. Find out what support groups exist in the community for older adult caregivers.

REFERENCES

Anderson MA et al; School-associated violent deaths in the United States, 1994-1999. *JAMA* 286:2695-702, 2001.

Alcohol abuse and violence against women, *J Psychosoc Nurs Ment Health Serv* 36(8):9, 1999.

Anderson RN, Smith BL: Deaths: leading causes for 2001, *Natl Vital Stat Rep* 52(9):1-86, 2003.

Arnetz JE, Arnetz BB: Implementation and evaluation of a practical intervention programme for dealing with violence toward healthcare workers. *J Adv Nurs* 31(3): 668-680, 2000.

Blow R, Gest E: A social disease: violence, *Mother Jones* 18:26, 1993.

Botash AS, Galloway AE, Booth T, Ploutz-Snyder R, Hoffman-Rosenfeld J, Cahill L: Continuing medical education in child sexual abuse: cognitive gains but not expertise. *Arch Pediatr Adolesc Med,* 159(6): 561-566, 2005.

Bureau of Justice, www.ojp.usdoj.gov/bjs/homicide/intimates.html.

Campbell J, Humphreys J: *Nursing care of survivors of family violence,* St. Louis, 1993, Mosby.

Carlton L: *Elder abuse prevention protocol,* San Francisco, 1983, San Francisco Task Force.

Centers for Disease Control and Prevention: Perceptions of child sexual abuse as a public health problem, Vermont, September 1995, *Morbid Mortal Wkly Rep* 46(34): 801, 1997.

Centers for Disease Control and Prevention: Suicide among black youths: United States, 1980-1995, *Morbid Mortal Wkly Rep* 47(10):193-196, 1998.

Centers for Disease Control and Prevention: Nonfatal and fatal firearm-related injuries:

United States, 1993-1997, *Morb Mortal Wkly Rep* 48(45):1029-1034, 1999a.

Centers for Disease Control and Prevention: Youth risk behavior surveillance: national alternative high school youth risk behavior survey, United States, 1998, *Morbid Mortal Wkly Rep* 48(SS07):1, 1999b.

Centers for Disease Control and Prevention: Youth risk behavior surveillance: United States 2003. *Morbid Mortal Wkly Rep* 53 (SS-2), 2004.

Centers for Disease Control and Prevention: Youth risk behavior surveillance: United States 2005 *Morbid Mortal Wkly Rep* 55 (SS-5), 2006.

Centers for Disease Control and Prevention, National Center for Health Statistics: *Assault/homicide fact sheet*, The Author, http://www.cdc.gov/nchs/fastats/homicide.html.

Centers for Disease Control and Prevention, National Center for Injury Prevention and Control: Fact sheet on dating violence, March 1, 2000a, The Author, http://www.cdc.gov/ncipc/dvp/yvpt/datviol.html.

Centers for Disease Control and Prevention, National Center for Injury Prevention and Control: Suicide in the United States, March 1, 2000b, The Author, http://www.cdc.gov/ncipc/factsheets/suifacts.html.

Centers for Disease Control and Prevention, National Center for Injury Prevention and Control: Addressing violence against women, Goodwin M, Bacak S, January 2004a, The Author, http://www.cdc.gov/ncipc/avaw/vaw.html.

Centers for Disease Control and Prevention, National Center for Injury Prevention and Control: Child maltreatment fact sheet, August 5, 2004b, The Author, http://www.cdc.gov/ncipc/factsheets/cmfacts.html.

Centers for Disease Control and Prevention, National Center for Injury Prevention and Control: Division of violence prevention, August 5, 2004c, The Author, http://www.cdc.gov/ncipc/dvp/dvp.html.

Centers for Disease Control and Prevention, National Center for Injury Prevention and Control: Intimate partner violence: fact sheet, August 5, 2004d, The Author, http://www.cdc.gov/ncipc/factsheets/ipvfacts.html.

Centers for Disease Control and Prevention, National Center for Injury Prevention and Control: Preventing Intimate Partner Violence, Sexual Violence, and Child Maltreatment. August 5, 2004e, The Author, http://www.cdc.gov/ncipc/pub-res/research_agenda/07_violence.html.

Centers for Disease Control and Prevention, National Center for Injury Prevention and Control: Sexual violence: fact sheet, September 22, 2004f, The Author, http://www.cdc.gov/ncipc/factsheets/svfacts.html.

Centers for Disease Control and Prevention, National Center for Injury Prevention and Control: Suicide fact sheet, July 26, 2004g, The Author, http://www.cdc.gov/ncipc/factsheets/suifacts.html.

Centers for Disease Control and Prevention, National Center for Injury Prevention and

Control: Youth violence: fact sheet, August 5, 2004h, The Author, http://www.cdc.gov/ncipc/factsheets/yvfacts.html.

Chan LS et al: *Preventing violence and related health-risking social behaviors in adolescents*, Agency for Healthcare Research and Quality 107, September 2004, http://www.ahrq.gov.

Cook PJ, Ludwig J: *Gun violence: the real costs*, New York: Oxford University Press, 2000.

Cook DE et al: *Joint statement on the impact of entertainment violence on children*, Congressional Public Health Summit, September 2000, http://www.dove.org/columns/2000/column0009.html.

Eberwine D: Violence pandemic: how public health can bring it under control. Pan American Health Organization, 2003, http://www.comminit.com/strategicthinking/st2004/thinking-820.html. 1/30/05

El Bassel N et al: Substance abuse, history of childhood abuse, and HIV risks, *AIDS Patient Care STDS* 15(1):41-51, 2001.

Federal Bureau of Investigation/Department of Justice (FBI/DOJ): *Crime in the U.S.: 2004*, 2005, The Author, http://www.fbi.gov/ucr/cius_04/documents/CIUS2004.pdf

Felitti VJ et al: Relationship of childhood abuse and household dysfunction to many of the leading causes of death in adults. *Am J Prev Med* 14(4).245-258, 1998.

Frattaroli S: Grassroots advocacy for gun violence prevention: a status report on mobilizing a movement, *J Public Health Policy* 24(3,4):380-385, 2003.

Gray HM, Foshee V: Adolescent dating violence: differences between one-sided and mutually violent profiles, *J Interpers Violence* 12(1):126, 1997.

Kellerman AL et al: Suicide in the home in relation to gun ownership, *N Engl J Med* 327:467-472, 1992.

Koop C, Lundberg G: Violence in America: a public health emergency, *JAMA* 267:3075-3076, 1992.

Krug EG et al: Moral report on violence and health, Serial online, May 2004. http://www.who.int/violence_injury_prevention/violence/moral_report/wazh1/en.

Lent B, Morris T, Rechnen S: The effect of domestic violence on pregnancy and labour. Commissioned by CFPC's Maternity and Newborn Care Committee. Jan. 28, 2000, http://www.cfpc.ca/English/efpc/prgrams/patient%20care/maternity/violence/default.asp?s=1.

Levine JM: Elder neglect and abuse: a primer for primary care physicians, *Geriatrics* 58(10):37-43, 2003.

Loring M, Smith R: Health care barriers and interventions for battered women, *Public Health Rep* 109:328-338, 1994.

Lyman SA, Hughes-McLain C, Thompson G: 'Date-rape drugs:' a growing concern, *Health Educ J* 29(5):271-274, 1998.

Mason J: Prevention of violence: a public health commitment, *Public Health Rep* 106:265, 1991.

McFarlane J, Parker B: Preventing abuse during pregnancy: an assessment and intervention

protocol, *MCN Am J Matern Child Nurs* 19(6):321-324, 1994.

McPhaul KP, Lipscomb J: Workplace violence in healthcare: recognized but not regulated. *Online J Issues Nurs* 9(3):6, 2004, http://www.nursingworld.org/ojin/topic25/tpc25_6.html.

Media Awareness Network: http://www.media-awareness.ca/English/issues/violence/violence_entertainment.cfm.

Michaels D: Reports of rape in prison increase, *Dallas Morning News* January 23, 2005, http://www.dallasnews.com/s/dws/dn/latestnews/stories/012405dntexprisonrape.3dbel.html.

Mid-Valley Women's Crisis Service: Safety plan, March 2000, The Author, http://www.mvwcs.com.

Miller CA: *Nursing for wellness in older adults: theory and practice*, ed 4, Philadelphia, 2004, Lippincott Williams and Wilkins.

Mother goose nursery rhymes, Bath, England, 2000, Robert Frederick Publishing.

National Center on Elder Abuse: Frequently asked questions, 2005, The Author, http://www.elderabusecenter.org/default.cfm?p=faqs.cfm.

National Institute of Justice: Toward safe and orderly schools: the National Study of Delinquency Prevention in Schools, November 2004, The Author, http://www.ojp.usdoj.gov/nij.

National Women's Health Information Center: Date rape drugs, 2004, The Author, http://www.4woman.gov/faq/rohypnol.html.

Nichols FH, Zwelling E: *Maternal-newborn nursing: theory and practice*, Philadelphia, 1997, WB Saunders.

Oregon Public Health Association, Public Health Nursing Section, Seattle–King County Department of Public Health, Washington State Public Health Association: *Public health nursing domestic violence protocol* (booklet), Seattle, Wash, and Salem, Ore, 1993, The Authors.

Ozmar B: Encountering victims of interpersonal violence, *Crit Care Nurs Clin North Am* 6:515-523, 1994.

Palestra: An epidemic of violence, July, 1999, http://www.oclc.org.

Palusci VJ: Shaken baby/shaken impact syndrome, 2004, http://www.kidshealth.org/parent/medical/brain/shaken.html.

Paulozzi LJ et al: Surveillance for homicide among intimate partners: United States—1981-1998. *MMWR Surveill Summ* 50(SS-3):1-16, Oct 12, 2001.

Pillado O: *The southern California center of excellence in youth violence prevention*, Fall 2004, University of California, Riverside, http://www.stopyouthviolence.ucr.edu/publications/childabuse.pdf.

Phillips LR: Domestic violence and aging women. *Geriatr Nurs* 4:188-193, 2000.

Rawlins P, Williams S, Beck C: *Mental-health psychiatric nursing: a holistic life-cycle approach*, St. Louis, 1993, Mosby.

Rosenberg M, O'Carroll P, Kenneth E: Let's be clear: violence is a public health problem, *JAMA* 267:3071-3072, 1992.

Ruttenberg H: The limited promise of public health methodologies to prevent youth violence, *Yale Law J* 103:1885-1912, 1994.

Simonowitz J: *Guidelines for security and safety of health care and community service workers*, San Diego, 1993, Medical Unit, Division of Occupational Safety and Health, Department of Industrial Relations.

Sonkin DJ, Durphy M: *Learning to live without violence: a handbook for men*, ed 4, Volcano, Calif, 1997, Volcano Press.

Stewart M: RNs confront causes and consequences of school violence, *Am Nurse* 30(5): 16-17, 1998.

Tjaden P, Thoennes N: *Prevalence, incidence and consequences of violence against women: findings for the National Violence Against Women Survey*, National Institute of Justice; Report NCJ 183781, 2000.

Treating violence as a public health problem, *BMJ* 325:726-727, 2002.

US Department of Health and Human Services: *Healthy People 2010,* Washington, DC, 2000, USDHHS, PHS.

US Department of Justice Federal Bureau of Investigation FBI Releases Crime Statistics for 2003 October 25, 2004, The Author, http://www.fbi.gov/pressrel/pressrel04/crimestat102504.htm.

US Department of Justice, Bureau of Justice Statistics: September 28, 2004, The Author, http://www.ojp.usdoj.gov/bjs/homicide/hmrt.htm.

US Department of Justice, National Drug Intelligence Center: Drug facilitated sexual assault: fast facts. April 2004, The Author, http://www.usdoj.gov/ndic/pubs8/8872/.

US Department of Justice Statistics: *Weapon use and violent crime,* Washington, DC, 2003, The Author, NCJ 194820.

US Department of Justice: *Stalking domestic violence: report to congress.* Washington, DC, 2001, The Author, NCJ 186157.

US Preventive Services Task Force: Screening for family and intimate partner violence: recommendation statement, *Ann Intern Med* 140(5):382-386, 2004.

Walker LE: *The battered woman,* New York, 1979, Harper & Row.

White JS, Koss MP: Courtship violence: incidence in a national sample of higher education students, *Violence Vict* 6(4):247-257, 1991.

Wilson SG: The tracks of her tears, *Bulletin,* March 1998, http://www.sbcms.org/southcal-physician/articles/art3e-98.html.

Winett LR: Constructing violence as a public health problem, *Public Health Rep* 113: 498-507, 1998.

26

Natural and Man-Made Disasters

Edith B. Summerlin

MEDIA RESOURCES

Additional Material for Study, Review, and Further Exploration

evolve Website at http://evolve.elsevier.com/Nies

❖ Quiz ❖ Case Studies ❖ Content Updates ❖ Glossary ❖ WebLinks

---

OBJECTIVES

Upon completion of this chapter, the reader will be able to:

1. Identify the types of disasters.
2. Discuss the characteristics of disasters.
3. Describe the stages of a disaster.
4. Discuss the stages of disaster management.
5. Describe the role of federal, state, local, and volunteer agencies involved in disaster management.
6. Identify potential bioterrorist chemical and biological agents.
7. Discuss the impact of disasters on a community.
8. Describe the role and responsibilities of nurses in relation to disasters.

KEY TERMS

American Red Cross
direct victim
disaster
disaster triage
displaced person
Federal Emergency
  Management Agency
  (FEMA)

first responder
frequency
imminence
indirect victim
mass casualty
multiple casualty
NA-TECH disaster

Office of Emergency
  Management
predictability
preventability
refugee
resource map
risk map

shelter in place
terrorism
U.S. Department of
  Homeland Security
weapons of mass
  destruction

CHAPTER OUTLINE

DISASTER DEFINITIONS

TYPES OF DISASTERS

CHARACTERISTICS OF DISASTERS
  Frequency
  Predictability
  Preventability
  Imminence
  Scope and Number of Casualties
  Intensity

DISASTER MANAGEMENT
  Local, State, and Federal Governmental Responsibilities
  Public Health System
  American Red Cross

DISASTER MANAGEMENT STAGES
  Prevention Stage
  Preparedness and Planning Stage
  Response Stage
  Recovery Stage

Communities throughout the world experience an emergency or disaster incident of one kind or another almost daily. The media may only mention these events or may report on them in great detail, depending on the number of dead or injured, the amount of devastation or damage to the area involved, and how much the event has disrupted normal activities within the community.

The health of a community can be affected significantly by disasters. Hurricane Katrina and Hurricane Rita, which hit the same geographical area (U.S. Gulf Coast) at nearly the same time (September 2005), are examples of how communities and their hospitals, clinics, nursing homes, and other health care facilities are directly affected as a result of a disaster. During these hurricanes, access to health care was impeded by physical barriers, such as road closures due to flooding, inadequate numbers of first responders, and limited transportation for search and rescue. Patients were evacuated from one hospital to another, sometimes not once but twice. Medical and nursing personnel, medicines, and needed supplies were unavailable, scarce, or depleted due to the increased demand. Temporary shelters and health care services were established in schools, churches and a variety of other facilities throughout the area. The wind damage and extensive flooding from Hurricane Katrina resulted in panic for food, water, and rescue in the gulf coast regions between New Orleans, Louisiana, and Biloxi, Mississippi. First responders and rescue teams were overwhelmed in their attempts to reach the victims.

The evacuation of Houston, Texas, and the surrounding coastal area due to Hurricane Rita created severe traffic jams, many lasting 18 to 20 hours, and resulted in travelers needing water, food, and gasoline before they reached shelter. As a result, many people suffered from dehydration and urinary tract infections. In addition, Hurricane Rita occurred during a period of record heat, and many travelers became victims of heat exhaustion caused by the high temperature and humidity. Among the lessons learned from these recent events is that detailed planning for evacuation can make the difference between life and death (McUsic, 2005).

Hurricanes, tornados, floods, wildfires, and industrial accidents occur yearly in some parts of the United States. Further, in recent years, terrorist attacks have become more common. The bombing of the World Trade Center in New York City in 1991 and the bombing of the Alfred P. Murrah Federal Building in 1995 occurred more than a decade ago, but the combined terrorist attacks on the twin towers of the World Trade Center in New York City, the Pentagon in Washington, DC, and the plane hijacking and crash in Pennsylvania in 2001 indicate that the potential is ever present. Additionally, terrorist attacks occur all over the world on an almost daily basis, and concerns about potential terrorist attacks have increased the focus on what needs to be done in terms of prevention, preparedness, response, and recovery—not only in the event of terrorist attacks but also in the event of disasters of all kinds.

Because of the recognition of the need to be prepared, programs have been created to address the national, state, and local management of disasters. President G.W. Bush established the **U.S. Department of Homeland Security** on March 1, 2003, and put into place the National Incident Management System on March 1, 2004. Local Citizen Corps Councils have been established throughout the country to provide volunteers an opportunity to support local fire, law enforcement, emergency medical services, and community public health efforts and to contribute to the four stages of emergency management: prevention, preparedness, response, and recovery (Texas Association of Regional Councils, 2005).

Efforts to prepare for disasters have also been significantly enhanced at the state level. In Texas, for example, the 78th Regular Session of the Texas Legislature passed HB 1483, which requires nurses to attend a continuing education program related to bioterrorism (Board of Nurse Examiners for the State of Texas, 2005). Further, the Ready Texas Nurses Emergency Response System (Ready Texas Nurses) was created to provide mobilization of volunteer nurses to support communities in times of crisis or disaster (Texas Department of Health and Texas Nurses Association, 2004). Similar actions are occurring throughout the country.

Nurses are uniquely positioned to provide valuable information for the development of plans for disaster prevention, preparedness, response, and recovery for communities. Nurses, as team members, can cooperate with health and social representatives, government bodies, community groups, and volunteer agencies in disaster planning and preparedness programs (i.e., drills). Nurses using their knowledge of nursing, public health, and cultural-familial structures, as well as their clinical skills and abilities, can actively assist or participate in all aspects and stages of an emergency or disaster, regardless of the setting in which the event may occur. Nurses have a significant role in meeting the health care needs of the community, not only on a day-to-day basis, but also in relation to disasters.

DISASTER DEFINITIONS

A **disaster** is any event that causes a level of destruction, death, or injury that affects the abilities of the community to respond to the incident using available resources. Emergencies differ from disasters in that the agency, community, family, or individual can manage an emergency using their own resources. But, a disaster event, depending on the characteristics of the disaster, may be beyond the ability of the community to respond and recover from the incident using their own resources. Disasters frequently require assistance from outside the immediate community, both to manage resulting issues and to recover.

Some disasters (e.g. a house fire) my affect only a few persons, while others (e.g. a hurricane) can impact thousands. A **mass casualty** event is one in which 100 or more individuals are involved; a **multiple casualty** event is one in which more than 2 but fewer than 100 individuals are involved. Casualties can be classified as a direct victim, indirect victim, displaced person or refugee. A **direct victim** is an individual who is immediately affected by the event; the **indirect victim** may be a family member or friend of the victim or a first responder. Displaced persons and refugees are special categories of direct victims. **Displaced persons** are those that have to evacuate their home, school, or business as a result of a disaster; **refugees** are a group of people who have fled their

The devastation of the tsunami that occurred in Indonesia in December, 2004. (Copyright Associated Press.)

The aftermath of a tornado in Moore, Oklahoma in May, 2003. (From the Federal Emergency Management Agency.)

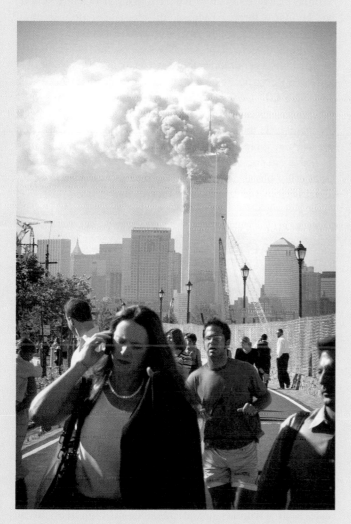

New York residents immediately after the September 11, 2001 World Trade Center terrorist attacks. (Copyright 2001 Thomas A. Ferrara/Corbis Sygma)

home or even their country as a result of famine, drought, natural disaster, war, or civil unrest.

TYPES OF DISASTERS

Disasters are identified as natural, man-made, or a combination of both. A **NA-TECH (natural-technological) disaster**

is a natural disaster that creates or results in a widespread technological problem. An example of a NA-TECH disaster is an earthquake that causes structural collapse of roadways or bridges that, in turn, cause downed electrical wires and subsequent fires. Another example is a chemical spill resulting from a flood. Types of natural disasters and man-made disasters are listed in Box 26-1.

BOX 26-1 Types of Disasters

NATURAL DISASTERS	MAN-MADE DISASTERS
Avalanches	Terrorism
Blizzards	Civil unrest (riots)
Communicable disease epidemics	Explosions, bombings
Droughts, wildfires	Fires
Earthquakes, tsunamis	Structural collapse (bridges)
Floods, mudslides	Toxic or hazardous spills
Hailstorms	Mass transit accidents
Heat waves	Pollution
Hurricanes	Wars
Tornados, cyclones	
Volcanic eruptions	

The American Public Health Association (2005) identified several types of disasters and their consequences. Types of disasters include blizzards, cold waves, heavy snowfalls, cyclones, tornados, drought, earthquakes, floods, heat waves, thunderstorms, volcanic eruptions, wildfires, man-made and technological events, explosions or blasts, and epidemics. It was noted in the report that injury or death from the disaster in question may be direct or indirect. For example, injuries from hurricanes occur because people fail to evacuate or take shelter, do not take precautions in securing their property despite adequate warning, and do not follow guidelines on food and water safety or injury prevention during recovery. Drowning, electrocution, lacerations or punctures from flying debris, and blunt trauma from falling trees or other objects are some of the morbidity concerns. Heart attacks and stress-related disorders also occur. Injuries also may occur from activities in the recovery phase, for example, from use of chain saws or other power equipment or from bites from animals, snakes, or insects.

Americans are familiar with most of the disasters listed in Box 26-1, but terrorism was largely unknown or unheeded prior to the bombing of the Alfred P. Murrah Federal Building in Oklahoma City in 1995. A study conducted by the U.S. Army in 1988 found 100 definitions of the word *terrorism*. The U.S. Code of Federal Regulations defines **terrorism** as "the unlawful use of force and violence against persons or property to intimidate or coerce a government, the civilian population, or any segment thereof, in furtherance of political or social objectives" (Wikipedia, 2005). The **Federal Emergency Management Agency (FEMA)** defines terrorism as "the use of force or violence against persons or property in violation of the criminal laws of the United States for purposes of intimidation, coercion, or ransom" (FEMA, 2005b). The Central Intelligence Agency (CIA) is guided by the definition of terrorism contained in Title 22 of the U.S. Code, Section 2656f(d), which states that terrorism "is premeditated, politically motivated violence perpetrated against noncombatant targets by sub-national groups or clandestine agents, usually intended to influence an audience" (Central Intelligence Agency, 2005, p. 1). In short, terrorists often use threats of acts of mass destruction to create fear among the public, to try to convince citizens that their government is powerless, and to seek immediate publicity (FEMA, 2005b).

Acts of terrorism include threats of terrorism, assassinations, kidnappings, hijackings, bomb scares and bombings, computer-based attacks, and the use of chemical, biological, nuclear, and radiological weapons. In addition to those mentioned earlier (i.e., September 11, 2001; bombing of the Alfred P. Murrah Federal Building, 1995), other examples of terrorist acts include the nerve gas (sarin) attack in the Tokyo subway in March 1995, which killed 12 and injured more than 6000 people; the bombing of the commuter train in Spain in March 2004, which killed 191 people; and the suicide bombing in the London subway in July 2005, which killed 52 commuters and 4 terrorists.

Concerns now are increasingly focused on **weapons of mass destruction.** Weapons of mass destruction refer to any weapon that is designed or intended to cause death or serious bodily injury through release, dissemination, or impact of toxic or poisonous chemicals, or their precursors; any weapon involving a disease organism; any weapon that is designed to release radiation or radioactivity at a level dangerous to human life; or any destructive device as defined in Section 921 of Title 18 of the U.S. Code. Biological organisms considered to be potential weapons of mass destruction are found in Table 26-1, and chemicals that are potential weapons of mass destruction are listed in Table 26-2. Chemical warfare agents are classified as nerve agents, vesicants, pulmonary agents, and cyanides (formerly "blood agents"). These tables also include information about the lethality, treatment, and impact related to each.

CHARACTERISTICS OF DISASTERS

Several characteristics have been used to describe disasters (Box 26-2). These characteristics are interdependent and therefore important to consider in plans for managing any disaster event. Each is discussed briefly.

Frequency
Frequency refers to how often a disaster occurs. Some disasters occur relatively often in certain parts of the world. Terrorist activities are occurring on an almost daily basis in Iraq and elsewhere in the world. Other examples are hurricanes, which occur with frequency between the months of June and November, and earthquakes, which occur periodically throughout the world. In the United States, earthquakes are generally considered to be a West Coast problem, but 45 states and territories are at moderate to high risk for an earthquake, and earthquakes have occurred in every region of the country (U.S. Department of Homeland Security, 2004). Other disasters, like volcanic eruptions, are far less frequent and are geographically limited to certain regions.

Predictability
Predictability relates to the ability to tell when and if a disaster event will occur. Some disasters, such as floods, may be predicted in the spring by monitoring the snowmelt. Weather forecasters can predict when conditions are right

TABLE 26-1 Biological Weapons of Mass Destruction

BIOLOGICAL ORGANISM	LETHALITY	PREVENTION	TREATMENT	POTENTIAL FOR USE
Smallpox (incubation 1-5 days)	High	Vaccine	Symptomatic; secondary infections	One person could possibly cause a national epidemic
Anthrax (incubation 2-60 days)	Very high	Vaccine	Antibiotics early; if late, nothing	Likely agent; resistant to weather; can be stored
Plague (Yersinia pestis) (incubation 1-3 days)	Very high; 100% if untreated	No vaccine	Antibiotics	Not considered a likely agent; difficult to turn into a weapon
Botulism	High	Vaccine being tested	Antitoxin; requires intensive supportive care	Not considered a likely weapon
Tularemia	Moderate	Vaccine being studied	Antibiotics	Difficult to stabilize for use as a weapon
Ebola	Very high	No vaccine	Minimal	Not considered a likely weapon; difficult to acquire; poorly understood
Brucellosis (incubation 5-21 days)	Low	No vaccine	Antibiotics; begin upon suspicion of disease	Not considered a likely weapon; low lethality
Q Fever (Coxiella burnetii) (incubation 14-26 days)	Low	Vaccine	Antibiotics; begin in incubation period	Not considered a likely weapon; low lethality
Other potentials: Viral Venezuelan equine encephalitis, cholera, salmonella, influenza, and staphylococcal enterotoxin B				

From Cieslak TJ, Eitzen EM: Bioterrorism: agents of concern, *J Public Health Manag Pract* 6(4):19-29, 2000.

TABLE 26-2 Chemical Agents of Mass Destruction

CHEMICAL AGENT	LETHALITY	TREATMENT	IMPACT
Sarin (nerve agent)	High	Move to fresh air; wash skin; drugs limited effectiveness	Likely nerve agent; chemicals needed to produce are banned by International Chemical Weapons Convention
VX (nerve agent)	Very high	Move to fresh air, wash skin, drugs limited effectiveness	Not likely weapon, difficult to manufacture
Tabun (nerve agent)	High	Move to fresh air; wash skin; drugs limited effectiveness	Easy to manufacture nerve agent; likely agent to be used
Chlorine (pulmonary agent)	Low	Move to fresh air; wash skin; no antidote	Readily available; likely agent because of availability; breaks down with water
Hydrogen cyanide (blood agent)	Low to moderate	Move to fresh air; wash skin; some drugs mitigate effects	Industrial product; some chemicals used to produce are banned; likely agent because of availability

From Cieslak TJ, Eitzen EM: Bioterrorism: agents of concern, *J Public Health Manag Pract* 6(4):19-29, 2000.

BOX 26-2 Characteristics of Disasters

Frequency
Predictability
Preventability
Imminence
Scope and number of casualties
Intensity

for the development of tornados; these generally occur between April and June, but they may occur at any time of the year or occur as a secondary result of hurricanes. Weather forecasters can predict hurricanes with increasing accuracy. Other disasters (e.g., fires and industrial explosions) may not be predictable at all.

Preventability

Preventability refers to actions taken to avoid a disaster. Some disasters (e.g., hurricanes, tornados, and earthquakes) are not preventable, whereas others can be easily controlled if not prevented entirely. For example, flooding can be controlled or prevented though construction of dams or levees or deepening bayous.

Primary prevention is aimed at preventing the occurrence of a disaster or limiting consequences when the event itself cannot be prevented. Primary prevention occurs in the nondisaster and predisaster stages. The nondisaster stage is the period before a disaster occurs and the predisaster stage refers to action(s) taken when a disaster is pending. Preventive actions during the nondisaster stage include assessing communities to determine potential disaster hazards; developing disaster plans at local, state, and federal levels; conducting drills to test the plan; training volunteers

FIGURE 26-1 Community risk map.

and health care providers; and providing educational programs of all kinds.

Risk maps and resource maps are developed to aid in planning. A **risk map** is a geographic map of an area that is analyzed for the impact of a potential disaster on the population and buildings in the area that would be involved (e.g., an area in a flood plain, an area covered if a nuclear explosion would occur. an area involved in an explosion of an industrial site) (Figure 26-1). A **resource map** is a geographic map that outlines the resources that would be available in or near the area affected by a potential disaster (e.g., potential shelter sites, potential medical sources, and location of equipment that might be needed) (Figure 26-2).

The disaster plan is initiated predisaster or when a disaster is imminent. Primary prevention actions during this stage include notification of the appropriate officials, warning the population, and advising what response to take (e.g., shelter in place or evacuate).

Secondary prevention strategies are implemented once the disaster occurs. Secondary prevention actions include search, rescue, and triage of victims and assessment of the destruction and devastation of the area involved.

Tertiary prevention focuses on recovery of the community, that is, restoring the community to its previous level of functioning and its residents to their maximum functioning. Tertiary prevention is aimed at preventing a recurrence or minimizing the effects of future disasters.

Nurses should be involved in all stages of prevention and related activities. In order to respond effectively, personally, and professionally during different types of disasters, nurses need to know (1) what kind of disasters threaten their communities, (2) what injuries to expect from different disaster scenarios, (3) evacuation routes, (4) location of shelters, and (5) warning systems. They must be able to educate others about disasters and how to prepare for and respond to them. Finally, nurses need to keep up-to-date on the latest recommendations and advances in lifesaving measures (e.g., basic first aid, CPR, and use of automated external defibrillators).

Imminence

Imminence is the speed of onset of an impending disaster, and relates to the extent of forewarning possible and the anticipated duration of the incident. Weather forecasters can

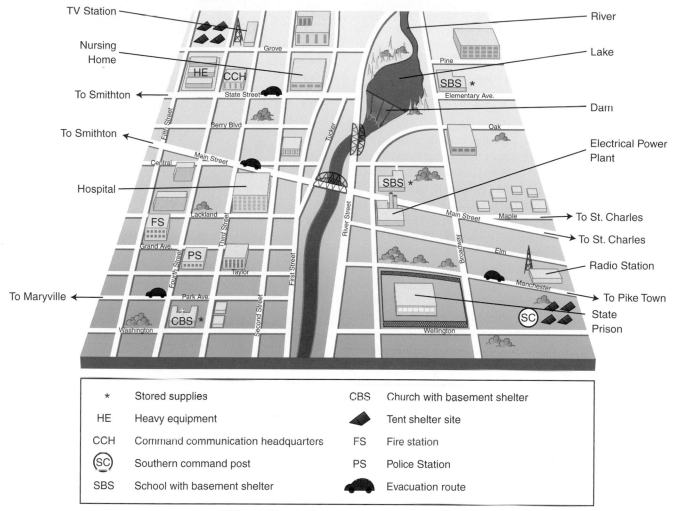

FIGURE 26-2 Community resource map.

*	Stored supplies	CBS	Church with basement shelter
HE	Heavy equipment		Tent shelter site
CCH	Command communication headquarters	FS	Fire station
(SC)	Southern command post	PS	Police Station
SBS	School with basement shelter		Evacuation route

tell when a hurricane may be developing days ahead of its expected arrival and can give the time of arrival, general direction it will take, and an approximate location for its landing and forward movement. Hurricanes, however, are subject to other weather variables and can change direction and intensity several times before actual landfall.

Some disastrous incidents (e.g., wildfires, explosions, and terrorist attacks) have no warning time. Bioterrorist attacks are generally silent, and the first awareness may be days or even weeks after exposure. For example, individuals exposed to a pathologic agent (e.g., anthrax, smallpox) may arrive at health care facilities at various times and to various providers making diagnosis and early treatment difficult. Nurses and medical personnel need to know the signs and symptoms of biological, chemical, radiation, and nuclear exposure in order to identify the nature of the threat and then to treat and control the spread of both biological and chemical agents (see Table 26-1 and Table 26-2).

Scope and Number of Casualties

The scope of a disaster indicates the range of its effect. The scope is described in terms of the geographical area involved and in terms of the number of individuals affected, injured, or killed. From a health care perspective, the location, type, and timing of a disaster event are predictors of the types of injuries and illnesses that might occur. For example, the October 1989 earthquake in San Francisco occurred while people were on their way to work. Overall, more than 60 people died from a multitude of causes, including a motorcycle officer who was killed following the collapse of a freeway, 16 people who were killed from building collapses, 5 who died as a result of falls, and 9 who died from heart attacks.

In contrast, the earthquake and tsunami in October 2004 killed over 174,000 people in South Asia, Southeast Asia, and East Africa; most died from drowning (Centers for Disease Control and Prevention, 2005). Another example of the horribly destructive power of earthquakes occurred in Pakistan in October 2005. That quake resulted in landslides that killed more than 73,000 people; many of the dead were children whose schools were buried from the mudslides.

Hurricanes generally affect a large geographical area. Despite this, they may cause few if any deaths if sufficient preventive measures are taken. The scope of Hurricane Katrina in September 2005 covered all of New Orleans, most of south Louisiana, and parts of Florida, Alabama, and Mississippi. Hurricane Rita, only a few days later, struck New Orleans again, as well as south Louisiana and much of eastern Texas. Remarkably, despite the widespread destruction caused by these storms, the number of dead from Katrina was slightly more than 1300, and the number of dead from Hurricane Rita was 58, including 23 elders who were killed in a bus accident while evacuating.

Intensity

Intensity is the characteristic describing the level of destruction and devastation of the disaster event. Factors contributing to the amount of damage from a disaster event such as a hurricane are the distance from the zone of maximum winds, how exposed the location is, building standards, vegetation type, and resultant flooding. Parts of New Orleans were under water from the primary and secondary effects of Hurricane Katrina. Some buildings and homes were completely destroyed, and others were left in terrible conditions due to flooding and wind damage.

Various hurricane and tornado scales have been developed based on wind intensity and predicted level of destruction. The Fujita Tornado Intensity Scale is one such scale. This measure uses the following values (Texas Department of Health, 1998b):

- *F-0:* A gale tornado with wind speed of 40 to 72 mph (chimney damage, broken tree limbs, small trees uprooted)
- *F-1:* A moderate tornado with wind speed of 73 to 112 mph (roof surfaces partially removed, mobile homes overturned, moving automobiles pushed from roads)
- *F-2:* A significant tornado with wind speed of 113 to 157 mph (roof surfaces removed, mobile homes demolished, railroad cars overturned, large trees uprooted or split, lightweight objects thrown)
- *F-3:* A severe tornado with wind speed of 158 to 206 mph (roofs and walls removed, trains overturned, most trees uprooted, heavy cars thrown)
- *F-4:* A devastating tornado with wind speed of 207 to 260 mph (houses leveled, structures with foundations moved, heavy cars and large objects thrown)
- *F-5:* An incredible tornado with wind speed of 261 to 318 mph (homes destroyed, trees debarked, cars thrown more than 100 yards, incredible phenomena occur).

The Saffir-Simpson Hurricane Scale lists hurricanes as Category 1, 2, 3, 4, or 5, depending on the amount of devastation that is likely to occur due to the sustained wind velocity and accompanying storm surge (Box 26-3). When comparing the wind speed of tornados with hurricanes, it is evident that potential damage form an F-4 or F-5 tornado is likely to be more severe and deadly than a Category 5 hurricane.

Geographical areas determined to be within a hurricane's path are divided into zones. The zone number identifies the anticipated degree of impact on a particular area. Criteria and guidelines associated with each zone number determine what actions the members of a community or area need to take. For example, for a Category 1 hurricane, the residents in Zone 1 would be required to evacuate to distant shelter locations on the recognized evacuation routes, and the residents in Zone 2 would need to take preventive actions. For a Category 2 storm, people living in Zones 1 and 2 would need to evacuate and protect their homes and businesses, and so on. Higher category

---

BOX 26-3 Saffir-Simpson Hurricane Scale

Category 1: 74-95 mph sustained winds resulting in minimal devastation

Category 2: 96-110 mph sustained winds resulting in moderate devastation

Category 3: 111-130 mph sustained winds resulting in extensive devastation

Category 4: 131-155 mph sustained winds resulting in extreme devastation

Category 5: greater than 155 mph sustained winds resulting in catastrophic devastation

---

hurricanes require more zones to evacuate due to the potential hurricane surge expected. Higher category hurricanes require more zones to evacuate due to the potential hurricane surge expected. Typically, it is the storm surge that causes the most damage and deaths attributed to hurricanes.

DISASTER MANAGEMENT

When one is aware of the types and characteristics of disasters, the question then becomes What can be done to prevent, prepare for, respond to, and recover from disasters? Disaster management requires an interdisciplinary, collaborative team effort and involves a network of agencies and individuals to develop a disaster plan that covers the multiple elements necessary for an effective plan. Communities can respond more quickly, more effectively, and with less confusion if the efforts needed in the event of a disaster have been anticipated and plans for meeting them identified. The result of planning is that more lives are saved and less property is damaged. Planning ensures that resources are available and that roles and responsibilities of all personnel and agencies, both official and unofficial, are delineated.

Nurses need to know their personal, professional, and community responsibilities. They should realize that conflicts may arise between their personal and professional responsibilities if these have not been considered and planned for in advance. Also, nurses may be direct or indirect victims and may even be displaced persons as a result of a disaster event. Recognizing this possibility, nurses need to plan, prepare, practice, and teach their family and significant others how to respond (Aucoin, 2005).

Local, State, and Federal Governmental Responsibilities

Local Government

The local government is responsible for the safety and welfare of its citizens. Emergencies and disaster incidents are handled at the lowest possible organizational and jurisdictional level. Police, fire, public health, public works, and medical emergency services are the **first responders** responsible for incident management at the local level. Local officials and agencies are responsible for preparing their citizens for all kinds of emergencies and disasters and for testing disaster plans with mock drills. They manage events during an incident by carrying out evacuation, search and rescue, and maintaining

Deciding Whether to Care for Family or Care for Patients

During a disaster, a nurse might face an ethical dilemma because of competing responsibilities to family, employer, and patients. For example, a nurse who is a single parent with young children and a limited support system may be forced to decide between her responsibility to care for her children or a mandate to report to work to care for patients. Choosing may result in loss of employment or danger to the children. Potential conflicts such as this should be considered, discussed, and decisions made in conjunction with the employer before a disaster event.

BOX 26-4 Guidelines for Early Detection for Biochemical Terrorist Incidents

- A rapidly increasing disease incidence (within hours or days) in a normally healthy population.
- An unusual increase in the number of people seeking care, especially with fever, respiratory, or gastrointestinal complaints.
- An endemic disease rapidly emerging at an uncharacteristic time or in an unusual pattern.
- Clusters of patients arriving from a single locale.
- Large numbers of rapidly fatal cases—patients who die within 72 hours after admission to the hospital.
- Any patient presenting with a disease that is relatively uncommon and has bioterrorism potential (e.g., pulmonary anthrax, smallpox, or plague).

From Chettle C: Recognizing bioterrorism: nurses on the frontline, *NurseWeek* 6:29-30, Nov 12, 2001.

public health and public works responsibilities. Local communities should have contingency operation plans for multiple disaster situations and for various aspects of the plan. For example, telephone service and cell phone service may not work, so other forms of communication need to be available.

In an incident other than a biological, chemical, radiation, or nuclear event, in most cases, it is the 911 communication center or the fire or police department that gets the initial message. The emergency communication center would then communicate the incident to the other first responders and the director of the **Office of Emergency Management,** who determines others who may be needed (e.g., ambulances, other officials, and voluntary group representatives). Local hospitals are notified of the incident and the predicted nature of impending casualties. The hospitals may begin to receive victims who have not been triaged at the site of the incident via private automobiles. According to the CDC, a hospital can assess the expected number of victims that they may receive by counting the number that arrives within the first hour and doubling that number.

For a biological or chemical terrorist incident, the process is very different. First responders generally are not involved. Rather, nurses and doctors in health care facilities may be the first to suspect that a biological or chemical agent has been released into the community. Box 26-4 lists the guidelines for detecting biochemical incidents. If any of these instances occur in a health care provider setting, the suspicion should be immediately reported to the infection control department, the administration of the facility, or both. Each setting should post, near the telephone, the numbers to be called if a biochemical incident (whether internal or external) is suspected. These numbers should include those of the CDC Bioterrorism Emergency Response the CDC Hospital Infections program, and the U.S. Army Medical Research Institute of Infectious Disease (Chettle, 2001).

The Office of Emergency Management involves representatives from all official and unofficial agencies in developing the community disaster plan, developing scenarios to test the plan through drills, and assessing the scope, intensity, and number of casualties (once an incident has occurred) in order to initiate the proper response. For those events that are not within the abilities of the local community or in the event of a terrorist-type incident, higher level agencies and resources must be requested and will become involved.

State Government

When a disaster overwhelms the local community's resources, then the State's Department or Office of Emergency Management is called for assistance. Prior to an event, state officials provide technical support for prevention, preparedness, response, and recovery. State officials visit local officials to assist and assess local emergency management plans, promote and conduct workshops and training courses, assist with training exercises, advise and support local government officials, and are on-scene at disaster events to facilitate coordination of state resources and to disseminate information. In some cases, the National Guard may be called in to aid the community. When the scope of the event is so great that local and state resources are not adequate to meet the needs, the state calls on the federal government; at that point, the President may declare the incident a "national disaster." Once the President declares a national disaster, federal aid is made available. At that point, the National Response Plan, the core operational plan for domestic incident management, would be initiated.

Federal Government

The policy of the federal government is to have a comprehensive and effective program in place to ensure continuity of essential federal functions across a wide array of incidents. The national strategy is to develop a system connecting all levels of government without duplicating efforts. More than 87,000 governmental jurisdictions at the federal, state, and local level have security responsibilities. All federal agencies are required to have in place a viable Continuity of Operations capability plan that ensures the performance of their essential functions during any incident that disrupts normal operations (FEMA, 2005d).

U.S. Department of Homeland Security

The U.S. Department of Homeland Security (DHS) was established on March 1, 2003, to realign the current systems into a single department, focusing on protecting the American people and their homeland. The DHS consolidated 22 agencies

FIGURE 26-3 Homeland Security Advisory System. (From US Department of Homeland Security: *Homeland Security Advisory System: current threat level*, 2005c, The Author, http://www.dhs.gov/dhspublic/display?theme=29&content=3927&print=true.)

and their 180,000 employees into a single agency (The White House, 2005).

The DHS has three primary missions: (1) prevent terrorist attacks within the United States, (2) reduce America's vulnerability to terrorism, and (3) minimize the damage from potential attacks and natural disasters (DHS, 2005a). The organizational structure of the DHS contains several divisions: the Office of the Secretary, Border and Transportation Security, Emergency Preparedness and Response Directorate, Information Analysis and Infrastructure Protection, Science and Technology, Office of Management, U.S. Citizenship and Immigration Services, U.S. Coast Guard, and the U.S. Secret Service. Within each of these divisions are multiple offices and centers (DHS, 2005b).

The DHS established its Homeland Security Advisory System for terrorist threats to the mass transit sector. This system was designed to combine threat information with vulnerability assessments and provide communications to public safety officials and the public. The color-coded threat level system communicates a level of threat for terrorist attacks so that protective measures can be implemented to reduce the likelihood or impact of an attack (Figure 26-3).

Preparation for a terrorist incident is similar to preparation for other crisis events. General guidelines from FEMA are to

be aware of surroundings; move or leave if you feel uncomfortable; take precautions when traveling; do not accept packages from strangers; report unusual behavior; learn where emergency exits are located in buildings; plan how to get out of buildings in the event of an emergency; be prepared to do without services normally dependent on (i.e., electricity, telephone, natural gas, gasoline pumps, cash ATMs, and Internet transactions). An additional guideline is to ensure the following items are available: a portable, battery-operated radio with extra batteries; several flashlights with extra batteries; a first aid kit and manual; hard hats and dust masks; and florescent tape to rope off dangerous areas (FEMA, 2005b).

In addition to the Homeland Security Advisory System, DHS has published other information for public use. The DHS pamphlet *Preparing Makes Sense: Get Ready Now* (DHS, 2005d) gives advice as to what plans need to be in place to survive without help for a period of time. Other publications are *Homeland Security Advice* and *What To Do in Different Types of Emergencies* (Boxes 26-5 and 26-6, respectively).

The National Response Plan

The National Response Plan (NRP) is a comprehensive, all-hazards approach to managing domestic incidents. The plan integrates practices and procedures from homeland security, emergency management, law enforcement, firefighting, public works, public health, responder and recovery worker health and safety, emergency medical services, and the private sector into a unified structure (DHS, 2004). The plan addresses prevention, preparedness, response, and recovery activities.

The DHS Emergency Preparedness and Response Directorate and FEMA, in conjunction with the DHS Office of the Secretary, function as the executive agent for NRP management and maintenance. The Secretary of DHS developed the National Incident Management System (NIMS), which integrates practices in disaster preparedness and response into a comprehensive national framework for incident management. The NIMS enables responders at all levels to work together effectively in managing domestic incidents, no matter what the cause, size, or complexity (FEMA, 2005c).

The Federal Emergency Management Agency

FEMA became part of DHS on March 1, 2003. FEMA's mission is "to lead the efforts to prepare the nation for all hazards and effectively manage federal response and recovery efforts following any national incident (FEMA, 2005a). FEMA also initiates proactive mitigation activities, trains first responders, and manages the National Flood Insurance Program and the U.S. Fire Administration.

Department of Health and Human Services/Centers for Disease Control and Prevention

After the rescue of survivors has been accomplished, the Department of Health and Human Services, Centers for Disease Control and Prevention steps in to ensure that clean drinking water, food, shelter, and medical care are available for those affected. Their involvement may be necessary depending on the type of disaster. For example, floods pose

BOX 26-5 Homeland Security Advice

Emergency Supplies
Food
➤ Store least a 3-day supply of nonperishable food.
➤ Have a manual can opener.
➤ Keep disposable plates/cups and utensils.

Clean Air
➤ Store snugly fitting face masks.
➤ Store plastic sheeting, duct tape, and scissors to seal off a room.

First Aid Kit
Sterile gloves, dressings, soap, antibiotic ointment, bandages, eye wash, nonprescription medications (e.g., aspirin).

Make a Plan
Create a Family Plan
➤ Plan on how to contact one another if the family is separated.
➤ Review plan for different situations.

At Work and School
➤ Schools, daycare providers, workplaces, apartment buildings, and neighborhoods should all have site-specific emergency plans.

In a High-Rise Bulding
➤ You may be in a high-rise building at the time of an attack.
➤ Plan for the possibility.
➤ Note where the closest **emergency exit** is.
➤ Be sure you know **another way out** in case your first choice is blocked.

➤ **Take cover** against a desk or table if things are falling.
➤ **Face away** from windows and glass.
➤ **Move away** from exterior walls.
➤ **Do not use elevators**.
➤ **Stay to the right** while going down stairwells to allow emergency workers to come up.

Water
➤ Store at least a 3-day supply; 1 gallon per day per person.
➤ Store water in clean plastic bottles.

Supply Checklist
➤ Basic supplies include flashlight, batteries, radio, garbage bags, map, moist towlettes, whistle, clothing, bedding and tools.

Special Needs Items
➤ Prescription medications; special items for infants (diapers, formula), elders, or persons with disabilities.

In a Moving Vehicle
➤ If the vehicle becomes difficult to control, pull over.
➤ Avoid road hazards.
➤ Obey barriers and signs.

Deciding to Stay or Go
➤ Depending on your circumstances and the nature of the attack, the first important decision is whether you stay put or get away.
➤ You should understand and plan for both possibilities.

From Department of Homeland Security. (2005). The Author, http://www.Ready.gov.

risks of contaminated water and food supplies; loss of shelter leaves people vulnerable to heat or cold and other environmental hazards (e.g., insects); earthquakes create traumatic injuries (e.g., broken bones, head injuries) that will need to be addressed.

Public Health System

The public health system's mission is the promotion of health, prevention of disease, and protection from threats to health. The *public health system* is a broad term used to describe all of the governmental and nongovernmental organizations and agencies that contribute to the improvement of the health of populations. Public health agencies are the primary agencies for the health and medical response to disaster incidents and therefore are a part of the initial response activities.

Public health officials provide advice and assistance to other public officials related to environment and health matters. Preparedness includes vigilance and reporting of suspicious illnesses (e.g., signs and symptoms of biological agents, food-borne diseases, and communicable diseases) in the community by physicians and nurses in local health care facilities or private offices and clinics. Public health officials then have the responsibility of detecting outbreaks, determining the cause of illness, identifying the risk factors for the population, implementing interventions to control the outbreak, and informing the public of the health risks and preventive

measures that need to be taken. These relate both directly and indirectly to the 10 essential public health services (Box 26-7).

American Red Cross

The **American Red Cross** (ARC) is not a governmental agency. The ARC, however, is chartered by Congress to provide disaster relief. It works in partnership with FEMA, DHS, the Centers for Disease Control and Prevention, and other federal agencies to provide and manage needed services.

The ARC is primarily a volunteer organization with chapters in all 50 states, Puerto Rico, the Virgin Islands, and the Pacific Rim; the national headquarters is in Falls Church, Virginia. Disaster Services is only one of the programs that the ARC provides. Other program services provided are International Services, Biomedical Services, Armed Forces Emergency Services, and Health, Safety and Community Services.

The ARC places great emphasis on preparedness and participates with communities in developing and testing their disaster plans, maintaining and training personnel for disaster response, and responding during an actual emergency or disaster. The ARC publishes many pamphlets and educational materials to help individuals, families, neighborhoods, schools, and businesses prepare for potential disasters. The key actions they recommend are (1) identify potential disaster events, (2) create a disaster plan for sheltering in place or for evacuation, (3) assemble a disaster supplies kit, and (4) prac-

BOX 26-6   What To Do in Different Types of Emergencies

Biological attack
➤ Quickly get away.
➤ Cover your mouth and nose to filter air.
➤ Wash with soap and water.

Nuclear blast
➤ Take cover quickly.
➤ Limit amount of radiation exposure by shielding, getting away from blast, and minimizing time exposed.

Chemical attack
➤ Quickly get away.
➤ If exposed, strip immediately and wash.
➤ Seek medical attention.

Radiation threat
➤ "Dirty bomb" uses common explosives to spread radioactive material.
➤ Limit exposure same as for nuclear blast.

Explosions
➤ Take shelter against a desk or sturdy table.
➤ Quickly exit building.
➤ Crawl if there is fire.

Trapped in debris
➤ Use flashlight, whistle, or tap on pipe or wall to signal rescuers.
➤ Unnecessary movement and shouting risk breathing unsafe dust.

From US Department of Homeland Security (2005). The Author, http://www.Ready.gov.

BOX 26-7   Essential Public Health Services

1. Monitor health status to identify community health problems.
2. Diagnose and investigate health problems and health hazards in the community.
3. Inform, educate, and empower people about health issues.
4. Mobilize community partnerships to identify and solve health problems.
5. Develop policies and plans that support individual and community health efforts.
6. Enforce laws and regulations that protect health and ensure safety.
7. Link people to needed personal health service and ensure the provision of health care when otherwise unavailable.
8. Ensure the existence of a competent public health and personal health care workforce.
9. Evaluate effectiveness, accessibility, and quality of personal and population-based health services.
10. Research and develop new insights and innovative solutions to health problem.

From Berkowitz B: Public health nursing practice: aftermath of September 11, 2001, *Online J Issues Nurs,* Sept 30, 2002, http://www.nursingworld.org/ojin/topic19/tpc19_4.htm.

tice and maintain the plan. The disaster plan should include an emergency communications plan, a predetermined meeting place for family members or significant others, and plans for care of pets in the event that evacuation is required.

If local authorities issue a **shelter-in-place** communication, instructions that address what actions to take if at home, at work, at school, or in a vehicle should be followed. There are

RESEARCH HIGHLIGHTS

School Nurses and Emergency Preparedness

A survey of 193 school nurses was recently conducted to assess knowledge of bioterrorism and educational needs for emergency preparedness (Evers and Puzniak, 2005). The researchers reported that although 80% of the respondents stated that their school had an emergency plan and an evacuation plan, only about half (48.5%) had a shelter-in-place plan. Further, although most (62%) stated that their school was "somewhat prepared" for a disaster, only 6.2% rated their school as "very prepared." Knowledge of specific information on bioterrorism was only fair. For example, it was noted that only 55% of survey respondents could distinguish between signs and symptoms of anthrax and influenza. Finally, slightly more than half of respondents believed that a biological or chemical attack was "somewhat likely," and nearly 40% believed that a nuclear attack was "somewhat likely." The researchers concluded that school nurses need more training and preparation to be able to respond appropriately to an emergency or disaster situation.

From Evers S, Puzniak L: Bioterrorism knowledge and emergency preparedness among school nurses, *J School Health* 75(6):232-237, 2005.

TABLE 26-3   American Red Cross Disaster Relief Hurricane Season, 2004

TYPE OF ASSISTANCE	NUMBER
Shelters and evacuation centers opened	1,828
Shelter population	424,428
Emergency aid stations opened	46
Service centers opened	329
Meals and snacks served	10,642,370
Outreach contacts	34,240
Health services contacts	46,511
Mental health contacts	78,606
Emergency response vehicles deployed	574
Total American Red Cross workers	34,771

American Red Cross: *America's disasters* 2004, 2005, The Author, from http://www.redcross.org/pubs/dspubs/amdisasters2004.pdf.

specific actions to take, depending on where you are at the time the shelter-in-place communication is issued. For example, during a disaster, such as hazardous gas emission from an industrial plant, if someone is at home, a business, or public building, they may be instructed to go inside and follow home or work shelter-in-place recommendations (e.g., close doors, turn off fans and air conditioning, bring children and pets inside, and stay inside until "all clear" has been called). In order to be prepared to assist during a disaster, the ARC recommends that individuals get trained and, if possible, volunteer and give blood (ARC, 2003b).

The Red Cross disaster response efforts focus on meeting the immediate disaster-related needs of affected people and providing support services to the emergency rescue and recovery workers (ARC, 2003b). The disaster response functions are to provide health services, mental health services, family services, and mass care, and to inquire about family well-being. Mass care includes feeding, sheltering, providing basic first aid, bulk distribution, and a Disaster Welfare Information system (ARC, 2005). Table 26-3 shows the breadth of services that the ARC provided for hurricane disaster relief in 2004.

DISASTER MANAGEMENT STAGES

Prevention Stage

The first stage in disaster management occurs before a disaster is imminent and is known as the *nondisaster stage*. Potential disaster risks should be identified and risk maps created (see Figure 26-1). The population demographics and vulnerabilities, as well as the community's capabilities, should be analyzed. Primary prevention measures include educating the public regarding what actions to take to prepare for disasters at the individual, family, and community levels. Further, based on the assessment of potential risks, the community must develop a plan for meeting the potential disasters identified.

With regard to bioterrorist attacks, prevention means that health care providers need to be knowledgeable about the biological and chemical agents that might be used. In addition, health care providers need to know the signs and symptoms of the various biological and chemical agents that have been recognized as potential threats. As mentioned, unlike other disasters, biochemical terrorist threats may only be identified when events raise suspicions of health care providers, rather than first responders at a particular site.

Early identification of ill or exposed persons, rapid implementation of preventive therapy, special infection control considerations, and collaboration or communication with the public are essential in controlling the spread of cases. Hospitals need to identify rooms that can be converted into isolation units to meet the demand. Nurses need to be instructed in decontamination and reminded of isolation techniques that might be needed, depending on the biological agent. Volunteers and professionals must remain current in first aid, CPR, and advanced lifesaving procedures.

Preparedness and Planning Stage

Individual and family preparedness includes training in first aid, assembling a disaster emergency kit, establishing a predetermined meeting place away from home, and making a family communication plan. Recommendations for what needs to be included in each of these are available from many sources (e.g., ARC, DHS, and FEMA). These are guidelines, and each individual and each family needs to modify the preparations to meet their individual needs.

Although there will be some variation according to the individual community's needs, all community disaster plans should address the following elements: authority, communication, control, logistical coordination of personnel, supplies and equipment, evacuation, rescue, and care of the dead. The plan should indicate who has the power to declare there is a disaster and who has the power to initiate the disaster plan.

Authority should be designated by the title of the person; it should not specify a person by name. There should also be backup positions identified in the event the first individual is not available. Every individual should be equally informed about the role and responsibilities that go with this authority. A clear chain of authority for carrying out the plan is critical for successful implementation of the plan. Authority may change, depending on whether the disaster is natural or man-made as a result of some criminal action, and change of authority should be addressed in the plan.

Communication is recognized as the biggest problem area in disasters. Reliance on telephone systems or cell phones should not be the sole planned means of communicating because these may not work or the systems might be overwhelmed. Misinformation and misinterpretation can occur when communication is ineffective. The communication section should address how the authority figure will be notified of the disaster, how the emergency management team members will be notified, how the community residents will be warned about the incident, and what actions to take. This section needs to address how communication between relief workers and authorities will be maintained. Also, it should include information on the role of the media in keeping people informed and in letting people know what assistance and supplies are needed.

The analysis of the population that was completed during the non-disaster stage should identify groups that need special attention as to how they will be notified. These people include those who speak different languages, are homeless or poor, are without television or other means of communication, and those in institutions like prisons, nursing homes, day care settings, or schools. Effective communication during a disaster must be credible, current, authoritative, and give some indication of future events.

The *logistical* section should specify where supplies and equipment are located or where additional supplies and equipment can be obtained, where these will be stored or found, and how they will be transported to the disaster site (see Figure 26-2). Essential *human resources* (e.g., emergency and disaster specialists, officials of governmental and voluntary agencies, engineers, weather specialists, and community leaders) should be identified and where they will be located together determined. The plan should include information about transportation for *evacuation and rescue* (particularly taking into account vulnerable groups), documentation and record keeping, and plans for evaluation of the success or failure of the plan.

A disaster plan is a dynamic entity. Planning is a continuous process, and plans change with circumstances and when gaps are identified during drills or from actual disaster incidents. The plan should set realistic expectations of effects and needs, should be brief and concise, and should establish priorities and timelines for actions. Plans should follow the disaster planning principles discussed in Box 26-8.

For a plan to be effective, it must be tested by having different disaster scenario drills. The more times realistic scenarios are created to test the plan in actual practice sessions, and not just table top or paper drills, the more problems with the plan will be identified and solutions for those problems can be found. Without practice drills, plans may have many unrecognized faults and as a result, many more individuals may be harmed and communities damaged when an actual disaster occurs.

Response Stage

This stage begins immediately after the disaster incident occurs. The community preparedness plans that have been

BOX 26-8 Disaster Planning Principles

1. Measures usually taken are not sufficient for major disasters.
2. Plans should be adjusted to people's needs.
3. Planning does not stop with development of a written plan.
4. Lack of information causes inappropriate responses by community members.
5. People should be able to respond with or without direction.
6. Plans should coordinate efforts of the entire community, so large segments of the citizenry should be involved in the planning.
7. Plans should be linked to surrounding areas.
8. Plans should be general enough to cover all potential disaster events.
9. As much as possible, plans should be based on everyday work methods and procedures.
10. Plans should specify a person's responsibility for implementing segments by position or title rather than by name.
11. Plans should develop a record-keeping system before a disaster occurs, regarding:
    Supplies and equipment
    Records of all present at any given time (to account for everyone and to identify the missing)
    Identification of victims and deceased, conditions and treatment documented, and to which facility victims are sent
12. Backup plans need to be in place for the following:
    Disruption of telephone and cell phone lines
    Disruption of computer data (should be downloaded weekly and stored off site)
    Protecting essential public health functions (e.g., vital records and communicable disease data)

TABLE 26-4 Shelter-in-Place Instructions

LOCATION	INSTRUCTIONS
Home	Close all windows, turn off all fans, go to above-ground room, take disaster supplies with you, and bring pets inside; go to room with a telephone, wet some towels and jam them in the space under the door, etc.
School	Close the school, activate emergency plan, and keep visitors in the building; provide for telephone inquiries from concerned parents; if children have cell phones, allow them to call a parent; select interior rooms above the ground floor, etc.
Work	Close the business, bring everyone into the one room, shut and lock the doors, keep customers in the building, turn on call-forwarding, change the recording to indicate the business is closed; if danger of explosion, close the window shades, blinds, or curtains, etc.
Vehicle	If close to home, office, or a public building, go there. If unable to get to a home or building, pull over to the safest place possible, turn off the engine, close windows and vents, listen to the radio regularly for updated advice, and follow directions from law enforcement officials.

From American Red Cross: *Disaster services: shelter in place*, 2003a, The Author, http://www.seattleredcross.org/prepare/shelter.htm.

developed are initiated. If a disaster occurs, people should remain calm and exert patience, follow the advice of local emergency officials, and listen to the radio or television for news and instructions. If people nearby are injured, one should give first aid, seek help, and check the area for dangerous hazards. Those at home should shut off any damaged utilities, confine or secure pets, call family contact(s), and check on neighbors, especially the elderly or disabled.

The plan may call for people to shelter in place, to evacuate, or for search and rescue to begin. If the only response needed is shelter in place, then people need to know what to do if they are at home, at work, at school, or in their vehicle.

Shelter in Place

The American Red Cross has provided explicit instructions for individuals and families to be followed when told by authorities to "shelter in place" in the event of a disaster. Table 26-4 shows these guidelines.

Evacuation

Each community has established evacuation routes for the residents to use if evacuation from the area is called for. In some instances, mandatory evacuation may be implemented. However, there are always some individuals who will not leave their home for any numbers of reasons (e.g., fear of vandalism, denial of the potential extent of the disaster, pride in their home and belongings, etc.). Education of residents as to the potential

damage, deaths, and injuries that will be incurred from the potential disasters that may affect their community needs to be done in the preparedness stage and not when evacuation is ordered. In some extreme cases, it may be necessary for hospitals and other facilities, such as nursing homes, to evacuate patients. This requires significant advance planning, as health practitioners must determine how to move seriously and even critically ill people and coordinate transportation and placement for their disposition to safe facilities.

Search and Rescue

Before search and rescue should begin, safety must be considered. In some instances, if a criminal action is suspected, law officials will be among the first to respond in order to secure the area and possibly gather evidence. While the area is being checked and then cleared of potential threats, a staging area can be set up at or near the site of the incident to direct on-site activities. Search and rescue of victims can begin once clearance is given, a disaster triage area is established, and an emergency treatment area is set up to provide first aid until transportation for victims to hospitals or health care facilities for treatment can be coordinated (Figure 26-4).

Staging Area

The staging area is the on-site command station. Disaster responders should report to this area to "check in" so that everyone is accounted for and can be given an assignment. This will allow for the most effective use of the skills and abilities of those responding. No one should go to the disaster site unless directed to do so by the staging area commander. The staging area is also where the authority rests for decisions as to additional resources to be called to the area in order to

**Initial triage
and rescue area**

**Treatment
and transportation/
evacuation area**

**Incident
command
staging area**

FIGURE 26-4   Areas of operation of disaster response.

manage the disaster incident. Resources may be construction equipment to move building materials, rescue dogs to locate humans that are buried in the debris, or more fire, police, or medical personnel.

Disaster Triage

Triage at the site and again at the treatment area is very different from triage that is routinely conducted in the emergency room. The focus of **disaster triage** is to do as little as possible, for the greatest number, in the shortest period of time. One triage system that is used by first responders is the START triage system. START stands for "simple triage and rapid treatment." This system describes what to do when first arriving at a multicasualty or mass casualty incident. Disaster triage of an injured person is to occur in less than 1 minute. This system also describes how to use people with minor injuries to assist. As a decision is made regarding the status of an individual, the person is tagged with a colored triage tag (Figure 26-5).

Green on the triage tag is for the walking wounded or those with minor injuries who can wait several hours before they receive treatment; yellow is for those with systemic but not yet life-threatening complications, who can wait 45 to 60 minutes; red is considered top priority and is for those with life-threatening conditions but who can be stabilized and have a high probability of survival; black is for the deceased or for those whose injuries are is so extensive that nothing can be done to save them.

A new classification of victim, those who are contaminated, will require a hazmat (for "hazardous materials") tag. To assess an individual within the 1-minute guideline, the system uses three characteristics. First, respirations are checked; if they are over 30, the individual is tagged immediately. If the

FIGURE 26-5   Disaster triage tag. Source: www.mettag.com.

When Hurricane Katrina hit the Gulf Coast in late August, 2005, thousands of evacuees from New Orleans and south Louisiana were sent to Houston. Two huge shelters were set up in the city to accommodate those displaced, and the needs, as was documented in the media, were massive.

Faculty, staff, and students from the University of Texas Health Science Center at Houston, personnel from the city and county health departments, and local EMS personnel were joined by thousands of volunteers to care for these disaster victims. Indeed, doctors, nurses, and other health care providers came from across Texas and the Gulf Coast area, and from as far away as California, Arizona, Illinois, and New York to help.

To care for the health needs of the evacuees, a clinic was established in the George R. Brown Convention Center. According to one of the officials at UT-Houston, "We got the call at 9 AM Friday [to create the clinic], and by 5 PM it was all set up." The clinic was modeled after army field hospitals, with a command center, triage areas, and various clinics. There were sections for trauma and acute care, adult medical care, women's/gynecological care, and pediatric care and an area for persons with mental health concerns. A full-service pharmacy was also set up.

During the next 17 days, more than 10,000 patient visits were logged, and there were more than 6000 volunteers. These photos depict how care was organized and shows the efforts of the many volunteers.

Organizational meeting.

Setting up the registration area to check in clinic clients.

Organizing medical supplies.

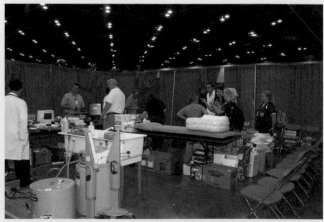

Setting up one of the client care areas (note the portable water supply)

Photos courtesy The University of Texas Health Science Center, Houston, Texas.

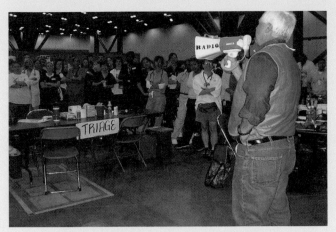

Final instructions before initiation of client care.

Registration and triage area as clients are being seen.

Client registration.

Triage area.

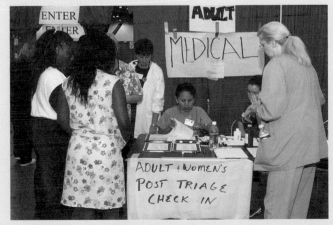

Check-in for the adult clinic.

Waiting area.

Nurses organizing client medications.

Examining an infant.

Caring for a family.

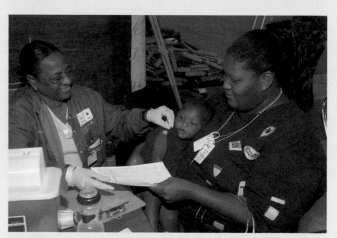
Immunizing a small child.

individual has fewer than 30 respirations, then the assessor moves to the second step—perfusion. Pinching the nail bed and observing the reaction are done to check perfusion; color should return to normal within 2 seconds. The third step is checking mental status. The assessor should ask the individual simple questions (e.g., Who are you?). By doing these steps, the individual responsible for triage can very quickly assess an individual and decide which color tag fits his or her condition. Further, the steps are easy to remember by thinking "30-2-can do," where "30" is the number of respirations, "2" is the number of seconds needed to check for perfusion, and "can do" relates to checking mental status.

Following triage, victims are then moved to the treatment area where their condition is checked again. First aid may be provided there, until transportation is available. Ambulances, helicopters, busses, or all three may be used to transport the victims to various hospitals or health care facilities. Some victims, such as those in the surrounding area that may have been affected by the incident, may even go by private vehicle to a hospital or medical facility. This process may go on for days as it did in the September 11 incidents, the 2005 tsunami in South Asia, and Hurricanes Katrina and Rita. Search and

rescue eventually will be called off, and the recovery stage will begin.

While search and rescue is going on, other agencies (e.g., public health agencies) are checking for threats such as contaminated water, vectors, and air quality. They also disseminate data on what has been found and relate health information to officials, the media, and the public as appropriate. Designated agencies measure the occurrence and distribution of health-related events associated with the disaster, describe factors contributing to health-related effects, and assess the needs of populations and facilities. They will allocate resources and work to prevent further adverse health problems that may result from the disaster. For example, following Hurricane Katrina, public health officials administered tetanus and hepatitis A immunizations to rescuers and victims.

Although triage of individuals exposed to chemical warfare agents is basically the same as for any multiple or mass casualty incident, it poses special challenges. For these events, the triage area is set up in the "hot zone" to assist in determining priorities for resuscitation, decontamination, pharmacological therapy, and site evacuation. Only specially trained emergency personnel who are familiar with chemical agents

---

TABLE 26-5 Common Reactions to a Disaster

EMOTIONAL REACTIONS	COGNITIVE REACTIONS	PHYSICAL REACTIONS	INTERPERSONAL REACTIONS
Shock	Impaired concentration	Fatigue	Alienation
Anger	Impaired decision making	Insomnia	Social withdrawal
Despair	Memory impairment	Sleep disturbance	School impairment
Emotional numbing	Disbelief	Hyperarousal	Increased conflict
Terror	Confusion	Headaches	Vocational impairment
Guilt	Distortion	Startle response	Social withdrawal
Grief or sadness	Decreased self-esteem	Somatic complaints	Alienation
Irritability	Decreased self-efficacy	Gastrointestinal problems	Increase interpersonal conflict
Helplessness	Self-blame	Decreased appetite	Social withdrawal
Dissociation	Worry	Decreased libido	Alienation
Loss of pleasure	Intrusive thoughts or memories	Impaired immune response	Social withdrawal

Modified from Young BH et al: *Disaster mental health services: a guidebook for clinicians and administrators*, Menlo Park, Calif, 1998, Department of Veterans Affairs, National Center for PTSD.

---

and the use of personal protection equipment should triage chemical agent victims. The same triage categories can be assigned to these victims.

Psychological triage presents the challenge of determining who most needs help and deciding what interventions will help. Mental health disorders related to disasters can include anxiety disorders, exacerbation of existing substance abuse problems, somatic complaints, depression, and later post-traumatic stress disorder (PTSD). Research has identified four keys to gauging the mental health impact of such events, any two of which may result in severe, lasting, and pervasive psychological effects. The key factors are (1) extreme and widespread property damage; (2) serious and ongoing financial problems; (3) high prevalence of trauma in the form of injuries, threat to life, and loss of life; and (4) when human intent caused the disaster. In addition, panic during the disaster, horror, separation from family, and relocation or displacement are factors that may play a part in psychological impairment. Nurses need to evaluate an individual's danger to self or others. Nurses need to know the symptoms to look for and know what resources are available for people who need help (Patterson, 2005).

Rapid Epidemiological Assessment

Rapid epidemiological assessment is a strategy or process designed and used by public health officials to provide reliable estimates of health hazards in an expedient manner. Investigations conducted provide information about the effects of a disaster on a population. An example of an epidemiological assessment is the one conducted by the Oklahoma Department of Health to provide a description of the physical injuries and fatalities resulting from the April 19, 1995, bombing of the Alfred P. Murrah Federal Building in Oklahoma City. The assessment included all persons injured by the bombing and all at-risk occupants of the building and the four adjacent buildings. A total of 759 persons sustained injuries; of these, 83 were hospitalized, 509 were treated as outpatients, and 167 died. Of the 361 individuals who were in the federal building, 319 were injured; of these, 163 died,

including 19 children. In the four adjacent buildings, injury rates varied, and three individuals died (Mallonee et al., 1996).

Community Responses to a Disaster

Heroic Phase

The classic four phases of a community's reaction to a disaster are the heroic phase, honeymoon phase, disillusionment phase, and reconstruction phase. During the heroic phase, nearly everyone feels the need to rush to help people survive the disaster. Medical personnel may work hours without sleep, under very dangerous and life-threatening conditions, in order to take care of their patients. Medical personnel may help out in areas with which they are not familiar and have no experience. Disaster Medical Assistance Teams, consisting of professionals and paraprofessional medical personnel, provide emergency relief during a disaster and may travel long distances to help out in a disaster. This was illustrated by the thousands of people who volunteered to help in the immediate aftermaths of September 11 and Hurricanes Katrina and Rita.

Honeymoon Phase

Individuals who have survived the disaster gather together with others who have simultaneously experienced the same event; this is known as the honeymoon phase. People begin to tell their stories and review over and over again what has occurred. Bonds are formed among victims and health care workers. Gratitude is expressed for being alive.

Disillusionment Phase

When time has elapsed and a delay in receiving help or failure to receive the promised aid has not occurred, feelings of despair arise. Medical personnel and other first responders may begin to experience depression due to exhaustion from many long days of long hours. Depression may set in as a result of knowledge of what has happened to the community, friends, and family. People realize the way things were before the disaster is not the way things are now and may never be the same again. They recognize that many things are different and much needs to be done to adjust to the current situation.

CASE STUDY   Application of the Community Assessment Process

ASSESSMENT

Deer Park, Texas, is a city 20 miles east of Houston, Texas. The population is approximately 30,000 people. The majority of the people are white (80.8%) and Hispanic (15.2%). The median age of the population is 34.7 years; the median income is $61,334. Eighty-nine percent of the population over 25 years has a high school diploma or higher education degree. The unemployment rate is 5.6%. The city consists of residential homes, apartment complexes, and retail and service businesses. There are nine schools and several churches of all denominations. Many AM and FM radio stations and TV broadcast stations are available to the Deer Park area.

The Federal Communications Commission (FCC) has developed the Emergency Alert System to warn of any emergency (nuclear attack, hurricane, tornado, flood, or chemical release). The FCC has designated KTRH 740 AM as the station for the Houston area. The city has a volunteer fire department (5 full-time employees) and a city police department (55 full-time employees). The city government consists of a mayor, city council, and city manager. The city has two emergency committees: the Community Awareness and Emergency Response Committee and the Local Emergency Planning Committee.

There are no hospitals in Deer Park. The closest hospitals are 6 to 7 miles away and take 20 minutes to reach. The closest Level 1 trauma center is 15 miles away and the nearest adult care burn center is 20 miles away; the pediatric burn center is in Galveston, Texas, which is about 45 miles away.

The city is also the home of the Shell Deer Park Chemical Plant and the Shell Deer Park Refining Company. The company processes 3% of the nation's oil supply into gasoline. The Shell plants are located on 1500 acres on the Houston Ship Channel. Shell employs approximately 1100 people and 2200 contract workers. The chemical plant and the refining company have their own fire stations, an internal railroad, docks and transportation networks, small medical facilities (one physician and four nurses, 7 days a week, 24 hours a day), first responder teams, two ambulances, and a vehicle that can handle 30 casualties.

DIAGNOSIS

Individual

Because of Deer Park's location on the Gulf Coast and the presence of the Shell Deer Park Refining Company and Shell Deer Park Chemical plant, the residents are at risk for injury or death due to hurricane disasters and potential industrial accidents from either accidental or terrorist causes.

Family

The families of Deer Park are at risk for losing their homes, separation from family members, and having to evacuate from their homes either temporarily or permanently due to hurricane damages or industrial accidents.

Community

The community of Deer Park is at risk for destruction of buildings and city public works due to hurricane disasters and potential explosions from either accidental or terrorist causes.

PLANNING

Disaster Management

Deer Park is in the storm surge zone that requires its residents to evacuate when a Category 1 hurricane is predicted to land in, or within a 100-mile radius of, the Deer Park area. The media sources available to the Deer Park area or the city officials are to give instructions about supplies and equipment to have ready and when to leave. There is only one evacuation route available to the community.

A survey was conducted during the nondisaster stage to identify vulnerable groups that would need help in evacuating.

Individual

Vulnerable individuals that would need to have special consideration for evacuation are the very young (4000 individuals between birth and 10 years), the elderly (2110 individuals ages 65 and over), and families below the poverty level (1200). It was determined that more than 7000 individuals might need some form of transportation in order for them to evacuate.

Long-Term Goal
- Residents will have disaster kit prepared according to ARC and FEMA guidelines.

Short-Term Goals
- Residents will follow official's instructions for sheltering in place or evacuation.
- Vulnerable individuals will know what to do in the event of an evacuation order or shelter in place announcement.

Family
Long-Term Goal
- Family members will continually update the family disaster plan according to family dynamics.

Short-Term Goals
- Families will have in place a disaster plan for communicating.
- Families will have disaster kit in place to accommodate each family member for a period of at least 3 days

Community
Long-Term Goals
- Additional evacuation routes will be identified for area residents.
- Central meeting locations will be identified for those needing transportation assistance for evacuation.

Short-Term Goal
- School buses will be used for evacuation of vulnerable invidduals and families who need transpiration.

- Identify other sources.
- Identify other sources that could be called upon to provide transportation.
- Allow school bus drivers to include their family members on the bus with others being evacuated, so they will not have to worry about their families.

If all individuals follow instructions, there should be no injuries to, or deaths of, Deer Park residents from a hurricane or related storm surge. Homes may be damaged or destroyed, but no lives should be lost. With the help of local, state, and possibly federal agencies, the community should recover.

Long-Term Goal

- City officials will continually update the community disaster plan as gaps are identified and keep the residents informed as plans change.

Onsight Management

The figure below summarizes the disaster plan in place for the Deer Park Shell plants for handling any industrial accident that occurs on their property.

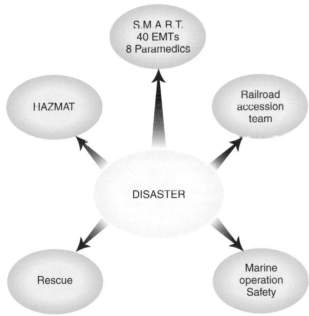

Shell has annual drills with the Harris County's Emergency Management and Channel Industries Mutual Aid organization to evaluate emergency response. This group is Shell's direct link to support in the event of a disaster. Many buildings on Shell property can serve as shelters, and no visitor or employee is allowed on the property without having a "safe shelter map" in his or her possession. If an explosion occurs that is confined to the property, and only minor casualties result, the resources available should be sufficient to manage the disaster.

Shell has developed a buffer zone between the plants and the city of Deer Park. However, if fumes escape as a result of the explosion, a shelter-in-place warning would be issued for Deer Park residents through a specific six sounding message system. Chemical products that are used and that might potentially escape are benzene, toluene, solvent xylene, iso-prene butadiene, sulfur, phenol, hydrogen sulfide, and asbestos. Citizens would be advised about actions to take according to the chemical released. Most plants have also installed dedicated, fiber-optic telephone lines so that the city and industry can stay in touch, even when normal phone circuits are overloaded or out of service.

Community and Local Response Preparedness

Deer Park's police and fire dispatchers have been trained how to handle calls from industries about a chemical release and how to quickly activate the city's emergency warning systems. The Local Emergency Planning Committee has adopted a three-level Community Awareness and Emergency Response system to categorize the severity of each chemical release. Level 1 is information only, Level 2 is standby alert, Level 3 is full emergency condition, with shelter in place required. The final level is "all clear." Deer Park has a website featuring Wally Wise Guy who gives instructions to the citizens about what to do if a shelter-in-place emergency is issued.

The Local Emergency Planning Committee hired a consulting group to study the impact of toxic substances on the community to ensure shelter-in-place procedures are adequate for protecting the residents. They recommended that each home in the region have a shelter-in-place kit containing 2- to 3-inch wide masking tape, plastic film or sheets, towels or sheets for sealing under doors, battery-powered radio and extra batteries, flashlight and extra batteries, and bottled water stored inside a designated shelter-in-place room.

The Deer Park Communications Subcommittee works with others to develop detailed procedures on how to notify and warn the public of a chemical release. The city and local industry have invested in six state-of-the-art systems to provide reliable and redundant warning to homes, schools, businesses, and visitors. Siren-type alarms have been mounted on utility poles throughout the city. This system is used only for chemical emergencies, not for tornados, hurricanes, or other types of emergencies. In addition, the city has contracted with First Call Interactive Network, an automated telephone notification network that can ring the telephones of homes and businesses in the immediate danger area, giving prerecorded instructions about what to do.

EVALUATION

Individuals and Families

- Before a hurricane, all residents will have evacuated.
- All vulnerable individuals and families will have been evacuated to shelters.
- All residents will know and respond to shelter-in-place warnings as indicated by the siren-type alarm system in place.

Community

- City officials will evaluate and continually update the community disaster plan as gaps are identified.
- Community residents will remain informed and prepared.

Continued

The City of Deer Park and the Dear Park Shell plants have detailed plans for prevention, preparedness, and response in the event of an industrial accident. In the event of an accident, evaluation of the plan will take place to identify gaps and make appropriate changes. A plan needs to be in place for hurricane preparedness of the plants to avoid accidental industrial accidents and the plan evaluated for effectiveness. Drills are conducted to test their industrial accident plans; they provide training of personnel; they have identified sites for shelters both on Shell property and in the city; and they have elaborate notification and warning systems in place.

Areas that need to be enhanced include city health resources readily available (lack of a nearby trauma hospital or burn center near to care for the type of injuries that would occur). Plans for preparing the plants for hurricanes and evacuation need to be developed and made available to the workers.

PREVENTION

Primary

- Perform periodic education of area residents regarding warning systems in place and appropriate response to take should they be implemented.
- Perform periodic review of plans in response to changing demographics.

Secondary

- Check credentials of first responders for currency.
- Screen first responders for training needs and preparedness to take action during disasters.

Tertiary

- Institute building codes that will reduce amount of damage to infrastructures.

Reconstruction Phase

Once the community has restored some of the buildings, businesses, homes, and services, and some sense of normalcy is returning, feelings of despair will subside. Counseling support for victims and helpers may need to be initiated to help people to recover more fully. During this phase, people begin to look to the future.

Common Reactions to a Disaster

The reactions by individuals to a disaster vary. Table 26-5 lists some of the more commonly encountered emotional, cognitive, physical, and interpersonal reactions to a disaster that may be experienced.

Posttraumatic Stress Disorder

The reactions mentioned usually resolve in 1 to 3 months after the disaster event but, in some cases, may lead to PTSD. PTSD is a psychiatric disorder that can occur following an individual's experiencing or witnessing a life-threatening event, such as a disaster. Men and women, adults and children, and all socioeconomic groups can experience PTSD. People who suffer from PTSD often relive the experience through nightmares and flashbacks. The social and psychological symptoms mentioned in Table 26-5 can be severe enough, and last long enough, to significantly impair a person's daily life. If PTSD occurs in conjunction with related disorders (e.g., depression, substance abuse, and other problems of physical and mental health), the situation becomes more complicated. Individuals experiencing PTSD require medical attention (National Center for PTSD, 2005).

Recovery Stage

The recovery stage begins when the danger from the disaster has passed and all local, state, and federal agencies are present in the area to help victims rebuild their lives and help the community restore public services.

Cleanup of the damage and repair of homes and businesses begin. Evaluation and revision of the disaster plans based on lessons learned from the experience are made. Understanding the financial impact on the community and agencies involved is essential in developing future public health policy.

Research is needed on all aspects of prevention, preparedness, response, and recovery stages of disasters. Research is also needed on the education and training needs of first responders, health care providers, and community populations. Nurse researchers, in partnership with researchers from other disciplines, can play a significant role in conducting research on disaster management.

SUMMARY

Communities, now more than ever, need to be aware of potential disasters that may affect their community. Comprehensive disaster plans at all levels of government and by all communities, families, and individuals need to be developed. Having disaster plans in place increases the likelihood of an effective response, resulting in saved lives and minimized destruction to the community.

Nurses have a role and contribution to make at every stage of disaster management. Nurses need to have personal and professional plans in place for any disaster. All medical personnel must keep their credentials current and must learn the signs and symptoms of the weapons of mass destruction so that they will recognize people who may have been exposed. They should learn what injuries may be sustained from various disasters and know which types of disasters are most likely to affect their communities, so that disaster triage and treatment can save lives. Finally, they must take drills in their respective health care facilities seriously. The more prepared the population and health care providers are for all kinds of disasters the fewer lives will be lost.

LEARNING ACTIVITIES

1. Assess the community where you live for potential disasters that could result in mass casualties. What disasters are predictable? Are there measures that can be taken to prevent or minimize injuries, death, or destruction?

2. Find out who is responsible for disaster management in your community. What plans are in place for warning people and for communicating which actions to take in the event of a disaster? Are the people aware of these plans?

3. What social and cultural factors need to be considered in disaster planning in your community? Are there vulnerable populations with special needs (e.g., homeless, prisoners, mobility impaired)? If evacuation of the community is mandated, have plans for evacuation of these groups been made?

4. Create an emergency plan for yourself, your family, or both. What factors would you consider in deciding whether to stay or leave your home? If evacuation were mandated, what important documents and mementos would you need to take with you?

5. Interview the person or persons in the American Red Cross responsible for disaster services in your area. What is the role of their disaster nurses? What are the requirements to become a disaster nurse for the American Red Cross?

6. Speak with police and fire department personnel about their responsibilities during a disaster. Do their roles during a disaster differ from their roles on a day-to-day basis? Do they have special teams and plans for biological, chemical, nuclear, or radiological incidents?

7. What emergency supplies does your health care facility have available in the event of a disaster? What provisions have been made available for vulnerable patients when there is no electricity? How would patients be evacuated from your facility to safe shelters?

REFERENCES

American Public Health Association: *Types of disasters and their consequences,* The Author, http://www.medscape.com/viewarticle/513258_print.

American Red Cross: *America's disasters 2004,* The Author, http://www.redcross.org/pubs/dspubs/amdisasters2004.pdf.

American Red Cross: *Disaster service,* The Author, http://www.redcross.org/services/disaster/0,1082,0_319_,00.html

American Red Cross: *Disaster services: shelter in place,* 2003a, The Author, http://www.seattleredcross.org/prepare/shelter.htm.

American Red Cross: *Disaster services: terrorism—preparing for the unexpected,* 2003b, The Author, http://www.seattleredcross.org/prepare/unexpected.htm.

Aucoin M: *Perfect performance. Memorial Hermann nurses rise above floodwater, relying on basic nursing care and providing effective patient evacuation,* http://www.advanceweb.com.

Berkowitz B: Public health nursing practice: aftermath of September 11, 2001, *Online J Issues Nurs* Sept 30, 2002, http://www.nursingworld.org/ojin/topic19/tpc19_4.htm.

Board of Nurse Examiners for the State of Texas: Legislative report: 78th Regular Texas Legislative Session, *RN Update* 34(5), 2005.

Centers for Disease Control and Prevention: *Tsunami disaster: health information for humanitarian workers,* Washington, DC, Jan 2, 2005, US Department of Health and Human Services.

Central Intelligence Agency: *The war on terrorism: terrorism FAQs,* The Author, http://www.cia.gov/terrorism/faqs.html.

Chettle C: Recognizing bioterrorism: nurses on the frontline, *NurseWeek* 6:29-30, Nov 12, 2001.

Cieslak TJ, Eitzen EM: Bioterrorism: agents of concern, *J Public Health Manag Pract* 6(4):19-29, 2000.

Evers S, Puzniak L: Bioterrorism knowledge and emergency preparedness among school nurses, *J School Health* 75(6):232-237, 2005.

Federal Emergency Management Agency: *About FEMA: what we do,* 2005a, The Author, http://www.fema.gov/about/.

Federal Emergency Management Agency: *Are you ready? General information about terrorism,* 2005b, The Author, http://www.fema.gov/areyouready/terrorism_general_info.shtm.

Federal Emergency Management Agency: *National Incident Management System,* 2005c, The Author, http://www.fema.gov/nims/.

Federal Emergency Management Agency: *Office of National Security coordinating agency,* 2005d, The Author, http://www.fema.gov/onsc/

James DC, Langan JC: *Nurses as heroes,* http://www.Advanceweb.com.

Hosley A: Relieving disaster: and loving it, *Reflect Nurs Leaders* 30:18-19, 2004.

International Council of Nurses: *Nurses and disaster preparedness: ICN position statement,* Geneva, 2001, The Author, http://www.icn.ch/psdisasterprep01.htm.

International Council of Nurses: *ICN recommendations: supporting the South Asia tsunami relief effort,* Press release, Jan 5, 2005, http://www.icn.ch/PR01_05.htm.

Mallonee S et al: Physical injuries and fatalities resulting from the Oklahoma City bombing, *JAMA* 276(5):382-287, 1996.

McUsic T: *Road readiness: with a hurricane on the horizon, and elderly patients as charges, careful preparation paid off amid the exodus from Houston,* http://community.nursingspectrum.com/MagazineArticles/article.cfm?AID=18167.

National Center for Post-Traumatic Stress Disorder: *What is posttraumatic stress disorder?* The Author, http://www.ncptsd.va.gov/facts/general/fs_what_is_ptsd.html.

Patterson K: *Psychological triage: in Katrina's wake, sorting out who will need mental health care the most won't be easy,* http://www.nursingspectrum.com/Katrina/PsychTriage.cfm.

Texas Association of Regional Councils: *Texas Citizen Corps: what is Citizen Corps?* The Author, http://www.txregionalcouncil.org/cc_cert/.

Texas Department of Health: The specter of chemical and biological terrorism. *Dis Prev News* 58(8):1-6, 1998a.

Texas Department of Health: Texas tornado disaster, *Dis Prev News* 58(17), 1998b.

Texas Department of Health and Texas Nurses Association: Strategic National Stockpile (SNS) volunteer nurses needed for Ready Texas Nurses Emergency Response System, *Texas Board Nurs Bull* 35(4), 2004.

US Department of Homeland Security: *National response plan,* Dec 2004, The Author, http://www.dhs.gov/dhspublic/display?theme=14&content=4264&print=true.

US Department of Homeland Security: *DHS organization: department subcomponents and agencies,* 2005a, The Author, http://www.dhs.gov/dhspublic/interapp/editorial/editorial_0515.xml.

US Department of Homeland Security: *DHS organization: the DHS transition,* 2005b, The Author, http://www.dhs.gov/dhspublic/display?theme=10.

US Department of Homeland Security: *Homeland Security Advisory System: current threat level,* 2005c, The Author, http://www.dhs.gov/dhspublic/display?theme=29&content=3927&print=true.

US Department of Homeland Security: *Preparing makes sense: get ready now,* 2005d, The Author, http://www.ready.gov/america/_downloads/Ready_Brochure_Screen_EN_20040129.pdf

The White House: *Improving homeland security,* The Author, http://www.whitehouse.gov/info-cus/homeland/index.html.

Wikipedia, the free encyclopedia: *Definition of terrorism,* The Author, http://en.wikipedia.org/wiki/Definition_of_terrorism.

Young BH et al: *Disaster mental health services: a guidebook for clinicians and administrators,* Menlo Park, Calif, 1998, Department of Veterans Affairs, National Center for PTSD.

UNIT 7

Community Health Settings

School Health

Cathi A. Pourciau ▪ Elaine C. Vallette

MEDIA RESOURCES

Additional Material for Study, Review, and Further Exploration

evolve Website at http://evolve.elsevier.com/Nies

❖ Quiz ❖ Case Studies ❖ Content Updates ❖ Glossary ❖ WebLinks ❖ Resource Tool
27A 2003 United States Youth Risk Behavior Survey Data

OBJECTIVES

Upon completion of this chapter, the reader will be able to do the following:

1. Discuss how *Healthy People 2010* can be used to shape the care given in a school health setting.
2. Identify and discuss the eight components of a comprehensive school health program.
3. Recognize the major stressors that can negatively affect an adolescent's mental and physical health.
4. Identify common health concerns of school-aged children and associated health interventions.
5. Explore the various roles of the nurse in the school setting.
6. Be familiar with the standards under which school nurses practice.
7. Cite several resources available to the school nurse.

KEY TERMS

Early and Periodic
  Screening, Diagnosis, and
  Treatment (EPSDT)
Family Educational Rights
  and Privacy Act (FERPA)

Health Insurance Portability
  and Accountability Act of
  1996 (HIPAA)
Individuals with Disabilities
  Education Act of 1990

Public Law 99-142
school-based health
  centers
school health
school nurse

Youth Risk Behavior
  Surveillance System
  (YRBSS)
Youth Risk Behavior
  Survey

CHAPTER OUTLINE

HISTORY OF SCHOOL HEALTH

SCHOOL HEALTH SERVICES
  Health Education
  Physical Education
  Health Services
  Nutrition
  Counseling, Psychological, and Social Services

  Healthy School Environment
  Health Promotion for School Staff
  Family and Community Involvement

SCHOOL NURSING PRACTICE

SCHOOL-BASED HEALTH CENTERS

FUTURE ISSUES AFFECTING THE SCHOOL NURSE

Schools could do more than perhaps any other single institution in society to help young people, and the adults they will become, to live healthier, longer, more satisfying, and more productive lives.
    (Carnegie Council on
    Adolescent Development,
    Centers for Disease Control
    and Prevention [CDC], p. 1,
    2006)

School-aged children and adolescents face increasingly difficult challenges related to health. Many of today's health challenges are different from those of the past and include behaviors and risks linked to the majority of the leading causes of death, such as heart disease, injuries, and cancer. The use of tobacco, alcohol, and drugs; poor nutritional habits; inadequate physical activity; irresponsible sexual behavior; violence; suicide; and reckless driving are examples of behaviors

BOX 27-1 Youth at Risk

> Every day, nearly 4000 young people start smoking.
> Daily participation in high school physical education classes dropped from 42% in 1991 to 28% in 2003.
> Almost 78% of young people do not eat the recommended number of servings of fruits and vegetables.
> Every year, almost 1 million adolescents become pregnant and about 4 million become infected with an STD (CDC, 2004b).

TABLE 27-1 Racial and Ethnic Breakdown of Uninsured Children in the United States in the Year 2000

RACE	NUMBER	PERCENT
White	3.6 million	39.5
Latino	3.3 million	35.3
Black	1.6 million	17.6
Asian and Pacific Islander	478,000	5.2
American Indian or Alaskan Native	221,000	2.4

From Children's Defense Fund: *Child health: key facts: the uninsured*, 2001, The Author, http://www.childrensdefense.org/childhealth/chip/key_facts.aspx.

that often begin during youth and increase the risk for serious health problems (Box 27-1).

In the United States, approximately 50 million children attend school every day. This creates a unique opportunity for the **school nurse** to make a positive impact on the nation's youth. The primary providers of health services in schools are school nurses, and there are between 50,000 and 60,000 registered nurses working in schools in the United States (National Association of School Nurses [NASN], 2003b). Although the NASN recommends one school nurse for every 750 students in the general population, one for every 225 students in mainstreamed special education populations, and one for every 125 severely chronically ill or developmentally disabled students, caseloads vary widely depending on mandated functions, socioeconomic status of the community, and service delivery model (NASN, 2004).

On a daily basis, school nurses see students with a variety of complaints. Increasing numbers of children are being seen in the school setting because they lack a source of regular medical care. According to the Children's Defense Fund (2001), in the United States there are 9.2 million children under the age of 19 years who do not have health insurance. This is a decrease from the nearly 12 million in previous years. Table 27-1 illustrates the racial and ethnic breakdown of uninsured children in the United States in the year 2000. Through education, counseling, advocacy, and direct care across all levels of prevention, the nurse can improve the immediate and long-term health of this population.

Seventeen percent of the nation's children are living in poverty and are less likely to have access to primary and preventive care (Annie E. Casey Foundation, 2002). Decreased

or inferior medical care has been linked to serious health problems resulting in an increase in absenteeism that may be correlated with failure in school. The school nurse can effectively manage many complaints and illnesses, allowing these children to return to or remain in class.

There is a need for mental and physical health services for students of all ages, in an effort to improve both their academic performance and their sense of well-being. This chapter provides an overview of **school health** and the role of the nurse in the provision of health services and health education. An in-depth look at the components of a successful school health program, related to the major problems of today's youth, is included.

HISTORY OF SCHOOL HEALTH

Before 1840, education of children in the United States did not exist or was uncoordinated and sparse. In 1840, Rhode Island passed legislation that made education mandatory and other states soon followed. In 1850 a teacher and school committee member, Lemuel Shattuck, spearheaded the legendary report that has become a public health classic. This report, known as the Shattuck Report, has had a profound impact on school health because it proposed that health education was a vital component in the prevention of disease.

Public health officials and others soon realized that schools played an important part in the prevention of communicable disease. When smallpox broke out in New York City in the 1860s, health officials were faced with trying to implement a widespread prevention program. They chose to target the schools and began vaccinating children. In 1870 this led to the requirement that all children be vaccinated against smallpox before entering school (Allensworth et al., 1997).

At that time, schools were poorly ventilated and lacked fresh air, effectively spreading diseases among the children. Late in the nineteenth century, a practice of inspecting schools began to identify children who were ill and exclude them until it was deemed they were no longer infectious. Soon thereafter compulsory vision examinations became a requirement to identify children who might have difficulty in school. In 1902, New York City hired the first nurses to help inspect children, educate families, and ensure follow-up treatment. Within a few years the renowned nurse Lillian Wald was able to show that the presence of school nurses could reduce absenteeism by 50%. By 1911 slightly over 100 cities were using school nurses; in 1913, New York City employed 176 school nurses (Allensworth et al., 1997).

As they became more comfortable in their positions, early school nurses began to take on a more active role in the assessment of children, treatment of minor conditions, and referral for more serious problems. In addition to identification, treatment, and exclusion for communicable diseases and screening for problems that might affect learning, other issues quickly became part of school nurse school practice. In the early part of the twentieth century the temperance movement led schools to teach about the effects of alcohol and tobacco. Also, early in the twentieth century "gymnastics" was introduced in schools in an effort to promote physical activity.

World War I was a pivotal point for school health services, and the call for a national effort to improve the health of schoolchildren emerged. In 1918 the National Education Association (NEA) joined forces with the American Medical Association (AMA) to form the Joint Committee on Health Problems and publish the report *Minimum Health Requirements for Rural Schools*. This group also called for the coordination of health education programs, medical supervision, and physical education that some authorities contend is still lacking. By 1921 nearly every state had laws that required physical and health education in schools. Additionally, fire drills became part of safety education programs introduced during and after World War I (Allensworth et al., 1997).

Even though emphasis was placed on health services in schools, barriers still existed. Many schools and cities were unwilling to take on the task of providing primary health care for all children. The idea that schools should simply identify and refer problems to physicians was a common practice that the AMA backed. By the 1920s, medical services and preventive health services were clearly separated in the public health arena and in the schools. Not surprisingly, school health became known as school health education. The federal government did not get involved with school health until the passage of the National School Lunch Program in 1946. The School Breakfast Program was implemented 30 years later (Allensworth et al., 1997).

There was no impetus to change the direction of school health programs until the 1960s and 1970s. During these decades there was increasing publicity about children living in poverty and the move to mainstream children with disabilities. These two issues, with an increase in the number of children of immigrants, contributed to changes in school health programs.

During the 1960s the first nurse practitioner training programs opened and made the inclusion of primary care services in schools possible. In 1976 the first National School Conference, supported by the Robert Wood Johnson Foundation, was held in Galveston, Texas. Following this conference a variety of school health service models began to emerge with new partnerships and ideas created to provide the most comprehensive health care services for school-aged children. In addition, the Education for the Handicapped Act in 1975 mandated that all children, regardless of disabilities, have access to educational services.

The 1980s and 1990s saw several measures aimed at improving the health of schoolchildren. The Drug Free Schools and Community Act was implemented in 1986 to fight substance abuse through education and was expanded in 1994 to include violence prevention measures. The Centers for Disease Control and Prevention (CDC), Division of Adolescent and School Health began funding state education agencies to develop and implement programs aimed at alcohol and tobacco use, physical education, and the reduction of sexually transmitted diseases (STDs) and human immunodeficiency virus (HIV) infection among the nation's youth. Also, the federal government encouraged states to use part of their maternal and child block grant monies to fund school-based health centers.

At the present time school health services vary widely among states and school districts. There continues to be a lack of coordination among providers, and no single agency is responsible for tracking services. Recognizing that there are differences among schools in the United States and that important health information must be delivered to children and adolescents, the United States Department of Health and Human Services (USDHHS) addressed many related issues in *Healthy People 2010*. Objectives targeting children and adolescents are written for diverse areas, including physical activity, sex education and HIV prevention, nutrition, smoking prevention, school absences related to asthma, and many others. The *Healthy People 2010* table lists a few of the objectives of *Healthy People 2010* related to school health.

SCHOOL HEALTH SERVICES

The School Health Policies and Programs Study (SHPPS) describes school health services as a "coordinated system that ensures a continuum of care from school to home to community health care provider and back" (Allensworth et al., 1997, p. 153). School health services goals and objectives vary from state to state, community to community, and school to school. These differences reflect wide variations in student needs, community resources, funding sources, and school leadership preferences. Many organizations, such as the American School Health Association (ASHA) and NASN, are involved in the care and welfare of school-aged children and have compiled and adopted definitions, standards, and statistics related to school health.

According to SHPPS (2000), 89% of states have at least one school-based health center, and 77% of schools in the United States have either a full- or part-time school nurse who provides health services that might include vision, hearing, and scoliosis screening; first aid care; and medication administration. Nearly all schools maintain a health record on every student and, at a minimum, monitor immunization status. Most authorities agree that comprehensive school health programs should include the following eight components (Figure 27-1): health education; physical education; health services; nutrition services; counseling, psychological, and social services; healthy school environment; health promotion for staff; and family and community involvement.

Health Education

An objective of *Healthy People 2010* sets a goal that 70% of middle, junior, and senior high schools provide health education courses in priority areas. The six behavioral categories or topics identified by the CDC (2004b) include the following negative behaviors that often start in childhood or adolescence and persist into adulthood:

1. Alcohol and drug use
2. Injury and violence (including suicide)
3. Tobacco use
4. Poor nutrition
5. Lack of physical activity
6. Sexual behavior that results in STDs or unwanted pregnancies

HEALTHY PEOPLE 2010 | Selected Objectives for School Health

Objective	Baseline (1998)	Target
6-9: Increase the proportion of children and youth with disabilities who spend at least 80% of their time in regular education programs	45%	60%
7-1: Increase high school completion	85%	90%
7-2e: Increase the proportion of schools that prevent health problems in tobacco use and addiction	86%	95%
7-4a: Increase the proportion of the nation's elementary, middle, junior high, and senior high schools that have a nurse-to-student ratio of at least 1:750	28%	50%
9-7: Reduce pregnancies among adolescent females 15 to 17 years old	68 % (1996)	43%
14-23g: Maintain measles vaccination coverage levels for children in kindergarten through the first grade	96%	95%
15-17: Reduce nonfatal injuries caused by motor vehicle crashes for people aged 16 to 20 years	3116 per 100,000	1000 per 100,000
15-19: Increase use of safety belts in 9th to 12th grade students	84%	92%
15-38: Reduce physical fighting among 9th to 12th grade students	36%	32%
15-39: Reduce weapon carrying by 9th to 12th grade students on school property	6.9%	4.9%
18-02: Reduce the rate of suicide attempts that required medical attention in 9th to 12th grade students	2.6%	1%
19-03: Reduce the proportion of children and adolescents aged 12 to 19 years who are overweight or obese	11%	5%
19-15: Increase the proportion of children and adolescents aged 6 to 19 years whose intake of meals and snacks at schools contributes proportionally to good overall dietary quality	NA	NA
21-13: Increase the proportion of school-based health centers with an oral health component	NA	NA
22-07: Increase the proportion of 9th to 12th grade students who engage in vigorous physical activity that promotes cardiorespiratory fitness, 3 or more days per week for at least 20 min	65%	85%
24-5: Reduce the number of school days missed by students because of asthma	NA	NA
25-11: Increase the proportion of 9th to 12th grade students who abstain from sexual intercourse or use condoms if currently sexually active	85%	95%
26 9c: Increase the proportion of high school seniors who never drink alcoholic beverages	19%	29%
26-10b: Reduce the proportion of adolescents reporting use of marijuana during the past 30 days	9.4%	0.7%
27-2: Reduce tobacco use by 9th to 12th grade students	40%	21%
27-4a: Increase the average age of first use of tobacco products among adolescents age 12 to 17 years	12 yr	14 yr

From US Department of Health and Human Services: *Healthy People 2010, conference edition*, Washington, DC, 2000, PHS.

These problems and behaviors are preventable and often coexist. They also lead to both social and educational problems that contribute to our nation's high drop-out and unemployment rates and crime statistics.

In a comprehensive health education program, students should be given the opportunity to practice decision-making and communication skills. To learn more about high-risk behaviors among youth, the CDC conducted the **Youth Risk Behavior Survey** (YRBS) (CDC, 2004b). This survey is conducted every 2 years among selected high school students throughout the United States. Box 27-2 lists the purposes of the YRBS. Reports from this study provide valuable information that can help improve health education programs in schools. See **Resource Tool 27A** on the book's website at http://evolve.elsevier.com/Nies/ for a summary of selected YRBS data.

Injury Prevention

Injury prevention should be taught very early in schools, and the information should be age appropriate. For example, bicycle safety, including the importance of wearing a helmet, as well as the proper use of backpacks must be stressed

FIGURE 27-1 The eight components of school health programs.

beginning in elementary schools. Safety on the schoolyard and playground is also important for this age-group, because approximately 200,000 children per year are injured on playgrounds in the United States. According to the National Program for Playground Safety (Tinsworth and McDonald, 2001), approximately 45% of these injuries occurred on school property. Motor vehicle safety should be included in programs for adolescents who are beginning to drive.

Sports safety is particularly important among adolescents because participation in sports continues to grow, especially among girls. Greater than 3.5 million children under the age of 15 receive medical treatment each year for sports-related injuries (National SAFE KIDS Campaign, 2004). Males are injured more frequently than females, and students in middle school have the highest incidence of injury. Injury rates are highest in basketball, followed by football, baseball, soccer, and softball (CDC, 2002). Injuries include orthopedic injuries (e.g., strains, sprains, fractures, and dislocations), dental injuries, neurological problems (e.g., head injury), ophthalmic injuries, cuts, abrasions, and bruises.

Use of proper equipment should be mandatory for children and adolescents. Fitted mouth guards, shin guards, pads, helmets, and other protective gear should be required to prevent injury. Regular hydration and frequent rest periods should be required to prevent heat-related illnesses, especially during hot weather. Effective warm-up and cool-down exercises should be encouraged to prevent muscle strain. Schools that participate in aquatic sports should include pool safety.

The sports physical is a good time for the school nurse to talk with and counsel the student about the risk of developing health problems related to physical activity. This is a perfect setting for the nurse to question girls about menstrual irregularities and to ask all students about their eating behaviors, feelings about their weight, and history of musculoskeletal injuries. It is also a good time for the nurse to stress the importance of stretching exercises to help prevent injuries. Additionally, this is an opportunity for the nurse to work with the coaching staff to promote positive health outcomes.

Many school districts have school safety committees that make recommendations for sports-related safety. These committees collect data on injuries, develop safety inspection policies, and plan staff training and student education related to school environmental factors. These committees should include school nurses.

Tobacco Use

For the past several decades, major concerns have been raised about long-term health problems associated with adolescents' use of tobacco, alcohol, and illegal substances. There is an increased likelihood that these youthful abusers will ultimately engage in other high-risk behaviors.

Smoking is a major problem in this country and is the single leading preventable cause of death in the United States. Prevention should be emphasized in young people because an estimated 80% of adults who use tobacco began before the age of 18 years. Although the overall percentage of high school students who report smoking has declined in recent years, rates remain high at 22% (CDC, 2004d). An estimated 4000 youths, aged 12 to 17 years, try their first cigarette each day. If this pattern of smoking continues, approximately 6.4 million children in this country can expect to die prematurely from a smoking-related disease, such as heart disease, chronic lung disease, or cancers of the lung, pharynx, esophagus, and bladder. Prevalence of smoking increases as the student progresses through the grade levels. White students have the highest rate of current cigarette use at 25%, followed by Hispanics at 18%, and blacks at 15% (CDC, 2004b).

Eleven percent of males and 2% of females report using smokeless tobacco, and studies show that adolescents who use smokeless tobacco are likely to become cigarette smokers. The use of smokeless tobacco can cause cancers of the mouth, esophagus, and pharynx, and can increase the risk of developing heart disease and stroke. Of particular interest is that 15% of students surveyed report having smoked cigars, cigarillos, or little cigars within the past month (CDC, 2004b).

Risk factors for developing oral cancer include the use of tobacco in all forms, and, to a lesser degree, alcohol (USDHHS, 2004b). Therefore all adolescents should be queried as to their use of both tobacco and alcohol. Education and counseling should be offered to students who use tobacco products. Limiting adolescents' exposure to tobacco advertising and teaching them the negative consequences associated with tobacco are essential in preventing its use.

Substance Abuse

The use of alcohol and other drugs is associated with problems in school, injuries, violence, and motor vehicle deaths. All fifty states and the District of Columbia have outlawed the sale of alcohol to anyone under the age of 21 years, yet it is still the most commonly used drug among children and adolescents. In 2004 statistics show that nearly 1 in 5 eighth graders had at least one drink within the past month, with increasing frequency as the adolescent progresses in school (Center on Alcohol Marketing and Youth, 2005). Males are more likely to drink than females. Additionally, alcohol use, defined as five or more drinks in a row on one or more of the past 30 days, is more prevalent among white twelfth graders (40.8%) and Hispanic twelfth graders (36.9%) than blacks (20.6%). The reported use of alcohol on school property remains relatively unchanged in the last 10 years, at 5.2%. Adolescents may become addicted to alcohol in as little as 6 to 18 months, as opposed to some adults who may not become addicted for 5 to 15 years. Research shows a direct correlation between alcohol abuse and liver disease, cancer, cardiovascular disease, as well as neurological and psychiatric problems.

BOX 27-3 Teen Pregnancy

➤ The United States teen pregnancy rate is one of the highest among developed countries, even though birth rates for teenagers have declined over the past 10 years.
➤ More than 870,000 teenagers become pregnant each year.
➤ Black and Hispanic youth are disproportionately affected.
➤ Teen mothers are less likely to complete high school.
➤ Teen mothers are more likely to be single parents and live in poverty.
➤ Birth rates among teenagers vary substantially from state to state (CDC, 2004c).

The use of illicit drugs, except for the use of inhalants, remains essentially unchanged over the past 10 years. The use of inhalants has actually declined from 20.3% in 1995 to 12.1% in 2003. Males are more likely to use illicit drugs than females. Eleven percent of students report having used ecstasy, also called MDMA, in 2003, whereas 40.2% report the use of marijuana one or more times in their life. The percentage of students who report marijuana use prior to the age of 13 years is 9.9%, while 5.8% of all students report using marijuana on school property, and 28.7% of students were offered, sold, or given marijuana (CDC, 2004b). Marijuana use has been linked to the same health problems as tobacco.

There are more than 100 different types of anabolic steroids, and each one requires a prescription. Most anabolic steroids users are athletes who believe that these drugs will produce an increase in strength and muscle mass. Approximately 1.9% of eighth grade students reported using these drugs in 2004, whereas 2.4% of tenth graders and 3.4% of twelfth graders reported using these drugs in the same time period (CDC, 2004b). Part of the problem is that students are trying to emulate professional sports figures, some of whom purportedly have used these drugs to enhance performance. Abuse or improper use of anabolic steroids can result in severe problems, including liver cancer, heart attacks, elevated cholesterol levels, and even stunted growth patterns (Office of National Drug Control Policy, 2004).

Sex Education

A number of objectives of *Healthy People 2010* address issues of human sexuality and prevention of pregnancy, STDs, and HIV. These issues are important when working with older children and adolescents.

Teens are becoming sexually active at earlier ages and despite recent declines, pregnancy rates continue to be high (Box 27-3). Data obtained from the **Youth Risk Behavior Surveillance System (YRBSS)** reveal a decrease from 48.4% in 1997 to 46.7% in 2003 of adolescents in grades 9 through 12 who have had sexual intercourse (CDC, 2004b). Even though 87.9% of students have been given HIV/AIDS education in school, AIDS remains high among adolescents and young adults. AIDS is now the seventh leading cause of death among people aged 13 to 24 years in the United States (National Institute of Allergy and Infectious Diseases, 2004). Research shows that HIV transmission is at least 2 to 5 times higher in the presence of a coexisting STD (USDHHS, 2004c). Therefore it is imperative that older children and adolescents have age-appropriate information on sexuality issues, including prevention of pregnancy and STDs, before becoming sexually active.

According to the CDC, 902,223 cases of AIDS had been reported through the end of 2003. Of these, 9348 were reported in children under age 13 years. During this same time there were 505,801 AIDS deaths and, of these, 5406 occurred in children under age 13 years (CDC, 2005). It is important to note that HIV reporting is not mandatory in all states and may underestimate the devastation of this illness on school-aged children.

School-based education related to sexual orientation is a controversial topic. Children with gender identity confusion must also face the same growth and developmental issues as other adolescents. However, there are unique health problems and risks for these children both emotionally and physically. The school nurse needs to be aware of these students be sensitive and understanding.

Sex education in the school setting is another controversial topic. Opponents of sex education in the schools believe that parents have the responsibility for teaching this content to their children. Laws in certain states prohibit or dramatically limit sex education in public schools. Proponents argue that for many children, sex education will not be addressed in the home. If this information is not taught in schools, children may receive inadequate or incorrect information from peers, media, or other sources. School nurses have been caught in the center of this controversy, but historically have advocated for education on normal human sexuality, encouraging discussion in an objective, nonjudgmental manner in which students are free to ask questions and receive correct answers.

Tattoos and Body Piercings

Tattoos and body piercings are a form of self-expression and attention-seeking behavior. This practice has risen dramatically in the last several years. Unfortunately, these procedures are often done at home, on the streets, or in parlors where sterile technique and safety precautions are not practiced. This presents a unique opportunity for the school nurse to educate students on the importance of making healthy decisions on whether to have this done, and if so, where and under what conditions it is performed.

Dental Health

One of the most frequent complaints of school-aged children is dental caries. There are numerous contributing factors, including poor oral hygiene, lack of fluoridated water, and lack of funds or insurance for dental care. By second grade more than half of all children will have at least one cavity, and 80% will have cavities by the time they complete high school (USDHHS, 2004b).

Proper brushing of teeth should be taught along with good nutritional habits and the importance of regular dental check-ups. Children should also be taught the relationship between high-sugar foods and dental caries. All children should be encouraged to see a dentist regularly.

Physical Education

One of the major objectives of *Healthy People 2010* is improvement of health and fitness through regular daily physical activity. Children today are less active today than children in the past. Daily enrollment among high school students in physical education classes has dropped from 42% in 1991 to 28% in 2003. With the advent of computers and television and the decreasing requirement of physical education in schools, children are becoming more sedentary. It was reported in 2001 that the proportion of children in grades 10 through 12 who engaged in strenuous physical activity was lower than in previous grades (CDC, 2004b).

A sedentary lifestyle is associated with obesity, hypertension, heart disease, and diabetes. Studies show that people who are active outlive those who are inactive, and that those who are active have a better quality of life. Habits in childhood are likely to continue into adulthood, making it imperative that children are taught the importance of being physically active at a young age. Studies also show that children and adolescents who are physically active have increased self-confidence and self-esteem, and decreased anxiety, stress, and depression (CDC, 2004b). Regular physical activity helps build and maintain healthy bones and muscles.

Physical education should focus on activities that children can continue into their adult years, such as walking, swimming, biking, and jogging. The educational content may change as the child ages. For example, what may appeal to a young child, such as playing on the playground with friends, is different from what motivates an adolescent, such as competitive spirit or weight control. The CDC has made 10 recommendations for the promotion of lifelong physical activity (Box 27-4).

Health Services

Health care provided in schools include such preventive services as immunizations and screenings. This component of a comprehensive school health program may include emergency care, management of acute and chronic health conditions, appropriate referrals, health counseling, education about healthy lifestyles, and medication administration. Care of children with special health needs is also included.

Immunizations

Immunizations are a vital component of routine health care. They provide long-lasting protection against many diseases. Vaccine-preventable deaths (VPD) are at or near record-low levels. According to the CDC (2005) most diseases have been reduced by greater than 95% as a result of immunizations. Undervaccination of children, especially those in large urban areas, is causing concern because of the potential for disease outbreaks.

All states now require proof of current immunization status or evidence of immunity before school entrance. Certain exceptions may apply based on religious and moral beliefs, or medical contraindications. The school nurse plays an important role in verifying compliance with immunization requirements and in educating children and parents about the benefits of immunization. School nurses play a vital role in coordi-

BOX **27-4** Guidelines for School and Community
Programs: Promoting Lifelong Physical
Activity

1. Establish policies that promote enjoyable, lifelong physical activity.
2. Provide physical and social environments that encourage and enable young people to engage in safe and enjoyable physical activity.
3. Implement sequential physical activity education curricula and instruction in grades K to 12.
4. Implement health education curricula.
5. Provide extracurricular physical activity programs that offer diverse, developmentally appropriate activities—both noncompetitive and competitive—for all students.
6. Encourage parents and guardians to support their children's participation in physical activity, to be physically active role models, and to include physical activity in family events.
7. Provide training to enable teachers, coaches, recreation and health care staff, and other school and community personnel to promote enjoyable, lifelong physical activity to young people.
8. Assess the physical activity patterns of young people, refer them to appropriate physical activity programs, and advocate for physical activity instruction and programs for young people.
9. Provide a range of developmentally appropriate community sports and recreation programs that are attractive to all young people.
10. Regularly evaluate physical activity instruction, programs, and facilities.

From Centers for Disease Control: *CDC's guidelines for school and community programs: promoting lifelong physical activity,* 1997, The Author, ftp://ftp.cdc.gov/pub/Publications/mmwr/rr/rr4606.pdf.

nating school immunization programs and teaching families about both infant and adult immunizations. See Chapter 23 for current immunization schedules.

Health Screenings

Unfortunately, many children in the United States are not appropriately screened for treatable conditions that then remain undetected. Impaired vision and hearing can result in poor academic performance, slowed emotional development, and stress-related disorders. Children are exposed to a variety of potentially harmful noises in school and at home. Identifying and treating these problems early is highly effective and less costly in the long run. Height, weight, vision, and hearing screenings are provided at most schools according to a schedule set by the state or school district. The American Academy of Pediatrics (AAP) recommends objective hearing testing at ages 4, 5, 6, 8, 10, 12, 15, and 18 years (AAP, 2000). Adolescents exposed to loud noises or those with recurrent ear infections may need yearly screening.

Vision screening is required in most states with referrals as needed. The standard Snellen vision chart is the usual screening tool. The AAP recommends routine objective vision screening for children and adolescents at ages 3, 4, 5, 6, 8, 10, 12, 15, and 18 years (AAP, 2000). Screening for strabismus is a nursing responsibility, and this condition must be identified and treated early to prevent amblyopia. If left untreated, amblyopia may result in loss of vision. Referral to an eye specialist is a critical component of all abnormal eye examinations.

Scoliosis or postural screening should be done to identify spinal deviations and intervene early to prevent related secondary problems. Spinal problems may lead to deformities that are cosmetic, functional, or both. Scoliosis screening in the school setting consists primarily of a visual inspection of the back. The AAP (2000) recommends biannual screening of all children 10 to 16 years of age, whereas the American Academy of Orthopedic Surgeons (1992) recommends screening of all girls at ages 10 and 12 years, and boys at either age 13 or 14 years.

The detection of high blood pressure during childhood is important in identifying children who have hypertension and who will benefit from early intervention and follow-up. Vascular and end-organ damage can begin in childhood. Periodic blood pressure measurements are inexpensive and should be performed routinely for all children..

The Children's Health Insurance Program (CHIP) is a national program designed for children of families who earn too much money to qualify for Medicaid but cannot afford the high cost of health insurance. Medicaid-eligible children are guaranteed access to comprehensive health care services and routine dental examinations. Medicaid created the **Early and Periodic Screening, Diagnostic and Treatment (EPSDT)** service because of the large number of uninsured children. EPSDT is a comprehensive child health program for uninsured people under the age of 21 years and includes health education and periodic screening. Services provided under the EPSDT program are often performed through the public health offices in each state, but may occur in community health clinics and schools. Screening services must include a comprehensive health and developmental history, an unclothed physical examination, plus immunizations and laboratory testing that are age appropriate (Centers for Medicare & Medicaid Services, 2006).

Emergency Care

Schools are a frequent site for student injuries that range from minor scrapes and bruises to serious injuries, such as fractures and seizures, to severe and life-threatening injuries, such as head injuries and severe asthma attacks. Injuries may occur in school buildings, classrooms, physical education classes, or during athletic events. Emergencies can include natural events such as hurricanes, tornadoes, and earthquakes, or man-made disasters, such as hazardous material spills, fires, and civil disobedience. Basic first aid equipment should be available in all schools. The school nurse must be knowledgeable about standard first aid and certified in CPR. Additionally, a procedure for activating an emergency management system (EMS) should be in place.

Care of the Ill Child

The school nurse is responsible for monitoring the health of all students. For students with acute or chronic illnesses administration of medications or treatments may be necessary. The nurse is often required to assess an ill child to determine the type of illness or health problem, identify the source of

BOX 27-5 Asthma Assessment Tool

1. Is the school free of tobacco smoke all of the time, including during school-sponsored events?
2. Does the school maintain good indoor air quality? Does it reduce or eliminate allergens and irritants that can make asthma worse?
3. Is a school nurse in the school all day, every day?
4. Can children take medicines at school as recommended by their doctor and parents? Are children allowed to carry their own asthma medicines?
5. Does the school have an emergency plan for taking care of a child with a severe asthma attack? Does it clearly explain what to do? Who to call? When to call?
6. Does someone teach school staff about asthma, asthma management plans, and asthma medicines? Does someone teach all students about asthma and how to help a classmate who has it?
7. Do students have good options for fully and safely participating in physical education class and recess? Do students have access to their medicine before exercise? Can they choose modified or alternative activities when medically necessary?

From National Heart, Lung, and Blood Institute, National Asthma Education and Prevention Program, School Asthma Education Subcommittee: How asthma friendly is your school? *J Sch Health* 68(4):167-168, 1998.

BOX 27-6 Expectations of the Child With Diabetes

Elementary school
➤ The child should be able to assist in all diabetes tasks at school.
➤ By the age of 8 years, the child is usually able to perform his or her own finger-stick glucose monitoring.

Middle school and junior high school
➤ The child should be able to perform self-monitoring of blood glucose.
➤ Most children should be able to administer their own insulin with supervision.

High school
➤ The child should be able to perform self-monitoring of blood glucose.
➤ Adolescents should be able to administer insulin with supervision.
➤ All children may need assistance with blood glucose testing when the glucose level is low.

From American Diabetes Association: Position statement: care of children with diabetes in the school and day care setting, *Diabetes Care* 27(suppl 1):SS122-SS128, 2004.

the illness, and determine how to manage the illness (i.e., contact the parent or send the child back to class).

In 2002 it was reported that 8.3% of children under the age of 17 years had asthma. Asthma is one of the most common chronic childhood conditions and accounts for some 14 million lost school days every year (CDC, 2004a). Because asthma is so prevalent, it is recommended that school-based support exist. Actions undertaken by some schools across the country include immediate access to asthma medications, development and implementation of asthma action plans, and student and staff education on asthma. An assessment tool (Box 27-5) has been developed to determine how well schools assist children with asthma. Answers to all the questions in the assessment tool should be "yes." "No" answers indicate that students may not be in an environment conducive to asthma control.

Diabetes is second only to asthma in prevalence in the school-aged child and affects 210,000 young people less than 20 years of age. Approximately 13,000 new cases of type 1 diabetes are diagnosed in children annually and the vast majority of these children attend school or day care (American Diabetes Association, 2002). Type 2 diabetes is now being diagnosed in children, a condition that has historically been diagnosed only in adults. Childhood obesity and the decline in physical activity are thought to be major factors in this development. In general, teachers are inadequately prepared to care for children with diabetes and must rely on the nurse. According to the American Diabetes Association (ADA), children should be able to participate in their care to the extent that they are able. The ADA has specific recommendations based on age as shown in Box 27-6.

Medication Administration

Administration of medications is a service provided almost universally by school districts across the country. The use of medications by school-aged children has increased over the last several years. This has allowed many children to attend school despite serious health problems.

Medication administration in the schools is a serious undertaking. Issues facing the school nurse include safety, monitoring of both therapeutic and side effects, proper documentation, confidentiality, and ongoing communication with the student and family. The nurse must comply with all legal regulations and school policies. Only those medications considered necessary are administered at school.

The following guidelines from NASN (2003a) indicate that medications should be:

- In containers that are properly labeled with all appropriate student and medication information
- Accompanied by a written request from the health care provider and parent or guardian
- Administered without violating standing orders or nursing protocols
- Kept in locked containers

Also, school nurses must monitor self-administration of medications and provide education as needed to both children and parents. Rescue medications such as albuterol must be available to the child with asthma, and the nurse must be familiar with its expected effects to properly assist the child. With the increasing number of diabetic children, it is imperative that the nurse recognize the signs and symptoms of hypoglycemia and hyperglycemia in order to assist the child in monitoring of glucose levels and insulin administration.

Medications commonly given in schools include analgesics and antipyretics (e.g., Tylenol or Advil), antacids, antitussives, anticonvulsants, antiemetics and antidiarrheals, antifungals, antihistamines, and antibiotics. Medications, such as Ritalin, Cylert, and Adderall, used to treat attention-deficit hyperactivity disorder (ADHD) are the most commonly adminis-

TABLE 27-2 Overview of Increase in Number of Students With Disabilities

TYPE OF DISABILITY	1976 TO 1977	1990 TO 1991	1996 TO 1997
All disabilities	8.33	11.55	12.98
Specific learning disabilities	1.80	5.17	5.81
Speech or language impairments	2.94	2.39	2.29
Mental retardation	2.16	1.30	1.27
Serious emotional disturbance	0.64	0.95	0.98
Hearing impairment	0.20	0.14	0.15
Orthopedic impairments	0.20	0.12	0.14
Other health impairments	0.32	0.13	0.35
Visual impairments	0.09	0.06	0.06
Multiple disabilities	—	0.23	0.21
Deafness-blindness	—	<0.005	<0.005
Autism and others	—	—	0.10
Preschool disabled	—	1.07	1.62

Children from birth to age 21 who were served by federally supported programs for students with disabilities, as a percentage of total public K to 12 enrollment; 1976 to 1977 to 1996 to 1997

From National Center for Education Statistics: *NCES fast facts: students with disabilities*, 2000, The Author, www.nces.ed.gov/fastfacts/display.asp/id=64.

tered, followed by nonprescription medications and medications used in the treatment of asthma (McCarthy, Kelly, Reed, 2000).

Alternative and complementary medicine includes practices and products outside the realm of conventional medicine. The NASN recommends that an advisory committee be formed in the community to address the administration of these products. NASN also recommends that the school not allow the child to carry or self-administer any products that could be considered a drug, without written orders from a health care provider, a written request from the parent, and verification that the product and dosage are safe. The request for the administration of any of these medications provides the nurse with an excellent health teaching opportunity (NASN, 2001).

Children With Special Health Needs

In 1976 **Public Law 99-142** was enacted, giving all students, including those who are severely handicapped, the right to public education in the least restrictive environment possible, regardless of mental or physical disabilities. The Education for All Handicapped Children Act of 1973 and the subsequent **Individuals with Disabilities Education Act (IDEA) of 1990** enhanced the opportunities for children previously served in acute care and long-term care settings to have access to public education (Duncan and Igoe, 1998). President George W. Bush signed the reauthorized IDEA into law on December 3, 2004, to support over 6 million children with disabilities in the U.S. school systems. Children affected by these laws include those who are hearing impaired, mentally retarded, multihandicapped, orthopedically impaired, "other" health impaired (e.g., chronic or acute health problems such as heart condition or epilepsy), seriously emotionally disturbed, speech impaired, visually handicapped, or have a specific learning disability.

The rapid development of medical technology has enabled students to attend public school when their conditions may have prevented them from leaving an institution or controlled environment in the past. These children need nursing services of varied types to continue their progression in school. Public Law 94-142 requires school nurses to screen or identify children in need of special education and related services, and complete an Individualized Education Program (IEP) that is developed by an interdisciplinary team and includes educational goals and specific services to be provided. It also requires provision of "designated instruction and services," which outlines services, including nursing care, required to help the child benefit from education. The nurse is responsible for the development of an individualized health plan (IHP) for all students requiring continuous nursing management while at school. Table 27-2 gives an overview of the increase in the number of students with disabilities.

Student Records

Health records should be maintained on all students according to individual school district policy. At a minimum, student health records should include immunization status, pertinent health concerns, results of screenings and examinations, health history, and individualized plans of care. The **Family Educational Rights and Privacy Act (FERPA),** a strong privacy protection act, protects student education records, including the health record. Student health records should be afforded the same level of confidentiality as that given to clients and patients in other settings (i.e., sharing confidential information with others, without approval, is considered unethical and improper except in emergency situations).

The **Health Insurance Portability and Accountability Act of 1996 (HIPAA)** was published in 2002 and instituted nationwide in 2003. A major component of HIPAA is ensuring confidentiality of personal health information. Public schools that provide health care services fall under HIPAA regulations. Private schools that do not receive federal funding but engage in HIPAA-related activities are also governed by this act.

Delegation of Tasks

Not every school has a full-time nurse available on site. Often, a nurse is assigned to three or four schools, resulting in delegation of certain tasks to unlicensed personnel. Each state's nurse practice act stipulates which procedures may be delegated. The responsibility for assessment may never be delegated. When tasks are delegated, the nurse must provide appropriate education, written procedures, and ongoing supervision and evaluation of the caregivers. The nurse is also responsible for periodic reassessment of the child.

Nutrition

School-aged children are undergoing periods of rapid growth and development and consequently have high nutritional needs. A variety of foods must be ingested to meet their daily requirements. Diets should include a proper balance of carbohydrate, protein, and fat, with sufficient intake of vitamins and minerals. However, children and adolescents share a well-known preference for junk food. Their diet is often high in fat and sugar and frequently consists of fast food items, such as hamburgers and French fries, instead of fruits and vegetables. Skipping meals, especially breakfast, and eating unhealthy snacks contributes to poor childhood nutrition. Identifying nutritional problems, counseling, and making appropriate referrals are important in the school setting.

Poor nutritional status is closely associated with poverty. Federally funded programs such as the School Breakfast Program and National School Lunch Program were initiated to ensure that all children have access to these meals during the school day.

VENDING MACHINE FOOD CHOICES

In 2002, the NASN addressed the issue of unhealthy foods found in school vending machines and sold in school fund-raising projects. They specifically resolved that schools should provide healthy food choices in school vending machines and for sale in fund-raising projects (NASN, 2002). ∎

Eating Disorders

Statistics have shown that few adolescents feel good about their bodies. Of those surveyed, 24% of boys and 36% of girls describe themselves as being overweight, and as many as 30% of boys and 59% of girls are dieting at any one time. It has been reported that 8% of girls in high school take laxatives or vomit to lose weight or keep from gaining weight, and approximately 11% take diet pills. These kinds of harmful practices have been reported in girls as young as 9 years old (CDC, 2004b).

It is imperative that the school nurse recognize the association between feelings of inadequacy (e.g., low self-esteem, anger, anxiety, and depression) and unhealthy eating practices in adolescents and young people. These self-perceptions begin early in life; therefore education and counseling must begin in elementary school. Prevention should concentrate on eliminating misconceptions surrounding nutrition, dieting, and body composition, and should stress optimal health and personal performance. Unfortunately, outside influences such as commercials and advertisements make this a serious problem;

adolescents and young children are bombarded with such messages as "you can never be too thin" and "life will be wonderful if you look and dress like a model."

Nurses must also be aware of eating disorders, such as anorexia nervosa and bulimia. Anorexia is a severely restricted intake of food based on an extreme fear of weight gain. Literature has shown that anorexia is multifactorial, is seen primarily in females, and is often correlated with family dysfunction or history of sexual abuse. Bulimia is a form of anorexia characterized by a chaotic eating pattern with recurrent episodes of binge eating followed by purging. Purging may take the form of self-induced vomiting, laxative or diuretic abuse, or excessive exercise. Health consequences of eating disorders may include reduction of bone density, severe dehydration, tooth decay, and potentially fatal electrolyte imbalances.

FEMALE ATHLETE TRIAD

The "female athlete triad" is a syndrome consisting of eating disorders, amenorrhea, and osteoporosis. Pressure to attain a particular body shape or weight considered desirable in a selected sport may place the female athlete in danger of developing this disorder. It is a complex problem with psychological and physiological factors. It can result in menstrual irregularities, premature osteoporosis, and decreased bone mineral density (BMD); if taken to the extreme, it can become life threatening (Sherman and Thompson, 2004). ∎

Obesity

Obesity is not considered an eating disorder and therefore many professionals, including nurses, overlook it. Obesity is the fastest rising public health concern in the nation and may overtake tobacco use as the single leading preventable cause of death. Nine million children over the age of 6 years are now considered obese, and this number is increasing. The childhood obesity rate has more than doubled for children aged 2 to 5 years and adolescents aged 12 to 19 years over the past 3 decades. It has more than tripled for children aged 6 to 11 years (Institute of Medicine, 2004). Obesity and its prevention or treatment must be of concern to the school nurse. Statistics show that obese children and adolescents are more likely to become obese adults.

Although many of the underlying causes of obesity are not well understood, several contributing factors have been identified that include reduced access and affordability of nutritious foods, decreased physical activity, and cultural and genetic influences. Obesity is associated with development of diabetes, dyslipidemia, hypertension, and other disorders, such as osteoarthritis, sleep apnea, and cholelithiasis. In addition, obesity may result in social and quality-of-life impairments related to physical endurance and possible job discrimination. Obese children are often labeled by their peers and ridiculed. Guidelines to Adolescent Preventative Services (GAPS) recommends the determination of body mass index (BMI) for all adolescents. A BMI greater than the 85th percentile for age and gender indicates the need for further assessment and referral. To be successful, the treatment of obesity must begin early and be multifaceted (Montalto, 1998).

BOX 27-7 Warning Signs of Stress

- Problems eating or sleeping
- Use of alcohol or other substances (e.g., sedatives, sleep enhancers)
- Problems making decisions
- Persistent angry or hostile feelings
- Inability to concentrate
- Increased boredom
- Frequent headaches and ailments
- Inconsistent school attendance

Nutritional Education Programs

Nutritional education is essential and must include parents, teachers, and the child. Children need to know and understand the food pyramid, how to make healthy snack choices, and the importance of balancing physical activity with food intake. Obesity, dental caries, anemia, and heart disease can be reduced or prevented with proper education and lifestyle changes. In addition, all adolescents and school-aged children should receive counseling regarding intake of saturated fat.

Congress enacted the Nutritional Education and Training (NET) Program in 1977. NET focuses on healthy nutritional choices and health promotion and disease prevention topics in school and child care settings. In addition, the American Dietetic Association, the American School Food Service Association, and the Society for Nutrition Education take the position that comprehensive school-based nutrition programs and services should be provided to all elementary and secondary students. The ultimate goal of these efforts is that children will make healthy nutritional choices in and out of the school setting.

Counseling, Psychological, and Social Services

The mental health of a child or adolescent is affected by physical, economic, social, psychological, and environmental factors. Children, like adults, often hide problems from themselves and from others. They may see problems as a sign of weakness or as a lack of control. Children may also be trying to protect themselves or someone they love and not seek help. This can have tragic results. Promotion of mental health and reduction or removal of threats to mental health are important to children and adolescents. Mental health is often difficult, yet essential, to assess.

Children and teens struggle with such issues as depression, substance abuse, conduct disorders, self-esteem issues, suicide ideation, and eating disorders. They may also have to cope with physical or mental abuse, pregnancy, and STDs. Warning signs of stress in children are presented in Box 27-7. Drugs and alcohol can enter a child's life as early as elementary school. Many children live in single-parent households with little social or economic support. They may not have enough to eat or a safe, warm place to sleep, yet they are expected to come to school each day, ready to learn. Services aimed at helping children cope with these problems are often lacking or are too costly for many families.

The nurse or teacher may be the only stable adult in the child's life who will listen without being judgmental. There-

BOX 27-8 Truths About Adolescent Suicides

1. Since 1950 the suicide rate for adolescents has more than tripled.
2. Most adolescents who attempt suicide are ambivalent and torn between wanting to die and wanting to live.
3. Any threat of suicide should be taken seriously.
4. There are usually warning signs preceding a suicide attempt, and these may include depression, substance abuse, decreased activity, isolation, and appetite and sleep changes.
5. Suicide is more common in adolescents than homicide.
6. Education concerning suicide does not lead to an increased number of attempts.
7. Females are more likely to consider or attempt suicide, and males are more likely to complete a suicide attempt.
8. One suicide attempt is more likely to result in a subsequent attempt.
9. Firearms and suffocation are the predominant modalities of completed suicides in children and adolescents.
10. Most adolescents who have attempted or completed suicide have not been diagnosed as having a mental disorder.
11. All socioeconomic groups are affected by suicide.

fore one of the most important roles of the school nurse is to act as counselor and confidante. Children may come to the school nurse with various vague complaints, such as recurrent stomachaches, headaches, or sexually promiscuous behavior, and the nurse must look beyond the initial complaint to identify underlying problems.

Major depressive disorders often have their onset in adolescence and are associated with an increased risk of suicide. Early detection and treatment may prevent untoward consequences. In 2001 the third leading cause of death among 10- to 19-year-olds was suicide, whereas homicide was the second leading cause of death in 15- to 19-year olds (CDC, 2004b). It is well known that suicide attempts are more common than completed suicides. A survey of students in grades 9 through 12 in 2003 showed that 8.5% attempted suicide in the preceding year. The rate for female students was higher than that of male students, at a rate of 11.5% versus 5.4%. The nurse and other school personnel must be on the alert for suicide clusters that are often known to follow a successful suicide. Results from the YRBSS indicate that almost 17% of students have seriously considered attempting suicide (CDC, 2004b). Many schools have implemented suicide prevention programs; however, myths continue to exist. Adolescents often approach school nurses and other school professionals for help before a suicide attempt. Therefore it is important for the school nurse to be cognizant of the warning signs associated with suicide and to recognize and refer at-risk adolescents to appropriate mental health professionals (Box 27-8).

Unfortunately, a large number of children are abused daily in this country. Physical and psychological abuse and neglect are usually a result of many interacting factors, such as poverty, social isolation, and drug and alcohol abuse. School nurses and other school personnel are mandated to report cases of child abuse and neglect. The nurse must be alert to subtle changes in behavior or physical appearance that may point to

BOX 27-9 Possible Signs of Abuse

Physical Abuse
➤ Unexplained burns, bites, bruises, black eyes, or broken bones
➤ Shrinks at the approach of adults
➤ Appears frightened of parents or other relatives and cries when it is time to go home

Neglect
➤ Is frequently absent from school
➤ Steals food or money
➤ Lacks adequate medical or dental care
➤ Appears dirty or disheveled or is underweight
➤ Does not have proper seasonal clothing

Sexual Abuse
➤ Has difficulty walking or sitting
➤ Reports new onset of nightmares or bedwetting
➤ Refuses to change into gym attire or participate in physical activities
➤ Runs away from home
➤ Becomes pregnant or develops an STD

Emotional Abuse
➤ Exhibits changes in behavior, such as acting out or extreme passivity
➤ Exhibits delay in either physical or emotional development
➤ Has attempted suicide
➤ Exhibits inappropriate adult or infantile behavior

From National Clearinghouse on Child Abuse and Neglect Information (DHHS): *Recognizing child abuse and neglect: signs and symptoms,* 2003, The Author, http://nccanch. acf.hhs.gov/pubs/factsheets/signs.cfm.

abuse. Box 27-9 outlines some of the signs and symptoms of different types of child abuse.

The school nurse may help the child learn how to solve problems, how to cope, and how to build self-esteem. The role of the nurse often extends outside the school campus. The family is an integral part of a child's well-being, and the nurse may need to work closely with families to develop an appropriate health plan for a particular child.

Healthy School Environment

A healthy school environment is one in which distractions are minimized and free of physical hazards and psychological threats. NASN believes that "all students and staff have a right to learn and work in a healthy school environment . . . ." and that the school nurse, as ". . . . an advocate for students, staff and community, will be actively involved in the development and maintenance of a plan for a healthy school environment" (NASN, 1998).

Violence

Violence is a major public health problem because it threatens the health and well-being, both physical and psychological, of many children and adolescents. According to the U.S. Department of Justice (2002), 15% of the almost 5 million crimes that occurred in 2002 took place inside a school building or on school grounds. The only place that had a higher incidence of crime was in the home. There were 309,000 instances of serious violence to students aged 12 to 18 years away from school, compared with approximately 88,000 instances at school (U.S. Department of Justice, 2004). Students, teachers, and staff may all be victims of violence, intentional or accidental. Students, when questioned, will frequently admit to feeling unsafe in schools. Greater than 5% of high school students admitted to skipping at least one day of school because of safety concerns in 2003. This number is up from 4.4% in 1993 (CDC, 2004b).

The number of violent crimes, such as locker thefts and destruction of school property, has declined over the last several years. The National Center for Education Statistics (NCES) (2004) reported that 1.1 million crimes of theft occurred at school in 2002. The U.S. Department of Justice (2004) reports that in 2003, 4% of students aged 12 to 18 years reported being a victim of a theft, and 5% reported being a victim of a nonfatal crime. According to the CDC (2004b), the percentage of students who reported being in a fight on school property declined from 16.2% in 1993 to 12.8% in 2003. This decline has been overshadowed by the increase in truly violent crimes, such as school shootings.

In recent years there have been a number of school shootings and other acts of serious violence in schools. The YRBSS data reveals that 9.2% of students in this country were either threatened or injured with a weapon while on school property in 2003 (CDC, 2004b). Serious violent behavior at school includes gang activity, bullying and intimidation, gun use, and assault. The school shooting at Columbine High School in Littleton, Colorado, in 1999 shocked the nation and was probably the first time that people in this country realized how unsafe schools could be. Two students attending Columbine killed 12 classmates, a teacher, and then themselves, making this the nation's worst school shooting. There were 48 violent school-related deaths in 2003-2004, making it one of the deadliest school years in history. A March 2005 school shooting in Red Lake, Minnesota, by a 16-year-old student resulted in the deaths of an unarmed school guard, five students, a teacher, and ended with the student's suicide.

School nurses and other school personnel should be aware of risk factors and signs that could indicate a tendency toward violence. Factors common in those who commit violent acts in school include being a male, coming from a disadvantaged or poor socioeconomic background, and having a history of abuse. Media influences that desensitize the impact of violence are being studied more closely as another cause of increased violence among children and adolescents. These children often have a need for instant gratification, easy access to guns, and may have a history of discipline problems. Most events occurred either at the beginning or end of the school day or during the lunch period (Anderson, et al, 2001).

Although the number of students who commit violent acts is small, these random acts are frightening, and school officials are struggling with ways to prevent their occurrence and to recognize the signs of troubled youth early. Violence prevention programs should begin in elementary schools. Children who exhibit aggressive behavior in elementary school are more likely to exhibit antisocial and violent behavior as adolescents and adults. Programs should target stress management, conflict and anger resolution, and personal and self-esteem development. Nurses should use data collected through the YRBSS and other local data as a means of assessment when developing violence policy and prevention programs in the school and community. Additionally, nurses should initiate and participate in research that examines the complex developmental, social, and psychological factors surrounding violence.

Terrorism

Even though schools may not be the primary target in an act of terrorism, they will be affected by terrorism. Events following the September 11, 2001, attack illustrated potential problems that face schools when an act of terrorism has occurred. These problems included direct exposure of students to the act or incident or being in the immediate vicinity, fear and panic among students, teachers, and parents, and enduring anxiety among those directly affected.

Every school is encouraged to develop an emergency management plan. In fact, many states mandate that schools develop plans to address the potential threat of another terrorist attack or a natural or man-made disaster. School nurses must be prepared to act after any form of terrorism has occurred, including a bioterrorist attack. The school nurse has an important role as a potential first responder in any emergency situation and should be an active participant in planning and policy development with local governments and health departments.

Health Promotion for School Staff

According to the National Center for Education Statistics (2003b), schools in the United States employ more than 2.9 million teachers and over 3 million other employees. Health promotion programs at the work site produce beneficial results, including positive effects on blood pressure control, daily physical activity, smoking cessation, and weight control. Staff that participate in health promotion programs increase their health knowledge and positively change their attitudes and behaviors relative to smoking practices, nutrition, physical activity, stress, and emotional health. Other studies show that health promotion programs improve morale, reduce job stress and absenteeism, and heighten interest in teaching health-related topics to students. School nurses play an important role in all levels of prevention through assessment, planning, intervention, and evaluation.

The American Association of School Administrators reports that as many as 50% of schoolteachers are overweight, therefore school health promotion activities for faculty and staff should center on exercise, nutrition education, and dietary management (Illuzzi and Cinelli, 2000). The school nurse can assist the faculty and staff by giving workshops on exercise and nutrition, screening for increased blood pressure, and establishing weight management programs.

Family and Community Involvement

School nurses are often asked to provide health content to family, parents, and the community, on a variety of topics, such as sexuality, STDs, HIV, communicable diseases, and substance abuse. Health education in the community should consist of programs that are designed to positively influence parents, staff, and others in matters related to health. School nurses are a ready resource to the community whenever health-related problems arise. They must step forward and volunteer their services and expertise in a way that can positively affect their community. Programs such as smoking cessation can include the entire community. The school nurse should be aware of the existence of these programs; they may also serve as a consultant during implementation and as an advocate for programs to remain in place.

Family Risk Index

Children living in families with four or more of the following characteristics are considered at "high risk" (Annie E. Casey Foundation, 2000):

- Child is not living with two parents.
- Household head is a high school dropout.
- Family income is below the poverty line.
- Child is living with parent(s) who do not have steady, full-time employment.
- Family is receiving welfare benefits.
- Child does not have health insurance.
- Percent of children living in "high-risk" families, based on definition above, is 10%. ■

Programs aimed at adolescent weight control may also need to be targeted to the parents. Parents may not be aware of the important role they play in helping to prevent obesity in their children. School nurses can help parents develop healthier eating habits in the home that will directly affect their families. The nurse can also help develop physical activity programs in the community that include both the child and the family.

Nurses should become adept at working in the public sphere by increasing their visibility and becoming skilled in working with the media and legislators. The media can be a useful tool in assisting school nurses with health education advocacy.

SCHOOL NURSING PRACTICE

School nursing is a specialty unto itself. School nurses need education in specific areas, such as growth and development, public health, mental health nursing, case management, program management, family theory, leadership, and cultural sensitivity to effectively perform their roles. They must be prepared to work with children of different ages and under highly variable circumstances. The nurse must also keep abreast of issues affecting children and participate in research that explores and expands the role. The school nurse's practice is relatively independent and autonomous, even though the school nurse functions as a member of an interdisciplinary team. For entry into school nursing, it is recommended that nurses hold a minimum of a bachelor's degree. Some univer-

TABLE 27-3 Standards of Professional School Nursing Practice

STANDARDS OF CARE	
Standard I: Assessment	The school nurse collects client data.
Standard II: Diagnosis	The school nurse analyzes the assessment data in determing nursing diagnoses.
Standard III: Outcome identification	The school nurse identifies expected outcomes individualized to the client.
Standard IV: Planning	The school nurse develops a plan of care and action that specifies interventions to attain expected outcomes.
Standard V: Implementation	The school nurse implements the interventions identified in the plan of care and action.
Standard VI: Evaluation	The school nurse evaluates the client's progress toward attainment of outcomes.

STANDARDS OF PROFESSIONAL PERFORMANCE	
Standard I: Quality of care	The school nurse systematically evaluates the quality and effectiveness of school nursing practice.
Standard II: Education	The school nurse evaluates his or her own nursing practice in relation to professional practice standards and relevant statutes, regulation, and policies.
Standard III: Education	The school nurse interacts with and contributes to the professional development of peers and school personnel as colleagues.
Standard IV: Collegiality	The school nurse interacts with and contributes to the professional development of peers and school personnel as colleagues.
Standard V: Ethics	The school nurse's decisions and actions on behalf of clients are determined in an ethical manner.
Standard VI: Collaboration	The school nurse collaborates with the student, family, school staff, community, and other providers in providing student care.
Standard VII: Research	The school nurse promotes use of research findings in school nursing practice.
Standard VIII: Resource utilization	The school nurse considers factors related to safety, effectiveness, and cost when planning and delivering care.
Standard IX: Communication	The school nurse uses effective written, verbal, and nonverbal communication skills.
Standard X: Program management	The school nurse manages school health services.
Standard XI: Health education	The school nurse assists students, families, school staff, and community to achieve optimal levels of wellness through appropriately designed and delivered health education.

From National Association of School Nurses: *Healthy school environment: NASN position statement, 1998*, The Author, www.nasn.org/issues/.

sities are now preparing school nurses at the master's level. The school nurse must be able to identify and access professional development in order to maintain competency in the care of children and adolescents.

Definition of School Nursing

School nursing is a specialized practice of professional nursing that advances the well-being, academic success, and lifelong achievement of students. To that end, school nurses facilitate positive student responses to normal development; promote health and safety; intervene with actual and potential health problems; provide case management services; and actively collaborate with others to build student and family capacity for adaptation, self-management, self-advocacy, and learning.

From National Association of School Nurses: *NASN board of directors meeting, Providence, Rhode Island, June 1999: definition of school nursing, J Sch Nurs 16(1):5, February 2000.* ■

School nurses function in many roles. Among these are care provider, student advocate, educator, community liaison, and case manager. Additional skills needed by the school nurses include the ability to supervise others, practice independently, and delegate care. Table 27-3 presents the standards of school nursing practice. These standards are currently being updated.

The school setting is a perfect place to conduct research on how children adapt to life transitions, such as divorce, illness or death of a loved one, illness of either themselves or a peer, domestic violence, and health-related behaviors of the young. Edwards (2002) reported on the establishment of research priorities for school nursing through the use of the Delphi

technique. The study resulted in the identification of the top 10 ranked research priorities for school nursing. See Research Highlights for details about the study and the Delphi process.

SCHOOL-BASED HEALTH CENTERS

School-based health centers are one of the best ways to offer comprehensive health care services to school-aged children and adolescents. The center or clinic works in collaboration with, but does not take the place of, the school nurse. The collaboration between the school nurse and the school-based health center staff prevents fragmented care and duplication of services. **School-based health centers** provide an interdisciplinary team approach with personnel, such as nurse practitioners, social workers, psychologists, and physicians, who provide services; they are usually employed by one or more local agencies, such as health departments, hospitals, or medical schools. Some of the services provided in these centers include nutrition education, injury treatment, general and sports physicals, prescriptions, pregnancy testing, laboratory services, immunizations, gynecological examinations, medication dispensing, social work services, and management of chronic illnesses. Close collaboration must exist within and among the community, the educational board, and the families for such a center to develop and flourish. The National Assembly on School-Based Health Care (2005) defines the Principles and Goals for School-Based Health Care that outline the essential elements of a school-based health care program.

RESEARCH HIGHLIGHTS

Research Priorities in School Nursing: A Delphi Process

School nurses have long been aware of the extensive nature of their role in implementing a comprehensive school health program. Lack of documentation of the benefits of their services, however, has frequently meant that their efforts go unrecognized, remain undervalued, and are often seen as expendable. Although the body of literature relative to school health services is not small, very little exists to validate the impact of outcome of those services.

The earliest set of formalized nursing research priorities was established in 1988, by the National Center for Nursing Research. These priorities led to the implementation of programs and interventions targeting low-birth-weight infants, HIV prevention, and prevention of obesity. The 1990s saw increasing recognition of the need to establish priorities and conduct research in school health. A Centers for Disease Control and Prevention (CDC) conference in 1994 identified seven critical issues that needed to be addressed to assist school nurses in meeting students' health needs. In 1996 the National Center for School Health Planning was established within the American Nurses Association (ANA). A second major force began with the convening in late 1994 of an Institute of Medicine (IOM) committee to study comprehensive school health programs.

The following two priority actions on research were identified in the 1996 conference: (1) draft a research agenda for school nursing, and (2) expand and improve access to the useable school nursing research information and data resources. The IOM report was selected as the basis upon which to set a research agenda. Convening a conference of researchers to frame a research agenda was one of the strategies to accomplish their priority actions. In March 1999, 24 leaders in nursing research and school nursing

met for an invitational summit about developing a school nursing research agenda. The summit participants developed eight recommendations for the development and implementation of a school nursing agenda. In subsequent meetings a list of research topics was developed. It was suggested that a Delphi approach be used to reach accord on the priorities for research. The Delphi study method uses a series of questionnaires for ranking priorities. In studies where consensus is desired, a three-round process is suggested. Original participants of the invitational meeting were asked to participate in the Delphi study.

The Delphi method proved to be a dynamic mechanism to bring together leaders in school nursing and research to agree on priority research issues about school nursing. The results of this study revealed a concern about outcomes. The 10 priority issues are as follows, in order of ranking:

1. Impact of school nurse services on student health
2. Relationship between school nurse practice and educational outcomes
3. Benefits and cost effectiveness of school health services
4. Value of school health services to the educational system
5. Predictors of outcomes for students, including special need students
6. Nursing interventions for mental health promotion
7. Characteristics of successful school nurse interventions
8. Prevention and interventions for children with chronic diseases
9. Core elements of school nursing practice
10. Nursing interventions in violence and substance abuse prevention

From LH Edwards: Research priorities in school nursing: a Delphi process, *J Sch Health* 72(5):173-177, 2002.

FUTURE ISSUES AFFECTING THE SCHOOL NURSE

Our nation's youth are our greatest asset and hope for the future. The school nurse's role must be constant evolving to meet the demands of the future. Issues that will face the school nurse of tomorrow include ethical dilemmas, use of telehealth, threat of bioterrorism, new and emerging infectious diseases, and increase in antibiotic-resistant diseases. The school nurse will need to adapt to understand and appreciate the multicultural community in which he or she will practice.

SUMMARY

Components of a comprehensive school health program have been clearly identified and discussed. Many of the *Healthy People 2010* objectives specifically relate to issues that can be addressed in the school setting. The role of the school nurse has changed dramatically since its inception and continues to evolve to meet the demands of school-aged children, their parents, and the communities in which they live. School nurses continue to reduce the number of days and the frequency with which students miss school related to illness. They have become child advocates, counselors, health promoters and collaborators, educators, researchers, and resources, both in the school and the community.

ETHICAL Insights

An Ethical Dilemma: What Would You Do?

You are working as the school nurse in a rural high school when Grace, a 15-year-old female student, enters the clinic. Grace appears very worried, and after several hesitant starts, she begins to cry and tells you that she is sexually active with a 17-year-old senior. She goes on to tell you that she has missed her last period and that her home pregnancy test is positive. She states that she is afraid to tell her parents because she feels that they will be very disappointed in her and because she is afraid of what her father will do. She asks you where she can go to get an abortion. You speak with Grace for quite a while and encourage her to speak with her parents. She leaves the clinic a little more composed and promises you that she will think about what you have said. The next day Jenny, Grace's mother, comes into the clinic and asks to speak with you. She confides that she is worried about Grace and asks if you know what is going on with her child. What would you do in this situation?

Although maintaining confidentiality and a professional relationship respectful of the student's wishes is vital, state laws and school district policies will determine what a school nurse may do, and in some cases is required to do, when providing care to minor children. When dealing with personal and sensitive information such as is described above, the school nurse should be well-versed in relevant laws and policies and follow them. When in doubt, contact a supervisor.

CASE STUDY Application of the Nursing Process

The nursing process is a systematic, organized approach to problem solving that nurses use when working with clients. It is neither fixed nor stagnant. It is a flexible process that allows for ongoing changes. This case study illustrates the use of the nursing process in a school setting.

Sandra Baker is a nurse at an elementary school in a small town. A second-grade teacher brought Carrie Broussard to the clinic and told Sandra that Carrie had been scratching her head all day and she was worried that Carrie might have an infection.

ASSESSMENT

Carrie is 7 years old. Her shoulder-length blond hair appeared neat and clean. When questioned by Sandra, Carrie replied that her head had been itching for 2 or 3 days, but she denied any pain or trauma. Sandra noted that Carrie did not have a fever or swollen lymph nodes, but examination of her scalp revealed multiple excoriated areas. Carrie's hair was examined with a Wood's light and Sandra saw adult lice at the base of her hair follicles on the back of her head near the nape of the neck. Multiple nits were also noted. Sandra learned that Carrie had two brothers in the school and one sister who was a toddler at home.

On Carrie's initial visit to the clinic, Sandra assessed the following:
- Temperature
- Lymph nodes
- Scalp for any abnormal findings

DIAGNOSIS

Individual
- Head lice

Family and Community (School)
- Potential for spread of infestation in both family and school
- Potential knowledge deficit related to spread and treatment of lice by teachers and family members

PLANNING

Sandra is familiar with the school district's policy that covers head lice in schoolchildren. According to the policy, the nurse must do the following:

Individual
Long-Term Goal
- Carrie's return to school after successful treatment

Short-Term Goals
- Contact Carrie's parents to tell them about the lice
- Inform Carrie's parents that she must be picked up from school

- Recommend treatment based on school protocol
- Provide guidelines for returning to school

Family and Community
Long-Term Goal
- Ensure that the teachers, staff, and family members have the necessary education relative to prevention and treatment of head lice

Short-Term Goals
- Examine the hair of all other children in Carrie's class for lice and treat each according to the school protocol
- Check the hair of all siblings who attend the school for lice
- Check the hair of all students in the siblings' classes if lice are identified

INTERVENTION

Family
Carrie's brothers, David and Paul, are brought to the clinic for examination. Both brothers have lice. Sandra contacted Mrs. Broussard, explained the situation to her, and requested that she come to the school to pick up her children. When Mrs. Broussard arrived at the school, Sandra gave her written information on treatment and prevention of lice and showed her what nits and lice look like. Mrs. Broussard was also instructed to check other members of the family not attending this school, especially those who share hairbrushes, pillowcases, and towels, because all family members with lice must be treated or the lice would continue to be passed from member to member. Sandra also explained procedures for cleaning combs and brushes and bedding and potentially contaminated clothing and toys. Finally, Mrs. Broussard was informed that the children could return to school the day after treatment.

It was obvious to Sandra that Mrs. Broussard was embarrassed. To ease her mind, Sandra carefully explained that head lice are highly contagious, easily passed from child to child, and are not an indication of poor hygiene. Mrs. Broussard repeated the instructions and left with her three children.

Community
Sandra examined all of the students from each of the Broussard children's classes for head lice.

From the three classes, she identified five more children with head lice and notified their parents. Those children had siblings in three additional classrooms and she repeated the procedure for each of them. At the end of the day, she had identified a total of 15 children with head lice and contacted all parents.

Sandra investigated whether the teachers and staff desired an information session on the transmission and spread of head lice because so many students had lice. She discovered that it had been 2 years since this was done and arranged a class for the coming week for the teachers and teachers' aides to learn how to identify and treat head lice.

CASE STUDY Application of the Nursing Process (cont'd)

EVALUATION

Individual and Family

Mrs. Broussard brought Carrie, David, and Paul to school the following day, and on examination Sandra found their hair to be free of lice and nits. Mrs. Broussard expressed her appreciation for the nurse's help and nonjudgmental approach to the problem.

COMMUNITY

Over the next 2 days, Sandra reexamined all of the children in the affected classrooms and found that the infected children had been successfully treated and that there were not any new cases. New cases were not identified during the remainder of the semester. The teachers and staff gave her positive feedback about the head lice education class and asked for it to be repeated at the beginning of each school year.

LEVELS OF PREVENTION AND SCHOOL HEALTH

School nursing encompasses all three levels of prevention (i.e., primary, secondary, and tertiary), and all three may be practiced individually or concurrently. Table 27-4 lists examples of school nursing interventions for each of the three levels of prevention.

TABLE 27-4 Examples of Prevention and the Role of the Nurse in the School Setting

EXAMPLE	NURSE'S ROLE
PRIMARY PREVENTION	
Nutrition education	Provide education to children and parent; consult with dietary staff
Immunizations	Provide for or refer to source(s) for immunizations; offer consultation for immunization in special circumstances
Safety	Provide safety education; inspect playgrounds and buildings for safety hazards
Health education	Teach healthy lifestyle education; develop health education curriculum for appropriate grade levels; provide health education to parents, faculty, and staff; develop suicide prevention programs and sex education materials
SECONDARY PREVENTION	
Screenings	Schedule routine screenings for scoliosis, vision and hearing problems, eating disorders, obesity, depression, anger, dental problems, abuse, and Early and Periodic Screening, Diagnostic and Treatment (EPSDT) program
Case finding	Identify at-risk students
Treatment	Administer medications; develop individualized health plan (IHP); implement procedures and tasks necessary for student with special health needs; administer first aid
Home visits	Assist with family counseling and assess special and at-risk students
TERTIARY PREVENTION	
Referral of student for substance abuse or behavior problems	Serve as an advocate; assist with resource referrals; assist parent, faculty, and staff; consult with neighborhood and law enforcement officials; initiate outreach programs
Prevention of complications and adverse effects	Follow-up and referral for student with eating disorders and obesity; participate with faculty and staff to reduce recurrence and risk factors; serve as a case manager
Faculty and staff monitoring	Follow-up for faculty and staff experiencing chronic or serious illness; follow-up of work-related injuries and accidents

---

LEARNING ACTIVITIES

1. Explain how the *Healthy People 2010* objectives can be used to shape school-based health care.
2. Attend a meeting of the school nurse association in the area. Identify the major pros and cons of being a school nurse. Look at factors such as working conditions, number of children assigned to each nurse, job functions, and job satisfaction.
3. Visit a comprehensive school-based clinic in the area. Discuss how the care given in this type of clinic differs from the care that a school nurse can provide. Review the protocols of both settings and see how they differ.
4. Purchase a 1-year subscription to a school health journal.
5. Interview a member of the local school board about controversial subjects in health education in the local school system (e.g., sex education).
6. Review the most common diseases and reported injuries in school-aged children in the area. Develop a plan for how the school and the community can work together to decrease their incidence.
7. Interview the parents of several school-aged children. Ask what health services they would like to see provided in the school setting.
8. Arrange with the principal of a local school to have a discussion session with children in a particular grade level. Ascertain what their eating habits are and then develop a class that can enhance healthy eating.

REFERENCES

Allensworth D et al, editors: *Schools and health: our nation's investment,* 1997, Institute of Medicine, Division of Medicine.

American Academy of Orthopedic Surgeons: *Position statement: school screening program for the early detection of scoliosis,* 1992, The Author, http://www.aaos.org/wordhtml/papers/position/1122.htm.

American Academy of Pediatrics: Committee on practice and ambulatory medicine: recommendations for preventive pediatric health care (RE9535), *Pediatrics* 105(3):645-646, 2000.

American Diabetes Association: *National diabetes fact sheet,* 2002, The Author. http://www.diabetes.org/uedocuments/NationalDiabetesFactSheetRev.pdf.

American Diabetes Association: Position statement: care of children with diabetes in the school and day care setting, *Diabetes Care* 27(suppl 1):SS122-SS128, 2004.

Anderson M et al: School-associated violent deaths in the United States: 1994-1999, *JAMA* 286(21):2695-2702, 2001.

Annie E. Casey Foundation: *Children at risk: state trends: 1990-2000,* 2002, The Author, http://www.aecf.org/kidscount/c2ss/.

Center on Alcohol Marketing and Youth: *Underage drinking in the United States: status report, 2004,* 2005, The Author, http://camy.org/research/underage2004/report.pdf#search='Underage%20drinking%20in%20the%20United%20States%3A%20status%20report'.

Centers for Disease Control and Prevention: Guidelines for school and community programs: promoting lifelong physical activity, *MMWR Morb Mortal Wkly Rep* 46(RR-6):1-42, 1997, ftp://ftp.cdc.gov/pub/Publications/mmwr/rr/rr4606.pdf

Centers for Disease Control and Prevention: Nonfatal sports and recreational-related injuries treated in emergency departments: United States, July 2000-June 2001, *MMWR Morb Mortal Wkly Rep* 51(33):736-740, 2002.

Centers for Disease Control: *School Health Policies and Program Study 2000: fact sheet—school based health centers and services provided at other sites,* The Author, http://www.cdc.gov/healthyyouth/shpps/factsheets/school_based_health.htm.

Centers for Disease Control and Prevention: *Strategies for addressing asthma within a coordinated school health program,* 2004a, The Author, http://www.cdc.gov/Healthy-Youth/asthma/strategies.htm.

Centers for Disease Control and Prevention: Youth Risk Behavior Surveillance: United State—2003, *MMWR Morb Mortal Wkly Rep* 53(SS02),1-96, 2004b, http://www.cdc.gov/mmwr/preview/mmwrhtml/ss5302a1.htm.

Centers for Disease Control and Prevention: *Health United States,* 2004c, The Author, http://www.cdc.gov/nchs/pressroom/04news/hus04.htm.

Centers for Disease Control and Prevention: *Tobacco use and the health of young people,* 2004d, The Author, http://www.cdc.gov/mmwr/preview/mmwrhtml/ss5302a1.htm.

Centers for Disease Control: Summary of notifiable diseases: United States, 2003; *MMWR Morb Mortal Wkly Rep* 52(54):1-95, 2005, http://www.cdc.gov/mmwr/preview/mmwrhtml/mm5254a1.htm.

Centers for Disease Control and Prevention: *Healthy youth: an investment in our nation's future,* 2006, The Author, http://www.cdc.gov/nccdphp/publications/aag/pdf/aag_dash2006.pdf.

Centers for Medicare and Medicaid Services: *Early and periodic screening diagnostic and treatment program (EPSDT): overview.* 2006, The Author, http://www.cms.hhs.gov/MedicaidEarlyPeriodicScrn/01_Overview.asp#TopOfPage.

Children's Defense Fund: *Child health: key facts—the uninsured. Children's health coverage in 2001,* The Author, http://www.childrensdefense.org/childhealth/chip/key_facts.aspx.

Duncan P, Igoe J: School health services. In Marx E, Wooley SF, Northrop D, editors: *Health is academic: a guide to coordinated school health programs,* New York, 1998, Teachers College Press.

Edwards L: Research priorities in school nursing: A Delphi process: *J Sch Health* 72(5):173-178, 2002.

Illuzzi S, Cinelli B: A coordinated school health program approach to adolescent obesity, *J Sch Nurs* 16(1):12-17, 2000.

Institute of Medicine: *Childhood obesity in the United States: facts and figures—fact sheet,* 2004, The Author, http://www.iom.edu/Object.File/Master/22/606/0.pdf#search='childhood%20obesity%20in%20the%20United%20States%3A%20Facts%20and%20Figures'.

McCarthy A, Kelly M, Reed D: Medication administration practices of school nurses, *J Sch Health* 70(9):371-376, 2000.

Montalto N: Implementing the guidelines for adolescent preventive services, *Am Fam Physician,* 57(9):2181-2190, 1998.

National Assembly on School-Based Health Care: *Principles and goals for school-based health care,* 2005, The Author, http://www.nasbhc.org/APP/NASBHC%20FINAL%20GOALS.pdf.

National Association of School Nurses: *Healthy school environment: NASN position statement,* 1998, The Author, http://www.nasn.org/Default.aspx?tabid=293.

National Association of School Nurses: NASN board of directors meeting, Providence Rhode Island, June 1999, Definition of school nursing, *J Sch Nurs* 16(1):5, 2000.

National Association of School Nurses: *Alternative medicine use in the school setting: NASN position statement,* 2001, The Author, http://www.nasn.org/Default.aspx?tabid=199.

National Association of School Nurses: *Position statement: soft drinks and candy in the school setting,* 2002, The Author, http://www.nasn.org/Default.aspx?tabid=248.

National Association of School Nurses: *Medication administration in the school setting: NASN position statement,* 2003a, The Author, http://www.nasn.org/Default.aspx?tabid=230.

National Association of School Nurses: *Access to a school nurse: NASN position statement,* 2003b, The Author, http://www.nasn.org/Portals/0/statements/resolutionaccess.pdf.

National Association of School Nurses: *Caseload assignments: NASN position statement,* July 2004, The Author, http://www.nasn.org/Default.aspx?tabid=209.

National Center for Education Statistics: *Indicators of school crime and safety: 2004,* The Author, http://www.nces.ed.gov/programs/crimeindicators/.

National Center for Education Statistics: *NCES fast facts: students with disabilities,* 2003, The Author, http://nces.ed.gov/fastfacts/display.asp?id=64.

National Center for Education Statistics: *Digest of education statistics,* 2003, The Author, http://www.nces.ed.gov/programs/digest/d03/.

National Clearinghouse on Child Abuse and Neglect Information (DHHS): *Recognizing child abuse and neglect: signs and symptoms,* 2003, The Author, http://nccanch.acf.hhs.gov/pubs/factsheets/signs.cfm.

National Heart, Lung, and Blood Institute, National Asthma Education and Prevention Program, School Asthma Education Subcommittee: How asthma friendly is your school? *J Sch Health* 68(4):167-168, 1998.

National Institute of Allergy and Infectious Diseases, National Institutes of Health: *HIV infection in adolescents and young adults,* 2004, The Author, http://www.niaid.nih.gov/factsheets/hivadolescent.htm.

National SAFE KIDS Campaign: *Sports injury fact sheet,* 2004, The Author, http://www.usa.safekids.org/content_documents/Sports_facts.pdf.

Office of National Drug Control Policy: *Drug Facts: steroids,* The Author, http://www.whitehousedrugpolicy.gov/drugfact/steroids/index.html.

Sherman R, and Thompson R: The female athlete triad, *J Sch Nurs,* 20(4):197-202, 2004.

Tinsworth D and McDonald J: *Special study: injuries and death associated with children's playground equipment,* Washington, DC, 2001, US Consumer Product Safety Commission.

US Department of Health and Human Services: *Healthy People 2010,* Washington, DC, 2004, PHS.

US Department of Health and Human Services: *Progress review: oral health,* 2004, The Author, http://www.healthypeople.gov/Data/2010prog/focus21/.

US Department of Health and Human Services: *Progress review: sexually transmitted diseases,* 2004, The Author, http://www.healthypeople.gov/Data/2010prog/focus25/.

US Department of Justice, Bureau of Justice Statistics: *Criminal victimization in the United States,* 2002, The Author, http://www.ojp.usdoj.gov/bjs/pub/pdf/cvus02.pdf.

US Department of Justice: *Indicators of school crime and safety,* 2004, The Author, http://www.ojp.usdoj.gov/bjs/pub/pdf/iscs04.pdf.

28

Occupational Health

Bonnie Rogers ▪ Patricia Hyland Travers

MEDIA RESOURCES

Additional Material for Study, Review, and Further Exploration

evolve Website at http://evolve.elsevier.com/Nies

❖ Quiz ❖ Case Studies ❖ Content Updates ❖ Glossary ❖ WebLinks ❖ Resource Tools
28A Preplacement Health Evaluation, **28B** Occupational Health History, **28C** Example of Screening and Surveillance: Guide to OSHA Standard for Benzene, **28D** Physical Demands Analysis

---

OBJECTIVES

Upon completion of this chapter, the reader will be able to do the following:

1. Describe the historical perspective of occupational health nursing.
2. Discuss emerging demographic trends that will influence occupational health nursing practice.
3. Identify the skills and competencies germane to occupational health nursing.
4. Apply the nursing process and public health principles to worker and workplace health issues.
5. Discuss federal and state regulations that affect occupational health.
6. Describe a multidisciplinary approach for resolution of occupational health issues.

KEY TERMS

Ada Mayo Stewart
Americans With Disabilities
   Act (ADA)
disability syndrome

ergonomics
industrial hygiene
occupational health nursing

Occupational Safety and
   Health Administration
   (OSHA)

safety
toxicology
Workers' Compensation Acts

CHAPTER OUTLINE

EVOLUTION OF OCCUPATIONAL HEALTH NURSING

**DEMOGRAPHIC TRENDS AND ACCESS ISSUES
   RELATED TO OCCUPATIONAL HEALTH CARE**

**OCCUPATIONAL HEALTH NURSING PRACTICE
   AND PROFESSIONALISM**

**OCCUPATIONAL HEALTH AND PREVENTION
   STRATEGIES**
   Healthy People 2010 and Occupational Health
   Prevention of Exposure to Potential Hazards
   Levels of Prevention and Occupational Health Nursing

**SKILLS AND COMPETENCIES OF THE OCCUPATIONAL
   HEALTH NURSE**
   Competent
   Proficient

   Expert
   Examples of Skills and Competencies for Occupational
      Health Nursing

**IMPACT OF FEDERAL LEGISLATION ON OCCUPATIONAL
   HEALTH**
   Occupational Safety and Health Act
   Workers' Compensation Acts
   Americans With Disabilities Act

LEGAL ISSUES IN OCCUPATIONAL HEALTH

MULTIDISCIPLINARY TEAMWORK

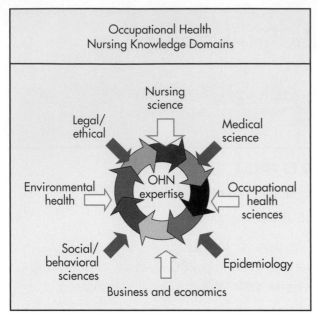

FIGURE 28-1 Occupational health nursing knowledge domains. (From Rogers B: Occupational health nursing expertise, *AAOHN J* 46:477-483, 1998. Copyright Bonnie Rogers, 1998.)

Occupational health nursing, a component of public health nursing, is defined by the American Association of Occupational Health Nurses (AAOHN) as the following:

> The specialty practice that focuses on the promotion, prevention, and restoration of health within the context of a safe and healthy environment. It includes the prevention of adverse health effects from occupational and environmental hazards. It provides for and delivers occupational and environmental health and safety programs and services to clients. Occupational and environmental health nursing is an autonomous specialty and nurses make independent nursing judgments in providing health care services (AAOHN, 2004b).

As depicted in Figure 28-1, occupational health nursing derives its theoretical, conceptual, and factual framework from a multidisciplinary base. Elements of this multidisciplinary base include the following (Rogers, 1998, 2003b):

- *Nursing science,* which provides the context for health care delivery and recognizes the needs of individuals, groups, and populations within the framework of prevention, health promotion, and illness and injury care management, including risk assessment, risk management, and risk communication
- *Medical science* specific to treatment and management of occupational health illness and injury, integrated with nursing health surveillance activities
- *Occupational health sciences,* including **toxicology,** to recognize routes of exposure, examine relationships between chemical exposures in the workplace and acute and latent health effects such as burns or cancer, and understand dose-response relationships; **industrial hygiene,** to identify and evaluate workplace hazards so control mechanisms can be implemented for exposure reduction; **safety,** to identify and control workplace injuries through active safeguards

and worker training and education programs about job safety; and **ergonomics,** to match the job to the worker, emphasizing capabilities and minimizing limitations

- *Epidemiology,* to study health and illness trends and characteristics of the worker population, investigate work-related illness and injury episodes, and apply epidemiological methods to analyze and interpret risk data to determine causal relationships and to participate in epidemiological research
- *Business and economic theories, concepts, and principles* for strategic and operational planning, valuing quality and cost-effective services, and for management of occupational health and safety programs
- *Social and behavioral sciences,* to explore influences of various environments (e.g., work and home), relationships, and lifestyle factors on worker health and determine the interactions affecting worker health
- *Environmental health,* to systematically examine interrelationships between the worker and the extended environment as a basis for the development of prevention and control strategies
- *Legal and ethical issues,* to ensure compliance with regulatory mandates and contend with ethical concerns that may arise in competitive environments

EVOLUTION OF OCCUPATIONAL HEALTH NURSING

The evolution of occupational health nursing in the United States has mirrored the societal changes in moving from an agrarian-based to an industrial-based economy and, entering the twenty-first century, a continuing move to a service-based economy. Occupational health nursing dates to the late 1800s with the employment of Betty Moulder and Ada Mayo Stewart (Parker-Conrad, 2002; Rogers, 2003b).

A group of coal-mining companies hired Betty Moulder in 1888 to care for coal miners and their families (American Association of Industrial Nurses [AAIN], 1976). Seven years later, the Vermont Marble Company hired **Ada Mayo Stewart** to care for workers and their families. Stewart is often referred to as the first "industrial nurse," and her activities are well documented (Parker-Conrad, 1988). In 1897, Anna B. Duncan was employed by the John Wanamaker Company to visit sick employees at home; then, in 1899, a nursing service was established for employees of the Frederick Loeser department store in Brooklyn, New York (AAIN, 1976).

At the turn of the twentieth century, the industrial revolution was well under way, and the concept of health care for employees spread rapidly (Travers, 1987). Companies hiring industrial nurses in the early 1900s included the Emporium in San Francisco; Plymouth Cordage Company in Massachusetts; Anaconda Mining Company in Montana; Broadway Store in Los Angeles; Chase Metal Works in Connecticut; Hale Brothers in San Francisco; Filene's in Boston; Carson, Pirie, and Scott in Chicago; Fulton Cotton Mills in Georgia; and Bullock's in Los Angeles (McGrath, 1946; Parker-Conrad, 1988). The cost-effectiveness of providing health care to employees was achieving increased recognition, and by 1912, after workers' compensation legislation had been instituted, 38 nurses were employed by business firms (McGrath, 1946; Parker-Conrad, 1988). The following year, a registry of industrial nurses was initiated, and in 1915, the Boston Industrial Nurses Club was formed, later evolving into the Massachusetts Industrial Nurses Organization.

In 1916, the Factory Nurses Conference was organized. This group was open only to graduate, state-registered nurses affiliated with the American Nurses Association (ANA), and their efforts identified the industrial nurses' need to explore the uniqueness of this evolving specialty area (AAIN, 1976). More important, industrial nurses were practicing in single-nurse settings and recognized the benefit of uniting as a group for the purpose of sharing ideas with peers practicing in the same nursing arena. In 1917, the first educational course for industrial nurses was offered at Boston University's College of Business Administration.

During and after the Great Depression, many nurses lost jobs because employers and business managers viewed industrial nursing as a nonessential aspect of business (Felton, 1985, 1986). The focus of health care for employees again changed as a result of many factors, including the impact of the two world wars. During World War I, the government demanded health services for workers at factories and ship yards holding defense contracts. Demographics in the workplace were also dramatically different during World War II because increased numbers of women entered the workforce. In 1942, the U.S. Surgeon General told an audience of nurses that the health conservation of the "industrial army" was the most urgent civilian need during the war (Felton, 1985).

From 1938 to 1943, the number of occupational health nurses increased by more than 10,000. In 1942, some 300 nurses from 16 states voted to create a national association for the specialty. Catherine R. Dempsey, a nurse at Simplex Wire and Cable Company in Cambridge, Massachusetts, was elected president of the national association. By 1943, approximately 11,000 nurses were employed in industry (AAIN, 1976).

Nine years later, members of AAIN voted to remain an independent, autonomous association rather than merge with the National League for Nursing or the ANA. In 1953, another important step was taken toward formalizing this specialty area of nursing practice when the *Industrial Nurses Journal* (i.e., now the *AAOHN Journal)* was published. In 1977, the organization changed its name to the AAOHN, reflecting a broader, more diverse scope of practice.

In the 1980s and 1990s, occupational health nursing moved rapidly into increased role expansion in health promotion, policy development, management, and research and maintained traditional occupational health nursing practice. In 1989, AAOHN developed its first research agenda, and in 1993, the Occupational Safety and Health Administration (OSHA) established the Office of Occupational Health Nursing, reenergizing the concept of occupational health into practice. In 1999, the AAOHN Foundation was established, and competencies in the specialty were delineated. In the twenty-first century, the AAOHN continues to expand specialty

borders, emphasizing the importance of occupational health concepts and population-based practice.

DEMOGRAPHIC TRENDS AND ACCESS ISSUES RELATED TO OCCUPATIONAL HEALTH CARE

At the beginning of the twenty-first century, sweeping transformations in industry are influencing the direction of occupational health nursing. These transformations include: changing workforce demographics, rising health care costs, diversity of health care systems with the integration of managed care, influence of the world economy, shift in production from goods to services, and proliferation of advanced technologies. The focus of U.S. industry is moving away from large manufacturing facilities to smaller, service-based businesses, and other changes are anticipated (Hecker, 2001). Work may be performed where and when the customer requires, which will force employers to make different demands on their employees. Flexible and varying work schedules and worksites may become more common than the daily trek to the same building for the 40-hour, 9-to-5 routine that has been the standard for decades. Of major importance will be the demand for an increase in skill level of all employees. The ability to read, follow directions, perform mathematical calculations, and be computer literate will be core skills for workers. The increasing availability of older workers, women, minorities, and immigrants will have far-reaching implications for employers and pose specific challenges for occupational health professionals.

In 2001, most U.S. workers (nearly 71.4%) fell within the prime working ages of 25 to 54; 15% were younger than 25, and 13.6% were 55 or older. By 2010, the baby boom generation will reach the ages of 45 to 64, and middle and older age-groups in the labor force will outnumber younger workers. Data for 2001 indicate that two major occupational groups (managerial and professional specialty; and technical, sales, and administrative support) account for more than 60% of employed persons in the United States. Among industry sectors, services employed the most workers in 2001 (37.4% of the labor force, or 50.5 million workers), followed by retail trade (16.7%) and manufacturing (14.0%). The Bureau of Labor Statistics estimates that these industrial sectors will have the greatest growth between 2000 and 2010: Employment will increase to 52.2 million for the service sector and to 34.2 million for wholesale and retail trade (National Institute for Occupational Safety and Health [NIOSH], 2004). These trends are important to understand because they have a direct impact on the national rate of economic growth, especially in the area of population-sensitive products such as food, automobiles, housing units, household goods, and education services, with concomitant hazards.

Within the context of these evolving organizational trends, key characteristics include a focus on a shared vision, strategy, and long-term objectives within an environment composed of individuals working in teams. In contrast to the past, occupational health nurses have opportunities to work on cross-

TABLE 28-1 Standards of Occupational and Environmental Health Nursing

Standard I: Assessment	The occupational and environmental health nurse systematically assesses the health status of the client(s).
Standard II: Diagnosis	The occupational and environmental health nurse analyzes assessment data to formulate diagnoses.
Standard III: Outcome identification	The occupational and environmental health nurse identifies outcomes specific to the client(s).
Standard IV: Planning	The occupational and environmental health nurse develops a goal-directed plan that is comprehensive and formulates interventions to attain expected outcomes.
Standard V: Implementation	The occupational and environmental health nurse implements interventions to attain desired outcomes identified in the plan.
Standard VI: Evaluation	The occupational and environmental health nurse systematically and continuously evaluates responses to interventions and progress toward the achievement of desired outcomes.
Standard VII: Resource management	The occupational and environmental health nurse secures and manages the resources that support occupational health and safety programs and services.
Standard VIII: Professional development	The occupational and environmental health nurse assumes accountability for professional development to enhance professional growth and maintain competency.
Standard IX: Collaboration	The occupational and environmental health nurse collaborates with the client(s) for the promotion, prevention, and restoration of health within the conduct of a safe and healthy environment.
Standard X: Research	The occupational and environmental health nurse uses research findings in practice and contributes to the scientific base in occupational and environmental health nursing to improve practice and advance the profession.
Standard XI: Ethics	The occupational and environmental health nurse uses an ethical framework for decision making in practice.

From American Association of Occupational Health Nurses: Standards of occupational and environmental health nursing, *AAOHN J* 52:270-274, 2004b.
Copyright American Association of Occupational Health Nurses, www.aaohn.org.

functional teams to shape decisions in areas such as benefits, research, safety, and legal matters. Specifically, occupational health nurses have opportunities to positively affect the transformation of the health care delivery system, establish policies within the managed care environment and within corporations, and assume leadership positions on legislative staffs and in governmental agencies.

Corporations have become driving forces in shaping the development of alternative approaches to health care. Rapidly increasing health care costs have spawned a number of alternative approaches to providing health care. Health maintenance organizations (HMOs) and preferred provider organizations (PPOs) are two of the more common health care management programs. In the late 1980s, Digital Equipment Corporation seized the opportunity to control escalating health care costs by becoming an active and creative value purchaser of health care services (Digital Equipment Corporation, 1995). This was accomplished by designing a model that identified well-organized and well-managed HMOs as the key delivery channel. A tremendous opportunity exists for occupational health nurses to draft similar performance standards and to participate in total quality management processes designed to improve the quality, efficiency, and value of the managed health care delivery system.

It is important that the occupational health nurse remain informed about the various health care options available to the workforce as rapid changes occur regarding corporate benefits. This is of particular importance when considering referral of an employee to a health resource. Participation in one of the managed care plans requires that treatment take place according to the organization's guidelines and within their health service delivery system. Managed care plans have almost replaced traditional indemnity plans. Access to care is closely managed and often limited. As this trend continues, the role of the occupational health nurse will take on added importance. The nurse must be prepared to accept increasing responsibilities as a primary care provider.

As businesses seek ways to maximize the value of their dollars spent on health care services, occupational health nurses and other health professionals face both an opportunity and a threat. The opportunity comes from being able to demonstrate that cost-effective, quality health programs do improve the health of employees and their dependents, positively influencing their company's attempts to control rising health care costs. The threat is that if health professionals cannot prove cost-effectiveness and value to companies, their functions may be eliminated or replaced by contract services (Intili and Laws, 2003).

OCCUPATIONAL HEALTH NURSING PRACTICE AND PROFESSIONALISM

As workplaces have continued to change over the past few decades, the role of the occupational health nurse has become even more diversified and complex. Often working as the only on-site health care professional, the occupational health nurse collaborates with workers, employers, and other professionals to identify health problems or needs, prioritize interventions, develop and implement programs, and evaluate services delivered. The occupational health nurse is in a unique and critical position to coordinate a holistic approach to the delivery of quality, comprehensive occupational health services. The Standards of Occupational and Environmental Health Nursing, the Code of Ethics, and AAOHN practice competencies guide the nurse.

AAOHN's Standards of Occupational and Environmental Health Nursing Practice (AAOHN, 2004b) form the basis by which the profession describes its responsibilities and accountabilities. The 11 Standard statements are listed in Table 28-1. For each standard, identifiable criteria are detailed that can be used to evaluate practice relative to the specific standard. Refer to the complete standards document from the AAOHN for this information.

BOX 28-1 AAOHN Code of Ethics

➤ Occupational health and environmental nurses provide health care in the work environment with regard for human dignity and client rights, unrestricted by considerations of social or economic status, personal attributes, or the nature of the health status.

➤ Occupational health and environmental nurses promote interdisciplinary collaboration with other professionals and community health agencies to meet the health needs of the client.

➤ Occupational health and environmental nurses strive to safeguard employees' rights to privacy by protecting confidential information and releasing information only upon written consent of the employee or as required or permitted by law.

➤ Occupational health and environmental nurses, through the provision of care, strive to provide quality care and to safeguard clients from unethical and illegal actions.

➤ Occupational health and environmental nurses, licensed to provide health care services, accept obligations to society as professional and responsible members of the community.

➤ Occupational health and environmental nurses maintain individual competence in nursing practice, based on scientific knowledge, and recognize and accept responsibility for individual judgments and actions, while complying with appropriate laws and regulations that impact the delivery of occupational and environmental health services.

➤ Occupational health and environmental nurses participate in activities that contribute to the ongoing development of the profession's body of knowledge, while protecting the rights of clients.

From American Association of Occupational Health Nurses: Standards of occupational and environmental health nursing, *AAOHN J* 52:270-274, 2004a.

ETHICAL Insights

Confidentiality of Employee Health Information

Occupational health nurses sometimes experience ethical dilemmas because of dual responsibility to both their employer and employees. In dealing with health information, the employee has a right to privacy and should "be protected from unauthorized and inappropriate disclosure of personal information" (AAOHN, 2004, p. 1). Exceptions can, and in some situations must, be made, however. These include: (1) life-threatening emergencies, (2) authorization by the employee to release information to others (e.g., insurance company, health care provider), (3) workers' compensation information, and (4) compliance with government laws and regulations.

The AAOHN identifies three "levels of confidentiality" of health information. Level I relates to information required by law (e.g., data on occupational illness and injuries, exposure data, and information derived from special examinations [i.e., tests given to food handlers]). Level II covers information that will assist in management of human resources (e.g., information obtained from job placement and other health examinations to determine "workability status" of the employee). Finally, Level III focuses on "personal Health Information." This includes non–job-related health problems or health counseling.

Disclosure of Levels I and II information to management should be allowed only on a "need-to-know" basis, generally with reference to workability status and regulatory compliance. Disclosure of Level III information to management and regulatory agencies should only be allowed as required by law. Finally, disclosure of Level III information health insurance providers should be made only with appropriate written authorization of the employee.

American Association of Occupational Health Nurses: *Position statement: confidentially of employee health information,* 2004, The Author, http://www.aaohn.org/practice/positions/upload/Confidentiality_of_Emp_Health_Info.pdf.

Guided by an ethical framework made explicit in the AAOHN Code of Ethics (AAOHN, 2004a), occupational health nurses encourage and enable individuals to make informed decisions about health care concerns (Box 28-1). The occupational health nurse is a worker advocate and has the responsibility to uphold professional standards and codes. The occupational health nurse is also responsible to management, is usually compensated by management, and must practice within a framework of company policies and guidelines (Rogers, 2003a). Ethical dilemmas arise because the nurse is loyal to both workers and management. Issues such as screening, drug testing, informing employees regarding hazardous exposures, and confidentiality of health information, which is integral and central to the practice base, often create ethical debates. As advocates for workers, occupational health nurses foster equitable and quality health care services and safe and healthy work environments.

Occupational health nurses now make up the largest professional group providing health care services to employees in highly complex work environments. The roles of occupational health nurses are changing as a result of many factors, including rising health care costs, increased recognition of health effects associated with various exposures, emphasis on health promotion and wellness, health surveillance, women's issues, ergonomics, reproductive issues, downsizing, trends in managed care, and multicultural workforces. Box 28-2 reflects this

growth in scope of practice and outlines occupational health nursing services currently mandated by state and federal regulations and occupational health nursing services generally mandated by company policies.

Approximately 30,000 nurses are practicing in the occupational health field in the United States (1.5% to 2% of the total nursing population). Approximately 60% of these 30,000 nurses work alone, making decisions regarding health and safety issues, influencing policy in health and safety, and planning and implementing myriad health programs. The majority of nurses practicing in occupational health are prepared at the baccalaureate level and have been practicing in the field of occupational health for at least 10 years (AAOHN, 1999).

Meeting the needs of employees in smaller businesses is another important practice priority. The integration of occupational health principles into the curricula of schools of nursing, engineering, and management is critical. Community health nurses may assume occupational health nursing roles; therefore community health nurses must be knowledgeable about the specialty area of occupational health nursing. Municipalities, smaller companies, visiting nurse associations, and home care agencies may provide opportunities for community health nurses to be involved in screening programs, health education activities, workplace hazard evaluations, and other occupational health-related activities (Konstantinos and Crespo, 1998).

BOX 28-2 Occupational Health Nursing Services

Services Mandated by Federal and State Regulations

Safe and healthful workplace
Emergency medical response
First aid responder selection and training
First aid space, supplies, protocols, and records
Designated medical resources for incident response
Workers' compensation
Confidentiality of medical records
Compliance with medical record retention requirements
OSHA compliance
Medical personnel requirement (29 CFR 1910.15)
Injury and illness reporting and recording
Accident and injury investigation
Cumulative trauma disorder prevention
Employee access to medical and exposure records
Medical surveillance and hazardous work qualification
Personal protective equipment evaluation and training
Infection control
Employee Right-to-Know Act notification and training
Community Right-to-Know Act compliance
ADA compliance
Rehabilitation Act: handicap, preplacement, fitness for duty evaluations, accommodations
Department of Defense, Department of Transportation, Nuclear Regulatory Commission, and Drug-Free Workplace Act compliance
Policy development
Drug awareness education
Drug testing and technical support
Employee Assistance Program services
Threat of violence and duty to warn
Video display terminal (VDT) local regulations

State and local public health regulations
Nursing practice acts
Board of Pharmacy and Drug Enforcement Agency regulations
Continuing professional education required for licensure

Services Often Mandated by Company Policy

Clinical supervision of on-site health services
Health strategy development
Health services standards
Space, staffing, and operational standards
Occupational illness and injury assessment, diagnosis, treatment, and referral
Nonoccupational illness and injury assessment, diagnosis, treatment, and referral
Disability and return-to-work evaluations and accommodations
Impaired employee fitness for duty evaluation
Preplacement evaluation and medical accommodation
Handicap evaluation, placement, and accommodation
Employee Assistance Program standards
International health: travel, medical advisory, and immunizations
Data collection and analysis
Medical consultation
Pregnancy placement in hazardous environments
Professional education and development
Audit and quality assurance

Optional Services

Health education and health promotion
Medical screening for early detection and disease prevention
Physical fitness programs
Allergy injection programs

ADA, Americans With Disabilities Act; *OSHA,* Occupational Safety and Health Administration.

The occupational health nurse's strengths are embedded in assessing, planning, implementing, and evaluating health programs for populations, care plans for individuals, and health education activities for worker aggregates. Often, lack of understanding or misconceptions about the occupational health nursing role have fostered the invisibility of the nurse, both within the nursing profession itself and within the business environment, thereby exacerbating the difficulties faced in being the sole guardian of health for workers in many companies. Empowered, well-trained, educated occupational and environmental health nurses can help bring about crucial changes in the areas of primary, secondary, and tertiary prevention in occupational health.

In response to societal changes and historical events, the practice of occupational health nursing has changed dramatically, demanding a sophisticated knowledge base and problem-solving skills that are empirically grounded and multidisciplinary in nature (Rogers, 2003b). The roles and responsibilities of the occupational health nurse must be clearly articulated to lay people; managers; workers; union representatives; and colleagues in occupational health, nursing, and medicine to ensure that occupational health nursing can continue to positively affect workers' health, contribute to decreasing health care costs, and foster reduction in health risks. Occupational health nurses must seize opportunities in areas such as program planning, research, and policy making during this era fraught with a health care system in crisis. Issues to be addressed and managed include nursing shortages in many areas of the country, dramatic changes in the business environment, employees' increasing awareness of workplace hazards, and the ever-increasing need to demonstrate the cost-effectiveness of occupational health nursing care and services (Richlin, 2003).

Research is an integral component of occupational and environmental health nursing practice because it provides the basis for scientific discovery that improves practice. In 1989, research priorities in occupational health nursing were first identified and published (Rogers, 1989). These priorities have been updated (Rogers, 2000) and will serve as the scientific basis to continue to build the body of knowledge in occupational and environmental health nursing for practice improvement and expansion (Box 28-3).

OCCUPATIONAL HEALTH AND PREVENTION STRATEGIES

Like the practice of all community health professionals, the occupational health nurse's practice is based on the concept

➤ Effectiveness of primary health care delivery at the worksite
➤ Effectiveness of health promotion nursing intervention strategies
➤ Methods for handling complex ethical issues related to occupational health
➤ Strategies that minimize work-related health outcomes (e.g., respiratory disease)
➤ Health effects resulting from chemical exposures in the workplace
➤ Occupational hazards of health care workers (e.g., latex allergy and blood-borne pathogens)
➤ Factors that influence workers' rehabilitation and return to work
➤ Effectiveness of ergonomic strategies to reduce worker injury and illness
➤ Effectiveness of case management approaches in occupational illness and injury
➤ Evaluation of critical pathways to effectively improve worker health and safety and enhance maximum recovery and safe return to work
➤ Effects of shift work on worker health and safety
➤ Strategies for increasing compliance with or motivating workers to use personal protective equipment

From Rogers B: Occupational health nursing research priorities, *AAOHN J* 48:9-16, 2000.

of prevention. Promotion, protection, maintenance, and restoration of worker health are priority goals set forth in the definition of occupational health nursing. This section describes prevention strategies, including objectives from *Healthy People 2010*. Prevention of exposure to occupational and environmental safety hazards and specific strategies for each level of prevention are described.

Healthy People 2010 and Occupational Health

Healthy People 2010 is the federal government initiative that focuses on health promotion and illness prevention. The stated goal of Priority Area 20 of *Healthy People 2010* is to "promote the health and safety of people at work through prevention and early intervention" (USDHHS, 2000). Objectives from this priority area cover work-related injuries and deaths, repetitive motion injuries, homicide, assault, lead exposure, skin disorders, stress, needle-stick injuries, and hearing loss. In addition, objectives from other priority areas also address issues related to occupational health and safety. The *Healthy People 2010* table lists objectives that deal with occupational health.

Prevention of Exposure to Potential Hazards

To prevent occupational and environmental safety hazards in the work environment, it is important to identify work-related agents and exposures that are potentially hazardous. These can be categorized as follows:

1. *Biological-infectious hazards:* Infectious-biological agents such as bacteria, viruses, fungi, or parasites that may be transmitted via contact with infected clients or contaminated objects or substances
2. *Chemical hazards:* Various forms of chemical agents,

including medications, solutions, and gases, that interact with body tissues and cells and are potentially toxic or irritating to body systems
3. *Enviromechanical hazards:* Factors encountered in work environments that cause accidents, injuries, strain, or discomfort (e.g., poor equipment or lifting devices and slippery floors)
4. *Physical hazards:* Agents within work environments such as radiation, electricity, extreme temperatures, and noise that can cause tissue trauma through transfer of energy from these sources
5. *Psychosocial hazards:* Factors and situations encountered or associated with the job or work environment that create stress, emotional strain, or interpersonal problems

Table 28-2 provides examples of work-related exposures in each of these areas. Having a good understanding of the nature of these hazards will allow for the development of health promotion and prevention strategies to mitigate exposure risk.

Levels of Prevention and Occupational Health Nursing

As occupational health nurses usually practice autonomously in their role as health care providers, the occupational health nurse's activities in primary, secondary, and tertiary prevention strategies are expected to assume an even more important role in the prevention and treatment of illness, injury, and chronic disease in the future (Rogers and Lawhorn, 2000). For example, a study by Rogers and Livsey (2000) examined the scope of independent and interdependent practice by occupational health nurses related to these activities and found 71% of occupational health nurses had overall responsibility for program management, and the majority performed surveillance, screening, and prevention functions as independent practice. Physician supervision for any of these activities ranged from only 0% to 8% in reporting. The results of this study validate the independent functioning in scope of occupational health nursing practice related to surveillance, screening, and prevention activities while recognizing the contributions all providers make to a healthy workforce.

Primary Prevention

In the area of primary prevention, the occupational health nurse is involved in both health promotion and disease prevention. O'Donnell and Harris (2002) describe health promotion as the following:

The science and art of helping people change their lifestyle to move toward a state of optimal health. Optimal health is defined as a balance of physical, emotional, social, spiritual and intellectual health. Lifestyle change can be facilitated through a combination of efforts to enhance awareness, change behavior and create environments that support good health practices. Of the three, supportive environments will probably have the greatest impact in producing lasting changes.

Disease prevention begins with recognition of a health risk, a disease, or an environmental hazard and is followed by measures to protect as many people as possible from harmful consequences of that risk.

HEALTHY PEOPLE 2010	Objectives for Some Areas of Occupational Health	
Objective	**Baseline (1998)**	**Target**
6-8: Eliminate disparities in employment rates between working-age adults with and without disabilities	52%	82%
7-6: Increase the proportion of employees who participate in employer-sponsored health promotion activities	28%	50%
8-17: Increase the number of office buildings that are managed using good indoor air quality practices	NA	NA
9-13: Increase the proportion of health insurance policies that cover contraceptive supplies and services	NA	NA
12-4: Increase the proportion of adults aged 20 years and older who call 911 and administer CPR when they witness an out-of-hospital cardiac arrest	NA	NA
14-28c: Increase Hep B coverage among occupationally exposed workers	71%	98%
19-16: Increase the proportion of work sites that offer nutrition or weight management classes or counseling	55%	85%
20-1: Reduce deaths from work-related injuries	4.5 per 100,000 workers	3.2 per 100,000 workers
20-3: Reduce the rate of injury and illness cases involving days away from work from overexertion or repetitive motion	675 per 100,000 workers	338 per 100,000 workers
20-8: Reduce occupational skin diseases or disorders among full-time workers	67 per 100,000 workers	47 per 100,000 workers
20-9: Increase the proportion of work sites employing 50 or more persons that provide programs to prevent or reduce employee stress	37%	50%
20-10: Reduce occupational needle-stick injuries among health care workers	600,000	420,000
22-13: Increase the proportion of work sites offering employer-sponsored physical activity and fitness programs	36%	75%
26-8: Reduce the cost of lost productivity in the workplace from alcohol and drug use	NA	NA
27-12: Increase the proportion of work sites with formal smoking policies that prohibit smoking or limit it to separately ventilated areas	79%	100%
28-8: Reduce occupational eye injury	NA	NA
28-16: Increase the use of appropriate ear protection devices, equipment, and practices	NA	NA

From US Department of Health and Human Services: *Healthy People 2010, conference ed,* Washington, DC, 2000, The Author.
CPR, Cardiopulmonary resuscitation; *Hep B,* hepatitis B, *NA,* not available.

The occupational health nurse uses a variety of primary prevention methods, with one-on-one interaction as an important strategy for evaluating risk reduction behavior for individuals (Rogers, 2000). The occupational health nurse has daily contact with numerous employees for many reasons (e.g., assessment and treatment of episodic illness or injury and health surveillance); therefore this is an important method of promoting health. The phrase "seize the moment" aptly describes the opportunity that exists with every employee encounter.

Occupational health nurses plan, develop, implement, and evaluate aggregate-focused intervention strategies. The occupational health nurse plans and implements programs such as weight and cholesterol reduction, AIDS awareness, ergonomics training, and smoking cessation (Rogers, 2000). Performing "walk-throughs" in the workplace on a regular basis, recognizing potential and existing hazards, and maintaining communications with safety and industrial hygiene resources to prevent illness and injury from occurring will continue to be critical work for the occupational health nurse (Levy et al., 2005).

For overall *health promotion,* the nurse may plan, implement, and evaluate a health fair, which is a multifaceted health promotion strategy that usually includes a number of community health resources to provide expertise on a wide range of health issues and community services. As part of an overall health and wellness strategy, the occupational health nurse may negotiate with the employer for an on-site fitness center or area with fitness equipment; if cost or space is prohibitive, the employer may choose to partially subsidize membership at a local fitness center (Blix, 1999).

Types of *nonoccupational programs* included in the area of primary prevention are cardiovascular health, cancer awareness, personal safety, immunization, prenatal and postpartum health, accident prevention, retirement health, stress management, and relaxation techniques. Occupational health programs could include topics such as emergency response, first aid and cardiopulmonary resuscitation training, right-to-know

TABLE 28-2 Types of Occupational Hazards and Associated Health Effects

CATEGORY	EXPOSURES	HEALTH EFFECTS
Biological	Blood or body fluids	Bacterial, fungal, and viral infections (e.g., hepatitis B)
Chemical	Solvents	Headache and central nervous system dysfunction
	Lead	Central nervous system disturbances
	Asbestos	Asbestosis
	Acids	Burns
	Glycol ethers	Reproductive effects
	Mercury	Ataxia
	Arsenic	Peripheral neuropathy
Enviromechanical	Static or nonneutral postures	Musculoskeletal disorders
	Repetitive or forceful exertions	Back injuries
	Lighting	Headache and eye strain
	Shift work	Sleep disorders
	Electrical	Electrocution
	Slips and falls	Musculoskeletal conditions
	Struck by or against object	Injury
Physical	Noise	Hearing loss
	Radiation	Reproductive effects and cancer
	Vibration	Raynaud's disease
	Heat	Heat exhaustion and heat stroke
Psychosocial	Stress	Anxiety reactions and a variety of physical symptoms
	Work-home balance	

training, immunization programs for international business travelers, prevention of back injury through knowledge of proper lifting techniques, ergonomics, and other programs targeted to the specific hazards identified in the workplace (Blix, 1999; Walz and Wehse, 2002).

Women's health and safety issues such as maternal-child health, reproductive health, breast cancer education and early detection, stress management, and work-home balance issues will achieve heightened significance as more women enter the workforce. Thirty percent of women currently in the workforce are between ages 16 and 44 years, and each year approximately one million infants are born to these women. Interest in workplace safety and the relationship to reproductive outcomes continues to grow as women of child-bearing age enter the workplace in greater proportions than ever before.

The occupational health nurse can play a key role in the development and delivery of prenatal, postpartum, and childhood programs in the workplace. Of primary importance will be the ability to serve as a change agent to initiate needed programs in the work environment. Employers must be educated regarding strategies not only to reduce health care costs for women and infants but also to improve the work environment for mothers (Wyatt, 2002). Women who believe their employers are interested in the well-being of themselves and their families are more apt to be productive and satisfied employees. The occupational health nurse can play a critical role in the shaping of supportive policies and practices to accommodate the needs of families, including flexible working hours, parental leave, and on-site child care (McGovern and Cossi, 1996).

By 2010, members of *racial and ethnic minority* groups will make up a large share of the expanded labor force (OSHA, 1999). Nonwhites accounted for 29% of the net addition to the workforce between 1985 and 2000 and more than 15% of the workforce in 2000 (OSHA, 1999). As the number of minority and ethnic workers in the workforce increases, so will the illnesses traditionally associated with these groups of workers (e.g., heart disease and stroke, hypertension, cancer, cirrhosis, and diabetes) (NIOSH, 2004). In addition to basic health concerns for this population, available statistics indicate that minority workers have been disproportionately concentrated in some of the most dangerous work, and they are at greater risk for experiencing many of the leading occupationally related diseases and injuries. Table 28-3 illustrates examples of common occupational diseases and injuries.

The occupational health nurse may face challenges in developing programs that are culturally and linguistically appropriate. The occupational health nurse may be in an advocacy role to negotiate with the employer for changes in the work environment that will reduce or eliminate existing or potential occupational exposure to risk factors.

Secondary Prevention

Secondary prevention strategies are aimed at early diagnosis, early treatment interventions, and attempts to limit disability. The focus at this level of prevention is on identification of health needs, health problems, and employees at risk.

As with primary prevention, the occupational health nurse uses a number of different secondary prevention strategies (Rogers, 2003b). By providing direct care for episodic illness and injury, the occupational health nurse is afforded the opportunity to conduct assessments and provide treatment and referrals for a variety of physical and psychological conditions. The occupational health nurse can offer health screenings, which are designed for early detection of disease, at the worksite with relative ease and at minimal cost. Screenings may focus on vision, cancer, cholesterol, hypertension, dia-

TABLE 28-3 Work-Related Diseases and Injuries

WORK-RELATED DISEASE OR INJURY	EXAMPLES OF EFFECT
Occupational lung disease	Cancer and asthma
Musculoskeletal injuries	Back, upper extremity, and musculoskeletal disorders
Occupational cancers	Leukemia, bladder, and skin
Trauma	Death, amputation, and fracture
Cardiovascular diseases	Hypertension and heart disease
Reproductive disorders	Infertility and miscarriage
Neurotoxic disorders	Neuropathy and toxic psychosis
Noise-induced hearing loss	Loss of hearing
Dermatological conditions	Chemical burns and allergies
Psychological disorders	Neurosis; alcohol or substance abuse

betes, tuberculosis, and pulmonary function. Other types of screening, such as mammography, may be contracted with a vendor who uses mobile equipment.

Secondary prevention efforts provided by the occupational health nurse include *preplacement, periodic,* and *job transfer evaluations* to ensure that the worker is being placed or is continuing to work in a job that is safe for that worker (Rogers, 2003b). The preplacement evaluation is performed before the worker begins employment in a new company or is placed in a different job (see **Resource Tool 28A,** Preplacement Health Evaluation, on the book's website at http://evolve. elsevier.com/Nies/). The evaluation is a baseline examination that consists of a medical history, an occupational health history, and a physical assessment that should target the type of work that the employee will be performing (Agency for Toxic Substances and Disease Registry, 1999) (see **Resource Tool 28B,** Occupational Health History, on the book's website at http://evolve.elsevier.com/Nies/). For example, if the employee is going to be lifting materials in a warehouse, special attention should be paid to any history of musculoskeletal problems. Strength testing and range of motion should be performed for all muscle groups.

The examination may also include medical tests to determine specific organ functions that may be affected by exposure to existing agents in the employee's workplace. For example, if the employee is working with a chemical that is a known liver toxin, baseline liver function tests may be appropriate to determine the current health status of the liver and its ability to handle this specific chemical exposure. However, the preplacement examination must be carefully evaluated to ensure compliance with the ADA, which is discussed later in the chapter.

Periodic assessments usually occur at a regular interval (e.g., annual and biannual) and are based on specific protocols for those exposed to substances or irritants such as lead, asbestos, noise, or various chemicals. Examinations of individuals transferring to other jobs are critical to document any changes in health that may have occurred while the employee was working in a specific area or with a specific process. This is usually done to comply with OSHA regulations or NIOSH recommendations (see **Resource Tool 28C** on the book's website at http://evolve.elsevier.com/Nies/ for an example of an OSHA screening and surveillance guide). For full details of compliance requirements, the OSHA standard must be consulted.

Activities must continue to focus on prevention and early detection by increasing awareness of the incidence of other health conditions such as breast cancer and providing accessible and affordable screening programs. Caplan (1998) provides a detailed review of breast cancer screening at the worksite. It is estimated that almost 213,000 women will be diagnosed with invasive breast cancer in 2006 and that about 41,000 women will die from the disease, making breast cancer one of the most commonly diagnosed malignancies among women in the United States and the second leading cause of cancer death (after lung cancer). Further, breast cancer accounts for about 15% of cancer deaths among women (ACS, 2006). By detecting early malignancies, breast cancer screening reduces the mortality rate in women between ages 50 and 69. Mammography is the most effective method for detecting these early malignancies. The occupational health nurse is in an excellent position to play a key role in reducing morbidity and mortality associated with breast cancer. Increasingly, the occupational health nurse will be expected to document the return on investment for these and other related activities in the workplace (Thomas et al., 2002).

Tertiary Prevention

On a tertiary level, the occupational health nurse plays a key role in the rehabilitation and restoration of the worker to an optimal level of functioning. Strategies include case management, negotiation of workplace accommodations, and counseling and support for workers who will continue to be affected by chronic disease (Pergola et al., 1999; Rogers, 2003b).

In industry, disability costs average 8.4% of payroll. Four percent of the gross national product, or $170 billion, is the figure cited for costs associated with total disability (Boden, Biddle, and Spieler, 2001). In the United States, it is estimated that more than 500,000 workers take an estimated 5 months of leave from work each year because of a physical disability; only 48% return to work (Fletcher, 2003). Research findings indicate the importance of developing strategies to reinforce the behavioral change of the individual to avoid what is often referred to as the **disability syndrome,** a state in which an individual chooses not to work when medical clearance has been granted (Curtis and Scott, 2004).

Knowledge of the workplace, the ability to negotiate with the employer for appropriate accommodations, early intervention, and comprehensive case management skills have been and will continue to be essential to the disabled employee's successful return to work. The process of returning an individual to work begins with the onset of injury or illness (Rogers, 1998, 2003b). Regardless of whether this involves an occupational or a nonoccupational condition, the occupational health nurse is the center of case management (Kalina, Haag, and Tourigan, 2004). The nurse works closely with the primary care provider to monitor the progress of the ill or injured worker and to identify and eliminate potential barriers in the return-to-work process. The nurse has a comprehensive understanding of the workplace and of the physical requirements necessary for the employee to work. The physical demands analysis (Randolph and Dalton, 1989) is a useful tool in objectively assessing the physical demands of any job (see **Resource Tool 28D,** Physical Demands Analysis, on the book's website at http://evolve.elsevier.com/Nies/). Once the assessment is completed, the occupational health nurse can relay this information to community health professionals caring for the employee.

For workers needing special accommodations, the occupational health nurse can negotiate and facilitate those appropriate to the employee's health limitations (Kalina et al., 2004). The nurse is often the driving force behind the employer's creating a transitional duty pool. The goal of this type of program is to provide temporary work that is less physically demanding in nature than the employee's regular work. This facilitates the employee's return to the workplace earlier than it required to wait until full strength is regained.

The occupational health nurse can monitor and support the health of employees returning to work who continue to experience adverse health effects of chronic disease. For example, the employee who is returning to work after sustaining a myocardial infarction may have blood pressure monitored on a routine basis. Counseling regarding adjustment to normal work life and support for behavior modification (e.g., smoking cessation) also may be provided (Byczek et al., 2004).

In addition, because the workforce is aging and because older workers are more prone to chronic disease, the occupational health nurse can implement and monitor treatment protocols and assist workers to live and work at their optimum comfort level while managing their disease (NIOSH, 2004). Responsibilities for the care of elderly parents or significant others will influence the balance of work and home for older workers. The occupational health nurse's role as counselor, referral resource for workers, and consultant to management can influence future beneficial changes.

SKILLS AND COMPETENCIES OF THE OCCUPATIONAL HEALTH NURSE

Although clinical and emergency care remains an important tenet of occupational health nursing, the current and future practice must focus on a proactive approach with the goal of preventing illness and injury and promoting health. Therefore

---

BOX 28-4 Competency Categories in Occupational and Environmental Health Nursing

1. Clinical and primary care
2. Case management
3. Workforce, workplace, and environmental issues
4. Regulatory and legislative
5. Management
6. Health promotion and disease prevention
7. Occupational and environmental health and safety education and training
8. Research
9. Professionalism

From American Association of Occupational Health Nurses: Competencies in occupational and environmental health nursing, *AAOHN J,* 51: 290-302, 2003.

---

the occupational health nurse must possess competencies necessary to recognize and evaluate potential and existing health hazards in the workplace. Management and budgeting skills and knowledge of legal and regulatory requirements, toxicology, ergonomics, epidemiology, environmental health, safety, counseling, and health promotion and education are essential to meet the present and future demands of occupational health nursing practice.

Competencies in occupational and environmental health nursing have been delineated in nine categories by AAOHN (Box 28-4) (AAOHN, 2003). Each competency delineates comprehensive performance criteria at the competent, proficient, and expert levels. Each level is described, followed by an example of occupational health nursing practice at that level.

Competent

At the "competent" level of practice, the nurse has gained confidence and his or her perception of the role is one of mastery and an ability to cope with specific situations. There is less of a need to rely on the judgments of peers and other professionals. Work habits tend to stress consistency rather than routinely tailoring care to encompass individual differences (Benner, 1984).

Occupational and environmental health nursing example: The competent nurse is an occupational and environmental health nurse with sufficient experience to recognize a range of practice issues and function comfortably in such roles as clinician, occupational health services coordinator, and case manager. This nurse follows company procedures and relies on assessment checklists and clinical protocols to provide treatment (Rees and Hays, 1996).

Proficient

The "proficient" nurse has an increased ability to perceive client situations as a whole based on past experiences, focusing on the relevant aspects of the situation. The nurse is able to predict the events to expect in a particular situation and can recognize that protocols sometimes must be altered to meet the needs of the client (Benner, 1984).

Occupational and environmental health nursing example: A proficient occupational and environmental health nurse is able to quickly obtain the information needed for accurate assessment and move rapidly to the critical aspects of the problem. Structured goals are replaced by priority setting in response to the situation. This nurse usually possesses sophisticated clinical or managerial skills in the occupational health setting (Rees and Hays, 1996).

Expert

The "expert" nurse has extensive experience and a broad knowledge base and is able to grasp a situation quickly and initiate appropriate action. The nurse has a sense of salience grounded in practice guiding actions and priorities (Benner, 1984).

Occupational and environmental health nursing example: Occupational and environmental health nurses at the expert level include those providing leadership in developing occupational and environmental health policy within an organization; those functioning in upper executive or management roles; those serving as consultants to business and government; and those designing and conducting significant research in the field (Rees and Hays, 1996).

Examples of Skills and Competencies for Occupational Health Nursing

As described, numerous skills and competencies are necessary for occupational health nursing practice. Examples of some of these are outlined here, according to the nine defined areas of competence.

Clinical and Primary Care
- Applying the nursing process in delivery of care
- Providing first aid and primary care according to treatment protocols
- Conducting a physical assessment
- Taking an occupational and environmental health history
- Diagnosing and treating
- Being knowledgeable about immunization protocols
- Identifying employees' emotional needs and providing support and counseling
- Using a multidisciplinary problem-solving approach to occupational health illness and injury
- Maintaining records
- Clinical testing and monitoring
- Responding to medical emergencies
- Being knowledgeable about trends in health-related issues

Case Management
- Identifying the need for case management services
- Conducting case management assessments using a multidisciplinary framework
- Developing case management care plans
- Evaluating resources and vendors for case management
- Implementing early return-to-work programs
- Monitoring and evaluating outcomes
- Developing policies and programs for case management
- Analyzing trends for case management services

- Designing disability management systems
- Conducting case management outcomes-based research

Workforce, Workplace, and Environmental Issues
- Having knowledge of worksite operations, manufacturing processes, and job tasks
- Identifying and monitoring potential and existing workplace exposures
- Influencing appropriate and targeted recommendations for control of workplace hazards
- Having knowledge of toxicological, epidemiological, and ergonomic principles
- Understanding appropriate engineering and administrative controls and personal protective equipment specific to preventing workplace health hazard exposures
- Understanding roles and collaboration with other cross-functional groups as an integral part of a core multidisciplinary team
- Performing risk assessments
- Managing health surveillance programs

Legal and Ethical Responsibilities
- Being knowledgeable of state nursing practice acts and ability to practice occupational health nursing within state guidelines
- Being knowledgeable of federal, state, and municipal regulations pertaining to occupational and environmental health
- Being knowledgeable of the ADA, associated guidelines, and other relevant occupational and environmental health laws
- Being knowledgeable of all aspects of medical record-keeping practices in compliance with nursing practice, state law, and standards of practice
- Being knowledgeable of current legal trends related to negligence and malpractice cases in professional nursing and in the occupational health setting
- Being knowledgeable of confidentiality parameters
- Influencing regulatory and legal processes related to occupational and environmental health

Management and Administration
- Managing budgets
- Hiring staff and management of staff performance
- Fostering professional development plans
- Developing program goals and objectives
- Developing business plans through knowledge of internal and external resources
- Providing comprehensive on-site services and programs
- Knowing needs of business and employees
- Writing reports
- Performing audits and quality assurance
- Handling workers' compensation and disability
- Performing cost-benefit analyses, cost-effectiveness analyses, and outcomes monitoring
- Allocating appropriate staff resources
- Providing leadership in health-related issues
- Negotiating

- Facilitating work accommodations and return-to-work processes
- Coordinating medical response activities and site disaster planning
- Being a resource expert on health issues for employees and management
- Participating in strategic operations planning

Health Promotion and Disease Prevention
- Conducting needs assessments
- Recognizing cultural differences and their relationship to health issues
- Using effective communication styles to match diverse employee and management audiences
- Making effective presentations
- Planning, developing, implementing, and evaluating health programs designed to meet the needs of specific employee groups or organizations
- Evaluating health promotion outcomes
- Applying adult learning theory and principles to health education programs
- Integrating all levels of prevention into company culture

Occupational and Environmental Health and Safety Education
- Creating effective professional and technical support networks both functionally and cross-functionally
- Developing and implementing training programs for workers and professionals

Research
- Identifying researchable problems
- Systematically collecting, analyzing, and interpreting data from different sources
- Recognizing trends in health outcomes by department, work area, or work process
- Planning, developing, and conducting research
- Developing and testing models and theories relative to occupational and environmental health nursing practice

Professionalism
- Engaging in a lifelong learning plan
- Being knowledgeable of AAOHN Standards of Occupational and Environmental Health Nursing and Code of Ethics
- Maintaining currency in practice
- Acting as a professional role model for students and colleagues
- Advancing the specialty through knowledge and science

IMPACT OF FEDERAL LEGISLATION ON OCCUPATIONAL HEALTH

Legislation and associated activities have influenced the practice of occupational health in the United States. Table 28-4 presents a historical perspective of some of the major pieces of legislation that have had, and will continue to have, a direct impact on the general practice of occupational and environmental health nursing. The Occupational Safety and Health Act, Workers' Compensation Acts, and the ADA are highlighted below.

Occupational Safety and Health Act

The Occupational Safety and Health Act of 1970 was enacted 2 years after a major coal-mining disaster in West Virginia. The passage of this legislation came about because there were concerns for workers' health, a burgeoning environmental awareness, union activities, and an increased knowledge about workplace hazards. The general duty clause of the Act states that employers must "furnish a place of employment free from recognized hazards that are causing or likely to cause death or serious physical harm to employees." The Act also identifies the roles of the various government agencies, provides for the establishment of federal occupational safety and health standards, and identifies a structure of penalties, fines, and sentences for violations of regulations. Under the Act, any state has the right to implement its own occupational safety and health administration. The only requirement is that the state standards meet or exceed federal standards. Currently, 25 states and the Virgin Islands operate state occupational safety and health administrations. The following organizations were formed under the provisions of the Act:

- Under the jurisdiction of the Department of Labor, the **Occupational Health and Safety Administration (OSHA)** is responsible for promulgating and enforcing occupational safety and health standards.
- Under the jurisdiction of the USDHHS, NIOSH is responsible for funding and conducting research, making recommendations for occupational safety and health standards to OSHA, and funding Occupational Safety and Health Education and Research Centers for the training of occupational health professionals
- The Occupational Safety and Health Review Commission, which is appointed by the president, is responsible for advising OSHA and NIOSH regarding the legal implications of decisions or actions in the course of performing their duties.
- The National Advisory Committee on Occupational Safety and Health, which is appointed by the president, is a group of consumers and professionals who are responsible for making recommendations to OSHA and NIOSH regarding occupational health and safety.
- The National Commission on State Workers' Compensation Laws, appointed by the president, studied the adequacy of state workers' compensation laws and made recommendations to the president on their findings. This commission's work ended as of October 30, 1972.

Since it was instituted, OSHA has promulgated occupational health and safety standards. These are published in the *Code of Federal Regulations* (CFR) and updated on a regular basis. Having access to the most recent publication of these standards is a crucial responsibility of the occupational health nurse.

The occupational health nurse must be knowledgeable of Title 29 of the code, part 1910 (29 CFR 1910), and other

TABLE 28-4   Historical Perspective of Legislation Affecting Occupational Health in the United States

YEAR	LEGISLATION
1836	First restrictive child labor law enacted (Massachusetts)
1877	State legislation passed requiring factory safeguards (Massachusetts)
1879	State legislation passed requiring factory inspections (Massachusetts)
1886	State legislation passed requiring reporting of industrial accidents (Massachusetts)
1910	State legislation passed requiring formation of an Occupational Disease Commission (Illinois)
1911	Workmen's Compensation Act passed (New Jersey)
1935	Social Security Act passed (state and federal unemployment insurance program)
1936	Walsh-Healy Act (federal legislation setting occupational safety and health standards for certain government contract workers)
1938	Fair Labor Standards Act (setting minimum age for child labor)
1948	All states have workers' compensation acts
1964	Civil Rights Act
1965	McNamara-O'Hara Act (extends protection of the Walsh-Healy Act to include suppliers of government services)
1966	Mine Safety Act (mandatory inspections and health and safety standards in mining industry)
1969	Coal Mine Health and Safety Act (mandatory health and safety standards for underground mines)
1970	Occupational Safety and Health Act
1970	Environmental Protection Agency established
1970	Consumer Protection Agency established
1972	Equal Employment Opportunity Act
1972	Noise Control Act
1972	Clean Water Act
1973	HMO Act
1973	Rehabilitation Act
1976	Toxic Substances Control Act
1976	Resources Conservation and Recovery Act
1977	Federal Mine Safety and Health Act
1990	Americans With Disabilities Act
1991	Bloodborne Pathogens Standard
1993	Family Medical Leave Act
2001	Needlestick Safety and Prevention Act
2002	Recordkeeping Rule Amended

sections of the code that apply to specific hazards in the workplace. For example, 29 CFR 1904 pertains to OSHA's record-keeping requirements and mandates the employer's responsibility to keep records of work-related injuries, illnesses, and deaths. These records must be posted in the workplace for 1 month per year and made available for review by OSHA at any time. In many cases, the occupational health nurse has full responsibility for compliance with this standard.

OSHA has 10 regional offices throughout the United States. Inspectors are assigned to each region to enforce the standards and to provide consultation to industries. An OSHA inspection can be initiated in one of several ways. Each office plans a schedule of routine visits to the industries in their respective regions. In the past, funding has been an issue, and inspections have not taken place in the quantity or frequency originally intended. An inspection will occur if a major health or safety problem, such as a death, occurs at the worksite, or if three or more workers are sent to the hospital as a result of the same incident. Inspection also may occur by employer request. This is not usually done unless the employer has an exemplary occupational health and safety program and wishes to participate in OSHA's voluntary inspection program. Inspection also may be initiated by an employee request if there is concern about a suspected hazardous condition. In this case, OSHA is mandated to respond, and it must keep the employee's name confidential at the employee's request. In the past, penalties have been inconsequential, and sentences have been served

rarely. However, recent events indicate that fines have increased, and OSHA has made public its intention to criminally prosecute company executives for serious and willful violations.

In many organizations, the occupational health nurse is the interface with the OSHA inspector. This requires the nurse to be knowledgeable about the potential hazards in the workplace and about the appropriate control measures designed to eliminate or minimize exposure. The nurse should know that employees or their union representatives have the right to accompany the OSHA investigators.

Workers' Compensation Acts

Workers' Compensation Acts are state mandated and state funded. These programs provide income replacement and pay for health care services for workers who sustain a work-related injury, temporary or permanent disability, or death. Workers' Compensation Acts also protect the employer if the compensation received by the employee precludes legal suits against the employer. Each state regulates its own workers' compensation program that is unique to that state. The employer can self-insure, contract with commercial insurance carriers, or purchase a policy with the state-operated insurance fund. Workers receive an average of 66% of their take-home pay before taxes and some disabled workers and their families are eligible for other benefit programs, including old age, survivors, disability, and health insurance; supplemental security income (SSI); or any other disability program that they may have purchased through the company or on an individual basis.

In an era of high health care costs and a propensity for injured workers to engage the services of lawyers to represent them in negotiating financial settlements, many employers are claiming that workers' compensation costs are crippling their ability to compete in an international marketplace. The occupational health nurse has a unique opportunity to support both the employee and employer in this arena. For the employee, the nurse may be the initial person to whom the work-related injury or illness is reported. Accurate assessment of the injury or illness and appropriate treatment are essential. Community resources must be identified to ensure the injured worker is provided with high-quality health care and appropriate medical follow-up.

The occupational health nurse educates the employee regarding benefits under the Workers' Compensation Act and is often the one who files the claim. If the employee is disabled from work for a period of time, the nurse provides case management support and remains in contact with the employee until return to work. If the employer uses an insurance carrier, the nurse works closely with the claims adjuster to manage the case. The need for light duty or other workplace accommodations is determined before the employee's return. In most cases, the nurse facilitates this process with the employer.

For the employer, the occupational health nurse provides the expertise in early intervention and case management. The goal is to limit the worker's disability and provide an opportunity for early return to work through appropriate workplace accommodations. The desired outcome is a productive employee with optimum health and productivity, with reduced health care and workers' compensation costs.

Americans With Disabilities Act

The **Americans With Disabilities Act (ADA)** enacted by Congress in July 1990, is a comprehensive act that prohibits discrimination on the basis of disability. The core of this law requires employers to adjust facilities and practices for the purpose of making "reasonable accommodations" to enhance opportunities for individuals with disabilities (Kaminshine, 1991). Employment provisions of this act began on July 26, 1992, for employers with 25 or more employees and were revised in July 1994 to include employers with 15 or more employees. Provisions regarding access to public transportation and accommodations became effective in January 1993.

The ADA defines disability as "physical or mental impairment that substantially limits one or more major life activities; having record of such an impairment; or being regarded as having such an impairment" (Kaminshine, 1991, p. 249). Physical or mental impairment guidelines are the same as those described in the Federal Rehabilitation Act and include "any physiologic disorder or condition, cosmetic disfigurement, anatomical loss affecting any of the major body systems, or any mental or psychological disorder" (Kaminshine, 1991, p. 249). Major life activities include caring for self, walking, seeing, hearing, and speaking. The ADA excludes conditions relating to sexual preference and gender identity, compulsive gambling, kleptomania, and pyromania. The ADA also denies protection for individuals who are currently involved in illegal drug use.

With regard to the ADA, the occupational health nurse has particular responsibility in two areas. The first involves the duty to provide or facilitate reasonable accommodations. This is facilitated by the nurse's familiarity with the physical requirements of jobs in the workplace. The second involves preplacement inquiries and health examinations. Preplacement health examinations will be permitted only if phrased in terms of the applicant's general ability to perform job-related functions rather than in terms of a disability and after a job offer has been made. The examination must be job related and consistently conducted for all applicants performing similar work.

As illustrated in this discussion of specific laws pertinent to occupational health, the legal context for occupational health nursing practice is broad and involves many arenas. The occupational health nurse must be knowledgeable about all laws and regulations that govern any industry where the nurse provides health care to employees (e.g., laboratories, transportation, and utilities).

LEGAL ISSUES IN OCCUPATIONAL HEALTH

In recognition of the dynamic nature of occupational health nursing practice, coupled with the influences and impact of larger policy issues, the occupational health nurse must know the legal parameters of practice and respond to legislative mandates that govern worker health and safety (AAOHN, 1999). The occupational health nurse is professionally primarily accountable to workers and worker populations and to the employer, the profession, and self (AAOHN, 1999). In particular, the occupational health nurse must be aware of liability and legal issues related to the following:

- The employee-nurse relationship
- The employment capacity of the occupational health nurse
- Any acts of negligence

The employee-nurse relationship can be confusing when the employer hires the nurse to provide services to the employee. The concern is whether a professional relationship exists under the law or the relationship is based on a coworker status.

MULTIDISCIPLINARY TEAMWORK

As workplaces have become more complex, a diverse array of expertise has emerged in many functional and technical areas. To be successful, the occupational health nurse must recognize the need to work as part of an interdisciplinary team. The nurse may interact with occupational medicine professionals, industrial hygienists, safety professionals, employee assistance counselors, personnel professionals, and union representatives (Figure 28-2). Community health professionals, insurance carriers, and other support agencies in the community are also critical links.

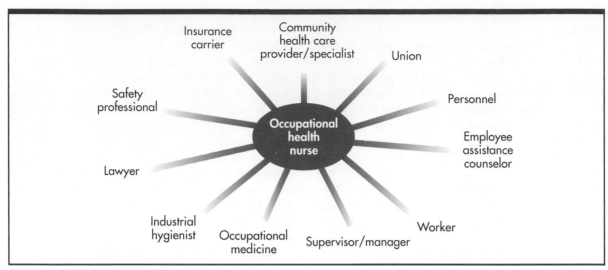

FIGURE 28-2 The occupational health nurse's professional links in the workplace and community.

SUMMARY

This chapter described the evolution of occupational health nursing during its first century of practice. Current and future demographics and business trends are highlighted as they relate to this nursing specialty area. Aging workers, escalating health care costs, increasing numbers of women and minorities in the workforce, and the competitive international marketplace are key factors shaping occupational health nursing practice.

The occupational health nursing role is challenging and can have a tremendous impact on the quality and delivery of health care to workers and their families. Nurses working in occupational settings should have an excellent understanding of all levels of prevention and possess the skills and competencies outlined here.

For the community health nurse who works in other settings such as home health, clinics, and schools, knowledge of occupational health nursing practice is also important. Many companies do not have on-site occupational health nurses and therefore must rely on community health nurses to support their occupational health and safety needs.

LEARNING ACTIVITIES

1. A large automobile manufacturer needs a program designed to control respiratory disease among foundry workers. Workers in different areas of ferrous foundries are exposed to different respiratory hazards. The main problems are exposure to silica and formaldehyde. The corporation would like to develop a pilot program for one of its foundries that will then be applied to its other foundries. Health and industrial hygiene data will be collected. Both the corporation and the workers support the project, and both see the project as having the following three purposes:
   - Detecting health effects in individuals who may benefit from intervention
   - Determining the relationship of health effects to environmental exposures
   - Identifying control strategies as appropriate
2. Outline a pilot program. Discuss the implications of discovering adverse health effects among current workers. Describe the roles of the occupational health nurse, physician, industrial hygienist, safety professional, manager, and employee.
3. A weight-loss program was conducted during August. Ten people participated in the 6-week program. The total weight loss for the group was 185 pounds. The following chart indicates the weight loss for the individuals:

Weight Before Program (lb)	Weight After Program (lb)
215	190
175	160
139	129
275	245
145	120
198	183
120	115
243	233
185	145
210	200

Is there a more effective way to show the results of the program? Assume a peer distributed this report for critique. Be creative, filling in any data, facts, figures, or other information that may be missing. Redesign a report to send to management.
4. Take an occupational history on five currently employed workers. Identify the occupation, associated job tasks, and potential health hazards. Describe control strategies that could minimize or eliminate the risk of adverse health effects.
5. Conduct a literature review to identify critical concepts in occupational health nursing, epidemiology, ergonomics, safety, industrial hygiene, and medicine and describe how these disciplines work together to achieve optimal ends.

CASE STUDY   Application of the Nursing Process

Leslie Johnston is a 23-year-old woman who was transferred by her employer into a job that required her to work with chemicals used in photolithography. Leslie became concerned when she noticed the label on one of the pieces of equipment warned of possible adverse effects on reproduction. Because of her concern and related issues, she went to the on-site health clinic to talk with Peter Mitchell, the occupational health nurse.

Peter invited Leslie into his office to ask her questions and do a brief health history. Leslie reported that her health had been "excellent" until recently, but that she had not felt well since transferring to her new position. She explained that she was newly married and thought she may be pregnant, but this was unconfirmed. She questioned whether her vague physical complaints (fatigue, headaches, occasional queasiness) might be related to working with chemicals, a pregnancy, or another reason.

Peter reassured Leslie that he had been employed at the company for 8 years, and he was aware that there were no restrictions in Leslie's work area for pregnant women. He pulled up her health file from his computerized database and gave her a set of health history forms to complete. He also had her read and sign several forms related to confidentiality and assured her that none of her health information would be shared with their employer without her consent.

ASSESSMENT

To obtain needed information, Peter:
- Completed general health and occupational health histories.
- Performed a modified physical assessment and discussed the symptoms Leslie was experiencing.
- Referred Leslie to her personal health care provider for further evaluation and to obtain a pregnancy test. (NOTE: In some cases, on-site clinics will be equipped for basic procedures such as this. If this is not a service provided by the occupational health nurse, referral must be made to the employee's health care provider. If the employee does not have one, referral must be made to an appropriate community health resource). Peter encouraged Leslie to inform her supervisor and himself should the pregnancy test be positive so they could adapt her assignments to her condition.
- Assessed Leslie's work area with an industrial hygienist to determine if there might be problems such as leaking equipment or problems with ventilation.
- Reviewed the most current industrial hygiene data appropriate to the area.

DIAGNOSIS

Individual
- At risk for chemical exposure
- Vague physical complaints of unknown etiology
- Possible pregnancy

- At risk for possible adverse pregnancy outcomes
- Stress related to concern regarding possible exposure to harmful chemicals

Community
- Potential for exposure of employees to unsafe chemicals and/or working conditions

PLANNING

Peter developed a plan of care based on Leslie's health history and concerns. Together they set the following goals:

Individual
Short-Term Goals
- Determine pregnancy status.
- Determine potential exposure levels and review side effects of chemicals.
- Determine reason for her vague physical complaints.
- Reduce stress experiences.

Long-Term Goals
- Ensure that the work environment is safe for future pregnancies (if Leslie is not pregnant at present).
- Collaborate with Leslie and her supervisor on possible work restrictions.

Community (Workplace)
Short-Term Goals
- Company personnel (e.g., the occupational health nurse, the industrial hygienist, and all others who are directly affected) will be knowledgeable in safe handling of all hazardous chemicals
- All company policies will be followed regarding safety and exposure.

Long-Term Goals
- Policies on handling of chemicals and related information will be reviewed periodically as required by law.
- All employees who work with and around potentially hazardous chemicals will undergo periodic instruction and check-off related to proper procedures.
- Work areas will be monitored per policy for compliance with safe practices.
- There will be no incidents involving worker exposure to chemicals.

INTERVENTION

Individual
Peter conducted a brief physical examination and did not identify any obvious physical abnormalities. Because Leslie's chief complaints were fatigue, occasional headaches, and queasiness, he encouraged her to make an appointment with her primary care provider or gynecologist for a more extensive workup and to assess for pregnancy.

Continued

CASE STUDY Application of the Nursing Process (cont'd)

With her permission, he called the industrial hygienist to counsel with Leslie regarding the policies of the company and to explain what chemicals might potentially be hazardous and to review procedures and restrictions. The hygienist also stated that he would send a team to Leslie's work area to take air samples, check lighting and perform other tests to ensure there were no problems.

Community (Workplace)

The assigned industrial hygiene team sampled the environment for chemical exposure per established procedure. They also set up a plan to add the area to more frequent observation pending the results of the tests. The hygienist assured Peter and Leslie that he would communicate any work restrictions or changes to the personnel department and Leslie's supervisor if needed.

EVALUATION

Individual

Following the meeting with Peter and the industrial hygienist, Leslie stated that she felt reassured. She agreed to make an appointment ASAP with her doctor for an evaluation and

pregnancy test. She also agreed to inform Peter and her direct supervisor if she learned that she was pregnant.

Community (Workplace)

The industrial hygienist and his assistants performed several tests in close proximity to Leslie's work station and found no abnormal readings and all equipment was in good working order. Per agency policy and following OHSA regulations, they charted all findings and submitted reports.

LEVELS OF PREVENTION

Primary

- Teach about chemicals, exposures, etc.
- Instruct about chemical avoidance.
- Remove employee from environment through work restrictions.

Secondary

- Assess employee for signs and symptoms.
- Assess work environment for exposure.
- Refer for evaluation of possible health problems as needed.

Tertiary

- Provide reproductive counseling.

REFERENCES

Agency for Toxic Substances and Disease Registry: Reproductive and developmental hazards: an overview for occupational and environmental health nurses, *AAOHN J* 46:57-66, 1999.

American Association of Industrial Nurses: *The nurse in industry,* New York, 1976, The Author.

American Association of Occupational Health Nurses: *Compensation and benefits study,* Atlanta, 1999, The Author.

American Association of Occupational Health Nurses: Competencies in occupational and environmental health nursing, *AAOHN J,* 51:290-302, 2003.

American Association of Occupational Health Nurses: AAOHN Code of ethics and interpretive statements, *AAOHN J* 52:140-142, 2004a.

American Association of Occupational Health Nurses: *Standards of occupational and environmental health nursing, AAOHN J* 52:270-274, 2004b.

American Cancer Society: *Cancer Statistics, 2006,* The Author, http://www.cancer.org/docroot/MED/content/MED_1_1_Most-Requested_Graphs_and_Figures_2006.asp.

Barlow R: Role of the occupational health nurse in the year 2000: perspective view, *AAOHN J* 40:463-467, 1992.

Benner P: *From novice to expert: excellence and power in clinical nursing practice,* Menlo Park, Calif, 1984, Addison-Wesley.

Blix A: Integrating occupational health protection and health promotion: theory and

program application, *AAOHN J* 47:168-174, 1999.

Boden LI, Biddle EA, Spieler EA: Social and economic impacts of workplace illness and injury, *Am J Ind Med* 40:398-402, 2001.

Byczek L et al: Cardiovascular risk factors, *AAOHN J* 52:66-76, 2004.

Caplan L: Worksite breast cancer screening programs: a review, *AAOHN J* 46:443-453, 1998.

Curtis J, Scott LR: Integrating disability management into strategic plans, *AAOHN J* 52:298-301, 2004.

Digital Equipment Corporation: *1995 HMO performance standards,* Maynard, Mass, 1995, The Author.

Felton JS: The genesis of occupational health nursing: part I, *Occup Health Nurse* 28:45-49, 1985.

Felton JS: The genesis of occupational health nursing: part II, *AAOHN J* 34:210-215, 1986.

Fletcher M: Careful integration, management of disabilities helps hospitals trim millions from its corporate costs, *Bus Insur* 37:26-28, 2003.

Hecker DE: Occupational employment practices to 2010, *Mon Labor Rev* 124:21-38, 2001.

Intili H, Laws C: Delivering health care in a large urban hotel: cost-effective, quality care for an underserved and uninsured population, *AAOHN J* 51:306-309, 2003.

Kalina CM, Haag A, Tourigan R: Challenges and solutions in case management, *AAOHN J* 52:143-145, 2004.

Kaminshine S: New rights for the disabled: the Americans with Disabilities Act of 1990, *AAOHN J* 39:249-251, 1991.

Konstantinos K, Crespo J: Cost effective, hospital based occupational health services: successful program, *AAOHN J* 46:127-132, 1998.

Levy BS et al: *Occupational and environmental health,* ed 5, Philadelphia: Lippincott Williams & Wilkins, 2005.

McGovern PM, Cossi DA: Work and family: policy and program options affecting occupational health, *AAOHN J* 44(8):408-418, 1996.

McGrath BJ: *Nursing in commerce and industry,* New York, 1946, The Commonwealth Fund.

National Institute for Occupational Safety and Health: *Worker health chartbook, 2004,* DHHS (NIOSH) Pub No 2004-146, 2004.

Occupational Safety and Health Administration: *The future of work,* Washington, DC, 1999, The Author.

O'Donnell M, Harris J: *Health promotion in the workplace,* ed 3 New York, 2002, Delmar.

Parker-Conrad JE: A century of practice: occupational health nursing, *AAOHN J* 36:156-161, 1988.

Parker-Conrad JE: Celebrating our past, *AAHON J* 50:537-541, 2002.

Pergola T et al: Case management services for injured workers: providers' perspectives, *AAOHN J* 47:397-404, 1999.

Randolph SA, Dalton PC: Limited duty work: an innovative approach to early return to work, *AAOHN J* 37:446-452, 1989.

Rees P, Hays B: Fostering expertise in occupational health nursing, *AAOHN J* 44:67-72, 1996.

Richlin D: *AAOHN guidelines for starting an occupational health and safety service,* Atlanta, 2003, The Author.

Rogers B: Establishing research priorities in occupational health nursing, *AAOHN J* 37: 493-500, 1989.

Rogers B: Occupational health nursing practice, education, and research: challenges for the future, *AAOHN J* 38:536-543, 1990.

Rogers B: Occupational health nursing expertise, *AAOHN J* 46:477-483, 1998.

Rogers B: Occupational health nursing research priorities, *AAOHN J* 48:9-16, 2000.

Rogers B: Nursing: an ethic of caring, *AAOHN J* 51:155-157, 2003a.

Rogers B: *Occupational health nursing: concepts and practice,* ed 2, Philadelphia: WB Saunders, 2003b.

Rogers B, Lawhorn E: Occupational health nursing strategies for health promotion. In Hickey J, Ovimetle R, Venegoni S, editors: *Advanced practice nursing,* Philadelphia, 2000, Lippincott Williams & Wilkins.

Rogers B, Livsey K: Occupational health surveillance, screening, and prevention activities in occupational health nursing practice, *AAOHN J* 48:92-99, 2000.

Thomas B et al: Breast health educational interventions: changes in beliefs and practices of working women, *AAOHN J* 50:460-467, 2002.

Travers PH: *A comprehensive guide for establishing an occupational health service,* Atlanta, 1987, AAOHN.

US Department of Health and Human Services: *Healthy People 2010, conference ed,* Washington, DC, 2000, The Author.

Walz JA, Wehse KL: Wellness for welders: prevention strategies, *AAOHN J* 50:303-306, 2002.

Wyatt SN: Challenges of the working breast feeding mother: workplace solutions, *AAOHN J* 52:61-66, 2002.

Forensic and Correctional Nursing

Angela Snow

MEDIA RESOURCES

Additional Material for Study, Review, and Further Exploration

evolve Website at http://evolve.elsevier.com/Nies

❖ Quiz ❖ Case Studies ❖ Content Updates ❖ Glossary ❖ WebLinks

OBJECTIVES

Upon completion of this chapter, the reader will be able to do the following:

1. Define forensic nursing.
2. Describe the specialties of forensic nurses.
3. Explain issues important to each of the subspecialty areas of forensic nursing.
4. Describe interventions and services forensic nurses perform.
5. Discuss factors affecting health and wellness in a correctional setting.

KEY TERMS

clinical forensic nurse
coroner
correctional nursing
elder abuse
forensic
forensic nurse death
   investigator

forensic nursing
forensic psychiatric nurse
geriatric forensic nurse
legal nurse consultant
living forensics

medical examiner
nurse attorney
nurse coroners
organ donation and
   transplant procurement

pediatric forensic nurse
prison culture
sexual assault nurse
   examiner (SANE)

CHAPTER OUTLINE

SUBSPECIALTIES OF FORENSIC NURSING
   Sexual Assault Nurse Examiner
   Death Investigation Examiner
   Legal Nurse Consultant and Nurse Attorney
   Clinical Forensic Nurse
   Forensic Psychiatric Nurse

CORRECTIONAL NURSING
   Maintenance of a Safe Environment
   Prison Culture

HEALTH ISSUES IN PRISON POPULATIONS
   Chronic and Communicable Diseases
   Women in Prison
   Adolescents in Prison

MENTAL HEALTH ISSUES IN CORRECTIONAL SETTINGS

STANDARDS OF NURSING PRACTICE IN CORRECTIONAL SETTINGS

EDUCATION AND FORENSIC NURSING

According to the Bureau of Justice Statistics National Crime Victimization Survey, in 2003 approximately 5,401,720 violent crimes were reported (USDoJ/BJS, 2004). These crimes ranged from vandalism and theft, to rape and sexual assault, to aggravated assault and murder. Because of the prevalence of violence and violent crimes in society, health care professionals are required to be able to identify victims of crime and provide proper care to them. Indeed, screening for violence is now considered to be a minimum standard of care for all clients (Sekula, 2005).

HEALTHY PEOPLE 2010 | Objectives Related to Forensic Nursing

Objective	Baseline	Target
15-6: Extend state-level child fatality review of deaths due to external causes for children aged 14 years and under.	NA	NA
15-10: Increase the number of States and the District of Columbia with statewide emergency department surveillance systems that collect data on external causes of injury.	12 states (1998)	All states and the District of Columbia
15-33: Reduce maltreatment and maltreatment fatalities of children.	NA	NA
15-34: Reduce the rate of physical assault by current or former intimate partners.	4.4 assaults per 1,000 persons aged 12 and older	3.3 assaults per 1,000 persons aged 12 and older
15-35: Reduce the annual rate of rape or attempted rape.	0.8 rapes or attempted rapes per 1,000 persons (1998)	0.7 rapes or attempted rapes per 1,000 persons
15-36: Reduce sexual assault other than rape.	0.6 sexual assaults other than rape per 1,000 persons aged 12 and older	0.4 sexual assaults other than rape per 1,000 persons aged 12 and older
26-19: (Developmental) Increase the proportion of inmates receiving substance abuse treatment in correctional institutions.	NA	NA

From US Department of Health and Human Services: *Healthy People 2010*, Washington, DC, 2000, US Government Printing Office.

The term **forensic** means "pertaining to the law; legal" (Venes, 2001). It refers to instances, activities, or information used in or suitable to courts of law. Health care providers, especially nurses, frequently care for both victims and perpetrators of crime (American Association of Colleges of Nursing, 1999); therefore they should be educated in forensic issues.

Forensic nursing is a field of nursing that combines aspects of forensic science, criminal justice, and nursing into a specialty practice area that assists victims of violence. Forensic nursing is one of the newest specialty areas recognized by the American Nurses Association (ANA) and is growing nationally and internationally. It was officially recognized by the ANA in 1995, and the *Scope and Standards of Forensic Nursing for Practice* was published in 1997 (Burgess, Berger, and Boersma, 2004).

The International Association of Forensic Nursing (IAFN) defines forensic nursing as "the application of forensic science combined with the bio-psychological education of the registered nurse, in the scientific investigation, evidence collection and preservation, analysis, prevention and treatment of trauma and/or death medical-legal issues" (ANA, 1997, p. v). Thus the forensic nurse's role as a clinical investigator provides a vital link between the health care system, the investigative process, and courts of law (Lynch, 2006).

Forensic nurses practice in multiple areas of client care and across a number of settings. Their responsibilities include collecting evidence from perpetrators and survivors in settings such as hospitals or death scenes and testifying in court as witnesses. In addition to working with victims of crime and perpetrators, forensic nurses may be involved in paternity disputes and cases involving workplace injuries, medical malpractice, vehicle accidents, food or drug tampering, and medical equipment defects (Burgess et al., 2004). The *Healthy*

BOX 29-1 Specialties of Forensic Nurses

➤ Sexual Assault Nurse Examiner
➤ Nurse Coroner and Death Investigator
➤ Legal Nurse Consultant and Nurse Attorney
➤ Forensic Nursing Educator and Consultant
➤ Forensic Psychiatric Nurse
➤ Clinical Nursing Specialist
  Transplant
  Pediatrics
  Gerontology
➤ Correctional Nurse

People 2010 table lists some objectives related to this highly specialized practice area.

SUBSPECIALTIES OF FORENSIC NURSING

The IAFN recognizes core specialties within forensic nursing (Box 29-1). Each of the subspecialties will be briefly discussed; the specialty area of correctional nursing will be examined in more detail because of its uniqueness and complexity.

Sexual Assault Nurse Examiner

Sexual assault nurse examiner (SANE) is the most widely recognized subspecialty in forensic nursing. In the 1970s, emergency department (ED) registered nurses identified a special client population—sexual assault or rape victims—who were not receiving the appropriate, compassionate care after a traumatic event (Ledray and Arndt, 1994). They observed that the sexual assault victim would enter the ED and in

---

BOX 29-2 Type of Evidence Collected From a Victim of Sexual Assault

- Pubic combings
- Pubic hair controls (from the victim)
- Genital and thigh swabs
- Vaginal swabs and smears
- Rectal swabs and smears
- Oral swabs and smears
- Head hair
- Blood sample
- Fingernail scrapings
- Urine specimen
- All clothing worn at the time of the attack

From Safertein R: Evidence collection and preservation. In Lynch VA, editor: *Forensic nursing,* St Louis, Mosby, 2006.

---

many cases, the staff did not know how to compassionately approach the situation, properly collect evidence, or testify in court; therefore the SANE was developed.

A SANE is a specially trained registered nurse who applies the nursing process during forensic examinations to victims of sexual assault. The SANE collects forensic evidence related to a reported crime and frequently testifies as a witness at subsequent trials (Girardin, 2001; IAFN, 1996; Ledray, 2006). SANEs are usually employed in EDs, labor and delivery departments, and clinics dedicated to victims of violence.

If the victim is medically stable, the SANE is responsible for conducting a thorough examination including obtaining a history, performing the physical assessment, and collecting evidence (Box 29-2). If the victim is medically unstable, he or she will be assessed and stabilized by a physician prior to the sexual assault examination (Antognoli-Toland, 1985). Other responsibilities of the SANE are crisis intervention, evaluation of the victim for sexually transmitted infection, pregnancy risk assessment and interception as needed, and client referral for additional support (Ledray, 2006).

SANE is the only forensic nursing subspecialty with a certification currently offered through the IAFN. The requirements for a registered nurse to be eligible for the SANE certification examination are that the nurse must (1) be in practice for a minimum of 2 years, (2) have successfully completed 40 hours of didactic instruction or 3 semester hours of academic credit from an accredited nursing program, and (3) demonstrate competency in sexual assault examinations (IAFN, 1998).

Death Investigation Examiner

In the United States, death investigation systems are divided into three types: medical examiner system, mixed medical examiner system, and coroner systems (Fulton, 2003; Hanzlick, 1996; Hanzlick and Combs, 1998; Lynch, 2006; Prahlow and Lantz, 1995) State law determines how each system is defined.

Medical examiners are licensed physicians with experience in forensic pathology, that is, specialized training in medicolegal death investigation and forensic autopsies (Hanzlick and Combs, 1998). Medical examiners are appointed for

an unspecified term and serve a county, district, region, or state as determined by law (Hanzlick, 1996).

The mixed medicolegal system is combination of medical examiner and coroner systems, depending on the law. The coroner system allows many nonmedical persons to certify cause and manner of death and to conduct death investigations. In most circumstances, **coroners** are laypeople without mandatory medicolegal training who are elected for a specific term (Fulton, 2003; Hanzlick, 1996).

Medical examiners and coroners are responsible for identifying the cause and manner of death. The cause of death is the event that initiated the progression of events that ended in death and can be categorized into two types, disease and trauma (Lynch, 2006). The National Association of Medical Examiners (NAME) identifies five acceptable options for recording manner of death: natural, accident, suicide, homicide and "undetermined" (Hanzlick, Hunsaker, and Davis, 2002).

Role of a Forensic Nurse in Death Investigation

Forensic nurses enter the death investigation arena possessing essential knowledge of anatomy, physiology, pharmacology, and growth and development that will be needed to conduct a comprehensive death investigation (Fulton, 2003). In most cases related to a death scene investigation, investigators are police officers and homicide detectives—professions without medical knowledge. The **forensic nurse death investigator** evaluates the death scene with a specialized, medically oriented perspective and might interpret the scene differently.

CLINICAL EXAMPLE

A police officer entering a house observes several pools of blood located throughout the residence and discovers a deceased male, nude and lying in bed; the police officer suspects murder. The forensic nurse death investigator entering the same death scene notices the same findings as the initial police officer, but also notes bloody emesis in the toilet, blood-soaked towels in the washing machine, and empty alcohol bottles in the trash. A preliminary examination of the decedent by the forensic nurse reveals ascites and multiple contusions at varying stages of healing. Following communication with family members, the forensic nurse discovers the decedent was an alcoholic with many health problems; she suspects that he suffered from ruptured esophageal varices. This was confirmed by an autopsy, and the manner of death was determined to be from natural causes rather than homicide as initially believed by the police officer. ■

Role of Nurse Coroner

Forensic nurses may be employed in a medical examiner system investigating deaths, both those deemed to be "natural" and those determined to be otherwise. In coroner systems, nurses may decide to run for the position of coroner or **nurse coroner,** and be responsible to perform death investigations and certify death certificates. A nurse coroner's medical background and knowledge enables them to identify disease processes that the lay coroner may not recognize or may misinterpret as foul play as in the clinical example.

Forensic nurse death investigators and nurse coroners exhibit crucial communication skills when dealing with grieving families. Nurses are trained in therapeutic communication. They use open-ended questions, attentively listen, and are fully present with the family. The use of these techniques allows the family to openly share the feelings and thoughts experienced with the death of a loved one (Potter and Perry, 2005).

Nurse coroners and forensic nurse death investigators complement the criminal justice system and forensic science field by linking the three disciplines together. The forensic nurse can contribute much needed expertise and speak for the decedent through the knowledge he or she has obtained in a more holistic manner.

Legal Nurse Consultant and Nurse Attorney

Legal nurse consultant (LNC) and **nurse attorney** are nurses who provide assistance within the legal system using specialized nursing knowledge and expertise when interaction of law and health issues arise (Geissler-Murr and Moorhouse, 2006; Saunders, 2000). Among many activities, LNCs evaluate, analyze, and render informed opinions on the delivery of health care and its outcomes (AALNC, 1999). Legal nurse consultants are hired by attorneys and insurers to review and interpret medical records and charts, provide objective opinions based on standards of care, and possibly to testify in court (Burgess et al., 2004; Raymond, 2002; Saunders, 2000).

Nurse attorneys are educated in both law and nursing. They are most often involved in medical error cases; this may be from a malpractice plaintiff's or defendant's perspective, may involve licensure disciplinary action, or may involve agency oversight (Collins and Halpern, 2005). Some practitioners have differing opinions regarding LNCs and nurse attorneys. They may be perceived as either defending the profession or prosecuting peers by testifying against professional colleagues. Haas and Bradshaw (1999) observe that by providing services as experts and testifying, nurses serving as legal consultants help hold accountable poor practitioners who are dangerous to clients. In contrast, meticulous practitioners who are wrongfully accused of negligence will be defended.

The number of legal nurse consultants is growing and totals around 4000 (Raymond, 2002). According to the American Association of Legal Nurse Consultants (1999), LNCs perform many different services and activities, including the following:

- Organizing and analyzing medical records and related materials
- Preparing chronologies of health care events
- Identifying standards of care
- Determining causation and damage issues
- Conducting literature research and summarizing medical literature
- Helping to determine the merits or defensibly of a case
- Providing education regarding facts and issues relevant to a case
- Identifying and determining damages and related costs of services
- Acting as a liaison among attorney, health care providers, clients, and experts

---

> **BOX 29-3** Tips for Testifying at a Deposition or in Court

> ➤ Dress professionally and conservatively.
> ➤ Tell the truth at all times.
> ➤ Listen to the complete question before responding.
> ➤ Speak slowly, clearly, and concisely when answering.
> ➤ Avoid saying "I think" or "I believe."
> ➤ Never interrupt.
> ➤ Take a few seconds to formulate an answer before responding.
> ➤ Minimize "ums" or "uhs" by pausing at the end of sentences.
> ➤ If there is an objection, stop talking and wait for the judge to make a ruling.
> ➤ When answering questions, make eye contact with the jury members.
> ➤ Remain calm.
> ➤ Respond confidently.
> ➤ Do not answer a question that you do not understand; ask the attorney to repeat questions as needed.
> ➤ Practice difficult words.
> ➤ Do not become defensive or angry.
> ➤ Avoid nervous gestures; keep your hands in your lap.

> Data from Ruiz-Contreras A: The nurse as an expert witness, *Top Emerg Med* 27(1): 27-35, 2005.

LNCs read reports and records and determine whether the standards of care were met or breached. In general, if working for a plaintiff in a malpractice case, the LNC will look for breaches in the standards of care; if working for the defense, the LNC will look for nursing care that is given within the standards of care related to the complaint. It is essential that the attorneys be kept informed of all findings—even those that might negatively affect their care (Meiner, 2005).

When providing services, the LNC may submit an affidavit, which is a written statement explaining the expert's credentials, background, and licensing or certification(s). It also provides a list of the materials read and considered in the case, and the findings of the review are summarized into a case analysis. Following the submission of an affidavit, the LNC may be asked to provide a deposition. The deposition is a pretrial discovery process that allows the attorneys on both sides to learn more about what the courtroom testimony will be. It is given to a court reporter, and the respondent is under oath.

During the deposition, the LNC will present the facts of the case and be questioned by attorneys from both sides. This process may be quite lengthy and stressful. It is essential that the LNC be prepared, having reviewed the case and all related materials very thoroughly. Following this process, the LNC will be given a written transcript of the deposition; this needs to be carefully reviewed for accuracy. If the case goes to trial, the LNC will then testify in court (Meiner, 2005; Ruiz-Contreras, 2005).

In some cases, the forensic nurse will be called upon to testify in court, not as an expert witness as described above, but as a factual witness—one who has firsthand knowledge of the case in question. In these cases, the forensic nurse is present to provide factual statements about the evidence collected and what was observed (Ruiz-Contreras, 2005). Box 29-3 lists tips that will be helpful for nurses to review prior to testifying in court.

Clinical Forensic Nurse
Emergency and Critical Care
Registered nurses may be employed in EDs and critical care units as **clinical forensic nurses**. In this role they deliver care to both living and dead clients who are somehow involved with the legal system, and their services may include several subspecialties. The term **living forensics** refers to individuals who are subject to forensic investigations, including but not limited to survivors of rape, drug and alcohol addiction, domestic violence, nonfatal assaults, motor vehicle and pedestrian accidents, and police detainees (Lynch, 2006; Saunders, 2000).

The ED is frequently the initial location of the medicolegal investigation involving these individuals, both living and deceased (Fulton and Assid, 2006). It is imperative that ED registered nurses identify forensic cases and initiate the proper collection, preservation, and chain of command of evidence and provide accurate documentation for this unique population (Lynch, 1991). This collection of evidence plays an important role in the investigation of crimes and can have a major impact on legal decisions.

Organ Donation and Transplant Procurement
Another area of clinical forensic nurse in an ED or unit relates to **organ donation and transplant procurement.** This area of care is incredibly complex and requires detailed understanding of related legal and ethical issues. When a patient is declared brain dead, the family may be approached for organ donation, and a forensic nurse specializing in this area may be vitally important to successful outcome. A thorough death investigation of the decedent at the hospital facility is required, and reviewing medical records and documenting injuries are essential to identifying acceptable candidates and potential organs and tissues for harvest. The nurse involved in this process must be knowledgeable about legal specifications related to organ donation and have familiarity with the criteria for brain death. The nurse must also have excellent communication skills as well as the ability to relate compassionately to grieving families. In this capacity, the forensic nurse working harmoniously with organ procurement agencies can obtain release authorization of lifesaving organs (Shafer, 2006).

Care of Vulnerable Populations
The youngest and oldest populations are the most vulnerable to abuse. Nurses dedicating their practice to these vulnerable populations have an essential role of advocacy for individuals that cannot protect themselves.

Child Abuse and Neglect
Child abuse and neglect are major concerns for society; therefore the role of a **pediatric forensic nurse** is especially imperative. The Federal Child Abuse Prevention and Treatment Act defines child abuse as

> *Any recent act or failure to act on the part of a parent or caretaker which results in death, serious physical or emotional harm, sexual abuse or exploitation; or an act or failure to act which presents an imminent risk of serious harm (National Clearinghouse on Child Abuse and Neglect Information, 2005a).*

In 2003, approximately 906,000 children suffered some type of abuse or neglect, and 80% of the perpetrators were the parents (National Clearinghouse on Child Abuse and Neglect Information, 2005b). Reported cases of child abuse or neglect resulting in death in 2003 were estimated to be 1500 children.

States have varying definitions of what constitutes or determines child abuse and neglect. The following definitions are provided by the National Clearinghouse on Child Abuse and Neglect Information (2005b):

* *Neglect:* Deprivation of adequate food, clothing, shelter or medical care for no apparent financial reasons
* *Sexual abuse:* Range of activities ranging from non-contact indecent exposure to fondling and genital contact to actual adult-child sexual intercourse
* *Physical abuse:* Intentional physical injury including striking, kicking, burning, or biting
* *Emotional abuse:* Injury to the psychological capacity of the child as evidenced by a change in the child's behavior

For the well-being and safety of the child, a pediatric forensic nurse ensures that abuse and neglect are swiftly identified and reported to proper authorities (LaSala and Lynch, 2006). The nurse obtains a thorough history and assessment, focusing on several facets of abuse and neglect. These include child-parent interaction, the child's appearance and behavior, child-child interaction, and the environment.

A pediatric forensic nurse may be employed in a variety of clinical settings that see and treat children. These settings may include pediatric or general emergency departments, hospitals, physician offices, school nurses, home health and child advocacy agencies.

Elder Abuse
Geriatric forensic nurses play an important role similar to that of pediatric forensic nurses. **Elder abuse** is thought to be one of the most underdiagnosed and underreported crimes in the United States (Pearsall, 2005). Unfortunately, there is no exact accounting of elder abuse cases due to a lack of standardized reporting systems, no consistent definition of elder abuse, and lack of national data collection (National Center on Elder Abuse, 2005). The 1998 National Elder Abuse Incidence Study discovered that when the perpetrator was known, 90% were family members residing with the elder and two thirds were adult children or spouses performing the abuse (National Center on Elder Abuse, 1998). Therefore the elderly client may be hesitant to report abuse, ask for assistance, or acknowledge the maltreatment because the abuser might be the son, daughter, or close relative (Moynihan, 2006) or the disclosure would possibly result in litigation and institutionalization (Pearsall, 2005). Geriatric forensics nurses may be employed in any setting treating or seeing elder clients. Some settings include emergency departments, hospitals, physician offices, nursing homes, home health agencies and geriatric daycare centers.

There are several types of elder abuse: physical, psychological or emotional, financial, neglect, and sexual abuse (McGann and Moynihan, 2006; Pearsall, 2005). Physical abuse is the intentional harm or injury of another person (McGann and Moynihan, 2006) resulting in bruises, abrasions, lacerations, fractures, or all of these (Pearsall, 2005). Psychological or emotional abuse occurs when there is mental or emotional anguish (e.g., humiliating, intimidating or threatening directed toward the elder) (National Center on Elder Abuse, 2005); this can be difficult to identify in an acute care setting. According to McGann and Moynihan (2006), more than 12% of verifiable elder abuse cases are financial abuse. Financial abuse occurs when the elder person's financial resources are utilized for another person's benefit without the elder's consent.

Neglect is the most common form of elder abuse, whether it is caregiver neglect or self-neglect. Caregiver neglect occurs when the caregiver does not provide appropriate clothing, food, or health services or in the case of abandonment of the elder client. Self-neglect occurs when the elder discounts personal well-being—this could be the result of medical or mental illnesses. Lastly, sexual abuse is the nonconsensual intimate contact between two people (Pearsall, 2005). The elder population is at risk for sexual abuse due to inability to resist pursuits or inability to recognize the abuse because of mental illness.

Forensic Psychiatric Nurse

The **forensic psychiatric nurse** connects the gap between the criminal justice, legal, and mental health systems (Saunders, 2000). Forensic psychiatric nurses apply the nursing process to clients pending a criminal hearing or trial while maintaining a neutral, objective, and detached position (Coram, 2006). Forensic psychiatric nurses collect evidence by determining intent or diminished capacity in the client's thinking at the time of the incident. To do this, they often spend several hours interviewing and observing the client, carefully documenting conversations and observations.

Forensic psychiatric nurses may be called to court to testify as an expert witness in mental health issues; therefore it is imperative that the nurse have an exceptional understanding of mental illnesses and personality disorders. Roles filled by or activities provided by psychiatric forensic nurses include the following (Coram, 2006):

- Sanity or competency evaluation (for legal purposes)
- Assessment of violence potential
- Assessment of capacity to formulate intent
- Parole and probation considerations
- Assessment of racial or cultural factors in crime
- Assistance in jury selection
- Sexual predator screening
- Provision of expert witness testimony

CORRECTIONAL NURSING

Correctional nursing is a very specialized sub-set of forensic nursing. It requires a significant amount of discrete knowledge as well as an understanding and awareness of the unique needs and perspective of the clients served. Several issues specific to correctional nursing and related issues are described in this section.

Unlike any other care setting, clients are inmates, and care is negotiated and provided with recognition of safety and security issues for the nurse and the constitutional right of prisoners to receive adequate and timely health care. The primary goals in correctional facilities are security and a safe and humane environment for inmates. Health care, including nursing care, is a necessary and essential part of that environment.

Maintenance of a Safe Environment

Correctional facilities are, by nature, violent environments, and nurses practicing in correctional settings must continually negotiate security *and* nursing care. Nurses in this setting must be aware that even medical supplies issued to inmates can be a threat to the security environment. For example, a simple elastic bandage can be used to improve the grip on a homemade weapon. Virtually any prescribed medication can have value on the prison "black market." Further, nurses and the health care environment are subject to manipulation by inmates, who may seek medical and nursing care for reasons other than health. Nurses may simply be someone to talk to in an inherently isolating environment. Nursing decisions can become avenues to a changed work assignment, different living arrangements, or supplemental diets. Perhaps the greatest challenge for nurses is interacting with inmates without assuming the worst but always being aware that it can happen.

As the following clinical example illustrates, in correctional settings, the nurse must maintain an escape route should a situation of personal violence be imminent. In addition, no nursing care situation in a correctional environment requires a nurse to be locked in an enclosed environment with an inmate. Although it might appear that providing humane, therapeutic nursing care in an environment of potential violence is contradictory, it is ultimately a prerequisite for nursing practice in correction settings (Bell and Allen, 1998).

CLINICAL EXAMPLE: SAFETY IN CORRECTIONAL FACILITIES

In a county jail in Georgia in 1996, two nurses were attacked and beaten by an inmate being held on aggravated assault charges. The deputy on duty responsible for protecting them was also subdued by the inmate. These nurses were locked inside the jail with the inmate with their freedom, mobility, and flight to safety limited. The nurses sued the sheriff and deputy for failing to protect them in their work environment. The lawsuit was dismissed because the court determined that the nurses did not have a constitutional right to protection from harm in the work environment (Cohen, 1999c, p. 34). ■

Prison Culture

Understanding the **prison culture** is essential to nursing practice in correctional settings. Where people are incarcerated, often for significant periods of time, a distinct way of life evolves. Prison culture has its own rules, language, and traditions. Prison language is often a form of expression that is not understandable to the outside world. It is a mechanism of communication that has evolved from a unique set of circumstances, perhaps to have ownership over something in a place where ownership is often denied or simply insider communication in a world where extreme surveillance is the norm.

Prison gangs are often associated with and held liable for prison violence. For many inmates, prison gangs are a source

RESEARCH HIGHLIGHTS

Hearing-impaired Prisoners

Miller, Vernon, and Capella (2005) compared the incidence and types of violent offenses of a deaf prison population to a hearing prison population in the Texas correctional system. A total of 99 individuals with severe-to-profound hearing loss were included in the study population. Of those 99 offenders, 64.6% were convicted of violent offenses including robbery, homicide, assault, and sexual assault.

The study found that compared with hearing violent offenders, a lower percentage of deaf violent offenders committed robberies. The authors speculated that this might be due to the circumstances involved in a robbery, such as communication issues. The findings also revealed that deaf offenders had a higher percentage of sexual assault convictions compared to hearing offenders. The researchers thought that one reason for this might be due to the offender being sexually assaulted as a child.

The authors proposed increasing education for the deaf population and developing regional centers for deaf defendants charged with a crime. It is hoped that the regional centers will allow the deaf defendant time to understand the linguistics of the criminal system and will allow for due process.

Miller KR, Vernon M, Capella, ME: Violent offenders in a deaf prison population, *J Deaf Stud Deaf Educ* 10(4):417-424, 2005.

of protection, which is consistent with the notion that being alone and surviving in a correctional facility is difficult. In many cases, gangs engage in specific activities within prisons; some are involved in drug trade, extortion, and gang-related violence.

HEALTH ISSUES IN PRISON POPULATIONS

Today's prison inmate often enters prison with significant health care issues. Nurses employed in the correctional setting are likely to see health care problems that are similar to those in an acute care community outpatient clinic. The daily operation of a correctional clinic includes management of acute and chronic illness. Most health care clinics in correctional environments screen each inmate upon entry into the facility. The health care triage process generally includes a physical health history and a mental health history. Many significant health care issues are recognized during the screening process, often for the first time.

Chronic and Communicable Diseases

The most critical health care issues among the incarcerated population are chronic and communicable diseases. Of particular concern are HIV, hepatitis, and tuberculosis (TB). According to the Bureau of Justice Statistics, the rate of HIV infection is 1.9% among male inmates and 2.8% among female inmates in the United States (Maruschak, 2005). The most recent data indicate that close to 6,000 inmates in the United States have confirmed AIDS; this rate is 3 times higher than the general U.S. population. Despite the high rates of HIV infection, the number of AIDS-related deaths actually decreased 73% from 1995 to 2003; during these years a total of 282 prisoners died from AIDS-related causes. The high rate of HIV infection in this population is associated with high-risk

behaviors common among inmates, including current and previous drug use, unprotected sexual intercourse, and tattooing (Hellard and Aitken, 2004; Macalino et al., 2004).

Hepatitis B and hepatitis C have become increasingly serious health care issues in correctional facilities. Although data are incomplete, the rate of hepatitis B and C infection is higher among inmates than in the general population. Prison inmates represent the population at highest risk for hepatitis (e.g., the medically underserved, injection drug users, people with tattoos, and immigrants or refugees from areas with a high incidence of hepatitis B and C). Hepatitis C infection is further associated with HIV infection and injection drug use. The National Commission on Correctional Health Care (NCCHC) recommends that all inmates be screened and, if indicated, treated for hepatitis upon incarceration. Approximately 1209 out of 1584 state public and private adult correctional facilities report testing inmates for hepatitis C between July 1999 and June 2000 (Beck and Maruschak, 2004b). Out of the facilities testing for hepatitis C, about 31% of these tests were positive. The NCCHC also recommends that all staff members and inmates receive education related to modes of transmission, prevention, treatment, and disease progression (NCCHC, 1999).

Although rates of TB are considerably higher among black and Hispanic prisoners, the overall rate of TB is only marginally higher among incarcerated people than in the general population. The rate of infection in correctional facilities is related to overcrowding, poor ventilation, and rapid movement of inmates into and out of jail, all conducive to the spread of the disease (Baillargeon et al., 2004). In 1996, the Centers for Disease Control and Prevention released general recommendations for the prevention and control of TB in correctional facilities, including the following:

- TB screening for all staff members and inmates
- Containment by preventing transmission and providing adequate treatment to inmates with the disease
- Ongoing monitoring and evaluation of screening and containment efforts

As in the public domain, TB, especially in its antibiotic-resistant forms, will continue to be a major threat to the health of incarcerated people in the foreseeable future.

Women in Prison

Almost two thirds of women in prison have at least one child under the age of 18 years old (Mumola, 2000). More than 4 in every 10 women in prison admit to being abused before the current imprisonment: 34% physically abused and 34% sexually abused (Snell and Morton, 1994). Almost half of the women in prison report being under the influence of drugs or alcohol at the time of the offense and using drugs months prior to the offense. Given these statistics, the fact that women use correctional health care services at twice the frequency of men is not surprising.

Drug use and victimization, combined with the stress associated with being separated from their children, place incarcerated women at risk for many mental and physical health problems, including the risk of HIV infection and other sexually transmitted diseases (Snell and Morton, 1994).

ETHICAL Insights

Inmates' Refusal of Medications

An inmate's right to refuse treatment is a legal and ethical issue that nurses working in a correctional environment will sometimes experience. The right to refuse treatment and the state's power to enforce treatment are both highly charged legal and political issues and have gained attention in state and local courts. The issue of forced medication and competence to stand trial is of particular concern. The legal and ethical principles that guide forced treatment against the will of an inmate have historically been potential for violence toward self or others and the capacity to understand the consequence of refusing medical treatment. A recent court decision determined that a judicial hearing is now required to forcibly treat a non-dangerous incompetent offender to render competence to stand trial. The court decision was based on the following three-factor analysis (Cohen, 1999b, p. 17):

1. Individual's interests
2. State's interest
3. Value of the suggested treatment

Unlike nursing practice with the general population, prison inmates who refuse health care do not leave the facility and return home. Nurses practicing in correctional facilities continue to provide care and address the consequences of an inmate's refusal of treatment. For example, an inmate who refuses to adhere to treatment protocols for HIV infection may experience declining health status. Nurses are obliged to treat any resultant health issues. Individuals who are incarcerated by the state have a constitutional right to refuse and receive health care. Nurses practicing in correctional settings must respect the right to refuse care even if the result is an adverse outcome.

Unfortunately, health care providers in correctional facilities have limited experience and training to meet the unique health care needs of women in prison, and quality of care is adversely affected. For example, women who have been sexually assaulted are often reticent about obtaining regular gynecological examinations. Health care providers unaware of this phenomenon might simply label this behavior as noncompliance or resistance to care. The NCCHC confirms that routine gynecological examinations are not consistently a part of health screening for women upon entry into a correctional facility or a routine part of ongoing health care. Given the unique health care issues for women who are incarcerated, the NCCHC (1999) offers the following to guide the provision of health care:

- Correctional institutions' health care intake procedures should include comprehensive gynecological examinations.
- Comprehensive health care services should be available to incarcerated women that give special consideration to the reproductive health needs of women, high rate of victimization among incarcerated women, counseling related to parenting issues, and accessibility to drug or alcohol treatment.

The correctional institute nurse must be mindful of the need to view incarcerated women holistically, realizing that many factors, such as early childhood trauma, violent victimization, gender discrimination, drug use, and a context of economic impoverishment, have often contributed to their current situations.

Adolescents in Prison

Increasing numbers of adolescents are committing violent crimes, and many states have lowered the age limit allowing adolescents to be tried and sentenced as adults. Consequently, adolescents who have been convicted of violent crimes are often incarcerated in adult facilities. Incarcerating adolescents in an adult population presents barriers to meeting the distinct developmental needs of adolescents. These developmental changes include rapid physical and emotional growth and unique nutritional needs, all influenced by environment, genetics, and family experiences. Adult correctional facilities are not generally equipped to deal with the challenges of adolescent development. Adolescents in an adult correctional facility are more likely to be sexually assaulted, attacked by other inmates, or threaten suicide than are adolescents in a juvenile facility (National Coalition of State Juvenile Justice Advisory Groups, 1993). Juveniles in detention and correctional facilities are 4 times greater than youths in the general public to commit suicide, and 50% to 75% have diagnosed mental illness (Coalition for Juvenile Justice, 2000).

To ensure the safety of adolescents in an adult facility, the nurse must be aware of their individual vulnerability. A mechanism for adolescents to access medical and mental health care is essential. Services and interventions should be provided considering the developmental stage and experience of adolescence.

MENTAL HEALTH ISSUES IN CORRECTIONAL SETTINGS

On any given day, approximately one in every eight prisoners is receiving mental health therapy or counseling during the year 2000 (Beck and Maruschak, 2001a). Being in prison with a mental illness such as schizophrenia, bipolar affective disorder, major depressive disorder, or personality disorder makes adjustment to incarceration extremely difficult. The great number of inmates with a mental illness in today's prisons makes it difficult to meet the needs of this population, yet the U.S. Constitution provides prisoners with the right to mental health care.

In the late 1950s and early 1960s, deinstitutionalization moved people with mental illness out of state hospitals into communities that were often ill prepared to care for them. As a result, many people with a mental illness reside in nursing homes, residential homes, prisons, or jails. People with mental illness are often jailed for crimes committed in response to the symptoms of mental illness. With community services declining and increasing numbers of people with mental illness being incarcerated, the "criminalization of the mentally ill" has become a highly charged political topic (National Alliance for the Mentally Ill [NAMI], 1999).

According to NAMI, most jail inmates with symptoms of mental illness are charged with minor crimes. A far lesser number of inmates with severe mental illness commit more serious crimes, again frequently a consequence of either inadequate or no treatment. NAMI takes the position that many dangerous or violent acts by people with a severe mental illness are a result of inappropriate or inadequate treatment. The following strategies have been suggested to reduce the number of incarcerated people with severe mental illness:

- Diverting nonviolent offenders with severe mental illness away from incarceration to adequate treatment
- Convening mental health courts to address all cases involving offenders with severe mental illness
- Educating court judges and personnel about severe mental illness

The use of psychotropic medications in correctional facilities has an obscure history. Psychiatric medications were frequently used to sedate inmate behavior rather than treat the symptoms of mental illness. In the past, antipsychotic medications were used as a means of chemical restraint because they have sedating properties. This practice reached the Texas courts in a case challenging the conditions of medical care in prisons. The courts specifically addressed the issue of psychiatric medication when describing minimally acceptable medical care. The court decision read as follows:

Prescriptions and administration of behavior altering medications in dangerous amounts, by dangerous methods or without appropriate supervision and periodic evaluation, is an unacceptable method of treatment (cited in Cohen, 1999c, p. 58).

Mental illness became increasingly understood as a neurobiological illness; therefore those prescribing psychiatric medications have changed their objective from attempting to control behavior to targeting the symptoms of mental illness. Antipsychotic medications, along with psychosocial support, have become the standard of treatment for people diagnosed with schizophrenia or other mental illnesses that result in alterations in perception. Access to mental health treatment, including psychiatric medication, is a right for prison inmates. Correctional facilities must supply inmates with psychotropic medication after discharge for a time reasonable to seek community mental health treatment. Consequently, the state's responsibility for providing psychiatric medication extends beyond discharge from a correctional facility into the community (Cohen, 1999a, 1999c).

Nurses employed in correctional settings must always be aware of the vulnerabilities of people with mental illness who are incarcerated. Depression, schizophrenia, bipolar disorder, and other neurobiological disorders can be readily treated with new-generation psychiatric medications that radically reduce or ameliorate symptoms, but the unique vulnerabilities of incarceration often remain.

STANDARDS OF NURSING PRACTICE IN CORRECTIONAL SETTINGS

Several accrediting bodies have issued standards of nursing practice applicable to correctional settings. The ANA *Scope and Standards of Nursing Practice in Correctional Facilities* (ANA, 1995) generally addresses the use of the nursing process in the correctional setting. The American Correctional Association and National Commission have written additional guidelines for nursing practice in correctional health care. These guidelines articulate standards of practice for specific populations and health care issues, including communicable

TABLE 29-1 Basic Curricula for Forensic Nursing Programs

SUBJECT	TOPIC
Fundamentals for Forensic Nursing	Evidence collection
	Documentation
	Interviewing skills
	Basic criminal, procedural, and constitutional law
	Scope of practice
	Interdisciplinary collaboration
	Testifying in court as an expert witness
Forensic Law	Legal concepts (culpability, burden of proof, rationale for punishment, mitigating circumstance)
	Defense issues (justification, insanity, entrapment, duress)
Forensic Science	Collection and preservation of evidence
	Interpretation of DNA and laboratory reports
	Forensic chemistry and toxicology
	Cause of death
	Blood spatter interpretation
	Manner and mechanism of injury; wound identification and cause

Data from Burgess AW, Berger AD, Boersma RR: Forensic nursing: investigating the career potential in this emerging graduate specialty, *Am J Nurs* 104(3):58-64, 2004.

diseases, health care service delivery systems, and standards of practice for vulnerable populations such as women, adolescents, and people with mental illness.

EDUCATION AND FORENSIC NURSING

According to Burgess and colleagues (2004), because of the amount and depth of knowledge and skills needed by forensic nurses, whatever their subspecialty area, simply completing a continuing education course is not adequate for practice. As a result, colleges and universities have begun to offer a variety of programs to educate practitioners. This is the direct result of the identified need and growing knowledge base for practice of this specialty area. Table 29-1 gives an overview of basic curricula for forensic nursing programs. In addition, during the formal programs of study, the student usually completes a minimum specified number of supervised clinical hours; a clinical internship also may be required.

For those interested in seeking additional education in the growing and interesting specialty of forensic nursing, Box 29-4 lists nursing colleges and universities that have programs in forensic nursing. It should be noted that some of these programs offer a certificate in forensic nursing, whereas others provide a minor or concentration, and still others grant a graduate degree (typically a Master of Science in Nursing degree).

SUMMARY

Forensic nursing is an innovative, stimulating specialty that combines multiple aspects of client care with forensic science and the legal process. Most often, the forensic nurse will be

CASE STUDY | Application of the Nursing Process: Correctional Nursing

Mr. Smith is a 65-year-old African-American male serving a sentence of 30 years for aggravated assault of a minor. He has served 15 years and is ineligible for parole. Mr. Smith has a medical history of diabetes mellitus, hypertension, coronary artery disease, and peripheral vascular disease. Three weeks ago, his right foot was amputated due to gangrene. Mr. Smith has been admitted to the infirmary 6 times since the surgery, stating, "I'm not feeling well; can you double-check my sugar?"

The incision site is healing well and his diabetes mellitus is under control with medication. Mr. Smith takes his medications as prescribed, and his doctor believes he is doing well and continues with his current medication regimen.

Mr. Smith's daughter visits him only once every 6 months because she lives out of state. His son is also in prison but at another location. Mr. Smith's wife recently died from a motor vehicle accident, and he was unable to attend the funeral.

ASSESSMENT

Mr. Smith has a flat affect and does not make eye contact. He constantly looks at the ground and does not speak clearly when asked questions. Many times he is asked to repeat himself. According to medical records, he has lost approximately 18 pounds since surgery and he says, "I'm not hungry, that's why I don't eat." When asked about his sleeping habits, Mr. Smith states he sleeps all day except when the guards make him get up. He says he hasn't played cards with his buddies in more than a week. He also reports that he has been buying soma "from them" and hasn't taken a bath in 3 days.

DIAGNOSIS

Individual
- Hopelessness related to deteriorating physiological condition
- Ineffective coping related to situational crises
- Powerlessness related to illness-related regimen

Family
- Ineffective coping related to situational crises

Community
- Lack of mental health services

PLANNING

Mr. Smith will set goals with the health care provider and will ask for assistance with communication with his daughter and son.

Individual
Long-Term Goal
- Client will reestablish positive relationships with fellow inmates within 2 weeks.

Short-Term Goal
- Client will verbalize and recognize his feelings.
- Client will participate in diversion activities of his choice (e.g., playing cards).

Family
Long-Term Goal
- Family will demonstrate coping skills appropriate to the situation.

Short-Term Goal
- Family will verbalize and recognize feelings.

Community
Long-Term Goal
- Program will be available for all individuals.

Short-Term Goal
- Begin mental health programs for individuals in need, utilizing forensic nurses.

INTERVENTION

Individual
- Mr. Smith will be encouraged to express his feelings in an open and nonjudgmental environment, allowing for the development of a therapeutic relationship.
- The forensic nurse will schedule several visits to the clinic and encourage Mr. Smith to participate in activities, such as card playing, with his friends.
- Mr. Smith will be encouraged to discuss past achievements and conduct a life review with assistance from the nurse.

Family
- Mr. Smith's daughter will be included in the plan of care and encouraged to express her thoughts and feelings relating to her father's imprisonment.
- Mr. Smith's daughter also will be supported to convey her thoughts about her mother's death.

Community
- The forensic nurse will arrange several activities for inmates suffering from mental illnesses, including group activities and group talk.

EVALUATION

Individual
Mr. Smith slowly engaged the forensic nurse individually and in group therapy. Mr. Smith gained 5 pounds over 2 weeks and was able to make eye contact. Mr. Smith expressed his grief for the death of his wife. He gradually stopped buying soma and spent more time with his friends.

Continued

CASE STUDY   Application of the Nursing Process: Correctional Nursing (*cont'd*)

Family

Mr. Smith's daughter continued to visit only once every 6 months, but was able to fully explain her thoughts and feelings about her father's incarceration and her mother's death. The time the daughter spent with her father increased and was more meaningful.

Community

A forensic nurse was on constant duty to assist inmates with mental health illnesses.

LEVELS OF PREVENTION

Primary
- Encourage interaction with colleagues and family.
- Promote participation in prison activities.

Secondary
- Screen for depression.
- Provide outreach services to inmates with mental illness.

Tertiary
- Encourage therapy to reduce symptoms of mental illness.

CASE STUDY   Application of the Nursing Process: Forensic Nursing

Transcript of a 911 telephone call:
Emergency operator: "This is 911, what is your emergency?"
Caller: "My son isn't breathing, he's not moving, I need help!"
Emergency operator: "We will send an ambulance and police to assist you."
Caller: "Thank you, please hurry!"

Emergency medical personnel arrived at the house to discover James Oats, a 14-year-old Caucasian male, lying face up on his bed. The young man was unresponsive and not breathing. Emergency medical personnel immediately began lifesaving interventions, but despite all efforts, they were unsuccessful. James Oats was pronounced dead at his house.

Police officers arrived at the residence during the rescue attempt and secured the scene. They then notified homicide detectives and the medical examiner's office. Teresa Fernandez, a forensic nurse death investigator (FNDI) employed by the medical examiner's office, was dispatched to the residence to work in collaboration with the homicide detective, Pete Smith, to investigate the house and crime scene.

The police determined that there was no indication of foul play: The house was in order, there was no ransacking of the residence, no evidence of a robbery, and all the doors and windows were locked. The decedent's room was typical for a 14-year-old boy. There was a Play Station attached to the television, various clothes strewn about the room, and schoolbooks on the desk.

The decedent's mother, Jane Oats, informed the FNDI that James was in fine health. She explained that he had undergone a physical exam last week for athletics and that the findings were unremarkable. James had an older brother and younger sister, both in excellent health. James's father has hypertension and a history of heart disease, and diabetes and cancer were present in grandparents, but James was healthy.

Teresa (the FNDI) tried to comfort Mrs. Oats, who was extremely upset; she was crying and hyperventilating. Teresa turned to Mr. Oats, who was also present. In answer to Teresa's questioning, Mr. Oats reported that other parents and teachers had been concerned about rumors of increasing use of "bars" in area schools. Teresa was alarmed by this admission and questioned him further about what he meant; he confirmed that the school kids were reportedly using the antianxiety medication Xanax.

ASSESSMENT

Teresa performed an initial assessment of the decedent. James was wearing blue jeans, a yellow shirt, and socks. Her findings: "Livor mortis is consistent with body position and blanchable; rigor mortis is breakable in the jaw, arms, and legs. There are no visible signs of trauma."

The decedent was removed from the residence by technicians from the medical examiner's office, and an autopsy was performed the following day. The pathologist reported that the physical findings from the autopsy were unremarkable. During the autopsy, toxicology samples were collected from the heart, liver, and stomach.

Toxicology results were returned in 3 weeks and were positive for an extremely large amount of alprazolam (Xanax). The final, official cause of death for James Oats was alprazolam toxicity; the manner of death was ruled an accident.

Along with James's parents and Detective Smith, Teresa was informed of the cause and manner of death. Mr. and Mrs. Oats were devastated by the news and, upon questioning, stated that they did not understand how James had obtained the Xanax pills. They assured the detective and the FNDI that the only prescription medications in the residence were locked in the master bedroom cabinet and that James had no access to them.

Mr. Oats reported that Mrs. Oats has not been eating and has lost 25 pounds in 3 weeks. She has not been able to return to work, cries continuously, and does not care for their other children. Mr. Oats reports the entire family is withdrawn; the younger child is misbehaving in school and has received detention several times. Mr. Oats expressed exasperation with the need to provide all child care, perform routine chores, and go to work; he admitted that he doesn't know how much more he can handle.

Mr. Oats told the investigators that community and church members have been extremely helpful and sensitive to the family. The school officials and area churches agreed to support and offer programs to encourage children to say no to drugs; these programs would focus more attention on prescription medications. Further, the school James attended is doing an investigation into drug and alcohol abuse. The school social worker told Mr. Oats that a support group is being formed to assist students with James's death.

CASE STUDY — Application of the Nursing Process: Forensic Nursing (cont'd)

Detective Smith interviewed several of James's classmates and discovered that Xanax is used by many of them. From the information that he was able to gather from other students, it appeared that this was the first time James had tried the drug. Detective Smith discovered that some of the students were obtaining Xanax from their parents and selling it in the schools to their peers. Further, he learned that students are trying the "bars" because "it's cool."

DIAGNOSIS

Family

- Anxiety related to death of a child
- Grieving, dysfunctional, related to death of a child
- Coping: compromised related to situational crisis
- Caregiver role strain related to situational crisis

Community

- Coping: readiness for enhanced related to social worker availability

PLANNING

Family

The Oats family will initiate counseling to assist with acceptance of and coping with James's death.

Long-Term Goal

- Family will identify need for outside support and seek such support.

Short-Term Goals

- Family will verbalize and recognize feelings surrounding the death.
- Family will express feelings honestly.

Community

Long-Term Goal

- Members of the community will establish a plan to deal with problems and stressors, including premature deaths.

Short-Term Goal

- Members of the community, including school personnel and students, will identify positive and negative factors affecting management of current and future problems and stressors.

INTERVENTION

Family

Teresa Fernandez:

- Listened to the family's comments, remarks, and expression of concerns, noting nonverbal behaviors and responses
- Encouraged family members to verbalize feelings openly and clearly

- Referred family to appropriate resources for assistance as indicated (e.g., counseling, psychotherapy, spiritual guidance)

Community

With police, school personnel, and community leaders, Ms. Fernandez:

- Reviewed community plan for dealing with substance abuse problems among school children and assessed related stressors
- Determined community's strengths and weaknesses
- Identified available resources
- Established mechanism for self-monitoring of community needs and evaluation of efforts

EVALUATION

Family

- The Oats family began family counseling and slowly accepted James's death.
- James's siblings began educating fellow classmates about the ill effects of abusing prescription medications.

Community

- The community implemented quarterly meetings for grieving families including licensed counselors.
- The community members employed "just say no" rallies focusing on school-age children.

LEVELS OF PREVENTION

Primary

- Initiate drug and prescription medication teaching in middle and high schools, focusing on long-term associated problems and side effects.
- Support programs that encourage students to role play and practice "just say no" to drugs.

Secondary

- Organize group sessions in school to discuss illegal prescription medication abuse.
- Provide information to school personnel and parents on how to identify or screen for evidence of use of drugs and alcohol among school-age children.
- Provide information on area groups that provide support for students who want to avoid using drugs or want to stop using drugs.

Tertiary

- Reduce risk of additional students abusing prescription medication.

BOX 29-4 Schools Offering Programs in Forensic Nursing (Graduate and Certificate Programs)*

California
University of California at Riverside
Riverside, California

Colorado
University of Colorado at Colorado Springs
Beth-El College of Nursing
Colorado Springs, Colorado

Connecticut
Quinnipac University
Hamden, Connecticut

Maryland
Johns Hopkins University
Baltimore, Maryland

Massachusetts
Fitchburg State College
Fitchburg, Massachusetts

New Jersey
Monmouth University
West Long Branch, New Jersey

Seaton Hall University
South Orange, New Jersey

New York
Kaplan College
New York, New York—Online

Ohio
Xavier University
Cincinnati, Ohio

Pennsylvania
Duquesne University
Pittsburgh, Pennsylvania

University of Pennsylvania
Philadelphia, Pennsylvania

University of Pittsburgh
Pittsburgh, Pennsylvania

University of Scranton
Scranton, Pennsylvania

Tennessee
Vanderbilt University
Nashville, Tennessee

Washington
Gonzaga University
Spokane, Washington

*As of 2005.

employed in a clinic, ED, or correctional facility, or by a city or county coroner's office. Specialized skills (e.g., evidence collection, testifying in court) and knowledge (e.g., legal requirements for determination of brain death) are essential to the practice and require advanced education and training.

As mentioned previously, assessing for evidence of violence and intervening as needed are fundamental requirements of care that all health professionals must perform. Therefore every nurse has the potential to be a forensic nurse, regardless of the client population or setting of care. With the increase in violence in society, forensic nurses are faced with the challenge of advocating for victims of violence, living or deceased, and the need for practitioners in this specialty area is expected to grow.

LEARNING ACTIVITIES

1. Spend a few hours of clinical time working with a forensic nurse in an ED. Observe the nurse's interventions and processes related to evidence collection and preservation and collaboration with, for example, police officers and court officials. Take note of the techniques used for interviewing and counseling.

2. Attend a session of local or state mental health court (court proceedings to determine the status of an individual's mental status and disposition—e.g., confinement to a mental institution or release in the care of a ward of family member). Report on the experience to classmates.

3. Spend a clinical day in a jail or correctional facility working with a correctional forensic nurse. Pay particular attention to differences in care delivery related to legal and ethical issues unique to this subspecialty. Develop impressions into a paper.

REFERENCES

American Association of Colleges of Nursing: *Violence as a public health problem,* 1999, http://www.aacn.nche.edu/Publications/positions/violence.htm.

American Association of Legal Nurse Consultants: *Getting started in legal nurse consulting: an introduction to the specialty,* ed 2, Chicago, 1999, The Author.

American Nurses Association: *Scope and standards of nursing practice in correctional facilities,* Washington, DC, 1995, American Nurses Publishing.

American Nurses Association: *Scope and standards of forensic nursing practice,* Washington, DC, 1997, American Nurses Publishing.

Antognoli-Toland P: Comprehensive program for examination of sexual assault victims by nurses: a hospital-based project in Texas, *J Emerg Nurs* 11(3):132-135, 1985.

Baillargeon J et al: The infectious disease profile of Texas prison inmates, *Prev Med* 38:607-612, 2004.

Beck AJ, Maruschak LM: *Mental health treatment in state prisons, 2000,* Bureau of Justice Statistics Special Rep No NCJ 188215, July 2001a, http://www.ojp.gov/bjs/pub/pdf/mhtsp00.pdf.

Beck AJ, Maruschak LM: *Hepatitis testing and treatment in state prisons,* Bureau of Justice Statistics Special report No NCJ 199173C, April 2004b, http://www.ojp.usdoj.gov/bjs/pub/pdf/httsp.pdf.

Bell K, Allen W: Healthcare workers must be on constant guard, *St. Louis Post-Dispatch* Sept 27, 1998:A-12.

Burgess AW, Berger AD, Boersma RR: Forensic nursing: investigating the career potential in this emerging graduate specialty, *Am J Nurs* 104(3):58-64, 2004.

Centers of Disease Control and Prevention, MMWR recommendations and reports: *Prevention and control of tuberculosis in correctional facilities recommendations of the advisory council for the elimination of tuberculosis,* 1996, The Author, http://www.cdc.gov/mmwr/preview/mmwrhtml/00042214.htm.

Coalition for Juvenile Justice: *Mental health needs of youth and young offenders,* 2000, The Author, http://www.juvjustice.org/resources/fs002.html.

Cohen F: Deliberate indifference to detainee's serious medical needs shown, *Corrections Mental Health Rep* 1(4):65, 1999a.

Cohen F: Judicial hearing and strict scrutiny required to forcibly medicate incompetent detainees, *Corrections Mental Health Rep* 1(2):17, 1999b.

Cohen F: Prisons' duty to provide psychotropic medication includes post-release supply, *Corrections Mental Health Rep* 1(4):49, 1999c.

Collins SE, Halpern KJ: Forensic nursing: a collaborative practice paradigm, *J Nurs Law* 10(1):11-19, 2005.

Coram JW: Psychiatric forensic nursing. In Lynch V, editor: *Forensic nursing,* St. Louis, 2006, Mosby.

Fulton DR, Assid P: Evidence collection in the emergency department. In Lynch V, editor: *Forensic nursing,* St. Louis, 2006, Mosby.

Fulton M: Forensic nurses as coroners and death investigators, *Forensic Nurse* Jan/Feb:15-16, 2003.

Geissler-Murr A, Moorhouse MF: Legal nurse consulting. In Lynch V, editor: *Forensic nursing,* St. Louis, 2006, Mosby.

Girardin B: Is this forensic specialty for you? *RN* 64(12):37-41, 2001.

Haas RE, Bradshaw MJ: The expert witness: defending the profession or prosecuting your peers, *CRNA* 10(2):71-79, 1999.

Hanzlick R: Coroner training needs, a numeric and geographic analysis, *JAMA* 276(21):1775-1778, 1996.

Hanzlick R, Combs D: Medical examiner and coroner systems, history and trends, *JAMA* 279(11):870-874, 1998.

Hanzlick R, Hunsaker JC, Davis GJ: *A guide for manner of death classification,* 2002, National Association of Medical Examiners.

Hellard ME, Aitken CK: HIV in prison: what are the risks and what can be done? *Sexual Health* 1(2):107-113, 2004.

International Association of Forensic Nurses: *Sexual assault nurse examiner standards of practice,* Pitman, NJ, 1996, The Author.

International Association of Forensic Nurses: *Sexual assault nurse examiner education guidelines,* Pitman, NJ, 1998, The Author.

LaSala KB, Lynch VA: Child abuse and neglect. In Lynch V, editor: *Forensic nursing,* St. Louis, 2006, Mosby.

Ledray LE: Sexual assault. In Lynch V, editor: *Forensic nursing,* St. Louis, 2006, Mosby.

Ledray LE, Arndt S: Examining the sexual assault victim: a new model for nursing care, *J Psychosoc Nurs* 32(2):7-12, 1994.

Lynch V: Forensic nursing in the emergency department: a new role of the 1990s, *Crit Care Nurs Q* 14(3).69-86, 1991.

Lynch V: The forensic investigation of death. In Lynch V, editor: *Forensic nursing,* St. Louis, 2006, Mosby.

Macalino G et al: Prevalence and incidence of HIV, hepatitis B virus, and hepatitis C virus infections among males in Rhode Island prisons, *Am J Public Health* 94(7):1218-1223, 2004.

Maruschak LA: *HIV in prisons, 2003,* Bureau of Justice Statistics Rep No NCJ 210344, Sept 2005, http://www.ojp.gov/bjs/pub/pdf/hivp03.pdf.

McGann E, Moynihan BA: Elder abuse. In Lynch V, editor: *Forensic nursing,* St. Louis, 2006, Mosby.

Meiner, SE: The legal nurse consultant, *Geriatr Nurs* 26(1):34-36, 2005.

Miller KR, Vernon M, Capella, ME: Violent offenders in a deaf prison population, *J Deaf Stud Deaf Educ* 10(4):417-424, 2005.

Moynihan BA: Domestic violence. In Lynch V, editor: *Forensic nursing,* St. Louis, 2006, Mosby.

Mumola CJ:: *Incarcerated parents and their children,* Bureau of Justice Statistics Special Rep No NCJ 182335, Aug 2000, http://www.ojp.usdoj.gov/bjs/pub/pdf/iptc.pdf.

National Alliance for the Mentally Ill: *Position papers on criminalization of the mentally ill,* 1999, The Author, http://www.nami.org.

National Center on Elder Abuse: *National elder abuse incidence study (NEAIS): Final report, 1998,* The Author, http://www.aoa.gov/eldfam/elder_rights/elder_abuse/ABuseReport_Full.pdf.

National Center on Elder Abuse: *Elder abuse prevalence and incidence,* 2005, The Author, http://www.elderabusecenter.org/pdf/publication/FinalStatistics050331.pdf.

National Clearinghouse on Child Abuse and Neglect Information: *Child maltreatment 2003: Summary of key findings,* Washington, DC, 2005a, The Author, http://nccanch.acf.hhs.gov/pubs/factsheets/canstats.pdf.

National Clearinghouse on Child Abuse and Neglect Information: *Definitions of child abuse and neglect,* Washington, DC, 2005b, The Author, http://nccanch.acf.hhs.gov/general/legal/statutes/define.cfm#fn1.

National Coalition of State Juvenile Justice Advisory Groups: *Myths and realities: meeting the challenge of serious, violent and chronic juvenile offenders,* 1992 Annual report, Washington, DC, 1993, The Author.

National Commission on Correctional Health Care: *Standards for health services in corrections,* Chicago, 1999, The Author.

Pearsall C: Forensic biomarkers of elder abuse: What clinicians need to know, *J Foren Nurs* 1(4):182-186, 2005.

Potter PA, Perry, AG: *Fundamentals of nursing,* St. Louis, 2005, Mosby.

Prahlow JA, Lantz, PE: Medical examiner/death investigator training requirements in state and medical examiner systems, *J Forensic Sci* 40(1): 55-58, 1995.

Raymond L: Is a legal career for you? *RN,* 65(3):63-64, 2002.

Ruiz-Contreras A: The nurse as an expert witness, *Top Emerg Med* 27(1):27-35, 2005.

Safertein R: Evidence collection and preservation. In Lynch VA, editor: *Forensic nursing,* St Louis, Mosby, 2006.

Saunders L: Forensic nursing: formalizing a new role or recognizing existing practice? *Aust Nurs J* 8(3):49-50, 2000.

Sekula, LK: The advance practice forensic nurse in the emergency department, *Top Emerg Med* 27(1):5-14, 2005.

Shafer TJ: Organ donation. In Lynch V, editor: *Forensic nursing,* St. Louis, 2006, Mosby.

Snell TL, Morton D: *Women in prison: survey of state inmates, 1991,* Bureau of Justice Statistics Special Rep No NCJ 145321, March 1994, http://www.ojp.gov/bjs/pub/pdf/wopris.pdf.

US Department of Health and Human Services: *Healthy People 2010,* Washington, DC, 2000, US Government Printing Office.

US Department of Justice/Bureau of Justice Statistics (USDoJ/BJS): *Criminal victimization, 2003,* Bureau of Justice Statistics Rep No 205455, http://www.ojp.usdoj.gov/bjs/pub/pdf/cv03.pdf.

Venes D, editor: *Taber's cyclopedic medical dictionary,* ed 19, Philadelphia, FA Davis, 2001.

30

Parish Health

Beverly Cook Siegrist

MEDIA RESOURCES

Additional Material for Study, Review, and Further Exploration

evolve Website at http://evolve.elsevier.com/Nies

❖ Quiz ❖ Case Studies ❖ Content Updates ❖ Glossary ❖ WebLinks ❖ Resource Tool
30A Guidelines for Simple Prayer Services

OBJECTIVES

Upon completion of this chapter, the reader will be able to do the following:

1. Understand the potential role of faith communities in improving the health of Americans.
2. Describe the philosophy and historical basis of parish nursing.
3. Define the roles, functions, and education of the parish nurse.
4. Discuss faith communities as clients of the community health nurse.

5. Describe the role of the parish nurse in the spiritual health and wellness of faith communities.
6. Discuss contemporary issues in parish nursing, such as working with vulnerable populations and facing ethical and legal issues.
7. Apply the nursing process to a case study related to parish nurse practice.

KEY TERMS

CIRCLE Model of Spiritual Care
coordinator of volunteers
developer support groups

facilitator
faith community
Granger Westberg
health advocate

health educator
integrator of health and healing
personal health counselor

referral agent
spiritual distress
spirituality

CHAPTER OUTLINE

FAITH COMMUNITIES: ROLE IN HEALTH AND WELLNESS

FOUNDATIONS OF PARISH NURSING

ROLES OF THE PARISH NURSE

EDUCATION OF THE PARISH NURSE

THE PARISH NURSE AND SPIRITUALITY

ISSUES IN PARISH NURSE PRACTICE
Providing Care to Vulnerable Populations
End-of-Life Issues: Grief and Loss
Family Violence Prevention
Confidentiality
Accountability

Nurses seem to have one foot in the sciences and one in the humanities; one foot in the spiritual world and one in the physical one. . . . they [nurses] have insight into the human condition (Maginnis and Associates, 1993, p. 1).

The purpose of this chapter is to present an overview of parish nursing as a role for the community health nurse in faith communities. Based on centuries-old philosophies from churches and religious groups, nurses are applying the science of nursing and caring to address the biopsychosocial health needs of individuals and groups in church congregations and faith communities across the country. The following scenarios illustrate models of parish nursing found in the

United States and suggest the unique ways that parish nurses provide nursing care.

CLINICAL EXAMPLES

PARISH NURSING MODEL 1

Sandra Mills began her parish nurse practice as a volunteer when her parish priest recruited her to help establish a cancer support group and coordinate classes for caregivers. Within 6 months, her church's social concerns committee established a paid position on their ministry team and employed her as a full-time, paid staff member. After completing a parish nurse program through a local university, she began to develop a parish nurse program in her church. She describes her days as full and rewarding. Each day, she visits ill or homebound parish members and provides support through prayer, education, and listening. Each day, she is challenged to locate and refer community resources, provide health education to church groups (e.g., mother's day out and the over 55 group), and coordinate the efforts of other volunteer nurses in the church. She is practicing holistic nursing for the first time in her 15 years of practice. She found that the church, as a healing community, allows her to focus on the body-mind-spirit connection she believes is necessary to improve the health of congregation members. ∎

PARISH NURSING MODEL 2

Marilyn Michaels is a former home care and hospice nurse who works as a parish nurse coordinator for St. Luke's Hospital, which is a 400-bed medical center serving a midwestern rural population. Her position was created to assist community churches in developing and maintaining parish nurse programs. She coordinates educational programs, including a 30-hour preparation program for beginning parish nurses, an advanced program for parish nurse coordinators in individual churches, and monthly educational topics offered through a parish nurse support group. Marilyn developed the support group and facilitates communication among the 200 parish nurses and 100 church communities that St. Luke's Hospital serves by editing St. Luke's bimonthly newsletter. She also assists parish nurse programs by connecting them with other services that the hospital and community agencies provide (e.g., screening, support groups, and speakers). The program at St. Luke's Hospital is self-supporting from grants and educational programs. ∎

PARISH NURSING MODEL 3

Sue James is a member of a parish nursing group from five inner-city churches in south-central Indiana. This group of nurses came together from five different church denominations to meet their congregation members' health needs. The nurses are unpaid parish nurses within their own congregations. They came together to share their resources because their churches are small in membership and they identified similar and unmet health needs in each of the churches. Primarily, the group serves an aging population that represents the few remaining individuals and families living in the inner-city area. Sue agreed to serve as the group coordinator, a position that has been shared among their group. In this position, she plans biweekly meetings for the nurses at alternating churches and serves as a community liaison for participating churches. The group's parish nurse effort began 2 years earlier, supported by a local hospital grant and matched with small donations from the participating churches. Each nurse volunteers at least 10 hours each week. Based on the health and wellness assessment completed in each church, they arranged a health fair that included health screening and referral information at one church and began educational classes on topics related to depression and healthy aging. They focus on health promotion, and their individual churches recognize them as the parish nurse, the congregational nurse, and the health minister. ∎

The three clinical examples illustrate how parish nursing is evolving in the United States. More than 3000 nurses provide nursing care to children, adults, and the elderly in churches, synagogues, and mosques. Parish nurse programs are also established in other countries such as Canada, Korea, and Australia (Berry, 2000; Granberg-Michaelson, 1997; McDermott, Solari-Twadell, and Matthews, 1998). The growing number of RNs in parish nursing documents this practice as a significant role for the community health nurse. Community health nursing has evolved from early church efforts to provide care for the sick and disenfranchised (O'Brien, 2003; Nies and McEwen, 2001). Modern parish nursing focuses on the global health and wellness issues of all people and has it roots in more recent efforts to encourage the reemergence and blending of health care roles into the healing ministry of churches (Joel, 1998; McDermott and Burke, 1993; Patterson, 2004; Solari-Twadell and McDermott, 1999).

FAITH COMMUNITIES: ROLE IN HEALTH AND WELLNESS

Former President Jimmy Carter, faculty and founding member of Strong Partners Interfaith Health Program at Emory University in Atlanta, Georgia, understands the importance of faith communities for Americans. President Carter is quoted on the Interfaith Health Program website (http://www.ihpnet.org),

> What if churches, mosques, and temples worked together to improve the health of their communities? If faith groups adopted one small area and made sure that every single child were immunized . . . that every person had a basic medical exam . . . that every woman who became pregnant would get prenatal care? Are these possible? We believe the answer is yes (Interfaith Health Program, 2005).

Throughout history, church communities have provided care for the indigent and disenfranchised, meeting basic human needs of food and clothing and basic health care. The majority of the world's populations belong to organized faith communities. Nearly one third of the people in the world identify themselves as Christians, followed by Muslims (1.2 to 1.3 billion), Hindus (800-900 million) and Buddhists (350-400 million) (International Parish Nurse Resource Center [IPNRC], 2004a). All of these religions have traditions and rituals related to health and healing, including specific prayers and practices. Some of the religions give specific guidelines for ministering to the ill, homebound, or dying members. All of the major religions describe the relationship between health, healing, and wholeness. The Old Testament discusses *Shalom*, or God's desire for health and wholeness for the earth and its people. The New Testament documents the healing activities

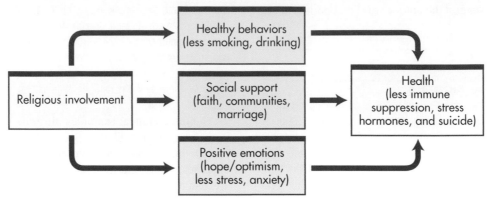

FIGURE 30-1 Possible explanations for the positive correlation between religious involvement and health and longevity. (From Myers DG: *Stress and health in psychology,* ed 7, New York, 2004, Worth Publishers.)

of Jesus, restoring health to people. The Talmud describes the importance of maintaining physical health and vigor so that Jewish people will understand God's will in their lives. Followers of Buddhism believe that healing and recovery are promoted by awakening to the teachings of Buddha (IPNRC, 2004).

The National Health Interview Survey, completed in 1999 and financed by the Centers for Disease Control and Prevention, attempted to identify predictors of health in religiously active people. They found that people who attended religious services weekly or more often had a life expectancy nearly 5 years greater than those people who never attended an organized religious meeting (Hunter et al., 1999). One reason for this variance may be that the people who reported the highest level of religious involvement also reported practicing healthier lifestyles, including exercising more and smoking less (Tsuang, Williams, and Lyons, 2002; Myers, 2004). Faith communities also fulfill the need for social support meeting another basic human need of belonging (Koenig and George, 2002). Loneliness is documented as a contributor to depression and isolation in the elderly. Myers (2004) and George (2004) suggest that faith communities contribute to the well-being of its members through support, prayer, and providing a sense of hope. The importance of stress management in health promotion and disease management is well documented. The interaction and possible explanation for the positive correlation between religious involvement and health is visualized in Figure 30-1.

Organized religions are attempting to meet the needs of members in many nontraditional ways including exploring Internet Church services, developing support groups, and including modern music and drama in traditional worship services to improve intergenerational communication. Parish nurses, because of their educational preparation and goals, are ideal health professionals to ensure that the health information provided in congregations is accurate and accessible. Parish nurses also understand the importance of **spirituality** in health and healing. The role of the parish nurse therefore complements the ministry of health found in faith communities.

FOUNDATIONS OF PARISH NURSING

Reverend **Granger Westberg,** a Lutheran minister, is considered the founder of the modern parish nurse movement. Westberg, educated as a chaplain and minister, worked with nurses in hospitals, medical schools, and church communities. Impressed with the nurse's perspective of health and wholeness in viewing the physical, emotional, and spiritual challenges of human illness, he described parish nursing as the culmination of his lifelong work in relating theology and health care. In 1984, he first proposed a parish nurse program to Lutheran General Hospital (LGH) in Chicago, Illinois. Westberg envisioned a partnership between the hospital and all church congregations in the hospital's community. He proposed that participating churches would make contributions to fund a nurse's salary and identified seven roles the nurse could use to provide services to faith communities (O'Brien, 2003; Patterson, 2004; Smith, 2003; Solari-Twadell and McDermott, 1999).

In 1985, six parish nurses were hired in the Chicago area. Initially, LGH and the participating churches' contributions primarily funded the nurses' salaries. The churches assumed increasing responsibility for the nurses' salaries over a 4-year period. Westberg supported the development of a parish nurse training program and required the nurses to participate in a weekly educational session. Teaching chaplains, nurse educators, and physicians led the sessions, which were aimed at enhancing nurses' skills in counseling, education, spiritual assessment, and related nursing interventions. The meetings evolved into an ongoing support group for the nurses as they developed the parish nurse programs and identified self-care needs. LGH continued to provide parish nurse leadership through the IPNRC. Located in Park Ridge, Illinois, the center offered education, development guidance, and contact with parish nurses nationally and internationally. In 2001, ownership of the IPNRC moved from the Lutheran-rooted Advocate Health Care System to the Deaconess Foundation of St. Louis, Missouri. The Deaconess ministries in the United States has its roots in the Deaconess service movement founded in Germany

RESEARCH **HIGHLIGHTS**

Parish Nurse Practice With Client Aggregates

Parish nursing practice is a recent innovative model of health care that aims to address the needs of the changing health care system, consistent with the shift from a cure orientation to that of a continuum of care. This purpose of this study was to describe parish nurses' practice with client aggregates to determine if existing classification systems could be used with aggregates or groups and to determine if these systems could be used to describe and document parish nurse practice. The two classification systems selected were the North American Nursing Diagnosis Association (NANDA) and the Nursing Interventions Classifications (NIC).

Nineteen parish nurses practicing in 22 faith communities (seven denominations represented) in a regional network made up the sample. Both qualitative and quantitative methods were used in this study. The data collection instrument was based on elements of the Nursing Minimum Data Set. Ten nurses from the original group of 19 volunteered to participate in a focus group.

During a 5-month study period, the parish nurses provided services to 51 client aggregates (as well as 700 individual clients). Of the group encounters, 56% focused on prevention, 10% on illness management, and 26% on "other." Prevention programs included support or counseling groups, teen pregnancy, safety, smoking cessation, sexually transmitted diseases (STD), HIV, and breast self-examination classes. Illness programming included arthritis and asthma management. Some examples of "other" were healing prayer service, children's worship service, health fair, and Bible reflection study. Members of aggregates receiving parish nurse services crossed the life span, from children through elders.

The most frequent NANDA diagnoses were health-seeking behaviors (28.7%), readiness for enhanced spiritual well-being (14.9%), and knowledge deficit (11.5%). The most frequent NIC intervention was active listening, followed by health screening and support system enhancement. A total of 12 NIC interventions were identified. Several interventions not part of NIC were also listed, such as health fair, bulletin board display, healing prayer service, and facilitating transportation.

This research identified that parish nursing practice with aggregates focused on health promotion and illness prevention as well as the psychosocial-spiritual dimension of care. Diagnostic labels and interventions usually could be selected from the existing framework provided by NANDA and NIC for aggregate health care. The parish nurse has the potential to become an important link in the health care shift to community-based care and an important partner in the seamless continuum of health care. Classification systems that can be used across the health care continuum will provide not only vital communication but also a vehicle for promoting evidence-based practice among parish nurses.

From Weis DM et al: Parish nurse practice with client aggregates, *J Community Health Nurs* 19(2):105-113, 2002.

in the mid 1800s Deaconess has been involved in parish nursing since the late 1980s and has established the Deaconess Parish Nurse Ministry as a leader in the specialty in the United States. The Deaconess Parish Nurse Ministries currently employs more than 25 parish nurses and serves more than 28 community churches. The Deaconess Parish Nurse Ministries is the current parent organization of the IPNRC (2004b).

Solari-Twadell and McDermott (1999) and Westberg (1999) described the philosophical basis of parish nursing as encompassing the following five key elements:

1. The spiritual dimension is central to the practice.
2. The role balances nursing science and technology with service and spiritual care.
3. The nurse's clients are members of the **faith community** defined by the church and its public service philosophy.
4. Parish nursing services are built upon principles of self-care and capacity building, with a focus on understanding the connection between health and the individual's relationship with God, faith traditions, nursing, and the broader society.
5. The parish nurse understands that holistic health is a dynamic process that requires connections among the person's spiritual, psychological, physical, and social dimensions.

These beliefs direct the parish nurse in planning nursing care and defining health not only as wellness but also as wholeness of body and spirit. They also emphasize spiritual health as a motivating factor in seeking wellness care, participating in education, and enhancing self-care capabilities (Berquist and King, 1994; Patterson, 2004; Smith, 2003).

A review of the historical foundations of community health nursing practice describes the significance of the church in early health care). In the Bible, the book of Romans (16:1-2) describes the early works of Phoebe, who is considered to be the first visiting nurse. In his 1786 sermon "On Visiting the Sick," John Wesley, the founder of the Methodist church, directed his believers to visit the sick to convey God's grace to others (Wesley, 1986). These selected examples illustrate the significance of the church as an influence on health and healing. The histories of all religions provide similar examples. The reemergence of these basic beliefs in health, healing, and spirituality are moving the church toward assisting members in wholeness; this is evidenced by the growing number of health ministries and parish nurse programs found in churches throughout the nation (Patterson, 2004; Smith, 2002). The defining characteristics and roles of the parish nurse in any church setting come from these philosophical foundations.

The title "parish nurse" has been maintained to honor the founder, Dr. Westberg. In faith communities across the United States, other titles can be found, including "church nurse," "congregational nurse," and "faith community nurse." The ANA is currently revising the parish nurse standards and has recommended the revised standards be titled "Nursing in Faith Communities."

The current mission statement for parish nurses was developed and approved in 2000 by more than 600 attendees at the 14th annual Westberg Symposium.

Parish nursing is the intentional integration of the practice of faith with the practice of nursing so that people can achieve wholeness in, with, and through communities of faith in which the parish nurse serves. Parish nurses educate, advocate, and activate people to take positive action regarding wellness, prevention, appropriate treatment of illness, and social and spiritual connections with God, members of their congregations, and their wider community (Patterson, 2004, p. 32).

| HEALTHY PEOPLE **2010** | Parish Nursing |

Objective 7: Educational and Community Based Programs

Goal: Increase the quality, availability, and effectiveness of education and community-based programs designed to prevent disease and improve health and quality of life.

Parish nurse practice may vary depending upon the needs of the faith community served. Programs and services may contribute to many *Healthy People 2010* goals. Objective 7—Educational and Community Based Programs—directs public health agencies to form partnerships with many community-based organizations, including faith communities, to improve the quality and effectiveness of health education programs.

From US Department of Health and Human Services: *Healthy People 2010,* Washington, DC, 2000, US Government Printing Office, http://www.healthypeople.gov/healthfinder.

ROLES OF THE PARISH NURSE

The parish nurse's practice focuses on health promotion and wellness. It is based on a holistic nursing practice that holds the spiritual dimension central to health and healing. In the nursing process, the parish nurse does not perform "hands-on nursing care," but improves the health of a faith community by implementing the seven interrelated roles of health educator, personal health counselor, referral agent, health advocate, coordinator of volunteers, developer of support groups and integrator of health and healing (Berry, 2000; IPNRC, 2004; Keller, 1994; McDermott and Burke, 1993; Solari-Twadell and McDermott, 1999).

As a **health educator,** the parish nurse provides or coordinates educational offerings for people of all ages and developmental stages. The educational efforts may target lifestyles, values, and wellness and incorporate the spiritual aspects of individual and community well-being. The educator role includes educating the church leaders and members about the roles and purposes of a parish nurse. Educational efforts are planned based on the church community's priorities and *Healthy People 2010* (US Department of Health and Human Services, 2000). Because the faith community membership includes people across the life span, church-based educational programs can address all 10 major health indicators (IPNRC, 2004). Early in the development of a parish nurse program, and periodically thereafter, the parish nurse should assess the health status and needs of the congregation members to determine educational priorities. Figure 30-2 presents an example of an adult congregational health and wellness survey. The parish nurse should complete an assessment on each population group served by the congregation and include children grouped by developmental stages. Examples of educational efforts are teaching CPR (cardiopulmonary resuscitation) to new mothers; teaching signs and symptoms of hypertension and stroke to adults in the congregation; educating lay church ministers in the signs and symptoms of acute illness when visiting homebound individuals; and teaching basic health and safety to school-age children.

In the role of **personal health counselor,** the parish nurse discusses health problems with individuals and families within the church community. The nurse may focus on self-care issues such as explaining a prescribed medical regimen; assessing the need for further resources and referrals; or making visits to homes, nursing homes, or hospitals.

The parish nurse is a **referral agent** and must be aware of community resources and be able to guide individuals as they access available resources. In this role, the nurse may function as a liaison and, with the client's approval, provide referrals to resources or health care providers. The parish nurse recognizes the difficulties encountered by vulnerable populations within the faith community and helps them maneuver the health care maze to access needed resources. These vulnerable populations may include non–English-speaking individuals, those who speak English as second language (ESL), individuals living in poverty, individuals without health care insurance, and individuals living with complicated chronic or catastrophic illness.

In the role of **health advocate,** the parish nurse "facilitates clients efforts in obtaining needed health services and appropriate care management plan, promotes community awareness of significant health problems, lobbies for beneficial public policy, and stimulates supportive action for health" (Clemon-Stone, McGuire, and Eigsti, 2002, p. 45). Advocacy can present challenges for the parish nurse. The nurse must always remember that the client (individual, family, or group) has the right to self-determination. The parish nurse's role may be that of educating clients to make the best choices or empowering them to speak for themselves. The nurse also must understand the policies and beliefs of the congregation related to specific health issues. Church doctrine may guide members to adopt values and beliefs that are in conflict with current health care recommendations. Individuals may request that the parish nurse provide education and support in making decisions related to issues of infertility, stem cell technology, birth control, and sex education for teens and youth. Although assuming the role of advocate implies a commitment to change, the parish nurse must understand that the politics of working within the faith system requires acceptance of individual and system values and beliefs.

The role of **coordinator of volunteers** includes recruiting, training, and directing volunteers to work with the parish nurse program or health ministry. The nurse may work with other nurses and lay people within the congregation. The parish nurse program may encompass all programs related to the health of the church community. For example, the parish needs assessment may identify the need for development of a transportation committee or respite program. These services affect the ability of church members to access health and related services; these programs may be delegated to the

Wellness Ministry Survey

Thank you for taking the time to complete this Wellness Survey. The results will be used to plan programs and activities that will meet the health care interests and needs of everyone in the congregation. Think of this as your survey to indicate the type of services you would like available to you, your family, and your brothers and sisters in Christ. Please do not sign your name. All information will be confidential.

Please complete the following:

My age is _____.

I am _____ female _____ male.

I am _____ White _____ Black _____ Hispanic _____ Asian.

I am _____ single _____ married _____ divorced _____ widowed.

I am _____ employed _____ unemployed _____ retired _____ homemaker _____ student.

I have health insurance. _____ yes _____ no

I have a family doctor. _____ yes _____ no

I think my health is _____ good _____ fair _____ poor.

Please place an "X" by those activities that you would benefit from now or might use in the future:

___ Visits to those individuals who are homebound

___ Visits to those who are experiencing loss

___ Visits to parishioners in hospitals or nursing homes

___ A nurse to assist parishioners in obtaining personal health counseling

___ Health education pamphlets or brochures

___ Classes held at church on health-related topics

___ Information on classes held elsewhere in our community

___ Health screening at our church

___ Flu shots or immunizations at our church

___ Volunteer training for parishioners to assist parishioners (e.g., respite and homebound visits)

___ Support groups at our church

___ Support groups elsewhere

___ Prayer and healing service

___ Other (please list):

Please place an "X" by those health topics listed below that you want to know more about

Heart Sense
___ Heart disease
___ Stroke
___ High blood pressure
___ Diet and cholesterol

Healthy Living
___ Nutrition and weight control
___ Exercise
___ Quitting smoking
___ Alcohol and drug issues

Emotional Health
___ Depression
___ Other mental illness
___ Reducing stress
___ Eating disorders
___ Self-esteem
___ Anger management

Women's Health
___ Breast cancer
___ Menopause
___ Estrogen replacement
___ Osteoporosis

An Ounce of Prevention
___ Cancer prevention
___ Protecting your back
___ Talking to your doctor
___ Understanding your medications
___ Safety at home and away
___ Understanding insurance

Healthy Families
___ Sexuality
___ Marriage
___ Pregnancy and childbirth
___ Parents through life stages
___ Teen issues
___ Single parenting

Chronic Concerns
___ Arthritis
___ Diabetes
___ Prostate trouble
___ HIV/AIDS
___ Pain management
___ Urinary incontinence
___ Life with a disability

As We Age
___ Our physical changes
___ Care of aging parents
___ Living well alone
___ Alzheimers
___ Loneliness
___ Getting "our affairs in order"

As Life Ends
___ Grief issues
___ Living wills and power of attorney
___ Hospice care
___ Organ donation

Other topics? _____

Put an "X" by days and times you would participate in an activity or class

Day of week	Mornings	Afternoon	Evenings
Monday	_____	_____	_____
Tuesday	_____	_____	_____
Wednesday	_____	_____	_____
Thursday	_____	_____	_____
Friday	_____	_____	_____
Saturday	_____	_____	_____
Sunday	_____	_____	_____

FIGURE 30-2 Parish health assessment form. (Courtesy Holy Spirit Catholic Church, Bowling Green, Kentucky.)

parish nurse. As a coordinator of volunteers, the nurse would plan, implement, and direct these programs. Many parish nurses work through existing health ministry frameworks within their churches, such as health or social welfare committees. The membership of these committees may be interdisciplinary or representative of the entire church congregation. The parish nurse may be delegated the responsibility of developing specific health-related programs and activities. In the **facilitator** role, the nurse would also connect the church with existing resources and programs to meet identified health and educational needs. For example, the nurse might facilitate available health screenings, flu shots, or immunizations through the local public health department. In the parish nurse role, the nurse would not directly provide or duplicate the available community services but would work with other agencies in providing care to the church community.

The role of **developer of support groups** requires skills in accessing, and the parish nurse uses community assessment and program evaluation skills. The parish nurse may practice within a community rich in resources and support groups or in a community with few health-related resources. Support groups are people who meet for support and sharing of issues related to common problems. Examples of support groups are bereavement groups or new mother groups. Support groups are different from self-help groups, which focus on personal growth (e.g., Alcoholics Anonymous). Some individuals prefer support groups be physically located within their faith community where they have existing support systems and can network with individuals who share common values and beliefs. The parish nurse must evaluate the need for a support or self-help group within the faith community. Situations that might indicate the need for support groups include the increased incidence of a sudden and shared experience by members, for example, five or more members dying of cancer in a short time frame; several incidences of suicide; or eating disorders within a teen group. A needs assessment of the faith community also might indicate the need for development of a support group. There are many models that the parish nurse may use as guidance in the development of groups. For example, I Can Cope is a program developed by the American Cancer Society that provides a series of educational programs related to cancer. This program can be adapted to meet the needs of individual groups (http://www.cancer.org). If acceptable to the client, an individual referral may be made to existing community groups. It is also important to remember that groups usually have an anticipated "life expectancy." After the needs of the groups are met through education or support, there may no longer be a need for a particular support group. The parish nurse should document the history of the group and move forward toward new goals.

As an **integrator of health and healing,** the parish nurse acknowledges and integrates spirituality as the basis of his or her nursing practice. For example, in teaching a class on healthy aging, the nurse will discuss lifestyle, compliance to prescribed medical treatment, attitudes, and values and their connections to well-being. In a home visit to a terminally ill person, the nurse will explore the meaning of healing versus cure and provide emotional support and encouragement. In certain churches or parishes, the nurse may lead, or contribute to, healing services as a member of the health ministry team. A basis for successful integration of health and healing in parish nurse practice is an understanding of spirituality as a foundation for parish nurse practice. The importance of spirituality to parish nurse practice and health is discussed later in this chapter.

These examples illustrate the diversity and autonomy found in parish nursing. Depending on the needs of the church community and its members, the roles may be implemented in a variety of ways and through various organizational structures. Some organizational models use volunteer and paid nurses in the role of parish nurse. Hospitals provide parish nurses to community churches through grants, contracts, and public service. Many faith communities have incorporated positions for part-time and full-time parish nurses within their ministerial teams. Job descriptions and programs vary; examples can be found online at websites for individual parish nurse programs or at the IPNRC website (http://www.ipnrc.parishnurses.org).

EDUCATION OF THE PARISH NURSE

A baccalaureate-prepared registered nurse with several years of experience in clinical practice is best prepared to implement the roles of the parish nurse; however, many schools of nursing provide parish nurse training in baccalaureate prelicensure, RN (registered nurse) to BSN (Bachelor of Science in Nursing), and MSN (Master of Science in Nursing) programs. The self-direction and independent decision making required by the autonomous roles of the parish nurse require a nurse experienced in clinical nursing and community-based nursing practice. The educational preparation of the baccalaureate nurse in community health nursing provides the theoretical basis needed to plan and implement programs for diverse populations in a congregational setting and to function as a beginning member of a pastoral team (IPNRC, 2004). All parish nurses should complete a formal program of study (IPNRC, 2004b, 1980; Smith, 2003; Solari-Twadell and McDermott, 1999; Westberg and McNamara, 1990). Universities, hospitals, or parish nurse programs now offer hundreds of parish nurse programs that nurses may take for college credit, continuing education, or postgraduate certification. Courses are offered online, in seminars, and in regular classrooms. More than 40 international educational partners offer parish nurse courses. A list of these educational providers can be found on the IPNRC website (http://www.ipnrc.parishnurses.org).

Many universities are incorporating existing certificate programs into advanced nursing degree programs. Programs are generally offered at beginning, intermediate, and advanced levels and consist of approximately 30 contact hours of planned classroom instruction, self-study, or clinical experiences at each level. Box 30-1 provides an example of the curriculum content for a beginning parish nurse program as suggested by the IPNRC. Intermediate parish nurse programs focus on the development of skills for parish nurse coordinators and include human resource development, grant writing, and developing budgets. A third level of education is available for nurse educators who plan to teach parish nursing or develop curricula for parish nurse programs.

As parish nurse programs grow in number and services provided to faith communities, continuing education programs will increase in availability and in diversity of content. The IPNRC conference held annually at the Westberg Symposium in St. Louis, Missouri, provides the greatest opportunity for education and networking among parish nurses in the world.

Implementation of the parish nurse's roles requires the use of the nursing process to plan nursing interventions in wellness and physical, emotional, and spiritual health (Bergquist and King, 1994). Other chapters in this text provide useful information concerning health promotion and planning activities to promote physical and mental health. Spirituality, as a major focus of nursing care, presents different challenges for the parish nurse.

THE PARISH NURSE AND SPIRITUALITY

Westberg (1988) described the ideal parish nurse as one who is spiritually mature and able to apply spiritual aspects to the health care of congregation members. Many parish nurses find the need for further education to develop spiritual assessment skills, acquire theological knowledge, and learn the nurse's role in healing.

Wright (2005) defines spirituality as "the human desire for a sense of meaning, purpose, connection, and fulfillment through intimate relationships and life experiences" (p. xviii). In nursing, **spiritual distress** is more often the focus of care. The North American Nursing Diagnosis Association

(1992) defines spiritual distress as "a disruption in the life principle that pervades a person's entire being and that integrates and transcends one's biological and psychosocial nature" (p. 46). Parish nurses provide nursing interventions related to the nursing diagnosis as connected to spiritual distress (e.g., loneliness, isolation, and hopelessness). Spirituality is the basis of nursing care in the church setting.

Schnorr (1988, 2003) suggests the **CIRCLE Model of Spiritual Care**. This model illustrates the following concepts of care that guide nursing practice and interventions:

C aring
I ntuition
R espect for religious beliefs and practices
C aution
L istening
E motional support

Caring includes caring practices and attitudes. Nurse theorist Jean Watson described caring as "professional, ethical, scientific, esthetic, personalized giving-receiving behaviors that allow for contact between the nurse and client" (quoted in Dossey, 1999, p. 45). Intuition requires acting on instinct, hunches, or "gut feelings." Benner (1984) described intuitive abilities as responses that expert nurses have after several years of experience; these abilities enable the nurse to "read between the lines." Schnorr (1988) described respect as understanding the importance of religious beliefs and practices. The nurse allows time for prayer and sacrament and supports and encourages religious activities. Caution in spiritual care advises the parish nurse to avoid proselytizing or "preaching" religion to clients. The ANA's (2003) Code for Nurses also provides the nurse with direction to avoid judgments and respect the client's right to self-determination. Listening is a skill that is highly developed in most experienced nurses. It allows an understanding of spoken and unspoken words and feelings, encourages open communication, and supports and empowers patients to communicate needs and desires. Emotional support is the link between the physical and spiritual. Among the emotional interventions, Schnorr (1988) includes working with feelings, showing love, and using appropriate touch and empathy.

Prayer is a commonly used spiritual intervention and can provide comfort and support. Many nurses are not comfortable with sharing individual or group prayer (see **Resource Tool 30A** on the book's website at http://evolve.elsevier.com/Nies/ for guidelines to assist nurses in the development of group prayer sessions). Clients may ask parish nurses to offer prayer for healing or recovery. Many faith traditions, such as catholic or Jewish, have traditional prayers which the parish nurse can read or memorize. A guideline to follow is to keep the prayer simple and offer the request to the client's higher power. The nurse may have a poem for healing that is meaningful, which may be also be used. The use of silence may also be used after a simple prayer or the nurse may request for the client to offer their own prayer. Carson and Koenig (2002) and Berquist and King (1994) suggest that through prayer, spiritual assessment, and hope and faith, the parish nurse facilitates important client outcomes for spiritual health and well-being, including self-esteem, self-actualization, hope, trust, and peace.

CLINICAL EXAMPLE

During a meeting of the health ministry committee, the parish nurse learned that Mrs. James, a church member, was diagnosed with end-stage breast cancer. Mrs. James is a 45-year-old wife and mother of two school-age children. She returned home following surgery and had to decide whether to seek further treatment within the following weeks. Her husband attended church with his family although he was a member of another faith community. A home health nurse was involved with Mrs. James's postoperative care, and it was possible that a referral to hospice would occur following her decisions regarding further treatment. The parish nurse called Mrs. James and offered to make a home visit to assess how the parish nurse and church community could support and care for the family's well-being. Mrs. James welcomed the visit. Showing respect for their faith beliefs, the nurse offered prayer and waited for a request from the couple. The nurse's instincts and experience working with cancer patients and families guided her in using listening as a nursing intervention during this initial visit and in using caution when Mrs. James asked for guidance in making treatment decisions. The nurse further explored the home situation, the needed educational support, and the physician's prognosis and treatment options with the patient. Emotional support was important for Mrs. James, and the parish nurse offered support through touch and words of concern. This model helped develop an initial nurse-client relationship of trust and open communication. ■

ISSUES IN PARISH NURSE PRACTICE

The practice of parish nursing is affected by many issues common to community health practice as well as issues specific to parish nursing. Selected issues, which are discussed in this section, include working with vulnerable populations and the legal and ethical issues of confidentiality and accountability. Other issues identified as important by the IPNRC are end-of-life and family violence issues; these are required content in parish nursing courses.

Providing Care to Vulnerable Populations

The philosophical foundations of faith communities related to caring, outreach, and support of vulnerable populations place the parish nurse in a position to positively influence the health of diverse groups. Historically, churches have been among the first groups to sponsor and support refugees, develop programs for homeless individuals and families, provide assistance and resources to low-income families, and provide resources to entire communities during disasters (e.g., floods and tornadoes). Parish nurses are able to provide care for diverse populations using skills in assessment, planning, and interventions.

Boss (1994, 1996, 1999) suggests that parish nurses can be instrumental in helping diverse populations access services; however, nurses should not attempt to meet the populations' many needs alone. She reminds the nurse that in using available health resources, "more is not necessarily better." The

A Hispanic church located in a rural community. Established churches may provide resources for Hispanic populations to form their own churches. The parish nurse may serve an outreach church in addition to the parent church.

nurse in the educator role can assess the needs of vulnerable populations and teach the faith community about the people and their spiritual, emotional, and physical needs. A community of caring that can collectively meet the many needs of vulnerable populations will emerge from the congregation. Boss (1999) called this the Nehemiah approach, which means that people collectively share their talents and desire to do the work. The parish nurse works as a member of a caring church community to meet the health and related needs of vulnerable populations.

End-of-Life Issues: Grief and Loss

Faith communities have long been the first line provider of support related to loss, grief, and dying. Timms (2003) suggests that changes in the U.S. health care system (a movement away from hospitals and toward ambulatory and community-based services) have resulted in an increased need for nurses to be knowledgeable in end-of-life issues. The aging population, increased prevalence in chronic diseases such as HIV and cancer, and public awareness have contributed to the need for improved end-of-life care. Parish nurses may become partners with hospice and home care nurses in providing palliative care to congregation members. The IPNRC suggests that parish nurses need a theoretical base that includes an understanding of grief and loss from a developmental and social perspective, knowledge of manifestations of normal and complicated grief, and nursing interventions to facilitate healthy grieving.

Parish nurse activities related to end-of-life care may include educational sessions on drawing up living wills, establishing health care surrogates, and understanding hospice and palliative care; providing home visits to dying congregational members and emotional support to family and survivors; and developing grief support groups.

Family Violence Prevention

Education and prevention of family violence directly relate to *Healthy People 2010* objectives, and parish nurses must be informed in this area (IPNRC, 2004, Smith, 2003). The parish nurse must have an understanding of risk factors for family, child, and elder abuse; knowledge of the cycle of abuse; and assessment skills to identify individuals and families at risk for violence. Family violence affects all racial, ethnic, religious, and socioeconomic classes in the United States.

In intimate partner violence (IPV) (also known as domestic abuse, spouse abuse, domestic violence, courtship violence, battering, marital rape, or date rape), it is important to understand that the main issue is an imbalance of power. There are no standard reporting laws (across the United States) related to IPV; however, it is essential that the parish nurse recognize signs and symptoms of IPV and have an intervention plan that includes providing support, establishing a trusting relationship, discussing safety issues, making appropriate referrals for shelter and counseling, and documenting the abuse according to policy (IPNRC, 2004; Saltzman et al, 2002).

Child abuse and neglect are reportable in all 50 states.
All 50 States, the District of Columbia, and the U.S. territories have enacted statutes specifying procedures that a mandatory reporter must follow when making a report of child abuse and neglect. Mandatory reporters are individuals who are required by law to report cases of suspected child abuse or neglect. In most States, the statutes require mandatory reporters to make a report immediately upon gaining their knowledge or suspicion of abusive or neglectful situations. In all jurisdictions, the initial report may be made orally to either the child protection services agency or to a law enforcement agency (National Clearinghouse on Child Abuse and Neglect Information, 2005).

Nursing interventions for suspected or actual child abuse include the following:
1. Report to the appropriate authority.
2. Provide resources and referrals.
3. Establish a trusting relationship with the child or adolescent.
4. Provide presence.
5. Listen.
6. Document according to policy, law, or both.

The U.S. Senate Special Committee on Aging estimates that as many as 5 million elders are victims of abuse each year (National Center on Elder Abuse, 2004). Elder abuse includes not only physical abuse but also psychological neglect, with or without verbal threats; violation of personal choice or rights; financial theft or misuse of the elder's money; and failing to provide basic needs (food, shelter, clothing, and medical care). The parish nurse or another church volunteer may be the first individual to identify signs and symptoms of elder abuse. The parish nurse's role may also include educating church volunteers on identifying abuse and making reports and referrals. The nurse must have skill in recognizing symptoms of abuse and must possess assessment or screening questions to identify specific problems. Specific nursing interventions include the following:

> ### ETHICAL Insights
>
> ### Principles of Applied Ethics in a Faith Community
>
> Applied ethics refers to the utilization of ethical principles in real-life situations. The values and beliefs of faith communities raise additional ethical considerations for the parish nurse. Actions of the parish nurse may result in a conflict between established nursing interventions and beliefs of the faith community. The IPNRC (2004a) identifies these potential areas of ethical conflict:
>
> ➤ Infertility treatment
> ➤ Organ donations
> ➤ Blood transfusions
> ➤ Proper dress or behavior
> ➤ Withdrawal of and withholding nutrition
> ➤ DNR (Do Not Resuscitate) orders
> ➤ Pro-Life versus Pro-Choice
> ➤ Use of advanced directives
> ➤ Distribution of scarce resources
> ➤ Competency for decision making
> ➤ Clergy sexual conduct (p. 319)
>
> The parish nurse's roles include understanding the scope of practice for parish nurses related to ethical practice and the values and beliefs of the community served. The nurse must understand his or her own beliefs and values that are in conflict with the faith community's beliefs. It is necessary that the parish nurse know when to seek help, when to refer, and when to remove himself or herself from the ethical decision-making process (O'Brien, 2003).

1. Recognizing that all states have laws against elder abuse but that reporting varies from state to state so must know state laws
2. Establishing a trusting relationship with the elder and a presence (being with the elder as needed)
3. Providing appropriate referral and resources
4. Documenting the abuse, according to policy, law, or both

Confidentiality

The *Code for Nurses* (ANA, 2003) and the *Scope and Standards of Parish Nursing Practice* (Health Ministries Association and ANA, 1998) provide ethical guidance to parish nurses. Parish nurses are accountable to state boards of nursing, employing agencies (i.e., including churches), and the faith communities they serve. Many ethical and legal issues are generic to clinical practice settings; however, confidentiality issues have the potential to be problematic in a church community.

Concerned church members may identify individuals in need and refer them to the parish nurse. In the role of health minister, the parish nurse may receive private and sensitive information. The nurse does not act in the role of minister or priest. Congregation members should not relate information in the form of confession or repentance; however, the connection with the church ministry team may put the nurse in a position to hear this type of sensitive information.

The nurse should protect the client's right to confidentiality in relation to information concerning their health or health-

Text continued p. 668

CASE STUDY   Application of the Nursing Process

Nancy Elliot, a parish nurse at Living Hope Baptist Church, recently completed a needs assessment of her faith community of 200 families. Nancy is new to the parish nurse role, having recently been hired as parish nurse. Living Hope, considered to be a moderate-size church, is located in a rural community of 40,000. Nancy decided to complete the needs assessment of the congregation and community prior to planning programs and services for the faith community.

ASSESSMENT

The community has one hospital and a variety of voluntary and official community agencies. Many private practitioners are available, either in the town or within a 1-hour drive of a larger city. Recently the city was awarded a grant to develop community parks and recreational facilities. Nancy is surprised by the demographic picture she finds following completion of the assessment. Young families with toddlers to young school-age children comprise more than 70% of the congregation. She notes that these families are in the childbearing developmental stage of family growth and development. The remaining 30% of the members are elders with more than half being 80 years of age or older. The survey indicates that the members are most interested in health screening and educational opportunities presented at the church. Only 3% of the members reported having no health insurance.

A discussion with the minister provides additional information. Two new industries have recently relocated to the area. The parent home of both of these industries was formerly located in distant states. Many new members have relocated to the area. Nancy understands that these young families may have decreased family and social support and little knowledge of existing community resources. The minister also identifies that the current church ministries focus on the elderly members and that new services are needed. Nancy schedules a meeting with the young parents following a church social gathering. Fifty mothers and fathers attend the session to discuss the health-related needs of the families. They identify that a "mothers-day-out" program is a priority and also request information on community resources, parenting classes, and health and wellness programs for the children and parents. Based upon the needs assessment and sessions with the parents, the parish nurse identifies the following goals, nursing diagnoses, and population-focused nursing interventions.

DIAGNOSIS

Individual

- Health-seeking behaviors, as evidenced by requests for health information related to parenting, health, and wellness
- Risk for altered parenting, as evidenced by developmental stage of families, requests for education, and presence of new community members with limited knowledge of community resources
- Risk for social isolation and role strain, as evidenced by individual concerns related to limited social support and lack of social networks

Family

- Altered growth and development, related to stage of family development
- Risk for ineffective family coping, related to recent relocation to new community and lack of social network

Community (Faith Community)

- Ineffective community coping, related to recent change in membership demographics, lack of developed resources, and new or developing parish nurse role

PLANNING

A plan of care is developed to address the needs of the individuals, families, and the Living Hope faith community. Goals suggested by the parish nurse are mutually agreed upon by the ministerial team and congregational members.

Individual

Long-Term Goals

- Monthly educational programs will be offered addressing current issues in parenting and health and wellness of young families.
- Congregation will establish a social network for young parents.
- Ministerial leaders will dedicate funds to increase resources for children and young adults.

Short-Term Goals

- Establish parent steering committee for educational program ideas, identification of parent talents (assist with education programs).
- Explore development of parents-day-out program.

Family

Long-Term Goals

- Parent members will report increased social networks.
- Parent members will identify adequate resources to support growing family.

Short-Term Goal

- Identify community and congregation support for new and growing families.

Community (Faith Community)

Long-Term Goal

- Programs will be established to support growing families

Short-Term Goal

- Implement one new program (educational, social) or resource for families each quarter of the church year.

INTERVENTIONS

Nancy utilizes all seven roles of the parish nurse to meet the goals established for families of Living Hope.

Individual

Nancy asked the parents (men and women) to complete a talent survey to identify the resources available within the families of Living Hope. From this survey Nancy identified two registered nurses willing to help provide educational programs and three previously certified early childhood teachers. The teachers were willing to develop a committee to explore the development of a "mothers-day-out" program, a playgroup, and a new parent support group. Additional members were willing to begin a ministry to provide meals to new parents. Community resources were identified at the local health department to help teach parenting classes and provide immunizations. A plan was established to begin the mothers-day-out program part time within 2 months. The playgroup and educational programs were implemented immediately.

Family

The ministerial team and a parent advisory group were formed to identify family needs. Family social events were planned, including a church picnic. Planning was made for age-appropriate activities such as the development of a soccer team for the youth, a softball team for the young adults, and a literary club for those interested. The advisory committee developed a budget to submit to the ministerial team requesting financial support to develop a playground for the children attending the "mothers-day-out" program and the hiring of a part-time employee to supervise the related activities. The families reported increased feelings of support from the faith community, increased social support and networks, and a feeling of belonging to the greater community.

Community (Faith Community)

The faith community developed a budget to support individual and family requests. Monthly health education programs became the standard, with topics noted on the monthly calendar. Members reported increased feelings of "community" not only among the young families but also across generational lines, as new members increasingly participated in leadership roles within the congregation. The minister has documented an increase in weekly attendance, which had a positive impact on the long-range goals identified by the congregational members.

EVALUATION

Individual and Family

Attendance at the health and wellness and parenting sessions increased with each educational session offered. Initial attendance was 5 to 7 people for each session, and after 6 months, the average attendance was 15 to 20 people for each session. The request from attendees changed from offering additional educational sessions to planning intervention programs such as a yoga class and a weight reduction program. The playground was completed in less than the planned time due to the increased budget. The "mothers-day-out" program, which began as a part-time, 3-day per week program, grew to a Monday-through-Friday program within 12 months. The program became self-sufficient by the end of the year due to established fees, parent volunteers, and donations. Men and women verbalized an increased satisfaction with their spiritual growth and support from the faith community. Nancy developed a health ministry committee of volunteers from within the church and was able to increase the number and variety of related parish nurse activities.

Community (Faith Community)

The health and wellness activities attracted the attention of sister churches, and a grant was offered to increase the number of family support services and wellness programs

Continued

CASE STUDY Application of the Nursing Process (cont'd)

offered within the church. Health and wellness programs were expanded to include additional methods for reaching congregational members, such as through a website. The increased attendance and participation of congregational members positively affected all members, who benefited from the leadership and positive environment. The educational offerings and intervention programs were developed based upon *Healthy People 2010* goals, in particular increasing activity and exercise, healthy eating and obesity prevention (U.S. Department of Health and Human Services, 2000).

LEVELS OF PREVENTION

The roles of the parish nurse direct the interventions and programs planned for faith communities. The following are examples of all three levels of prevention applied to this case study.

Primary

- Assessment and teaching about parenting, health, and wellness.
- Development of programs and social support systems to prevent social isolation and increase resources for successful parenting and healthy behaviors.

Secondary

- Parish nurse assessment and screening to identify individuals and families at risk.
- Congregational resources and educational programs developed to meet individual and family needs.

Tertiary

- Parish nurse provides, or refers to, resources for rehabilitation, for families coping with children with disabilities or chronic health problems (parents and children).

---

related condition. Although the nurse must share information with the church minister in certain instances, the nurse should share confidential information with other church ministry leaders (or prayer groups) only when given permission by the client. Exceptions are found in religious sects or congregations that require the public confession of members' behaviors or conditions so that members may benefit from divine intervention and forgiveness. As a care provider, the parish nurse should be aware of these rituals and practices before counseling members of the faith community (Fowler, 1999). General guidelines for medical record management should be followed by the parish nurse. Policies and procedures for managing and storing records and sharing and requesting medical information must be established. Parish nurse programs within faith communities generally are not required to follow Health Insurance Portability and Accountability Act (HIPAA) guidelines related to medical records and confidentiality because churches are not in the category of identified health care providers. An exception is parish nurse services provided by a licensed health care provider such as a hospital; in this instance, HIPAA regulations do apply (IPNRC, 2004).

Accountability

Sister Mary Angela Shaughnessy (1998) provides direction for the parish nurse by listing the following information related to church law:

1. Volunteers in a church are held to the same degree of accountability as are paid employees.
2. The doctrine of separation of church and state does not exempt churches from discrimination laws.
3. Ministers, both ordained and nonordained, may be required to disclose confidential information in court.

As volunteers or paid employees, nurses are accountable to the nursing standards and civil laws designed to protect individuals from abuse, neglect, and discrimination. Parish nurses, as nonordained ministers, do not have client-professional privileges and should be aware of appropriate standards in documenting provided services. In documenting parish nurse services, "less is better." Many churches may not have the facilities to store medical records in a secure locked area. In this instance the nurse should have a file storage system that locks and can be kept in a secure location. Simple records of blood pressure screenings, or health education programs could include only numbers of attendees or blood pressure results categorized by American Heart Association Standards as hypertensive, borderline, or normal. Also included in the documentation could be numbers of individuals referred for services. Faith community governing boards or committees need not have the names of individual clients but will be interested in the type of services and numbers of clients served. Individual client services will require a nurses note or assessment and development of a nursing care plan. Prior to beginning a parish nurse program, the nurse should develop and follow general policies and guidelines for record keeping and storage. Shaughnessy (1998) provides further information related to contract law. The handbooks, brochures, or programs that church-related institutions offer are contracts. The parish nurse should ensure that health information is current and based on accepted practices and standards. These suggestions are not intended to limit the parish nurse's creativity or scope; rather, they emphasize that the professional nurse is accountable for his or her practice in any role.

SUMMARY

This chapter provided an overview of the parish nurse's role in providing nursing care for faith communities, and it explored the historical and philosophical foundations of the modern parish nurse practice. Traditional nurse roles of the nurse are used in unique ways to allow the parish nurse to provide nursing care to church communities in the seven roles of the parish nurse: health educator, personal health counselor, referral agent, health advocate, coordinator of volunteers, developer of support groups, and integrater of health and healing. The parish nurse's role in the development of spiritual health and well-being becomes significant and requires the nurse to focus on the spiritual needs of congregation members. The CIRCLE model for planning spiritual nursing may be used to guide nursing interventions. Parish nursing offers new opportunities for increasing the health and wellness of clients and requires the nurse to refocus skills and knowledge.

Many educational programs are available throughout the United States to provide parish nurse education and certification through three levels of education: beginning, intermediate, and advanced parish nurse practice. These programs are offered as continuing education and through formal university courses as part of degree programs. Church law, nursing ethics, and standards are the basis for the legal and ethical parish nursing practice. As a relatively new area of community health nurse practice, parish nursing offers the RN many opportunities to improve the health of faith communities through a holistic nursing practice that connects the body, mind, and spirit in the celebration of health and healing.

LEARNING ACTIVITIES

1. Speak with a parish nurse in the community. Ask the nurse about congregational health needs and discuss how the roles of the parish nurse are implemented through the parish nurse programs and ministry. Observe the nurse in his or her daily activities and identify how spirituality is a basis for parish nursing care.

2. Speak with a minister or priest in the community from a faith belief system different from your own. Explore the philosophical basis for the church's role in health and healing.

3. Visit websites devoted to parish nursing and identify the models of parish nursing programs or read parish nurses' descriptions of their practice. Share these with the clinical group.

REFERENCES

American Nurses Association: *Code for nurses with interpretative statements*, Washington, DC, 2003, The Author.

Benner P: *From novice to expert*, Menlo Park, Calif, 1984, Addison-Wesley.

Berry RA: Community health nurse as parish nurse and block nurse. In Stanhope M, Lancaster J, editors: *Community and public health nursing*, ed 5, St. Louis, 2000, Mosby.

Boss J: Being a professional caregiver can be dangerous to your health, *Health Dev* 4:10-14, 1994.

Boss J: Lesson learned over time: great teachers—St Francis, St. Clare, and Eleanor, *Health Dev* 2:7-19, 1996.

Boss J: Parish nursing with underorganized, underserved, and marginalized clients. In Solari-Twadell PA, McDermott MA, editors: *Parish nursing: promoting whole persons health within faith communities*, Thousand Oaks, Calif, 1999, Sage.

Clemon-Stone S, McGuire S, Eigsti D: *Comprehensive community health nursing*, ed 6, St. Louis, 2002, Mosby.

Deaconess Parish Nurse Ministries: *What is parish nursing?* St. Louis, 2005, The Author, http://www.parishnurses.org/whatis.phtml.

Dossey MD: Dynamics of healing and the transpersonal self. In Dossey MD et al, editors: *Holistic nursing: a handbook for practice*, Gaithersburg, Md, 1999, Aspen.

Granberg-Michaelson K: Staying healthy: the spiritual dimension, *Contact* 155:3, 1997.

Health Ministries Association and American Nurses Association: *Scope and standards of parish nursing practice*, Washington, DC, 1998, American Nurses Association.

Hunter RA et al: Religious involvement and adult mortality, *Demography*, 36:273-285, 1999.

Interfaith Health Program: *Strong Partners: Interfaith Health Program*, Atlanta, Ga, 2005, Emory University, http://www.ihpnet.org.

International Parish Nurse Resource Center: *Basic parish nurse preparation curriculum*, St. Louis, 2004a, Deaconess Parish Nurse Ministries.

International Parish Nurse Resource Center: *Role of parish nurse, mission and resources*, Ridge Park, Ill, 2004b, The Author.

Joel AJ: Parish nursing: as old as faith communities, *Am J Nurs* 98:7, 1998.

Keller B: Parish nursing: a holistic approach, *Ky Med News* May-June 1994.

Koenig HG, George L: Religion, spirituality, and health in hospitalized older patients, *J Am Geriatr Soc* 52A:532-541, 2004.

Koenig HG et al: Does religious attendance prolong survival? A six-year followup study of 3,968 older adults, *J Gerontol Med Sci* 54A:370-377, 1999.

Maginnis and Associates: *Combining health care and theology: the parish nurse*, Maginnis Communique, Louisville, Ky, Sept 1993, The Author.

McDermott MA, Burke J: When the population is a congregation: the emerging role of the parish nurse, *J Community Health Nurs* 10: 179-190, 1993.

McDermott MA, Solari-Twadell PA, Matthews R: Promoting quality education for the parish nurse and parish nurse coordinator, *Nurs Health Care Perspect* 19:4, 1998.

Myers DG: On assessing prayer, faith and health, *Reform Rev* 53(2):119-126, 2000.

Myers DG: Stress and health: spirituality and faith communities. In Myers DG, editor: *Stress and health, psychology*, ed 7, New York, 2004, Worth Publishers.

National Center on Elder Abuse 2003, http://www.elderabusecenter.org/pdf/basics/fact2.pdf.

National Clearinghouse on Child Abuse and Neglect Information http://childwelfare.gov/systemwide/laws_politics/statutes/nnpproc.pdf.

Nies MA, McEwen M: *Community health nursing: promoting the health of populations*, Philadelphia, 2002, WB Saunders.

North American Nursing Diagnosis Association: *NANDA nursing diagnosis: definitions and defining characteristics*, ed 3, Philadelphia, 2001, The Author.

O'Brien ME: *Parish nursing: healthcare ministry within the church*, Sudbury, Mass, 2003, Jones and Bartlett.

Patterson D: *Parish nursing: a beneficial partner for clergy*, The Clergy Journal, Sept 2004, 32-33.

Saltzman LE et al: Intimate partner violence surveillance: uniform definitions and recommended data elements, Atlanta, 2002, Centers for Disease Control and Prevention, NCIPC.

Schnorr MA: Parish nurse pedagogy or nandragogy, *Proceedings of the 17th Annual Westberg Parish Nurse Symposium*, St. Louis, 2003, IPNSC.

Schnorr MA: Spiritual nursing care: theory and curriculum development, Doctoral dissertation, Northern Illinois University, *Dissert Abstr Int* 50:601-A, DA8912525, 1988.

Shaughnessy MA: *Ministry and the law: what you need to know*, New York, 1998, Paulist Press.

Smith SD: *Parish nursing: a handbook for the new millennium*, New York, 2003, Haworth Pastoral Press.

Solari-Twadell PA, McDermott MA: *Parish nursing: promoting whole person health within faith communities*, Thousand Oaks, Calif, 1999, Sage.

Timms J: A role for the nurse in end-of-life care. In Smith SD: *Parish nursing: a handbook for the new millennium*, New York, 2003, The Haworth Pastoral Press.

Tsuang MT, Williams WM, Lyons MJ: Pilot Study of Spiritual and Mental Health in Twins, *Am J Psychiatry* 159:486-488, 2002.

US Department of Health and Human Services: *Healthy People 2010*, Washington, DC, 2000, US Government Printing Office, http://www.healthypeople.gov.

Weis DM et al: Parish nurse practice with client aggregates, *J Community Health Nurs* 19(2):105-113, 2002.

Wesley J: On visiting the sick, 1786. In Outler AC, editor: *The works of John Wesley*, Nashville, 1986, Abingdon.

Westberg G: Parishes, nurses, and health care, *Lutheran Partners* Nov-Dec 1988, 34-36.

Westberg G: A personal historical perspective of whole person health and the congregation. In Sloari-Twadell PA, McDermott MA, editors: *Parish nursing: promoting health within faith communities*, Thousand Oaks, Calif, 1999, Sage.

Westberg G: Parishes, nurses, and health care, *Lutheran Partners*, Nov-Dec, 1988, pp. 34-36.

Westberg G, McNamara JW: *The parish nurse: providing a minister of health for your congregation*, 1990, Minneapolis, Minn, Augsburg Fortress.

Wright LM: *Spirituality, suffering and illness*, Philadelphia, 2005, FA Davis.

Home Health and Hospice

Carrie L. Motyka ▪ Mary A. Nies

MEDIA RESOURCES

Additional Material for Study, Review, and Further Exploration

evolve Website at http://evolve.elsevier.com/Nies

❖ Quiz ❖ Case Studies ❖ Content Updates ❖ Glossary ❖ WebLinks ❖ Resource Tools
31A Outcome Assessment and Information Set (OASIS B-1), **31B** Case Study—Public Health Visit:
Communicable Disease Follow-up, **31C** Case Study—Public Health Visit: Antepartum Client

OBJECTIVES

Upon completion of this chapter, the reader will be able to do the following:
1. Discuss the purpose of home health services.
2. Define home health care.
3. Differentiate between the purpose of a public health nursing visit and that of a home health and hospice nursing visit.
4. Use the nursing process in outlining the steps involved in conducting a home visit.
5. Identify the types of home health agencies.
6. Apply the nursing process to a home health client situation.

KEY TERMS

advance directive
durable power of attorney

home health care
living will

CHAPTER OUTLINE

HOME HEALTH CARE
    Purpose of Home Health Services

TYPES OF HOME HEALTH AGENCIES
    Official Agencies
    Nonprofit Agencies
    Proprietary Agencies
    Chains
    Hospital-Based Agencies

CERTIFIED AND NONCERTIFIED AGENCIES

SPECIAL HOME HEALTH PROGRAMS

REIMBURSEMENT FOR HOME CARE

OUTCOME AND ASSESSMENT INFORMATION SET (OASIS)

NURSING STANDARDS AND EDUCATIONAL PREPARATION OF HOME HEALTH NURSES

CONDUCTING A HOME VISIT
    Visit Preparation
    The Referral

    Initial Telephone Contact
    Environment
    Improving Communication
    Building Trust

DOCUMENTATION OF HOME CARE

APPLICATION OF THE NURSING PROCESS
    Assessment
    Diagnosis and Planning
    Intervention
    Evaluation

FORMAL AND INFORMAL CAREGIVERS

HOSPICE HOME CARE
    Caring for the Caregiver
    Pain Control and Symptom Management

The purposes of home health services are to provide nursing care to individuals and their families in their homes and to maximize the self-care abilities and functional capacity of clients. The specific objectives and services nurses provide vary depending on the type of agency providing services and the population served. Nurses who work for public health departments, visiting nurse associations, home health agencies, hospice agencies, or school districts usually provide home visits.

Nurses from clinics or health departments often conduct home visits as part of client follow-up. These public health nurses make visits to follow clients with communicable diseases and provide health education and community referrals to clients with identified health problems. Home health nurses who work for home health agencies that are affiliated with hospitals or nursing registries often make home visits to assist clients in their transition from hospital to home. However, health care providers in private practice also order these visits when clients experience exacerbation of chronic conditions.

The focus of all home visits is on the individual for whom the referral is received. In addition, the nurse assesses the individual-family interaction and provides education and interventions for the family and the client. The nurse evaluates how the individual and family interact as part of an aggregate group in the community. The nurse identifies the need for referrals to community services and performs the referrals as necessary.

Nurses who make home visits receive referrals from a variety of sources, including the client's physician, nurse practitioner or nurse midwife, hospital discharge planner or case manager, schoolteacher, or clinic health care provider. The client or the client's family can also originate requests for nursing visits to assess and assist in the client's health care.

Home visits have been an integral part of nursing for more than a century, originating with Florence Nightingale's "health nurses" in England. In the United States in 1877, the Women's Branch of the New York City Mission sent the first trained nurses into the homes of the poor to provide nursing care. Under the direction of Lillian Wald, pioneering efforts were initiated to provide services to the poor in their homes in the late nineteenth century (Kelly and Joel, 1995).

HOME HEALTH CARE

The term *home health care* describes a system in which health care and social services are provided to homebound or disabled people in their homes rather than in medical facilities

(U.S. Department of Commerce and International Trade Administration, 1990). The U.S. Department of Health and Human Services (USDHHS) set forth the following definition of home health care that an interdepartmental work group developed:

Home health care is that component of a continuum of comprehensive health care, whereby health services are provided to individuals and families in their places of residence for the purpose of promoting, maintaining or restoring health, or maximizing the level of independence, while minimizing the effects of disability and illness, including terminal illness. Services appropriate to the needs of the individual client and family are planned, coordinated, and made available by providers organized for the delivery of home care through the use of employed staff, contractual arrangements, or a combination of the two patterns (Warhola, 1980).

Purpose of Home Health Services

The primary purpose of home health services is to allow individuals to remain at home and receive health care services that would otherwise be offered in a health care institution, such as a hospital or nursing home. The home health industry grew tremendously in the 1980s and in early 1990; it has declined slightly since 1997, because of changes in Medicare home health reimbursement (National Association for Home Care and Hospice [NAHC], 2004). Numerous factors generated the growth of home health services, including the increasing costs of hospital care and the subsequent introduction of the prospective payment system (PPS) by the Social Security Amendments in 1983. Under the PPS, hospitals receive a fixed amount of money based on the relative cost of resources used to treat Medicare clients within each type of diagnosis-related group (Guterman and Dobson, 1986). Moreover, many other third-party payers negotiate preferred provider programs or managed care systems. In a managed care arrangement, the health care provider is paid a set fee for providing care to clients enrolled in the program. Providing home care services contributes to cost containment in a managed care environment. This cost containment is accomplished through timely hospital discharges by providing nursing services in the home setting and supporting clients at home rather than in skilled facilities. Home care is also popular with consumers, who prefer to receive care in their own homes rather than in an institution.

Home health care services have changed to address the needs of the population. Home health nurses visit acutely ill clients, clients with AIDS, the elderly, terminally ill clients, women with high-risk pregnancies, and ill infants and children

(Feldman, 1993). Home health care continues to focus on the care of sick clients and could expand to include health promotion and disease prevention interventions. Currently, most reimbursement for nursing services is based on the client's need for skilled nursing. On each client visit the nurse must document that the care provided is of a skilled nature that requires the knowledge and assessment skills of a nurse. The nurse must also verify that the client or a family member could not provide the same level of care.

Services coordinated in the home include not only skilled nursing care provided by RNs, such as administering IV antibiotics or performing dressing changes, but also the services of physical, occupational, and speech therapists; social workers; and home health aides. This team of health care professionals working together is essential for the client's success in reaching their maximal functional capacity. Each member of the team is accountable to the rest of the team and must provide high quality care for the team to function effectively. The broader industry definition of home health care includes supportive social services, respite care, community nursing centers, group boarding homes, homeless shelters, adult day care, intermediate skilled extended care facilities, and assisted living facilities (American Nurses Association, 1999).

TYPES OF HOME HEALTH AGENCIES

Home health agencies differ in their financial structures, organizational structures, governing boards, and populations served. The most common types of home health agencies are official (i.e., public), nonprofit, proprietary, chains, and hospital-based agencies. The number of freestanding proprietary agencies has grown faster than any other type of Medicare-certified home health agency. Freestanding proprietary agencies now comprise 40% of all home health agencies and hospital-based agencies comprise 30% of all certified home health agencies (NAHC, 2001).

The number of managed care agencies, which may have any type of financial structure, continues to increase. Managed care agencies contract with payers, such as insurance companies, to provide specified services to the enrolled clients at a predetermined price. Managed care agencies receive payment before offering services and are responsible for taking the financial risk of providing care to clients within the budgeted allotment. This works well with large numbers of enrolled clients, where the financial risk is spread across a larger number of people, many of whom are healthy and will not require skilled services.

Official Agencies

Local or state governments organize, operate, and fund official (i.e., public) home health agencies. These agencies may be part of a county public health nursing service or a home health agency that operates separately from the public health nursing service but is located within the county public health system. Taxpayers fund official home health agencies, but they also receive reimbursement from third-party payers such as Medicare, Medicaid, and private insurance companies.

Nonprofit Agencies

Nonprofit home health agencies include all agencies that are not required to pay federal taxes because they have tax exempt status. Nonprofit groups reinvest any profits into the agency. Nonprofit home health agencies include independent home health agencies or hospital-based home health agencies. Not all hospital-based home health agencies are nonprofit, even if the hospital is nonprofit. The home health agency can be established as a profit-generating service and serve as a source of revenue for the hospital or medical center. In this situation, the home health agency is categorized organizationally as for-profit, and they pay federal taxes on the profits.

Proprietary Agencies

Proprietary home health agencies are classified for-profit and pay federal taxes on the profits generated. Proprietary agencies can be individual-owned agencies, profit partnerships, or profit corporations. Providing the agencies make a profit, investors in corporate proprietary partnerships receive financial returns on their investments in the agencies. A percentage of the profits generated are also reinvested into the agency.

Chains

A growing number of home health agencies are owned and operated by corporate chains. These chains are usually classified as proprietary agencies and may be part of a proprietary hospital chain. Agencies within chains have a financial advantage over single agencies. The chains have lower administrative costs because a larger single corporate structure provides many services. For example, a multiagency corporation has greater purchasing power for supplies and equipment because they purchase a larger volume. A single corporate office can provide administrative services, such as payroll and employee benefits, for all chain employees, thereby reducing duplication of these services. Criticism of proprietary and chain agencies includes concerns over the quality of agency services that are profit driven.

Hospital-Based Agencies

Since the implementation of PPS in 1983, the number of hospital-based home health agencies has more than doubled (NAHC, 2001). This trend is not surprising in light of the fixed reimbursement under PPS and the hospitals' incentive to decrease length of stay. By establishing home health agencies, hospitals are able to discharge clients who have skilled health care needs, provide the necessary services to the client, and receive reimbursement through third-party payers, such as Medicare, Medicaid, and private insurance companies. The increasing number of home health agencies indicates that these agencies are profitable endeavors and provide hospitals with an additional revenue source.

CERTIFIED AND NONCERTIFIED AGENCIES

Certified home health agencies meet federal standards; therefore they are able to receive Medicare payments for services provided to eligible individuals. Not all home health agencies are certified. The number of Medicare-certified home health agencies increased to approximately 10,444 in 1997. This number is double the existing 5,695 Medicare-certified home health agencies in 1990. However, that number fell to approximately 7,152 in 2000 (NAHC, 2001).

The noncertified home care agencies, home care aide organizations, and hospices remain outside the Medicare system. Some operate outside the system because they provide non–Medicare-covered services. For example, they do not provide skilled nursing care and are not eligible to receive Medicare reimbursement.

SPECIAL HOME HEALTH PROGRAMS

Many home health agencies offer special, high-tech home care services. Offering high-technological services at home is both beneficial to the client's health and financially advantageous. Through the implementation of these special programs, clients who require continuous skilled care in an acute or skilled nursing institution are able to return to their homes and receive care at home. From the financial perspective, skilled services provided at home are less costly than hospitalization.

Examples of special services include home intravenous therapy programs for clients who require daily infusions of total parenteral nutrition or antibiotic therapy, pediatric services for children with chronic health problems, follow-up for premature infants who are at risk for complications, ventilator therapy, and home dialysis programs. The key to the success of all these programs is the client's, family's, or caregiver's ability to learn the care necessary for a successful home program and the motivation of these individuals to provide the care. If family or caregiver support is not available in the home, the client cannot be a candidate for any of these programs and other arrangements for care must be found.

REIMBURSEMENT FOR HOME CARE

Before the establishment of Medicare in 1965, individuals who required home health services paid cash for the services; donations to the service agency providers helped subsidize care services for clients who were unable to pay (Kent and Hanley, 1990). Since 1965, individuals who are eligible for Medicare benefits under Title XVIII of the Social Security Act, for Medicaid benefits under Title XIX, or have private health insurance are reimbursed by the federal government through the Medicare program to receive short-term, skilled health care services in their homes. Provided services include nursing care, social service, physical therapy, occupational therapy, and speech therapy, and the program is individualized to meet the client's needs.

Any individual over the age of 65 years who is homebound, under the care of a physician, and requires medically necessary skilled nursing care or therapy services may be eligible for home care through a Medicare-certified home health agency. These services must be intermittent or part-time, and they require physician authorization and periodic review of the plan

of care. The only exception is hospice care. Any individual over 65 years old who is terminally ill with a life expectancy of 6 months certified by a physician is eligible to receive the Medicare Hospice Benefit. There is no requirement for the individual to be homebound or in need of skilled care or for the services to be intermittent or part-time. The physician must recertify the client every 6 months to determine if he or she is still eligible for hospice care (NAHC, 1996).

The rapid growth of the home health market is reflective of the following:

- Increasing proportion of people aged 65 years and older
- Lower average cost of home health care compared with institutional costs ($750 per month for routine skilled nursing care at home, compared with $2000 for care in an institution)
- Active insurer support for home care
- Medicare promotion of home health care as an alternative to institutionalization (NAHC, 2001)

Client or family payments comprised 46% of the private financing (12% of total spending) for home health services. Private health insurance and nonclient revenue paid the remaining private financing.

Between 1967 and 1985, the number of home health agencies certified to provide care to Medicare recipients tripled from 1753 to 5983. In the mid 1980s this number leveled off at 5900, resulting from an increase in the volume of paperwork required and unreliable payment policies. This led to a lawsuit against the Health Care Financing Administration HCFA, charged by Representatives Harley Staggers (D-WV), Claude Pepper (D-FL), a coalition of members of the U.S. Congress, consumer groups, and the NAHC. The successful conclusion of the lawsuit gave NAHC the opportunity to participate in rewriting the Medicare home care payment policies. New payment policies brought an increase in the home health benefit, and increased the number of Medicare-certified home health agencies to over 10,000. The number is now declining as a direct result of the changes in Medicare home health reimbursement, enacted as part of the Balanced Budget Act BBA 97 (NAHC, 2004). Under this new payment system, home care agencies are reimbursed on a PPS based on the client's diagnosis and the projected time skilled services are needed. The amount provided to home health agencies is based on the average national cost of treating a home health client for 60 days (NAHC, 2004). The goal of this system is to encourage efficient use of home health services without sacrificing quality (NAHC, 2004).

OUTCOME AND ASSESSMENT INFORMATION SET (OASIS)

The Outcome and Assessment Information Set (OASIS) is a data set that measures outcomes of adult home care clients to monitor outcome-based quality improvement. The data set includes sociodemographic, environmental, support system, health status, and functional status attributes of adult clients, as well as information about service utilization. These items are used to monitor outcomes, plan client care, provide reports on client characteristics for each agency, and evaluate and improve clinical performance. The use of OASIS is mandatory for all Medicare and Medicaid clients receiving skilled care (Centers for Medicare and Medicaid Services, 2006).

See Resource Tool 31A on the book's website at: http://evolve.elsevier.com/Nies/.

NURSING STANDARDS AND EDUCATIONAL PREPARATION OF HOME HEALTH NURSES

The American Nurses Association (ANA, 1999) has revised its standards for home health nursing practice. These standards are differentiated into the following levels of practice: that of the generalist home health nurse, who is prepared at the baccalaureate level; and that of the advanced practice nurse, who is prepared at the graduate level. According to the ANA, the generalist nurse provides care to individuals and their families and caregivers. The generalist home health nurse must have community health assessment skills to assess client and caregiver needs, provide client and caregiver education, perform nursing actions following the client's plan of care, manage resources to facilitate the best possible outcomes, provide and monitor care, collaborate with other disciplines and providers to coordinate client care, and supervise ancillary staff and caregivers. The responsibilities of the generalist home health nurse include, but are not limited to, performing holistic, periodic assessments of client and family and caregiver resources; participating in performance improvement activities; collecting and using research findings to evaluate the plan of care; educating clients and families on health promotion and self-care activities; being a client advocate; promoting continuity of care; using the *Scope and Standards of Home Health Nursing Practice* to guide clinical practice; and identifying ethical issues and exploring options with the necessary individuals and staff members to achieve resolution (ANA, 1999).

The advanced practice home health nurse can, and sometimes does, perform all of the duties of the generalist home health nurse. In addition, the advanced practice nurse contributes significant clinical expertise to home health clients and their families, demonstrates proficiency in care management and consultation, and expertly implements and evaluates health programs, resources, services, and research for clients with complex conditions. The duties of the advanced practice home health nurse include, but are not limited to, providing consultation and serving as a resource to the generalist home health nurse, participating at all levels of quality improvement and research, educating all members of the health care team about emerging trends in home health care, performing direct care of the client and family, managing and evaluating the care the client is receiving from caregivers, monitoring trends in reimbursement for home health services, consulting with staff about any ethical issues that may arise, managing an interdisciplinary team, and disseminating practice and research findings to colleagues (ANA, 1999).

RNs with less than a baccalaureate degree are not educationally prepared to meet the professional standards for home health nursing. They are encouraged to use the standards in providing care and pursuing professional development. Unfortunately, many home health agencies have not adopted the ANA's standards for home health nursing and have hired nurses without baccalaureate preparation. Some of these home health agencies offer salaries that are lower than those the acute hospital setting offers and they cannot recruit educationally qualified nurses.

Albrecht's conceptual model (1990) for home care clearly identifies educational content areas for students in undergraduate and graduate nursing programs that have specialties in home health care. An underlying premise of the model is that professional satisfaction and effective client outcomes depend on the education and experience of the home health nurse. Implications that are apparent in the model include the following:

- Nursing programs at the undergraduate and graduate levels must prepare competent providers of home health care.
- Curricula must include concepts related to the suprasystem, health service delivery system, and home subsystem, which includes structural, process, and outcome elements.
- Students at the undergraduate level need at least one clinical observation or experience in a home care agency.
- Graduate-level students need specific courses that cover concepts present in the model, including knowledge of education; preventive, supportive, therapeutic, and high-tech nursing interventions for home health care; a multidisciplinary approach to home health care; health law and ethics; systems theory; economics covering supply, demand, and productivity; and case management and coordination (Albrecht, 1990, p. 125).

The home health nurse serves as a case manager for clients who receive care from the staff of the home health agency or receive care through contract services. The success of the case management plan is contingent upon the nurse's ability to use the nursing process to develop a plan of treatment that best fits the individual needs of the client, the client's family, or the caregiver. Client and family assessment is the first step in developing the treatment plan and nursing care plan.

The Albrecht nursing model for home health care (Figure 31-1) provides a framework for nurses, clients, and their families to interact and identify mutual goals of interventions and promote the client's self-care capability at home (Albrecht, 1990). Three major elements for measuring the quality of home health care client outcomes include structural, process, and outcome elements.

Structural elements include the client, family, provider agency, health team, and professional nurse. The process elements include the type of care, coordination of care, and intervention. Outcome elements consist of client and family satisfaction with care, quality of care, cost-effectiveness of care, health status, and self-care capability.

In the Albrecht model for home care, the relationship between the structural elements and the process elements directs the interventions. The nurse executes the nursing process; including assessment, nursing diagnosis, planning, intervention, and evaluation, and then the nurse coordinates client care (Albrecht, 1990).

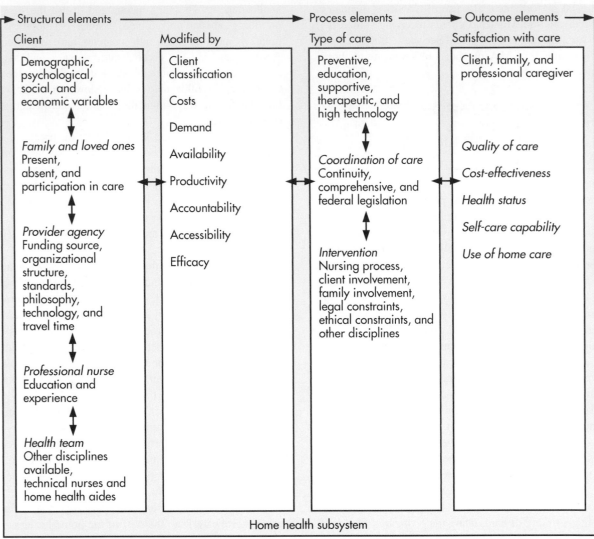

FIGURE 31-1   Albrecht nursing model for home health care. (Based on Albrecht MN: The Albrecht model for home health care: implications for research, practice, and education, *Public Health Nurs* 7:118-126, 1990. Reprinted by permission of Blackwell Scientific Publications, Inc.)

CONDUCTING A HOME VISIT

Visit Preparation

It is important that the nurse prepare for the home visit by reviewing the referral form, including the purpose of the visit, the geographical residence of the family, and any other pertinent information. The first home visit gives the nurse the opportunity to establish a trust relationship with the client and family to establish credibility as a resource for health information and community referrals in a nonthreatening environment.

The Referral

The referral (Figure 31-2) is a formal request for a home visit. Referrals come from a variety of sources, including hospitals, clinics, health care providers, individuals, and families. The type of agency that receives the referral will vary, depending on the necessary client services. Public health referrals are made for clients who are in need of health education (e.g.,

infant care education and resource allocation) or for clients with communicable diseases who need a follow-up visit.

Home health referrals are requested to provide clients with short-term, intermittent, skilled services and rehabilitation. Visits can last from 30 to 90 minutes and are scheduled on an intermittent basis depending on the specific needs of the client. For example, a client who had a stroke requires skilled nursing assessments, physical therapy visits for gait training, speech therapy for speech deficit improvement, and occupational therapy for retraining in activities of daily living ADL, such as bathing and cooking.

By reviewing the referral form before the first visit, the community health nurse (CHN), which includes the home health nurse and the public health nurse, obtains basic information about the client, such as name, age, diagnosis or health status, address, telephone number, insurance coverage, and reason for the referral. The form also specifies the source of the referral, such as a clinician, health care provider, communicable disease service, hospital, client, or client's family.

Patient number	☐ New ☐ Readmit **Intake**	Date last seen by MD	Case manager

Name: Last   First   M.I. | **Telephone no.:** | **Sex** M F | **Birthdate** | **Age** | **Date of first visit**   **MD auth.** Yes____ No____

Street address: **City:**   **State:**   **Zip:**

Hosp/snf:
Adm. date:
Dis. date:

Directions:

Diagnoses: Primary #
1.
2.
3.
4.
     DX known to pt?_____

Physician name: Specialty:
Address:
Tel. no:

Hosp/snf:
Adm. date:
Dis. date:

Physician name: Specialty:
Address:
Tel. no:

Medicare no.
Medical no./ss#.

History:

Agency worker: Tel. no:

Pay sources/service request:

PHN	PT	ST	OT
MSW	HHA	HCA	PD

Ins. co.:
Policy #:
Grp:. #:
Cov. code:
Tel. no:

Religious/cultural patterns/ language/psychosocial

Medications

Emergency/family contacts (by priority)
   Name   Rel.   Home#   Work#
#1
Address
#2
Address

Contact person:

Pertinent hospital information

Diet/fluids

Allergies

Equipment: DME Yes_____ No_____

Date/time:_____
Skilled orders per:_____

Intake source name	Agency	Tel. no:
How did you learn about our services?		
Intake received by	Date	

FIGURE 31-2   Referral form. (Courtesy Home Calls, Oakland, California.)

Public health referrals usually provide information on the client's condition that necessitates public health nurse (PHN) visits. For example, for a client who is positive for tuberculosis (TB), the PHN is notified of the client's place of residence, type and location of employment, and any known contacts, including family and friends. Another example of a public health referral is a 16-year-old girl who is referred for antepartum visits because she is 7 months pregnant and has just initiated prenatal care.

Additional information provided in the home health referral includes current client medications, prescribed diet, physician's orders, care plan goals, and other disciplines involved in the client's care. This information is important because it helps the nurse become familiar with the client's condition.

Initial Telephone Contact

The nurse contacts the client and informs him or her about the service referral. The first telephone contact with the client or family consists of an exchange of essential information, including an introduction by the nurse, identification of the agency that received the referral, and the purpose of the visit. After the initial exchange of information, the nurse informs the client of his or her desire to make the home visit, the client gives permission, and the group sets a mutually acceptable time for the visit. The nurse is a guest in the client's home; therefore it is important that the client agrees to the visit. The nurse then verifies the client's address and asks for specific directions to the client's home.

During a home health visit, the nurse requests proof of insurance, such as a Medicare, Medicaid, HMO membership, or insurance card. The nurse should forewarn the client so the client or family can locate the information before the visit. If the client is unable to provide this verification, the nurse assists with locating the information during the visit. Clients who receive a public health home visit do not require evidence of insurance coverage, because these services are not billed directly. A county public health budget or state or federally funded programs generally cover these visits.

Not all clients have a telephone. If this is the case, the nurse should check the referral for a telephone number where messages can be left. It is also worthwhile to contact the health care provider who made the referral, to see whether the telephone number was omitted unintentionally. If the client does not have a telephone, the nurse may choose to make a drop-in visit. This type of visit consists of an unannounced visit to the client's home, during which the nurse explains the purpose of the referral, receives the client's permission for the visit, and appoints a time for a future visit with the client. The client may agree to the first visit while the nurse is there.

If the client is not at home for the drop-in visit, the nurse should leave an official agency card and a brief message asking the client to contact the agency to schedule a nursing visit. The nurse informs the referring agency that the visit was attempted, but that the client was not available for contact. A formal agency letter, identifying the agency and the reason for the referral, is often sent to clients who are difficult to contact. The nurse's primary responsibility when unsuccessful in locating the client is to keep the clinic, physician, or referring agency informed of efforts to establish contact with the client.

Environment

An environmental assessment begins as the nurse leaves the agency en route to the client's home. The nurse should make specific observations to answer the following questions (Keating and Kelman, 1998):

- How does the client's neighborhood compare with other neighborhoods in the area?
- Are there adequate shopping facilities, such as grocery stores, close to the client's home?

The nurse should also note the client's dwelling, to determine, for example, whether the client lives in a single-family home, in a single room in a home or hotel, in an apartment, or in a shared apartment or house. Specific assessments include answering the following questions:

- Is the client's residence easily accessible by the client, given the client's age and functional ability? For example,

if the client has limited endurance, can he or she negotiate several flights of stairs when entering or leaving the dwelling?
- Are handicapped facilities available as necessary?
- Is the dwelling in an area with high rates of drug abuse or crime?
- Is the building or home secure? Does the client live alone? If so, how does the client get to the physician or clinic? How does the client purchase groceries?
- Does the client have food in the home? If so, who prepares the client's meals? Are the meals nutritious?
- Are there rodents, cockroaches, or other potential vectors of disease present in the client's home?
- Does the client's home have hot running water, heat, sanitation facilities, and adequate ventilation?
- Is the client's residence safe relative to the client's physical status, or is the home cluttered with debris and furniture?

Improving Communication

When the nurse meets with the client, whether in the home or at another mutually agreeable location, the initial conversation revolves around social topics. The nurse assumes a friendly manner and asks general questions about the client, the client's family, and health care services that will benefit the client. These questions help the nurse assess the client's needs and create a comfortable atmosphere for communication. If there is a lot of noise such as a loud TV, the nurse should ask the client if the TV can be turned down for the duration of the nurse's visit to facilitate good communication and an accurate assessment.

Building Trust

Many clients in need of nursing visits do not trust the health care system and are uncomfortable with the representative from an agency visiting their home. For example, a client who is pregnant and does not have legal status in the United States will most likely be hesitant to allow a nurse to visit; she will likely be afraid of being reported to immigration authorities. The nurse's role in visiting this client is to focus on the health and safety of the client and her fetus. The nurse must build a trust relationship early in the visit or the client will not allow additional visits. If a trust relationship is not established and the client believes that the nurse will report her to immigration, it is highly probable that the client will move to another location to avoid future contact.

DOCUMENTATION OF HOME CARE

The nurse documents assessment data and interventions for all home visits. The client record also contains a copy of the nursing care plan.

Many home health nurses would probably identify documentation issues as the most frustrating part of providing home health care. Medicare holds a prominent position as a home health care payer; therefore the HCFA's regulations determine the home health industry's documentation. Correct and accurate completion of required Medicare forms is the key to reimbursement. Payment or denial for visits is based on the information presented on the forms. If the nurse does not clearly document the provided skilled care in the nursing notes, the fiscal intermediaries will argue that the care was either unnecessary or not performed and will deny reimbursement. The home health nurse must have an excellent clinical foundation and the ability to identify and document actual and potential client problems that require skilled nursing interventions (ANA, 1999).

Documenting the care provided to record the client's quality of care is just as important as documenting for reimbursement purposes. The documentation of home visits records the nurse's observations, assessments of the client's condition, provided interventions, and the client's and family's ability to manage the care at home. In addition, documentation of client visits serves as a formal communication system among other home health professionals who also interact with the client and family.

APPLICATION OF THE NURSING PROCESS

Assessment

During the first home visit the type of client assessment will vary with the purpose of the home visit. The home health nurse assesses the client's knowledge of his or her health status. The nurse identifies knowledge deficits and uses this information to develop a care plan.

Subjective information is obtained from the client and the client's family, including the client's perception of the situation and what the client identifies as problems. The nurse assesses whether the client is isolated from others physically or socially and whether the client is a member of a close-knit, nurturing, supportive family or kinship network. The amount of support the client perceives as available may or may not be accurate; therefore the nurse asks several questions about the client's family, friends, and daily routine to assess the client's level of social support.

The home health nurse assesses the client's health knowledge; his or her physical, functional, and psychosocial status; physical environment; and social support during the first home visit. The nurse collects information through observations and questions the client, family, and other possible caregivers in the home environment. It is not unusual to find inconsistencies between information the client provides during hospitalization concerning the amount of physical and emotional support available to the client in the home, and the actual amount of help available to the client in the home. The nurse validates or modifies the referral information to reflect the true home situation. Home health nurses often use contracts that the nurse, client, and family jointly develop to delineate the responsibilities of the client in the home.

The client's physical assessment is generally performed during the home health visit and includes a review of all systems, with an emphasis on the systems affected by the client's present condition. The nurse obtains objective data through the use of essential physical assessment skills, such as observation, palpation, auscultation, and percussion. The physical assessment also includes information regarding the client's functional status. Assessment of the functional status is important for obtaining Medicare reimbursement and for developing an individualized plan of care. This assessment includes the client's ability to ambulate, perform ADLs independently, and use assist devices, such as a cane or wheelchair. Specific functional limitations, such as shortness of breath or muscle weakness, are assessed at this time. For example, the nurse can assess the clients' mobility by watching them move around the home during the visit. Do they use a walker? Do they have to hold on to furniture to move through the house? Do they have to rest frequently? These are all important questions to consider when assessing mobility. It is also important to evaluate the home environment for potential safety hazards such as loose carpeting or visible cords that could cause a client to trip and fall.

Information obtained during the assessment phase is used to identify nursing diagnoses and develop a plan of care. Data collection continues while the client receives home health services. Changes in the client's condition, environment, or social structure necessitate modifications in the treatment plan and the nursing care plan.

There are differences between the treatment plan and the nursing care plan. The plan of treatment includes the type of home health services received, the projected frequency of visits by each discipline (Albrecht, 1991), and the necessary interventions. The nursing care plan addresses specific nursing interventions designed to treat the client's actual or potential problems and includes identified goals with measurable outcomes.

Diagnosis and Planning
Develop a Plan for the Client and Family

After the assessment phase of the home visit, the nurse identifies the nursing diagnoses that address the client's problems and identifies actual or potential problems. The identification of nursing diagnoses serves as the basis for the nursing care plan. This plan is developed in consultation with the client and the family. The plan identifies short-term and long-term goals and measurable outcomes for the client. The plan identifies necessary nursing interventions and additional home health services that are appropriate to help the client achieve the identified goals. To maximize the plan's success, it is important that the client and family are involved in the planning process and access community resources. Planning is a dynamic process that continues while the client receives nursing services. The plan is modified as needed, depending on the client's condition, until the identified goals are met.

Often the nurse will develop a contract with the client that delineates the roles and responsibilities of the nurse, the family, and the client in carrying out the nursing care plan (Spradley, 1990). If the client expresses a disinterest in contracting to improve health during the planning phase, the nurse will be limited in possible interventions. Goals are identified that the client is willing to work toward with the nurse's assistance.

The goal of home visits for both public health and home health nursing is to involve the client and family in taking an active role in health promotion. The nurse is careful not to allow the client to become dependent on the nurse's interventions, because the nurse's involvement is short term.

Outline the Client and Family Roles

Written contracts are helpful for both the nurse and the client, because the client's role and the nurse's role in implementing the plan are clearly delineated (Spradley, 1990). If either the client or the nurse forgets their role in the plan, the written contract becomes a reference. The client and the nurse can modify the contract by mutual agreement.

Intervention

Implementation of the care plan begins during the first home visit. The nurse begins to provide the client and family with health information concerning the client's health status and informs them about the availability of and access to community resources. In the case of the home health visit, the nurse provides skilled nursing care. At the end of the initial home visit, the nurse discusses the need for another home visit. The nurse and client discuss the goal of the next visit; specifically, they discuss what the client should do before the visit. The nurse informs the client and family about any information or skills he or she will provide during the next visit, and the nurse and client agree on a day for the next visit.

Referral for Community Services

During the first visit, the nurse provides the client and family with information regarding community resources, including the purpose of the resources, their eligibility for the services provided, possible expenses, and agency telephone numbers. Referrals depend on the availability of community resources, the client's eligibility for the services, the client's and the family's willingness to use the services, and the suitability of resources for the client and family. Examples of such services include information about immunization clinics for children in the family; adult day care or senior centers for elderly clients who could benefit from socialization; adult education classes or continuation of high school for pregnant teen clients who have dropped out of high school; Meals on Wheels (MOW) services for clients who are not able to prepare meals; homeless shelters for men, women, and families; soup kitchens; resources for clothing and housing; mental health clinics; resources for battered spouses; and primary care clinics for low-income clients with and without insurance.

If necessary, the client or client's family may request the nurse's assistance in contacting the community resources. The client and family are encouraged to make the contacts, but if the client and family are unable to make the calls or do not speak English, the nurse needs to intervene on behalf of the client. By providing referral information during the first home visit, the nurse can follow up on the client's or the family's success in contacting and using community services.

Terminating the Visit

The nurse terminates the first visit when the assessment is completed and a care plan is established with the client. The average visit should not exceed one hour. The client receives a great deal of information during that hour, and the nurse collects a great deal of information. Most clients are tired at the end of a 1-hour visit and often cannot retain additional information. It is preferable to set a date for another home visit to reinforce the information provided and work progressively toward achieving goals.

Evaluation
Evaluation of Progress Toward Goals

The evaluation phase occurs when the nurse can determine whether the mutually established goals are realistic and achievable for the client and the client's family. The evaluation process is continuous and allows the nurse to determine the success or progress toward the client's identified goals. The nurse can identify the need for revisions in the nursing care plan and treatment plan through the collection of additional data during the evaluation phase. The nurse can intervene to make necessary changes. An example is an elderly wife who, during the initial home visit, stated that she preferred to provide the physical care for her frail, nonambulatory husband. On a subsequent visit, the nurse assessed that the client was not receiving the care required for the client's personal care, specifically bathing. The nurse discussed the problem with the wife and presented her with available options. These included the services of a home health aide to provide personal care and bathing three times a week. A new plan was developed and it included the home health aide. The plan was implemented and evaluated during future visits. Input from the client is critical to determine whether the goals established are realistic and achievable for the client.

Modification of the Plan as Needed

The evaluation process also allows the nurse, client, and family to discuss what is working well and where modifications are necessary in the plan. Evaluation occurs through open communication between the nurse and client, and the nurse asks questions about specific parts of the care plan. If a trust relationship exists, the client feels comfortable telling the nurse about problems in the care plan.

When Goals Are Achieved

The overall purpose of home visits is to assist the client with necessary information and nursing care to enable the client to function successfully without nursing interventions. When the care plan goals are achieved, the client does not need the nurse any longer. The client knows what community resources are available and how to access health care services for primary, secondary, and tertiary interventions.

FORMAL AND INFORMAL CAREGIVERS

Formal caregivers include professionals and paraprofessionals who provide in-home health care and personal services. They are compensated for the services they provide. The Bureau of Labor Statistics estimates that more than 500,000 people were employed in home health care agencies in 1998 (U.S. Department of Labor, Bureau of Labor Statistics, 2000). The largest number of employees consists of home care aides and RNs.

Informal caregivers are family members who are caring for the client. The presence or absence of an involved family member can make the difference between the successful completion of the plan of treatment, with the client remaining in the home, and the need to transfer the client to an extended-care facility or board-and-care facility. When a capable family member or caregiver is available to assist the client, the home health nurse spends much of the visit assessing the skills of the caregiver. The home health nurse instructs the caregiver in the correct procedures for providing care and in recognizing the signs and symptoms of problems that must be reported to the health care provider. The goal of the home health nurse's instruction is to provide the caregiver with the skills necessary to care for the client successfully in the home without intervention of the nurse or other members of the home health team.

The home health nurse faces a special challenge in those clients who lack a family member or caregiver capable of learning and providing necessary care. When the client lives alone and does not have caregivers, the nurse explores other resources available to supplement the client's self-care activities in the home. For example, if the client has extensive physical care needs and sufficient financial resources, the nurse may suggest hiring an attendant. Medicare and private insurance companies do not pay for attendant care. If the client's income is low enough, in-home county support services may be an option. The nurse may consider other services for the client such as MOW for nutritious meals delivered to the client's home. Friendly Visitors, a volunteer service, sends a volunteer to the client's home once a week or more to provide socialization for the client. Other options that are available in some communities include adult day health centers or senior service centers. Both of these options require arranged client transportation to and from the centers. A variety of transportation methods are available in different communities; volunteers may transport clients to the centers or public transportation systems may be available such as minivans that provide door-to-door service. Selected services and referrals are based on the client's individual needs and on the client's level of functional ability.

HOSPICE HOME CARE

Hospice and palliative nursing care is becoming increasingly important as there is a tremendous need to improve end-of-life care for the terminally ill. Nurses that work with the terminally ill seek to enhance the client's quality of life by focusing on relieving suffering throughout the illness, supporting the client and family through the dying process, and providing grief support to the family after the client has died (ANA, 2002). Hospice and palliative care nurses have a holistic approach to their clients. They are responsible for

---

ETHICAL Insights

Ethics: Home Health and Hospice Care

➤ Most legal and ethical issues in home health care involve the care of terminally ill clients.

➤ Early education about these issues is essential in the prevention of problems.

➤ Early education also gives clients the opportunity to make decisions for themselves and communicate those decisions to family members and health care providers.

➤ All competent adults have the right to make decisions that will direct health care providers in the type of care they administer.

➤ This communication can occur through the completion of advance directives, durable power of attorney for health care, and living wills.

Advance Directive

➤ An **advance directive** is a written document in which a competent person gives instructions about future health care, in the event that the individual is unable to make decisions. These directives are completed on a voluntary basis. All Medicare-certified health care agencies are obligated to ask clients about advance directives and provide clients with the advance directive form if the client is interested in completing the document (Department of Health and Human Services, 2000).

Durable Power of Attorney for Health Care

➤ A **durable power of attorney** for health care is one type of advance directive. Also called a health care proxy, the durable power of attorney for health care gives another person the power to make medical decisions related to care. This person, as identified by the client, acts as the client's agent in all decisions regarding health care, personal care, and custody, in the event that the client becomes incompetent or disabled and unable to make decisions.

Living Will

➤ A **living will** is a written document in which a client voluntarily informs doctors and family members about the type of medical care desired should the client become terminally ill or permanently unconscious and unable to communicate. In the living will, the client can describe the type of care desired, depending on the clinical situation. For example, if the client is terminally ill and unconscious, the client can direct the health care team to perform only those measures that will provide comfort and nothing further. The client can specifically indicate his or her opposition to life-saving measures; for example, the client may request the denial of cardiopulmonary life support in the event of a cardiac arrest. Other examples include indicating the exclusion of chemotherapy, blood transfusions, and respirator use in an attempt to prolong life.

---

taking a comprehensive health history and physical exam, including evaluating mental status and functional abilities; performing appropriate lab and diagnostic studies; determining effective pharmacological and nonpharmacological therapies to manage symptoms; identifying client, family, and caregiver goals; providing culturally competent care that is consistent with the client's health beliefs, values, and practices; evaluating the client's emotional state and the response to their illness and impending death; identifying coping strategies and support systems; evaluating financial resources; and conducting a spiritual assessment (ANA, 2002).

Hospice and palliative nursing care is provided in a variety of settings including hospitals, nursing homes, residential homes, and palliative care clinics. For those clients receiving hospice services in the home, the goal is to keep the client as comfortable at home as long as possible and to provide support and instruction to caregivers. When the client becomes terminally ill, the focus shifts from cure to comfort care. Some clients insist on staying home until they die and others allow their caregivers to decide if they should remain at home or be admitted to an extended care facility or a hospital. Each family unit has different needs and must be supported in their decisions. Home death should not be the standard that determines excellence in any case, nor should home death be the ultimate measure of "successful" home care. It is vital to realize that caring for a terminally ill person also includes caring for the family or caregivers. Not all caregivers want their loved one to die at home and not all caregivers are capable of allowing that to happen. The goal of having a home death must be the goal of the client and family, regardless of the nurse's personal preference.

When caring for a terminally ill person at home, the hospice nurse must be skilled in physical and psychosocial care for both the client and the caregiver. The client is viewed as a whole person, not as an isolated disease. Caring for a terminally ill person at home demands that the nurse view the family system as a unit. In addition, the nurse is not the only member of the hospice team assigned to each client. Each client has a physician, a nurse, a social worker, a nurse assistant, and a spiritual counselor to provide a multidisciplinary, holistic approach to caring for that client and his or her family. Furthermore, many hospice agencies have weekly interdisciplinary meetings where the various members of the hospice team meet to discuss the clients and work together to resolve issues and make sure the clients are receiving the best possible care. This team approach is essential to promoting quality of life (QOL) among hospice clients because of the complexity of issues that arise during a terminal illness. For example, a client may have physical, emotional, spiritual, and financial concerns that are negatively affecting their QOL. It will take the entire hospice team working together to help this client in all areas.

Caring for the Caregiver

Although the dying client is the focus of all skilled nursing care, the experienced home care nurse knows that a careful assessment of the caregiver's mental and physical health is important. The spouse, lover, children, friends, and neighbors who have made the commitment to stay until the end need the nurse's time and attention as much as, if not more than, the client. Although the client's wishes are important, all decisions regarding care are made considering the health of the caregivers. Gaynor (1990) found that women with more caregiving experience had increased physical health problems than those with less caregiving experience; younger women found caregiving more psychologically burdensome than

RESEARCH HIGHLIGHTS

Preventive Health Practices: Comparison of Family Caregivers Age 50 and Older

Nurses and other health professionals are encouraged to address the health promotion and disease prevention behaviors of their clients, even those who are not the direct recipients of their services. Family caregivers are a population accessible to clinicians. Family caregivers may suffer ill health effects from the burden of their responsibilities and also may neglect themselves over time. The purpose of this study was to describe adherence to recommended preventive health practices among middle-aged and older male and female family caregivers of individuals receiving home health services.

This study described selected health promotion and disease prevention behaviors among male and female family caregivers, age 50 years and older, of individuals receiving home health services. Selected variables used to explore such behaviors included family caregivers' prior preventive health practices, their current adherence to recommended guidelines, and their ability to attend to their own health-related needs. Perceptions of the burden and benefit of caregiving, amount of social interaction, and use of community resources were also studies. Because morbidity is more frequently observed among caregiving women than men, it was hypothesized that gender differences would be found in each of these selected variables.

A sample of participants was recruited during a 21-month period from family caregivers of clients of a Medicare-certified home health agency in southwestern Pennsylvania. Family caregivers took part in a telephone survey, and over 300 caregivers were interviewed. Women participants tended to care for either a parent or a spouse, whereas men most often were caring for their wives. Few were employed; most were retired. Fifty-six percent were solo caregivers, on average spending 11 hours per day aiding the care-receiver. They used a variety of community resources, most frequent home nursing, a home health aide or companion, and physical therapy.

Feeling needed was the most positive aspect of caregiving for both men and women. Men were more likely than women to indicate that caregiving make them feel useful and appreciated. Their daily lives revolved largely around the care-receiver's unique rituals and needs, and they had limited interaction with others. On average, both male and female caregivers had engaged in 86% of preventive health practices under investigation at least once in their lives. However, they were current with just 63% of these practices. They tended to have health concerns of their own and rate their health as worse than the public at large. Health promoting behaviors were performed at rates similar to those observed among middle-aged and older adults in general. Women tended to take a more active role in gathering health information. Men tended to have greater participation in exercise and leisure-time activities.

The study demonstrated that family caregivers aged 50 years and older do participate in an array of age- and gender-appropriate health promotion and disease prevention behaviors, despite their often time-consuming responsibilities. However, the marked disparity between their past and current adherence is worrisome. Nurses who interact with family caregivers are well positioned to encourage their health promotion and disease prevention behaviors.

Matthews JT et al: Preventive health practices: comparison of family caregivers 50 and older, *J Gerontol Nurs* 30(2): 46-54, 2004.

older women. Nursing interventions must be directed toward preventing a decline in the caregiver's health.

Caregivers need reassurance that their judgment is sound, and they need reminders that they cannot do anything

Home health nurses and some community health nurses (CHNs) make visits to families with health problems. A referral for this home visit is received from a client's nurse practitioner. The client was discharged from the hospital with a primary diagnosis of noninsulin-dependent diabetes mellitus (NIDDM) and a secondary diagnosis of hypertension and S/P cerebrovascular accident (CVA), which occurred 10 months ago.

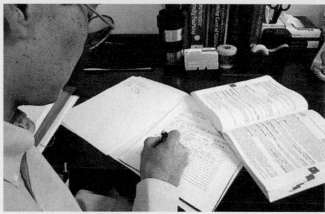

The nurse reviews the information on the referral from. The referral reveals the client is newly diagnosed with NIDDM and has a history of hypertension and CVA with left-sided weakness. The client's insurance is Medicaid. The current medications listed are: 25 mg hydrochlorothiazide q.d., 5 mg Isordil q.i.d., and 5 mg Micronase b.i.d. The prescribed diet is a low-fat, 1200-calorie diet with no added salt. If there is information missing, it is important to obtain it before making initial client contact.

The nurse brings to the community health setting experience and knowledge from a variety of specialties such as maternity, mental health, medical-surgical, pediatrics, pharmacology, and epidemiology.

The nurse usually makes the initial contact by phone. It is important to introduce yourself and the agency you represent and to explain the purpose of he visit. You will need to obtain permission and arrange a date and time for the visit. Occasionally, the client may not have a phone. This may a require a drop-in visit. Attempt a home visit and be prepared for a full visit if the client is at home and requests your services. If the client is not at home, the nurse should leave a business card with a note requesting a call to arrange a home visit.

The assessment process begins as soon as the nurse leaves the office on the way to the home visit. Transportation may be a problem for the client. Is it available? What is the cost and hours of operation? Are there safety concerns about using public transportation?

It is important to assess the availability of services, such as a pharmacy and a bank. Where does the client go to get cash or deposit a check and to fill a prescription? Is the area safe for these transactions for the client?

Is there a grocery store nearby? What types of foods are available?

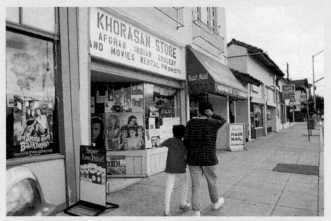

The nurse notices an Afghan-Indian grocery store that provides for ethnic communities.

The school in the area provides evidence of diverse families in the community.

Assessment of the type of neighborhood in which the client resides is also important. Is it residential, business, or mixed; high- or low-density housing, single-family homes, or apartments? Is the neighborhood safe or unsafe, for example, high crime or drug area?

It is extremely important for the nurse to be aware of the environment and surroundings as you approach and observe the residence. You are not to disregard personal safety to make a home visit. If it is unsafe, arrange another time and place for the home visit.

When you knock at the door, be sure to state your name, role, agency you represent, and the purpose of the visit.

You should always wear your identification badge.

Business cards with the agency name, address, and phone number should be available to give to clients. Building trust provides the foundation for a therapeutic relationship with the client. Clients may be hesitant to trust the health care/social system.

It is important to establish a comfortable atmosphere. This may be accomplished by initiating social conversation. It moves from general questions about the client and family to more sensitive health issues. The purpose of the visit is to provide health care services, and this should be clearly communicated to the client. This home visit includes a health history and limited physical examination.

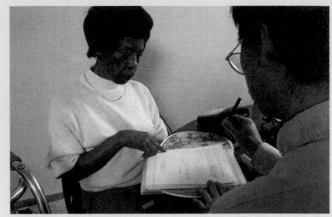

Agencies vary in the type of paperwork required. A consent form is often required prior to providing services. The form should be explained so the client may make an informed consent.

Medical insurance should also be verified so that the service may be billed properly.

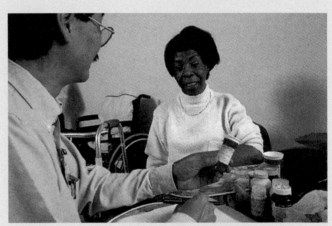

The client may have several prescriptions from different health care providers. These medications may have expired or may no longer be necessary. This is an opportunity for the nurse to provide instructions pertaining to the use of medications.

Inquiring about the diet provides an opportunity to explore compliance and cultural implications. It is helpful to have a diet plan that includes culturally relevant food. Teaching the client how and why to maintain a diet log will assist in evaluating compliance with the low-fat, 1200-calorie diet.

Health history includes a functional assessment of the client. Physical limitations of the client in performing activities of daily living are important health assessment data. The nurse has already noted any physical barriers to ambulation, both exterior and interior, that may exist. The nurse has already observed the use of a walker by the client at the door and a wheelchair nearby.

It is important to do a family assessment. Observation of the interaction between the client and family will be helpful in developing a nursing care plan. The family should be incorporated into the nursing care plan for the client.

Equipment for talking vital signs may not be provided by the client. The nurse should always have a stethoscope and have access to a sphygmomanometer. To many clients, the taking of a blood pressure is a reassuring initial step in a health examination. It provides nurses a window of opportunity to obtain important health history data and provide health teaching.

A focused physical examination is done on the client. This will provide the baseline data of the client's health status. This information will be used on subsequent visits to assess progress toward the identified nursing goals.

Since the client is newly diagnosed with NIDDM, it would be important to teach proper foot care.

The use of a glucometer may help the provider in making clinical decisions regarding treatment. This is another opportunity to provide health teaching for the client. Review the proper use of the glucometer and have the client do a demonstration. It is helpful to incorporate the family members in the teaching plan.

The establishment of a nursing care plan requires input from the client and family. An agreed-upon goal is following a low-fat, 1200-calorie diet. The family will help in preparing the food and doing blood glucose monitoring. The nurse will provide a culturally relevant diet and contact the local American Diabetes Association (ADA) chapter for a support group for the family. A return visit is scheduled for the following week.

At the end of the visit, always ask if there is anything else you could assist with. It provides an opening for the client and family to ask for assistance that may not have been covered during the home visit. Remind the client of the business card and ask the client to call if there are any problems. Also advise the client you will be contacting the health care provider regarding outcomes of the home visit.

The nurse continues to note environmental conditions that impact the client, family, and community. The nurse can then begin to advocate for health promotion and prevention interventions surrounding the environmental issues confronting the community.

The nurse charts according to agency policy as soon as possible to ensure accurate, clear, and concise notes of the home visit. This may be done at the office or between home visits.

It is the responsibility of the nurse to inform the referral source of the home results. This is especially important if the nurse has been unable to locate the client. The result of the home visit may be provided in a written or verbal format.

The nurse acts as a referral resource for the community. The nurse continuously searches for community resources and develops a resource database. The nurse calls the local ADA chapter to find out about the services provided. The agency does indeed have a culturally sensitive diet available for the client as well as a support group for family members. The nurse calls the client with the information.

CASE STUDY 1   Application of the Nursing Process—Home Health Visit

Susan Brown is a 40-year-old woman who was the driver in a single-car, rollover accident. She was airlifted to a trauma center and treated for multiple lacerations and abrasions, including a severe laceration to the left inner aspect of her arm. The hospital made a referral for home health services at the time of discharge. The referral requested the home health nurse to perform daily wound care to the infected left arm laceration. The specific wound care medical orders consisted of removing the arm brace, performing wet-to-dry dressing changes using one-fourth strength Dakin's solution, wrapping the arm with gauze, and reapplying the brace. Medications included 1 or 2 Vicodin tablets every 6 hours as needed for pain, and 500 mg of Keflex, 4 times a day.

ASSESSMENT

The home health nurses assessed the following related to Susan's wound:

- Amount, color, and odor of wound drainage (Susan had a moderate to large amount of yellow drainage from the laceration on her left arm.)
- Pain assessment, including history, character, severity, location, effects on quality of life, precipitating factors, and relieving factors
- Client's understanding of the wound care and the appropriate administration of the medication

The home health nurse assessed Susan's support network and found that Susan has a large, supportive family, and a caregiver was available to assist her every day. However, there were problems between Susan's husband and Susan's sister that created tension and stress for Susan. Her family coordinated transportation to and from physician appointments without the nurse's intervention.

DIAGNOSIS

In this case, the care plan revolves around Susan and her family. A community intervention was not necessary.

Individual

- High risk for infection related to left arm laceration as evidenced by large amounts of yellow drainage
- Severe arm pain related to the injury
- Knowledge deficit related to inadequate understanding of the self-administration of antibiotic

When the home health nurse asked Susan when she took the Keflex, Susan explained that she took the medication at 9:00 AM, 1:00 PM, 5:00 PM, and 9:00 PM, because the drug was prescribed to be taken 4 times a day.

Family

- Anxiety related to family communication problems

PLANNING

Individual

Long-Term Goals

- Healed laceration without drainage or infection within 1 week
- Full range of motion of the affected arm within 2 weeks
- Pain-free when arm injury is healed
- Infection resolved within 1 week

Short-Term Goals

- Keep the laceration clean, and debride the wound with daily wet-to-dry dressing changes
- Encourage self-care in dressing changes within 24 to 48 hours
- Pain control initiated through medication and relaxation techniques within 24 hours
- Client will demonstrate correct self-administration of antibiotic within 24 hours

Family

Long-Term Goals

- Anxiety resolved or controlled within 1 week
- Support network will remain intact and will provide care to client as needed until injury is healed

Short-Term Goal

- Decreased anxiety through verbalization of feelings within 24 to 48 hours

INTERVENTION

Individual

Dressing changes were performed as ordered and the nurse monitored the wound daily. When the large amount of drainage persisted more than 3 days after initiating the antibiotic therapy, and the client continued to have low-grade fevers (temperature 99.2° to 99.8° F), the home health nurse notified the physician and took a culture of the drainage. An alternative antibiotic was prescribed based on the culture results. The nurse taught Susan and her mother how to change the dressings and the nurse supervised them.

The assessment of Susan's arm pain included a history of when the pain was most severe and the frequency of pain medicine administration. The home health nurse assessed that the pain was most severe at night and recommended that Susan take 2 Vicodin tablets before going to bed and place her left arm in a position of comfort, supported by pillows to decrease edema. The nurse instructed Susan to lie down, rest, and listen to relaxing music during the day when the pain was intense to decrease the amount of arm pain through relaxation. In addition, the nurse explained the purpose of the antibiotic and the importance of taking it every 6 hours to

Continued

CASE STUDY 1   Application of the Nursing Process—Home Health Visit (cont'd)

maintain an optimum blood level. Susan and the nurse agreed on a schedule of 6:00 AM, 12:00 noon, 6:00 PM, and bedtime.

Family

Susan's sister arrived from out of state to assist with her care after the accident. Within 3 days of her arrival, Susan's husband and sister got into an argument and the sister left abruptly and returned home. This altercation was very upsetting to Susan, who was distraught over the communication problems between her husband and sister. The home health nurse encouraged Susan to express her feelings concerning the dysfunctional relationship and discuss how she would address the situation with both her husband and her sister. The nurse stressed that the problem was between the husband and her sister and that Susan should not feel guilty or responsible for the disagreement.

EVALUATION

Individual

The nurse remained involved with Susan until the infection cleared and the family learned how to provide the necessary wound care. Susan's pain was adequately controlled until the infection resolved and the arm healed. Susan took her antibiotics and pain medication as prescribed. Susan's internist and orthopedist referred her for follow-up. She was

also referred for a gynecological appointment for evaluation of sudden onset of slight vaginal bleeding.

Family

Susan's sister returned to her home and further confrontations did not occur. The nurse suggested counseling for Susan if the hostile relationship persisted between her husband and sister, or if it continued to cause Susan anxiety.

LEVELS OF PREVENTION

The following are examples of the three levels of prevention as applied to the individual and the family in this case.

Primary
- Intervening to ensure that the wound did not get infected, by regularly changing the dressing to keep the wound clean and monitoring the wound for signs and symptoms of infection

Secondary
- Recognizing that the wound was infected and ensuring that the antibiotics were administered correctly

Tertiary
- The home health nurse taking steps to ensure that the infection does not spread and resolves in a timely manner

---

"wrong" if it is done for the client's comfort. The caregivers must understand that they will not mistakenly overdose the client, and they must be reminded repeatedly that the client will not die from something they did or did not do. Caring for the terminally ill requires that the home care nurse is willing to nurse the entire family. In addition, the nurse must involve all members of the hospice team to ensure that the caregivers receive the care they need.

Pain Control and Symptom Management

Pain control is an important goal for hospice nurses and their clients. Hospice nurses perform regular pain assessments, which involve gathering the following information about their client's pain: history; character, such as sharp, dull, or aching; severity or intensity, which is most commonly rated on a pain intensity scale from 0 to 10, with 0 being no pain and 10 being the worst pain imaginable; location; effects on quality of life; precipitating factors; and relieving factors (Norlander, 2001). It is vital that the hospice nurse not only performs regular pain assessments, but also remembers that pain is highly subjective and every person experiences pain differently and uniquely; therefore the client's pain is whatever he or she says it is regardless of the nurse's objective evaluation of the situation.

Pain medication is administered in doses sufficient to keep the client free of pain, and on a regular schedule to prevent

pain from recurring before the next dose. Hospice methods of pain control are particularly well suited to home care. The vast majority of clients can be pain free until their deaths. The key to successful pain control for the terminally ill is to convince clients to take their medications on a regular basis, not just when they "cannot stand it any longer." Generally these medications are long acting and are administered every 8 to 12 hours. In addition, clients will also have a fast acting pain medication to take for "breakthrough pain," which happens when the client experiences an increase in pain before it is time for their next dose of scheduled pain medication. The fast acting medications are generally administered every 1 to 2 hours as needed.

Many clients, especially the elderly, are afraid of becoming "junkies" or "druggies" and want to delay using pain medication until they "get really bad." Many people believe that using these medications signals "the end of the line" and they are amazed to learn that clients do well while receiving this drug for months, even years, before death occurs. Almost every family must learn that addiction is not the same as tolerance and that if the client eventually needs a higher dose to achieve the same level of pain control that indicates tolerance to the drug, not addiction to the drug. The goal is to achieve adequate pain control without making the client too lethargic.

In addition to pain control, hospice nurses help manage other symptoms, such as nausea and vomiting, constipation,

CASE STUDY 2   Application of the Nursing Process—Hospice Home Visit

Anne McMillan is 80 years old and is terminally ill with metastatic breast cancer. She has been a widow for 5 years and has three daughters and two sons. All of her children are married with kids of their own, except one son who is handicapped and lives with Anne. Anne is too weak to care for herself and is moving in with her youngest daughter. Her daughter's house is a colonial with all bedrooms upstairs. There is a first floor bathroom. During her first visit, the hospice nurse talks with Anne and her daughter and explains what hospice is all about. The nurse then admits Anne into the hospice program and begins her initial assessment. Anne's primary physical complaints are back pain and constipation. She is still eating and drinking regularly. The nurse immediately recognizes that Anne will need a hospital bed. Anne already has a walker, but the nurse informed Anne and her daughter that they could have a bedside commode if needed in the future, as Anne becomes weaker. Anne's biggest concern is her handicapped son. "He can't be by himself for long and I don't know where he can go now that I can't take care of him." Except for the handicapped son, all of her children and many of her grandchildren are active in her care.

ASSESSMENT

On her initial visit the hospice nurse collects the following data about Anne, her family, and her community. In this case, the community consists of Anne's social support outside of her family, such as her neighborhood and church.

- Pain assessment, including history, character, severity, location, effects on quality of life, precipitating factors, and relieving factors
- Other physical symptoms, such as fatigue, nausea, vomiting, constipation, diarrhea, decreased appetite, and decreased mobility
- Client and family fears, anxiety about dying, and the dying process
- Support network and family dynamics
- Client's anxiety about situation concerning handicapped son
- Additional support network outside of family
- Effect of diagnosis and prognosis on Anne's social support, including her neighbors and her church community

DIAGNOSIS

Individual
- Pain related to disease process
- Constipation related to decreased mobility
- Anxiety related to concerns about safety and well-being of handicapped son

Family
- Effective family coping as evidenced by active family participation in Anne's care

Community
- Anticipatory grieving related to social isolation secondary to leaving neighborhood and moving in with daughter

PLANNING

Individual
Long-Term Goals
- Pain will remain controlled until client dies.
- Client will have regular bowel movements for the next 2 months.
- Client will verbalize satisfaction about resolution of situation concerning handicapped son.

Short-Term Goals
- Pain will be well controlled within 24 to 48 hours.
- Client will have a bowel movement within 24 to 48 hours.
- Client will have decreased anxiety about handicapped son within 24 to 48 hours, as the social worker will have found a place for the son to live.

Family
Long-Term Goals
- Family will remain active in Anne's care until she is buried.
- Family will provide a support network for each other and use hospice services for continued support through Anne's death and burial and for months afterward.

Short-Term Goal
- Family will actively participate in Anne's care.

Community
Long-Term Goal
- Client will continue to receive support from friends.

Short-Term Goal
- Client will verbalize feelings about moving in with daughter and leaving friends behind.

INTERVENTION

Individual
After talking with the doctor, the hospice nurse starts Anne on methadone, 10 mg every 8 hours, and Roxanol, 5 mg as needed for breakthrough pain. The nurse explains to Anne and her daughter that she is constipated because of her decrease in mobility. The nurse obtains an order for a stool softener and instructs Anne to take it twice daily. The nurse also explains to Anne and her daughter that as Anne declines, her appetite will decrease and she will eat less and less and may not have bowel movements very frequently. Anne should let the nurse know if she every feels uncomfortable because she has not had a bowel movement in a few days. The nurse talks to the social worker who finds a group home for Anne's handicapped son.

Continued

CASE STUDY 2 Application of the Nursing Process—Hospice Home Visit (cont'd)

Family

The nurse and social worker talk with the family and help them develop a system so that Anne always has someone with her, and so that the responsibility for Anne's care does not fall on one person. They also inform the family about resources to support the family.

Community

Anne has a nurse, social worker, spiritual counselor, and nurse assistant assigned to her care. Each of these hospice workers helps Anne discuss her feelings about her situation and works with her to continue to receive support from her friends and neighbors.

EVALUATION

Individual

All of Anne's goals are met as she has good pain control until she dies, she no longer experiences discomfort and problems with constipation, and she expresses less anxiety and worries about her handicapped son. Although she still has some concerns, she feels much better about the situation.

Family

The family's goals are met as they remain active in Anne's care until she dies. In addition, they use hospice resources appropriately and as necessary, and they support each other through the entire process.

Community

The goals are met as Anne expresses her feelings about her situation and her closest friends remain supportive to Anne through visits and phone calls.

LEVELS OF PREVENTION

In this case the three levels of prevention focus on assisting the client and family through all phases of hospice care, from admission until death. Some examples are listed below.

Primary

- Anticipating needs and intervening early on to prevent problems, such as skin breakdown and lack of pain control
- Educating the client and family about hospice and the dying process

Secondary

- Responding quickly to needs as they arise
- Continued education about the hospice and dying experience

Tertiary

- Assisting the client and family through the active phase of dying
- Providing follow-up bereavement support to the family

---

diarrhea, fatigue, and decreased appetite. Nurses assist clients in managing these symptoms through medications, strategies to help cope with the symptoms, or both. Strategies include increasing fluids to prevent constipation, resting frequently to minimize fatigue, and eating small amounts as desired to cope with the decrease in appetite. In addition, the nurse educates the client and family that some of these symptoms, such as fatigue and decreased appetite, are related to the dying process and are signs that the client is declining.

Furthermore, the nurse, along with other members of the hospice team, provides emotional support to clients and families as they adjust to the client's impending death. The nurse educates the client and family about what physical symptoms the client will most likely experience as he or she approaches death. In addition, the nurse, along with the social worker and spiritual counselor, provides emotional support and helps the client and family work through any anxiety or fears they have about dying. Finally, the nurse is there to support the family immediately after the client dies, and hospice provides bereavement support to families up to a year after the client's death.

See Resource Tools 31B and 31C on the book's website at http://evolve.elsevier.com/Nies/ for additional case studies.

SUMMARY

This chapter presented information on performing public health, home health, and hospice nursing visits to clients in their homes. A general overview of the nursing process for clients in the home setting was presented and expanded to include the individual, family, and community. Case studies illustrating a typical home health visit and a typical hospice visit have been presented. The home visit is the foundation of community health nursing and provides a forum for important interventions with individuals, families, and communities. The CHN is responsible for bringing the concerns of individuals and families into the community.

LEARNING ACTIVITIES

1. Make arrangements to accompany a public health nurse, a home health nurse, and a hospice nurse on home visits.
2. Interview a public health nurse about the types of client referrals received and ask what interventions are usually performed. Repeat this activity with a home health nurse and a hospice nurse. Ask the nurses what they like best about their jobs.

3. Contact a local home health agency and interview the agency director. Ask what type of agency it is, the profit status, and whether it is Medicare certified. Report findings to classmates.
4. Attend a team meeting in a home health agency or a hospice program to see how the roles of the various team members blend together to provide family-centered care.
5. Interview a public health nurse and home health nurse and ask how the community influences the care they provide.

REFERENCES

Albrecht MN: The Albrecht nursing model for home health care: implications for research, practice, and education, *Public Health Nurs* 7:118-126, 1990.

Albrecht MN: Home health care: reliability and validity testing of a patient-classification instrument, *Public Health Nurs* 8:124-131, 1991.

American Nurses Association: *Scope and standards of home health nursing practice.* Washington, DC, 1999, American Nurses Association.

Centers for Medicare and Medicaid Services, *OASIS overview*, 2006, The Author, http://www.cms.hhs.gov/HomeHealthQualityInits/01_Overview.asp#TopOfPage.

Department of Health and Human Services: *Medicare state operations manual provider certification*, The Author, http://www.cms.hhs.gov/transmittals/downloads/R17SOM.pdf.

Feldman R: Meeting the educational needs of home health care nurses, *J Home Health Care Pract* 5:12-19, 1993.

Gaynor SE: The long haul: the effects of home care on caregivers, *Image J Nurs Sch* 22:208-212, 1990.

Guterman S, Dobson A: Impact of the Medicare prospective payment system for hospitals, *Health Care Financ Rev* 7:97-114, 1986.

Keating SB, Kelman GB: *Home health care nursing: concepts and practice*, Philadelphia, 1998, JB Lippincott.

Kelly L, Joel L: *Dimensions of professional nursing*, ed 8, New York, 1995, McGraw-Hill.

Kent V, Hanley B: Home health care, *Nurs Health Care* 11:234-240, 1990.

National Association for Home Care and Hospice: *How to choose a home care provider: who pays for home care services?* 1996, The Author, http://www.nahc.org/Consumer/wpfhcs.html#26.

National Association for Home Care and Hospice: *Basic statistics about home care*, 2001, The Author, http://www.nahc.org/Consumer/hcstats.html.

National Association for Home Care and Hospice: *Crisis in home care: dismantling of the Medicare home health benefit*, 2004. The Author, http://www.nahc.org/NAHC/LegReg/Crisis/crisishh.html.

Norlander, L: *To comfort always: a nurse's guide to end of life care*, Washington, DC, 2001.

Spradley BW: *Community health nursing: concepts and practice*, ed 3, Glenview, Ill, 1990, Scott, Foresman and Little, Brown.

US Department of Health and Human Services: *Healthy People 2010*, 2001, The Author, http://www.healthypeople.gov/Document/tableofcontents.htm.

US Department of Labor, Bureau of Labor Statistics: *National industry-occupation employment matrix, data for 1996*, 2000, The Author, http://www.bls.gov/oes/current/oessrci.htm.

Warhola C: *Planning for home health services: a resource handbook*, USDHHS Pub No HRA 80-14017, Washington, DC, 1980, PHS, USDHHS.

UNIT 8

The Future of Community Health Nursing

32

Health in the Global Community

Julie Cowan Novak

MEDIA RESOURCES

Additional Material for Study, Review, and Further Exploration

evolve Website at http://evolve.elsevier.com/Nies

❖ Quiz ❖ Case Studies ❖ Content Updates ❖ Glossary ❖ WebLinks

---

OBJECTIVES

Upon completion of this chapter, the reader will be able to do the following:

1. Describe population characteristics and international patterns of health and disease.
2. Discuss the World Health Organization (WHO) concepts of "Health for All" and primary health care.
3. Identify international health care organizations.
4. Describe the role of the community or public health nurse in international care.
5. Discuss the tobacco use pandemic and local to global prevention and cessation responses.

KEY TERMS

Centers for Disease Control and Prevention (CDC)
developed country
International Council of Nurses (ICN)

lesser developed country
Pan American Health Care Organization (PAHO)
primary care
primary health care

tobacco use pandemic
United Nations International Children's Fund (UNICEF)
World Bank

World Health Organization (WHO)
WHO Tobacco Free Initiative (TFI)

CHAPTER OUTLINE

POPULATION CHARACTERISTICS

ENVIRONMENTAL FACTORS

PATTERNS OF HEALTH AND DISEASE

INTERNATIONAL ORGANIZATIONS

INTERNATIONAL HEALTH CARE DELIVERY SYSTEMS
The Role of the Community Health Nurse in International Health Care

RESEARCH IN INTERNATIONAL HEALTH

Human health and its influence on every aspect of life are at the center of the global agenda (World Health Organization [WHO], 2004). Health, the most valuable possession, is a primary concern throughout the world. Nurses, as first responders, expert care providers, and leaders in international health care, promote and restore health in individuals, families, and communities in frontier, rural and urban settings. Community public health nurses must be aware of forces that threaten health in the global community. Nurses must study models of community assessment, community empowerment, and health care delivery in the United States and other countries to promote health.

This chapter highlights population characteristics; international patterns of health and disease; social, cultural, and economic factors; international health organizations, including WHO; health care providers; health care delivery systems; and the community public health nurse's role in the global community. The chapter presents the most recent evidence related to the worldwide **tobacco use pandemic,** that kills 4.9 million people each year, and describes local to global responses and interventions. These intervention models provide a framework for international research, education, service, practice, policy, and systems design.

Population characteristics, including patterns of growth and demographics, are among the many health issues that merit attention and study because they have global effects and threaten human life. This chapter also explores these issues and other environmental factors, including identified stressors and patterns of health and disease.

POPULATION CHARACTERISTICS

More than 1 billion people entered the twenty-first century without benefiting from the health care revolution. Enormous population growth presents a threat to the health and the economy of many nations. The exponential nature of world population growth is evident. In 1804, after 2 to 5 million years of human existence, the world population exceeded 1 billion. Between 1804 and 1927, the population reached 2 billion and between 1927 and 1960, 3 billion. The population soared to 4 billion between 1960 and 1974 and 5 billion between 1974 and 1987. In 1999, the world population grew to 6 billion and, in 2005, nearly 7 billion (WHO, 2005). The Central Intelligence Agency (2005) estimated the world population to be 6,446,131,400 as of July 2005. World population in the mid twenty-first century is expected to reach 10 to 12 billion (WHO, 2005).

In any society, large populations create pressure. For example, feeding a population becomes problematic in developing countries if famine, international trade problems, or war occurs. Malnutrition, disease, or death may be the outcome. Pressures from population growth are also felt in industrialized nations. Although food may be plentiful, overcrowding leads to pollution, stress, disease, and violence. Each of these challenges represents a major barrier to economic growth. The poor suffer this burden of excess mortality and morbidity disproportionately. Thus improving quality of life (QOL) through health promotion, effective health care delivery systems, and the enhancement of the environmental infrastructure will address the origins of poverty and ultimately increase productivity and improve QOL.

World population distribution is uneven. Over 50% of the population lives in China, India, the former Soviet Union, the United States, and Indonesia. In 2004, 40% of the world population consisted of children, 12% of elderly, 80 million lived in developing countries, and approximately 6 million lived in developed countries (WHO, 2004). In developed countries, the life expectancy was 70 to 84 years of age and in developing countries, it was 39 to 65 years of age (WHO, 1999). Malcolm Potts, a world-renowned population theorist, predicted that "by the twenty-first century the world may end up divided not into political or economic groups but by demographic structure," where countries will be classified into slow-growth or fast-growth countries instead of rich or poor countries. This will eventually further divide the rich and poor (Potts, 1994).

As the world population grows, a global trend toward urbanization occurs; people live closer together and migrate to urban areas for employment. For example, in 1975, 38.5% of the world's population lived in urban areas. By 1994, the proportion of urban dwellers swelled to 45%; this proportion is expected to reach 50% by 2015 (United Nations Population Fund, 1998). With increasingly dense living arrangements and global travel, the health of the general population is threatened by environmental factors and disease (e.g., the avian influenza pandemic).

ENVIRONMENTAL FACTORS

The relationship between humans and their environment is an important component of individual and global health. The field of environmental health and sustainable development has exploded since 1990. Environmental stressors are categorized into five types. First, stressors such as lead poisoning and air pollution directly assault human health. Second, stressors such as the effects of air pollution on products and structures damage society's goods and services. Third, stressors such as noise and litter affect QOL. Fourth, stressors such as global warming interfere with the ecological balance. Finally, natural disasters, terrorism, and war affect all of the above.

Air, water, and land pollution are among the consequences of environmental stressors. For example, 50% of the worldwide air pollution problem is attributable to the chemical pollutant carbon monoxide. Other primary pollutants, such as nitrogen monoxide, sulfur oxides, particulate matter, and hydrocarbons, combine with carbon monoxide to create 90% of the world's pollution. In developing countries, only 75% of the urban population and 50% of the rural population have sanitation facilities, which is a significant contributing factor to water pollution.

Agricultural, industrial, residential, and commercial wastes increase land pollution. For example, chemical fertilizers have displaced natural fertilizers; synthetic pesticides have displaced natural means of pest control; and petrochemical products, such as detergents, synthetic fiber, and plastics, have replaced soap, cotton, and paper. Disposable goods have replaced reusable goods, resulting in increased waste. Production technologies are contributing to worldwide environmental and ecological stress.

PATTERNS OF HEALTH AND DISEASE

Lifestyles, health and cultural beliefs, infrastructure, economics, and politics affect existing illnesses and society's commitment to prevention. Disease patterns vary throughout the world; therefore primary causes of mortality differ in developed and developing countries. Cardiovascular disease (CVD), cancer, respiratory disease, stroke, violence, and traumatic injury are the primary causes of mortality in developed countries. Infections, malnutrition, and violence are the primary causes of mortality in developing countries; however, CVDs are becoming more prevalent (Labarthe, 1998). Once plagued with high rates of infectious disease, developed countries significantly reduced high mortality rates from these diseases through improved sanitation, nutrition, immunization, and improved medical care. A **developed country** has a more stable economy and a wide range of industrial and technological development. These countries experience an epidemiological transition, for example, the morbidity and mortality profile of a country changes from **a lesser developed country** profile to a developed country profile. For example, many developed countries experienced an epidemiological transition from having an infectious disease profile to having a chronic disease profile and are now plagued by chronic diseases such as CVD, respiratory disease, and cancer, secondary to air pollution and the tobacco use pandemic. This altered profile has created a demographic transition from traditional societies, where almost everyone is young, to societies with rapidly increasing numbers of middle-age and elderly people.

Among the infectious diseases that contribute to high rates of mortality in developing countries are AIDS, TB, endemic malaria, hepatitis B, rheumatic heart disease, parasitic infection, and dengue fever. These diseases claim the lives of millions, yet the World Bank (2002) estimated that these diseases could be reduced by up to 50% through effective public health interventions. Many of these diseases will join smallpox as a disease known only to history through the development and implementation of immunization programs or to the twenty-first century threats of bioterrorism. Immunization is the most powerful and cost-effective strategy at our disposal for many infectious diseases (Centers for Disease Control, 2005). TB recommendations included in the "Commission for Africa" report were presented to world leaders attending the G8 summit in Scotland in 2005. The paper calls for wealthy nations to double their aid to Africa in order to rebuild systems to deliver public health services, provide staff training, develop new medicines, and provide better sexual and reproductive health services. The WHO "two diseases, one patient" strategy should be supported to provide integrated TB and HIV care; 70% of the 14 million people worldwide who have both HIV and TB are in Africa (WHO, 2005b). The bacille Calmette-Guérin (BCG) vaccine series induces active immunity, but it does not reduce the transmission of infectious types of TB. At least one third of the world's population harbors the TB pathogen, *Mycobacterium tuberculosis*. The WHO programs "Roll Back Malaria," "Stop TB," "HIV/AIDS Control," and "Tobacco Free Initiative (TFI)" and more recently, "Avian Influenza Pandemic Preparedness" target key infectious and chronic disease issues of the twenty-first century.

AIDS is an enormous global concern. The WHO "3 by 5 Initiative" proposed treating 3 million people living with HIV/AIDS by the end of 2005. In 2004, over 28.5 million adults and children were estimated to be living with AIDS in sub-Saharan Africa, and 40 million adults and children worldwide were living with this disease. The total number of AIDS deaths since the beginning of the epidemic is 30 million; 40 million more are infected (WHO, 2003).

Although AIDS is a global epidemic, it varies demographically in different parts of the world. For example, the estimated male-female ratio of HIV infections in North America is 5:2, whereas in Africa the ratio is 1:1 (WHO, 2004). Urbanization and within-country migration also play a role in the spread of AIDS. For instance, in Rwanda the HIV seroprevalence is 14 to 20 times higher in urban areas versus rural areas. Annually, HIV threatens more lives as more people migrate to the world's largest cities. The United Nations estimates that by the year 2010, 50% of the developing world will live in cities. This is an increase from 25% in 1970.

Malaria is a life-threatening parasitic disease transmitted by mosquitoes. Today approximately 40% of the world's population is at risk for malaria. Malaria is found throughout the tropical and subtropical regions of the world and causes more than 300 million acute illnesses and at least 1 million deaths annually. Malaria kills an African child every 30 seconds. Effective low-cost strategies are available for its prevention, treatment, and control, including insecticide-treated nets and new generation medications, including artemisinin-based combination therapies (WHO, 2005a). Efforts are ongoing to develop an antitrust malarial vaccine.

With over 450,000 tobacco-related deaths in the United States each year and 4.9 million worldwide, tobacco control is a critical component of the international health care agenda. By 2020, an estimated one in seven deaths will be tobacco related. Since 1990, tobacco policies have been implemented at various political levels in the United States and abroad with 20 states and 10 countries enacting smoke-free worksites and public places and 300 communities approving secondhand smoke ordinances and policies. The magnitude and consequences of the tobacco pandemic, however, were unexpected. Smoking prevention and cessation programs, state and federal mandates, tobacco taxation, the tobacco settlement, antitobacco media campaigns, strict licensing of tobacco retailers, the elimination of tobacco vending machines and point-of-sale advertising, and the elimination of tobacco sales by pharmacies have made an impact on tobacco sales in the United States. Due to health concerns and cost, many countries from Ireland to New Zealand have developed tobacco-free policies. Although American adults have enrolled in cessation programs, the tobacco industry has targeted youth (young adults 18 to 24 years of age), increasing smoking rates in this population from 22% in 1996 to 29% in 2002. The industry has dramatically increased international exports as well (Novak, 2005). A global commitment to tobacco control can avert millions of premature deaths in the next half century.

The **WHO Tobacco Free Initiative (TFI)** group, in furthering the aims and objectives of the WHO Framework Convention on Tobacco Control (tobacco product regulation provisions) and upon the recommendation of the WHO Study Group on Tobacco Product Regulation, convened the first meeting of the WHO Tobacco Laboratory Network in The Hague on April 28-29, 2005. Proposed activities include the following:

- Assess capabilities of each member and make an inventory.
- Conduct collaborative study on smokeless tobacco.
- Initiate a quality management program that will lead to accreditation in the future.
- Develop and initiate training programs and capacity building.
- Establish a communication channel for network members, including a website and an expert panel for assistance.
- Develop a compendium of expanded testing methods for tobacco product emissions and contents.
- Participate in international standardization activities.
- Define periodic meetings for scientific research, exchange of information, and to identify research priorities and agendas.

- Exchange information with policy makers and regulators (WHO, 2005).

The global approach to tobacco control can guide the development of effective interventions based upon best evidence and best practice. Countering potential threats to health resulting from economic crises, unhealthful environments, or risky behavior is critical. Promotion of a healthy lifestyle underpins a proactive strategy for risk reduction, tobacco use prevention and cessation, immunization provision, cleaner air and water, adequate sanitation, healthful diets, fitness and exercise programs, and safe transportation.

INTERNATIONAL ORGANIZATIONS

Promoting worldwide health is humankind's greatest challenge. Several global agencies, such as the **World Health Organization (WHO),** the **Pan American Health Organization (PAHO), United Nations International Children's Fund (UNICEF),** the **World Bank,** and the **Centers for Disease Control and Prevention (CDC),** play important roles in improving the health of all nations. Founded in 1948, WHO is an international health agency of the United Nations that consists of countries working toward "health for all by the year 2000." This goal was instituted at the Alma-Ata conference in the USSR in 1978. The conference defined "health for all" as "the attainment by all citizens of the world by the year 2000 of a level of health that will permit them to lead a socially and economically productive life" (WHO, 1999, p. 65). The central goal of health for all was not attained; therefore the target year for achievement has been extended to 2010.

The Alma-Ata conference on primary heath care expressed the need for urgent action by all governments. The WHO statement of beliefs, goals, and objectives are outlined in the Declaration of Alma-Ata, which is presented in Box 32-1. The concept of primary health care stresses health as a fundamental human right for individuals, families, and communities; the unacceptability of the gross inequalities and disparities in health status; the importance of community involvement; and the active role of all sectors. Primary health care seeks to obtain the highest level of health care for all people. The program promotes seven elements of primary health care, including health education regarding disease prevention and cure, proper food supply and nutrition, adequate supply of safe drinking water and sanitation, maternal and child health care, immunizations, control of endemic diseases, and the provision of essential drugs.

According to WHO, a primary health care system should provide the entire population with the following: universal coverage; relevant, acceptable, affordable, and effective services; a spectrum of comprehensive services that provide for primary, secondary, and tertiary care and prevention; active community involvement in the planning and delivery of services; and integration of health services with development activities to ensure that complete nutritional, educational, occupational, environmental, and safe housing needs are met (Bryant, 1984).

PAHO is an international public health agency with nearly a century of experience in working to improve the health and living standards of the Americas. It serves as the regional office of WHO and is recognized as part of the United Nations system.

UNICEF is another important global health organization. Founded in 1946 to assist children in war-ravaged Europe, UNICEF works for children's survival, development, and protection by developing and implementing community-based programs. UNICEF achievements are well documented in child health, nutrition, education, water, sanitation, and progress for women. UNICEF collaborates with WHO as an advocate for child health and women's health.

The major goal of the World Bank is to facilitate significant interventions to improve the health status of individuals living in areas that lack economic development. Projects range from safe water to effective sanitation to affordable housing. Financial assistance for the education of health care providers; the improvement of internal infrastructures; and funding for projects related to health status, disease control, and prevention has been provided.

The CDC is located in Atlanta, Georgia. The CDC is one of the 13 major operating components of the U.S. Department of Health and Human Services (USDHHS), which is the principal agency in the U.S. government for protecting the health and safety of all Americans and for providing essential human services, especially for those people who are least able to help themselves.

Since it was founded in 1946 to help control malaria, CDC has remained at the forefront of public health efforts to prevent and control infectious and chronic diseases, injuries, workplace hazards, disabilities, and environmental health threats. Today, CDC is globally recognized for conducting research and investigations and for its action-oriented approach. CDC applies research and findings to improve people's daily lives and responds to health emergencies—something that distinguishes CDC from many of its peer agencies. The CDC is committed to achieving true improvements in people's health. To do this, the agency is defining specific health impact goals to prioritize and focus its work and investments and measure progress (CDC, 2005).

Through the **International Council of Nurses (ICN),** nursing has been internationally involved at a professional level for more than 100 years. The ICN and its member associations have addressed current and future nursing and health care needs. Nursing research, advanced practice nursing, doctoral education, first responder, disaster preparedness, mass casualty, policy, and advocacy have received increased emphasis over the past decade in ICN and other nursing organizations worldwide.

INTERNATIONAL HEALTH CARE DELIVERY SYSTEMS

When comparing health care systems, developed and developing countries can learn much from each other. Although transferring specialized medical technologies from developed to developing countries may not always be appropriate,

BOX 32-1 Declaration of Alma-Ata

The International Conference on Primary Health Care, meeting in Alma-Ata this twelfth day of September in the year Nineteen hundred and seventy-eight, expressing the need for urgent action by all governments, all health and development workers, and the world community to protect and promote the health of all the people of the world, hereby makes the following Declaration:

I. The Conference strongly reaffirms that health, which is a state of complete physical, mental, and social well-being and not merely the absence of disease or infirmity, is a fundamental human right and that the attainment of the highest possible level of health is a most important worldwide social goal, whose realization requires the action of many other social and economic sectors in addition to the health sector.

II. The existing gross inequality in the health status of the people, particularly between developed and developing countries and within countries, is politically, socially, and economically unacceptable and is therefore of common concern to all countries.

III. Economic and social development, based on a New International Economic Order, is of basic importance to the fullest attainment of health for all and to the reduction of the gap between the health status of developing and developed countries. The promotion and protection of the health of the people are essential to sustained economic and social development and contribute to a better quality of life and to world peace.

IV. The people have the right and duty to participate individually and collectively in the planning and implementation of their health care.

V. Governments have a responsibility for the health of their people, which can be fulfilled only by the provision of adequate health and social measures. In the coming decades, a main social target of governments, international organizations, and the whole world community should be the attainment by all peoples of the world by the year 2000 of a level of health that will permit them to lead a socially and economically productive life. Primary health care is the key to attaining this target as part of development in the spirit of social justice.

VI. Primary health care is essential health care based on practical, scientifically sound, and socially acceptable methods and technology made universally accessible to individuals and families in the community through their full participation and at a cost that the community and country can afford to maintain at every stage of their development in the spirit of self-reliance and self-determination. It forms an integral part both of the country's health system, of which primary health care is the central function and main focus, and of the overall social and economic development of the community. It is the first level of contact for individuals, the family, and the community with the national health system bringing health care as close as possible to where people live and work and it constitutes the first element of a continuing health care process.

VII. Primary health care:

1. reflects and evolves from the economic conditions and sociocultural and political characteristics of the country and its communities and is based on the application of the relevant results of social, biomedical, and health services research and public health experience;

2. addresses the main health problems in the community, providing promotive, preventive, curative, and rehabilitative services accordingly;

3. includes at least education concerning prevailing health problems and the methods of preventing and controlling them; promotion of food supply and proper nutrition; an adequate supply of safe water and basic sanitation; maternal and child health care, including family planning; immunization against the major infectious diseases; prevention and control of locally endemic diseases; appropriate treatment of common diseases and injuries; and provision of essential drugs;

4. involves, in addition to health sector, all related sectors and aspects of national and community development, in particular agriculture, animal husbandry, food industry, education, housing, public works, communication, and other sectors; and demands the coordinated efforts of all those sectors;

5. requires and promotes maximum community and individual self-reliance and participation in the planning, organization, operation, and control of primary health care making fullest use of local, national, and other available resources; and to this end, develops through appropriate education the ability of communities to participate;

6. should be sustained by integrated, functional, and mutually supportive referral levels, on health workers, including physicians, nurses, midwives, auxiliaries, and community workers, as applicable, and on traditional practitioners as needed, suitably trained socially and technically to work as a health team and to respond to the expressed health needs of the community; and

7. relies, at local and referral levels, on health workers, including physicians, nurses, midwives, auxiliaries, and community workers, as applicable, and on traditional practitioners as needed, suitably trained socially and technically to work as a health team and to respond to the expressed health needs of the community.

VIII. All governments should formulate national policies, strategies, and plans of action to launch and sustain primary health care as part of a comprehensive national health system and in coordination with other sectors. To this end, it will be necessary to exercise political will, to mobilize the country's resources, and to use available external resources rationally.

IX. All countries should cooperate in a spirit of partnership and service to ensure primary health care for all people because the attainment of health by people in any one country directly concerns and benefits every other country. In this context the joint WHO-UNICEF report on primary health care constitutes a solid basis for the further development and operation of Primary Health Care through the world.

X. An acceptable level of health for all the people of the world by the year 2000 can be attained through a fuller and better use of the world's resources, a considerable part of which is now spent on armaments and military conflicts. A genuine policy of independence, peace, détente, and disarmament could and should release additional resources that could well be devoted to peaceful aims and in particular to the acceleration of social and economic development of which primary health care, as an essential part, should be allotted its proper share.

The International Conference on Primary Health Care calls for urgent and effective national and international action to develop and implement primary health care throughout the world and particularly in developing countries in a spirit of technical cooperation and in keeping with a New International Economic Order. It urges governments, WHO and UNICEF, and other international organizations, and multilateral and bilateral agencies, non-governmental organizations, funding agencies, all health workers and the whole world community to support national and international commitment to primary health care and to channel increased technical and financial support to it, particularly in developing countries. The Conference calls on all the aforementioned to collaborate in introducing, developing and maintaining primary health care in accordance with the spirit and content of this Declaration.

Reprinted, by permission, from Alma-Ata: *Primary health care, report of the international conference on primary health care,* "Health for All" Series, No 1, pp. 2-6, Geneva, Sept 6-12, 1978, World Health Organization.

developing countries are currently learning from health care reform policies and the technological revolution in developed countries. Likewise, developed countries have much to learn about low-technology initiatives such as oral rehydration therapy for the treatment of diarrhea and the delivery of primary health care as defined by the WHO. Participatory approaches to health care delivery, such as community involvement in health and education, are also essential. This exchange is important given the state of the current health care policy in developed countries. Many developed countries have made health care inaccessible to portions of their general public.

Even in countries with socialized medicine, medical costs increase annually and citizens are faced with paying supplemental medical fees or copayment. There is a need to expand the knowledge base that made the twentieth-century health care revolution possible. In the twenty-first century, it is critical to provide research and development that is relevant to infectious diseases that overwhelmingly affect the poor. In addition, it is necessary to systematically generate an information base that countries can use to shape the future of their health care system (WHO, 2004). Nurses must think more broadly about potential collaborators in solving the problems of the health care delivery system. Disciplines such as industrial engineering have much to offer nursing and the other health care professionals, as engineering principles are applied to information technology, system design, patient safety, medication administration, simulated learning, chronic disease management, and hospital and clinic development, design and renovation. The Doctor of Nursing Practice (DNP) was developed by nursing leaders and endorsed by the American Association of Colleges of Nursing in order to reengineer health care (Wall, Novak, and Wilkerson, 2005). Eleven programs have admitted DNP students with 190 programs in developmental phase.

The Lalonde report (1974) proposed the "health field concept" as a useful way to consider the determinants of health such as biology, lifestyle, environment, and health services. This report emphasized lifestyle and environment as determinants of health outside the traditional medical sphere. It became the basis for rethinking new paradigms for health care delivery. "The Lalonde report signified the beginning of a paradigm shift in health care away from the traditional medical model to a more holistic system-environment perspective" (Boothroyd and Eberle, 1990, p. 2). However, in the subsequent decade, policy makers focused more attention on individual lifestyle change (Hoffman and Dupont, 1985) and implemented health education programs targeting healthier personal lifestyles. Using both education and income levels as measures of socioeconomic status, strong, positive relationships have been observed for various health indicators, including QOL, health status, and preventive health practices (Adams, 1993).

In the 1980s and 1990s, the rising costs of health care were a major catalyst for change, focusing attention on the need to provide alternative models of care. Day surgery and outpatient services, nurse-managed clinics, ambulatory care, and home care provide alternatives to hospital-based care. In each of these areas, the nurse plays a prominent role and has the potential to bring a needed dimension of health promotion and disease prevention to individuals, families, communities, and systems.

In 2004, U.S. expenditures for health care made up 14.6% of the gross domestic product (American Public Health Association, 2004). However, more than 48 million Americans under the age of 65 are uninsured and cannot afford health care (National Center for Health Statistics, 2005). A market-based developed country such as the United States treats health care as a market commodity; therefore it focuses on curative medicine rather than preventive medicine because it creates more capital. A market-based health care system could lead to a goal opposite that of health for all. Theoretically, the advent of the managed care system in the United States proposed a capitated model to cut health care costs. Few managed care models, however, propose universal access or the comprehensive primary health care that WHO advocates.

Given the two basic health care systems, market-based and population-based, and the fact that countries at different levels of development need to learn from each other, it is evident that a single model of health care delivery is not appropriate for every country. For example, in 1985, Cuba was recognized for reaching WHO's goal of "health for all." Cuba began to demonstrate to the world that health care could be provided as a basic human right rather than a privilege. In addition, Canada developed a universal health care system and Canadian community health nurses (CHNs) created innovative models for practice. Canada's Achieving Health for All provided a health promotion framework that includes fostering public participation in decisions that affect health, strengthening community health service networks with the disadvantaged communities they serve, and coordinating public health policy efforts (Epp, 1996).

The pressure for change provides the opportunity for reform and the broad goal of health for all should guide this reform. Effective health care delivery systems must increase access and efficiency; improve health status through health promotion and disease prevention; eliminate health disparities; and protect individuals and families from financial loss due to catastrophic illness.

The Role of the Community Health Nurse in International Health Care

In a rapidly changing health care environment, the nursing role is becoming less traditional and much more diverse. The traditional structure of provider roles is challenged as professional disciplines are recruited to provide expanded and diverse health care services. The nursing role is reciprocal, and it is interdependent with clients and families, physicians, and other health care professionals. The nurse's role expectations and societal expectations influence the formation of behavior patterns specific to the professional nursing role. These expectations provide the basis for the role of the community health nurse (CHN) in international health care.

Florence Nightingale was the first nurse to establish international links and networks that became vastly important to her own country and to nursing throughout the world. Every

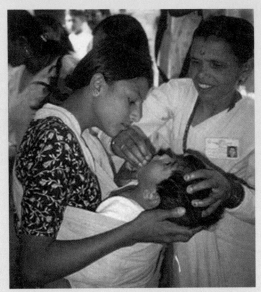

Nepalese child receives vitamin A supplement. Over 3 million Nepali children are now receiving twice-yearly vitamin A supplements in a program instituted by the U.S. Agency for International Development (USAID). Approximately 15,000 child deaths are averted each year in Nepal as a result of this program. (From U.S. Agency for International Development, Washington, DC [http://www.usaid.gov.])

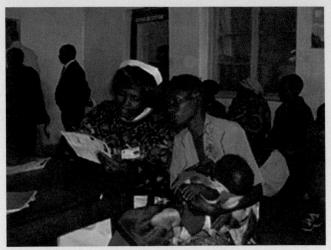

Malaria is the number one killer among children in Tanzania. A child health nurse consults with a mother at a maternal-child health clinic in Iringa, Tanzania. (From U.S. Agency for International Development, Washington, DC [http://www.usaid.gov.] John Dunlop.)

India has the second largest number of HIV-infected people in the world. The *Saadhan* (meaning "key" or "solution") clinics in India, supported by the U.S. Agency for International Development (USAID) in partnership with Population Services International, offer high-quality voluntary counseling and testing services and appropriate follow-up, all key factors in reducing HIV transmission. This *Saadhan* mobile clinic, which serves transient populations, provides HIV counseling and testing, and treatment of sexually transmitted infections. (From U.S. Agency for International Development, Washington, DC [http://www.usaid.gov.])

obstacle to health and wellness confronted her. She confronted these obstacles and overcame them systematically. This legacy serves as the foundation for CHNs in the global health care arena. Nightingale channeled her energies into all aspects of health from the care of wounded soldiers at Scutari in the Crimea to the broad public policies that affected health in her time (Splane and Splane, 1997).

CHNs seek to ensure the attainment of health for all in a cost-effective health care system. They must be involved in research, community assessment, planning, implementation, management, evaluation, health services delivery, disaster preparedness and emergency response, health policy, advocacy, and legislation. Nurses in all countries coordinate their work with other health care personnel and community leaders. Health for all requires attitudes, levels of competence, knowledge, and skills that differ substantially from those required in traditional nursing. The changes in the health environment, such as technological advancements, changes in the morbidity and mortality patterns of the population, and social and political changes, all form the basis for the nursing role.

Community health nursing is similar in both developed and developing countries; it has similar components of physical care, safety, social norms, interpersonal processes, economic factors, and community cohesion (Kupina, 1995). With the development of the nurse practitioner (NP) role over the past 40 years in the United States and over the past 20 years abroad, nurses with advanced degrees and areas of specialization have strengthened the community-based health care system. The development of the new Doctor of Nursing Practice (DNP) in the United States and PhDs in nursing in a variety of countries further elevates the knowledge and skill base for nursing's role in reengineering health care (Wall, Novak, and Wilkerson, 2005).

As primary health care and primary care may be practiced differently in other countries, the NP and the CHN face a challenge (Barnes et al., 1995). **Primary health care** refers to essential services that support a healthy life. It involves access, availability, service delivery, community participation, and the citizen's right to health care. In contrast, **primary care** refers to first line or point-of-access medical and nursing care controlled by providers and focused on the individual. Primary care may not be the norm, particularly in communities in developing or lesser developed countries that have overwhelming needs for basic necessities such as safe drinking water and sanitation. The needs of the group outweigh the needs of the individual.

Nurses can make a difference in helping solve the existing and emerging health problems in countries throughout the world. The advent of technology has enhanced global communication and facilitated travel. It is important that nurses throughout the world understand each other and learn from each another. Nurses are the most valuable assets of any health care system. Community health nursing can improve access to care for the most vulnerable and hard-to-reach groups in any country. Community health nursing, in its many forms, continues to be relevant and will expand in the future. The future will demand an increase in information technology, international projects, educational endeavors, and research. CHNs are a key factor in the cost-effective delivery of care to individuals, families, and communities.

RESEARCH IN INTERNATIONAL HEALTH

Since 1990, international nursing research has focused predominantly on the following three areas: (1) student and faculty educational exchange programs, (2) diverse clinical experiences, and (3) the international development of home care or transition from hospital to home.

WHO collaborating centers in nursing provide a framework for research, education, and service delivery partnerships. Duquesne University, an affiliate of George Mason University's WHO Collaborating Center in Nursing, developed an education and service partnership model for their work in Nicaragua (White and Smith, 1998). Purdue University and the University of Virginia, both affiliates of Case Western Reserve University and the University of Mexico WHO Collaborating Centers, contributed to a partnership for educational programming, clinical practice, and research for graduate students in Primary Health Care Nursing and Community Health.

Crigger et al. (2004) focused on ethical issues related to introducing antibiotic resistance into the second and third world community assessment and clinic development in Honduras while O'Neil and Altman immerse their Spanish for Health Care Professionals nursing students in orphanages and clinics in Nicaragua (2006). Squires (1998) described models that focus on chronic conditions such as hypertension, diabetes, and cancer. Land (1998) described projects in Latin America and the Caribbean that focus on health promotion, epidemiology, surveillance, mental health, and refugee care.

U.S. models of home health care are developing in many countries. These models provide a variety of services to bridge the gap between the hospital and community-based care. Sources of home care include home visits by nurses from official government public health agencies, nonprofit voluntary agencies, and for-profit home care agencies. Examples of home care services include assistance with activities of daily living, treatment, rehabilitation, transportation, and respite for caregivers.

Home care service providers in the United States and abroad face many challenges. Estimating financial implications and calculating potential caseloads are complex factors in the design of effective delivery systems. Inadequate hospital assessment, insufficient discharge planning and referral, restrictive or irrelevant policies regarding eligibility, failure to discharge clients from home care when services are unnecessary, and an inability to find less costly service as clients gain independence are other significant influencing variables (Gagnon, 1994). Barkauskas and Seskivicius (1998) described the development of home health care in Lithuania. Milstead, Keller, and Miller (1998) focused on similarities and differences in community and home health care in Holland, and Ross (1998) described a transcultural home health experience between Nicaraguan and U.S. nursing students, with an emphasis on program planning with limited resources.

CASE STUDY   Application of International Community Assessment

INTERNATIONAL COMMUNITY ASSESSMENT MODEL (ICAM): A COLLABORATIVE MODEL FOR COMMUNITY ASSESSMENT, EDUCATION, AND HEALTH CARE DELIVERY

In Mexico and Nicaragua, the provision of equitable health care services to a population that is geographically and educationally disparate is both economically and logistically challenging. Rural Mexico and Nicaragua are further challenged by a lack of infrastructure necessary for health promotion, protection, and maintenance. Smoking rates have increased over the past two decades in both countries. In planning intervention programs for the tobacco use problem, nurses need a globally diverse assessment tool and methodology to empower communities in developing countries to achieve health care goals and reduce health care costs. U.S. nursing students gaining international health care experience in a community in rural developing countries, including Mexico and Nicaragua, can implement the International Community Assessment Model (ICAM) (Figure 32-1) prior to planning targeted programs with local community leaders. The ICAM is currently being tested in rural Mexico and

Nicaragua as part of an ongoing project. U.S. nursing students are studying tobacco use prevention and effective cessation and would like to compare and contrast practices in various countries.

Nurses can collaborate with health and environmental experts in implementing a community empowerment framework (Querreno et al., 1998). In community empowerment, the community identifies its problems and a plan of action, and environmental experts and nurses remain consultants and team members to assist community members (May, Mendelson, and Ferketich, 1995). This process aids the community in developing interventions that are culturally acceptable, breaking down cultural barriers. In developing countries, health-promotion programs that do not involve community participation and education often fail after the experts leave the community (Yates, 1997).

ASSESSMENT

During the assessment phase, the nurse identifies key influential community members and leaders and encourages them to join a board of community members with the goal of assessing community health. The community board members may choose to use the ICAM for the purpose of providing

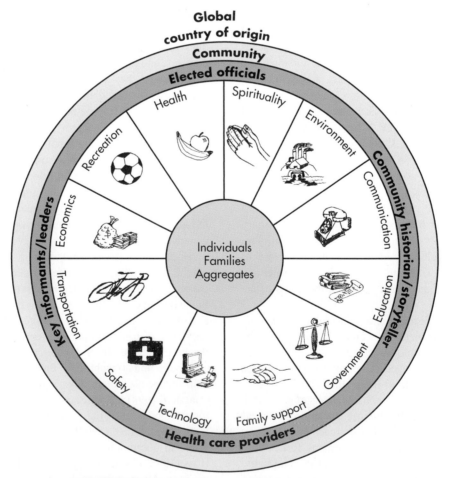

FIGURE 32-1 International Community Assessment Model.

a globally diverse assessment framework. Assessment of community culture helps identify potential cultural barriers to nursing interventions. The center of the model assesses the heart of the community's culture by identifying individual, family, and community characteristics, including their history, demographics, values, beliefs, rituals, and the effect of these characteristics on social and economic conditions.

The ICAM assesses the following:

- *Recreation:* Community cardiovascular fitness; stress management; energy renewal; and relaxation through sports, hobbies, and games.
- *Perceptions:* Community perceptions of health, including community members' physical, social, and mental balance and lifestyle choices related to tobacco use.
- *Spirituality:* The community's religious beliefs and practices.
- *Support systems:* Family support systems, including parental support of children and adult children, adult children's support of their parents, and support among extended family members. (*Family* is defined as a group of individuals who share common experiences and goals and are often linked together by genetics, marriage, living situation, or a common emotional bond.)

The physical environment encompasses the community's infrastructure, including homes, water sources, waste disposal sites, roadways, buildings for businesses and shops, factories, power lines, and considerations related to occupational health including exposure to secondhand smoke.

The ICAM also assesses the following:

- *Education:* The concept of education reflects the community's knowledge, skills, level of schooling or training, and literacy rate.
- *Transportation:* Transportation is defined as how community members travel from point A to point B.
- *Safety:* Evaluation of the community's safety includes examining potential dangers in the community that could lead to injury or death and examining safety measures and plans developed by the community to prevent these problems.
- *Government and politics:* How the community is governed or ruled is examined.
- *Economy:* The efficacy of economic resources are analyzed. (*Economy* is defined in terms of the "production, dispersal, and expenditure of resources," Neufeldt and Guralnik, 1997, p. 429.)
- *Communication:* Communication is evaluated by examining face-to-face and communitywide information exchange through speech, body language, writing, and drawings. Key components of the community's communication are native languages and forms of communication, such as letters, telephone, computer networks, the Internet, fax machines, television, billboards, signs, magazines, newspapers, and telegrams.
- *Access:* Electricity, public sanitation, public water systems, radio, television, technology, fax machines, libraries, computers, Internet, industrial machinery, and

agricultural practices and technology access also must be examined.

The ICAM will allow the board to examine all the public health threats to the community and additional barriers to an effective, culturally tailored campaign related to tobacco use education, prevention, and cessation.

The ICAM also reflects the importance of assessing the country of origin and global effects on the community. When assessing a community, the nurse must consider the external factors affecting the community. For example, the economy depends upon vendors, other Mexican states, and the international purchasing of their main exports. The marketing strategies of the tobacco industry must also be considered for effective counter intervention design.

After the community assessment, the collaborative team should develop an educational program that identifies potential problems with a tobacco education, prevention and cessation campaign. This program should motivate board members to identify these problems and then search for effective solutions. As board members become further aware of the health hazards of individual tobacco use, employee exposure, and other types of secondhand smoke, resources should be provided that will aid in their response.

Next, the community board members should be assisted in completing a survey and offering focus groups related to needs assessment and attitudes related to tobacco use.

The nursing team, local experts, key community informants, and the board need to establish the diagnosis in a collaborative manner.

PLANNING AND INTERVENTION

If tobacco use and health care costs remain the central issue for the board and community, the board will enter the planning phase of the campaign. Community board members can collaborate with environmental experts and the nurse to identify individual, family, and community goals and objectives to education and interventions related to tobacco use prevention and cessation based upon best evidence and practice.

The collaborative team will subsequently analyze possible interventions. This body of knowledge will allow the community board members to determine which, if any, of the proposed interventions would be relevant and appropriate for their community. In addition, they may be able to apply these ideas in creating their own interventions. When the community board members have selected or developed an intervention for their project, they can be encouraged to create strategies to educate the community.

IMPLEMENTATION

Before the project is implemented, the community awareness of the need for the campaign must be clear. The community must be given the opportunity to provide the board with feedback on proposed interventions. The board should be willing to compromise to meet the community's needs. After

Continued

CASE STUDY   Application of International Community Assessment (cont'd)

the communitywide education has occurred and necessary consensus and compromise have been achieved, the project can be implemented. At this point, the community members are trained to maintain the project. Once the implementation is completed, evaluation of the project can begin to ensure that the goals and objectives of the board are met.

EVALUATION

The collaborative team should evaluate the project in a formative and summative manner monthly and annually. In addition, the nurse should conduct community surveys to determine if members continue to recognize the need for the campaign and to provide feedback related to progress. The ICAM is being tested in rural Mexico and Nicaragua as part of an ongoing project. The targeted communities have a high incidence of poverty. As a result, 80% of the communities reside in crowded living conditions. Many factors in the community pose serious health threats, secondhand smoke, farm chemicals, air pollution from nearby cities, and so on.

Field workers are often powerless and have minimal recourse when exposed to unhealthy environmental contaminants causing increased morbidity and mortality.

The top three causes of mortality in the communities are cardiac disorders, diabetes, and automobile accidents. The leading causes of morbidity are respiratory infections, diabetes, hypertension, and gastrointestinal illnesses. The community's high rate of gastrointestinal illness is related to poor access to potable water. The community historians, community political leaders, key employers, full-time staff at nurse-run clinics, local community health faculty, and the *pasantes* (i.e., nursing graduates who have completed 1 year of community service at nurse-run clinics and public health agencies) are critical to the success of the project.

A multidisciplinary team of key influential community members, environmental experts, and nurses will further assess the community using the ICAM model. The goal of this assessment will be to assist the community members in further diagnosing the community's health care needs related to tobacco use and other issues as they are identified. Nurses will collaborate with community board members to develop culturally acceptable interventions. After the interventions are developed, the community board, clinic staff, and *pasantes* will continue to evaluate the effectiveness of these interventions, promoting a sense of ownership of the project in the community and helping to ensure improvements in health care long after the multidisciplinary team leaves the community.

SUMMARY

Community public health nurses face many exciting challenges in health care reform and designing effective systems of health care delivery. These include being responsive to emerging needs and health issues in the population, developing multidisciplinary practice models that adhere to the principles of primary health care in the context of a reengineered health care system, and mobilizing research dissemination and practice implementation strategies to ensure evidence-based practice as the norm rather than the exception. There is still much to be done to meet the challenge of WHO's goal of "Health for All by the Year 2010." Studying the progress achieved in other countries is critical; however, success will ultimately depend on society's commitment to achieve higher levels of health and well-being for all.

LEARNING ACTIVITIES

1. Discuss population characteristics and the threat of population growth on health and health care systems.
2. Compare and contrast the incidence and treatment of people living with AIDS, TB, and malaria. Discuss methods of prevention.
3. Explain the incidence of death from AIDS in Africa, Mexico, and the United States. What might account for the differences?
4. Compare population-focused nursing in a developing country with community health nursing in the community. How are they the same and how do they differ?
5. Conduct research and compare the rates of life expectancy and infant mortality in Africa, Mexico, and the United States. What factors might account for the similarities in rates between the developing and the developed countries?
6. Describe the key elements of an effective health care delivery system. Will the focus of future health care services reflect downstream thinking, or will the orientation uphold models of prevention and promotion that deal with root causes of health problems?
7. Test the International Community Assessment Model (ICAM) in a community. Evaluate its effectiveness.
8. Describe the worldwide tobacco use pandemic and local to global interventions for prevention and cessation of tobacco use.

REFERENCES

Adams O: Health status. In Stephens T, Fowler-Graham D, editors: *Canada's health promotion survey, 1990,* Technical Report, Ottawa, 1993, Ministry of Supply and Services.

Alma-Ata: *Primary health care, report of the international conference on primary health care,* "Health for All" Series, No 1, pp. 2-6, Geneva, Sept 6-12, 1978, World Health Organization.

American Public Health Association: *The nation's health,* The Author, http://www.apha.org/journal/nation/tnhsept99.htm.

Anderson ET, McFarlane JM: *Community-as-partner: theory and practice in nursing,* Philadelphia, 1995, Lippincott Williams & Wilkins.

Barkauskas VH, Seskevicius A: Development of home health care in Lithuania: current status and key development issues, *Home Health Care Manage Pract* 11(1):10-17, 1998.

Barnes D et al: Primary health care and primary care: a confusion of philosophies, *Nurs Outlook* 43:7-16, 1995.

Boothroyd P, Eberle M: *Healthy communities: what they are, how they're made,* CHS Research Bulletin, UBC Centre for Human Settlements, Vancouver, 1990, University of British Columbia.

Bryant J: Health services, manpower and universities in relation to health for all: an historical and future perspective, *Am J Public Health* 74:714-719, 1984.

Centers for Disease Control and Prevention: 2005, http://www.cdc.org.

Central Intelligence Agency: *World factbook,* 2005, The Author, http://www.cia.gov/cia/publications/factbook/fields/2119.html.

Crigger N et al: A model of antibiotic use in a lay Honduran population, *Int J Nurs Stud* 41(7):745-53, 2004

Epp J: *Achieving health for all: a framework for health promotion,* Ottawa, 1996, Health and Welfare Canada.

Gagnon AJ: *The effect of an early postpartum discharge program on competence in mothering: a randomized controlled trial,* doctoral dissertation, Montreal, 1994, McGill University.

Hanson BD: *Water and sanitation technologies: a trainer's manual,* Peace Corporations Information Collection and Exchange Training Manual T-32, 1985.

Hoffman K, Dupont JM: *Community health centres and community development,* Ottawa, 1985, Department of Health and Welfare of Canada, Minister of Supply and Services Canada.

Kupina PS: Community health CNSs and health care in the year 2000, *Clin Nurs Specialist* 9:188-198, 1995.

Labarthe DR: *Epidemiology and prevention of cardiovascular disease: a global challenge,* Gaithersburg, Md, 1998, Aspen.

Lalonde M: *A new perspective on the health of Canadians,* Ottawa, 1974, Minister of Supply and Services.

Land S: Community nursing in Latin America and the Caribbean home health care manager practice, *Nurs Outlook* 11(1):1-9, 1998.

May KM, Mendelson C, Ferketich S: Community empowerment in rural healthcare, *Public Health Nurs* 12(1):25-30, 1995.

Milstead JA, Keller AM, Miller MC: Focus on community: American and Dutch nurses share expertise, *Home Health Care Manage Pract* 11(1):18-23, 1998.

National Center for Health Statistics: *Health, United States: 1998,* Washington, DC, 1998, US Government Printing Office.

Neufeldt V, Guralnik DB, editors: *Webster's new world college dictionary,* ed 3, New York, MacMillan.

Novak J: Effective smoking cessation strategies, *Clin Lett Nurs Pract* 2(1):1-5, 1998.

O'Neil E and Altman M: Nicaragua experience, *Purdue Nurse,* Lafayette, Ind, 2006, Hayword Publishing.

Potts M: Common sense prevailing at population conference, *Lancet* 344:809, 1994.

Querreno R et al: *Key issues in health development: poverty and ill-health,* 1998, Division of Intensified Cooperation with Countries and People in Greatest Need, http://www.who.int/ico/key.htm.

Reiff FM et al: Low cost safe water for the world, a practical interim solution, *J Public Health Policy* 17(4):389-408, 1996.

Rosenkoetter MM: A framework for international healthcare consultations, *Nurs Outlook* 45(4):182-187, 1997.

Ross CA: Preparing American and Nicaraguan nurses to practice home health nursing in a transcultural experience, *Home Health Care Manage Pract* 11(1):66-70, 1998.

Rothman J: Three models of community organization practice, their mixing and phasing. In Cox FM et al, editors: *Strategies of community organization,* ed 3, Itasca, Ill, 1979, FE Peacock Publishers.

Splane VH, Splane R: *International nursing leaders past and present: current issues in nursing,* ed 5, St. Louis, 1997, Mosby.

Squires AP: Home health care in Mexico: an overview, *Home Health Care Manage Pract* 11(1):38-45, 1998.

UNAIDS: *HIV/AIDS report,* 1998, The Author, http://www.who.int/emc-hiv/.

United Nations Population Fund: *The state of world population 1995: decisions for development: women, empowerment and reproductive health,* Oxford, England, 1998, New Internationalist Publications.

Universidad Nacional Autonoma de Mexico Escuelo Nacional Enfermeria y Obstetrica; *San Luis community assessment,* unpublished document, 1998.

Wall B, Novak J, Wilkerson S: The Doctor of Nursing practice: reengineering healthcare, *J Nurs Educ* 44(9):396-403, 2005.

White JF, Smith CW: Developing an international nursing partnership in Nicaragua, *Int Nurs Rev* 44(1):13-18, 1998.

World Bank: *World Development Report 2002: investing in health,* Washington, DC, 2002, Oxford University Press.

World Health Organization: *The World Health Report 1999: making a difference,* Geneva, 1999, The Author.

World Health Organization: *Roll back malaria info sheet,* Geneva, 2005a, The Author, http://www.who.int/malaria/docs/Basicfacts.pdf.

World Health Organization: TB recommendations included in the "Commission for Africa" report, 2005b, The Author, http://www.who.int/tb/commission_for_africa/en/print.html.

World Health Organization: *The 3 by 5 initiative,* The Author, http://www.who.int/3by5/about/initiative/en/index.html.

33

Community Health Nursing: Making a Difference

Mary A. Nies ▪ Melanie McEwen ▪ Joan Bickes

MEDIA RESOURCES

Additional Material for Study, Review, and Further Exploration

evolve Website at http://evolve.elsevier.com/Nies

❖ Quiz ❖ Case Studies ❖ Content Updates ❖ Glossary ❖ WebLinks

OBJECTIVES

Upon completion of this chapter, the reader will be able to do the following:

1. Discuss how being a member of a population influences health.
2. Predict future community health issues based on shared population characteristics.
3. Describe the actions community health nurses (CHNs) may take to ensure that future trends and changes in the health care system will benefit the health care consumer.

CHAPTER OUTLINE

For most individuals, "medical care" focuses on a diagnosed disease process. However, nursing's focus goes beyond the traditional concept of health as the absence of disease, a definition that reflects health in medical or disease terms. Nurses are concerned with illness prevention and health promotion activities that serve individual patients, their families, and groups (e.g., childbirth preparation, parenting classes, or diabetes classes). Community health nursing extends the definition of health and nursing action to social units or aggregates at the community and population levels (e.g., schools, churches, workplaces).

Considering the individual in terms of his or her population is important in community health nursing. Many people in the community share common characteristics such as sex, age, education, income level, and occupation. These characteristics affect the health of families and communities and are important in determining their needs. Shared population characteristics also aid in determining interventions to meet the health needs of populations. Social interaction, political activity, values, and knowledge influence health priorities and resource allocation that affects the health of populations from local to national levels. CHNs can intervene and make a difference in these areas.

POPULATION VARIABLES THAT AFFECT HEALTH

Being a member of a population with shared characteristics may have a marked effect on health, whether these characteristics are age, ethnicity, environmental, or geographical factors. Shared population characteristics that may negatively influence health are deemed risk factors because they place a population at risk. These factors are important to public health and to community health nursing as they form the basis for assessment, planning, intervention, and evaluation. Although using the nursing process on behalf of individuals is important, implementing the nursing process at the population level has the potential to make positive changes based on an understanding of population characteristics.

Whether the needs or risks are based on age, social, or environmental characteristics, change at the population level will make the broadest impact on population health. For example, residents of a low-income neighborhood near a refinery in south Louisiana appealed to state and federal authorities to ensure safe air quality for their community. Likewise, the disabled population in San Francisco organized to advocate for their rights to equal opportunity in housing, education, and employment. Such activities require organized community planning and political activity.

This section illustrates how being a member of a population group can influence health. Areas described include socioeconomic status, gender, age, race and ethnicity, social interaction, environment, and geography and politics.

Socioeconomic Status

Socioeconomic status (SES) affects health in several ways. Those of lower SES have higher rates of morbidity and mortality than counterparts with higher SES. According to the World Health Organization, poverty reduces life expectancy through increased rates of infant mortality, developmental limitations, chronic disease, and traumatic death.

In the United States, the incidence of heart disease is 25% higher for people with low income, and the likelihood of developing cancer increases as family income decreases. Rates of infectious disease, including HIV infection, are more common among those of lower SES (U.S. Department of Health and Human Services [USDHHS], 2000). Also, adult males and females with a high school education or less (associated with lower SES) had death rates more than twice as high as the rates for those with more than a high school education in 2002 (NCHS, 2005a).

In 2002, Americans living in poverty increased to 12.1%, up from 11.7% in 2001 and 11.3% in 2000, reflecting the recession that started in spring 2000 and the economic fallout of the September 11, 2001, terrorist attacks. Children's poverty rate was 17% in 2002 (NCHS, 2005a).

In 2002, the percentage of persons living in poverty continued to differ significantly by age, race, and ethnicity. At all ages, a higher percentage of Hispanic and black persons were poor. In 2002, 29% to 32% of Hispanic and black children were poor, compared to 10% to 12% of Asian and non-Hispanic white children. Similarly, among persons 65 years and over, one fifth of Hispanics and nearly one quarter of blacks were poor, compared with 8% Asians and white non-Hispanics. In 2000-2002 more than 1 in 5 American Indians and Alaska Natives lived in poverty (NCHS, 2005a).

Gender

Gender affects health in the United States. Generally, women have higher morbidity, or disease rates, whereas men have higher mortality, or death rates. During the twentieth century, life expectancy at birth increased from 48 to 74 years for men and from 51 to almost 80 for women. Life expectancy increases were largely related to improvements in nutrition, housing, hygiene, medical care, and prevention and control of infectious disease in the first half of the twentieth century.

Life expectancy at age 65 also increased in the last century. The life expectancy of men 65 years of age rose from 12 to 16 years and that of women age 65 rose from 12 to 19 years. Women's life expectancy generally exceeded men's until the 1970s when there was a widening of the gap of life expectancy between men and women. The increasing gap was attributed to increases in male mortality due to ischemic heart disease and lung cancer, both of which increased largely as a result of men's early and widespread adoption of cigarette smoking. After the 1970s, the gender gap began to narrow. Between 1990 and 2001, the total gain in life expectancy for women was 1 year compared with more than 2 years for men, reflecting a proportionately greater decrease in heart disease and cancer mortality for men than women and a proportionally larger increase in chronic respiratory mortality among women (NCHS, 2005a).

Age

Age is an important health determinant and is closely linked to mortality. In 2002, there were a total of 2.4 million deaths in the United States. The overall age-adjusted death rate was 42% lower in 2002 than in 1950. This decrease in mortality in the second half of the twentieth century was related to declines in death from heart disease, stroke, and unintentional injuries.

Throughout the second half of the twentieth century, heart disease was the leading cause of death and stroke was the third leading cause. In 2002, death from heart disease was 59% lower than the rate in 1950. Stroke rate of death has declined 69% since 1950 (NCHS, 2005a).

Cancer was the second leading cause of death during the second half of the twentieth centry. Overall cancer death rates rose between 1960 and 1990 and then reversed direction. Between 1990 and 2002, overall death rates for cancer declined more than 10%. The death rates from cancer for males were 63% higher than rates for females in 1980 and 46% higher than females in 2002. This trend reflects the trend in death rates for lung cancer (NCHS, 2005a). Since 1970, the death rates for lung cancer for the total population have been higher than the death rates for any other cancer site. Lung cancer is strongly associated with cigarette smoking.

Chronic lower respiratory disease was the fourth leading cause of death in 2002. This was an increase of 54% from the rate in 1980. This upward trend is the result of steadily increasing death rates for females, which increased more than 150% between 1980 and 2002, whereas rates for men increased only 70%. This increasing trend is most noticeable for females age 55 years and older. It is strongly associated with smoking (USDHHS, 2005).

The fifth leading cause of death in 2002 was unintentional injuries. Death rates decreased from 1950 to 1992. Since 1992, however, unintentional injury deaths have increased slightly. Despite recent increases, the rate for unintentional injury deaths in 2002 is still 53% less than the 1950 rate. This rate is greater in males than in females. Risk varies with age. For males ages 15 to 64 in 2002, the death rates were 2 to 3 times the risk for females. Gender disparity is smaller between ages 15 and 64, but after age 64 for males and females, the rates increase steadily (NCHS, 2005a).

Overall, the death rate from unintentional injuries has increased slightly since early 1990s; however, the trend in motor vehicle–related injury mortality, which accounts for approximately half of all unintentional injury mortality, has decreased since the 1970s. The decline in motor vehicle–related deaths is attributed to safer vehicles and highways and behavioral changes such as increased use of seat belts and motorcycle helmets and decreased drinking and driving (NCHS, 2005a).

According to National Center for Health Statistics (NCHS) (2005a), the leading cause of death in childhood is unintentional injuries. This is also true for adolescents, for whom 33% of deaths are related to motor vehicle accidents (CDC, 1999h). Furthermore, over 22% of deaths in this age-group involve alcohol use (Insurance Institute for Highway Safety, Highway Loss Data Institute, 2000).

Morbidity patterns also vary with age. In 2000, 14.3% of U.S. residents were age 65 and older. It is estimated that in 2010, that figure will increase to 20.7%. In 2010, more than half the U.S. population will be age 55 and older.

Only around 5% of all elderly persons live in nursing homes. Many elderly people prefer to live on their own or with other family members. Eighty-two percent of those who live in nursing homes are 70 years or older, 65% of them are female, 66% are widowed, and 89% are white. The majority of those in nursing homes have serious illness or disabilities (Social Work Practice With the Elderly, 2004). Nursing homes serve mostly the frail elderly and are designed according to an acute care model that focuses on meeting the patients' physical needs rather than interpersonal, social, and environmental needs. The health and surveillance needs of this population will continue to grow.

Race and Ethnicity

Although differences in health status and health service access are partially attributed to inequalities of income and, education; race, and ethnicity also are factors. Heart disease death rates are over 40% higher for African Americans than for whites, and the death rate for all cancers is 30% higher for African Americans than for whites. Furthermore, Hispanics are almost twice as likely to die from diabetes as are whites (USDHHS, 2000).

Death rates increase with age for individuals with chronic diseases such as heart disease, cancer, stroke, and chronic lower respiratory disease, as well as for unintentional injuries. Death rates for black persons exceed those for white persons of the same gender from each of these causes.

Infant mortality rates have declined for all racial and ethnic groups, but large disparities remain. During the years 1999-2001, the infant mortality rate was highest for infants of black mothers. Infant mortality rates were also high among infants of American Indian, Alaska Native, Puerto Rican, and Hawaiian mothers. Infants of mothers of Chinese origin had the lowest infant mortality rate (NCHS, 2005a).

Communicable diseases, particularly sexually transmitted diseases, HIV, and AIDS, are found disproportionately in nonwhites. Although African Americans comprise only 12.3% of the total U.S. population, 50% of the AIDS cases reported between 2001 and 2004 were from that group. AIDS is the leading cause of death for all African Americans ages 25 to 44 years, the second leading cause of death among African American females, and the leading cause of death among African American males in that age-group. In 2004, the AIDS case rate among African Americans (66.4 per 100,000) was 8 times the rate for whites (8.2 per 100,000) and over twice the rate for Hispanics (28.1 per 100,000) (CDC, 2006) (see Chapter 12).

Social Interaction

Relationships also are important to health. Social support is a necessary factor in promoting health and functional independence. Retirement, the loss of a spouse or close friend, or a change in roles can affect support systems and social contact; all are risk factors for disease and functional dependence (USDHHS, 2000).

Social interactions dramatically influence behaviors and risk factors for disease. For example, in the 1992 to 1999 U.S. Current Population Surveys, Harris and Lopez-Valcarcel (2004) analyzed cigarette smoking among people ages 15 to 24 in approximately 90,000 households. They found that the prosmoking influence of a fellow smoker markedly exceeded the deterrent effect of a nonsmoking peer. This phenomenon has implications for financial markets, educational performance, criminal behavior, and other areas of inquiry where peer influence is important. Similarly, alcohol consumption and initiation of use of drugs and cigarettes among teenagers is frequently associated with social interaction and peer use (CDC, 2006b).

Geography and Politics

Where an individual lives may have an impact on population health. Traditional geographically related phenomena (e.g., earthquakes, weather, or lack of certain minerals in the soil) also contribute to population health. Significant health problems are attributable to floods, extreme temperatures, and other natural events and man-made hazards (e.g., chemical plants and terrorists) (see Chapters 13 and 26).

With the Oklahoma City bombing of the Alfred P. Murrah Federal Building on April 19, 1995, the terrorist attacks on New York and Washington, DC, on September 11, 2001, and the devastating hurricanes of 2005, United States residents have became acutely aware of their vulnerability. Life for the American public changed forever after September 11, 2001. Nursing also changed in the face of the terrorist

ETHICAL Insights

Ethical Issues With Terrorism

In 2001 a set of core Emergency and Disaster Preparedness Competencies for Nurses was prepared by Dr. Gebbie from the Columbia University School of Nursing, Center for Health Policy (Langan and James, 2005). Nurses are now contemplating ethical obligations in relation to the threat of international terrorism. What does this mean for nurses? Are we obligated to receive smallpox vaccine? What are our obligations as nurse educators, researchers, and clinicians in relation to terrorism (Laabs, 2003)?

threat. Nurses at every level are now dealing with disaster management and bioterrorism and disaster preparedness.

Political Factors and the Delivery of Health Care

Political factors also have an impact on the delivery of health care services at all levels. For example, Medicaid coverage and availability vary from state to state, depending on the local political climate. As a consequence, Medicaid assistance to citizens varies widely. Residency in a state with minimal Medicaid assistance may affect the health of that population. Medicaid is the largest program providing medical and health-related services to America's poorest people (Centers for Medicare and Medicaid Services, 2004).

For example, in 2004, Michigan's Medicaid program paid for 70% of all nursing home care in the state and more than 40,000 births (40% of the total number of births in the state) and provided health care services for one out of every seven people. Approximately 85% of Michigan's Medicaid dollars cover services for senior citizens, disabled persons, and children (Bucholz, 2005).

Environment

Asthma is a leading cause of childhood illness and a leading cause of disability and health care expenditures for adults. Asthma attack prevalence has remained fairly stable during 1997 to 2001 (39 to 43 per 1000 population). Asthma rates decrease with age and are higher among non-Hispanic blacks than among either non-Hispanic whites or Hispanics (NCHS, 2005a). It is a concern that the environmental pollutants may be causing this disease to increase.

The stressful lifestyle and hectic pace of life in the United States are also environmental factors that can contribute to the growing rates of depression and an increased use of antidepressants. Depression and other forms of mental illness are critical public health issues in America today. In 2001 to 2002, more than 1 in 10 noninstitutionalized adults in America were estimated to have a major depressive disorder at some point in their lifetime, with 6.6% having had a major depressive episode during the preceding 12 months. During this period, antidepressant use among adults in all age-groups doubled or tripled. In 1999 to 2000, 13% of women 45 to 64 years of age reported antidepressant use in the preceding month (NSHS, 2005a).

The environment may also contribute to the growing problem of obesity. Indeed, the prevalence of overweight children and adolescents in the United States between 1999

BOX 33-1   Ten Great Public Health Achievements: United States, 1900 to 2000

1. Vaccination
2. Motor vehicle safety
3. Safer workplaces
4. Control of infectious diseases
5. Decline in deaths from coronary heart disease and stroke
6. Safer and healthier foods
7. Healthier mothers and babies
8. Family planning
9. Fluoridation of drinking water
10. Recognition of tobacco use as a health hazard

Centers for Disease Control and Prevention: Ten great public health achievements: United States, 1900-1999, *Morb Mortal Wkly Rep* 48(12): 241-243, 1999k.

and 2002 indicates that an estimated 16% of children and adolescents ages 6 to 19 are overweight. This represents a 45% increase from the overweight estimates of 11% obtained from the National Health and Nutrition Survey in 1988 to 1994 (NCHS, 2005b). These data are related to the sedentary lifestyle of the children today. Video games and television occupy many hours of children and adolescents' leisure time. Fast food with high fat and sugar content make up a large portion of the American diet.

PUBLIC HEALTH: THE PAST

During the 1900s, the average American life span lengthened by more than 30 years, and 25 years of that gain was attributable to public health advances. Throughout 1999, the CDC published a series of reports outlining the "Ten Great Public Health Achievements" in the United States that contributed to improved health during the twentieth century (CDC, 1999k). Box 33-1 lists these remarkable achievements, and the following sections briefly describe each achievement.

Impact of Vaccines Universally Recommended for Children

At the beginning of the twentieth century, infectious diseases were widely prevalent in the United States. At that time, 5 of the 10 leading causes of death were attributed to infectious disease. Vaccination has greatly affected these statistics and has resulted in the eradication of smallpox, the elimination of polio in the Americas, and the control of many other diseases including measles, rubella, tetanus, and diphtheria.

National efforts to promote the vaccination of children began with the appropriation of federal funds for the polio vaccine in 1955. Since that time, federal, state, and local governments and private health care providers have worked to encourage vaccination coverage for all children. The task is daunting because approximately 11,000 children are born in the United States each day, and each child requires 15 to 19 injections by age 19 months for protection against 11 childhood diseases. Despite this number of vaccines and complicated immunization schedule, U.S. vaccine data for 2002 indicate that recommendations are being followed. The percentage of children 19 to 35 months old receiving vaccine for DPT is 82%, polio 90%, measles-mumps-rubella 92%, HiB 93%, hepatitis B 90%, and chickenpox 81% (NCHS, 2005a). The 2003 to 2004 school year coverage for school entrance was even higher: polio 93% to 95%, DPT 90% to 95%, measles 92% to 95%, mumps 92% to 95%, rubella 92% to 95%, hepatitis B 93% to 95%, and chickenpox 87% to 94% (National Immunization Program, 2005).

Motor Vehicle Safety

The reduction of the death rate attributable to motor vehicle crashes in the United States is a result of a public health response to one of the greatest technological advances of the twentieth century—the motorization of America (CDC, 1999h). Systematic motor vehicle safety efforts began in the 1960s with the passage of the Highway Safety Act and the National Traffic and Motor Vehicle Safety Act in 1966. These Acts authorized the federal government to set and regulate standards for motor vehicles and highways.

As a result of this legislation, vehicles were built with new safety features, including head rests, energy-absorbing steering wheels, shatter-resistant windshields, and safety belts. Furthermore, roads were vastly improved. Other efforts were encouraged to alter driver and passenger behaviors. Enactment and enforcement of traffic safety laws (e.g., speed limits, laws against driving while intoxicated, and the enforcement of safety belts and child safety seats) have reduced the number of injuries and deaths attributable to vehicle accidents. Safety belt use cuts the risk of death by 45% for people riding in cars and by as much as 60% for those traveling in trucks or SUVs. Seat belts save 14,000 lives each year, and every state has a law mandating the use of seat belts and child safety seats. Despite the known benefits of using seat belts and potential legal ramifications for failure to do so, 20% of Americans still fail to buckle up (U.S. Department of Labor, OSHA, 2005).

These efforts and the resulting improvements should lead to more measures to improve motor vehicle safety and driving habits and patterns in the United States. The ultimate goal is to further reduce the total number of deaths each year.

Improvements in Workplace Safety

At the beginning of the twentieth century, workers in the United States faced high health and safety risks on the job. In 1912, it was estimated that more than 20,000 workers died from work-related injuries. Employment in mining, agriculture, forestry, and fishing, construction, transportation, communications, and public utilities yielded the highest average death and injury rates (CDC, 1999g).

During the 1900s, deaths from work-related injuries declined 90% (from 37 per 100,000 workers to 4 per 100,000 workers) (CDC, 1999g). This decline in occupational fatalities is the result of collaborative efforts to identify and correct factors that contribute to occupational health risks. Declines are attributed to labor and management efforts to improve worker safety through research, education, and regulatory activities.

Despite accomplishments, workers continue to die from preventable injuries sustained on the job. The health of the U.S.

economy depends on a healthy and productive workforce. Yet, there were 5,524 occupational fatalities in 2002. The estimated direct costs for occupational injuries and illnesses reached $40.1 billion in 1999, with over $200 billion of indirect costs.

Lifestyle behaviors related to physical activities, nutrition, tobacco smoking, and substance abuse have a significant impact on people's health. These lifestyle exposures contribute to many diseases, including type 2 diabetes mellitus, hypertension, heart disease, stroke, some forms of cancer, and obesity. Investments in preventing occupational and non-occupational illness, injury, and disability experienced by the U.S. workforce can have a significant impact on the health-related productivity of American businesses. There are many programs, interventions and initiatives that allow both the occupational safety and health community and the health promotion community to develop and implement workplace programs collaboratively that prevent workplace illness and injury, promote health, and optimize the health of the U.S. workforce (National Institute of Occupational Safety and Health, 2005) (see Chapter 28).

Control of Infectious Diseases

The number of deaths from infectious diseases declined markedly in the United States during the twentieth century. In 1900, the three leading causes of death were pneumonia, tuberculosis (TB), and diarrhea and enteritis. Combined with diphtheria, these diseases caused one third of all deaths at that time. Of these, 40% were among children age 5 years and younger (CDC, 1999a). Successful public health efforts for infectious disease control resulted from improvements in the following areas: sanitation and hygiene, discovery of antibiotics, and implementation of childhood vaccination programs.

Sanitation and hygiene efforts included the provision of clean drinking water through chlorination and other treatments, which began in the early 1900s and became widespread over the next few decades. Other important sanitation and hygiene activities that began early in the century were sewage disposal, food safety, solid waste disposal, and public education about hygienic practices.

Penicillin was discovered in 1928, but it was not used for medical purposes until the 1940s. Since the 1940s, antimicrobials have provided quick and complete treatment for previously incurable bacterial illnesses and have saved many lives.

Vaccination campaigns have been highly successful in preventing the diseases that were previously common and often deadly. The success of vaccination programs in the United States and Europe inspired the concept of "disease eradication." The eradication of smallpox in the 1970s was a major public health triumph. A number of other diseases, including measles and polio, are slated for eradication in the next few years (see Chapter 23).

Decline in Deaths From Heart Disease and Stroke

Since 1921, heart disease has been the leading cause of death in the United States. Since 1938, stroke has been the third leading cause of death. Together they account for approximately 40% of all deaths. However, death from heart disease was 59% lower in 2002 than in 1950 and death from stroke was 69% lower (USDHHS, 2005). Reasons cited for this dramatic decline include epidemiological investigations that established major risk factors for heart disease and stroke including tobacco use, high blood cholesterol, high blood pressure, dietary factors, and sedentary lifestyle. Therefore improved mortality rates have been attributed to lowering risk factor levels through antismoking campaigns, antihypertensive and lipid-lowering drugs, and improved nutrition. Improvements in medical care, including advances in diagnosing and treating heart disease and stroke, also are important in the decline in death rates from heart disease and stroke (CDC, 1999b).

Safer and Healthier Food

Early in the twentieth century, contaminated food, milk, and water caused many food-borne infections, including typhoid fever, botulism, and many forms of dysentery. The passage of the Pure Food and Drug Act in 1906 created awareness of food-borne disease sources. Successful prevention methods include hand washing, sanitation, refrigeration, pasteurization, and pesticide application (CDC, 1999i).

The discovery of essential nutrients and their role in disease prevention dramatically reduced nutritional deficiencies such as goiter, rickets, and pellagra (e.g., dietary niacin deficiency). Later in the twentieth century, food and nutrition labeling and consumer information programs stimulated the development of products low in fat, cholesterol, and sodium. Efforts to increase the intake of fruits, vegetables, and fiber in the American diet have also been promoted to combat the growing problems associated with obesity (CDC, 1999i).

Although spread of disease through contaminated food has declined dramatically, outbreaks continue. Salmonella is the most common food borne illness in the United States (CDC, 2006c) and outbreaks are fairly commonplace. In mid-2004, for example, a series of salmonella infections linked to Roma tomatoes were reported in the United States and Canada, and almost 500 individuals became ill (CDC, 2005b). Many other organisms (e.g., *Campylobacter, Shigella, Listeria*) commonly cause food-borne disease. Recently, outbreaks of hepatitis A have occurred. For example, in 2001, 46 people were sickened by hepatitis A linked to an infected restaurant worker in Massachusetts (CDC 2003b). More seriously, 555 people in Pennsylvania were infected with hepatitis A; that outbreak was eventually traced to contaminated green onions (CDC, 2003c).

Improved surveillance, applied research, and outbreak investigations have brought an awareness of the mechanisms of contamination that are leading to new control measures for food-borne pathogens. New diagnostic techniques and the rapid exchange of information through use of electronic networks and the Internet will accelerate twenty-first century improvements. PulseNet, for example, is a network of laboratories in state health departments, CDC, and food regulatory agencies. In this network, the genetic DNA fingerprints of specific pathogens can be identified and shared electronically among laboratories, enhancing the ability to detect, investigate, and control geographically distant yet related outbreaks. Another example of technology is DPDx, a computer network

that identifies parasitic pathogens. By combining PulseNet and DPDx with field epidemiological investigations, the public health system can rapidly identify and control outbreaks. The CDC, the Food and Drug Administration, the U.S. Department of Agriculture (USDA), other federal agencies, and private organizations are enhancing food safety by collaborating in education, training, research, technology, and transfer of information and by considering food safety as a whole—from farm to table (CDC, 2001).

Healthier Mothers and Babies

For every 1000 live births in 1900, six to nine women in the United States died of pregnancy-related complications, and approximately 100 infants died before they reached 1 year of age. Between 1915 and 1997, the infant mortality rate declined more than 90% to 7.2 per 1000. Likewise, between 1900 and 1997, the maternal mortality rate declined almost 99% to less than 0.1 deaths per 1000 live births (CDC, 1999e). Factors in the dramatic improvement of maternal and infant mortality include environmental interventions, improvements in nutrition, advances in clinical medicine, improvements in access to health care, improvements in surveillance and monitoring of disease, increases in education levels, and improvements in standards of living.

Despite these improvements, the United States spends more money per capita on health care than any other country in the world, yet it is ranked 28th in infant mortality and morbidity rates and 15th in maternal mortality rate, that latter of which has not improved in 20 years.

Maternal mortality is nearly 4 times higher for African-American women than for white women. The U.S. cesarean birth rate is 24.4% and is highest for African-American women. This ranking is due, in large part, to disparities that continue to exist among various racial and ethnic groups in the United States, particularly African Americans (CDC, Office of Minority Health, 2005).

Research shows that midwives are the safest birth attendants for most mothers, with lower infant and maternal mortality rates and fewer invasive interventions such as episiotomies and caesareans. In developed countries where midwives are the primary care providers for pregnant women, mortality and surgical birth rates are much lower than in the United States. However, legal, regulatory, and financial barriers to practicing midwives can make it difficult to access a midwife in the United States (Citizens for Midwifery, 2005).

Family Planning

During the twentieth century, family planning in the United States improved to allow desired birth spacing and family size. A number of factors have been identified which contributed to having fewer children per family, including a reduction in infant and child mortality, urbanization of communities, and the increase in age at first marriage (CDC, 1999c). Smaller families and longer birth intervals have led to improvement in the health of infants, children, and women and have improved women's social and economic role. Family planning safeguards individual health and rights, preserves the world resources, and improves the quality of life for women, partners, and children.

But, economic factors in the late twentieth and early twenty-first centuries have necessitated that many mothers work outside the home. With a labor force participation rate of 59.2%, women represented 46% of the total U.S. labor force in 2004 (U.S. Department of Labor, Women's Bureau, 2005).

Margaret Sanger, a public health nurse concerned with the adverse health effects of frequent childbirth, miscarriage, and abortion, began the modern birth-control movement in the United States in 1912. Sanger initiated efforts to circulate information about and provide access to contraception. Her work became widespread throughout the 1920s and 1930s.

Beginning in the 1960s, birth control pills and intrauterine devices dramatically altered birth control efforts. In 1970, federal funding for family planning was established under the Family Planning Services and Population Research Act. Since the 1970s, family planning care has become widely available in the United States. As a result, modern contraception and reproductive health care systems help prevent an estimated 1.3 million unintended pregnancies in the United States every year (CDC, 1999c). In 1994, approximately half of the pregnancies in the United States were unintended, and the United States has set a goal to decrease the number of unintended pregnancies to 30% by 2010 (Global Health Options, 2004) (see Chapter 15).

Fluoridation of Drinking Water

The fluoridation of community drinking water was a major factor in the decline of dental caries during the second half of the twentieth century. At the beginning of the twentieth century, dental caries were extremely common in the United States. At that time, effective measures for preventing tooth decay were nonexistent, and the most common treatment was tooth extraction.

In 1901, Dr. F. S. McKay, a dentist in Colorado Springs, Colorado, noted that many of his patients had permanent stains on their teeth. He concluded that an agent in the public water supply was responsible for the mottled enamel. He also noted that teeth affected by this condition seemed less susceptible to dental decay. Over the next two decades, other dentists made similar discoveries; in the early 1930s, observational research began to assess the impact of fluoride on the development of dental caries (CDC, 1999d).

Studies in the mid 1940s showed that communities with fluoridated water experienced a 50% to 70% reduction in caries among children. As a result of ongoing research, a recommended optimum range of fluoride concentration was established in 1962. Since community water fluoridation efforts began in the second half of the twentieth century, dental caries have declined some 68% (CDC, 1999d). Among the most striking results of fluoridation is that tooth loss is no longer considered inevitable. Adults in the United States are retaining most of their teeth for a lifetime (CDC, 2001).

Tobacco as a Health Hazard

During the first few decades of the twentieth century, lung cancer was rare. However, as tobacco use became increasingly popular, the incidence of lung cancer became epidemic. For example, the lung cancer death rate for men was 4.9 per 100,000 in 1930; in 1990, the rate increased to 75.6 per 100,000

(CDC, 1999j). In 2001, the total number of deaths among men with lung, trachea, and bronchus cancers was 90,426 (National Center for Chronic Disease Prevention and Health Promotion, Cancer Prevention and Control, 2005). Other diseases and conditions caused or exacerbated by tobacco use increased dramatically during the century. These include heart disease, peripheral vascular disease, laryngeal cancer, oral cancer, esophageal cancer, chronic obstructive pulmonary disease, intrauterine growth retardation, and low birthweight.

In the 1940s and 1950s, scientists began to link cigarette smoking and lung cancer. In 1964, on the basis of some 7000 articles relating to smoking and disease, the U.S. Surgeon General concluded that cigarette smoking is a cause of lung and laryngeal cancer and a probable cause of chronic bronchitis. It was determined that "cigarette smoking is a health hazard." In 2003, the median prevalence of cigarette smoking among adults was 22.1%. For men, the median prevalence was 24.8% and for women, 20.3% (CDC, 2004).

An important accomplishment in the second half of the twentieth century was the reduction of smoking prevalence among those age 18 years or younger from 42.4% in 1965 to 24.7% in 1997. Additionally, the percentage of adults who never smoked increased from 44% in the mid 1960s to 55% in 1997 (CDC, 1999j). Since the late 1990s, smoking rates have continued to decrease. Indeed, in 2003, the median prevalence of cigarette smoking among adults was 22.1%. For men, the median prevalence was 24.8% and for women, 20.3% (CDC, 2004). Smoking reduction results from many factors. These factors include the following: scientific evidence linking disease and tobacco use, dissemination of this information to the public, prevention and cessation programs, campaigns by advocates for nonsmoker's rights, restrictions on cigarette advertising, counter-advertising, policy changes (e.g., enforcement of minors' access laws, legislation restricting smoking in public places, and increased taxation), improvements in treatment and prevention programs, and an increased understanding of the economic costs of tobacco (CDC, 1999j). However, according to the CDC, 28.7% of young adults ages 18 to 24 years are smokers. Smoking prevalence increased between 1996 and 2001 among 18- to 24-year-olds in the United States. It is believed that the tobacco companies are now targeting this age-group. Despite 18- to 24-year-olds having strong antismoking attitudes, they are also the most likely adult age-group to be susceptible to tobacco industry marketing (California Department of Health Services Tobacco Section, 2005).

PUBLIC HEALTH: THE FUTURE

On January 25, 2000, Surgeon General David Satcher presented the American people with *Healthy People 2010,* which outlined the national health goals (see Chapter 1). In this document and in related activities, there has been a push for living a healthier lifestyle and improving equal assess to health care. Furthermore, the document establishes a goal that, by 2010, most adults and children will have five 30-minute workouts each week. Developed objectives encourage more people to quit smoking, abstain from drugs, and abstain from engaging in casual sex without condoms.

HEALTHY PEOPLE 2010 | Health Indicators

Leading Health Indicators for Americans

➤ Physical activity

➤ Overweight and obesity

➤ Tobacco use

➤ Substance abuse

➤ Responsible sexual behavior

➤ Mental health

➤ Injury and violence

➤ Environmental quality

➤ Immunization

➤ Access to health care

US Department of Health and Human Services: *Healthy People, 2010: conference edition,* Washington, DC, 2000, US Government Printing Office.

Healthy People 2010 determined 10 leading health indicators to measure progress toward meeting the goals (see *Healthy People 2010* box). These health indicators reflect the major public health concerns in the United States and illuminate individual behaviors, physical and social environmental factors, and important health system issues that affect the health of individuals, groups, and communities. Applying the healthy community model standards to these 10 health indicators, communities can plan community public health services. The emphasis is on health outcomes and programs rather than professional practice.

In implementing the model standards, the community is encouraged to adapt a process to meet their specific needs. With *Healthy People 2010,* there may be a tendency to use the national objective targets as targets for community standards. Each community should compare its status in relation to the national targets, and then the community should translate national objectives into community action plans tailored to meet community needs. Efforts should be made to encourage the communication and coordination of public health efforts and to present plans for programs or interventions to the appropriate individual, agency, or legislative body (see Chapter 11). In all of these areas, the CHN can be a valuable player (USDHHS, 2000).

Continued efforts by public health systems, including CHNs, can dramatically affect the health of individuals, families, and communities for the next century. Areas in which the public health system will continue to be involved include the following (CDC, 2000):

- Monitoring community health status to identify potential hazards
- Investigating disease outbreaks and safety hazards
- Informing, educating, and empowering the public regarding health issues
- Mobilizing community partnerships to solve health problems
- Developing policies and plans that support individual and community health efforts
- Enforcing laws and regulations that protect health and ensure safety
- Linking populations with needed personal health services
- Ensuring a competent public health and personal health care workforce
- Evaluating effectiveness, accessibility, and quality of personal and population-based health services

RESEARCH HIGHLIGHTS

Increasing the Number of Public Health Nurses

The number of nurses interested in working in public health departments has declined significantly over the last decade. As a result, it has been recognized that efforts must be made to expose nursing students to public health nursing and to better prepare them with skills needed to practice in health departments. In Virginia, nurses from the State Department of Health teamed with Virginia Commonwealth University faculty to increase the number of nursing students choosing a career in public health nursing.

From this project, the researchers learned that the greatest barrier to ensuring appropriate public health preparation for nursing students was finding preceptors who were willing to provide practical experiences. To address this problem, they focused on strengthening communication between faculty and public health nurses, and determined that holding face-to-face discussions with public health nurses worked well to encourage them to take on the role of preceptor. They also noted that enhancing public health nursing concepts in the curriculum and providing well-planned field experiences dramatically increased students' interest in pursuing a career in public health nursing.

As a result of this collaborative effort, the number of students placed in public health settings for clinical experiences more than doubled. And, significantly, 40% of the students surveyed indicated that they would consider a career in public health nursing; this represented a dramatic increase.

From Moon MW, Henry JK, Connelly K, Kirsch P: Public health nurses for Virginia's future: A collaborative project to increase the number of nursing students choosing a career in public health nursing. *Am J Public Health* 95(7):11-2-1106, 2005.

COMMUNITY HEALTH NURSES MAKE A DIFFERENCE

CHNs can make a difference. Efforts at the individual, family, aggregate, and community levels can dramatically affect health and well-being. The following examples illustrate how CHN have greatly influenced the lives of many individuals and families, in very varied circumstances.

Nurses Taking Action

MAKING A DIFFERENCE THROUGHOUT THE WORLD

The world's most powerful earthquake in more than 40 years erupted underwater off the Indonesian island of Sumatra on December 26, 2004, creating a tsunami that sent a wall of water over thousands of miles of land. The number of deaths was estimated at 221,100 (Sengupta, 2005). The following is an adapted summary of the work of two nurses, Carrie Randall and Jeanie Schmidt, who volunteered in the aftermath (Dryden, 2004).

Our International Medical Corps (IMC) group was sent to Banda Aceh, Indonesia, the hardest hit area. Chaos from the aftermath of the disaster resulted in plans changing hourly. As we arrived, we witnessed soldiers from the Australian and German Armies shoveling out mud in what was left of the Zainal Abidin University Hospital ER in central Banda Aceh. They moved on to create water and sewer systems, an operating room, laboratories, and x-ray facility, and we helped to staff the emergency room.

A unique challenge was blending medications and supplies from six countries, none researchable in U.S. references. Charts, if any, were scraps of paper written in several different languages. In a 12- × 15-foot room, health care providers from Switzerland, China, Korea, Indonesia, Belgium, and Spain worked together to treat 200 patients a day. As patients backed up, the innovative Singaporeans shoveled out debris and silt to help create a hospital unit.

After the earthquake and tsunami, no infrastructure was left. The environment was harsh and filthy, with no usable water or toilets. There were no bedpans; urinals were made out of water bottles. There was no way to clean up patients. Mosquitoes and flies were rampant and cats were everywhere, including in the emergency room eating mice. The place was overwhelmingly hot and extremely humid, and there was no ventilation or lighting. Despite mud, blood, and excrement, per custom, the nurses and doctors worked shoeless. With limited equipment, supplies, and medication, and an overabundance of doctors and not enough nurses, it was almost impossible to give adequate care. In the chaotic frenzy of a small room with five cots, there was no privacy.

Even in tragedy, the human spirit prevailed in camaraderie among nations. The world responded and was there to help, and we all worked well together despite language barriers and cultural differences. Any mild suffering on our part was worth the effort.

Carrie Randall, RN, BS, helped provide emergency mental health services and assisted in disaster relief operations at Ground Zero in New York City after the September 11, 2001, terrorist attacks. Following that experience, she chose to change careers and entered the nursing profession. She is currently pursuing a master's degree in a family nurse practitioner program.

Jeanie Schmidt, RN, BSN, was a critical care nurse for 16 years in various settings, including the emergency department, intensive care unit, and postanesthesia care unit. She is currently preparing to attend medical school (Dryden, 2004). ■

MAKING A DIFFERENCE DURING A DISASTER

Hurricane Katrina hit the United States Gulf Coast in late August, 2005 causing widespread devastation. Many of those displaced by the storm were taken to Houston for shelter, food, and medical care. The University of Texas Health Science Center at Houston (UTHSC-H) was charged with opening a clinic for a "super shelter" at the George R. Brown Convention Center to help care for the influx of hurricane survivors.

The UTHSC-H-led clinic opened on September 3 and remained operational for nearly 3 weeks. During that time, an estimated 4000 volunteers assisted with more than 11,000 patient visits. Volunteer

health providers, many of them nurses, came from across Texas and the Gulf Coast region, as well as from across the country. Volunteers registered from Oregon, Arizona, New York, Hawaii, Illinois and many other states.

Elda Ramirez, RN, MSN, PhD-C, a UTHSC School of Nursing faculty member and Emergency Nurse Practitioner, was credited for designing the triage area (Brown, 2005). According to Ms Ramirez, "This is an unbelievable collaborative effort" with "every single service from ER to OB/GYN. We have mental health services and a full pharmacy."

Ms Ramirez was also largely responsible for staffing the clinic with nurses. For 18 days, her graduate ER students, and other faculty and students from UT helped in the clinic, serving as charge nurses, coordinating the nursing volunteers, and overseeing the nursing portion of clinic operations 24 hours a day. Describing the clinic, Elda noted, "We have worked together . . . side-by-side and seamlessly."

The nurses and other medical personnel did what they could to manage the health needs as well as the pain and devastation among the survivors of Hurricane Katrina. Reflecting on the clients seen and the needs encountered, Ms Ramirez observed, "What's gotten to me the most—the lost children. I've got a one little one who can't find his family. It just breaks your heart." Elda Ramirez, September 4, 2005 (UTHSC-H, 2005). ■

MAKING A DIFFERENCE AMONG UNDERSERVED POPULATIONS

The Agape Clinic is located in the basement of Grace United Methodist Church near downtown Dallas. Since 2000, the clinic has operated as a joint ministry of Grace Church and Baylor Community Care, a service-learning program of Baylor University's Louise Herrington School of Nursing (LHSON). The Agape Clinic provides health care to immigrants, including many from Mexico and other Latin American countries as well as refugees from such diverse areas as Cambodia, Sudan, and Iraq and to the working poor who have no health insurance (Wormser, 2005).

Charles Kemp, RN, MSN, FNP-C, FAAN, is a faculty member of LHSON and is the clinic coordinator and primary fund raiser. An expert in hospice and palliative care (Kemp, 1999) and refugee and immigrant health (Kemp, 2004), Kemp has been providing health care to immigrants for more than two decades. At the Agape Clinic, he has been able to successfully combine clinical experiences for more than 400 CHN students, with meeting the health needs of this seriously underserved aggregate.

At Agape, senior BSN students use the knowledge and skills they have learned to provide care to 30 to 60 patients per clinic day. With clinic staff and volunteers including, nurses, nurse practitioners, and physicians, the students provide well and sick child care, diagnose and treat acute illnesses, give immunizations, and manage chronic conditions such as hypertension and diabetes. They have diagnosed tuberculosis, chickenpox, and a host of other communicable diseases and have conducted follow-up home visits. Opportunities for health promotion and health education are varied, and include screening programs (e.g., mammography, hypertension, diabetes) and a collaborative teaching program serving the parents and students from area elementary schools.

The Agape Clinic is growing in scope and programs offered. Indeed, in 2004, almost 5400 patients were served there (Agape,

2004). This effort shows how nurses committed to proving care to underserved individuals, families, and groups can make a difference in people's lives. ∎

SUMMARY

Factors such as childbearing, aging, SES, crime, and chronic disease affect the health of individuals, families, and communities. These factors are complex in nature, and the associated nursing interventions to address family and community needs are also complex. Identifying and meeting individual, family, and community health needs from traditional medical and health care settings (e.g., hospitals, offices, and clinics) is a limited, if not impossible, task. Likewise, identifying and meeting individual, family, and community health needs while only making home visits are also difficult.

The complex problems facing the health of today's community require actions that result in social change through community organizations, political activity, a coalition, or groups of people. Although hospital, office, clinic, and home visits are important, the complexity of health problems that practitioners encounter has an impact on the family and the community; at times, the impact extends to the state, national, and international level. Health teaching and monitoring a medical regimen are necessary, but they are not sufficient interventions to ensure the health of an individual, family, and community. This is true for many reasons, including the following:

- Health is a complex, dynamic, multifaceted phenomenon.
- Individuals are members of groups and populations such as families, neighborhoods, schools, churches, and other institutions that make up communities.

- The community organization has an impact on the health of individuals, families, communities, and populations.
- To increase the health of populations, the community must identify its needs and organize to meet its needs.
- CHNs help promote the health of the community by working with families and other populations in the community to identify needs and organize to meet their needs.

Today more than ever, community health nursing can make a difference as the cornerstone of health care delivery. In the United States, the change to a prospective reimbursement system based on diagnosis-related groups and capitation have shortened hospital stays and increased the need for community-based health care. Groups and populations served in the community now require a broad range of nursing services. Fiscal realities and social demands are likely to mandate the continued growth of community-based care for the foreseeable future. Health care reform that results in upstream care will mandate the continued growth of community-based care over the long term.

LEARNING ACTIVITIES

1. Discuss with classmates how being a member of a population influences an aspect of personal health. Give an example.
2. Discuss why and how CHNs make a difference. Give examples of possible community health nursing interventions for the three Clinical Examples at the individual level, family level, and population or community level.
3. With classmates, identify the interventions, inventions, or developments that might become the "Greatest Health Achievements" of the twenty-first century.

REFERENCES

Agape: Agape clinic activities summary, 2004, The Author, http://www3.baylor.edu/~Charles_Kemp/2004_report.htm.

Brown D: Unity, hope and healing in the hour of need. *UT-Houston Magazine,* Fall, 2005, http://www.med.uth.tmc.edu/alumniMag/Fall05/Unity,%20hope%20story.html.

Bryer-Chuonroong L, Deaver P: Meeting the Preteen Vaccine Law: a pilot program in urban middle schools, *J Sch Health* 70:39-44, 2000.

Bucholz TJ: *Granholm to Congress: preserve Medicaid, maintain safety net for Michigan's citizens,* 2005, State of Michigan, http://www.michigan.gov/som/0,1607,7-192–115493–,00.html.

California Department of Health Services Tobacco Control Section, *18-24 Year Olds,* 2005, http://www.dhs.ca.gov/tobacco/documents/18-24YearOlds.pdf.

Centers for Disease Control and Prevention: Achievements in public health, 1900-1999: control of infectious disease, *Morb Mortal Wkly Rep* 48(29):621-629, 1999a.

Centers for Disease Control and Prevention: Achievements in public health, 1900-1999: decline in deaths from heart diseases and stroke: United States, 1990-1999, *Morb Mortal Wkly Rep* 48(30):649-656, 1999b.

Centers for Disease Control and Prevention: Achievements in public health, 1900-1999: family planning, *Morb Mortal Wkly Rep* 48(47):1073-1080, 1999c.

Centers for Disease Control and Prevention: Achievements in public health, 1900-1999: fluoridation of drinking water to prevent dental caries, *Morb Mortal Wkly Rep* 48(41):933-940, 1999d.

Centers for Disease Control and Prevention: Achievements in public health, 1900-1999: healthier mothers and babies, *Morb Mortal Wkly Rep* 48(38):849-858, 1999e.

Centers for Disease Control and Prevention: Achievements in public health, 1900-1999: impact of vaccines universally recommended for children: United States, 1990-1998, *Morb Mortal Wkly Rep* 48(12):243-249, 1999f.

Centers for Disease Control and Prevention: Achievements in public health, 1900-1999: improvements in workplace safety: United States, 1900-1999, *Morb Mortal Wkly Rep* 48(22):461-469, 1999g.

Centers for Disease Control and Prevention: Achievements in public health, 1900-1999: motor-vehicle safety: a 20th century public health achievement, *Morb Mortal Wkly Rep* 48(18):369-374, 1999h.

Centers for Disease Control and Prevention: Achievements in public health, 1900-1999: safer and healthier foods, *Morb Mortal Wkly Rep* 48(40):905-913, 1999i.

Centers for Disease Control and Prevention: Achievements in public health, 1900-1999: tobacco use: United States, 1990-1999, *Morb Mortal Wkly Rep* 48(43):986-993, 1999j.

Centers for Disease Control and Prevention: Ten great public health achievements: United States, 1900-1999, *Morb Mortal Wkly Rep* 48(12):241-243, 1999k.

Centers for Disease Control and Prevention: *About a century of success,* 2000, The Author, http://www.cdc.gov/phtn/tenachievements/about/about3.htm.

Centers for Disease Control and Prevention: Achievements in public health, 1900-1999: fluoridation of drinking water to prevent dental caries, 2001, *Morb Mortal Wkly*

Rep, http://www.cdc.gov/mmwr/preview/mmwrhtml/mm4841al.htm.

Centers for Disease Control and Prevention: Achievements in public health, 1900-1999: safer and healthier foods, 2001, *Morb Mortal Wkly Rep,* http://www.cdc.gov/mmwr/preview/mmwrhtml/mm4840a1.htm.

Centers for Disease Control and Prevention: Preventing tobacco use among young people: a report of the Surgeon General (Executive Summary), *Morb Mortal Wkly Rep,* 2003a, http://wonder.cdc.gov/wonder/prevguid/m0030927/m0030927.asp.

Centers for Disease Control and Prevention: Foodborne transmission of hepatitis A: Massachusetts, 2001, *Morb Mortal Wkly Rep* 52(24):565-567, 2003b.

Centers for Disease Control and Prevention: Hepatitis A outbreak associated with green onions at a restaurant: Monaca, Pennsylvania, 2003, *Morb Mortal Wkly Rep* 52(4):1155-1157, 2003c

Centers for Disease Control and Prevention: *Effect of ending an antitobacco youth campaign on adolescent susceptibility to cigarette smoking: Minnesota, 2002–2003, Morb Mortal Wkly Rep* 53(14):2004, http://www.cdc.gov/mmwr/PDF/wk/mm5314.pdf.

Centers for Disease Control and Prevention, Office of Minority Health: *Eliminate disparities in infant mortality,* 2005a, http://www.cdc.gov/omh/AMH/factsheets/infant.htm.

Centers for Disease control and Prevention: Outbreaks of salmonella infections associated with eating Roma tomatoes: United States and Canada, 2004, *Morb Mortal Wkly Rep* 54(13):325-326, 2005b.

Centers for Disease Control and Prevention: HIV/AIDS among African Americans: fact sheet. 2006a, The Author, http://www.cdc.gov/hiv/topics/aa/resources/factsheets/pdf/aa.pdf.

Centers for Disease Control and Prevention: Youth risk behavior surveillance, United States 2005. *Morb Mortal Wkly Rep* 55(SS05):1-108, 2006b, http://www.cdc.gov/mmwr/preview/mmwrhtml/ss5505a1.htm.

Centers for Disease Control and Prevention: Preliminary FoodNet data on the incidence of infection with pathogens transmitted commonly through food: 10 States, United States, 2005. *Morb Mortal Wkly Rep* 55(14):392-395, 2006c.

Centers for Medicare and Medicaid Services: *State Medicaid websites,* 2004, The Author, http://www.cms.hhs.gov/medicaid/stwebsites.asp.

Citizens for Midwifery: *Learn, connect, take action,* 2005, The Author, http://www.cfmidwifery.org.

Dryden P: When nothing is left: disaster nursing after the tsunami, 2004, *Washington Post,* http://www.washingtonpost.com/wpsrv/world/daily/graphics/tsunami_122804.html>referrer=emaillink.

Global Health Options: *Birth control and unintended pregnancies,* 2004, The Author, http://www.g-h-o.co.uk/id30.htm.

Harris JE, Lopez-Valcarcel B: *Asymmetric social interaction in economics: cigarette smoking among people in the United States, 1992-1999,* 2004, http://ideas.repec.org/p/nbr/nberwo/10409.html.

Insurance Institute for Highway Safety, Highway Loss Data Institute, *Safety facts: teenagers,* 2000, The Author, http://www.hwysafety.org/safety_facts/teens/teenager.htm.

Kemp CE: *Refugee and immigrant health.* London, 2004, Cambridge University Press.

Kemp CE: *Terminal illness: a guide to nursing care,* ed 2, Philadelphia, 1999, Lippincott.

Laabs C: Ethics and terrorism: September 11, 2001 and its aftermath, *Online J Issues Nurs* Jan 31, 2003, http://www.nursingworld.org/ojin/ethicl/ethics_11.htm.

Langan J, James D: *Preparing nurses for disaster management,* Upper Saddle River, NJ, 2005, Prentice Hall.

National Center for Chronic Disease Prevention and Health Promotion, Cancer Prevention and Control: *Lung cancer statistics,* 2005, The Author, http://www.cd.gov/cancer/lung/statistics.htm#trends.

National Center for Health Statistics: *FAST STATS A to Z: Immunization,* 2002, The Author, http://www.cdc.gov/nchs/fastats/immunize.htm.

National Center for Health Statistics: *Health, United States, 2004 with chartbook on trends in the health of Americans with special feature on drugs,* 2005a, The Author, http://www.cdc/nchs/data/hus/hus04chart.pdf.

National Center for Health Statistics: *Prevalence of overweight among children and adolescents: United States, 1999-2002,* 2005b, The Author, http://www.cdc.gov/nchs/products/pubs/pubd/hestats/overwght99.htm.

National Immunization Program: *Coverage estimates for school entry vaccinations 2003-2004 school year,* 2005, The Author, http://www.cdc.gov/mmwr/preview/mmwrhtml/mm5344a4.htm

National Institute for Occupational Safety and Health: *Steps to a healthier US workforce,* 2005, The Author, http://www.cdc.gov/niosh/steps/about.html.

Noble R: *United States HIV & AIDS statistics summary,* 2004, http://www.avert.org/statsum.htm.

Peavey L et al: Notes from the field, *Am J Public Health* 89:412, 1999.

Schmidt J: *Jeannie Schmidt's story,* 2005, onyxs@earthlink.net.

Sengupta S: Powerful quake jolts the seabed near Indonesia, *New York Times,* 2005, http://www.nytimes.com/pages/world/worldspecial4/.

State of Arizona: *AHCCCS fact sheet: Medicaid and AHCCCS acute care,* March 2005, http://www.ahcccs.state.az.us/Community/FactSheets/factsheet_Acute.pdf.

University of Texas Health Science Center at Houston: *Reflections of relief 2005,* The Author, http://publicaffairs.uth.tmc.edu/media/newsreleases/nrSpecial/katrina/relief_reflections.html.

US Department of Health and Human Services: *Healthy People, 2010: conference edition,* Washington, DC, 2000, US Government Printing Office.

US Department of Labor, Occupational Health and Safety Administration: *Motor vehicle safety,* 2005, The Author, http://www.osha.gov/SLTC/motorvehiclesafety.

US Department of Labor, Women's Bureau: *Quick stats 2004,* 2005, The Author, http://www.dol.gov/wb/stats/main.htm.

Zerwekh JW: The practice of empowerment and coercion by expert public health nurses, *Image J Nurs Sch* 24:101-105, 1992.

Wormser D: Do not grow weary in doing good: *Baylor Magazine,* 3(4): 2005, http://www.baylormag.com/story.php?story=005607.

Index

Special Features

CASE STUDY — Application of the Nursing Process

HEALTHY PEOPLE 2010 — Objectives Related to

RESEARCH HIGHLIGHTS